MEDICAL-SURGICAL NURSING

Patient-Centered Collaborative Care

MEDICAL-SURGICAL NURSING

Patient-Centered Collaborative Care

EIGHTH EDITION

Donna D. Ignatavicius, MS, RN, ANEF
Speaker and Curriculum Consultant for Academic
  Nursing Programs
Founder, Boot Camp for Nurse Educators®
President, DI Associates, Inc.
Placitas, New Mexico

M. Linda Workman, PhD, RN, FAAN
Senior Volunteer Faculty
College of Nursing
University of Cincinnati
Cincinnati, Ohio;
Formerly Gertrude Perkins Oliva Professor of Oncology
Frances Payne Bolton School of Nursing
Case Western Reserve University
Cleveland, Ohio

Section Editors:

Meg Blair, PhD, MSN, RN, CEN
Professor
Nebraska Methodist College
Omaha, Nebraska

Cherie Rebar, PhD, MBA, RN, FNP, COI
Director, Division of Nursing
Chair, Prelicensure Nursing Programs
Kettering College
Kettering, Ohio

Chris Winkelman, RN, PhD, CCRN, ACNP, CNE, FCCM, FANP
Associate Professor
Frances Payne Bolton School of Nursing
Case Western Reserve University
Cleveland, Ohio

ELSEVIER

ELSEVIER

3251 Riverport Lane
St. Louis, Missouri 63043

MEDICAL-SURGICAL NURSING:
PATIENT-CENTERED COLLABORATIVE CARE,
EIGHTH EDITION

ISBN (single volume): 978-1-4557-7255-1
ISBN (2-volume set): 978-1-4557-7258-2

Notices

Knowledge and best practice in this field are constantly changing. As new research and experience broaden our understanding, changes in research methods, professional practices, or medical treatment may become necessary.

Practitioners and researchers must always rely on their own experience and knowledge in evaluating and using any information, methods, compounds, or experiments described herein. In using such information or methods they should be mindful of their own safety and the safety of others, including parties for whom they have a professional responsibility.

With respect to any drug or pharmaceutical products identified, readers are advised to check the most current information provided (i) on procedures featured or (ii) by the manufacturer of each product to be administered, to verify the recommended dose or formula, the method and duration of administration, and contraindications. It is the responsibility of practitioners, relying on their own experience and knowledge of their patients, to make diagnoses, to determine dosages and the best treatment for each individual patient, and to take all appropriate safety precautions.

To the fullest extent of the law, neither the Publisher nor the authors, contributors, or editors, assume any liability for any injury and/or damage to persons or property as a matter of products liability, negligence or otherwise, or from any use or operation of any methods, products, instructions, or ideas contained in the material herein.

Previous editions copyrighted 2013, 2010, 2006, 2002, 1999, 1995, 1991

International Standard Book Number (single volume): 978-1-4557-7255-1
International Standard Book Number (2-volume set): 978-1-4557-7258-2

Executive Content Strategist: Lee Henderson
Traditional Content Development Manager: Billie C. Sharp
Senior Content Development Specialist: Rae L. Robertson
Publishing Services Manager: Deborah L. Vogel
Senior Project Manager: Jodi M. Willard
Design Direction: Margaret Reid

Printed in Canada

Last digit is the print number: 9 8 7 6 5 4 3

Working together
to grow libraries in
developing countries

www.elsevier.com • www.bookaid.org

CONSULTANTS AND CONTRIBUTORS

CONSULTANTS

Richard Lintner, RT(R), (CV), (CT), (MR)
Clinical Instructor
Interventional Radiology
Kansas University Hospital
Kansas City, Kansas

Deanne Blach, MSN, RN
President, Nursing Education
DB Productions of NW AR, Inc.
Green Forest, Arkansas

Stephanie Ignatavicius, MA
Phoenix, Arizona

CONTRIBUTORS

Katherine L. Byar, MSN, APN, BC
Hematological Nurse Practitioner
Department of Internal Medicine/
   Oncology-Hematology
University of Nebraska Medical Center
Omaha, Nebraska

Lara L. Carver, PhD, RN, CNE
Associate Professor
Department of Nursing
National University
Las Vegas, Nevada

Robin Chard, PhD, RN, CNOR
Associate Professor
College of Nursing
Nova Southeastern University
Fort Lauderdale, Florida

Tammy Coffee, MSN, RN, ACNP
Preceptor
Department of Nursing
Case Western Reserve University;
Nurse Practitioner
Department of Surgery
MetroHealth Medical Center
Cleveland, Ohio

Janice Zeigler Cuzzell, RN, MA, CWS
Senior Rheumatology Clinical Coordinator
Immunology and Ophthalmology
Genentech, Inc.
San Francisco, California

Barbara J. Daly, PhD, RN, FAAN
Professor
School of Nursing
Case Western Reserve University;
Director
Clinical Ethics
University Hospitals Case Medical Center
Cleveland, Ohio

**Laura M. Dechant, APN, MSN, CCRN,
   CCNS**
Clinical Nurse Specialist
Heart, Vascular, and Interventional Services
Christiana Care Health System
Newark, Delaware

Cheryl Dumont, PhD, RN, CRNI
Director, Nursing Research and Vascular
   Access Team
Nursing Administration
Winchester Medical Center
Winchester, Virginia

June Eilers, PhD, APRN-CNS, BC
Research Associate Professor
College of Nursing
University of Nebraska
Omaha, Nebraska

Rachel L. Gallagher, MS, ANP-BC
Staff Officer
Physical Disability Board of Review
Diversified Technical Services, Inc.
El Paso, Texas

Nicole M. Heimgartner, RN, MSN
Assistant Professor
Division of Nursing
Kettering College
Kettering, Ohio

Stephanie Ignatavicius, MA
Phoenix, Arizona

Mary F. Justice, MSN, RN, CNE
Associate Professor
Department of Nursing
University of Cincinnati Blue Ash College
Cincinnati, Ohio

Mary Kazanowski, PhD, APRN, ACHPN
Palliative and Hospice Nurse Practitioner
VNA Hospice of Manchester and Southern
   New Hampshire
Manchester, New Hampshire;
Palliative Care Nurse Practitioner
Palliative Care Team
Concord Hospital
Concord, New Hampshire

Linda A. LaCharity, PhD, RN
Assistant Professor (Retired)
Adult Health
University of Cincinnati
Cincinnati, Ohio

**Linda Laskowski-Jones, MS, RN, ACNS-BC,
   CEN, FAWM**
Vice President
Emergency & Trauma Services
Christiana Care Health System
Wilmington, Delaware

Rona F. Levin, PhD, RN
Clinical Professor and Director, Doctor of
   Nursing Practice Program
College of Nursing
New York University;
Visiting Faculty
Quality Management Services
Visiting Nurse Service of New York
New York, New York;
Professor Emeritus
Felician College
Lodi, New Jersey

**Margaret Elaine McLeod, MSN, APN,
   BC-ADM, ACNS-BC, CDE**
Clinical Nurse Specialist
Department of Nursing
Tennessee Valley Health Care System
Nashville, Tennessee

Chris Pasero, MS, RN-BC, FAAN
Pain Management Educator and Clinical
   Consultant
El Dorado Hills, California

Jennifer Powers, MSN, FNP-BC
Clinical Assistant Professor
School of Health and Human Services
National University
San Diego, California;
Family Nurse Practitioner
Health Care Partners
Las Vegas, Nevada

Cherie Rebar, PhD, MBA, RN, FNP, COI
Director, Division of Nursing;
Chair, Prelicensure Nursing Programs
Division of Nursing
Kettering College
Kettering, Ohio

Harry C. Rees, III, MSN, ACNP-BC
Acute Care Nurse Practitioner
Cleveland Clinic Health System;
Metro Life Flight
MetroHealth Medical Center
Cleveland, Ohio

James G. Sampson, DNP, NP-C
Adjunct Assistant Professor
College of Nursing
University of Colorado
Aurora, Colorado;
Clinical Supervisor, Adult Nurse
    Practitioner
Department of Internal Medicine
Denver Health Medical Center
Denver, Colorado

Karen Toulson, RN, MSN, MBA, CEN, NE-BC
Nurse Manager
Emergency Department, Christiana Hospital
Christiana Care Health Services
Newark, Delaware

Shirley E. Van Zandt, MS, MPH, CRNP
Assistant Professor
School of Nursing
Boise State University
Boise, Idaho

Laura M. Willis, MSN, RN
Assistant Professor, Service Learning
    Coordinator
Department of Nursing, Service Learning
Kettering College
Kettering, Ohio

Chris Winkelman, RN, PhD, CCRN, ACNP, CNE, FCCM, FANP
Associate Professor
Frances Payne Bolton School of Nursing
Case Western Reserve University;
Clinical Nurse
Trauma/Critical Care
MetroHealth Medical Center
Cleveland, Ohio

Fay Wright, MS, RN, APRN-BC
Doctoral Student
The Florence S. Downs PhD Program in
    Nursing Research and Theory
    Development
New York University College of Nursing
New York, New York

CONTRIBUTORS TO TEACHING/LEARNING RESOURCES

PowerPoint® Slides
Nicole Heimgartner, RN, MSN, COI
Associate Professor of Nursing
Kettering College
Kettering, Ohio

Cherie Rebar, PhD, MBA, RN, FNP, COI
Director, Division of Nursing;
Chair, Prelicensure Nursing Programs
Division of Nursing
Kettering College
Kettering, Ohio

Laura M. Willis, MSN, APRN, FNP-C
Adjunct Professor
Kettering College
Kettering, Ohio;
Family Nurse Practitioner
The Little Clinic;
President, Connect RN2ED
Englewood, Ohio

TEACH® for Nurses Lesson Plans
Carolyn Gersch, PhDc, MSN, RN, CNE
Associate Director, Division of Nursing
Kettering College
Kettering, Ohio

Cherie Rebar, PhD, MBA, RN, FNP, COI
Director, Division of Nursing;
Chair, Prelicensure Nursing Programs
Division of Nursing
Kettering College
Kettering, Ohio

Test Bank
Meg Blair, PhD, MSN, RN, CEN
Professor
Nursing Division
Nebraska Methodist College
Omaha, Nebraska

Linda Hughes, PhD, RN, BSN, MS
Dean of Nursing
Nebraska Methodist College
Omaha, Nebraska

Tami Kathleen Little, RN, DNP, CNE
Dean of Nursing
Brookline College
Albuquerque, New Mexico

Case Studies
Candice Kumagai, RN, MSN
Formerly Clinical Instructor
University of Texas at Austin
Austin, Texas

Linda A. LaCharity, PhD, RN, MN, BSN
Adjunct Faculty
Formerly Accelerated Program Director and
    Assistant Professor
College of Nursing
University of Cincinnati
Cincinnati, Ohio

Concept Maps
Deanne A. Blach, MSN, RN
President, Nursing Education
DB Productions of NW AR, Inc.
Green Forest, Arkansas

Review Questions for the NCLEX® Examination
Lisa A. Hollett, RN, BSN, MA, MICN, Certified Forensic Nurse
Stroke Coordinator
Hillcrest Medical Center
Tulsa, Oklahoma

Mary Beth Flynn Makic, PhD, RN, CNS, CCNS, FAAN
Research Nurse Scientist
University of Colorado Hospital;
Critical Care and Associate Professor
College of Nursing
University of Colorado
Aurora, Colorado

Andrea R. Mann, MSN, RN, CNE
Interim Dean, Third Level Chair
Aria Health School of Nursing
Trevose, Pennsylvania

Denise Robinson, RN, MS, CNE
Assistant Professor of Nursing
Monroe County Community College
Monroe, Michigan

Kathryn Schartz, RN, MSN, PPCPNP-BC
Assistant Professor of Nursing
School of Nursing
Baker University
Topeka, Kansas

Mitch Seal, RN, EdD, Med-IT, BSN
Director of Strategic Planning &
    Partnerships
Medical Education and Training Campus
    Joint Base
San Antonio, Texas

Peggy Slota, DNP, RN, FAAN
Associate Professor of Nursing
Carlow University
Pittsburgh, Pennsylvania

CONTENT REVIEW PANEL

Diane K. Daddario, MSN, ACNS-BC, RN, BC, CMSRN
Adjunct Faculty, School of Nursing
Pennsylvania State University
University Park, Pennsylvania

Denise A. Foster, MSN, RN, CNE
Associate Professor
Sentara College of Health Sciences
Chesapeake, Virginia

Bradley Harrell, DNP, APRN, ACNP-BC, CCRN
Chair and Associate Professor
Germantown Undergraduate Nursing
Union University School of Nursing
Jackson, Tennessee

LaWanda Herron, PhD, MSA, MSN, FNP-BC
Director of Nursing
Holmes Community College
Grenada, Mississippi

Jamie Lynn Jones, MSN, RN, CNE
Assistant Professor
University of Arkansas at Little Rock
Little Rock, Arkansas

Tamara Kear, PhD, RN, CNS, CNN
Assistant Professor of Nursing
College of Nursing
Villanova University
Villanova, Pennsylvania

Melissa S. McNulty, PhD, ARNP
Professor
Pasco-Hernando State College
Wesley Chapel, Florida

Jason Mott, PhD, RN
Instructor of Nursing
Bellin College
Green Bay, Wisconsin

CLINICAL CHAPTER REVIEWERS

Sameeya N. Ahmed-Winston, RN, MSN, CPNP, CPHON
Pediatric Nurse Practitioner
Children's National Medical Center
Washington, D.C.

Margaret-Ann Carno, PhD, RN, MBA, CPNP, FAAN
Associate Professor of Clinical Nursing and Pediatrics
University of Rochester, School of Nursing
Rochester, New York

Laura M. Dechant, APN, MSN, CCRN, CCNS
Clinical Nursing Specialist
Christiana Care Health System
Newark, Delaware

Kathleen Sanders Jordan, DNP, MS, RN, FNP-BC, ENP-BC, SANE-P
Clinical Assistant Professor
School of Nursing
University of North Carolina Charlotte;
Nurse Practitioner
Mid-Atlantic Emergency Medicine Association
Charlotte, North Carolina

Kari Jean Ksar, RN, MS, CPNP
Pediatric Nurse Practitioner
Pediatric Gastroenterology, Hepatology, and Nutrition
Lucile Packard Children's Hospital at Stanford
Palo Alto, California

Martha E. Langhorne, MSN, RN, FNP, AOCN
Nurse Practitioner
Binghamton Gastroenterology
Binghamton, New York

Casey Norris, MSN, BSN, APRN, BC
Nursing Instructor
ITT Technical Institute
Madison, Alabama

Charles D. Rogers, MSN, RN
Assistant Professor of Nursing
Morehead State University
Morehead, Kentucky

Mark Stevens, MSN, RN, CNS, CEN, MICN
Professor of Nursing
National University
Fresno, California

Laura C. Williams, MSN, CNS, ONC, CCNS
Orthopedic Clinical Nurse Specialist
Orlando Regional Medical Center
Orlando, Florida

PREFACE

The first edition of this textbook, entitled *Medical-Surgical Nursing: A Nursing Process Approach,* was in many ways a groundbreaking work. The following six editions built on that achievement and further solidified the book's position as a major trendsetter for the practice of adult health nursing. Now in its eighth edition, "Iggy" charts an essential course for the future of adult nursing practice—a course reflected in its current title: *Medical-Surgical Nursing: Patient-Centered Collaborative Care.* The focus of this new edition continues to be to help students learn how to provide safe, quality care that is patient-centered, evidence-based, and collaborative. In addition to print formats as single- and two-volume texts, this edition is now available in a variety of electronic formats, including Pageburst on VST, Pageburst on Kno, and e-book formats for Kindle, Nook, and other e-readers.

The book's subtitle was carefully chosen to emphasize the nurse's role in providing care in collaboration with the patient, family, and members of the interdisciplinary team in both acute care and community-based settings. The Institute of Medicine (IOM), The Joint Commission, the Quality and Safety Education for Nurses (QSEN) Institute, and the 2010 IOM *Future of Nursing* report have called for all health professionals to coordinate and deliver evidence-based patient care as a collaborative care team.

KEY THEMES FOR THE 8TH EDITION

The key themes for this edition strengthen the book's focus on safety, quality care, and clinical judgment to best prepare the student for collaborative patient-centered practice in medical-surgical health settings. Each theme is outlined and described below.

- **New Focus on Concepts.** Enhanced compatibility with the concept-based nursing curriculum in pre-licensure programs and a conceptual approach to teaching and learning is the key feature that sets this edition apart. To help students connect previously-learned concepts with new information in the text, six Concept Overviews introduce groups of content units. These unique features review basic concepts learned in nursing fundamentals courses—such as oxygenation and protection—to help students make connections between foundational concepts and patient care for medical-surgical conditions. The Concept Overviews are now even more accessible with color sidebars to identify these pages. For continuity and reinforcement, a list of more specific Priority Nursing Concepts has been added at the beginning of each chapter. This placement is designed to help students better understand the role of the nurse when caring for patients with selected health problems. When these concepts are explicated in the body of each chapter, they are presented in small capital letters (e.g., OXYGENATION) to help students relate and apply essential concepts to provide more focused nursing care. Nursing Concepts and Clinical Judgment Reviews at the end of most chapters apply these same concepts to the health problems presented in the chapter.
- **Improved Focus on the Core Body of Knowledge and QSEN Competencies.** This edition not only continues to emphasize need-to-know content for the RN level of practice, but also includes an increased emphasis on Quality and Safety Education for Nurses (QSEN) Institute core competencies. Clinical practice settings emphasize the essential need for safe practices and quality improvement to provide collaborative patient-centered care that is evidence-based. Many hospitals and other health care agencies have formally adopted these QSEN competencies as core values and goals for patient care. To help prepare students for the work environment as new graduates, as well as to highlight the integration of safety and quality into all nursing actions, this edition incorporates an enhanced focus on these competencies.
- **Emphasis on Patient Safety.** Patient safety is emphasized throughout this edition, not only in the narrative but also in **Nursing Safety Priority boxes** that enable students to immediately identify the most important care needed for patients with specific health problems. These highlighted features are further classified as Action Alerts, Drug Alerts, or Critical Rescue. We also continue to include our leading-edge Best Practice for Patient Safety & Quality Care charts to emphasize the most important nursing care. Highlighted yellow text also demonstrates the application of The Joint Commission's National Patient Safety Goals initiative (http://www.jointcommission.org/standards_information/npsgs.aspx) and Core Measures content into every day nursing practice.
- **Focus on Patient-Centered Care.** Patient-centered care is enhanced in the eighth edition in several ways. The eighth edition continues to use the term "patient" instead of "client" throughout. Although the use of these terms remains a subject of discussion among nursing educators, we have not defined the patient as a dependent person. Rather, the patient can be an individual, a family, or a group—all of whom have rights that are respected in a mutually trusting nurse-patient relationship. Most health care agencies and professional organizations use "patient" in their practice and publications. In addition, most nursing organizations support the term.
- **New Focus on Gender Considerations.** To increase our emphasis on patient-centered care, we delineated **Gender Health Considerations** rather than restricting our emphasis on Women's Health Considerations as we did in previous editions. To further expand that focus on differences in patient values, preferences, and beliefs, we have added new, cutting-edge **Chapter 73, Care of Transgender Patients,** dedicated to transgender patient care. Along with other individuals in the lesbian, gay, bisexual, and questioning population, the health needs of transgender patients have gained national attention through their inclusion in *Healthy People 2020* and The Joint Commission's standards. This new chapter provides tools to help prepare students and faculty to care for transgender patients who are considering or who have undergone the gender transition process.
- **Emphasis on Evidence-Based Practice.** The updated **Chapter 5, Evidence-Based Practice in Medical-Surgical Nursing** (written by evidence-based practice (EBP) experts Dr. Rona F. Levin and Fay Wright), discusses the importance of *using best current evidence in nursing practice* and how to locate and use this evidence to improve patient care. This chapter, along with the **Evidence-Based Practice boxes** throughout the book, offers a solid foundation in this

essential aspect of nursing practice. Each box summarizes a useful research article and explains the implications of its findings for practice and further research, as well as a rating of the level of evidence based on a well-respected scale.

- **New Focus on Quality Improvement.** The QSEN Institute and clinical practice agencies require that all nurses have *quality improvement* knowledge and skills. To help prepare students for that role, this edition includes new and unique **Quality Improvement boxes.** Each box summarizes a quality improvement project published in the health care literature and the implications of the project's success in improving nursing care. The inclusion of these boxes, in addition to disseminating information and research, helps students understand that quality improvement has its underpinnings in practice change at the "grass roots" level. It also emphasizes the role of the bedside nurse in identifying potential solutions to practice problems.

- **Refocused Emphasis on Clinical Judgment.** Stressing the importance of clinical judgment skills, including an enhanced emphasis on prioritization and delegation, helps to best prepare students for practice and the NCLEX® Examination. As in the seventh edition, the eighth edition emphasizes the importance of nursing judgment to make timely and appropriate clinical decisions and prioritize care. To help achieve that focus, all-new case-based **Clinical Judgment Challenges** (formerly called "Decision-Making Challenges"), based primarily on the QSEN core competencies, have been integrated throughout the text. Selected Clinical Judgment Challenges highlight ethical dilemmas and delegation and supervision issues. These exercises provide clinical situations in which students can use on-the-spot nursing judgment to help prepare them for the fast-paced world of medical-surgical nursing and become competent nurses. Suggested answer guidelines for these Clinical Judgment Challenges are provided on the book's Evolve website (http://evolve.elsevier.com/Iggy/). In addition, Dr. Christine Tanner's clinical judgment framework (Tanner, 2006) is used to help students apply selected concepts in the **Nursing Concepts and Clinical Judgment Reviews** at the end of most chapters. The components of this model include that clinical nurses use nursing judgment to provide safe, quality care by:
  - Noticing
  - Interpreting
  - Responding
  - Reflecting

- **Emphasis on Preparation for the NCLEX® Examination.** An enhanced emphasis on the NCLEX Examination and consistency with the 2013 NCLEX-RN® test plan has been refined in this edition. Like the seventh edition, the eighth edition also emphasizes "readiness"—readiness for the NCLEX® Examination, readiness for major emergencies such as those we see with all-too-frequent mass casualty events, readiness for safe drug administration, and readiness for the new and continually unfolding world of genetics and genomics. An increased number of new **NCLEX® Examination Challenges** are interspersed throughout the text to allow students the opportunity for practice in test-taking and decision-making. Answers to these Challenges are provided in the back of the book, and their rationales are provided on the Evolve website (http://evolve.elsevier.com/Iggy). As the NCLEX® Examination becomes more challenging, it is more critical than ever that students be ready to pass the licensure

exam on the first try. To help both students and faculty achieve that outcome, chapter-opening **Learning Outcomes** are now more consistent with the competencies outlined in the detailed 2013 NCLEX-RN Test Plan. The eighth edition also continues to include an innovative end-of-chapter feature called **Get Ready for the NCLEX® Examination!** This unique and effective learning aid consists of a list of **Key Points** *organized by Client Needs Category* as found in the NCLEX-RN® Test Plan. Relevant QSEN competency categories are identified for selected Key Points.

- **Expanded Content on Community-Based Care.** Expanded coverage on this important nursing area, including long-term care, is included in this edition. A recent editorial article in the journal *Medical-Surgical Nursing* stated that the future of medical-surgical nurses will change to an increased role in care coordination and transition management between acute care and community-based care (Lattavo, 2014). To help students prepare for this new role, the eighth edition of our text expands coverage of community-based care, including essential collaborative management that is needed in home, long-term, rehabilitation, and ambulatory settings.

- **Collaborative Problems and NANDA-I Nursing Diagnoses.** This edition also features an improved delineation of **NANDA-I nursing diagnoses and collaborative patient problems.** As health care becomes increasingly more collaborative, nurses need to be able to communicate with other members of the health care team, including the patient and family. To help students learn how to facilitate that communication, the eighth edition identifies patient problems and specifies which actual and potential problems are NANDA-I nursing diagnoses and which are collaborative health problems.

CLINICAL CURRENCY AND ACCURACY

To ensure the book's currency and accuracy, we listened to students and faculty who have used the previous editions, focusing on their impressions of and experiences with the book. We reviewed documents crafted by a variety of health care organizations, including the Institute of Medicine (IOM), The Joint Commission (TJC), and the Institute for Healthcare Improvement (IHI). Recent nursing education publications were also examined, such as those authored by the National League for Nursing (NLN), the American Association of Colleges of Nursing (AACN), and Dr. Patricia Benner and her colleagues in their book *Educating Nurses: A Call for Radical Transformation* (2010). A thorough nursing education literature search of best current evidence helped us validate best practices and national health care trends to help shape the focus of the eighth edition.

We also commissioned in-depth reviews of every chapter by a dedicated panel of instructors and clinicians across the United States, and we used their reviews to guide us in revising the chapters into their final form. A well-respected interventional radiologist ensured the accuracy of selected diagnostic testing procedures and associated patient care.

The results of these efforts are reflected in the eighth edition's:

- Strong, consistent focus on NCLEX-RN® Examination preparation, clinical judgment, patient-centered collaborative care, pathophysiology, drug therapy, evidence-based clinical practice, and community-based care

- Foundation of relevant research and best practice guidelines
- Emphasis on the critical "need to know" information that beginning nurses must master to provide safe patient care

With today's knowledge explosion, it is easy for a book to become larger with each new edition. However, today's nursing students have a limited time to absorb and begin to apply the information essential for medical-surgical nursing care. Therefore in this eighth edition we eliminated some of the content found in previous foundation courses or other specialty textbooks. We limited our discussions to how this content is *used* in adult nursing and focused on content that was "need to know" for safe, patient-centered, quality nursing practice.

OUTSTANDING READABILITY

Today's students need to be able to read information once and understand it; they do not have time to repeatedly read the same information. To achieve this level of readability, the text employs a direct-address style (wherever appropriate) that speaks directly to the reader, and sentences are as short as possible without sacrificing essential content. In addition, we ensured that this new edition has improved consistency of difficulty level from chapter to chapter.

Reading level is highly influenced by the length of sentences and the length of words. Although we can control the length of the sentences, medical terms are often 4 to 5 syllables long and tend to skew a chapter's reading level. Nevertheless, the result of our efforts is a med-surg text of consistently outstanding readability. The average reading level is 10th to 11th grade. It is important to note that reducing the reading level of this edition did not reduce the quality or depth of content that students need to know. Instead, the content is clear, focused, and accessible.

EASE OF ACCESS

To make the text as easy to use as possible, we have maintained the previous editions' approach of smaller chapters of more uniform length. Consistent with our focus on the "need to know," we eliminated some of the less foundational content in the first unit of the last edition and added one new chapter. The more focused eighth edition contains 74 chapters.

The overall presentation of the eighth edition has been updated, including more recent and high-quality photographs for realism, and design change features to improve content access. The design of the eighth edition includes better placement of display elements (e.g., figures, tables, boxes, and charts) for a chapter flow that enhances text reading without splintering content or confusing the reader. Additional ease-of-access features for this edition include tabbed markings for the glossary, index, illustration credits, and bibliography for quick reference. To increase the smoothness of flow and reader concentration, side-turned tables and charts have been reduced throughout the text, as have tables and charts covering multiple pages. Tables and charts now feature an alternating pattern of light and dark shading to ensure essential content for a specific topic or characteristic is not confused with another topic or characteristic.

We also have maintained the unit structure of previous editions, with vital body systems (cardiovascular, respiratory, and neurologic) appearing earlier in the book. In these three units we continue to provide complex care content in separate chapters that discuss managing critically ill patients with coronary artery disease, respiratory health problems, and neurologic health problems.

To help break up long blocks of text and also to highlight key information, we continue to include streamlined yet eye-catching headings, bulleted lists, tables, charts, and in-text highlights. Key Terms are in boldface color type and are defined in the text to foster the learning of need-to-know vocabulary. A glossary is located in the back of the book. Chapter bibliographies have been moved to the back of the book to save space in chapters for need-to-know content. These current bibliographic resources include research articles, nationally accepted clinical guidelines, and other sources of evidence when available for each chapter. Classic sources from before 2011 are noted with an asterisk (*).

A PATIENT-CENTERED COLLABORATIVE CARE APPROACH

As in all previous editions, we take a collaborative care approach to patient care. We believe that in the real world of health care, nurses, patients, and other health care providers (including physicians, advanced-practice nurses, and physician's assistants) *share* responsibility for the management of patient problems. Thus we present patient care in a collaborative care framework. In this framework we make no *artificial* distinctions between medical treatment and nursing care. Instead, under each Patient-Centered Collaborative Care heading we discuss how the nurse coordinates care and interacts with members of the health care team as appropriate for the patient's health problems, including health promotion and illness prevention.

This edition includes newly redesigned patient-centered Concept Maps that underscore this collaborative care approach. Each Concept Map contains a case scenario. It then shows how a selected complex health problem is addressed. Each Concept Map spells out the steps of the nursing process and related concepts to illustrate the relationships among disease processes, priority patient problems, collaborative management, and more.

Although our approach is collaborative, the text is first and foremost a *nursing* text. We therefore use a nursing process approach as a tool to organize discussions of patient health problems and their management. Discussions of *major* health problems follow a full nursing process format using this structure:

[Health problem]
Pathophysiology
    Etiology (and Genetic Risk when appropriate)
    Incidence and Prevalence
Health Promotion and Maintenance (when appropriate)
Patient-Centered Collaborative Care
    Assessment
    Analysis
    Planning and Implementation
        [Collaborative Intervention Statement (based on priority patient problems)]
        Planning: Expected Outcomes
        Interventions
    Community-Based Care
        Home Care Management
        Self-Management Education
        Health Care Resources
Evaluation: Outcomes

The Analysis sections list the priority patient problems (collaborative problems and nursing diagnoses) associated with major health problems and disorders. This eighth edition uses official NANDA-I nursing diagnosis language where it applies; however, most health care agencies prefer to identify collaborative patient problems or needs as the basis for the interdisciplinary plan of care rather than being restricted to NANDA-I language, which addresses primarily nursing-oriented patient problems. With its more flexible interweaving of NANDA-I diagnoses and collaborative patient problems or needs, the eighth edition more closely aligns with the language of clinical practice. The nursing diagnoses used in this edition are the 2012-2014 NANDA-I diagnoses—the most recently approved diagnoses at the time of publication of this edition. Health Promotion and Maintenance sections are found in selected discussions.

Discussions of less common or less complex disorders, although not given this complete subhead structure, nonetheless follow the same basic format: a discussion of the problem itself (including pertinent information on pathophysiology) followed by a section on patient-centered collaborative care of patients with the disorder. To demonstrate our commitment to providing the content foundational to nursing education and consistent with the recommendations of Benner and colleagues through the Carnegie Foundation for the Future of Nursing Education, we highlight throughout this edition essential pathophysiologic concepts that are key to understanding the basis for collaborative management.

Integral to this collaborative care approach is a clear delineation of just who is responsible for what. When a responsibility is primarily the nurse's, the text says so. When a decision must be made jointly by the patient, nurse, physician, and physical therapist, for example, this is clearly stated. When different health care practitioners in different care settings might be involved in the patient's care, this is stated.

ORGANIZATION

The 74 chapters of *Medical-Surgical Nursing: Patient-Centered Collaborative Care* are grouped into 16 units. Unit 1, Foundations for Medical-Surgical Nursing, lays the foundation for the health care concepts incorporated throughout the text. Unit 2 consists of three chapters on concepts of emergency and trauma care and disaster preparedness.

Unit 3 consists of three chapters on the management of patients with fluid, electrolyte, and acid-base imbalances. Chapters 11 and 12 review key assessments and related patient care in a clear, concise discussion. The chapter on infusion therapy (Chapter 13) is supplemented with an online Fluids & Electrolytes Tutorial on the companion Evolve website.

Unit 4 presents the perioperative nursing content that medical-surgical nurses need to know. This content provides a solid foundation to help the student better understand the collaborative care required for the surgical patient regardless of surgical setting. Even more emphasis is placed on continuous assessment during the perioperative period to prevent complications and improve outcomes in this era of increased ambulatory care.

Unit 5 provides core content on health problems related to immune system function. This content includes normal inflammation and the immune response, altered cell growth and cancer development, and interventions for patients with connective tissue disease, HIV infection, and other immunologic disorders, cancers, and infections.

The remaining 11 units, subdivided and introduced by the six Concept Overviews, cover medical-surgical content by body system. Each of these units begins with an Assessment chapter and continues with one or more Nursing Care chapters for patients with selected health problems in that body system. This framework is familiar to students who learn the body systems in preclinical foundational science courses such as anatomy and physiology.

MULTINATIONAL, MULTICULTURAL, MULTIGENERATIONAL FOCUS

To reflect the increasing diversity of our society, *Medical-Surgical Nursing: Patient-Centered Collaborative Care* takes a multinational, multicultural, and multigenerational focus. Addressing the needs of both U.S. and Canadian readers, we have included examples of trade names of drugs available in the United States and in Canada. Drugs that are available only in Canada are designated with a ✤ symbol. When appropriate, we identify specific Canadian health care resources, including their websites. In many areas, Canadian health statistics are combined with those of the United States for provide an accurate "North American" picture.

To help nurses provide quality care for patients whose preferences, beliefs, and values may differ from their own, numerous **Cultural Considerations** and **Gender Health Considerations boxes** highlight important aspects of culturally competent care throughout the text. In addition, a new chapter (Chapter 73) is dedicated to the special health care needs of transgender patients.

Increases in life expectancy and the "graying" of the baby-boom generation add up to a steadily increasing older adult population. To help equip nurses for this challenge, the eighth edition continues to provide thorough coverage of the care of older adults. Chapter 2 offers content on the role of the nurse and health care team in promoting health for older adults in the community. It also provides coverage of common health problems that older adults may have in the health care setting, such as falls and inadequate nutrition. The text includes many **Nursing Focus on the Older Adult charts.** Laboratory values and drug dosages typical for older patients are also included throughout the book. Charts specifying normal physiologic changes to expect in the older population are found in each Assessment chapter. In addition, **Considerations for Older Adults boxes** are included throughout the text to emphasize key points to consider when caring for these patients.

ADDITIONAL LEARNING AIDS

As in previous editions, the eighth edition continues to include a rich array of learning aids geared toward adult learners to help students quickly identify and understand key information and to serve as study aids.

- Written in "patient-friendly" language, **Patient and Family Education: Preparing for Self-Management charts** provide the types of instructions that nurses must learn to provide to patients and their families to help them cope with life changes caused by illness.
- **Laboratory Profile charts** summarize important information on laboratory tests commonly used to evaluate

health problems. Information typically includes normal ranges of laboratory values (including differences for older adults, when appropriate) and the possible significance of abnormal findings.

- **Common Examples of Drug Therapy charts** summarize important information about commonly used drugs. Most charts include both U.S. and Canadian trade names for typically used drugs, usual dosages (including dosages for older patients, as appropriate), and nursing interventions with rationales.
- **Key Features charts** highlight the clinical manifestations of important health problems based on pathophysiologic concepts.
- **Evidence-Based Practice boxes**, provided in many chapters, give synopses of recent nursing research articles and other scientific articles applicable to nursing. Each box provides a brief summary of the research, its level of evidence (LOE), and a brief commentary with implications for nursing practice and future research. The purpose of this feature is to help students identify the strengths and weaknesses of the research and to see how research guides nursing practice.
- New to this edition, **Quality Improvement boxes** offer anecdotes of recent nursing articles that focus on this important QSEN competency. These features, similar to the Evidence-Based Practice boxes, provide a brief summary of the research with commentary on the implications for nursing practice and research.
- As in the previous editions, **Home Care Assessment charts** serve as a convenient summary of essential assessment points for patients who need follow-up home health nursing care.
- Subtypes of **Clinical Judgment Challenges** (CJCs) emphasize the six QSEN core competencies: Patient-Centered Care, Teamwork and Collaboration, Evidence-Based Practice, Quality Improvement, Safety, and Informatics.

AN INTEGRATED MULTIMEDIA RESOURCE BASED ON PROVEN STRATEGIES FOR STUDENT ENGAGEMENT AND LEARNING

Medical-Surgical Nursing: Patient-Centered Collaborative Care, 8th edition, is the centerpiece of a comprehensive package of electronic and print learning resources that break new ground in the application of proven strategies for student engagement, learning, and evidence-based educational practice. This integrated multimedia resource actively engages the student in problem solving and practicing clinical decision-making skills.

Resources for Instructors

For the convenience of faculty, all Instructor Resources are available on a streamlined, secure instructor area of the Evolve website (http://evolve.elsevier.com/Iggy/). Included among these Instructor Resources are the reorganized *TEACH for Nurses* Lesson Plans. These Lesson Plans focus on the most important content from each chapter and provide innovative strategies for student engagement and learning. Lesson Plans are provided for each chapter and are categorized into several parts:
Learning Outcomes
Teaching Focus

Key Terms
Nursing Curriculum Standards
   QSEN
   Concepts
   BSN Essentials
Student Chapter Resources
Instructor Chapter Resources
Teaching Strategies
Additional Instructor Resources provided on the Evolve website include:

- A completely revised, updated, high-quality **Test Bank** consisting of more than 1750 items, both traditional multiple-choice and NCLEX-RN® "alternate" item types. Each question is coded for correct answer, rationale, cognitive level, NCLEX Integrated Process, NCLEX Client Needs Category, and new Keywords to facilitate question searches. Page references are provided for Remembering (Knowledge)- and Understanding (Comprehension)-level questions. (Questions at the Applying [Application] and above cognitive level require the student to draw on understanding of multiple or broader concepts not limited to a single textbook page, so page cross references are not provided for these higher-level critical thinking questions.) The Test Bank is provided in the Evolve Assessment Manager and in ExamView and ParTest formats.
- An electronic **Image Collection** containing all images from the book (approximately 550 images), delivered in a format that makes incorporation into lectures, presentations, and online courses easier than ever.
- **PowerPoint Presentations**—a revised collection of more than 2000 slides corresponding to each chapter in the text and highlighting key content with integrated images and Unfolding Case Studies. Audience Response System Questions (three discussion-oriented questions per chapter for use with iClicker and other audience response systems) are included in these slide presentations. Answers and rationales to the Audience Response System Questions and Unfolding Case Studies are found in the "Notes" section of each slide.

Also available for adoption and separate purchase:

- Corresponding chapter-by-chapter to the textbook, *Elsevier Adaptive Quizzing (EAQ)* integrates seamlessly into your course to help students of all skill levels focus their study time and effectively prepare for class, course exams, and the NCLEX® certification exam. *EAQ* is comprised of a bank of high-quality practice questions that allows students to advance at their own pace—based on their performance—through multiple mastery levels for each chapter. A comprehensive dashboard allows students to view their progress and stay motivated. The educator dashboard, grade book, and reporting capabilities enable faculty to monitor the activity of individual students, assess overall class performance, and identify areas of strength and weakness, ultimately helping to achieve improved learning outcomes.
- *Simulation Learning System (SLS) for Medical-Surgical Nursing* is an online toolkit designed to help you effectively incorporate simulation into your nursing curriculum, with scenarios that promote and enhance the clinical decision-making skills of students at all levels. It offers detailed instructions for preparation and implementation

of the simulation experience, debriefing questions that encourage critical thinking, and learning resources to reinforce student comprehension. Modularized simulation scenarios correspond to Elsevier's leading medical-surgical nursing texts, reinforcing students' classroom knowledge base, synthesizing lecture and clinicals, and offering remediation content that's critical to debriefing.

Resources for Students

Resources for students include a revised, updated, and retitled Clinical Nursing Judgment Study Guide, a Clinical Companion, Elsevier Adaptive Learning (EAL), Virtual Clinical Excursions (VCE), and Evolve Learning Resources.

The ***Clinical Nursing Judgment Study Guide*** has been completely revised and updated and features a fresh emphasis on clinical decision making, priorities of delegation, management of care, and pharmacology.

The pocket-sized ***Clinical Companion*** is a handy clinical resource that retains its easy-to-use alphabetical organization and streamlined format. It includes "Critical Rescue," "Drug Alert," and "Action Alert" highlights throughout based on the Nursing Safety Priority features in the textbook. National Patient Safety Goals highlights have been expanded as a QSEN feature, focusing on one of six QSEN core competencies, while still underscoring the importance of observing vital patient safety standards. This "pocket-sized Iggy" has been tailored to the special needs of students preparing for clinicals and clinical practice.

Corresponding chapter-by-chapter to the textbook, ***Elsevier Adaptive Learning (EAL)*** combines the power of brain science with sophisticated, patented Cerego algorithms to help students to learn faster and remember longer. It's fun, it's engaging, and it's constantly tracking student performance and adapting to deliver content precisely when it's needed to ensure core information is transformed into lasting knowledge.

Virtual Clinical Excursions, featuring an updated and easy-to-navigate "virtual" clinical setting, is once again available for the eighth edition. This unique learning tool guides students through a virtual clinical environment and helps them "learn by doing" in the safety of a "virtual" hospital.

Also available for students is a dynamic collection of Evolve Student Resources, available at http://evolve.elsevier.com/Iggy/. The Evolve Student Resources include the following:

- Review Questions for the NCLEX® Examination
- Answer Guidelines for NCLEX® Examination and Clinical Judgment Challenges
- Interactive Case Studies
- Concept Maps (digital versions of the 12 Concept Maps from the text)
- Concept Map Creator (a handy tool for creating customized Concept Maps)
- Fluid & Electrolyte Tutorial (a complete self-paced tutorial on this perennially difficult content)
- Key Points (downloadable expanded chapter reviews for each chapter)
- Audio Glossary
- Audio Clips and Video Clips
- Content Updates

In summary, *Medical-Surgical Nursing: Patient-Centered Collaborative Care,* 8th edition, together with its fully integrated multimedia ancillary package, provides the tools you will need to equip nursing students to meet the challenges of nursing practice both now and in an emerging healthcare environment that may look very different from today's. The only elements that remain to be added to this package are those that you alone can provide—your diligence, your commitment, your innovation, *your nursing expertise.*

Donna D. Ignatavicius
M. Linda Workman

To all the nursing educators who are passionate about teaching and all the nursing students who are passionate about learning.

Also, to my husband, Charles, who has endured countless hours of loneliness while I've worked on this project and to Stephanie, my daughter, who has educated me about the LGBTQ community's special needs. Thank you!

Donna

To students everywhere.
To John, still my one.

Linda

Donna D. Ignatavicius received her diploma in nursing from the Peninsula General School of Nursing in Salisbury, Maryland. After working as a charge nurse in medical-surgical nursing, she became an instructor in staff development at the University of Maryland Medical Center. She then received her BSN from the University of Maryland School of Nursing. For 5 years she taught in several schools of nursing while working toward her MS in Nursing, which she received in 1981. Donna then taught in the BSN program at the University of Maryland, after which she continued to pursue her interest in gerontology and accepted the position of Director of Nursing of a major skilled-nursing facility in her home state of Maryland. Since that time, she has served as an instructor in several associate degree nursing programs. Through her consulting activities and faculty development workshops, Donna has gained national recognition in nursing education. She is currently the President of DI Associates, Inc. (http://www.diassociates.com/), a company dedicated to improving health care through education and consultation for faculty. In recognition of her contributions to the field, she was inducted as a charter Fellow of the prestigious Academy of Nursing Education in 2007.

M. Linda Workman, a native of Canada, received her BSN from the University of Cincinnati College of Nursing and Health. After serving in the U.S. Army Nurse Corps and working as an Assistant Head Nurse and Head Nurse in civilian hospitals, Linda earned her MSN from the University of Cincinnati College of Nursing and a PhD in Developmental Biology from the University of Cincinnati College of Arts and Sciences. Linda's 30-plus years of academic experience include teaching at the diploma, associate degree, baccalaureate, and master's levels. Her areas of teaching expertise include medical-surgical nursing, physiology, pathophysiology, genetics, oncology, and immunology. Linda has been recognized nationally for her teaching expertise and was inducted as a Fellow into the American Academy of Nursing in 1992. She received Excellence in Teaching awards at the University of Cincinnati and at Case Western Reserve University. She is a former American Cancer Society Professor of Oncology Nursing and held an endowed chair in oncology for 5 years. In addition to authoring several textbooks and serving as a consult for major universities, she is Senior Volunteer Faculty at the College of Nursing, University of Cincinnati.

ACKNOWLEDGMENTS

Publishing a textbook and ancillary package of this depth and breadth would not be possible without the combined efforts of many people. Stephanie M. Ignatavicius assisted with literature searches. For this eighth edition, we welcomed three section editors to assist in our revision process: Meg Blair, Cherie Rebar, and Chris Winkelman. Each of these nursing educators worked with us on our seventh edition as contributors and/or ancillary material authors. For this eighth edition they updated and reviewed selected units of the text to provide their expertise.

Our contributing authors once again provided consistently excellent manuscripts in a timely fashion. Special thanks to Deanne Blach, who revised our Concept Maps, and Dr. Richard Lintner, who again provided expertise in interventional radiologic procedures and associated care. Our reviewers—expert clinicians and instructors from around the United States and Canada—provided invaluable suggestions and encouragement throughout the book's development.

The staff of Elsevier/Saunders once again provided us with crucial guidance and support throughout the planning, writing, revision, and production of the eighth edition. In particular, Executive Content Strategist Lee Henderson worked closely with us from the early stages of this edition to help us hone and focus our revision plan, and Lee coordinated the project from start to finish. Senior Content Development Specialist Rae Robertson then worked with us step-by-step to bring the eighth edition from vision to publication. Rae, Julia Curcio, and Kelly McGowan held the reins of our complex ancillary package and worked with a gifted group of writers and content experts to provide an outstanding library of resources to complement and enhance the text. Special thanks to Content Coordinators/Content Development Specialists Courtney Daniels and Samantha Taylor, who not only managed the *Clinical Companion* but also handled the countless administrative details associated with a project of this size.

Senior Project Manager Jodi Willard was once again a joy to work with. If, as is said, the mark of a good editor is that her work is invisible to the reader, then Jodi is the consummate editor. Her unwavering attention to detail, flexibility, and conscientiousness not only helped to make this edition the most consistently readable ever, but also made the entire production process incredibly smooth.

Special thanks also to Publishing Services Manager Debbie Vogel. For four editions now, Debbie has worked quietly behind the scenes to help bring the book to publication precisely on schedule and with a very high level of quality.

Designer Margaret Reid is responsible for the beautiful cover and the new interior design of the eighth edition. The praise of a book designer's work is often unsung, but Margaret's work on this edition has cast important features in exactly the right light, with neither too much nor too little emphasis, making this edition not only practical and easy to read, but also beautiful.

Our acknowledgments would not be complete without recognizing our dedicated team of Educational Solutions Consultants and other key members of the Sales and Marketing staff who helped to put this book into your hands.

Finally, we wish to thank John Danaher (President, Education) and Loren Wilson (Senior Vice President and General Manager, Content) for their ongoing vision, direction, and support for state-of-the-art educational resources for nurses.

Donna D. Ignatavicius
M. Linda Workman

CONTENTS

**CONCEPT OVERVIEW:
Urinary Elimination, 1342**

Unit XV Problems of Excretion: Management of Patients with Problems of the Renal/Urinary System

**CONCEPT OVERVIEW:
Sexuality, 1448**

Unit XVI Problems of Reproduction: Management of Patients with Problems of the Reproductive System

GUIDE TO SPECIAL FEATURES

COMMON EXAMPLES OF DRUG THERAPY

CONCEPT MAP

EVIDENCE-BASED PRACTICE

LABORATORY PROFILE

NURSING FOCUS ON THE OLDER ADULT

PATIENT AND FAMILY EDUCATION: PREPARING FOR SELF-MANAGEMENT

QUALITY IMPROVEMENT

CHAPTER | 1

Introduction to Medical-Surgical Nursing Practice

Donna D. Ignatavicius

http//evolve.elsevier.com/Iggy/

PRIORITY CONCEPTS

- SAFETY
- PATIENT-CENTERED CARE
- TEAMWORK AND COLLABORATION
- EVIDENCE-BASED PRACTICE
- QUALITY IMPROVEMENT
- INFORMATICS

LEARNING OUTCOMES

Safe and Effective Care Environment

1. Briefly describe the scope of medical-surgical nursing.
2. Explain the current priority focus on patient SAFETY and quality of care.
3. Identify the purpose and function of the Rapid Response Team (RRT).
4. Differentiate the six core Quality and Safety Education for Nurses (QSEN) competencies that health care professionals need to provide safe, PATIENT-CENTERED health care.
5. Identify six major ethical principles that help guide decision making and clinical judgment.
6. Communicate patient values, preferences, and expressed needs to other members of the health care team for effective COLLABORATION.
7. Outline the five rights of the delegation and supervision process.
8. Describe the SBAR procedure for successful hand-off communication in health care agencies.
9. Describe the nurse's role in the systematic QUALITY IMPROVEMENT process.
10. Identify three ways that INFORMATICS and technology are used in health care.

Medical-surgical nursing, sometimes called *adult health nursing,* is a specialty practice area in which nurses promote, restore, or maintain optimal health for patients from 18 to older than 100 years of age (Academy of Medical-Surgical Nurses [AMSN], 2012). A separate chapter on care of older adults is part of this textbook because the majority of medical-surgical patients are older than 65 years (see Chapter 2). To be consistent with the most recent health care literature, the authors use the term *patient* rather than *client* (except in NCLEX Examination Challenge questions). The *family* refers to the patient's relatives and significant others in the patient's life.

SCOPE OF MEDICAL-SURGICAL NURSING PRACTICE

The practice of medical-surgical nursing requires "specialized knowledge and clinical skills to manage actual or potential health problems that affect individuals, their significant others,

and the community" (AMSN, 2012, p. 4). Therefore medical-surgical nursing is practiced in many types of health care settings, such as acute care facilities, skilled nursing facilities, home care agencies, and ambulatory care clinics. The role of the nurse in these settings includes care coordinator, caregiver, patient educator, and patient and family advocate (Fig. 1-1).

The nursing process and critical thinking are tools that help the medical-surgical nurse make decisions using clinical judgment while being respectful of the patient's and family's cultural diversity, age, gender, and lifestyle choices (AMSN, 2012). Most fundamentals textbooks have information on cultural diversity and competence. This textbook presents many *Clinical Judgment Challenges* and *NCLEX Examination Challenges* to help you practice how to use clinical judgment to make appropriate decisions for diverse patients.

Medical-surgical health problems occur when a patient's basic needs are not met. These needs, also called *concepts,* were introduced in your fundamentals of nursing course. This

FIG. 1-1 A medical-surgical nurse providing care in an acute care hospital.

textbook builds on those concepts but focuses most on the role of nurses in safely meeting biologic (physiologic) needs for patients with selected medical-surgical health problems. Discussions of psychosocial (emotional), cultural, and spiritual needs are presented when appropriate to describe a holistic approach to patient care. For example, *Cultural Considerations* features highlight important content related to culture.

To further build a bridge between your basic fundamentals course and medical-surgical nursing care, several special features at the beginning of each textbook section review these selected concepts:

- Protection
- Oxygenation and Tissue Perfusion
- Mobility, Sensory Perception, and Cognition
- Nutrition, Metabolism, and Bowel Elimination
- Urinary Elimination
- Sexuality

Then, at the beginning of each chapter, a priority list highlights additional nursing concepts that apply to specific content in the chapter. These concepts are also emphasized in the concept maps for selected health problems. In addition to specified nursing concepts for each chapter, the QSEN core competency areas (professional nursing concepts) are integrated throughout the text.

PRIORITY FOCUS ON SAFETY AND QUALITY OF CARE

Nurses who practice medical-surgical nursing must have a broad knowledge base to meet the needs of patients. Rapid advances in technology, massive increases in available knowledge, and dramatic changes in the health care delivery system require that medical-surgical nurses use expert clinical judgment *to ensure patient safety as the priority in practice.*

Health care errors by physicians, nurses, and other health care professionals have been widely publicized for the past 20 years. Many of these errors have resulted in patient deaths and injuries and increased health care costs. As a result of these errors, a number of national and international organizations have implemented new programs and standards to combat this growing problem.

In 2000, the Institute of Medicine (IOM) stated in its *To Err Is Human: Building a Safer Health Care System* publication that between 44,000 and 98,000 patient *deaths* result each year from preventable errors in acute care hospitals. The report identified several factors that contributed to these findings and motivated other national bodies to examine ways they could improve patient safety and quality care. One of these groups, The Joint

TABLE 1-1	IHI Interventions to Save Patient Lives and Prevent Patient Harm	
INTERVENTIONS TO SAVE PATIENT LIVES	**INTERVENTIONS TO PREVENT PATIENT HARM**
Deploy Rapid Response Teams.	Prevent harm from High-Alert Drugs (e.g., anticoagulants, insulin, opioids).
Provide reliable, evidence-based care for acute myocardial infarction.	Reduce surgical complications.
Prevent central line infections.	Prevent pressure ulcers.
Prevent adverse drug events (ADEs).	Reduce methicillin-resistant *Staphylococcus aureus* (MRSA) infections.
Prevent surgical site infections (SSIs).	Provide reliable, evidence-based care for congestive heart failure.
Prevent ventilator-associated pneumonia (VAP).	Get boards of health care organizations to support measures to promote safe patient care.

IHI, Institute for Healthcare Improvement.

Commission (TJC), requires that health care organizations create a culture of SAFETY and encourage patients and families to become safety partners in protecting patients from harm.

The Joint Commission is one of several national organizations that offer peer evaluation for accreditation every 3 years for all types of U.S. health care agencies that meet their standards. Although acute care hospitals are accredited more often than other types of settings, many home care agencies, nursing homes, and ambulatory care centers are also TJC-accredited. Some agencies chose accreditation by organizations other than TJC (e.g., DNV Healthcare), but SAFETY is a major focus for all of them.

In 2002, TJC published its first annual **National Patient Safety Goals (NPSGs).** These goals require health care organizations to focus on specific priority safety practices, many of which involve establishing nursing and health system approaches to care. Since that time, TJC continues to add new goals each year. NPSGs address high-risk issues such as safe drug administration, health care–associated infections, and communication effectiveness among health care team members. When appropriate, this textbook highlights related NPSGs. A complete list of these 2015 goals can be found on the TJC website at www.jointcommission.org.

Protecting Five Million Lives from Harm

As a result of the IOM report and other data from national studies, the Institute for Healthcare Improvement (IHI) concluded that there are millions of health care errors in U.S. hospitals each year. In 2004, the IHI and its partner health care organizations launched the *100,000 Lives Campaign*—an effort to save patient lives over an 18-month targeted time frame. Six interventions for QUALITY IMPROVEMENT changes in care were implemented by partnering health care agencies (Table 1-1). As a result of this project, an estimated 122,000 patient lives were saved!

The next IHI objective was to *protect patients from five million incidents of medical harm* over a 2-year period (December 2006 to December 2008) (Institute for Healthcare Improvement [IHI], 2005). **Medical harm** refers not only to physician incidents but also to errors caused by *all* members of the health care team or system that lead to patient injury or death. To meet this IHI objective, six interventions for changes in care were added to the original list. As seen in Table 1-1, many of these interventions are within the scope of nursing practice and are therefore emphasized throughout this textbook. Some interventions, such as pressure ulcer prevention and adverse drug event reduction, are also part of TJC's NPSGs.

One of the most successful IHI initiatives was the creation of the Rapid Response Team (RRT), also called the *Medical Emergency Team (MET)*. Rapid Response Teams save lives and decrease the risk for harm by providing care to patients *before* a respiratory or cardiac arrest occurs. Although the RRT does not replace the Code Team who responds to patient arrests, it intervenes rapidly when needed for those who are *beginning* to clinically decline.

! NURSING SAFETY PRIORITY (QSEN)

Critical Rescue

Early clinical changes in condition occur in most patients for up to 48 hours before a "Code Blue." Therefore observe for, document, and report early indicators of patient decline, including decreasing blood pressure, increasing heart rate, increasing pain, and changes in mental status.

Members of an RRT are critical care experts who are on-site and available at any time. Although membership varies among facilities, the team may consist of an intensive care unit (ICU) nurse, respiratory therapist, intensivist (physician who specializes in critical care), and/or hospitalist (family practice physician or internist employed by the hospital). In other hospitals, acute care nurse practitioners or medical residents may be part of the team. The team responds to emergency calls, usually from nurses, according to established agency protocols and policies. Patient families may also activate the RRT. Outcome data demonstrate that the RRT approach to emergency care reduces medical complications and decreases the number of cardiac and respiratory arrests (Bogert et al., 2010).

TJC's NPSGs also include the need for early intervention for patients who are clinically changing. They require each health care organization to establish criteria for patients, families, or staff to call for additional assistance in response to an actual or perceived change in the patient's condition. NPSGs are highlighted in yellow throughout this text as they apply to the content.

Quality and Safety Education for Nurses Core Competencies

The IOM published many reports during the past 15 years suggesting ways to improve patient safety and quality care. One of its reports, *Health Professions Education: A Bridge to Quality*, identified five broad core competencies for health care professionals to ensure patient safety and quality care (Institute of Medicine [IOM], 2003). All of these competencies are interrelated and include:

- Provide patient-centered care.
- Collaborate with the interdisciplinary health care team.
- Implement evidence-based practice.
- Use quality improvement in patient care.
- Use informatics in patient care.

Several years later, the QSEN initiative, now called the *QSEN Institute*, validated the IOM competencies for nursing practice and added SAFETY as a separate competency to emphasize its importance. In addition, the QSEN project team created specific knowledge, skills, and attitudes (KSAs) needed to develop each core competency, using a Delphi research approach. More information about the QSEN Institute can be found on its website at www.qsen.org. QSEN core competency areas are identified in the Key Points at the end of each chapter of this text as appropriate.

This text also highlights the QSEN competencies in its *Clinical Judgment Challenges*. Teaching/learning activities to help students develop specific KSAs can be found in the *Instructor Resources* on the Evolve website and accompanying *Clinical Nursing Judgment Study Guide*. Each QSEN competency is briefly described in the following six sections.

Patient-Centered Care

To be competent in PATIENT-CENTERED CARE, the medical-surgical nurse recognizes "the patient or designee as the source of control and full partner in providing compassionate and coordinated care based on respect for [the] patient's preferences, values, and needs" (Quality and Safety Education for Nurses [QSEN], 2011). The KSAs for competence in patient-centered care focus on communication, compassion, culture, patient education and empowerment, and respect for patients and their families (Table 1-2).

TABLE 1-2	Examples of Knowledge, Skills, and Attitudes (KSAs) Needed to Develop the IOM/QSEN Patient-Centered Care Competency	
KNOWLEDGE	**SKILLS**	**ATTITUDES**
Describe how diverse cultural, ethnic, and social backgrounds function as sources of patient, family, and community values.	Provide patient-centered care with sensitivity and respect for the diversity of human experience.	Recognize personally held attitudes about working with different ethnic, cultural, and social backgrounds.
Demonstrate comprehensive understanding of the concepts of pain and suffering, including physiologic models of pain and comfort.	Assess presence and extent of pain and suffering.	Recognize personally held values and beliefs about the management of pain and suffering.
Examine how the safety, quality, and cost-effectiveness of health care can be improved through the active involvement of patients and families.	Engage patients or designated surrogates in active partnerships that promote health, safety and well-being, and self-care management.	Respect patient preferences for degree of active engagement in care processes.
Explore ethical and legal implications of patient-centered care.	Facilitate informed patient consent for care.	Respect and encourage individual expression of patient values, preferences, and expressed needs.

Data from Quality and Safety Education for Nurses, 2011 (www.qsen.org).
IOM, Institute of Medicine; *QSEN,* Quality and Safety Education for Nurses.

Nurses also provide family-centered care. As an advocate for the patient and family, teach them how to be empowered and have more control over their care. To assist in this process, TJC recommends a Speak Up™ campaign to provide information to patients and families to increase their empowerment (TJC, 2011). The basic framework of the campaign urges patients and their families to:

- **S**peak up if you have questions or concerns, and if you don't understand, ask again. It's your body and you have a right to know.
- **P**ay attention to the care you are receiving. Make sure you're getting the right treatments and medications by the right health care professionals. Don't assume anything.
- **E**ducate yourself about your diagnosis, the medical tests you are undergoing, and your treatment plan.
- **A**sk a trusted family member or friend to be your advocate.
- **K**now what medications you take and why you take them. Medication errors are the most common health care errors.
- **U**se a hospital, clinic, surgery center, or other type of health care organization that has undergone a rigorous on-site evaluation against established state-of-the-art quality and safety standards, such as that provided by TJC.
- **P**articipate in all decisions about your treatment. You are the center of the health care team.

Patient and family empowerment is one way to demonstrate respect for patients in their ability to be care partners.

Ethical Principles. Respect for people is the basis for six essential *ethical principles* that nurses and other health care professionals should use as a guide for clinical decision making. Respect implies that patients are treated as autonomous individuals capable of making informed decisions about their care. This patient **autonomy** is also referred to as *self-determination* or *self-management.* When the patient is not capable of self-determination, you are ethically obligated to protect him or her as an advocate within the professional scope of practice, according to the American Nurses Association (ANA) Code of Ethics for Nurses (ANA, 2010).

The second ethical principle is **beneficence**, which promotes positive actions to help others. In other words, it encourages the nurse to do good for the patient. **Nonmaleficence** emphasizes the importance of preventing harm and ensuring the patient's well-being. Harm can be avoided only if its causes or possible causes are identified. As described earlier in this chapter, patient safety is currently a major national focus to prevent deaths and injuries.

Fidelity refers to the agreement that nurses will keep their obligations or promises to patients to follow through with care. **Veracity** is a related principle in which the nurse is obligated to tell the truth to the best of his or her knowledge. If you are not truthful with a patient, his or her respect for you will diminish and your credibility as a health care professional will be damaged.

Social justice, the last principle, refers to equality and fairness; that is, all patients should be treated equally and fairly, regardless of age, gender identity, sexual orientation, religion, race, ethnicity, or education. For example, a patient who cannot afford health care receives the same quality and level of care as one who has extensive insurance coverage. An older patient with dementia is shown the same respect as a younger patient who can communicate. A Hispanic patient who can communicate only in Spanish receives the same level of care as a Euro-American patient whose primary language is English. More information on ethics and ethical principles can be found in your fundamentals textbook.

The ANA recognizes the need for nurses to provide culturally competent care, emphasizing that nurses should practice with respect and compassion to ensure the dignity and uniqueness of every person (ANA, 2010). The individual's unique values, preferences, and needs must be communicated to each member of the health care team. Some of the *Clinical Judgment Challenges* in this textbook focus on ethical issues.

Special Needs of the LGBTQ Population. Nurses today have been made aware of cultural variations and learned how to incorporate those differences to individualize patient care. However, one group that is rarely addressed in the nursing literature is the lesbian, gay, bisexual, transgender, and queer and/or questioning (LGBTQ) population (Pettinato, 2012). This terminology is widely accepted by the LGBTQ community and is commonly used, although *LGBT* may be seen more often in health care literature. Queer and/or questioning individuals prefer not having strict labels on their sexualities or genders. Another term that may also be used is *LGBTQI* to include intersex individuals. Intersex individuals have sexual or reproductive organs that are not clearly male or female or may have a combination of both male and female organs.

Many studies provide evidence that LGBTQ individuals do not feel comfortable with or trust health care professionals because of previous discrimination (IOM, 2011). The *Healthy People 2020* initiative added a category for these individuals because of health disparities in this population and the need in the United States to improve LGBTQ health. The complete document can be found on www.healthypeople.gov/2020. This textbook includes special health needs of this population as part of its *Gender Health Considerations* features. A new chapter on transgender health has also been added to this edition of the text to help students learn about the special needs of transgender patients.

The health care system, like other facets of society, often overlooks sexualities and genders that are alternative to the standard of heterosexuality and clearly delineated maleness or femaleness. As a health care professional, it is essential to not be restricted by rigid standards of identity. A good way of rethinking concepts of sexuality and gender is to think of each as existing along a spectrum as opposed to the confinement of heterosexual/homosexual and male/female.

To begin to gain trust and show respect for the LGBTQ patient, health care professionals need to know their patient's sexual orientation and gender identity. Do not assume that every patient is heterosexual or clearly gendered. *Include questions about gender identity and sexual activity as part of your patient's health assessment.* Table 1-3 lists recommended patient interview questions about sexual orientation, gender identity, and health care.

Teamwork and Collaboration

To provide patient- and family-centered care, the nurse "functions effectively within nursing and inter-professional teams, fostering open communication, mutual respect, and shared decision-making to achieve quality patient care" (QSEN, 2011). Therefore the KSAs for this competency emphasize the importance of communication and team functioning. Communication is an essential process for successful collaboration. **Collaboration** entails planning, implementing, and evaluating patient care together using an interdisciplinary (ID) plan of care. To help meet this purpose, health care agencies have frequent and regular ID meetings and conduct ID patient care rounds.

Electronic mail (e-mail) allows for quick communication among health care professionals to enhance collaboration and coordination of care. *However, it should not replace face-to-face and phone communication.*

Although there are many health care team members, some caregivers work more closely with nurses than others. For example, the physician or other health care provider and medical-surgical nurse collaborate frequently in a given day regarding patient care. The occupational therapist may not work as closely with the nurse unless the patient is receiving rehabilitation services. Collaboration with the rehabilitation team is discussed in Chapter 6.

One of the most important members of the ID team is the case manager (CM) or discharge planner, who is typically a nurse or social worker in health care agencies. The purpose of the case management process is to provide quality and cost-effective services and resources to achieve positive patient outcomes. In collaboration with the nurse, the CM coordinates inpatient and community-based care before discharge from a hospital or other facility. Part of that process may involve communicating with other CMs who are employed by third-party health care payers (e.g., Medicare) to keep patients from being readmitted to the hospital.

Communication. Poor communication between professional caregivers and health care agencies causes many medical errors and patient safety risks. In 2006, The Joint Commission began to require systematic strategies for improving communication. Two years later, another National Patient Safety Goal mandated that nurses communicate continuing patient care needs, such as pain management or respiratory support, to post-discharge caregivers.

To improve communication between staff members and health care agencies, procedures for hand-off communication were established. An effective procedure used in many agencies today is called *SBAR* (pronounced S-Bar). SBAR is a formal method of communication between two or more members of the health care team. The SBAR process includes these four steps:

- **S**ituation: Describe what is happening at the time to require this communication.
- **B**ackground: Explain any relevant background information that relates to the situation.
- **A**ssessment: Provide an analysis of the problem or patient need based on assessment data.
- **R**ecommendation: State what is needed or what the desired outcome is.

Several modifications of SBAR include I-SBAR and I-SBAR-R. In these procedures, the "I" reminds the individual to *identify* himself or herself. The last "R" stands for the *response* that the receiver provides based on the information given. Be sure to follow the established documentation and reporting protocols in your agency.

One of the most recent projects to improve communication was provided in 2010 by the Center for Transforming Health Care (www.centerfortransforminghealthcare.org). Every transition of care is potentially risky for patients because vital information needs to be communicated among caregivers and from one health care agency to another to keep patients safe. This QUALITY IMPROVEMENT (QI) project recommends these targeted solutions to ensure successful communication using the acronym SHARE as outlined in Table 1-4.

TABLE 1-3 Recommended Patient Interview Questions about Sexual Orientation, Gender Identity, and Health Care
• Do you have sex with men, women, both, or neither?
• Does anyone live with you in your household?
• Are you in a relationship with someone who does not live with you?
• If you have a sexual partner, have you or your partner been evaluated about the possibility of transmitting infections to each other?
• If you have more than one sexual partner, how are you protecting both of you from infections, such as hepatitis B or hepatitis C or HIV?
• Have you disclosed your gender identity and sexual orientation to your health care provider?
• If you have not, may I have your permission to provide that information to members of the health care team who are involved in your care?
• Who do you consider as your closest family members?

HIV, Human immune deficiency virus.

TABLE 1-4 Center for Transforming Health Care Targeted Solutions to Enhance Successful Hand-Off Communication and Collaboration: SHARE	
TARGETED SOLUTION	**DESCRIPTION OF SOLUTION**
Standardize critical content.	Providing details of the patient's history to the receiver, emphasizing key information about the patient, and synthesizing information from various sources before passing it on.
Hardwire within your system.	Developing standardized forms, tools, and methods, such as checklists; identifying new and existing technologies to assist in successful hand-off; and stating expectations about how to conduct a successful hand-off.
Allow opportunity to ask questions.	Using critical-thinking skills when discussing a patient's case as well as sharing and receiving Information as an interdisciplinary team ("pit crew"). Receivers should expect to receive all key information about the patient, scrutinize and question the data, and exchange contact information with the sender for additional questions.
Reinforce quality and measurement.	Demonstrating leadership commitment to successful hand-offs, such as holding staff accountable, monitoring compliance with use of standardized forms, and using data to determine a systematic approach for improvement.
Educate and coach.	Teaching staff throughout the organization about what constitutes a successful hand-off, standardizing training on how to conduct a hand-off, providing performance feedback at the time of the hand-off, and making successful hand-offs an organizational priority.

Data from the Joint Commission Center for Transforming Healthcare. (2010). *Joint Commission Center for Transforming Healthcare tackles miscommunication among caregivers.* Retrieved January 15, 2013, from www.centerfortransforminghealthcare.org.

Specific examples of ways to improve communication among nurses and other health care professionals using the SHARE principles have been cited in recent nursing literature. For instance, Maxson et al. (2012) reported a process for shift reporting from one nurse to another in which both shift nurses made bedside rounds during each patient's report. In this way, the patient and family were included in the communication process and patient safety was improved (see Evidence-Based Practice box). Burns (2011) reported a pilot study on a medical unit in which the unit's nurse, hospitalist physician, and physician's nurse made patient rounds as a team to improve health team communication and increase the patient's perception of and satisfaction with his or her care.

Delegation and Supervision. As a nursing leader, you will delegate certain nursing tasks and activities to unlicensed assistive personnel (UAP), such as patient care technicians (PCTs) or patient care assistants (PCAs). **Delegation** is the process of transferring to a competent person the authority to perform a selected nursing task or activity in a selected patient care situation. This process requires precise and accurate communication. *The nurse is always accountable for the task or activity that is delegated!*

An important process that is sometimes not consistently performed by busy medical-surgical nurses is supervision of the UAP to whom the task or activity has been delegated. **Supervision** is guidance or direction, evaluation, and follow-up by the nurse to ensure that the task or activity is performed appropriately. Examples of delegated tasks are turning and positioning, vital signs, and intake and output measurements.

Be sure to follow these five rights when you delegate and supervise a nursing task or activity to a UAP:

- *Right task:* The task is within the UAP's scope of practice and competence.
- *Right circumstances:* The patient care setting and resources are appropriate for the delegation.
- *Right person:* The UAP is competent to perform the delegated task or activity.
- *Right communication:* The nurse provides a clear and concise explanation of the task or activity, including limits and expectations.
- *Right supervision:* The nurse appropriately monitors, evaluates, intervenes, and provides feedback on the delegation process as needed.

Other activities or patient care responsibilities may be assigned by a registered nurse (RN) to another RN or to a licensed practical or vocational nurse (LPN/LVN). Each state designates which tasks may be safely delegated and assigned to nursing team members. Interventions that you can typically delegate or assign in any state are indicated throughout this text. Some of the *Clinical Judgment and NCLEX Examination Challenges* throughout this book will test your understanding of the delegation and supervision process.

Evidence-Based Practice

Evidence-based practice (EBP) is the integration of the best current evidence to make decisions about patient care. It considers the patient's preferences and values as well as one's own clinical expertise for the delivery of optimal health care (Melnyk & Fineout-Overholt, 2011; QSEN, 2011). Health care agencies follow the Core Measures developed by the Centers for Medicare & Medicaid (CMS) in collaboration with TJC to ensure that best practices are followed. Examples of Core Measures are highlighted throughout this textbook, such as those related to heart failure, stroke, and acute myocardial infarction.

The best source of evidence is research. However, available nursing research is limited and in some areas may not reflect the highest or best level of evidence. Some nursing research is designed as small, descriptive studies to explore new concepts. The findings of these studies cannot be generalized, but they provide a basis for future larger and better-controlled research.

As we did in the last edition of our text, this edition devotes a chapter to EBP (Chapter 5). In addition, *Evidence-Based Practice* boxes are found throughout the text to provide the most current research that serves as a basis for nursing practice. Each of these features presents a brief summary of the research, identifies the level (strength) of evidence using the scale in Chapter 5, and concludes with a "Commentary: Implications for Practice and Research" discussion to help you apply the findings of the study to your daily practice.

Quality Improvement

Ensuring patient and staff safety requires individual and systematic evaluation and change. To meet the **quality improvement** competency, nurses are expected to "use data to monitor the outcomes of care processes and use improvement methods

---

EVIDENCE-BASED PRACTICE [QSEN]

Does a Bedside Nurse Reporting Process Promote Patient Safety?

Maxson, P.M., Derby, K.M., Wrobleski, D.M., & Foss, D.M. (2012). Bedside nurse-to-nurse handoff promotes patient safety. *MEDSURG Nursing, 21,* 140-144.

Patient handoff at shift change in most hospitals has typically included a verbal or taped report, allowing nurses to communicate necessary patient information for continuity of care. Bedside handoff between shifts allows the patient and family to have an opportunity for input into the plan of care. This process helps meet the Joint Commission's National Patient Safety Goals and encourages patients to be an active part of their own care.

A convenience sample of 60 patients was used in a small study to examine the effects of bedside nurse-to-nurse handoff on a hospital unit. Thirty (30) patients were enrolled before the change in shift reporting, and 30 were enrolled after the change to bedside handoff. All nursing staff were invited to participate. Patients and staff completed surveys before and after the practice change. Fifteen nurses completed the pre- and post-survey indicating that they were more satisfied with the bedside handoff method when compared with the previous method of reporting. Patient satisfaction also increased as a result of the bedside nurse-to-nurse handoff process.

Level of Evidence: 4

This research was a small descriptive study that used a convenience sample.

Commentary: Implications for Practice and Research

Use of bedside nursing handoff increases patient and staff satisfaction and standardizes the shift report. This process also improves patient safety because both nurses see the patient during the change-of-shift period. Patients feel they are more active partners in their care and have the opportunity to ask questions and provide information during the handoff time. Additional studies using larger samples are needed to demonstrate the advantages and possible disadvantages of the shift change nurse-to-nurse handoff.

to design and test changes to continuously improve the quality and safety of health care systems" (QSEN, 2011). The KSAs stress the importance of learning how to use specific QI tools, participating in root cause analyses, and impacting changes in care processes.

As a medical-surgical nurse, you will be expected to:

- Identify indicators to monitor quality and effectiveness of health care.
- Access and evaluate data to monitor the quality and effectiveness of health care.
- Recommend ways to improve care processes.
- Implement activities to improve care processes.

A new feature for this edition of our textbook is *Quality Improvement* boxes that summarize articles on QI projects and end with a "Commentary: Implications for Practice and Research" discussion. Additional information about the QI process can be found in nursing leadership and management resources.

Informatics

Informatics involves using information and technology to communicate, manage knowledge, mitigate error, and support decision making (QSEN, 2011; Yoder-Wise, 2011). The emphasis of the KSAs for informatics is documentation, electronic data access, and data utilization.

Although most health care settings have information technology (IT) departments, nurses retrieve and use valuable information for patient care. The largest application of health care informatics is use of the electronic health record (EHR) (also called *electronic patient record [EPR]* or *electronic medical record [EMR]*) for documenting nursing and interdisciplinary care. Computers may be located at the nurses' work station or at the patient's bedside (point of care [POC]) (Fig. 1-2) or near the nurses' station. Handheld mobile devices are also popular because of their ease of use and portability.

FIG. 1-2 An electronic documentation system that is used at the bedside (point of care).

Another major purpose of informatics is for retrieval of data for the evidence-based practice process described in Chapter 5. The Internet provides ways to search for multiple sources of information very efficiently. However, all data sources must be evaluated for their credibility and reliability. Some health care agencies provide handheld mobile devices, such as the iPod Touch™, to health care professionals for data access and team communication via text or e-mail.

New technologies for patient, staff, and resource (inventory) management are emerging in health care agencies to promote patient safety and improve efficiency. An example of these technologies is radio frequency identification (RFID). RFID allows any person or object to be tracked electronically. For example, patients wear electronic identification wristbands.

Nurses need to be involved in decisions about introducing new or advanced health care technologies into the health care agency. They should also be included in designing technology that improves the effectiveness and efficiency of health care while providing for patient and staff privacy.

Safety

As discussed earlier in this chapter, nurses play a key role in promoting safety and preventing errors, including "missed nursing care," the necessary care that should have been provided by one or more nurses. The nurse "minimizes risk of harm to patients and providers through both system effectiveness and individual performance" (QSEN, 2011). The KSAs for safety stress the importance of examining care processes (QI), integrating national patient resources, and using appropriate tools to reduce reliance on memory, such as checklists.

The National Council of State Boards of Nursing (NCSBN) published findings of an extensive study of nursing practice breakdowns (Benner et al., 2010). These results identified nine key areas where nursing practice should be improved, including:

- Medication administration
- Clearly communicating patient data and clinical assessments
- Attentiveness/surveillance of patients
- Clinical reasoning or judgment
- Prevention of errors or complications
- Intervention (carrying out nursing actions in an appropriate and timely manner)
- Interpretation of authorized provider orders
- Professional responsibility and patient advocacy
- Mandatory reporting

The research report also provided case examples and analyses to assist in the development of quality improvement processes.

Three types of *Nursing Safety Priority* boxes are found throughout this text to emphasize the importance of safety when in daily practice. These features delineate safety based on patient need. For example, *Nursing Safety Priority: Critical Rescue* emphasizes the need for action for potential or actual life-threatening problems. *Nursing Safety Priority: Action Alert* boxes focus on the need for action but not necessarily for life-threatening situations. These safety alerts are essential, though, to ensure optimal patient outcomes. As the name implies, *Nursing Safety Priority: Drug Alert* boxes specify actions needed to ensure safety related to drug administration, monitoring, or related patient and family education.

GET READY FOR THE NCLEX® EXAMINATION!

KEY POINTS

Review these Key Points for each NCLEX Examination Client Needs Category.

Safe and Effective Care Environment

- Medical-surgical nursing is a specialty practice that requires a broad knowledge base and clinical skills to meet the needs of adult patients in a variety of settings.
- Medical-surgical nurses help meet human needs of adult patients, such as mobility and oxygenation, in a caring, respectful relationship.
- The Joint Commission requires that health care organizations create a culture of SAFETY by following the National Patient Safety Goals (NPSGs). **Safety** QSEN
- The Institute for Healthcare Improvement (IHI) interventions to save lives and prevent patient harm are listed in Table 1-1. **Safety** QSEN
- Rapid Response Teams (RRTs) save lives and decrease the risk for patient harm before a respiratory or cardiac arrest occurs. **Safety** QSEN
- Remember to always observe for slow and sudden changes in patient condition, especially changes in vital signs and mental status. **Safety** QSEN
- A vital role of the nurse is as an advocate to empower patients and their families to have control over their health care and function as safety partners.
- The six core competencies for health care professionals based on research by the Institute of Medicine (IOM) and Quality and Safety Education for Nurses (QSEN) are PATIENT-CENTERED CARE, TEAMWORK AND COLLABORATION, EVIDENCE-BASED PRACTICE, QUALITY IMPROVEMENT, INFORMATICS, and SAFETY.
- Examples of the knowledge, skills, and attitudes needed for patient-centered care are found in Table 1-2. **Patient-Centered Care** QSEN

- Six essential ethical principles to consider when making clinical decisions are autonomy, beneficence, nonmaleficence, fidelity, veracity, and social justice.
- Nurses must show respect and compassion for the uniqueness of every individual to ensure PATIENT-CENTERED CARE.
- The lesbian, gay, bisexual, transgender, queer and/or questioning (LGBTQ) population typically does not trust health care professionals; use sensitive questioning about sexual orientation and gender identity as part of your interview with patients in this group (see Table 1-3). **Patient-Centered Care** QSEN
- Nurses COLLABORATE by communicating patient's needs and preferences with members of the health care team to establish an individualized approach to care. **Teamwork and Collaboration** QSEN
- The SBAR procedure or similar established protocol is used for successful hand-off communication between caregivers and between health care agencies as part of the SHARE collaborative process (see Table 1-4).
- When delegating a nursing task to unlicensed assistive personnel (UAP), the nurse is always accountable to ensure that the task was performed safely and accurately. **Safety** QSEN
- EVIDENCE-BASED PRACTICE (EBP) is the integration of best current evidence to make decisions about patient care. It considers the patient's preferences and values, as well as one's own clinical expertise. **Evidence-Based Practice** QSEN
- Nurses are active participants in the systematic QUALITY IMPROVEMENT process in their health care agency. **Quality Improvement** QSEN
- INFORMATICS and technology are used for patient documentation, electronic data access, and health care resource tracking. **Informatics** QSEN

CHAPTER 2

Common Health Problems of Older Adults

Donna D. Ignatavicius

e http//evolve.elsevier.com/Iggy/

PRIORITY CONCEPTS

- NUTRITION
- MOBILITY
- SENSORY PERCEPTION
- COGNITION
- ELIMINATION
- TISSUE INTEGRITY

LEARNING OUTCOMES

Safe and Effective Care Environment

1. Explain the need to collaborate with members of the health care team to help the patient/family achieve health goals.
2. Identify risk factors for falls and impaired driving ability, including problems with MOBILITY, in older adults who live in the community or are hospitalized.
3. Explain evidence-based falls risk and prevention interventions for older adults in the hospital and community.
4. Describe best practices to promote patient safety when using restraints.

Health Promotion and Maintenance

5. Teach selected evidence-based lifestyle practices to promote healthy activities in older adults.
6. Conduct a medication assessment for potential risks for adverse drug events in older adults.

Psychosocial Integrity

7. Assess the older patient's risk for and signs of neglect and abuse.
8. Use valid and reliable assessment tools to document mental/behavioral health problems in the older adult.
9. Compare characteristics of common problems of COGNITION: depression, delirium, and dementia.
10. Develop a plan of care to assist the older adult to cope with relocation stress syndrome.

Physiological Integrity

11. Identify four subgroups of older adults.
12. Explain factors that contribute to NUTRITION-related problems among older adults in the community and inpatient facilities.
13. Describe the effects of drugs on the older adult.
14. Identify key interventions to prevent problems related to TISSUE INTEGRITY in older adults.

About 13% of the people in the United States are older than 65 years, but this number is expected to grow to 25% by 2050 (U.S. Census Bureau, 2013). In general, women live longer than men, although the exact reason for this difference is not known. Most patients on adult acute care and nursing home units are older than 65 years; many of these patients are discharged for home health services. Therefore nurses and other health care professionals need to know about the special needs of older adults to care for them in a variety of settings.

This chapter describes the major health issues, sometimes referred to as geriatric syndromes, associated with late adulthood in community and inpatient settings (Brown-O'Hara, 2013). The care of older adults (sometimes referred to as *elders*) with specific acute and chronic health problems is discussed as appropriate throughout this text. *Nursing Focus on the Older Adult* charts and *Considerations for Older Adults* boxes highlight the most important information. A brief review of major

physiologic changes of aging are listed in the Assessment chapter of each body system unit. A number of gerontologic nursing textbooks and journals are available for additional information about older adult care.

OVERVIEW

Late adulthood can be divided into four subgroups:
- 65 to 74 years of age: the young old
- 75 to 84 years of age: the middle old
- 85 to 99 years of age: the old old
- 100 years of age or older: the elite old

The fastest growing subgroup is the old old, sometimes referred to as the advanced older adult population. Members of this subgroup are sometimes referred to as the "frail elderly," although a number of 85- to 95-year-olds are very healthy and do not meet the criteria for being frail. *Frailty* is a geriatric syndrome in which the older adult has unintentional weight loss, weakness and exhaustion, and slowed physical activity, including walking. Frail older adults are also at high risk for adverse outcomes (Brown-O'Hara, 2013; Rocchiccioli & Sanford, 2009).

The vast majority of older adults live in the community at home, in assisted-living facilities, or in retirement or independent living complexes. Of all older adults, only about 5% live in long-term care (LTC) facilities (mostly nursing homes) and another 10% to 15% are ill but are cared for at home. Older adults from any setting usually experience one or more hospitalizations in their lifetime. About half of all older adults will likely be admitted at some time during their life for short-term stays in a skilled unit of a LTC facility, usually for rehabilitation or complex medical-surgical follow-up care.

Other institutions also have an increase in aging adults. For example, men older than 50 years are the fastest growing group of prisoners today. Like the rest of the older population, older prisoners have multiple chronic health problems. However, these problems are often complicated by a history of alcohol and substance abuse and poor NUTRITION that require deliberate management strategies. Nurses who work in these settings must have expertise in care of older adults.

The number of homeless people older than 60 years is also growing. The inability to pay for housing and family/partner relationship problems are primary factors that contribute to this trend. Most homeless adults have one or more chronic health problems, including mental/behavioral health disorders (Gerber, 2013). A growing number are veterans of war.

HEALTH ISSUES FOR OLDER ADULTS IN COMMUNITY-BASED SETTINGS

Health is a major concern for many older adults. Health status can affect the ability to perform ADLs and to participate in social roles. A failure to perform these activities may increase dependence on others and may have a negative effect on morale and life satisfaction. When older adults lose the ability to function independently, they often feel empty and worthless. Loss of autonomy is a painful event related to the physical and mental changes of aging.

Older adults may also experience a number of losses that can affect a sense of control over their lives, such as the death of a spouse and friends or the loss of social and work roles. Nurses need to support older adults' self-esteem and feelings of independence by encouraging them to maintain as much control as possible over their lives, to participate in decision making, and to perform as many tasks as possible.

Like younger and middle-aged adults, older adults need to practice health promotion and illness prevention to maintain or achieve a high level of wellness. Teach them the importance of promoting wellness and strategies for meeting this outcome (Chart 2-1).

Common health issues and geriatric syndromes that often affect older adults in the community include:
- Decreased NUTRITION and hydration
- Decreased MOBILITY
- Stress and loss
- Accidents
- Drug use and misuse
- Mental health/COGNITION problems (including substance abuse)
- Elder neglect and abuse

CHART 2-1   Patient and Family Education: Preparing for Self-Management

Lifestyles and Practices to Promote Wellness

Health-Protecting Behaviors
- Have yearly influenza vaccinations (after October 1).
- Obtain a pneumococcal vaccination.
- Obtain a shingles vaccination.
- Have a tetanus immunization, and get a booster every 10 years.
- Wear seat belts when you are in an automobile.
- Use alcohol in moderation or not at all.
- Avoid smoking; if you do smoke, do not smoke in bed.
- Install and maintain working smoke detectors and/or sprinklers.
- Create a hazard-free environment to prevent falls; eliminate hazards such as scatter rugs and waxed floors.
- Use medications, herbs, and nutritional supplements according to your health care provider's prescription.
- Avoid over-the-counter medications unless your physician directs you to use them.

Health-Enhancing Behaviors
- Have a yearly physical examination; see your health care provider more often if health problems occur.
- Reduce dietary fat to not more than 30% of calories; saturated fat should provide less than 10% of your calories.
- Increase your daily dietary intake of complex carbohydrate– and fiber-containing food to five or more servings of fruits and vegetables and six or more servings of grain products.
- Increase calcium intake to between 1000 and 1500 mg daily; take a vitamin D supplement every day if not exposed daily to sunlight.
- Allow at least 10 to 15 minutes of sun exposure two or three times weekly for vitamin D intake; avoid prolonged sun exposure.
- Exercise regularly three to five times a week.
- Manage stress through coping mechanisms that have been successful in the past.
- Get together with people in different settings to socialize.
- Reminisce about your life through reflective discussions or journaling.

Decreased Nutrition and Hydration

The minimum nutritional requirements of the human body remain consistent from youth through old age, with a few exceptions. Older adults need an increased dietary intake of calcium, vitamin D, vitamin C, and vitamin A because aging changes disrupt the ability to store, use, and absorb these substances. For older adults who have a sedentary lifestyle and reduced metabolic rate, a reduction in total caloric intake to maintain an ideal body weight is needed. NUTRITION-related problems can occur in older adults when these needs are not met.

Many physical aging changes influence nutritional status or the ability to consume needed nutrients. Diminished senses of taste and smell often result in a loss of desire for food. Older adults have less ability to taste sweet and salt than to taste bitter and sour. This aging change may result in an overuse of table sugar and salt to compensate. Some older adults consume numerous desserts and other sweet foods, which can cause them to become overweight or obese. Teach older adults how to balance their diets with healthy food selections. Remind them to substitute herbs and spices to season food and vary the textures of food substances to feel satisfied.

Tooth loss and poorly fitting dentures from inadequate dental care or calcium loss can also cause the older adult to avoid important nutritious foods. Unlike today, dental preventive programs were not readily available or stressed as being important when today's older adults were younger. Older people with dentition problems may eat soft, high-calorie foods such as ice cream and mashed potatoes, which lack roughage and fiber. Unless the person carefully chooses more nutritious soft foods, vitamin deficiencies, constipation, and other problems can result. The extensive use of prescribed and over-the-counter (OTC) drugs, including herbal supplements, may decrease appetite, affect food tolerances and food absorption, and cause constipation.

Constipation can reduce quality of life for older adults and cause pain, depression, anxiety, and decreased social activities (Toner & Claros, 2012). In some cases, it leads to a small or large bowel obstruction, potentially life-threatening events. Constipation is common among older adults and can be caused by multiple risk factors, including foods, drugs, and diseases.

> ### ! NURSING SAFETY PRIORITY (QSEN)
> #### Action Alert
>
> Teach older adults to increase fiber and fluid intake, exercise regularly, and avoid risk factors that contribute to constipation. Older adults should consume 35 to 50 g of fiber each day and drink at least 2 L a day unless medically contraindicated. Some people may also add a "colon cocktail" of equal portions of prune juice, applesauce, and psyllium (e.g., Metamucil) to their daily diet. Remind older adults to take 1 to 2 tablespoons of the mixture daily. If these measures do not prevent constipation, teach them to take a stool softener. For opioid-induced constipation (OIC), methylnaltrexone (Relistor) may be prescribed. This drug is given subcutaneously once every other day as needed and tends to have quick results (Toner & Claros, 2012).

Reduced income, chronic disease, fatigue, and decreased ability to perform ADLs are other factors that contribute to inadequate NUTRITION and constipation among older adults. "Fast food" is often inexpensive and requires no preparation. However, it is usually high in fat, carbohydrates, and calories but lacking in healthy nutrients. Older adults can become overweight or obese when they consume a diet high in fast food.

Other older adults may reduce their intake of food to near-starvation levels, even with the availability of programs such as food stamps (Supplemental Nutritional Assistance Program [SNAP]), community food banks, and Meals on Wheels. Many senior centers and homeless shelters offer meals, as well as group social activities. The lack of transportation, the necessity of traveling to obtain such services, and the inability to carry large or heavy groceries prevent some older adults from taking advantage of food programs. Others are too proud to accept free services.

Inadequate NUTRITION may also be related to loneliness. Older adults may respond to loneliness, depression, and boredom by not eating, which can lead to weight loss. Many who live alone lose the incentive to prepare or eat balanced diets, especially if they do not "feel well." Men who live at home alone are especially at risk for not eating enough calories to maintain their weight.

Some older adults are at risk for **geriatric failure to thrive (GFTT)**—a complex syndrome including under-nutrition, impaired physical functioning, depression, and cognitive impairment (Rocchiccioli & Sanford, 2009). However, drug therapy, chronic diseases, major losses, and poor socioeconomic

> ### ! NURSING SAFETY PRIORITY (QSEN)
> #### Action Alert
>
> Perform nutritional screening for older adults in the community who are at risk for inadequate NUTRITION—either weight loss or obesity. Ask the person about unintentional weight loss or gain, eating habits, appetite, prescribed and over-the-counter drugs, and current health problems. Determine contributing factors for older adults who have or are at risk for poor NUTRITION, such as transportation issues or loneliness. Based on these data, develop and implement a plan of care in collaboration with the registered dietitian, pharmacist, and/or case manager to manage these problems. Chapter 60 describes nutritional assessment and management of NUTRITION problems in detail.

status can cause these same health problems. Be sure to consider these factors when screening for GFTT. For those at risk for or who have GFTT, collaborate with the older adult and family to plan referral to his or her primary care provider for extensive evaluation. Early supportive intervention can help prevent advanced levels of deterioration.

People older than 65 years are also at risk for dehydration because they have less body water content than younger adults. In severe cases, they require emergency department visits or hospital stays.

> ### ! NURSING SAFETY PRIORITY (QSEN)
> #### Action Alert
>
> Older adults sometimes limit their fluid intake, especially in the evening, because of problems associated with MOBILITY, prescribed diuretics, and urinary incontinence. *Teach older adults that fluid restrictions make them susceptible to dehydration and electrolyte imbalances (especially sodium and potassium) that can cause serious illness or death.*
>
> Incontinence may actually increase because the urine becomes more concentrated and irritating to the bladder and urinary sphincter. Teach older adults the importance of drinking 2 liters of water a day plus other fluids as desired. Remind them to avoid excessive caffeine and alcohol because they can cause dehydration. Chapter 11 discusses fluid and electrolyte imbalances in detail.

Decreased Mobility

Exercise and activity are important for older adults as a means of promoting and maintaining MOBILITY and overall health (Fig. 2-1). Physical activity can help keep the body in shape and maintain an optimal level of functioning. Regular exercise has many benefits for older adults in community-based settings. The advantages of maintaining appropriate levels of physical activity include:

- Decreased risk for falls
- Increased muscle strength and balance
- Increased MOBILITY
- Increased sleep
- Reduced or maintained weight
- Improved sense of well-being and self-esteem
- Decreased depression symptoms
- Improved longevity
- Reduced risks for diabetes, coronary artery disease, and dementia

Assess older adults in any setting regarding their history of exercise and any health concerns they may have. For independent older adults, remind them to check with their health care provider to implement a supervised plan for regular

FIG. 2-1 Exercise is important to older adults for health promotion and maintenance.

physical activity. Teach all older adults about the value of physical activity.

For people who are homebound, focus on functional fitness, such as performing ADLs. For those who are not homebound, teach the importance of other types of exercise. Resistance exercise, for example, maintains muscle mass. Aerobic exercise, like walking, improves strength and endurance. One of the best exercises is walking at least 30 minutes, 3 to 5 times a week. During the winter, indoor shopping centers and other public places can be used. In addition, many senior centers and community centers offer exercise programs for older adults. For those who have limited MOBILITY, chair exercises are provided.

Swimming is also recommended but does not offer the weight-bearing advantage of walking. Weight bearing helps build bone, an especially important advantage for older women to prevent osteoporosis (see Chapter 50). Teach older adults who have been sedentary to start their exercise programs slowly and gradually increase the frequency and duration of activity over time, under the direction of their health care provider.

Stress and Loss

Stress can speed up the aging process over time, or it can lead to diseases that increase the rate of degeneration. It can also impair the reserve capacity of older adults and lessen their ability to respond and adapt to changes in their environment.

Although no period of the life cycle is free from stress, the later years can be a time of especially high risk. Frequent sources of stress and anxiety for the older population include:

- Rapid environmental changes that require immediate reaction
- Changes in lifestyle resulting from retirement or physical incapacity
- Acute or chronic illness
- Loss of significant others
- Financial hardships
- Relocation

How people react to these stresses depends on their personal coping skills and support networks. For instance, losses leave many older adults without friends for support and help. As a result, many must rely solely on their personal resources to maintain their mental health/behavioral health. A combination of poor physical health and social problems leaves older adults susceptible to stress overload, which can result in illness and premature death.

The ways in which people adapt to old age depend largely on the personality traits and coping strategies that have characterized them throughout their lives. Establishing and maintaining relationships with others throughout life are especially important to the older person's happiness. Even more important than having friends is the nature of the friendships. People who have close, intimate, stable relationships with others in whom they confide are more likely to cope with crisis.

Some older adults have chosen to return to work at least on a part-time basis to increase their income and socialize with other people. If a person retired between the ages of 55 and 65 years and lives into his or her 80s, funds can deplete; additional income is needed to meet basic needs, including money for prescription drugs. Although U.S. government Medicare Part A pays for inpatient hospital care, older adults pay for Medicare Part B to reimburse for 80% of most ambulatory care services, Medicare Part D for prescription drugs, and often a private Medi-Gap insurance (e.g., United or Blue Cross/Blue Shield) to cover the costs not paid for by Medicare. The premiums for these insurances are very expensive and may still require that older adults pay out-of-pocket copayments for health care services and prescription drugs.

Fortunately, most older adults are relatively healthy and live in and own their own homes. Physical and/or mental health problems may force some to relocate to a retirement center or an assisted-living facility, although these facilities can be very expensive. Others move in with family members or to apartment buildings funded and designated for seniors. Older adults usually have more difficulty adjusting to major change when compared with younger and middle-aged adults. Being admitted to a hospital or nursing home is a particularly traumatic experience. Older adults often suffer from relocation stress syndrome, also known as *relocation trauma.* Relocation stress syndrome is the physical and emotional distress that occurs after the person moves from one setting to another. Examples of physiologic behaviors are sleep disturbance and increased physical symptoms, such as GI distress. Examples of emotional manifestations are withdrawal, anxiety, anger, and depression. Chart 2-2 lists nursing interventions that may help decrease the effects of relocation.

Family members and facility staff need to be aware that older adults need personal space in their new surroundings. Older adults need to participate in deciding how the space will be arranged and what they can keep in their new home to help offset potential feelings of powerlessness. Suggest that the patient or family bring in personal items, such as pictures of

Minimizing the Effects of Relocation Stress in Older Adults

- Provide opportunities for the patient to assist in decision making.
- Carefully explain all procedures and routines to the patient before they occur.
- Ask the family or significant other to provide familiar or special keepsakes to keep at the patient's bedside (e.g., family picture, favorite hairbrush).
- Reorient the patient frequently to his or her location.
- Ask the patient about his or her expectations during hospitalization or assisted-living or nursing home stay.
- Encourage the patient's family and friends to visit often.
- Establish a trusting relationship with the patient as early as possible.
- Assess the patient's usual lifestyle and daily activities, including food likes and dislikes and preferred time for bathing.
- Avoid unnecessary room changes.
- If possible, have a family member, significant other, staff member, or volunteer accompany the patient when leaving the unit for special procedures or therapies.

relatives and friends, favorite clothing, and valued knickknacks, to assist in making the new setting seem more familiar and comfortable. This same intervention can be carried out in a hospital setting.

Accidents

Accidents are very common among older adults; falls are the most common. Motor vehicle crashes increase as well because of physiologic changes of aging or chronic diseases like Alzheimer's or peripheral neuropathy.

Fall Prevention

Most accidents occur at home. Teach older adults about the need to be aware of safety precautions to prevent accidents, such as falls. Incapacitating accidents are a primary cause of decreased MOBILITY and chronic pain in old age. Some people develop fallophobia (fear of falling) and avoid leaving their homes.

Home modifications may help prevent falls. Collaborate with family and significant others when recommending useful changes to prevent older adult injury. Safeguards such as handrails, slip-proof pads for rugs, and adequate lighting are essential in the home. Avoiding scatter rugs, slippery floors, and clutter is also important to prevent falls. Installing grab bars and using non-slip bathmats can help prevent falls in the bathroom. Raised toilet seats are also important. Remind older adults to avoid going out on days when steps are wet or icy and to ask for help when ambulating. To minimize sensory overload, advise the older adult to concentrate on one activity at a time.

Changes in SENSORY PERCEPTION and MOBILITY can create challenges for older adults in any environment. For example, presbyopia (farsightedness that worsens with aging) may make walking more difficult; the person is less aware of the location of each step. In addition, the older adult may have disorders that affect visual acuity, such as macular degeneration, cataracts, glaucoma, or diabetic retinopathy. Teach the person to look down at where he or she is walking and have frequent eye examinations to update glasses or contact lenses to improve vision. Drug therapy or surgery may be needed to correct glaucoma or cataracts.

A reduced sense of touch decreases the awareness of body orientation (e.g., whether the foot is squarely on the step). The decreased reaction time that commonly results from age-related changes in the neurologic system may also impair the ability to recognize or move from a dangerous setting. Chronic diseases such as peripheral neuropathy and arthritis can affect MOBILITY and SENSORY PERCEPTION in the older adult as well. If needed, encourage the use of visual, hearing, or ambulatory assistive devices. High costs and a fear of appearing old sometimes prevent older adults from obtaining or using hearing aids, eyeglasses, walkers, or canes.

Once an older person has been identified as being at high risk for falls, choose interventions that help prevent falls and possible serious injury. For example, for those in the community, tai chi exercise is very helpful to improve balance and functional MOBILITY, as well as to decrease the fear of falling, especially among older women (Wooten, 2010).

Driving Safety

Motor vehicle crashes are the most common cause of injury-related death in the young-old population—those between 65 and 74 years of age. Increased national concerns about this growing problem have prompted many states to require more frequent testing for older drivers. As one ages, reaction time and the ability to multitask decrease. Sleep disturbances, especially insomnia, are also common in older adults but are *not* part of normal aging. Some crashes occur because the person falls asleep while driving.

The older the person, the more likely he or she will have chronic diseases and the drugs needed to manage them. These health problems and treatments can contribute to motor vehicle crashes. For instance, drugs used for hypertension can cause orthostatic hypotension (low blood pressure when changing body position from a supine to sitting or standing position).

Physicians and other health care professionals play a major role in identifying driver safety issues. Yet, many are reluctant to intervene because older patients feel they will lose their independence if they cannot drive. They may also be angry and resistant to the idea of giving up perhaps their only means of transportation. As an alternative, health care professionals can recommend driving refresher courses and suggest that high-risk driving conditions, like wet roads, be avoided. Newer vehicles have some safety features to help older adults, such as large-print digital readouts for speed and other data. Chart 2-3 lists additional ways to improve older adult driver safety.

Drug Use and Misuse

Drug therapy for the older population is another major health issue. Because of the multiple chronic and acute health problems that occur in this age-group, drugs for older adults account for about one third of all prescription drug costs. The term polymedicine has been used to describe the use of many drugs to treat multiple health problems for older adults. Polypharmacy is the use of multiple drugs, duplicative drug therapy, high-dosage medications, and drugs prescribed for too long a period of time (Planton & Edlund, 2010). Another term, hyperpharmacy, has also been used to describe the excessive use of drugs to treat disease (Messina & Escallier, 2011).

Older adults commonly take multiple nonprescription (OTC) drugs, such as analgesics, antacids, cold and cough preparations, laxatives, and herbal/nutritional supplements, often without consulting a health care provider. Therefore this

CHART 2-3 Best Practice for Patient Safety & Quality Care QSEN

Recommendations for Improving Older Adult Driver Safety

- Discuss driving ability with the patient to assess his or her perception.
- Assess physical and mental deficits that could affect driving ability.
- Consult with appropriate health care providers to treat health problems that could interfere with driving.
- Suggest community-based transportation options, if available, instead of driving.
- Discuss driving concerns with patients and their families.
- Remind the patient to wear glasses and hearing aids, if prescribed.
- Encourage driver refresher classes, often offered by AARP (formerly the American Association of Retired Persons).
- Consult a certified driving specialist for an on-road driving assessment.
- Encourage avoiding high-risk driving locations or conditions, such as busy urban interstates and wet or icy weather conditions.
- Report unsafe drivers to the state department of motor vehicles if they continue to drive.

TABLE 2-1 Common Adverse Drug Events (ADEs) in Older Adults

• Edema	• Dizziness
• Severe nausea and vomiting	• Syncope
• Anorexia	• Urinary retention
• Dehydration	• Diarrhea
• Dysrhythmias	• Constipation/impaction
• Fatigue	• Hypotension
• Weakness	• Acute confusion

Data from Berryman, S.N., Jennings, J., Ragsdale, S., Lofton, T., Huff, D.C., & Rooker, J.S. (2012). Beers criteria for potentially inappropriate medication use in older adults. *MEDSURG Nursing, 21,* 129-133.

population is at high risk for adverse drug events (ADEs) directly related to the number of drugs taken and the frequency with which they are taken. Drug-drug, food-drug, drug-herb, and drug-disease interactions are common ADEs that often lead to hospital admission.

Effects of Drugs on Older Adults

Older adults often do not tolerate the standard dosage of drugs traditionally prescribed for younger adults. The physiologic changes related to aging make drug therapy more complex and challenging. These changes affect the absorption, distribution, metabolism, and excretion of drugs from the body. Even common antibiotics can lead to temporary memory loss or acute confusion. More commonly, antibiotic therapy can cause a *Clostridium difficile* infection, as discussed in Chapter 23.

Age-related changes that can potentially affect drug *absorption* from an oral route include an increase in gastric pH, a decrease in gastric blood flow, and a decrease in GI motility. Despite these changes, older adults do not have major absorption difficulties because of age-related changes alone.

Age-related changes that affect drug *distribution* include smaller amounts of total body water, an increased ratio of adipose tissue to lean body mass, a decreased albumin level, and a decreased cardiac output. Increased adipose tissue in proportion to lean body mass can cause increased storage of lipid-soluble drugs. This leads to a decreased concentration of the drug in plasma but an increased concentration in tissue.

Drug *metabolism* often occurs in the liver. Age-related changes affecting metabolism include a decrease in liver size, a decrease in liver blood flow, and a decrease in serum liver enzyme activity. These changes can result in increased plasma concentrations of a drug (Lilley, Collins, & Snyder, 2014). Monitor liver function studies, and teach older adults to have regular physical examinations.

Changes in the kidneys can also result in high plasma concentrations of drugs. The *excretion* of drugs usually involves the renal system. Age-related changes of the renal system include decreased renal blood flow and reduced glomerular filtration rate. These changes result in a decreased creatinine clearance and thus a slower excretion time for medications. Consequently,

serum drug levels can become toxic and the patient can become extremely ill or die. *Monitor renal studies, especially serum creatinine and creatinine clearance, when giving drugs to older adults!*

A creatinine clearance test measures the glomerular filtration rate of the kidneys. A commonly used formula for calculating creatinine clearance for men rather than directly measuring it is:

$$\frac{(140 - \text{Age in years}) \times \text{Lean body weight in kg}}{\text{Serum creatinine in mg/dL} \times 72}$$

For women, use this formula and multiply the answer by 0.85. A normal creatinine clearance for men is 107 to 139 mL/min and for women is 87 to 107 mL/min. Values decrease by 6.5 mL/min for each decade of life after 20 years of age (Pagana & Pagana, 2014).

When chronic disease is added to the physiologic changes of aging, drug reactions have a more dramatic effect and take longer to correct. Often a lower dose of a drug is necessary to prevent ADEs. The policy of "start low, go slow" is essential when health care providers prescribe drugs for older adults. The physiologic changes of aging are highly individual. Alterations in drug therapy should always be individualized according to the actual physiologic changes present and the occurrence and severity of chronic disease. Common ADEs are listed in Table 2-1.

Self-Administration of Drugs

Most people older than 65 years take their own medications. Because the risk for drug toxicity is considerably increased in the older population, assist patients in assuming this task responsibly. Teach patients and their caregivers, providing clear and concise directions and developing ways to assist them in overcoming difficulties with self-administration.

Older adults may make errors in self-administration or do not adhere to the drug regimen for several reasons. First, they may simply forget. In the rush of daily activities, they may not take their drugs or may take them too often because they cannot remember when or whether they have taken the medications. It is often helpful if they associate pill taking with daily events (e.g., meals) or keep a simple chart or calendar. Pill boxes are available for a daily, weekly, or monthly supply of medicine that can be placed in small compartments (Fig. 2-2). Egg cartons can be very cost-effective pill boxes. Large print on the drug label assists patients who have poor vision. Writing the drug regimen on the top of the bottle with large letters and numbers is helpful for some older adults. Colored labels or dots can also be applied. Easy-open bottle caps help older adults with limited hand mobility or strength.

FIG. 2-2 A medication system for safe self-administration.

TABLE 2-2 Examples of Beers Criteria for Potentially Inappropriate Medication Use in Older Adults

• meperidine (Demerol)	• promethazine (Phenergan)
• cyclobenzaprine (Flexeril)	• ketorolac (Toradol)
• digoxin (Lanoxin) (Should not exceed 0.125 mg daily except for atrial fibrillation)	• short-acting nifedipine (e.g., Procardia)
• ticlopidine (Ticlid)	• ferrous sulfate (Iron) (Should not exceed 325 mg daily)
• fluoxetine (Prozac)	• chlorpropamide (Diabinese)
• amitriptyline (Elavil)	• diphenhydramine (Benadryl)
• diazepam (Valium)	

Data from Berryman, S.N., Jennings, J., Ragsdale, S., Lofton, T., Huff, D.C., & Rooker, J.S. (2012). Beers criteria for potentially inappropriate medication use in older adults. *MEDSURG Nursing, 21,* 129-133.

A second reason for drug errors is poor communication with health care professionals. These problems result from poor explanations that are not understood because of educational limitations, language barriers, or difficulty with hearing and vision. Health care professionals often presume that their patients have learned the information if they have taught them about the drugs. Assist older adults in planning their drug therapy schedules as needed.

Complementary and Alternative Therapies. A third reason for errors is the varying ways that older adults take their medications. Many people older than 65 years use a multitude of complementary and alternative therapies. Some add to their drug regimen by taking OTC drugs, which can interact with prescription drugs and cause serious problems (Vitale, 2012). For example, a patient receiving warfarin (Coumadin, Warfilone ♣) for anticoagulation may take ibuprofen (Motrin) regularly for arthritis or garlic for hypertension. Because ibuprofen and garlic can inhibit clotting, this combination can cause serious bleeding. When obtaining a drug history, ask patients about all OTC drugs, including herbal and food supplements.

Some other older adults avoid taking their prescribed drugs. The fear of dependency or the cost of the drugs may cause many to discontinue their drug therapy too soon or not begin taking the drug. In addition, the actions or side effects of some drugs may not be desirable. For example, diuretics may cause incontinence when patients cannot get to the bathroom quickly enough. Others may think that two pills are twice as effective and, therefore, better than taking just one. Some older adults take drugs that are leftover from a previous illness or one that is borrowed from someone else. Teach patients to take their medications exactly as prescribed by their health care providers.

Medication Assessment and Health Teaching

The *Healthy People 2020* initiative recommends that older adults be interviewed regarding their medication use and include these questions:

- Do you take five or more prescription medications?
- Do you take herbs, vitamins, or other dietary supplements, or OTC medications?
- Do you have your prescriptions filled at more than one pharmacy?
- Is more than one health care practitioner prescribing your medications?
- Do you take your medications more than once a day?
- Do you have trouble opening your medication bottles?
- Do you have poor eyesight or hearing?
- Do you live alone?

- Do you have a hard time remembering to take your medications?

The Beers Criteria for Potentially Inappropriate Medication Use in Older Adults assessment tool, simply known as the *Beers criteria,* is also very useful in screening for medication-related risks in older adults who have chronic health problems (Berryman et al., 2012). The tool lists multiple medications and related concerns. Examples of these "at-risk" drugs are listed in Table 2-2.

To reduce drug-related risks in older adults, perform a medication assessment every 6 months or more often if an acute illness or exacerbation of a chronic disease occurs. Be sure to:

- Obtain a list of all medications taken on a regular and as-needed basis; include OTC and prescribed drugs, herbs, and nutritional supplements. If a list is not available, ask the older adult or family to gather all ointments, pills, lotions, eyedrops, inhalers, injectable solutions, vitamins, minerals, herbs, and other OTC medications and place into a bag for review.
- Highlight all medications that are part of the Beers criteria; highlight any medication for which the indication for its use is not clear, inappropriate, or could be discontinued (e.g., duplicative drug).
- Collaborate with the older adult, family, pharmacist, and primary health care provider if appropriate to determine the need for medication changes. Suggest once-a-day dosing if possible.
- Give older adults verbal and written information (at the appropriate reading level) regarding any change or new medication prescribed.
- Promote adherence to the drug therapy regimen exactly as prescribed; remind older adults to check with their primary care provider if they want to change their regimen or add an OTC medication or natural product (nutritional or herbal supplement, or probiotic).

? NCLEX EXAMINATION CHALLENGE

Physiological Integrity

A home care nurse conducts an assessment of an older woman's medications and herbal/nutritional supplements. Which supplement is most likely to cause an interaction with prescribed medications?
A. Calcium
B. Vitamin C
C. St. John's wort
D. Vitamin B complex

- Encourage lifestyle changes and other nonpharmacologic interventions to help manage or prevent health problems.
- Remind older adults not to share or borrow medications.

Mental Health/Behavioral Health Problems

Older adults are usually mentally sound and competent. Some changes in COGNITION have been identified as age related and are linked to specific cognitive functions rather than intellectual capacity. These changes include a decreased reaction time to stimuli and an impaired memory for recent events. *However, severe cognitive impairment, depression, hallucinations, and delusions are not common.*

Two forms of competence exist: legal competence and clinical competence. A person is **legally competent** if he or she is:
- 18 years of age or older
- Pregnant or a married minor
- A legally emancipated (free) minor who is self-supporting
- Not declared incompetent by a court of law

If a court determines that an older adult is not legally competent, a **guardian** is appointed to make health care decisions. Guardians may be family members or a person who is not related to the patient. When no one is available, a guardian may be appointed from a local Area Agency on Aging, an organization with comprehensive services and resources for older adults.

A person is **clinically competent** if he or she is legally competent and can make clinical decisions. Decisional capacity is determined by a person's ability to identify problems, recognize options, make decisions, and provide the rationale supporting the decisions. Selected behavioral/mental illnesses often affect both legal and clinical competence.

Nurses are in a unique position to teach older adults about ways to promote cognitive health. In a recent systematic literature review, Williams and Kemper (2010) found that collaborative interventions targeting cognitive training (e.g., learning a new skill), physical activity, social engagement, and NUTRITION were the most helpful in optimizing cognitive aging.

As older adults age, they are at increasing risk for severe mental health problems—depression, delirium, and dementia, often referred to as the *3Ds*. Many older veterans of the Korean and Vietnam wars also suffer from chronic pain, depression, post-traumatic stress disorder (PTSD), and severe anxiety. Substance abuse, especially alcoholism, is common among veterans and older adults in general. Alcoholism can contribute to cognitive decline and may be used as a coping mechanism for loss. Several mental health problems are discussed briefly here; more comprehensive discussions can be found in mental health/behavioral health textbooks.

Depression

Depression is the most common mental health/behavioral health problem among older adults in the community, affecting 15 of every 100 older adults (National Institute of Mental Health [NIMH], 2011). It increases in incidence when older adults are admitted to the hospital or nursing home. **Depression** is broadly defined as a mood disorder that can have cognitive, affective, and physical manifestations. It can be primary or secondary and can range from mild to severe, or major. As a *primary* problem, depression is thought to result from a lack of the neurotransmitters *norepinephrine* and *serotonin* in the brain. *Secondary* depression, sometimes called *situational* depression, can result when there is a sudden change in the person's life, such as an illness or loss. Common illnesses that can cause secondary depression include stroke, arthritis, and cardiac disease. It is often underdiagnosed by physicians and is therefore undertreated.

Families and nurses are in the best position to suspect depression in an older adult. Several screening tools are available to help determine if the patient has clinical depression. The **Geriatric Depression Scale—Short Form (GDS-SF)** is a valid and reliable screening tool and is available in multiple languages. The patient selects "yes" or "no" to 15 questions, or a nurse or other health care professional can ask the questions to the patient. A score of 10 or greater is consistent with a possible diagnosis of clinical depression (Fig. 2-3). These patients are then evaluated more thoroughly by the health care provider for treatment. Without diagnosis and treatment, depression can result in:
- Worsening of medical conditions
- Risk for physical illness
- Alcoholism and drug abuse
- Increased pain and disability
- Delayed recovery from illness
- Suicide

Older adults with depression may have early morning insomnia, excessive daytime sleeping, poor appetite, a lack of energy, and an unwillingness to participate in social and recreational activities. The primary treatment for depression usually includes drug therapy and psychotherapy. Selective serotonin reuptake inhibitors (SSRIs) are the first choice for drug therapy but take 2 to 3 weeks to work. They act by increasing the amount of serotonin and norepinephrine at nerve synapses in the brain.

> **! NURSING SAFETY PRIORITY** (QSEN)
>
> **Drug Alert**
>
> Tricyclic antidepressants should not be used because they have anticholinergic properties that can cause acute confusion, severe constipation, and urinary incontinence. For older adults who may be prescribed this group of drugs, question the health care provider and request an SSRI or other treatment.

Recent research has demonstrated that reminiscence or reflective therapies also help older adults overcome feelings of depression and despair. A study by McCaffrey et al. (2010) determined that frequent walking through a large garden and reflective journaling decreased depression as measured by the Geriatric Depression Scale (see the Evidence-Based Practice box). More information about depression, including strategies for preventing depression, is available in mental health/behavioral health nursing textbooks.

Dementia

Dementia is a broad term used for a syndrome that involves a slowly progressive cognitive decline, sometimes referred to as *chronic confusion*. This syndrome represents a global impairment of intellectual function and is generally chronic and progressive. There are many types of dementia, the most common being Alzheimer's disease. Multi-infarct dementia, the second most common dementia, results from a vascular disorder. Chapter 42 discusses dementias in detail, with a focus on Alzheimer's disease.

Geriatric Depression Scale—Short Form

Choose the best answer for how you have felt over the past week:

1. Are you basically satisfied with your life? YES / **NO**
2. Have you dropped many of your activities and interests? **YES** / NO
3. Do you feel that your life is empty? **YES** / NO
4. Do you often get bored? **YES** / NO
5. Are you in good spirits most of the time? YES / **NO**
6. Are you afraid that something bad is going to happen to you? **YES** / NO
7. Do you feel happy most of the time? YES / **NO**
8. Do you often feel helpless? **YES** / NO
9. Do you prefer to stay at home, rather than going out and doing new things? **YES** / NO
10. Do you feel you have more problems with memory than most? **YES** / NO
11. Do you think it is wonderful to be alive now? YES / **NO**
12. Do you feel pretty worthless the way you are now? **YES** / NO
13. Do you feel full of energy? YES / **NO**
14. Do you feel that your situation is hopeless? **YES** / NO
15. Do you think that most people are better off than you are? **YES** / NO

Answers in bold indicate depression. Score 1 point for each bolded answer.

A score > 5 points is suggestive of depression.
A score ≥ 10 points is almost always indicative of depression.
A score > 5 points should warrant a follow-up comprehensive assessment.

FIG. 2-3 The Geriatric Depression Scale—Short Form.

EVIDENCE-BASED PRACTICE (QSEN)

Do Reflective Activities Improve Symptoms of Depression and Despair in Older Adults?

McCaffrey, R., Hanson, C., & McCaffrey, W. (2010). Garden walking for depression: A research report. *Holistic Nursing Practice, 24*(5), 252-259.

Depression affects 15 of every 100 older adults at some point in their later years, which leads to physical, mental, and social dysfunction. In this mixed-method design study, the researchers created a walking guide and reflective journal entitled *Stroll for Well-Being: Garden Walks at the Morikami Museum* (Stroll) to be used by 40 community-dwelling older adults at their convenience for 12 visits over a period of 6 months. The participants were either self-diagnosed or were being treated by a health care provider for depression. The sample was 62.5% white and 12.5% African American. The remaining group was a mix of ethnic backgrounds. Most participants were educated at a high school level or higher.

The *Stroll* was structured so that they would spend about 2 hours each at 6 stops in the Morikami Museum and Japanese Gardens. At each stop, the participants made entries into a reflective journal to share their lived experience.

Using the short-form Geriatric Depression Scale (GDS) as a quantitative measure before and after the intervention, the researchers found a statistically significant change in depression scores, with lower scores indicating less depression. For the qualitative aspect of the study, a 4-step thematic analysis of the journal entries included:

- Being forced to spend time away from pressures of the day
- A sense of the beauty of nature
- Using the gardens to provide insight and depth to the experience
- Gratitude for the beauty of nature and the "life I have led"

Level of Evidence: 4

This study is a small descriptive study but includes both quantitative and qualitative methods to study the effect of the intervention for a selected convenience sample.

Commentary: Implications for Practice and Research

Depression is usually treated with psychotherapy and drugs, which often cause adverse drug effects in older adults. When nurses care for older adults with depression, they need to recommend alternative and complementary interventions that may help relieve depressive symptoms and possibly decrease dependence on drug therapy. Using the findings of this study, it is clear that enjoying the beauty of nature and reflecting on life experiences can benefit patients who have been diagnosed with or suspect that they have depression.

Delirium

Whereas dementia is a chronic, progressive disorder, **delirium** is an *acute* state of confusion. Delirium also differs from dementia in that it is often short-term and reversible within a month or less. It is often seen among older adults in a setting with which they are unfamiliar. It occurs in up to 50% of older adults who are hospitalized (Sendelbach & Guthrie, 2009). In addition to cognitive changes, some patients have physical and emotional manifestations. The types of delirium are *hyperactive, hypoactive, mixed,* and *unclassifiable. Hyperactive* patients may try to climb out of bed or become agitated, restless, and aggressive. *Hypoactive* patients are quiet, apathetic, and withdrawn. *Mixed* delirium patients have a combination of hyperactive and hypoactive manifestations. Others cannot be classified in one of these categories.

Some of the multiple factors that can cause delirium are:

- Drug therapy (especially anticholinergic and psychoactive drugs)
- Electrolyte imbalances
- Infections, especially urinary tract, pneumonia, and sepsis
- Fecal impaction or severe diarrhea
- Surgery
- Metabolic problems, such as hypoglycemia
- Neurologic disorders, such as tumors
- Circulatory, renal, and pulmonary disorders
- Nutritional deficiencies
- Hypoxemia (decreased arterial oxygen level)
- Relocation
- Major loss

> **! NURSING SAFETY PRIORITY** (QSEN)
>
> *Action Alert*
>
> Acutely confused patients who are discharged from the hospital are at an increased risk for functional decline, falls, and incontinence at home. Therefore carefully assess older patients in any setting for acute confusion so that it can be managed.

A number of tools have been developed for point-of-care screening for delirium, including the Confusion Assessment Method (CAM), Delirium Index (DI), NEECHAM Confusion Scale, and Mini-Cog (Sendelbach & Guthrie, 2009). The CAM consists of nine open-ended questions and a diagnostic algorithm for determining delirium (Table 2-3). This screening tool is easily adaptable for computerized point-of-care charting (Swan et al., 2011).

TABLE 2-3 The Confusion Assessment Method (CAM)

1. Acute onset and fluctuating course (e.g., Is there evidence of an acute change in mental status from the patient's baseline?)
2. Inattention (e.g., Does the patient have difficulty focusing attention or keeping track of what is being said?)
3. Disorganized thinking (e.g., Is the patient's thinking and conversation disorganized or incoherent?)
4. Altered level of consciousness (e.g., Is the patient lethargic, hyperalert, or difficult to arouse?)

The diagnosis of delirium by the CAM is the presence of features 1 and 2 *and* either 3 *or* 4.

Data from Sendelbach, S., & Guthrie, P.F. (2009). Evidence-based guideline—Acute confusion/delirium: Identification, assessment, treatment, and prevention. *Journal of Gerontological Nursing, 35*(11), 11-17.

Collaborate with the health care team to remove or treat risk or causative factors for acute confusion. For example, if the patient has a low oxygen saturation level, provide supplemental oxygen therapy to increase oxygen to the brain. If the patient has a urinary tract infection (UTI), it is treated. The primary clinical manifestation of UTIs in older adults is acute confusion.

To help prevent and manage delirium, use a calm voice to frequently reorient the patient. For example, playing tapes of soothing music may have a calming effect. Providing a doll or stuffed animal to "fidget" with may prevent the patient from removing important medical tubes or equipment. Some nurses believe that providing dolls and stuffed animals is treating the adult like a child, but this intervention can sometimes be very effective when used for therapeutic purposes. If the patient has a favorite item, such as an afghan blanket or a picture, ask the family or significant others to provide it for the same purpose.

Table 2-4 highlights the major differences between delirium and dementia and lists the major nursing considerations for each. The most difficult challenge is caring for a patient who is experiencing both problems at the same time.

Alcohol Use and Abuse

Excessive alcohol consumption increases the risk for falls and other accidents, affects mood and COGNITION, and leads to complications of chronic diseases like diabetes mellitus, hypertension, and gastroesophageal reflux disease (GERD). Isolation, depression, and delirium can result from alcohol abuse. The National Institute on Alcohol Abuse and Alcoholism (NIAAA) recommends that people older than 65 years have no more than one alcoholic drink a day or seven drinks in a week (NIAAA, 2011).

The Short Michigan Alcoholism Screening Test—Geriatric Version (SMAST-G) is often used by nurses and other health care professionals in ambulatory care settings to detect alcohol abuse or alcoholism. The 10 yes/no question test is available in English and Spanish and can be either self-administered

TABLE 2-4 Differences in the Characteristics of Delirium and Dementia

VARIABLE	DEMENTIA	DELIRIUM
Description	A chronic, progressive cognitive decline	An acute confusional state
Onset	Slow	Fast
Duration	Months to years	Hours to less than 1 month
Cause	Unknown, possibly familial, chemical	Multiple, such as surgery, infection, drugs
Reversibility	None	Usually
Management	Treat signs and symptoms	Remove or treat the cause
Nursing interventions	Reorientation not effective in the late stages; use validation therapy (acknowledge the patient's feelings, and do not argue); provide a safe environment; observe for associated behaviors, such as delusions and hallucinations	Reorient the patient to reality; provide a safe environment

or administered by a clinician. Examples of questions on the tool are:

- Do you drink to take your mind off your problems?
- When you feel lonely, does having a drink help?

A "yes" answer is worth one point. A total score of two or more points indicates that the person has a problem with alcohol.

Other screening tools for alcohol misuse in older adults include the CAGE questionnaire and the Alcohol-Related Problems Survey (ARPS) and the Short ARPS (shARPS). The acronym *CAGE* comes from four questions:

- Have you ever tried to <u>c</u>ut down on your drinking?
- Have people <u>a</u>nnoyed you by criticizing your drinking?
- Have you ever felt bad or <u>g</u>uilty about your drinking?
- Have you ever had a drink first thing in the morning to settle your nerves to get rid of a hangover (<u>e</u>ye-opener)?

The ARPS and shARPS were created specifically for use with older adults. In a classic study by Fink et al. (2002), these tools were shown to be more sensitive than the SMAST-G and CAGE screening tests in identifying older adults at risk for alcohol abuse. Those who were identified as non-hazardous and harmful drinkers by the ARPS tool were not identified by other tools. These groups were not diagnosed as having alcoholism but were at risk for this problem.

🔎 CLINICAL JUDGMENT CHALLENGE

Patient-Centered Care; Safety **QSEN**

A 67-year-old man recently lost his wife after being married for 42 years. He met his wife shortly after he returned from Vietnam as a combat soldier. He visits his physician and reports decreased appetite, moodiness, and extreme fatigue, even though he sleeps 10 to 12 hours a night. When giving his medical history, he admits that he drinks 4 or 5 beers and smokes marijuana almost every day.

1. What do you think caused this man's new symptoms and why?
2. As this man's office nurse, what other assessment data do you need to collect? What screening tools might you use?
3. For what safety issues is this older adult at risk and why?
4. With whom might you collaborate to develop his plan of care?

Elder Neglect and Abuse

Another problem for some older adults is neglect and abuse, both verbal and physical. Some older adults are more vulnerable to these problems than others, especially widows who may have difficulty being assertive. Elder abuse and neglect is a serious problem that affects an estimated 2 million older adults each year (U.S. Census Bureau, 2013). Older persons who are neglected or abused are often physically dependent. The abuser is often a family member who becomes frustrated or distraught over the burden of caring for the older adult. Unfortunately, only a few cases of elder abuse are reported (Stark, 2012).

Prolonged caregiving by a family member is a new and unexpected role for adult children, usually women. This new role may result in role fatigue, conflict, and strain. As a result, neglect can occur when a caregiver fails to provide for an older adult's basic needs, such as food, clothing, medications, or assistance with ADLs. The caregiver refuses to let other people, like nursing assistants or home care nurses, into the home. Whether intentional or unintentional, neglect accounts for almost half of all cases of actual elder abuse.

Physical abuse is the use of physical force that results in bodily injury, especially in the "bathing suit" zone (abdomen, buttocks, genital area, upper thighs). Examples of physical abuse are hitting, burning, pushing, and molesting the patient. Sedating the older adult is also abusive. Financial abuse occurs when the older adult's property or resources are mismanaged or misused; this is more common than physical abuse. Emotional abuse is the intentional use of threats, humiliation, intimidation, and isolation toward older adults.

Carefully assess the patient for signs of abuse, such as bruises in clusters or regular patterns; burns, commonly to the buttocks or the soles of the feet; unusual hair loss; or multiple injuries, especially fractures. If the older adult is too weak or has no other resources or support systems, he or she may not admit that abuse is occurring. Neglect may be manifested by pressure ulcers, contractures, dehydration or malnutrition, urine burns, excessive body odor, and listlessness. Depression and dementia are common in community older adults who are abused or neglected.

Be sure to screen for abuse and neglect of older adults using an appropriate assessment tool. Table 2-5 lists tools that can be used by nurses and other health care professionals to screen for elder abuse and neglect (Stark, 2012). The older adult should be referred to the appropriate service when there is:

- Evidence of mistreatment without sufficient clinical explanation
- Report by an older adult of being abused or neglected
- A belief by the health care professional that there is a high risk for or probable abuse, neglect, abandonment, or exploitation

All states in the United States and other Western countries have laws requiring health care professionals to report suspected elder abuse. In the community, if physical abuse or neglect is suspected, notify the local Adult Protective Services agency. In a hospital or nursing home, notify the social worker or case manager, who then will report the problem to the appropriate agency.

HEALTH CARE ISSUES FOR OLDER ADULTS IN HOSPITALS AND LONG-TERM CARE SETTINGS

Older adults who are admitted to hospitals and long-term care settings such as nursing homes have special needs and potential health problems. Many of these problems are similar to those seen among community older adults as discussed in this chapter. The Joint Commission and other agencies have addressed some of the most common problems seen in older adults. In addition, since 1996, the Hartford Institute for Gerontological Nursing has worked to ensure that all hospitalized patients 65 years of age and older be given quality care.

Nurses may not be aware that the needs of older adults differ from those of younger adults. Some health care systems have designated Acute Care of the Elderly (ACE) units with geriatric

---

TABLE 2-5 Examples of Elder Abuse Screening Tools

- Elder Abuse Suspicion Index
- Elder Assessment Instrument
- Indicators of Abuse Screen
- Questions to Elicit Elder Abuse
- Hwalek-Sengstock Elder Abuse Screening Tool
- Caregiver Abuse Screen
- Brief Abuse Screen for the Elderly
- Vulnerability to Abuse Screening Scale

CULTURAL CONSIDERATIONS

Patient-Centered Care QSEN

The health of Hispanic older adults continues to lag behind that for non-Hispanic whites due to a number of factors, such as language barriers, inadequate health insurance, and lack of health care access. To add to this health disparity, most nurses and other health care professionals are not trained in the language or culture of Hispanic older adults. Some older Hispanic patients may have beliefs and values that conflict with traditional Western health care views. Be respectful of these differences and incorporate them into your patient's plan of care. Become educated about the Hispanic culture and learn to speak basic medical Spanish to foster communication and trust (Strunk et al., 2013).

GENDER HEALTH CONSIDERATIONS

Patient-Centered Care QSEN

Significant health disparities are also associated with the lesbian, gay, bisexual, transgender, and questioning (LGBTQ) older adult population. Compared with heterosexual adults, LGBTQ older adults are at an elevated risk for disability from chronic disease and mental distress (Fredriksen-Goldsen, 2011). When admitted to the hospital or nursing home, they may hide their gender identity and sexual orientation from the nurse and other health care providers because of fear of rejection, discrimination, or lack of adequate health care.

Do not assume that your older patients or visitors are heterosexual. Establish a safe and trusting relationship with the patient and discuss sexual orientation and gender issues in a private setting to emphasize confidentiality. Do not force patients to answer any questions with which they feel uncomfortable. Teach direct caregivers, such as nursing assistants, that they may observe patients with sexual organs that conflict with the patient's gender identity. If this situation occurs, remind them not to be offensive or judgmental but, rather, carry out the task as planned. Chapter 73 in this text describes care of transgender patients in detail.

resources nurses and geriatric clinical nurse specialists. The patients are cared for by geriatricians who specialize in the care of older adults.

Other hospitals have developed interdisciplinary programs system-wide to meet the special needs of older patients. The incentive for these new programs is the Nurses Improving Care for Healthsystem Elders (NICHE) project, which continues to generate evidence-based practice guidelines for older adult care.

The purpose of all of these programs and units is to focus on the special health care issues or geriatric syndromes seen in the older population (Brown-O'Hara, 2013). The **Fulmer SPICES** framework was developed as part of the NICHE project and identifies six serious "marker conditions" that can lead to longer hospital stays, higher medical costs, and even deaths. These conditions are:

- **S**leep disorders
- **P**roblems with eating or feeding
- **I**ncontinence
- **C**onfusion
- **E**vidence of falls
- **S**kin breakdown

Each of these problems is briefly described here and also is discussed in more detail in other parts of this chapter and the textbook. Other problems, such as depression and constipation, are also common in older hospitalized patients. Rather than being fully comprehensive, the SPICES framework is intended to be an easy tool that has been called "geriatric vital signs" (Fulmer, 2007).

Problems of Sleep, Nutrition, and Continence

Sleep disorders are common in hospitalized patients, especially older adults. Adequate rest is important for healing, as well as for physical and mental functioning. Pain, chronic disease, environmental noise and lighting, and staff conversations are a few of the many contributing factors to insomnia in the acute and long-term care setting. Assess the patient, and ask how he or she is sleeping. If the patient is not able to answer, observe for restlessness and other behaviors that could indicate lack of adequate rest. Manage the patient's pain by giving pain medication before bedtime. Attempt to keep patients awake during the day to prevent insomnia. Keep staff conversations as quiet as possible and away from patients' rooms. Dim the lights to make the patient area as dark as possible. Avoid making loud noises such as slamming doors. Postpone treatments until waking hours or early morning if they can be delayed safely. If possible, place a "Do not Disturb" sign on the patient's door to avoid unnecessary interruptions in sleep.

Problems with eating and feeding prevent the older patient from receiving adequate NUTRITION. Malnutrition is common among older adults and is associated with poor clinical outcomes, including death. In a study by Volkert et al. (2010), NUTRITION-related problems were present in half of 205 older patients admitted to a community hospital, but only 8.3% of them received enteral nutrition supplements. The researchers concluded that nutritional screenings and standard protocols should be implemented for older patients in all hospitals. Nurses need to perform nutritional screenings on the first day of patient admission, including a thorough nutritional history, weight, height, and body mass index (BMI) calculation. Chapter 60 describes nutritional screening in more detail.

Collaborate with the registered dietitian (RD) about the patient's nutritional status as needed to achieve health goals. Consider cultural preferences, and determine what foods the patient likes. Manage symptoms such as pain, nausea, and vomiting. If the patient has difficulty chewing or swallowing, coordinate a plan of care with the speech-language pathologist and dietitian. If there are no dietary restrictions, encourage family members or friends to bring in food that the patient might enjoy. Additional interventions to prevent nutrition-related problems are discussed in Chapter 60.

Urinary and bowel ELIMINATION *issues* vary in type and severity and may be caused by many factors, including acute or chronic disease, ADL ability, and available staff. Assess the patient to identify causes for incontinence or retention. *These problems are not physiologic changes of aging but are very common in both the hospital and long-term care setting.* Place the patient on a toileting schedule or a bowel or bladder training program, if appropriate. Delegate and supervise this activity to unlicensed assistive personnel. Chapters 6 and 66 discuss bladder training in detail; Chapter 6 describes bowel training as well. Constipation was described earlier in this chapter.

Confusion, Falls, and Skin Breakdown

Acute and chronic confusion affect many older patients in both the hospital and nursing home. Whereas chronic confusion states such as dementia are not reversible, acute confusion, or delirium, may be avoidable and is often reversible when the cause is resolved or removed (see Table 2-4). For example, avoiding multiple drugs and promoting adequate sleep can help prevent acute confusion. Help the patient by reorienting him or her to reality as much as needed. Keep the patient as

🔍 NCLEX EXAMINATION CHALLENGE
Physiological Integrity

An older adult returns to the orthopedic unit after an open reduction, internal fixation surgery for a fractured hip. Upon admission, she is combative and screaming profane language. What is the nurse's first action?
A. Increase the client's rate of intravenous fluids.
B. Give the client IV morphine stat.
C. Start oxygen via mask at 6 L/min.
D. Assess for risk factors that could cause her behaviors.

comfortable as possible; for example, provide interventions to control pain. Delirium is discussed earlier in this chapter. Chapter 42 describes dementia in detail.

The most common accident among older patients in a hospital or nursing home setting is falling. A **fall** is an unintentional change in body position that results in the patient's body coming to rest on the floor or ground. Some falls result in serious injuries such as fractures and head trauma. The Joint Commission's **National Patient Safety Goals (NPSGs)** require that all inpatient health care settings have admission and daily fall risk assessment tools and a fall reduction program for patients who are at high risk.

Assess all older patients for risk for falls. Many evidence-based assessment tools, such as the Morse Fall Scale, STRATIFY, and the Hendrich II Fall Risk Model (HIIFRM), have been developed to help the nurse focus on factors that increase an older person's risk for falling. Some of these tools also recommend selected interventions depending on the patient's fall risk score (Swartzell et al., 2013). Chart 2-4 lists some of the common risk factors that should be assessed and evidence-based, collaborative interventions for preventing falls in high-risk patients. *A recent history of falling is the single most important predictor for falls.*

Toileting-related falls are very common, especially at night (Tzeng & Yin, 2012). Older patients often have **nocturia** (urination at night) and get out of bed to go to the bathroom. They may forget to ask for assistance and may subsequently fall as a result of disorientation in the darkness in an unfamiliar environment. In some cases, they may crawl over the siderail, which can make the fall more serious. Because of this, full or split siderails are used far less often in both hospitals and nursing homes. In both settings, siderails are classified as restraints unless the use of rails helps patients increase mobility.

A **restraint** is any device or drug that prevents the patient from moving freely and must be prescribed by a health care provider. In 1990, the federal government enforced a law that gives nursing home residents the right to be restraint free. Removing physical restraints from nursing home residents has reduced serious injuries, although falls and minor injuries have increased in some cases. Mattresses placed on floors next to patient beds or "low beds" have helped reduce injury.

Hospitals have also reduced the use of physical restraints. The Joint Commission has specific standards that limit the use of physical restraints in hospitals and nursing homes. Chemical restraints (psychoactive drugs) such as haloperidol (Haldol) have sometimes been used in place of physical restraints.

Experts agree that older adults should not be placed in a physical restraint or sedated just because they are old. Use alternatives before applying any type of restraint (Chart 2-5). However, if all other interventions (e.g., reminding patients to

CHART 2-4   Best Practice for Patient Safety & Quality Care   QSEN

Assessing Risk Factors and Preventing Falls in Older Adults

Assess for the presence of these risk factors:
- History of falls
- Advanced age (>80 years)
- Multiple illnesses
- Generalized weakness or decreased mobility
- Gait and postural instability
- Disorientation or confusion
- Use of drugs that can cause increased confusion, mobility limitations, or orthostatic hypotension
- Urinary incontinence
- Communication impairments
- Major visual impairment or visual impairment without correction
- Alcohol or other substance abuse
- Location of patient's room away from the nurses' station (in the hospital or nursing home)
- Change of shift or mealtime (in the hospital or nursing home)

Implement these nursing interventions for all patients, regardless of risk:
- Monitor the patient's activities and behavior as often as possible, preferably every 30 to 60 minutes.
- Teach the patient and family about the fall prevention program to become safety partners.
- Remind the patient to call for help before getting out of bed or a chair.
- Help the patient to get out of bed or a chair if needed; lock all equipment, such as beds and wheelchairs, before transferring patients.
- Teach patients to use the grab bars when walking in the hall without assistive devices or when using the bathroom.
- Provide or remind the patient to use a walker or cane for ambulating if needed; educate him or her on how to use these devices.
- Remind the patient to wear eyeglasses or a hearing aid if needed.
- Help the incontinent patient to toilet every 1 to 2 hours.
- Clean up spills immediately.
- Arrange the furniture in the patient's room or hallway to eliminate clutter or obstacles that could contribute to a fall.
- Provide adequate lighting at all times, especially at night.
- Observe for side effects and toxic effects of drug therapy.
- Orient the patient to the environment.
- Keep the call light and patient care articles within reach; ensure that the patient can use the call light.
- Place the bed in the lowest position with the brakes locked.
- Place objects that the patient needs within reach.
- Ensure that adequate handrails are present in the patient's room, bathroom, and hall.
- Have the physical therapist assess the patient for mobility and safety.

For patients at a high risk for falls:
- Implement all assessments and interventions listed above.
- Relocate the patient for best visibility and supervision.
- Encourage family members or significant other to stay with the patient.
- Collaborate with other members of the health care team, especially the rehabilitative services.
- Use technologic devices to alert staff to patients getting out of bed, such as mattress sensor pads and chair alarms.
- Use low beds or futon-type beds to prevent injury if the patient falls out of bed.

call for assistance when needed; asking a family member to stay with patients) are not effective in fall prevention, a physical restraint may be required for a limited period. Applying a restraint is a serious intervention and should be analyzed for its risk versus its benefit. Check the patient in a restraint every 30 to 60 minutes, and release the restraint at least every 2 hours for turning, repositioning, and toileting. Physical restraints such

---

CHART 2-5 Best Practice for Patient Safety & Quality Care (QSEN)

Using Restraint Alternatives

- If the patient is acutely confused, reorient him or her to reality as often as possible.
- If the patient has dementia, use validation to reaffirm his or her feelings and concerns.
- Check the patient often, at least every hour.
- If the patient pulls tubes and lines, cover them with roller gauze or another protective device; be sure that IV insertion sites are visible for assessment.
- Keep the patient busy, with an activity, pillow or apron, puzzle, or art project.
- Provide soft, calming music.
- Place the patient in an area where he or she can be supervised. (If the patient is agitated, do not place him or her in a noisy area.)
- Turn off the television if the patient is agitated.
- Ask a family member or friend to stay with the patient at night.
- Help the patient to toilet every 2 to 3 hours, including during the night.
- Be sure that the patient's needs for food, fluids, and comfort are met.
- If agency policy allows, provide the patient with a pet visit.
- Provide familiar objects or cherished items that the patient can touch.
- Document the use of all alternative interventions.
- If a restraint is applied, use the least restrictive device (e.g., mitts rather than wrist restraints, a roller belt rather than a vest).

---

as vests have caused serious injury and even death. *If restraint is needed, use the least restrictive device first. Be sure to follow your facility's policy and procedure for using restraints.*

Chemical restraints are often overused in hospital settings. Examples include:

- Antipsychotic drugs
- Antianxiety drugs
- Antidepressant drugs
- Sedative-hypnotic drugs

The most potent group of psychoactive drugs is the antipsychotics. These drugs are appropriate only for the control of certain behavioral problems, such as delusions, acute psychosis, and schizophrenia. Typical antipsychotic drugs include haloperidol (Haldol, Peridol ♦) and thiothixene (Navane). These drugs should not be used to treat anxiety or induce sedation.

! NURSING SAFETY PRIORITY (QSEN)

Drug Alert

Closely monitor older adults receiving antipsychotics for adverse drug events (ADEs). Assess patients for:
- Anticholinergic effects, the most common problem, causing constipation, dry mouth, and urinary retention
- Orthostatic hypotension, which increases the patient's risk for falls and fractures
- Parkinsonism, including tremors, bradycardia, and a shuffling gait
- Restlessness and the inability to stay still in any one position
- Hyperglycemia and diabetes mellitus, which occur more with drugs like risperidone (Risperdal) and quetiapine (Seroquel)

If any of these ADEs occur, notify the health care provider immediately.

Skin breakdown, especially pressure ulcers, is a major TISSUE INTEGRITY problem among older adults in hospitals and nursing homes. In some cases, these wounds cause death from infection. Therefore prevention is the best approach. The Joint

Commission's NPSGs require that all health care agencies have a program to prevent agency-associated pressure ulcers. The program should include these evidence-based interventions:
- Nutritional support
- Avoidance of skin injury from friction or shearing forces
- Repositioning and support surfaces
- A plan to increase MOBILITY and activity level, when appropriate
- Skin cleansing and use of moisture barriers

Assess older adults for their risk for pressure ulcers, using an assessment tool such as the Braden Scale for Predicting Pressure Sore Risk (see Chapter 25). Implement evidence-based interventions to prevent agency-acquired pressure ulcers and maintain TISSUE INTEGRITY. Coordinate these interventions with members of the health care team, including the dietitian and wound care specialist.

! NURSING SAFETY PRIORITY (QSEN)

Action Alert

Supervise unlicensed assistive personnel (UAP) for frequent turning and repositioning for the patient who is immobile. Assess the skin every 8 hours for reddened areas that do not blanch. Remind UAP to keep the skin clean and dry. Use pressure-relieving mattresses, and avoid briefs or absorbent pads that can cause skin irritation and excess moisture. Chapter 25 describes in detail additional interventions for prevention and management of pressure ulcers.

Skin tears are also common in older adults, especially the old-old group and those who are on chronic steroid therapy. Teach UAP to use extreme caution when handling these patients. Use a gentle touch, and report any open areas. Avoid bruising because older adults have increased capillary fragility.

Care Transition from the Hospital or Long-Term Care Setting to Home

Some older adults and their families experience a breakdown in communication and coordination of care when transitioning from the hospital or long-term care (LTC) setting (nursing home) to the home setting. If the transition is not optimal, older adults experience high readmission rates and an increase in visits to the emergency department or health care provider's office.

A qualitative study by Dossa et al. (2012) showed that health care professionals, especially nurses, did not communicate effectively as they prepared for the discharge of older adults. Care was not coordinated among health care professionals, which led to confusion for the older adult and family caregivers. To help prevent these problems, the authors recommended that a system needs to be in place to address patients' communication needs. The system should include follow-up phone calls after discharge to home and having one case manager to coordinate care during and after the transition from the inpatient agency to home. A home care nurse or other health care professional can serve as a "health coach" to ensure understanding of discharge instructions, consistent follow-up appointments, and a designated emergency contact for the patient and family. Discharge instructions should be easy to read, in large print, and accurate. Continuity of care for high quality transition between settings is essential to achieve positive outcomes for older adults.

GET READY FOR THE NCLEX® EXAMINATION!

KEY POINTS

Review these Key Points for each NCLEX Examination Client Needs Category.

Safe and Effective Care Environment

- Collaborate with members of the health care team when providing care to older adults in the community or inpatient setting. For example, consult with the registered dietitian for problems with NUTRITION; consult with the pharmacist to discuss the patient's drug regimen. **Teamwork and Collaboration** QSEN
- Assess all older adults for risk factors for impaired driving ability, such as decreased MOBILITY, SENSORY PERCEPTION, and COGNITION (see Chart 2-3).
- Assess older adults in the community and inpatient settings for falls risk factors (e.g., cognitive decline and vision impairment) and implement interventions as delineated in Chart 2-4. **Safety** QSEN
- Physical and chemical restraints should not be used for older adults until all other alternatives have been tried (see Chart 2-5).
- Follow The Joint Commission's National Patient Safety Goals and federal/state standards when using patient restraints to maintain patient safety. **Safety** QSEN

Health Promotion and Maintenance

- Teach older adults about the benefits of regular physical exercise.
- Provide information regarding community resources for older adults to help them meet their basic needs.
- Teach health promotion practices as listed in Chart 2-1.
- Conduct a medication assessment for potential risks in older adults using the Beers criteria.

Psychosocial Integrity

- Depression is the most common yet most underdiagnosed and undertreated mental health/behavioral health disorder among older adults.
- Delirium is acute confusion; dementia is chronic confusion (see Tables 2-3 and 2-4). Confusion is not part of the normal aging process.
- Screen older adults for alcohol abuse or alcoholism, and refer those with identified problems to appropriate resources. **Evidence-Based Practice** QSEN
- Screen older adults for neglect and abuse, which are serious problems; family caregivers are usually the abusers (see Table 2-5). **Safety** QSEN
- Relocation stress syndrome is the reaction of an older adult when transferred to a different environment; ways to minimize this problem are listed in Chart 2-2.

Physiological Integrity

- The four subgroups of the older adult population are the young old, middle old, old old, and elite old.
- The biggest concern regarding accidents among older adults in both the community and inpatient setting is falls. **Safety** QSEN
- Physiologic changes of aging predispose older adults to toxic effects of medication; drugs are absorbed, metabolized, and distributed more slowly than in younger people. They are also excreted more slowly by the kidneys.
- Medication use in older adults is often a problem when they commit errors when self-medicating, avoid needed medications, or have problems understanding their medication regimen. **Evidence-Based Practice** QSEN
- Follow The Joint Commission's National Patient Safety Goals and best practice guidelines to prevent agency-acquired pressure ulcers.
- Promote sleep and rest for older adults to decrease the incidence of delirium and to prevent falls.
- Use the SPICES assessment tool for identifying serious health problems that can be prevented or managed early.

Assessment and Care of Patients with Pain

Chris Pasero and Donna D. Ignatavicius

http//evolve.elsevier.com/Iggy/

PRIORITY CONCEPTS

- PAIN
- COGNITION
- SENSORY PERCEPTION

LEARNING OUTCOMES

Safe and Effective Care Environment

1. Identify the role of the nurse as an advocate for patients with acute pain or chronic cancer or non-cancer pain.
2. Explain the importance of collaborating with the health care team in developing the pain management plan of care.

Health Promotion and Maintenance

3. Develop a teaching plan for patients to include complementary and alternative therapies for pain management.
4. Incorporate special considerations for older adults related to pain assessment and management.
5. Describe how to provide patient-centered care by respecting patients' preferences, values, and beliefs regarding pain and its management.

Psychosocial Integrity

6. Discuss the attitudes and knowledge of patients and their families regarding pain assessment and management.
7. Explain the importance of assessing expectations of patient and family for relief of pain, discomfort, or suffering.

Physiological Integrity

8. Demonstrate comprehensive understanding of the concepts of pain and suffering, including physiologic models of PAIN and comfort.
9. Perform a complete pain assessment, and document per agency policy.
10. Compare and contrast the characteristics of the major types of PAIN and examples of each.
11. Explain the role of the three analgesic groups in pain management.
12. Differentiate between addiction, pseudoaddiction, tolerance, and physical dependence.
13. Develop a plan of care to prevent common side effects of opioid analgesics.
14. Compare the advantages and disadvantages of drug administration routes.
15. Describe the benefits and limitations of selected safety-enhancing technologies used in pain management.
16. Prioritize care for the patient receiving patient-controlled analgesia.
17. Outline care for a patient receiving epidural analgesia.
18. Identify the importance of incorporating nonpharmacologic interventions into the patient's plan of care as needed to control pain.

OVERVIEW

PAIN is a universal, complex, and personal experience that everyone has at some point in life. It is the most common reason people seek medical care and the number-one reason people take medication. Unrelieved pain can alter or diminish quality of life more than any other single health-related problem. Despite more than 30 years of education and dissemination of guideline recommendations, the failure to adequately manage pain remains a major health problem worldwide.

In response to mandates by many professional organizations and The Joint Commission (TJC), many hospitals and other health care agencies in the United States have implemented interdisciplinary PAIN initiatives to help ensure patients receive the best possible treatment. Some hospitals address this by establishing pain resource nurse (PRN) programs. As the name implies, one or more nurses per clinical unit are trained to serve as a resource to other members of the health care team in managing pain. Other hospitals have a formal team or pain service consisting of one or more nurses, pharmacists, case managers, and/or physicians. In larger facilities, pain services may specialize by type of pain (e.g., acute pain service or pain and palliative care team). Although a large part of the team's plan may center on drug therapy, these groups also recommend nonpharmacologic measures when appropriate.

SCOPE OF THE PROBLEM

PAIN is a major economic problem and a leading cause of disability that hampers the lives of many people, especially older adults. Chronic non-cancer pain, such as osteoarthritis, rheumatoid arthritis, diabetic neuropathy, and post-stroke pain syndrome, is the most common cause of long-term disability, affecting millions of Americans and others throughout the world.

Pain is inadequately treated in all health care settings. Populations at the highest risk in medical-surgical nursing are older adults, substance abusers, and those whose primary language differs from that of the health care professional. Older adults in nursing homes are at especially high risk because many residents are unable to report their PAIN. In addition, there often is a lack of staff members who have been trained to manage pain in the older adult population.

Inadequate PAIN management can lead to many adverse consequences affecting the patient and family members (Table 3-1). Therefore nurses have a legal and ethical responsibility to ensure that patients receive adequate pain control. Many professional organizations, including the American Society for Pain Management Nursing (ASPMN), the American Pain Society (APS), and TJC state that patients in all health care settings, including home care, have a right to effective pain management.

Patients rely on nurses and other health care professionals to adequately assess and manage their PAIN. As the coordinator of patient care, be sure to accurately document your assessments and actions, including patient and caregiver teaching. Communication and collaboration among the patient and members of the interdisciplinary health care team about the patient's pain, expectations, and progress toward control are equally important.

DEFINITIONS OF PAIN

Pain is defined as an unpleasant sensory and emotional experience associated with actual or potential tissue damage. McCaffery (1968) offered a more personal definition when she stated that PAIN is whatever the experiencing person says it is and exists whenever he or she says it exists. This has become the clinical definition of PAIN worldwide and reflects an understanding that the patient is the authority on the PAIN and the *only* one who can describe the experience. *In other words, self-report is always the most reliable indication of pain.* Nurses who approach pain from this perspective can help the patient achieve

effective management by advocating for proper control. If the patient cannot provide self-report, a variety of other methods, such as observation of behavioral indicators, are used to assess the PAIN (see later in this chapter).

CATEGORIZATION OF PAIN BY DURATION

PAIN is often described as being acute or chronic based on its duration (Table 3-2). *Acute pain* is usually short-lived, whereas *chronic pain* can last a person's lifetime. *Acute pain* often results from sudden, accidental trauma (e.g., fractures, burns, lacerations) or from surgery, ischemia, or acute inflammation. *Chronic pain or persistent pain* is further divided into two subtypes. *Chronic cancer pain* is pain associated with cancer and is usually the result of tissue changes from tumor growth. *Chronic non-cancer pain* is associated with past or ongoing tissue damage, such as chronic back or neck pain or osteoarthritis pain. *Non-cancer pain is the most common type of chronic pain.*

Acute Pain

Almost everyone experiences acute PAIN at some time. Brief acute pain serves a biologic purpose in that it acts as a warning signal by activating the sympathetic nervous system and causing various physiologic responses. Although not consistent in all people, when acute PAIN is severe, you may see responses similar to those found in "fight-or-flight" reactions, such as increased vital signs, sweating, and dilated pupils. Most people protect themselves by drawing away from the painful stimulus. Behavioral signs may include restlessness (especially among cognitively impaired older adults who sometimes fidget and pick at clothing), an inability to concentrate, apprehension, and overall distress of varying degrees. These heightened physiologic and behavioral responses are often referred to as the *acute pain model*. It is important to remember that the response to pain is highly individual and that humans quickly adapt physiologically and behaviorally to pain. Be careful not to expect certain responses when assessing any type of pain. *The absence of the*

TABLE 3-1 Impact of Unrelieved Pain

Physiologic Impact
- Prolongs stress response
- Increases heart rate, blood pressure, and oxygen demand
- Decreases GI motility
- Causes immobility
- Decreases immune response
- Delays healing
- Poorly managed acute pain increases risk for development of chronic pain

Quality-of-Life Impact
- Interferes with ADLs
- Causes anxiety, depression, hopelessness, fear, anger, and sleeplessness
- Impairs family, work, and social relationships

Financial Impact
- Costs Americans billions of dollars per year
- Increases hospital length of stay
- Leads to lost income and productivity

TABLE 3-2 Characteristics of Acute Pain and Chronic Pain

ACUTE	CHRONIC* (OR PERSISTENT)
• Has short duration	• Usually lasts longer than 3 months
• Usually has a well-defined cause	• May or may not have well-defined cause
• Decreases with healing	• Usually begins gradually and persists
• Is usually reversible	• Serves no useful purpose
• Initially serves a biologic purpose (warning sign to withdraw from painful stimuli or seek help)	• Ranges from mild to severe intensity
• When prolonged, serves no useful purpose	• Often accompanied by multiple quality-of-life and functional adverse effects, including depression, fatigue, financial burden, and increased dependence on family, friends, and the health care system
• Ranges from mild to severe intensity	
• May be accompanied by anxiety and restlessness	
• When unrelieved, can increase morbidity and mortality and prolong hospital length of stay	• Can impact the quality of life of family members and friends

*Includes chronic cancer pain and chronic non-cancer pain.

physiologic and behavioral responses does not mean the absence of pain.

Acute pain is usually temporary, has a sudden onset, and is easily localized. The PAIN is typically confined to the injured area and may subside with or without treatment. As the injured area heals, the SENSORY PERCEPTION of pain changes and, in most cases, diminishes and resolves. Both the caregiver and the patient can see an end to the pain, which usually makes coping somewhat easier.

PAIN that accompanies surgery is one of the most common examples of acute pain, but it is not always well managed. *The response to pain after surgery is highly individual and variable.* There is no evidence that shows one type of surgery is consistently more or less painful than another. Usually, poorly managed postoperative pain is a result of inadequate drug (analgesic) therapy. Poorly managed and prolonged acute pain serves no useful purpose and has many adverse effects including inability of the patient to participate in the recovery process with subsequent increased disability. The severity of early postoperative pain may be a predictor of long-term PAIN. Those who experience unrelieved severe postoperative pain are at high risk for the development of chronic persistent postsurgical PAIN (Pasero, 2011).

Chronic Pain

Chronic pain (also called *persistent pain*) is often defined as PAIN that lasts or recurs for an indefinite period, usually for more than 3 months. The onset is gradual, and the character and quality of the pain often change over time. *Chronic pain serves no biologic purpose.* Because it persists for an extended period, it can interfere with personal relationships and performance of ADLs. Chronic pain can also result in emotional and financial burdens, depression, and hopelessness for patients and their families. It is important to remember that the body adapts to persistent pain, and thus vital signs, such as pulse and blood pressure, may actually be lower than normal in people with chronic pain. *Although many characteristics of chronic pain are similar in different patients, be aware that each patient is unique and requires a highly individualized plan of care.*

Chronic Cancer Pain

Many patients with cancer report PAIN at the time of diagnosis, which increases in advanced stages of the disease. Most cancer pain can be successfully managed by giving adequate amounts of oral opioids around the clock, yet patients with cancer are often inadequately treated for what can be persistent, excruciating pain and suffering.

Most cancer PAIN is the result of tumor growth, including nerve compression, invasion of tissue, and/or bone metastasis, an extremely painful condition. Cancer treatments also can cause *acute pain* (e.g., from repetitive blood draws and other procedures, surgery, and toxicities from chemotherapy and radiation therapy).

Patients with cancer PAIN generally have pain in two or more areas of the body but usually talk about only the primary area. Be sure to perform a complete pain assessment to ensure an effective plan of care (see the Concept Map).

Chronic Non-Cancer Pain

Chronic non-cancer PAIN is a global health problem, occurring most often in people older than 65 years. This type of pain was formerly called *chronic nonmalignant* PAIN. However, most experts, and certainly patients who suffer daily, believe that all pain is malignant. There are many sources and types of chronic non-cancer PAIN. Among the most common are neck, shoulder, and low back pain following injury. Chronic conditions, such as diabetes, rheumatoid arthritis, Crohn's disease, and interstitial cystitis, often are associated with chronic pain. People who have had a stroke or are paralyzed may report persistent pain as a result of central nervous system (CNS) damage. Sometimes the exact cause of the pain is unclear as with fibromyalgia.

CATEGORIZATION OF PAIN BY UNDERLYING MECHANISMS

PAIN is more commonly categorized as either nociceptive (normal pain processing) or neuropathic (abnormal pain processing) (Table 3-3). The duration of nociceptive and neuropathic pain can be either acute (short-lived) or chronic (persistent), and a person can have both types.

Nociceptive Pain

The classic *gate control theory* is credited with stimulating intense research that led to discoveries that form the basis of what is known about PAIN transmission today. According to this theory, a gating mechanism exists in the spinal cord. It was proposed that when the gate is open, pain impulses ascend to the brain where the person perceives that PAIN is present (Pasero & McCaffery, 2011). When the gate is closed, the impulses are blocked and PAIN is not perceived. It is no longer necessary to discuss pain transmission in terms of theories because much is known today about this phenomenon, known as *nociception*.

Nociception is the term that is used to describe how PAIN becomes a conscious experience. It involves the *normal functioning of physiologic systems* that process noxious stimuli with the ultimate result being that the stimuli are perceived to be painful. In short, nociception means "normal" pain transmission and is generally discussed in terms of four processes: transduction, transmission, perception, and modulation (Fig. 3-1). Although it is helpful to consider nociception in the context of these four processes, it is important to understand that they do not occur as four separate and distinct entities. They are continuous, and the processes overlap as they flow from one to another.

Transduction is the first process of nociception and refers to the means by which noxious events activate neurons that exist throughout the body (skin, subcutaneous tissue, and visceral, or somatic, structures) and have the ability to respond selectively to specific noxious stimuli. These neurons are called *nociceptors*. When they are stimulated directly, a number of excitatory compounds (e.g., serotonin, bradykinin, histamine, substance P, and prostaglandins) are released that further activate more nociceptors (see Fig. 3-1) (Yaksh & Wallace, 2011).

Transmission is the second process involved in nociception. Nociceptors have small-diameter axons—either A-delta or C fibers (see Fig. 3-1). Effective transduction generates an electric signal (action potential) that is transmitted in these nerve fibers from the periphery toward the CNS. *A-delta fibers* are lightly myelinated and faster conducting than unmyelinated C fibers. The endings of A-delta fibers detect thermal and mechanical injury. The SENSORY PERCEPTION accompanying A-delta fiber activation is sharp and well-localized and leads to an appropriately rapid protective response, such as reflex withdrawal from

CONCEPT MAP

SENSORY PERCEPTION

PAIN

COGNITION

CHRONIC CANCER PAIN

HISTORY

62-year-old Jack Brown is receiving end-of-life PALLIATIVE care with metastasis of colon cancer. Palliative surgery removed an obstructive cancerous tumor but he continues to have persistent abdominal pain described as dull with an intensity of 7/10. He is receiving hydromorphone (Dilaudid) via PCA pump for pain control and Fentora lozenges are available for breakthrough pain.

PAIN Assessment →

- Grimacing, crying at times
- Verbalization of pain
- Restlessness
- Changes in interpersonal interaction—irritable with family interventions
- Changes in activity pattern/routine; hesitant to get out of bed

← Data Synthesis

PATIENT PROBLEMS

Pain – metastasis of colon cancer requiring palliation for end-of-life care

SENSORY PERCEPTION – pain interfering with clear thought, family relations, and ADLs

Data Synthesis →

PAIN Management →

- Hydromorphone-basal infusion 0.5 mg/hr, demand dose of 0.2 mg with lockout interval of 10 min and 4-hr limit of 6 mg
- Fentora: oral transmucosal lozenge, one lozenge as needed
- Massage therapy daily

Planning →

EXPECTED OUTCOMES

- Maintain level of pain control that allows patient to function and have acceptable quality of life
- Maximize independence and ability to perform ADLs
- Not experience unsafe effects from pharmacologic pain management
- Feel safe and well-cared for with physical/psychosocial needs met; provide closure with earthly life

← Planning

INTERVENTIONS

1 Comprehensive Pain Assessment
- Perform complete pain assessment and document findings. Ask patient to point to **area(s)** of pain on the body; rank **severity** of pain using the NRS; document using patient's own description, what makes pain better/worse, and how it impacts daily life. *Assesses sensory perception of pain and determines effectiveness of pain management for palliative therapy.*
- **Assess** impact of pain on performing ADLs. *Determines whether chronic pain interferes with ADLs.*
- Collaborate with interdisciplinary team about patient's pain, expectations, and progress toward control. *Coordinated efforts achieve effective pain management and palliation.*

2 Pharmacologic Pain Management
- Develop treatment plan to clarify outcomes, discussing options with patient and family. *Individualizes safe and effective use of analgesics based on comprehensive assessment.*
- Monitor effectiveness of around-the-clock dosing of analgesics. Give Fentora lozenges for breakthrough pain. *Successfully manages cancer pain.*
- Prevent common side effects: give antiemetics and fluids for nausea/vomiting; give a daily stool softener plus a mild peristaltic stimulant for constipation. *Side effects are a primary reason people stop taking pain medication.*

3 Nursing Safety Priority: Action Alert!
Teach patient how to use the PCA device and to report side effects. Monitor sedation level and respiratory status at least every 2 hours. Promptly decrease dose if increased sedation is detected. *Ensures patient is able to understand relationships between pain, accepting an analgesic dose, and pain relief. Ensures patient is cognitively and physically able to use the equipment.*

4 Nonpharmacologic Pain Management
- Explore nonpharmacologic interventions to complement drug therapy. *Cognitive-behavioral therapy, distraction, and imagery may strongly influence pain perception.*
- Teach alternative methods: heat, cold, pressure; Therapeutic Touch; massage; vibration; TENS unit; distraction; imagery; relaxation; hypnosis. *Facilitates relaxation and reduces anxiety, stress, and depression.*

5 Psychosocial Assessment
- Assist patient to verbalize concerns about body image, self-concept, role performance, self-esteem, sexuality. *Sets realistic goals based on patient preferences and values of palliative care at end of life.*
- Have patient describe personal attitudes about pain. *Prevents worries about addiction, death, or body mutilation, and thoughts of being punished or a spiritual significance to lingering pain.*
- Respect patient's verbal and nonverbal expressions of pain. *Avoids depression and hopelessness arising from uncontrolled chronic pain.*
- Explore support systems and coping strategies. *Helps keep unpredictability and uncertainty of terminal disease from affecting the entire family.*

6 Self-Management Education
- Teach patient and family about drug therapy. *Maximizes relief and symptom control at home, and eliminates unnecessary hospital readmissions.*
- Help patient establish an analgesic regimen that helps with sleep, rest, appetite, and activity level. *Helps patient identify and plan important activities with adequate rest periods.*
- Evaluate family support systems to assist patient in adhering to proposed treatment and plan of care. *Includes family members in activities during and after hospitalization.*

Concept Map by Deanne A. Blach, MSN, RN

TABLE 3-3   Physiologic Sources of Nociceptive Pain and Neuropathic Pain

PHYSIOLOGIC STRUCTURE	CHARACTERISTICS OF PAIN	SOURCES OF ACUTE POSTOPERATIVE PAIN	SOURCES OF CHRONIC PAIN SYNDROMES
Nociceptive Pain (normal pain processing)			
Somatic Pain			
Cutaneous or superficial: skin and subcutaneous tissues	Sharp, burning	Incisional pain, pain at insertion sites of tubes and drains, wound complications, orthopedic procedures, skeletal muscle spasms	Bony metastases, osteoarthritis and rheumatoid arthritis, low back pain, peripheral vascular diseases
Deep somatic: bone, muscle, blood vessels, connective tissues	Dull, aching, cramping		
Visceral Pain			
Organs and the linings of the body cavities	Poorly localized	Chest tubes, abdominal tubes and drains, bladder distention or spasms, intestinal distention	Pancreatitis, liver metastases, colitis, appendicitis
	Diffuse, deep cramping or splitting, sharp, stabbing		
Neuropathic Pain (abnormal pain processing)			
Peripheral or central nervous system: nerve fibers, spinal cord, and higher central nervous system	Poorly localized	Phantom limb pain, postmastectomy pain, nerve compression	HIV-related pain, diabetic neuropathy, postherpetic neuralgia, chemotherapy-induced neuropathies, cancer-related nerve injury, radiculopathies
	Shooting, burning, fiery, shocklike, sharp, painful numbness		

HIV, Human immune deficiency virus.

the painful stimuli. *C fibers* are unmyelinated or poorly myelinated slow conductors and respond to mechanical, thermal, and chemical stimuli. Activation after acute injury yields a poorly localized (more widely distributed) typically aching or burning pain. In contrast to the intermittent nature of A-delta sensations, C fibers usually produce more continuous pain.

Perception is the third broad process involved in nociception. Perception, which may be viewed as the end result of the neural activity associated with transmission of information about noxious events, involves the conscious awareness of PAIN (see Fig. 3-1). It requires the activation of higher brain structures, including the cortex, and involves both awareness and the occurrence of emotions and drives associated with pain. The physiology of pain perception is very poorly understood but presumably can be targeted by therapies that activate higher cortical functions to achieve pain control or coping. Cognitive-behavioral therapy and specific approaches such as distraction and imagery (discussed later in the chapter) have been developed based on evidence that brain processes can strongly influence pain perception.

Modulation of afferent input generated in response to noxious stimuli happens at every level from the periphery to the cortex (see Fig. 3-1). The neurochemistry of modulation is complex and not yet fully understood, but it is known that multiple peripheral and central systems and dozens of neurochemicals are involved. For example, the endogenous opioids (endorphins) are found throughout the peripheral nervous system (PNS) and CNS and, like the exogenous opioids administered therapeutically, they inhibit neuronal activity by binding to opioid receptors. Other central inhibitory neurotransmitters important in the modulation of pain include serotonin and norepinephrine, which are released in the spinal cord and brainstem by the descending fibers of the modulatory system to inhibit pain.

Nociceptive pain is the result of actual or potential tissue damage or inflammation and is often categorized as being somatic or visceral. *Somatic pain* arises from the skin and musculoskeletal structures, and *visceral pain* arises from organs. Examples include PAIN-associated trauma, surgery, burns, and tumor growth.

Neuropathic Pain

Neuropathic pain is a descriptive term used to refer to PAIN that is believed to be sustained by a set of mechanisms that is driven by damage to or dysfunction of the PNS and/or CNS. In contrast to nociceptive pain, which is sustained by ongoing activation of essentially *normal* neural systems, neuropathic pain is sustained by the *abnormal* processing of stimuli. Whereas nociceptive pain involves tissue damage or inflammation, neuropathic pain may occur in the absence of either.

It is not clear why noxious stimuli result in neuropathic PAIN in some people and not in others and why some treatments work in some and not in others. Neuropathic pain is difficult to treat and often resistant to first-line analgesics. Asking patients to describe it is the best way to identify the presence of neuropathic pain. Common distinctive descriptors include "burning," "shooting," "stabbing," and feeling "pins and needles." Much is unknown about what causes and maintains neuropathic pain; it is the subject of intense ongoing research.

PATIENT-CENTERED COLLABORATIVE CARE

Pain Assessment

All accepted guidelines identify the patient's self-report as the gold standard for assessing the existence and intensity of PAIN (Pasero & McCaffery, 2011). Because pain is such a private and personal experience, it may be difficult for the person to describe or explain it to others. However, subjective descriptions of the experience and measurement of pain intensity are more reliable and accurate than observable qualities of pain. The amount of pain and responses to it vary from person to person; therefore interpreting it solely on actions or behaviors can be misleading and is not recommended. Patients may report pain in the absence of any observable or documented physiologic changes.

Although nurses are entitled to their doubts and opinions about a patient's PAIN, those doubts and opinions cannot be allowed to interfere with appropriate patient care. The nurse's primary role in PAIN management is to advocate for patients by *accepting* their reports of pain and acting promptly to relieve it,

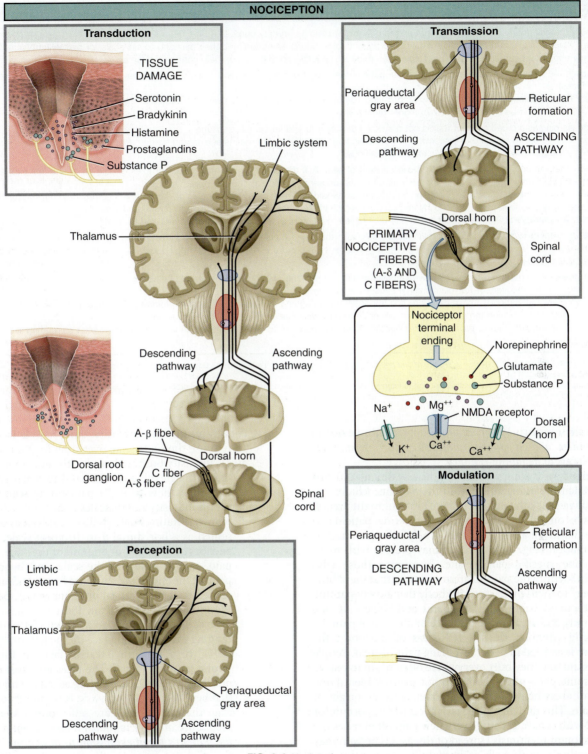

NOCICEPTION

Transduction

TISSUE DAMAGE
- Serotonin
- Bradykinin
- Histamine
- Prostaglandins
- Substance P

Limbic system

Thalamus

Descending pathway

Ascending pathway

A-β fiber

Dorsal root ganglion

C fiber

A-δ fiber

Dorsal horn

Spinal cord

Transmission

Periaqueductal gray area

Reticular formation

Descending pathway

ASCENDING PATHWAY

Dorsal horn

PRIMARY NOCICEPTIVE FIBERS (A-δ AND C FIBERS)

Spinal cord

Nociceptor terminal ending

Norepinephrine

Glutamate

Substance P

Na^+

Mg^{++}

NMDA receptor

Dorsal horn

K^+

Ca^{++}

Ca^{++}

Modulation

Periaqueductal gray area

Reticular formation

DESCENDING PATHWAY

Ascending pathway

Perception

Limbic system

Thalamus

Periaqueductal gray area

Descending pathway

Ascending pathway

FIG. 3-1 Nociception.

while respecting patients' preferences and values (Quality and Safety Education for Nurses [QSEN], 2011).

To be patient-centered, always respect the patient's verbal and nonverbal expressions of PAIN without making judgments or inferences about the reality of it. If patients perceive that health care professionals doubt the existence of their pain, mistrust and other negative feelings can arise and interfere with a therapeutic nurse-patient relationship.

The Comprehensive Pain Assessment

A comprehensive pain assessment should be conducted during the initial interview with the patient, with each new report of pain, and whenever indicated by changes in the patient's condition or treatment plan during the course of care. PAIN assessment at these intervals serves as the foundation for developing and evaluating the effectiveness of the treatment plan. Remember that patients' personal preferences and values affect how

TABLE 3-4   **Teaching Patients and Their Families How to Use A Pain Rating Scale***
Step 1. Show the pain rating scale to the patient and family, and explain its primary purpose.   *Example:* "This is a pain rating scale that many of our patients use to help us understand their pain and to set goals for pain relief. We will ask you regularly about pain, but any time you have pain you must let us know so that we can help control it. We don't always know when you hurt."
Step 2. Explain the parts of the pain rating scale. If the patient does not like it or understand it, switch to another scale (e.g., vertical presentation, VDS, or faces).   *Example:* "On this pain rating scale, 0 means no pain and 10 means the worst possible pain. The middle of the scale, around 5, means moderate pain. A 2 or 3 would be mild pain, but 7 or higher means severe pain."
Step 3. Discuss pain as a broad concept that is not restricted to a severe and intolerable sensation.   *Example:* "Pain refers to any kind of discomfort anywhere in your body. Pain also means aching and hurting. Pain can include pulling, tightness, burning, knifelike feelings, and other unpleasant sensations."
Step 4. Verify that the patient understands the broad concept of pain. Ask the patient to mention two examples of pain he or she has experienced. If the patient is already in pain that requires treatment, use the present situation as the example.   *Example:* "I want to be sure that I've explained this clearly, so would you give me two examples of pain you've had recently?" If the patient examples include various parts of the body and various pain characteristics, that indicates that he or she understands pain as a fairly broad concept. An example of what a patient might say is "I have a mild, sort of throbbing headache now, and yesterday my back was aching."
Step 5. Ask the patient to practice using the pain rating scale with the present pain or select one of the examples mentioned.   *Example:* "Using the scale, what is your pain right now? What is it at its worst?" OR "Using the pain rating scale and one of your examples of pain, what is that pain usually? What is it at its worst?"
Step 6. Set goals for comfort and function/recovery/quality of life. Ask patients what pain rating would be acceptable or satisfactory, considering the activities required for recovery or for maintaining a satisfactory quality of life.   *Example for a surgical patient:* "I have explained the importance of coughing and deep breathing to prevent pneumonia and other complications. Now we need to determine the pain rating that will not interfere with this so that you may recover quickly."   *Example for patient with chronic pain or terminal illness:* "What do you want to do that pain keeps you from doing? What pain rating would allow you to do this?"

From Pasero, C., & McCaffery, M. (2011). *Pain assessment and pharmacologic management.* St. Louis: Mosby. Copyright 2011, McCaffery, M., & Pasero, C. Used with permission.
VDS, Verbal descriptor scale.
*When a patient is obviously in pain or not focused enough to learn to use a pain rating scale, pain treatment should proceed without pain ratings. Teaching can be undertaken when pain is reduced to a level that facilitates understanding how to use a pain scale.

they report their history. *When culturally appropriate, be sure to include families and significant others in this information-gathering process to be family-centered.*

Components of a comprehensive PAIN assessment and tips on how to elicit the information from the patient include:

- *Location(s):* Ask the patient to state or point to the area(s) of PAIN on the body. Sometimes allowing patients to make marks on a body diagram is helpful in gaining this information (Fig. 3-2). Patients may present with more than one specific painful site. Encourage those who cannot identify the painful areas and state that they "hurt all over" to focus on parts of the body that are not painful. Ask them to begin with the hand and fingers of one extremity and identify the presence or absence of pain. By focusing attention on selected areas of the body, the patient is assisted in better localizing painful areas. People who state that they hurt everywhere often begin to realize that some parts of the body are not painful. Identifying painful areas helps the patient understand the origin of the pain. This understanding is particularly important for those with cancer, because every new pain often raises the suspicion of metastasis (spread of disease). The pain may have other causes, such as immobility or constipation. Pain may be described as belonging to one of four categories related to its location:

  1. Localized pain is confined to the site of origin.
  2. Projected pain is diffuse around the site of origin and is not well localized.
  3. Referred pain is felt in an area distant from the site of painful stimuli.
  4. Radiating pain is felt along a specific nerve or nerves.

- *Intensity:* Ask the patient to rate the severity of the PAIN using a reliable and valid assessment tool. Various self-report scales have been developed to help patients

communicate PAIN intensity. Once a scale is selected, be sure to use the *same* scale over time for that patient, and assess intensity both with and without activity. See Table 3-4 for strategies that can be used to teach patients and their families how to use a pain rating scale. The most common intensity rating scales are:

- Numeric Rating Scale (NRS): The NRS is usually presented as a horizontal 0-to-10 point scale, with word anchors of "no pain" at one end of the scale, "moderate pain" in the middle of the scale, and "worst possible pain" at the end of the scale (see Fig. 3-3). Some patients relate better to a vertical presentation of the scale.
- Wong-Baker FACES® Pain Rating Scale: The FACES scale consists of 6 cartoon faces with word descriptors, ranging from a smiling face on the left for "no pain (or hurt)" to a frowning, tearful face on the right for "worst pain (or hurt)." The faces are most commonly numbered 0 to 10. Patients are asked to choose the face that best describes their PAIN. It is important to appreciate that faces scales are self-report tools; *clinicians should not attempt to match a face shown on a scale to the patient's facial expression to determine pain intensity.* Fig. 3-3 provides the Wong-Baker FACES scale combined with the NRS.
- Faces Pain Scale-Revised (FPS-R): The FPS-R has 7 faces to make it consistent with other scales using the 0 to 10 metric. The faces range from a neutral facial expression to one of intense pain. As with the Wong-Baker FACES® scale, patients are asked to choose the face that best reflects their PAIN. Some research shows that the FPS-R is preferred by both cognitively intact and impaired older adults.
- Verbal Descriptor Scale (VDS): A VDS uses different words or phrases to describe the intensity of PAIN,

McGill-Melzack
PAIN QUESTIONNAIRE

Patient's name _____ Age _____

File No. _____ Date _____

Clinical category (e.g., cardiac, neurologic)

Diagnosis: _____

_____

_____

Analgesic (if already administered):

1. Type _____

2. Dosage _____

3. Time given in relation to this test _____

Patient's intelligence: circle number that represents best estimate.

1 (low)   2   3   4   5 (high)

****

This questionnaire has been designed to tell us more about your pain. Four major questions we ask are

1. Where is your pain?
2. What does it feel like?
3. How does it change with time?
4. How strong is it?

It is important that you tell us how your pain feels now. Please follow the instructions at the beginning of each part.

_____

© R. Melzack, Oct. 1970

Part 1. Where Is Your Pain?

Please mark, on the drawings below, the areas where you feel pain. Put E if external, or I if internal, near the areas you mark. Put EI if both external and internal.

Part 2. What Does Your Pain Feel Like?

Some of the words below describe your *present* pain. Circle *ONLY* those words that best describe it. Leave out any category that is not suitable. Use only a single word in each appropriate category—the one that applies best.

1	6	11	16
Flickering	Tugging	Tiring	Annoying
Quivering	Pulling	Exhausting	Troublesome
Pulsing	Wrenching	**12**	Miserable
Throbbing	**7**	Sickening	Intense
Beating	Hot	Suffocat-	Unbearable
Pounding	Burning	ing	
2	Scalding	**13**	**17**
Jumping	Searing	Fearful	Spreading
Flashing	**8**	Frightful	Radiating
Shooting	Tingling	Terrifying	Penetrating
3	Itchy	**14**	Piercing
Pricking	Smarting	Punishing	**18**
Boring	Stinging	Grueling	Tight
Drilling	**9**	Cruel	Numb
Stabbing	Dull	Vicious	Drawing
Lancinating	Sore	Killing	Squeezing
4	Hurting	**15**	Tearing
Sharp	Aching	Wretched	**19**
Cutting	Heavy	Blinding	Cool
Lacerating	**10**		Cold
5	Tender		Freezing
Pinching	Taut		**20**
Pressing	Rasping		Nagging
Gnawing	Splitting		Nauseating
Cramping			Agonizing
Crushing			Dreadful
			Torturing

Part 3. How Does Your Pain Change With Time?

1. Which word or words would you use to describe the *pattern* of your pain?

1	2	3
Continuous	Rhythmic	Brief
Steady	Periodic	Momentary
Constant	Intermittent	Transient

2. What kind of things *relieve* your pain?

3. What kind of things *increase* your pain?

Part 4. How Strong Is Your Pain?

People agree that the following 5 words represent pain of increasing intensity. They are:

1	2	3	4	5
Mild	Discomforting	Distressing	Horrible	Excruciating

To answer each question below, write the number of the most appropriate word in the space beside the question.

1. Which word describes your pain right now? _____
2. Which word describes it at its worst? _____
3. Which word describes it when it is least? _____
4. Which word describes the worst toothache you ever had? _____
5. Which word describes the worst headache you ever had? _____
6. Which word describes the worst stomachache you ever had? _____

FIG. 3-2 The McGill-Melzack Pain Questionnaire.

Wong-Baker FACES® Pain Rating Scale

0	2	4	6	8	10
No Hurt	Hurts Little Bit	Hurts Little More	Hurts Even More	Hurts Whole Lot	Hurts Worst

©1983 Wong-Baker FACES® Foundation. Visit us at www.wongbakerFACES.org.
Used with permission. Originally published in Whaley & Wong's Nursing Care of Infants and Children. ©Elsevier Inc.

FIG. 3-3 Wong-Baker FACES® pain rating scale.

such as "*no pain, mild pain, moderate pain, severe pain very severe pain,* and *worst possible pain.*" The patient is asked to select the phrase that best describes the pain intensity.

- *Quality:* Ask the patient to describe how the PAIN feels. He or she may use one word or a group of words to convey the SENSORY PERCEPTION of the pain. *Avoid suggesting descriptive words for the pain; allow patients to use their own words to describe the pain.* Descriptors such as "sharp," "shooting," or "burning" may help identify the presence of neuropathic pain. Ask the patient whether the pain is superficial or deep. In general, those with pain involving superficial or cutaneous (skin) structures describe it as superficial and can often localize the pain to a specific area.
- *Onset and duration:* Ask the patient when the PAIN started and whether it is constant or intermittent.
- *Aggravating and relieving factors:* Ask the patient what makes the PAIN worse and what makes it better. Ask about strategies the patient has used before to manage pain.
- *Effect of pain on function and quality of life:* The effect of PAIN on the ability to perform recovery activities should be regularly evaluated. It is particularly important to ask patients with persistent pain about how it has affected their lives. Ask what they could do before the pain began that they can no longer do and what they want to do but cannot do.
- *Comfort-function (pain intensity) outcomes:* For patients with *acute pain,* identify expected short-term functional outcomes. Reinforce to the patient that adequate PAIN control will lead to more successful achievement of those outcomes. For example, tell surgical patients that they will be expected to ambulate or participate in physical therapy postoperatively. Ask patients to identify a level of pain that will allow accomplishment of the expected outcomes. A realistic outcome for most patients is 2 or 3 on a scale of 0 to 10. Pain intensity that is consistently above the desired level requires further evaluation and consideration of possible adjustment of the treatment plan.
- *Other information:* Consider the patient's culture, past PAIN experiences, and pertinent medical history such as comorbidities. Current treatments and diagnostic studies are considered when performing an assessment. For example, patients who are intubated may be awake and alert but unable to speak. Strategies to assess the presence and severity of PAIN in these patients include (Tate et al., 2012):

CONSIDERATIONS FOR OLDER ADULTS
Patient-Centered Care QSEN

PAIN is not an inevitable consequence of aging; however, the incidence is higher in older adults. Sensitivity to pain does not diminish with age. Many older adults, even those with mild to moderate dementia, are able to use a self-report assessment tool if nurses and other caregivers take the time to administer it. Many older adults are reluctant to report pain for a variety of reasons including the belief that it is normal and that they are bothering the nurse. It is essential that attempts be made to elicit the patient's self-report and pain be assessed frequently with a focus on functional and quality-of-life indicators in this vulnerable population.

Psychosocial Assessment

PAIN holds unique meaning for the person experiencing it. Patients having *acute pain* from surgery may interpret it as necessary and expected. It may be viewed with relief as a sign that some greater problem has been resolved or alleviated by the surgery. Knowing that the duration of the pain is limited may be reassuring for a patient. In contrast, acute chest pain associated with angina may mark the beginning of a life of fear and uncertainty.

Various psychosocial factors influence *chronic* PAIN. Some factors are similar to those found in the acute pain experience, such as anxiety or fear related to the meaning of the pain. Because chronic pain persists or is perhaps only partially relieved, the patient may feel powerless, angry, hostile, or desperate. He or she is also vulnerable to labels such as "chronic complainer" or "faker." Remember that it is unprofessional and inappropriate to label or stereotype patients. *Remain objective, and advocate for proper pain control for all patients.*

Assess the status of family and other close relationships, along with the range of social resources available to the patient with chronic pain. The existence of a pain-specific conflict with a spouse or significant other may affect or limit coping strategies. Other people may react to chronic pain with depression, social withdrawal, and preoccupation with physical symptoms. Refer the patient and family to self-help groups, such as the American Chronic Pain Association (http://theacpa.org), which provides the "10-Step Program from Patient to Person."

If the chronic PAIN is associated with a progressive disease such as cancer, rheumatoid arthritis, or peripheral vascular disease, the patient may have worries and concerns about the consequences of the illness. People with cancer-related pain may fear death or body mutilation. Some may think they are being punished for some wrongdoing in life. Others may attach a religious or spiritual significance to lingering pain.

Ask open-ended questions (e.g., "Tell me how your pain has affected your job or your role as a mother.") to allow the patient to describe personal attitudes about PAIN and its influence on life. This opportunity can help someone whose life has been changed by pain. However, some patients choose not to share their private information or fears. As a patient-centered nurse, always respect patients' preferences and values.

❓ NCLEX EXAMINATION CHALLENGE
Physiological Integrity

A client who had a laminectomy reports new onset of severe back pain. What responses by the nurse are most appropriate for the client at this time? **Select all that apply.**
A. "How is your pain on a 0-10 scale with 10 being the worst possible pain you've had?"
B. "Could you describe the pain in your back?"
C. "When you had visitors, you seemed to be laughing and not in any pain."
D. "I'll get you some pain medication that the surgeon ordered."
E. "Can you tell me what positions make the pain feel worse and better?"

Assessment Challenges

Patients who are unable to report their PAIN using the customary self-report assessment tools are at higher risk for undertreated pain than those who can report. These include patients who are cognitively impaired, critically ill (intubated, unresponsive), comatose, or imminently dying. Patients who are receiving neuromuscular blocking agents or are sedated from general anesthetics and other drugs given during surgery are also among this at-risk population.

First suggested in 1999 by McCaffery and Pasero, the *Hierarchy of Pain Measures* is recommended by many professional organizations today as a framework for assessing PAIN in patients who cannot self-report. The key components of the Hierarchy require the nurse to (1) attempt to obtain self-report; (2) consider underlying pathology or conditions and procedures that might be painful (e.g., surgery); (3) observe behaviors; (4) evaluate physiologic indicators; and (5) conduct an analgesic trial. See Table 3-5 for detailed information on each component of the Hierarchy of Pain Measures.

Patients with problems of COGNITION are among those at highest risk for undertreated PAIN because they are unable or have difficulty reporting their pain. The Hierarchy of Pain Measures (Table 3-5) lists several strategies to use when obtaining self-report is a challenge. When these are ineffective, the Hierarchy suggests that a number of behaviors have been shown to be indicators of pain. Behavioral pain assessment tools are often used to systematically evaluate behaviors to help determine the presence of pain. Improvement in the behavioral pain score helps confirm suspicions that pain is present and provides a reference point for assessing the effectiveness of interventions.

It is important for nurses to remember that *a score obtained from the use of a behavioral tool is not the same as a self-reported pain intensity score.* Although it may seem logical to assume that the higher the behavioral score, the more intense the pain, this cannot be proven without the patient's report. Some patients remain nonverbal and lie completely still (which would yield a

---

TABLE 3-5 Hierarchy of Pain Measures

1. Attempt to obtain the patient's self-report, the single most reliable indicator of pain. Do not assume a patient cannot provide a report of pain; many cognitively impaired patients are able to use a self-report tool if simple actions are taken.
   - Try using a standard pain assessment tool (see Fig. 3-3).
   - Ensure eyeglasses and hearing aids are functioning.
   - Increase the size of the font and other features of the scale.
   - Present the tool in vertical format (rather than the frequently used horizontal).
   - Try using alternative words, such as "ache," "hurt," and "sore" when discussing pain.
   - Ask about pain in the present.
   - Repeat instructions and questions more than once.
   - Allow ample time to respond.
   - Remember that head nodding and eye blinking or squeezing the eyes tightly can also be used to signal presence of pain and sometimes used to rate intensity.
   - Ask awake and oriented ventilated patients to point to a number on the numeric scale if they are able.
   - Repeat instructions and show the scale each time pain is assessed.
2. Consider the patient's condition or exposure to a procedure that is thought to be painful. If appropriate, *assume pain is present* (APP) and document APP when approved by institution policy and procedure. As an example, pain should be assumed to be present in an unresponsive, mechanically ventilated, critically ill trauma patient. Nurses should assume that certain procedures are painful and premedicate based on that assumption.
3. Observe behavioral signs (e.g., facial expressions, crying, restlessness, and changes in activity). A pain behavior in one patient may not be in another. Try to identify pain behaviors that are unique to the patient ("pain signature"). Many behavioral pain assessment tools are available that will yield a pain behavior score and may help determine if pain is present. However, it is important to remember that a behavioral score is not the same as a pain intensity score. Behavioral tools are used to help identify the presence of pain and whether an intervention is effective, but the pain intensity is unknown if the patient is unable to provide it.
   - A surrogate who knows the patient well (e.g., parent, spouse, or caregiver) may be able to provide information about underlying painful pathology or behaviors that may indicate pain.
   - Although surrogates may be helpful in identifying behaviors that may indicate pain, research has shown that they commonly underestimate or overestimate the intensity of the pain. Therefore they should not be asked to rate the patient's pain intensity.
4. Evaluate physiologic indicators with the understanding that they are the *least* sensitive indicators of pain and may signal the existence of conditions other than pain or a lack of it (e.g., hypovolemia, blood loss). Patients quickly adapt physiologically despite pain and may have normal or below normal vital signs in the presence of severe pain. The overriding principle is that the absence of an elevated blood pressure or heart rate does not mean the absence of pain.
5. Conduct an analgesic trial to confirm the presence of pain and to establish a basis for developing a treatment plan if pain is thought to be present. An analgesic trial involves administering a low dose of analgesic and observing patient response. The initial low dose may not be enough to illicit a change in behavior and should be increased if the previous dose was tolerated, or another analgesic may be added. If behaviors continue despite optimal analgesic doses, other possible causes should be investigated.
   - In patients who are unresponsive, no change in behavior will be evident and the optimized analgesic dose should be continued.

From Pasero, C., & McCaffery, M. (2011). *Pain assessment and pharmacologic management.* St. Louis: Mosby.

low behavioral score) despite having severe PAIN. The reality is that if a patient cannot report the intensity of pain, the exact intensity is unknown. Two of the most commonly used behavioral assessment tools that are used for patients with problems of COGNITION such as delirium (acute confusion) or dementia (chronic confusion) are:

- Checklist of Nonverbal Pain Indicators (CNPI) has been tested in the acute care setting in patients with varying levels of cognitive impairment. The tool groups behavioral indicators of PAIN into six categories. Each category allows a score of 0 if the behavior is not observed and a 1 if the behavior occurred even briefly during activity or rest:
  - Facial expression (e.g., grimacing, crying)
  - Verbalizations or vocalizations (e.g., screaming)
  - Body movements (e.g., restlessness)
  - Changes in interpersonal interactions
  - Changes in activity patterns or routines
  - Mental status changes (e.g., confusion, increased confusion)
- Pain Assessment in Advanced Dementia (PAINAD) scale, which has been tested in patients with severe dementia (Herr et al., 2011). The tool groups behavioral indicators into five categories for scoring using a graduated scale of 0 (least intense behaviors) to 2 (most intense behaviors) per category for a maximum behavioral score of 10:
  - Breathing (independent of vocalization)
  - Negative vocalization
  - Facial expression
  - Body language
  - Consolability (ability to calm the patient)

❓ NCLEX EXAMINATION CHALLENGE

Psychosocial Integrity

> An older client who has advanced Alzheimer's disease is admitted to the clinical unit after abdominal surgery and is guarding her abdomen and moaning. What action will the nurse take?
> A. Ask the client's family to rate the intensity of the client's pain using the 0-to-10 scale.
> B. Use a behavioral pain assessment tool to determine the presence of pain.
> C. Ask the client to rate the intensity of her pain using the 0-to-10 scale.
> D. Contact the primary health care provider to request an order for an antianxiety drug.

For patients who are mechanically ventilated or may not be able to use other tools for communication, you can use these interventions:

- Establishing a reliable yes-no signal (e.g., thumbs up or down, head nods, or eye blinks) may be appropriate in some patients to establish the presence of pain.
- Use of communication boards, alphabet boards, computer, or picture boards with word labels may be helpful for patients with COGNITION problems.
- Correctly interpreting lip reading by maintaining eye contact, encouraging the patient to speak slowly, and using dentures if required are recommended.

Pharmacologic Management of Pain

Safe and effective use of analgesics requires the development of an individualized treatment plan based on a comprehensive assessment. This plan includes clarifying the desired outcomes of treatment and discussing options and preferences with the patient and family. Desired outcomes are periodically re-evaluated and changes made depending on patient response and, in some cases, disease progression.

Multimodal Analgesia

PAIN is complex, which explains why there is no single, universal treatment for it. Its complexity is also the basis for the widespread recommendation that a multimodal analgesic approach be used regardless of the type of pain (American Society of Anesthesiologists [ASA], 2012; Pasero & McCaffery, 2011; Portenoy, 2011; Turk et al., 2011; Wu & Raja, 2011). Multimodal treatment involves the use of two or more classes of analgesics to target different pain mechanisms in the PNS or CNS. It relies on the thoughtful and rational combination of analgesics to maximize relief and prevent analgesic gaps that may lead to worsening pain or unnecessary episodes of uncontrolled pain.

A multimodal approach may allow lower doses of each of the drugs in the treatment plan. Lower doses have the potential to produce fewer side effects. Further, multimodal analgesia can result in comparable or greater relief than can be achieved with any single analgesic. For postoperative PAIN, the use of combination therapy to prevent both inflammatory and neuropathic pain is likely to yield the best immediate results. It also offers the promise of reducing the incidence of prolonged or persistent postsurgical pain.

The multimodal strategy also has a role in the management of persistent PAIN. The complex nature of the many chronic conditions indicates the need for appropriate combinations of analgesics, such as anticonvulsants, antidepressants, and local anesthetics, to target differing underlying mechanisms.

Preemptive analgesia involves the administration of local anesthetics, opioids, and other drugs (multimodal analgesia) along the continuum of care, during the preoperative, intraoperative, and postoperative periods. This continuous approach is designed to decrease PAIN severity in the postoperative period, reduce analgesic dose requirements, prevent morbidity, shorten hospital stay, and avoid complications after discharge. Continuous multimodal analgesia may inhibit changes in the spinal cord that can lead to changes in the peripheral and central nervous systems that initiate and sustain chronic persistent postsurgical pain (see Nociception earlier in the chapter).

Routes of Administration

The oral route is the preferred route of analgesic administration and should be used whenever feasible because it is generally the least expensive, best tolerated, and easiest to administer. Other routes of administration are used when the oral route is not possible, such as in patients who are NPO, nauseated, or unable to swallow. For example, early postoperative pain and pain that is severe and escalating is managed with the IV route of administration. Then patients are transitioned to oral analgesics when they are able to tolerate oral intake.

Around-the-Clock Dosing

Two basic principles of providing effective management are (1) preventing PAIN and (2) maintaining a level of pain control that allows the patient to function and have an acceptable quality of life. Accomplishment of these desired outcomes may require the mainstay analgesic to be administered on a scheduled around-the-clock (ATC) basis, rather than PRN ("as needed"), to maintain stable analgesic levels. *ATC dosing regimens are designed to control pain for patients who report it being present 12 hours or more during a 24-hour period*, such as that associated with most chronic syndromes and pain during the first 24 to 48 hours after surgery or other tissue injury. PRN dosing of analgesics is appropriate for intermittent PAIN, such as before painful procedures and breakthrough pain (additional pain that "breaks through" the pain being managed by the mainstay analgesic), for which supplemental doses of analgesic are provided.

Patient-Controlled Analgesia

Patient-controlled analgesia (PCA) is an interactive method of management that allows patients to treat their pain by self-administering doses of analgesics. It is used to manage all types of PAIN and given by multiple routes of administration, including IV, subcutaneous, epidural, and perineural. A PCA infusion device ("pump") is used when PCA is delivered by invasive routes of administration and is programmed so that the patient can press a button ("pendant") to self-administer a set dose of analgesic ("PCA dose") at a set time interval ("demand" or "lockout") as needed. *Patients who use PCA must be able to understand the relationships between pain, pressing the PCA button and taking the analgesic, and pain relief. They must also be cognitively and physically able to use any equipment that is used to administer the therapy.*

PCA may be given with or without a basal rate (continuous infusion). The use of a basal rate is common when patient-controlled epidural analgesia (PCEA) is used. It is often added for opioid-tolerant patients and occasionally for opioid-naïve patients receiving IV PCA to allow them to achieve pain control. Remember that the patient has no control over the delivery of a continuous infusion. Essential to the safe use of a basal rate is prompt discontinuation of the basal rate if increased sedation or respiratory depression occurs.

> ### ❗ NURSING SAFETY PRIORITY (QSEN)
> #### Action Alert
>
> Teach patients how to use the PCA device and to report side effects, such as dizziness, nausea and vomiting, and excessive sedation. As with all opioids, monitor the patient's sedation level and respiratory status at least every 2 hours. Promptly decrease the opioid dose (i.e., discontinue basal rate) if increased sedation is detected.

The primary benefit of PCA is that it recognizes that only the patient can feel the PAIN and only the patient knows how much analgesic will relieve it. This fact reinforces that *PCA is for patient use only and that unauthorized activation of the PCA button (called "PCA by proxy") can be very dangerous.* Instruct staff, family, and other visitors to contact the nurse if they have concerns about pain control rather than pressing the PCA button for the patient.

The Three Analgesic Groups

Analgesics are categorized into three main groups: (1) non-opioid analgesics, which include acetaminophen and the NSAIDs; (2) opioid analgesics, such as morphine, hydromorphone, fentanyl, and oxycodone; and (3) adjuvant analgesics (sometimes referred to as *co-analgesics*), which make up the largest group and include a variety of agents with unique and widely differing mechanisms of action. Examples are local anesthetics and some anticonvulsants and antidepressants. Table 3-6 lists the three analgesic groups and examples of drugs in each group.

Non-opioid Analgesics. Acetaminophen and NSAIDs make up the non-opioid analgesic group. *Acetaminophen* is thought to relieve PAIN by underlying mechanisms in the CNS. It has analgesic and antipyretic properties but is not effective to treat inflammation. In contrast, *NSAIDs* have analgesic, antipyretic, and anti-inflammatory properties. These drugs produce pain relief by blocking prostaglandins through inhibition of the enzyme *cyclooxygenase (COX)* in the peripheral nervous system (see Nociception and Fig. 3-1 earlier in the chapter).

Non-opioids are available in a variety of formulations and given by multiple routes of administration. They are also flexible analgesics used for a wide range of conditions. Non-opioid drugs are appropriate alone for mild to moderate nociceptive pain (e.g., from surgery, trauma, or osteoarthritis) or are added to opioids, local anesthetics, and/or anticonvulsants as part of a multimodal analgesic regimen for more severe nociceptive pain. *However, they are not effective for neuropathic pain.*

Acetaminophen and an NSAID may be given together, and there is no need for staggered doses. Unless contraindicated, all surgical patients should routinely be given acetaminophen and an NSAID in scheduled doses as the foundation of the pain treatment plan throughout the postoperative course, preferably initiated preoperatively.

The non-opioids are often combined in a single tablet with opioids, such as oxycodone (Percocet) or hydrocodone (Vicodin, Lortab, Vicoprofen), and are very popular for the treatment of mild to moderate acute pain. Many people with persistent pain also take a combination non-opioid/opioid analgesic. However, it is important to remember that these combination drugs are not appropriate for severe pain of any type because the maximum daily dose of the non-opioid limits the escalation of the opioid dose.

Acetaminophen. Oral acetaminophen (Tylenol, Abenol ✦) has a long history of safety in recommended doses in all age-groups and most patient populations. It is recommended as first-line for musculoskeletal pain (e.g., osteoarthritis) in older adults but has no inflammatory properties so is less effective than NSAIDs for chronic inflammatory pain (e.g., rheumatoid arthritis). IV acetaminophen (Ofirmev) is approved for treatment of pain and fever in adults and children age 2 years and older and is given by a 15-minute infusion in single or repeated doses. It is given alone for mild to moderate pain or in combination with opioid analgesics for more severe pain and has been shown to be well tolerated and to produce a significant opioid dose-sparing effect and superior pain relief compared with placebo (Pasero & Stannard, 2012).

The most serious complication of acetaminophen is hepatotoxicity (liver damage) as a result of overdose. Patient's hepatic risk factors must always be considered before administration of acetaminophen. In the healthy adult, a maximum daily dose below 4000 mg is rarely associated with liver toxicity (Pasero & Stannard, 2012). Many experts recommend reducing the daily dose (e.g., 2500-3000 mg daily) when used for *long-term* treatment in older adults. Acetaminophen does not increase bleeding time and has a low incidence of GI adverse effects, making it the analgesic of choice in many people with comorbidities.

TABLE 3-6   The Three Analgesic Groups

Non-Opioid Analgesics

Advantages

- Versatile with multiple agents, formulations, and routes of administration available
- Flexible and useful for a wide variety of mild to moderate nociceptive-type pain conditions
- Identified as the foundation of a multimodal approach for nociceptive-type pain
- Can produce opioid dose-sparing effects
- Available in combination with opioids

Disadvantages

- Wide inter-individual differences in response
- Ineffective for neuropathic pain
- Acetaminophen adverse effects require careful consideration of patient's hepatic status before administration and care not to exceed recommended daily dose
- NSAID adverse effects prohibit use or suggest cautionary use in some patient populations, including older adults, patients with high CV and/or GI risk factors, and those with bleeding disorders
- All of the non-opioids and combination non-opioid/opioid formulations have a maximum daily dose that should not be exceeded

Examples

- Acetaminophen (Tylenol)
- Nonselective NSAIDs:
  - Aspirin
  - Diclofenac (Voltaren; Voltaren gel; Flector patch)
  - Ibuprofen (Motrin)
  - Ketoprofen (Orudis)
  - Ketorolac (Toradol)
  - Meloxicam (Mobic)
  - Naproxen (Naprosyn)
- COX-2-selective NSAIDs:
  - Celecoxib (Celebrex)

Opioid Analgesics

Advantages

- Cornerstone of moderate to severe nociceptive-type pain
- Mu agonists have no ceiling on analgesia
- Opioid rotation can be initiated for development of tolerance
- With the exception of constipation, tolerance develops to side effects with regular daily doses over several days

Disadvantages

- Constipation is an almost universal opioid side effect and the number-one reason people stop taking pain medication
- Although most side effects are manageable, undetected excessive sedation and respiratory depression are life threatening
- Close monitoring of sedation and respiratory status is indicated during at least the first 24 hours of opioid therapy
- Screening for appropriateness and ongoing monitoring via a therapeutic relationship between the patient and prescriber are required for safe and effective long-term opioid therapy
- Some opioids produce metabolites that can accumulate and produce toxicity, for example, morphine (morphine 3-glucuronide [M3G])

Examples of Mu Opioid Agonists

- Morphine (MS Contin; Kadian; Avinza; Roxanol; Duramorph; Astramorph)
- Fentanyl (Sublimaze; Duragesic; Actiq; Fentora; Onsolis)
- Hydromorphone (Dilaudid; Hydromorph; Exalgo)
- Hydrocodone (Zogenix ER; Lortab; Vicodin [also contain acetaminophen]; Vicoprofen [also contains ibuprofen])
- Oxycodone (OxyIR; OxyContin; Percocet [also contains acetaminophen]; Percodan [also contains aspirin])
- Oxymorphone (Opana; Opana ER)
- Methadone (Dolophine; Methadose)

Adjuvant Analgesics

Advantages

- Largest and most diverse analgesic group; wide variety of agents, formulations, and routes of administration available depending on agent
- Side effects often are responsive to dose reduction
- Tolerance develops to most of the adverse effects

Disadvantages

- Contain the agents that are recommended for treatment of neuropathic pain
- Considerable variability among people in their response to agents used to treat chronic neuropathic pain, including to agents within the same class; a "trial and error" strategy must be used, and multiple analgesic trials are sometimes necessary
- Most require titration of dose over several weeks to evaluate effectiveness; patients must be forewarned of delayed onset of analgesia
- Most have a maximum daily dose
- Side effects can be significant and may limit dose escalation

Examples

- Anticonvulsants:
  - Gabapentin (Neurontin)
  - Pregabalin (Lyrica)
- Antidepressants:
  - Tricyclic antidepressants:
    Nortriptyline (Aventyl; Pamelor)
    Desipramine (Norpramin)
  - Serotonin-norepinephrine reuptake inhibitors (SNRIs):
    Duloxetine (Cymbalta)
    Venlafaxine (Effexor)
- Alpha$_2$-adrenergic agonists:
  - Clonidine (Catapres, Duraclon)
  - Tizanidine (Zanaflex)
- Local anesthetics:
  - Bupivacaine (Marcaine)
  - Ropivacaine (Naropin)
  - Lidocaine injectable
  - Lidocaine patch 5% (Lidoderm)
- Muscle relaxants/antispasmodics:
  - Baclofen (Lioresal)
  - Cyclobenzaprine (Flexeril)
- NMDA antagonists:
  - Ketamine (Ketalar)

CV, Cardiovascular; *NMDA, N-*methyl-D-aspartate.

NSAIDs. A benefit of the NSAID group is the availability of a wide variety of agents for administration via noninvasive routes. Ibuprofen (Motrin, Novo-Profen✦), naproxen (Naprosyn, Nu-Naprox✦), and celecoxib (Celebrex) are the most widely used oral NSAIDs in the United States and Canada (see Table 3-6). Diclofenac (Voltaren) is prescribed in patch and gel form for topical administration. An intranasal patient-controlled formulation of ketorolac (Sprix) has been approved for short-term treatment of acute PAIN. IV formulations of ketorolac (Toradol) and ibuprofen (Caldolor) are also used to manage acute pain. Both have been shown to produce excellent analgesia alone for mild to moderate nociceptive pain and significant opioid dose-sparing effects when administered as part of a multimodal analgesic plan for more severe pain (Pasero & McCaffery, 2011).

NSAIDs have more adverse effects than acetaminophen, with gastric toxicity and ulceration being the most common of the adverse effects. Risk factors for NSAID adverse effects include being older than 60 years or having a history of peptic ulcer or cardiovascular (CV) disease. An important principle of NSAID use is to administer the lowest dose for the shortest time necessary.

All NSAIDs carry a risk for CV adverse effects through prostaglandin inhibition. The U.S. Food and Drug Administration (FDA) cautions against the use of any NSAIDs after high-risk open heart surgery because of an elevated CV risk with NSAIDs in this population. Prostaglandins also affect renal function. Be sure that the patient is adequately hydrated when administering NSAIDs to prevent acute renal failure.

Health Teaching. When taking a patient history, ask about the use of non-opioids, keeping in mind that most people do not understand the difference between the generic and brand names of over-the-counter (OTC) drugs. Patients may be taking both a generic non-opioid (e.g., acetaminophen, naproxen, or ibuprofen) and a brand name of the same non-opioid (e.g., Tylenol, Naprosyn, or Advil) at the same time and exceeding the safe maximum daily dose. They also may not realize that many OTC medications, such as sleep and cold remedies, contain non-opioids. Ask the patient or patient's family to provide the name of each drug (prescription and OTC) that the patient is taking, as well as the daily dose. Teach patients to be aware of the amount of non-opioid in combination products such as hydrocodone (e.g., Vicodin, Vicoprofen) and oxycodone (e.g., Percocet). Stress to patients that exceeding the safe maximum daily non-opioid dose places the patient at a high risk for adverse effects, such as liver toxicity (acetaminophen) and GI bleeding and CV complications (NSAIDs).

CONSIDERATIONS FOR OLDER ADULTS

Patient-Centered Care (QSEN)

Older adults are at increased risk for NSAID-induced GI toxicity. Acetaminophen should be used for mild pain. If an NSAID is needed for inflammatory pain or additional analgesia, the least ulcerogenic NSAID is recommended. The addition of a proton pump inhibitor (e.g., lansoprazole, omeprazole) to NSAID therapy, or opioid analgesics rather than an NSAID, is recommended for high-risk patients.

? NCLEX EXAMINATION CHALLENGE

Physiological Integrity

An older client takes acetaminophen (Tylenol) 2000 mg daily for osteoarthritis. What health teaching will the nurse provide for the client related to this medication?
A. "Be sure and take your medication with food to prevent stomach ulcers."
B. "Take your medication only when you need it for chronic pain."
C. "Avoid any over-the-counter medications that may contain acetaminophen."
D. "Take your blood pressure often because acetaminophen can cause it to go up."

Opioid Analgesics. Opioid analgesics are the mainstay in the management of moderate to severe nociceptive types of PAIN, such as postoperative, surgical, trauma, and burn pain (see Table 3-6). Although it is often used, the term "narcotic" is considered obsolete and inaccurate when discussing the use of opioids for pain management. "Narcotic" is used loosely by law enforcement and the media to refer to a variety of substances of potential abuse. Legally, controlled substances classified as narcotics include opioids, cocaine, and others. *The preferred term is "opioid analgesics" when discussing these agents in the context of pain management.* Some patients prefer the term "pain medications" or "pain medicine."

GENETIC/GENOMIC CONSIDERATIONS

Patient-Centered Care (QSEN)

It has long been known that the cytochrome (CY) *P450* enzyme system is important to the metabolism of some opioids. Interethnic variations in phenotypes of the *CYP450* enzymes are common, causing decreased metabolism of selected analgesics in a small percentage of Caucasians and Asians. These variations have clinical implications when the opioid *codeine*, which is metabolized by the *CYP450* enzyme system, is administered. Slow metabolizers may not respond well to codeine, and ultra-rapid metabolizers may have an exaggerated response (Pasero & McCaffery, 2011).

Opioids produce their effects by interacting with opioid receptor sites located throughout the body, including in the peripheral tissues, in the GI system, and in the spinal cord and brain (Yaksh & Wallace, 2011). When an opioid binds to the opioid receptor sites, it produces analgesia as well as unwanted effects, such as constipation, nausea, sedation, and respiratory depression. There are three classifications of opioids:

- Full or *mu agonists* ("morphine-like") bind primarily to the mu type opioid receptors in the CNS and, among other actions, block the release of the neurotransmitter *substance P,* which prevents the opening of calcium channels and the transmission of PAIN (Yaksh & Wallace, 2011). A major benefit of the mu opioid agonists is that they have no ceiling on analgesia. This means that increases in dose produce increases in pain relief and that there is no maximum dose (see Physical Tolerance later in the chapter). This property makes the mu opioid agonists the first-line opioid analgesics for moderate to severe nociceptive pain. Examples are morphine, fentanyl, hydromorphone, oxycodone, and hydrocodone.
- *Mixed agonists antagonists* bind to more than one type of opioid receptor. They bind as agonists to the kappa opioid receptors to produce analgesia and other effects and to the mu opioid receptors as antagonists. This antagonistic property explains why these drugs can trigger severe PAIN and opioid withdrawal syndrome characterized by rhinitis, abdominal cramping, nausea, agitation, and restlessness in patients who have been taking regular daily doses of a mu agonist opioid for several days. Another undesirable effect of these drugs is that they produce a dose-ceiling effect, which means further increases in dose will not produce further relief. This latter property limits their usefulness in pain management. Occasionally, these drugs are used in very low doses to antagonize (in hopes of relieving) opioid-induced side effects, such as pruritus. However, this approach risks reversing analgesia, so patients must be assessed frequently to ensure adequate PAIN control is maintained. Examples are butorphanol (Stadol) and nalbuphine (Nubain).
- *Partial agonists* have some kappa and mu opioid receptor activity but produce an analgesia plateau and are not easily reversed by opioid antagonists, such as naloxone (Narcan). These properties limit their role in PAIN management. Buprenorphine is a partial agonist opioid, available in a transdermal patch (Butrans) for stable pain management. The drug has been formulated alone (Subutex) and with naloxone (Suboxone) for the treatment of the disease of addiction.

Opioid antagonists (e.g., naloxone [Narcan], naltrexone [Revia]) are drugs that also bind to opioid receptors but produce no analgesia (Yaksh & Wallace, 2011). If an antagonist is present, it competes with opioid molecules for binding sites on the opioid receptors and has the potential to block analgesia and other effects. They are used most often to reverse opioid effects, such as excessive sedation and respiratory depression.

Key Principles of Opioid Administration. Many factors are considered when determining the appropriate opioid analgesic for the patient with pain. These include the unique characteristics of the various opioids and patient factors, such as type of pain, pain intensity, age, gender, coexisting disease, current drug regimen and potential drug interactions, prior treatment outcomes, and patient preference.

Titration (dose increases or decreases) of the opioid dose is usually required at the start and throughout the course of treatment when opioids are administered. Whereas patients with cancer pain most often are titrated upward over time for

GENDER HEALTH CONSIDERATIONS
Patient-Centered Care QSEN

Research has identified differences between females and males in a number of factors that influence the pharmacokinetics (absorption, distribution, metabolism, and excretion) and pharmacodynamics (effects on the body) of drugs. Some of these factors are organ physiology, body composition, gastric emptying time, enzyme activity, and drug clearance (Snidvongs, 2008). Abundant research shows that women are at substantially greater risk for more pain conditions than men and that they may experience more postoperative and procedural pain than men (Fillingim et al., 2009). In the immediate postoperative period, women seem to have a higher opioid requirement but men demonstrate higher opioid consumption after the initial recovery period. This difference may be partly explained by the faster recovery after general anesthesia in women. Side effects and complications associated with opioid and non-opioid analgesics appear to be more prevalent in women than in men. Creatinine clearance (drug excretion) is generally higher in men than in women due to increased muscle mass, and clearance varies with the menstrual cycle in women.

progressive pain, patients with acute pain, particularly postoperative pain, are eventually titrated downward as pain resolves. Although the dose and analgesic effect of mu agonist opioids have no ceiling, the dose may be limited by side effects. The absolute dose administered is unimportant as long as a balance between pain relief and side effects is favorable. *The desired outcome of titration is to use the smallest dose that provides satisfactory pain relief with the fewest side effects.*

When an increase in the opioid dose is necessary and safe, the increase can be titrated by percentages. When a slight improvement in analgesia is needed, a 25% increase in the opioid dose may be sufficient; a 50% increase for moderate improvement; and a 100% increase may be indicated for strong improvement, such as when treating severe, escalating pain (Pasero & McCaffery, 2011). The time at which the dose can be increased is determined by the onset and peak effects of the opioid and its formulation. For example, the frequency of IV opioid doses during initial titration may be as often as every 5 to 15 minutes (see later discussion of specific opioids). In contrast, at least 24 hours should elapse before the dose of transdermal fentanyl is increased after the first patch application.

CONSIDERATIONS FOR OLDER ADULTS
Patient-Centered Care QSEN

Although the patient's weight is not a good indicator of analgesic requirement, *age is considered an important factor to consider when selecting an opioid dose.* For older adults, the guideline is to "start low and go slow" with all drug dosing. For example, the starting opioid dose should be reduced by 25% to 50% in older adults because they are more sensitive to opioid side effects than are younger adults. The amount of subsequent doses is based on patient response, which should be evaluated frequently. Monitor sedation level and respiratory status, and promptly reduce the drug dose if sedation occurs or the respiratory rate is markedly decreased, depending on agency policy. Chart 3-1 describes best practices for pain assessment and management in the older adult.

Physical Dependence, Tolerance, and Addiction. The terms *physical dependence* and *tolerance* often are confused with *addiction,* so clarification of definitions is important. The most widely accepted definitions of these terms are:

- *Physical dependence is a normal response* that occurs with repeated administration of an opioid for several days. It

CHART 3-1 Nursing Focus on the Older Adult

Pain

Prevalence of Pain
- Recognize that older adults are at high risk for undertreated pain and those with cognitive impairment are at even higher risk.
- Common caregiver and health care team misconceptions, such as that pain sensitivity decreases with aging and older adults cannot tolerate analgesics without significant adverse effects, contribute to the undertreatment of pain in older adults.

Beliefs About Pain
- Older adults tend to report pain less often than younger adults, which frequently results in members of the health care team administering suboptimal analgesics and doses. The failure of older adults to report pain may be related to common beliefs and concerns they have about pain and the reporting of pain, such as:
  - Pain is an inevitable consequence of aging and little can be done to relieve it.
  - Expressing pain is unacceptable or is a sign of weakness.
  - Reporting pain will result in being labeled as a "bad" patient or a "complainer."
  - Nurses and physicians are too busy to listen to reports of pain.
  - Pain signifies a serious illness or impending death.
- Be aware of the common beliefs of older patients regarding pain and its management and correct misconceptions to help prevent barriers to achieving optimal pain relief.
- Nurses and other caregivers can overcome their reluctance to administer prescribed analgesics in adequate doses by following the principles of pain management in older persons (see *Management of Pain section*).

Assessment of Pain
- Ask the patient to provide his or her own report of pain; even mild to some moderate cognitively impaired older adults are able to provide self-report if nurses and caregivers take the time to obtain it.
  - Offer various self-report pain tools.
  - Always show tools in hard copy with large lettering, adequate space between lines, non-glossy paper, and color for increased visualization.
  - Be sure the patient is wearing glasses and hearing aids if needed and available.
  - Provide adequate lighting and privacy to avoid distracting background noise.
  - Repeat questions more than once, and allow adequate time for response.
  - Use verbal descriptions such as "ache," "sore," and "hurt" if the patient seems to have difficulty relating to the word "pain."
  - Ask about present pain only.
  - If the patient is able to use a self-report tool, use the same tool and reteach the tool each time pain is assessed.

Considerations for Cognitively Impaired Patients (also see Table 3-5)
- Remember to "assume pain is present" in patients with diseases and conditions or procedures commonly associated with pain (see discussion below on *analgesic trial*).
- If the patient is unable to provide self-report, look for behaviors that may indicate the presence of pain.

- Someone who knows the patient well, such as a family member or caregiver, may be helpful in identifying behaviors that might indicate pain. Do not ask others to rate pain intensity, and do not attempt to rate it yourself. Only the patient knows how severe the pain is, and if he or she cannot rate or describe the intensity, the exact intensity is unknown.
- Assess using a reliable and valid behavioral pain assessment tool.
  - Remember that behavioral tools tell us that pain might be present and provide a reference point to help determine the effectiveness of interventions, but the scores on behavioral tools have not been correlated with the ratings on pain intensity scales. A behavioral score is not a pain intensity rating.
  - Use the same behavioral assessment tool each time pain is assessed.
- Consider an analgesic trial to help determine the presence of pain and to establish an ongoing treatment plan in patients who are thought to have pain. This involves the administration of a low-dose analgesic; changes or decreases in the intensity of behaviors indicate that pain may be the cause of the behaviors. Doses should be increased or additional analgesics added as appropriate.

Management of Pain
- Use a multimodal approach that combines analgesics with different underlying mechanisms with the desired outcome of achieving optimal pain relief with lower doses than would be possible with a single analgesic; lower doses result in fewer side effects.
- Consider the type of pain, and begin therapy with the first-line analgesics that are recommended for that type of pain.
  - Non-opioids (acetaminophen, NSAIDs), opioids, and local anesthetics are first-line analgesics for nociceptive-type pain (e.g., postoperative pain, osteoarthritis pain, cancer pain).
  - Antidepressants, anticonvulsants, and local anesthetics are first-line analgesics for neuropathic-type pain (e.g., postherpetic neuralgia, diabetic neuropathy, phantom limb pain, post-stroke pain).
- Do not give meperidine to older adults because most have decreased renal function and are unable to efficiently eliminate its CNS-toxic metabolite *normeperidine*.
- Use around-the-clock (ATC) dosing of analgesics for pain that is of a continuous nature (e.g., chronic osteoarthritis or cancer pain; chronic neuropathic pain, first 24 to 48 hours after surgery).
- Use as needed (PRN) dosing for intermittent pain and before painful activities, such as before ambulation and physical therapy.
- Be aware of the main side effects of the analgesics that are administered and that they may be more likely to occur or be more severe in older than in younger adults.
- *Start low and go slow* with drug dosing; increase doses to achieve adequate analgesia based on patient's response to the previous dose.
- Teach the patient and family or other caregiver about the pain management plan (analgesics and nonpharmacologic strategies) and when to notify the primary health care provider for unrelieved pain or unmanageable or intolerable drug side effects.
- To promote adherence to the pain management plan in the home setting, suggest using a pillbox to organize each day's medications and keeping a diary to identify times of the day or activities that increase pain. The diary can be presented to the primary health care provider who can use it to make necessary adjustments in the treatment plan.

---

is manifested by the occurrence of withdrawal symptoms when the opioid is suddenly stopped or rapidly reduced or an antagonist such as naloxone is given. Withdrawal symptoms may be suppressed by the natural, gradual reduction of the opioid as pain decreases or by gradual, systematic reduction, referred to as *tapering. Physical dependence is not the same as addictive disease.*

- *Tolerance is also a normal response* that occurs with regular administration of an opioid and consists of a decrease in

one or more effects of the opioid (e.g., decreased analgesia, sedation, or respiratory depression). Like physical dependence, *tolerance is not the same as addictive disease.* Tolerance to analgesia usually occurs in the first days to 2 weeks of opioid therapy but is uncommon after that. It may be treated with increases in dose or rotation to a different opioid. However, disease progression, not tolerance to analgesia, appears to be the reason for most dose escalations. Stable pain usually results in stable opioid

TABLE 3-7 Equianalgesic Dose Chart for Common MU Opioid Analgesics

- *Equianalgesic* means approximately the same pain relief.
- The equianalgesic chart is a guideline for selecting doses for opioid-naïve patients. Doses and intervals between doses are titrated according to each person's responses.
- The equianalgesic chart is helpful when switching from one drug or route of administration to another.

OPIOID	ORAL	PARENTERAL	COMMENTS
Morphine	30 mg	10 mg	Standard for comparison; first-line opioid via multiple routes of administration; once-daily and twice-daily oral formulations; clinically significant metabolites.
Fentanyl	No formulation	100 mcg IV 100 mcg/hr of transdermal fentanyl is approximately equal to 4 mg/hr of IV morphine; 1 mcg/hr of transdermal fentanyl is approximately equal to 2 mg/24 hr of oral morphine	First-line opioid via IV, transdermal, and intraspinal routes; available in oral transmucosal and buccal formulations for breakthrough pain in opioid-tolerant patients; no clinically relevant metabolites.
Hydrocodone	30 mg (NR)	No formulation	Available only in combination with non-opioid and as such is appropriate only for mild to some moderate pain.
Hydromorphone (Dilaudid)	7.5 mg	1.5 mg	First-line opioid via multiple routes of administration; once-daily oral formulation; clinically significant metabolites noted with long-term, high-dose infusion.
Oxycodone	20 mg	No formulation in the United States	Short-acting and twice-daily oral formulations.
Oxymorphone	10 mg	1 mg	Parenteral and short-acting and twice-daily oral formulations.

Data from Pasero, C., & McCaffery, M. (2011). *Pain assessment and pharmacologic management.* St. Louis: Mosby.
NR, Not recommended.

doses. With the exception of constipation, tolerance to the opioid side effects develops with regular daily dosing of opioids over several days.

- *Opioid addiction is a chronic neurologic and biologic disease.* The development and characteristics of addiction are influenced by genetic, psychosocial, and environmental factors. No single cause of addiction, such as taking an opioid for pain relief, has been found. It is characterized by one or more of these behaviors: impaired control over drug use, compulsive use, continued use despite harm, and craving. *The disease of addiction is a treatable disease; as for any other suspected disease, refer the patient to an expert for diagnosis and treatment.*
- *Pseudoaddiction* is a mistaken diagnosis of addictive disease. When a patient's PAIN is not well controlled, the patient may begin to manifest symptoms suggestive of addictive disease. For example, in an effort to obtain adequate pain relief, the patient may respond with demanding behavior, escalating demands for more or different medications, and repeated requests for opioids on time or before the prescribed interval between doses has elapsed. PAIN relief typically eliminates these behaviors and is often accomplished by increasing opioid doses or decreasing intervals between doses.

Opioid Naïve versus Opioid Tolerant. Patients are often characterized as being either opioid naïve or opioid tolerant. An *opioid-naïve* person has not recently taken enough opioid on a regular basis to become tolerant to the effects of an opioid. An *opioid-tolerant* person has taken an opioid long enough at doses high enough to develop tolerance to many of the effects, including analgesia and the undesirable effects, such as nausea and sedation. There is no set time for the development of tolerance with wide individual variation among people. Some patients do not develop tolerance at all. Patients who have taken opioids regularly for about 7 days or longer are considered to be opioid tolerant.

Equianalgesia. The term *equianalgesia* means approximately "equal analgesia." An equianalgesic chart provides a list of analgesic doses, both oral and parenteral (IV, subcutaneous, and IM), that are approximately equal to each other in ability to provide pain relief (Table 3-7). Equianalgesic conversion of doses is used to help ensure patients receive approximately the same pain relief when they are switched from one opioid or route of administration to another. It requires a series of calculations based on the daily dose of the current opioid to determine the equianalgesic dose of the opioid to which the patient is to be switched. Consult and collaborate with the pharmacist whenever equianalgesic conversion is indicated.

Relative potency is the ratio of drug doses required to produce the same effect. For example, note in Table 3-7 that a single dose of 1.5 mg of parenteral hydromorphone produces approximately the same analgesia as 10 mg of parenteral morphine. This means that hydromorphone is more potent than morphine, but increased potency does not mean the drug is therapeutically superior or that it provides any advantage. Safe and effective pain management requires nurses to appreciate the differences in the potencies of the various opioids and apply the principles of equianalgesia when administering opioids.

Drug Formulation Terminology. The terms *short acting, fast acting, immediate release (IR),* and *normal release* have been used interchangeably to describe oral opioids that have an onset of action of about 30 minutes and a relatively short duration of 3 to 4 hours. The term *immediate release* is misleading because none of the oral analgesics have an immediate or even a fast onset of analgesia. The term *short acting* is preferred to reflect the short duration of oral opioids. Oral transmucosal and intranasal formulations are appropriately referred to as *ultra fast acting* because they have a peak effect of 5 to 15 minutes, depending on formulation.

The terms *modified-release, extended release (ER), sustained release (SR),* and *controlled release* are used to describe opioids that are formulated to release over a prolonged period of time.

For the purposes of this chapter, the term *modified-release* will be used when discussing these opioid formulations. *Long-acting* is applied to drugs with a long *half-life*, such as methadone. A drug's half-life provides an estimate of how fast the drug leaves the body. By definition, half-life is the time it takes for the amount of drug in the body to be reduced by 50%.

! NURSING SAFETY PRIORITY (QSEN)
Drug Alert

Modified-release opioids should never be crushed, broken, or chewed because doing so alters the formulation of the drug and can result in adverse events, including death from respiratory depression if consumed. Teach the patient to swallow the drug whole and allow the "time release" function of the drug to take effect. Intact modified-release tablets may be administered rectally in some patients who cannot swallow.

Selected Opioid Analgesics. *Morphine* is the standard against which all other opioid drugs are compared. It is the most widely used opioid throughout the world, particularly for cancer pain, and its use is established by extensive research and clinical experience. Morphine is a *hydrophilic* drug (readily absorbed in aqueous solution), which accounts for its slow onset and long duration of action when compared with other opioid analgesics (Table 3-8). It is available in a wide variety of short-acting and modified-release oral formulations and is given by multiple other routes of administration, including rectal, subcutaneous, and IV.

Fentanyl (Sublimaze) differs from morphine significantly in characteristics. It is a *lipophilic* (readily absorbed in fatty tissue) opioid and, as such, has a fast onset and short duration of action (see Table 3-8). These characteristics make it the most commonly used IV opioid when rapid analgesia is desired, such as for the treatment of severe, escalating acute PAIN and for procedural pain when a short duration of action is desirable. Fentanyl is the recommended opioid for patients with end-organ failure because it has no clinically relevant metabolites (Pasero & McCaffery, 2011). It also produces fewer hemodynamic adverse effects than other opioids so is often preferred in patients who are hemodynamically unstable, such as the critically ill.

Its lipophilicity makes fentanyl ideal for drug delivery by transdermal patch (Duragesic) for long-term opioid therapy and by the oral transmucosal (Actiq) and buccal (Fentora)

routes for breakthrough PAIN treatment in opioid-tolerant patients. After application of the transdermal patch, a subcutaneous depot of fentanyl is established in the skin near the patch. After absorption from the depot into the systemic circulation, the drug distributes to fat and muscle. When the first patch is applied, 12 to 18 hours are required for clinically significant analgesia to be obtained. Be aware that the patient may need adequate supplemental analgesia during that time. Change the patch every 48 to 72 hours depending on patient response.

! NURSING SAFETY PRIORITY (QSEN)
Drug Alert

Teach patients taking transdermal fentanyl not to apply heat (e.g., hot packs, heating pads) directly over the patch because heat increases absorption of the drug and can result in adverse events, including death from fentanyl-induced respiratory depression. Ask patients about the presence of patches on admission, and document and communicate this information to other members of the interdisciplinary health care team.

Hydromorphone (Dilaudid) is less hydrophilic than morphine but less lipophilic than fentanyl, which contributes to an onset and duration of action that is intermediate between morphine and fentanyl (see Table 3-8). The drug is often used as an alternative to morphine, especially for acute PAIN, most likely because the two drugs produce similar analgesia and have comparable side effects. It is a first- or second-choice opioid (after morphine) for postoperative management via IV PCA and is available in a once-daily modified-release oral formulation for long-term opioid treatment.

? NCLEX EXAMINATION CHALLENGE
Physiological Integrity

A client has a one-time order for morphine 2 mg IV push. The drug is available as 5 mg/mL. The nurse administers _____ mL of morphine for one dose.

Oxycodone is available in the United States for administration by the oral route only and is used to treat all types of PAIN. In combination with acetaminophen or ibuprofen, it is appropriate for mild to some moderate pain. Single-entity, short-acting (OxyIR) and modified-release (OxyContin) oxycodone formulations are used most often for moderate to severe cancer PAIN and in some patients with moderate to severe non-cancer pain. It has been used successfully as part of a multimodal treatment plan for postoperative pain as well. Like morphine, it is available in liquid form for patients who are unable to swallow tablets.

Hydrocodone in combination with non-opioids limits its use to the treatment of mild to some moderate PAIN. It is one of the most commonly prescribed analgesics in the United States, but its prescription for treatment of persistent pain (except for breakthrough dosing) should be carefully evaluated because of its ceiling on efficacy and safety related to the non-opioid constituent (ingredient).

Methadone (Dolophine) is a unique opioid analgesic that may have advantages over other opioids in carefully selected patients. In addition to being a mu opioid, it is an antagonist at the NMDA (*N*-methyl-D-aspartate) receptor site and thus has

TABLE 3-8 Characteristics of Selected First-Line Opioid Analgesics*

OPIOID	ONSET (MINUTES)	PEAK (MINUTES)	DURATION (HOURS)
Morphine	30-45 (oral)	60-90 (oral)	3-4 (oral)
	5-10 (IV)	15-30 (IV)	3-4 (IV)
Fentanyl	5 (OT)	15 (OT)	2 (OT)
	3-5 (IV)	10-20 (IV)	2 (IV)
Hydromorphone	15-30 (oral)	30-90 (oral)	3-4 (oral)
	5 (IV)	10-30 (IV)	3-4 (IV)

Data from Pasero, C., & McCaffery, M. (2011). *Pain assessment and pharmacologic management.* St. Louis: Mosby.

IV, Intravenous; *OT,* oral transmucosal.

*Characteristics do not apply to modified-release formulations.

the potential to produce analgesic effects as a second- or third-line option for some neuropathic pain states (Dworkin et al., 2010). It may be given as an alternative when it is necessary to switch a patient to a new opioid because of inadequate analgesia or unacceptable side effects during long-term opioid therapy.

Although it has no active metabolites, methadone has a very long and highly variable half-life (5 to 100+ hours; average is 20 hours). Watch patients closely for excessive sedation—a sign of drug accumulation during the titration period. Other limitations are its tendency to interact with a large number of medications and prolong QTc interval.

Dual Mechanism Analgesics. The dual mechanism analgesics, *tramadol* (Ultram) and *tapentadol* (Nucynta), are relatively new to the PAIN management arena. These drugs bind weakly to the mu opioid receptor site and block the reuptake (resorption) of the inhibitory neurotransmitters *serotonin* and/or *norepinephrine* in the spinal cord and brainstem of the modulatory descending PAIN pathway (see Nociception earlier in this chapter). This makes these neurotransmitters more available to fight pain. Because they have the opioid receptor binding property, they are discussed in the Opioid Analgesics section of this chapter. However, they are usually referred to as dual mechanism rather than opioid analgesics.

Tramadol is used for both acute and chronic PAIN and is available in oral short-acting (Ultram) and modified-release (Ultram ER) formulations, including a short-acting tablet in combination with acetaminophen (Ultracet). It is appropriate for acute pain and has been designated as a second-line analgesic for the treatment of neuropathic pain (Dworkin et al., 2010). Side effects are similar to those of opioids. The drug can lower seizure threshold and interact with other drugs that block the reuptake of serotonin, such as the selective serotonin reuptake inhibitor (SSRI) antidepressants. Although rare, this combination can have an additive effect and result in serotonin syndrome, characterized by agitation, diarrhea, heart and blood pressure changes, and loss of coordination.

The newer dual mechanism analgesic *tapentadol* is also available in short-acting (Nucynta) and modified-release (Nucynta ER) formulations and is appropriate for both acute and chronic PAIN. Major benefits of tapentadol are that it has no active metabolites and a significantly more favorable side effect profile (particularly GI effects) compared with opioid analgesics.

Opioids to Avoid. *Meperidine* (Demerol) was once the most widely used opioid analgesic in the inpatient setting. In recent years, it has either been removed from or severely restricted on U.S. hospital formularies for the treatment of pain in an effort to improve patient safety. A major drawback to the use of meperidine is its active metabolite, *normeperidine*, a CNS stimulant that can cause delirium, irritability, tremors, myoclonus, and generalized seizures. It is a particularly poor choice in older adults because they have decreased renal function, which prevents the elimination of the toxic metabolite. Meperidine has no advantages over any other opioid, and it has no place in the treatment of persistent pain or in delivery systems, such as PCA. If prescribed, meperidine should not be used for more than 48 hours or at doses exceeding 600 mg/24 hours (Pasero & McCaffery, 2011).

Codeine in combination with non-opioids (e.g., with acetaminophen in Tylenol #3) has been used for many years for the management of mild to moderate pain; however, it has largely been replaced by analgesics that are more efficacious and better tolerated (e.g., Percocet, Vicodin). Research has shown that codeine/acetaminophen is less effective and associated with more adverse effects than NSAIDs, such as ibuprofen and naproxen, for acute pain.

Intraspinal Analgesia. Intraspinal analgesia involves the administration of analgesics via a needle or catheter placed in the epidural space or the intrathecal (subarachnoid) space by an anesthesia provider. The intraspinal routes of administration are used to manage both acute pain, such as postoperative pain, and some chronic cancer and non-cancer pain.

Epidural analgesia can be delivered by intermittent bolus technique, continuous infusion, or patient-controlled epidural analgesia (PCEA) with or without continuous infusion. The most commonly administered analgesics by the epidural route are the opioids *morphine, hydromorphone,* and *fentanyl* in combination with a long-acting local anesthetic, such as bupivacaine (Marcaine) or ropivacaine (Naropin). This multimodal approach allows lower doses of both the opioid and local anesthetic and produces fewer side effects. A single epidural injection of preservative-free morphine (Duramorph) is effective for about 24 hours. An extended-release formulation of preservative-free epidural morphine (DepoDur) is effective for 48 hours.

Intrathecal (spinal) analgesia is usually delivered via single bolus technique for patients with acute pain (e.g., hysterectomy) or continuous infusion via an implanted device for the treatment of chronic pain. Because the drug is delivered directly into the aqueous cerebral spinal fluid (CSF), morphine with its hydrophilic nature is used most often for intrathecal analgesia. Extremely small amounts of drug are administered by the intrathecal route (about 10 times less than by the epidural route) because the drug is so close to the spinal action site.

The side effects of intraspinal analgesia depend on the type of drug administered. In other words, if opioids are administered, the same opioid-induced side effects that occur with other routes of administration can occur with intraspinal administration. If local anesthetics are administered, common side effects are urinary retention, hypotension, and numbness and weakness of lower extremities. The latter can occur on a continuum (mild and localized) to a complete block (undesirable and requires prompt anesthesia evaluation). In most cases, the side effects that occur during continuous infusion or PCEA can be managed by decreasing the dose.

Complications of intraspinal analgesia are rare but can be life threatening. Perform frequent neurologic assessments and promptly report abnormal findings to the anesthesiologist or nurse anesthetist.

> ## ❗ NURSING SAFETY PRIORITY (QSEN)
> ### Drug Alert
>
> Assess patients receiving epidural local anesthetic for their ability to bend their knees and lift their buttocks off the mattress (if not prohibited by surgical procedure). Ask them to point to any areas of numbness and tingling. Mild, transient lower extremity motor weakness and orthostatic hypotension may be present, necessitating assistance with ambulation. Most undesirable effects can be managed with a reduction in local anesthetic dose. Promptly report areas of numbness outside of the surgical site, inability to bear weight, and severe hypotension to the anesthesia provider. *Do not delegate assessment of local anesthetic effects to unlicensed assistive personnel!*

SENSORY PERCEPTION manifestations (e.g., increasing numbness and tingling of extremities), decreasing ability to bear weight, and/or changes in bowel or bladder function can indicate the development of an epidural hematoma or abscess. If not detected, a hematoma or abscess can cause spinal cord compression and paralysis.

Nurses have an extensive role in the management and monitoring of intraspinal techniques, including infusion device operation, replacing empty drug reservoirs, checking and protecting infusion sites and systems, treating side effects, preventing complications, discontinuing therapy, and removing catheters.

Adverse Effects of Opioid Analgesics. The most common side effects of opioid analgesics are constipation, nausea, vomiting, pruritus, and sedation (Pasero & McCaffery, 2011). Respiratory depression is less common but the most feared of the opioid side effects. *Most of the opioid side effects are dose-related, so simply decreasing the opioid dose is sufficient to eliminate or make most of the side effects tolerable for most patients.* Table 3-9 lists interventions to prevent and manage opioid-induced side effects.

Opioids can result in delayed gastric emptying, slowed bowel motility, and decreased peristalsis, all of which can result in slow-moving, hard stool that is difficult to pass. Risk for *constipation* is elevated with opioid use, advanced age, and immobility, but it is an almost universal opioid side effect in all populations (i.e., tolerance rarely develops). Constipation is a primary reason people stop taking their pain medication. Therefore teach the importance of taking a preventive approach and aggressive management if symptoms occur. To prevent constipation, remind patients to take a daily stool softener plus a mild peristaltic stimulant, such as senna, for as long as they are taking an opioid.

Postoperative nausea and vomiting (PONV) are among the most unpleasant of the side effects associated with surgery. It is less common in older than younger adults. Evaluate patients for PONV risk, reduce risk factors if possible, and provide multimodal analgesia so that the lowest effective opioid dose can be given.

Pruritus (itching) is a side effect, not an allergic reaction to opioids. Although antihistamines such as diphenhydramine (Benadryl) are commonly used, there is no strong evidence that they relieve opioid-induced pruritus. Patients may report being less bothered by itching after taking an antihistamine, but this is likely the result of sedating effects. Sedation can be problematic in those already at risk for excessive sedation, such as postoperative patients. This problem can lead to life-threatening respiratory depression (Jarzyna et al., 2011; Pasero & McCaffery, 2011). *Remember that the single most effective, safest, and least expensive treatment for pruritus is opioid dose reduction.*

As patients become opioid tolerant, *tolerance to the opioid side effects (with the exception of constipation) develops.* It is reassuring for patients receiving long-term opioid therapy to know that most of the side effects will subside with regular daily doses of opioids over several days.

Most patients experience sedation at the beginning of opioid therapy and whenever the opioid dose is increased significantly. *If undetected or left untreated, excessive sedation can progress to clinically significant respiratory depression.* Like most of the other opioid side effects, sedation and respiratory depression are dose-related. Prevention of clinically significant opioid-induced respiratory depression begins with administration of the lowest effective opioid dose (multimodal analgesia with a non-opioid foundation), careful titration, and close monitoring of sedation and respiratory status throughout therapy. *Unless the patient is at*

TABLE 3-9 Nursing Interventions to Prevent and Treat Selected Opioid Side Effects*

Constipation
- Assess previous bowel habits.
- Keep a record of bowel movements.
- Remind patients that tolerance to this side effect does not develop, so *a preventive approach must be used*; administer a stool softener plus mild stimulant laxative for duration of opioid therapy; do not give bulk laxatives because these can result in obstruction in some patients.
- Provide privacy, encourage adequate fluids and activity, and give foods high in roughage.
- If ineffective, try suppository or Fleet's enema.

Nausea and Vomiting (N/V)
- Use a multimodal antiemetic preventive approach (e.g., dexamethasone plus ondansetron in moderate- to high-risk patients).
- Assess cause of nausea and eliminate contributing factors if possible.
- Reduce opioid dose if possible.
- Reassure patients taking long-term opioid therapy that tolerance to this side effect develops with regular daily opioid doses.
- Treat with antiemetic drug as prescribed.
- Consider switching to another opioid for unresolved N/V.

Sedation
- Remember that sedation precedes opioid-induced respiratory depression; identify patient and iatrogenic risk factors and monitor sedation level and respiratory status frequently during the first 24 hours of opioid therapy.
- Use a simple sedation scale to monitor for unwanted sedation (see Table 3-10).
- If excessive sedation is detected, reduce opioid dose to prevent respiratory depression.
- Eliminate unnecessary sedating drugs such as antihistamines, anxiolytics, muscle relaxants, and hypnotics. If it is necessary to administer these drugs during opioid therapy, monitor sedation and respiratory status closely.
- Reassure patients taking long-term opioid therapy that tolerance to this side effect develops with regular daily opioid doses.
- Be aware that stimulants such as caffeine may counteract opioid-induced sedation.
- Consider switching to another opioid for unresolved excessive sedation during long-term opioid therapy.

Respiratory Depression
- Be aware that counting respiratory rate alone does not constitute a comprehensive respiratory assessment. Proper assessment of respiratory status includes observation of the rise and fall of the patient's chest to determine depth and quality in addition to counting respiratory rate for 60 seconds.
- Recognize that *snoring is respiratory obstruction* and an ominous sign (see text).
- Remember that sedation precedes opioid-induced respiratory depression; identify patient and iatrogenic risk factors and monitor sedation level and respiratory status frequently during the first 24 hours of opioid therapy (see Sedation section).
- Stop opioid administration immediately for clinically significant respiratory depression, stay with patient, continue attempts to arouse patient, support respirations, call for help (consider Rapid Response Team or Code Blue), and consider giving naloxone.
- Reassure patients taking long-term opioid therapy that tolerance to this side effect develops with regular daily opioid doses.

*With the exception of constipation, opioid side effects are dose-related. This means that a multimodal analgesic approach that incorporates non-opioid analgesics as its foundation and administers the lowest effective opioid dose should be used. The simplest and most effective method for managing opioid side effects when they occur is to reduce the opioid dose.

the end of life, promptly reduce opioid dose or stop titration whenever increased sedation is detected to prevent respiratory depression. In some patients (e.g., those with obstructive sleep apnea, pulmonary dysfunction, multiple comorbidities), mechanical monitoring, such as capnography (to measure exhaled carbon dioxide) and pulse oximetry (to measure oxygen saturation), is needed (Jarzyna et al., 2011; Pasero & McCaffery, 2011).

Occasionally, drugs that produce significant sedation are used to treat side effects and other conditions that accompany the PAIN experience. For example, *antianxiety agents* (anxiolytics), such as alprazolam (Xanax) and lorazepam (Ativan), are prescribed to reduce anxiety. Many of the drugs used to treat opioid side effects are sedating, such as the antihistamines (diphenhydramine) for pruritus and the antiemetics *promethazine (Phenergan)* and *hydroxyzine (Vistaril)* for nausea. It is important to recognize that administration of these drugs together has an additive sedating effect. If administered, closely monitor for sedation and assess respiratory status frequently.

To assess sedation, use a simple, easy-to-understand sedation scale developed for assessment of *unwanted* sedation that includes what should be done at each level of sedation (Jarzyna et al., 2011; Pasero & McCaffery, 2011). Table 3-10 presents a widely used sedation scale. The key to assessing sedation is to determine how easy it is to arouse the patient. Assess each person's response to the first dose of an opioid. If opioids are administered by bolus technique, assess sedation level and respiratory status at the opioid's peak time after each bolus. *If a patient is difficult to arouse, always stop the opioid, stay with the patient, continue vigorous attempts to arouse, and call for help!*

Respiratory depression is assessed on the basis of what is normal for a particular person and is usually described as clinically significant when there is a decrease in the rate, depth, and regularity of respirations from baseline, rather than just by a specific number of respirations per minute. Risk factors for opioid-induced respiratory depression include age 55 years or older, obesity, obstructive sleep apnea, and pre-existing pulmonary dysfunction or other comorbidities.

! **NURSING SAFETY PRIORITY** (QSEN)

Critical Rescue

An accurate respiratory assessment requires watching the rise and fall of the patient's chest to determine depth and regularity of respirations in addition to counting the respiratory rate for 60 seconds. Listening to the sound of the patient's respiration is critical as well—*snoring indicates airway obstruction and must be attended to promptly* with repositioning and, depending on severity, a request for respiratory therapy consultation and further evaluation (Pasero & McCaffery, 2011). For accuracy, respiratory assessment is done before arousing the sleeping patient.

CONSIDERATIONS FOR OLDER ADULTS

Patient-Centered Care (QSEN)

The incidence of opioid side effects in the older adult population varies depending on the side effect. Older adults are sensitive to the sedating effects of opioids, making them higher risk for respiratory depression than younger adults.

? **NCLEX EXAMINATION CHALLENGE**

Physiological Integrity

A nursing technician reports that a postoperative client who is receiving IV PCA morphine is very drowsy, unable to complete a sentence without falling asleep, and has a respiratory rate of 12 breaths per minute. What is the nurse's first action at this time?
A. Arouse the client and raise the head of the bed to a 90-degree angle.
B. Promptly call the primary health care provider to request an order to reduce the dose.
C. Take away the client's PCA button and tell the family to notify staff when pain returns.
D. Reduce environmental stimuli by darkening the room so that the client can sleep.

! **NURSING SAFETY PRIORITY** (QSEN)

Drug Alert

Unless the patient is at the end of life, promptly administer the opioid antagonist *naloxone (Narcan)* IV to reverse clinically significant opioid-induced respiratory depression. When giving the opioid antagonist *naloxone,* administer it slowly until the patient is more arousable and respirations increase to an acceptable rate. The desired outcome is to reverse just the sedative and respiratory depressant effects of the opioid but not the analgesic effects. Giving too much naloxone too fast not only can cause severe PAIN but also can lead to ventricular dysrhythmias, pulmonary edema, and even death. Continue to closely monitor the patient after giving naloxone because the duration of naloxone is shorter than the duration of most opioids and respiratory depression can recur. Sometimes more than one dose of naloxone is needed.

TABLE 3-10 Pasero Opioid-Induced Sedation Scale (POSS) with Interventions*

S = Sleep, easy to arouse
  Acceptable; no action necessary; may increase opioid dose if needed.
1 = Awake and alert
  Acceptable; no action necessary; may increase opioid dose if needed.
2 = Slightly drowsy, easily aroused
  Acceptable; no action necessary; may increase opioid dose if needed.
3 = Frequently drowsy, arousable, drifts off to sleep during conversation
  Unacceptable; monitor respiratory status and sedation level closely until sedation level is stable at less than 3 and respiratory status is satisfactory; decrease opioid dose 25% to 50%[1] or notify primary[2] or anesthesia provider for orders; consider administering a non-sedating, opioid-sparing non-opioid, such as acetaminophen or a NSAID, if not contraindicated; ask patient to take deep breaths every 15-30 minutes.
4 = Somnolent, minimal or no response to verbal and physical stimulation
  Unacceptable; stop opioid; consider administering naloxone[3,4]; call Rapid Response Team (Code Blue); stay with patient, stimulate, and support respiration as indicated by patient status; notify primary[2] or anesthesia provider; monitor respiratory status and sedation level closely until sedation level is stable at less than 3 and respiratory status is satisfactory.

From Pasero, C., & McCaffery, M. (2011). *Pain assessment and pharmacologic management.* St. Louis: Mosby. Copyright 1994. Used with permission.
*Appropriate action is given in italics at each level of sedation.
[1]Opioid analgesic orders or a hospital protocol should include the expectation that a nurse will decrease the opioid dose if a patient is excessively sedated.
[2]For example, the physician, nurse practitioner, advanced practice nurse, or physician assistant responsible for the pain management prescription.
[3]For adults experiencing respiratory depression, administer dilute solution (0.4 mg of naloxone in 10 mL of normal saline) very slowly (0.5 mL over 2 minutes) while observing the patient's response (titrate to effect).
[4]Hospital protocols should include the expectation that a nurse will administer naloxone to any patient suspected of having life-threatening opioid-induced sedation and respiratory depression.

Adjuvant Analgesics. Adjuvant analgesics (sometimes called *co-analgesics*) are drugs that have a primary indication other than PAIN but are analgesic for some painful conditions (see Table 3-6). For example, the primary indication for antidepressants is depression, but some antidepressants help relieve some types of pain. The adjuvant analgesics are the largest and most diverse of the three analgesic groups. Drug selection and dosing are based on both experience and evidence-based practice guidelines (Dworkin et al., 2010).

Anticonvulsants and Antidepressants. *Anticonvulsants* (also called *antiepileptic drugs [AEDs]* when used for seizure management) produce analgesia by blocking sodium and calcium channels in the CNS, thereby diminishing the transmission of PAIN. The gabapentinoids *gabapentin (Neurontin)* and *pregabalin (Lyrica)* are recommended as first-line analgesics for persistent neuropathic pain (Dworkin et al., 2010). They are increasingly being added to postoperative treatment plans to address the neuropathic component of surgical pain. Primary side effects are sedation and dizziness, which are usually transient and most notable during the titration phase of treatment.

Antidepressants relieve PAIN on the descending modulatory pathway by blocking the body's reuptake of the inhibitory neurochemicals *norepinephrine* and *serotonin*. Antidepressant adjuvant analgesics are divided into two major groups: the *tricyclic antidepressants* (TCAs) and the newer *serotonin and norepinephrine reuptake inhibitors* (SNRIs). Evidence-based guidelines recommend the TCAs *desipramine (Norpramin)* and *nortriptyline (Aventyl, Pamelor)* and the SNRIs *duloxetine (Cymbalta)* and *venlafaxine (Effexor)* as first-line options for neuropathic pain treatment (Dworkin et al., 2010).

The most common side effects of the TCAs are dry mouth, sedation, dizziness, mental clouding, weight gain, and constipation. Orthostatic hypotension is a potentially serious TCA side effect making TCAs a poor choice for older adults. The most serious adverse effect is cardiotoxicity, especially for patients with existing significant heart disease. The SNRIs have a more favorable side effect profile and are better tolerated than the TCAs. The most common SNRI side effects are nausea, headache, sedation, insomnia, weight gain, impaired memory, sweating, and tremors.

CONSIDERATIONS FOR OLDER ADULTS
Patient-Centered Care QSEN

Older adults are often sensitive to the effects of the adjuvant analgesics that produce sedation and other CNS effects, such as anticonvulsants and antidepressants. Therapy should be initiated with low doses, and titration should proceed slowly with systematic assessment of patient response. Caregivers in the home setting must be taught to take preventive measures to reduce the likelihood of falls and other accidents. A home safety assessment is highly recommended and can be arranged by social services before discharge.

Local Anesthetics. Local anesthetics relieve PAIN by blocking the generation and conduction of the nerve impulses necessary to transmit pain (Catterall & Mackie, 2011). The local anesthetic effect is dose-related. A high enough dose of local anesthetic can produce complete anesthesia, and a low enough dose (subanesthetic) can produce analgesia.

Local anesthetics have a long history of safe and effective use for the treatment of all types of PAIN. Allergy to local anesthetics is rare, and side effects are dose-related. CNS signs of systemic toxicity include ringing in the ears, metallic taste, irritability, and seizures. Signs of cardiotoxicity include circumoral tingling and numbness, bradycardia, cardiac dysrhythmias, and CV collapse.

The *lidocaine patch 5%* (Lidoderm) is 10 cm by 14 cm and contains 700 mg of lidocaine. The patch is placed directly over or adjacent to the painful area for absorption into the tissues directly below. A major benefit of the drug is that it produces minimal systemic absorption and side effects. The patch is left in place for 12 hours and then removed for 12 hours (12-hours-on, 12-hours-off regimen). This application process is repeated as needed for continuous analgesia.

Topical local anesthetic creams for superficial procedures, such as IV insertion, include *EMLA* (eutectic mixture of local anesthetics) *and LMX-4. EMLA* contains a combination of lidocaine 2.5% and prilocaine 2.5% and is applied to intact skin for 60 to 120 minutes before the procedure. *LMX-4* contains 4% lidocaine and is applied 30 minutes before the procedure. EMLA has a longer duration of action (2 hours) than LMX-4 (30 minutes) after cream removal. Topical local anesthetic side effects are rare and usually transient, with local skin reactions being the most common.

For many years, *regional anesthesia* has been administered by single-injection peripheral nerve blocks using a long-acting local anesthetic, such as bupivacaine or ropivacaine, to target a specific nerve or nerve plexus. This technique is highly effective in producing PAIN relief, but the effect is temporary (4-12 hours). *Continuous peripheral nerve block* (also called *perineural regional analgesia*) offers an alternative with longer lasting analgesia. A continuous peripheral nerve block involves establishment by an anesthesia provider of an initial block followed by placement of a catheter through which an infusion of local anesthetic is administered continuously, with or without PCA capability. When PCA capability is added, this is referred to as *PCRA* (patient-controlled regional analgesia). Just as with epidural and intrathecal analgesia, nurses are responsible for monitoring and managing the therapy (Pasero & McCaffery, 2011).

Use of Placebos

A placebo is defined as any medication or procedure, including surgery, which produces an effect in a patient because of its implicit or explicit intent, not because of its specific physical or chemical properties. A saline injection is one example of a placebo. Administration of a medication at a known subtherapeutic dose (e.g., 0.05 mg of morphine in an adult) is also considered a placebo.

Placebos are appropriately used as controls in research evaluating the effects of a new medication. Patients or volunteers who participate in placebo-controlled research must be able to give informed consent or have a guardian who can provide informed consent. Unfortunately, occasionally placebos are used clinically in a deceitful manner and without informed consent. This is often done when the clinician does not accept the patient's report of pain. Pain relief resulting from a placebo, should it occur, is mistakenly believed to invalidate a patient's report of pain. This typically results in the patient being deprived of pain-relief measures despite research showing that many patients who have obvious physical stimuli for pain (e.g., abdominal surgery) report pain relief after placebo administration. The use of placebos has both ethical and legal implications, violates the nurse-patient relationship, and deprives patients of more appropriate methods of assessment or treatment.

NURSING SAFETY PRIORITY (QSEN)
Drug Alert

Deceitful administration of a placebo violates informed consent law and jeopardizes the nurse-patient therapeutic relationship. Never administer a placebo to a patient. Promptly contact your nursing supervisor if you are given an order to do so.

Nonpharmacologic Management of Pain

Most people use self-management and nonpharmacologic strategies to deal with their health issues and promote well-being (Bruckenthal, 2010). Nonpharmacologic methods are appropriate alone for mild- and some moderate-intensity PAIN and should be used to complement, not replace, pharmacologic therapies for more severe pain. The effectiveness of nonpharmacologic methods can be unpredictable. Although not all have been shown to relieve pain, they offer many benefits to some patients of all ages (see Evidence-Based Practice box). For example, research has shown that nonpharmacologic methods can facilitate relaxation and reduce anxiety, stress, and depression, which often accompany the pain experience (Bruckenthal, 2010). Many patients find the use of nonpharmacologic methods helps them cope better and feel greater control over the pain experience. Nurses play an important role in providing and teaching their patients about nonpharmacologic strategies. Many of the methods are relatively easy for nurses to incorporate into daily clinical practice and may be used individually or in combination with other nonpharmacologic therapies.

Nonpharmacologic interventions are categorized as being body-based (physical) modalities; mind-body (cognitive-behavioral) methods; biologically based therapies; and energy therapies (Bruckenthal, 2010). Biologically based and energy therapies are used most often in the ambulatory care setting and are beyond the scope of this chapter.

Physical Modalities

The physical modalities have the best evidence for reducing pain. In the acute care setting, the physical modalities are used most often because of their ease in implementation and their role in postoperative recovery. In the ambulatory care setting, sustained physical regimens, such as regular low-impact exercise, in combination with analgesics improve outcomes for people with chronic pain. Many of the physical modalities require a prescription for use and reimbursement. Some require a trained expert to administer the technique (e.g., acupuncture). Among the most effective physical modalities used to manage or prevent pain are:

- Physical therapy
- Occupational therapy
- Aquatherapy
- Functional restoration (also has cognitive-behavioral components)
- Acupuncture
- Low-impact exercise programs, such as slow walking and yoga

The physical modalities are often administered using an interdisciplinary approach. The assistance of physical and occupational therapists to help design and implement an individualized plan with realistic goal setting promotes effectiveness of these methods. Coordinate with the therapist to implement strategies to decrease pain before therapy sessions with the purpose of

EVIDENCE-BASED PRACTICE (QSEN)
Does Education About the Use of Nonpharmacologic Methods Improve Pain Management in Rural Community-Dwelling Older Adults?

Fouladbakhsh, J.M., Szczesny, S., Jenuwine, E.S., & Vallerand, A.H. (2011). Nondrug therapies for pain management among rural older adults. *Pain Management Nursing, 12*(2), 70-81.

Researchers used a quasi-experimental two-group (experimental and control) design to test an educational intervention aimed at educating older adults in a rural community about the appropriate use of nonpharmacologic treatments for pain relief. The interventions were (1) the application of a moist hot pack and/or (2) cold pack to a part of the body for a specified period of time, and/or (3) the use of relaxation breathing exercises while experiencing pain. The sample consisted of 55 adult volunteers who were 60 years of age or older, English-speaking, and had experienced pain in the past 2 weeks. The subjects enrolled in an educational session by date and location that were convenient to them. Surveys to establish baseline pain, pain-related distress, and perception of control over pain were conducted before intervention to establish baseline levels. Participants were randomized to receive either a 30-minute (control) or 60-minute (experimental) education program and a follow-up evaluation session 2 weeks later. Both groups received an additional 30-minute session focused on safe use of over-the-counter (OTC) analgesics. The experimental group received an additional 30-minute session on the safe and appropriate use of the three nonpharmacologic treatments, and each participant in the experimental group was given one hot pack and one cold pack to take home after the education sessions.

At follow-up, there was a significant increase in the use of all three of the nonpharmacologic interventions in the experimental group with two to three times more participants reporting their use than those in the control group. The most frequently used nonpharmacologic therapy was topical application of heat and cold in both groups.

Level of Evidence: 3
The researchers used a quasi-experimental two-group (experimental and control) design to test the interventions.

Commentary: Implications for Practice and Research
This study suggests that older adults with pain may benefit from the use of simple nonpharmacologic interventions and that a structured educational program is helpful in increasing their use of these methods. However, further research and a larger sample size are needed to detect statistically significant changes over time.

increasing function and preventing further deterioration. Teach patients to adhere to their drug regimen to maximize effectiveness of the treatment plan. Expected patient outcomes include an increase in the range of motion, strength, and function of the affected area and an improved quality of life. The occupational therapist may also help decrease pain by making one or more splints to rest severely inflamed joints.

A number of *cutaneous (skin) stimulation* strategies, which apply mild stimulation to the skin and subcutaneous tissues, have been used for many years to relieve pain. Examples of cutaneous stimulation include:

- Application of heat, cold, or pressure
- Therapeutic massage
- Vibration
- Transcutaneous electrical nerve stimulation (TENS)

Cold applications are especially helpful for inflamed areas, such as for patients with rheumatoid arthritis and those who have knee surgery. Heat is appropriate when an increased blood flow is desired, such as for patients with osteoarthritis pain. Paraffin dips for the hands can be helpful to increase movement for those patients as well. Warm showers and compresses that can be done at home are useful in reducing stiffness and promoting movement in patients with arthritis, especially after awakening. Local short-acting gels and creams may provide *cryotherapy (cold treatment)* to relieve muscle aches and pains. These products can often be bought over the counter (OTC) (e.g., Bengay, Icy Hot). The effects of this type of application can last up to 2 hours. Discuss this information with the patient before the use of a cutaneous method:

- The benefits of these techniques are highly unpredictable and may vary from application to application.
- PAIN relief is generally sustained only as long as the stimulation continues.
- Multiple trials may be necessary to establish the desired effects.
- Stimulation itself may aggravate pre-existing pain or may produce new pain.

Despite these potential drawbacks, cutaneous stimulation can be effective in the management of both acute and chronic PAIN in selected patients. A major benefit of these methods is that many are easy for patients to self-administer.

TENS is used occasionally as an adjunctive treatment for PAIN. Although there are several types of TENS units, each involves the use of a battery-operated device capable of delivering small electrical currents through electrodes applied to the painful area. The voltage or current is regulated by adjusting a dial to the point at which the patient perceives a prickly "pins-and-needles" SENSORY PERCEPTION rather than the pain. The current is adjusted based on the degree of desired relief. TENS requires the person to be skilled in the use of the necessary equipment and to be able to apply leads to the correct areas of the body. These factors are cited by patients as drawbacks and can be barriers to older adults who live alone and who may have difficulty with lead application.

Spinal cord stimulation is an *invasive* stimulation technique that provides PAIN control by applying an electrical field over the spinal cord. A trial with a percutaneous epidural stimulator is conducted to determine whether permanent placement of the device is appropriate. If the trial is successful, electrodes are surgically placed in the epidural space and connected to an external or implanted programmable generator. The patient is taught to program and adjust the device to maximize comfort. Spinal cord stimulation can be extremely effective in selected patients but is reserved for intractable neuropathic pain syndromes that have been unresponsive to less invasive methods.

Cognitive-Behavioral Strategies

Cognitive-behavioral strategies are less effective in relieving PAIN than physical modalities. However, they help patients feel more in control and cope better with pain and the conditions that often accompany it, such as depression, anxiety, and stress. Cognitive-behavioral strategies are useful in reducing the patient's focus on pain but do not physiologically block pain transmission. They are most appropriate as an adjunct to pharmacologic therapy for more severe pain. In addition to potential benefits, the limitations of cognitive-behavioral methods should be explained to patients to prevent unrealistic expectations.

Cognitive-behavioral methods range from simple (e.g., prayer, relaxation breathing, artwork, reading, and watching television) to more complex (e.g., meditation, guided imagery, hypnosis, biofeedback, and virtual reality). It is important to recognize that many of the methods require patient teaching and subsequent patient participation. Therefore it is inappropriate to attempt to teach the more complex cognitive-behavioral methods to patients who are unfamiliar with them and are experiencing severe pain, anxiety, or agitation. Not all patients are receptive to the use of these methods. To respect their wishes, values, and preferences as part of patient-centered care, do not insist that patients use any method.

Distraction is probably the most commonly used cognitive-behavioral method. All of us use simple distraction measures in our daily life when we watch television or read a book. Nurses often observe that patients request less PAIN medication when family members are present and when talking on the phone. After visiting hours, it is not unusual for patients to request pain medication because they are no longer distracted.

Visual distracters (e.g., looking at a picture, watching television, playing a video game) can divert the attention to something pleasant or interesting. Auditory distracters (e.g., listening to music or relaxation tapes) can have a calming effect. Changing the environment involves removing or reducing unpleasant stressors that can interfere with the patient's ability to cope with pain, such as loud noise and bright lights. Ask patients if they use any cognitive-behavioral techniques in their daily life. Encourage them to apply those methods to their current pain experience.

Imagery is a more complex form of distraction in which the patient is encouraged to visualize or think about a pleasant or desirable feeling, sensation, or event. The person is encouraged to sustain a sequence of thoughts aimed at diverting attention away from the pain. Patients who practice this technique can mentally and vividly experience sights, sounds, smells, events, or other sensations. Intense concentration is required to visualize images; therefore patients must have fairly well-controlled pain to participate.

Before suggesting imagery, assess the patient's level of concentration to determine whether he or she can sustain a particular thought or thoughts for a desired time. The time interval for mental imagery can vary from 5 to 60 minutes. Behaviors that may be helpful in assessing whether a patient is a candidate for teaching guided imagery include that the patient is able to:

- Read and comprehend a newspaper or magazine article
- Tap to a rhythm or sing while listening to music
- Follow the logic and participate in sustained conversation
- Have an interest in environmental surroundings

When the patient has demonstrated ability to concentrate, assist him or her in identifying a pleasant or favorable thought. Encourage the patient to focus on this thought to divert attention away from painful stimuli. CDs or other audio recordings, either commercial or created by the patient and family, may help form and maintain images. This is an example of guided imagery instructions:

Imagine being on the beach of a deserted island. You can hear the sound of waves rushing onto the shore, the cry of seagulls flying high above, and the rustling of trees as they are brushed gently by the wind. You can feel the warmth of the sun over your body and the cooling breeze.

Patients may also use *relaxation techniques* to reduce anxiety, tension, and emotional stress, all of which can exacerbate pain. For example, before and during a painful procedure, patients can be reminded to breathe slowly, deeply, and rhythmically to divert attention and promote relaxation. Relaxation techniques can be both physical and psychological. Physical relaxation techniques include:

- Relaxation breathing
- Receiving a body massage, back rub, or warm bath
- Modifying the environment to reduce distractions
- Moving into a comfortable position

Psychological relaxation techniques include:

- Pleasant conversation
- Laughter and humor
- Music (provide a range of choices)
- Relaxation tapes

⑨ CLINICAL JUDGMENT CHALLENGE

Patient-Centered Care; Evidence-Based Practice QSEN

An older woman visits the neurologist for low back pain that she has had for several months. She has been taking high doses of ibuprofen and acetaminophen every day with some pain relief. After a thorough physical examination, the neurologist starts her on pregabalin (Lyrica) 75 mg twice daily for pain. As her office nurse, you are preparing for health teaching.

1. What questions will you ask the patient at this time in preparation for teaching?
2. How might you find the best evidence to help prepare her teaching plan?
3. What are the concerns about her current pain management regimen?
4. What nonpharmacologic methods might benefit her? How will you determine if they are appropriate for her values and beliefs?

Community-Based Care

Before patients are discharged from an acute care setting, collaborate with members of the health care team to optimize PAIN control. Before discharge or transfer from a hospital, ensure that the patient, especially one who will receive opioid analgesia, has appropriate prescriptions and enough doses to last at least until the first follow-up visit with the primary health care provider.

Home Care Management

Fatigue exacerbates PAIN. If physical modifications in the home (e.g., installing a downstairs bathroom) are unrealistic, suggest changes in schedules, role responsibilities, and daily routines to help prevent or reduce fatigue.

At home, patients may require a referral for physical therapy, especially to start or continue exercise regimens or treatment with cutaneous stimulation or heat or cold techniques. Patients may need a social worker to assist them develop coping strategies or maintain adequate family dynamics. A hospice or palliative care referral (hospital- or community-based) can help maintain continuity of care in the management of terminally ill patients and those who require treatment of some chronic conditions.

Home infusion therapy programs provide a wide variety of services to patients who require technology-supported PAIN care at home. Many of these services depend on approval by the insurance carrier, usually before analgesic options are considered and therapy is started. Case managers can be helpful in answering insurance and other payment questions. Well-defined home agency practices and professional support at home are required if patients leave the hospital with infusion therapy for pain management. Often, family members are taught to assume the responsibilities of home infusion therapy.

Self-Management Education

Teach the patient and family about analgesic regimens, including any technical skills needed to administer the analgesic; the purpose and action of various drugs, their side effects, and complications; and the importance of correct dosing and dosing intervals. Explain how to prevent or treat the constipation commonly associated with taking opioid analgesics and other medications. Inform the patient about what to do and who to contact if the prescribed management regimen is not controlling pain well or when side effects are intolerable or unmanageable.

Help the patient establish an analgesic regimen that does not interfere with sleep, rest, appetite, and level of physical mobility. Ensure that patients are aware of any dangers associated with driving or operating mechanical equipment. Tell patients to ask their primary health care provider when these activities are safe to perform. Older patients and others at risk for falls or accidents in the home setting may benefit from a home safety assessment.

In patients with PAIN from advanced cancer, all efforts are directed toward maximizing relief and symptom control at home and eliminating unnecessary hospital re-admissions. This may mean that the primary health care provider prescribes a flexible analgesic schedule that allows the patient to adjust analgesics according to the amount of pain. Teach the patient and family how to safely treat breakthrough pain and increase drug doses within the prescribed dosing guidelines. If painful ambulatory care treatments or procedures are expected, tell the patient how important it is to talk with his or her primary health care provider to determine available options for preventing procedural pain (e.g., premedicating).

Evaluate family support systems to assist the patient in adhering to and continuing the proposed medical treatment and nursing plan of care. Inform and include family members in activities during and after hospitalization. To achieve a reasonable level of involvement in life activities for the patient, suggest ways to continue participation in household, social, sexual, and work-oriented activities after discharge. Help the patient identify important activities and plan to do them with adequate rest periods.

The patient with chronic pain needs continued support to cope with the anxiety, fear, and powerlessness that often accompany this type of pain. Help the patient and family or significant others identify coping strategies that have worked in the past. Outside support systems are often extremely helpful, such as organizations like the *American Chronic Pain Association* (http://theacpa.org). This organization has the "10-Step Program from Patient to Person" and provides numerous educational materials and facilitates the establishment of local support groups for people with chronic PAIN.

Health Care Resources

Ask the prescriber for a home health care or hospice referral, as appropriate, for patients who require assistance or supervision with the PAIN management regimen at home. Important information to provide to the home health care nurse includes the

patient's condition, level of sedation, weakness or fatigue, possible constipation or nutritional problem, sleep patterns, and functional status. Detailed information about the patient's current pain management regimen and how well it has been tolerated is essential. Use a structured procedure such as SBAR (**s**ituation, **b**ackground, **a**ssessment, **r**ecommendations) to communicate this information.

In addition to explaining the patient's physical status to the home health care nurse, describe the patient's level of anxiety and general expectations about PAIN after discharge. Close relationships and available support networks are important factors in providing ongoing support for effective pain intervention strategies.

Referral to an advanced practice nurse pain specialist, social worker, or psychologist may be necessary for some patients and families to provide continued support, reinforce instructions for complex pharmacologic or nonpharmacologic strategies, or evaluate overall physical and emotional adaptation after discharge. When severe chronic or intractable pain exists, health care professionals should direct the patient and family to appropriate resources such as pain centers or health care providers who specialize in long-term PAIN management.

GET READY FOR THE NCLEX® EXAMINATION!

KEY POINTS

Review these Key Points for each NCLEX Examination Client Needs Category.

Safe and Effective Care Environment
- The nurse is legally and ethically responsible for acting as an advocate for patients experiencing PAIN.
- Coordinate the patient's plan of care as he or she transfers between health care agencies; be sure to clearly communicate the plan of care to the new agency. **Teamwork and Collaboration** QSEN

Health Promotion and Maintenance
- Provide information to the patient and family about nonpharmacologic therapies such as ice and heat; these modalities are additions to, not replacements for, the established plan of care.
- Consider the special needs of older adults when assessing and managing their PAIN (see Chart 3-1). **Patient-Centered Care** QSEN
- Assess and meet the patient's need for PAIN management promptly to promote relief; be sensitive to the cultural preferences and values of the patient and family. **Patient-Centered Care** QSEN

Psychosocial Integrity
- Be aware that some nurses and physicians may have biases about pain assessment and management; be objective when caring for patients with PAIN.
- Assess and document the patient's and family's expectations for management of PAIN. **Patient-Centered Care** QSEN
- Provide accurate information to patients who have misconceptions and misunderstandings about PAIN and pain management to prevent these from becoming barriers to effective pain management.

Physiological Integrity
- Remember that PAIN is what the patient says it is; self-report is always the most reliable indicator of pain. **Patient-Centered Care** QSEN
- Perform and document a complete PAIN assessment, including duration, location, intensity, and quality of pain. **Informatics** QSEN
- Never use placebos to assess the presence of PAIN; their deceitful use is prohibited by state boards of nursing and numerous professional organizations.

- Factors that affect PAIN and its management include age, gender, race, genetics, and culture. **Patient-Centered Care** QSEN
- The two major types of PAIN are nociceptive pain and neuropathic pain. Pain is also classified by its duration as acute or chronic. Chronic pain is further classified as cancer or non-cancer chronic pain.
- Examples of causes for acute PAIN include surgery and trauma; arthritis and cancer are common causes of chronic pain.
- Multimodal analgesia is the recommended approach for the management of all types of pain (see Table 3-6). Multimodal analgesia combines different drugs with different underlying mechanisms of action with the goal of producing better pain relief at lower analgesic doses than would be possible with any single analgesic alone. Lower doses result in fewer side effects. Non-opioid analgesics (acetaminophen, NSAIDs) are the first-line therapy for mild to moderate nociceptive pain and the foundation for a multimodal treatment plan for more severe nociceptive pain. **Evidence-Based Practice** QSEN
- Assess patients on acetaminophen for clinical manifestations of hepatotoxicity and nephrotoxicity; these adverse drug effects may occur when the medication is taken in higher than recommended daily doses. **Safety** QSEN
- Recall that NSAIDs should be used with caution in older adults because of adverse effects, such as GI toxicity, bleeding, and fluid retention, for which they are at higher risk than younger adults. **Safety** QSEN
- The mu opioid agonists are first-line therapy for moderate to severe nociceptive pain. Morphine, fentanyl, hydromorphone, and oxycodone are the most commonly used mu opioid agonists and are available in a wide variety of formulations for administration by a variety of routes of administration for both acute and chronic PAIN. **Evidence-Based Practice** QSEN
- Meperidine is not recommended for the treatment of any type of PAIN. Its toxic metabolite (normeperidine) can accumulate and cause confusion, seizures, and even death. It is a particularly poor choice in older adults and those with decreased renal clearance. **Evidence-Based Practice** QSEN
- Physical dependence is a normal response that occurs with repeated administration of an opioid for several days. It is manifested by the occurrence of withdrawal symptoms when

the opioid is suddenly stopped or rapidly reduced or an antagonist such as naloxone is given. It cannot be equated with addictive disease.

- Tolerance is a normal response that occurs with regular administration of an opioid and consists of a decrease in one or more effects of the opioid (e.g., decreased analgesia, sedation, or respiratory depression). It cannot be equated with addictive disease. With the exception of constipation, tolerance to the opioid side effects develops with regular daily dosing of opioids over several days.

- Opioid addiction is a chronic neurologic and biologic disease. The development and characteristics of addiction are influenced by genetic, psychosocial, and environmental factors. No single cause of addiction, such as taking an opioid for PAIN relief, has been found. It is characterized by one or more of these behaviors: impaired control over drug use, compulsive use, continued use despite harm, and craving.

- Use an equianalgesic chart (see Table 3-7 when changing from one opioid or route of administration to another to help ensure the patient receives about the same relief with the new opioid or route as with the previous. **Evidence-Based Practice** QSEN

- Be aware of the advantages and disadvantages of the various routes of analgesic administration.

- Observe for and prevent common side effects of analgesics (see Table 3-9). Remember that the single most effective treatment of most side effects is to decrease the dose of the drug causing the side effect.

- Remember that sedation precedes opioid-induced respiratory depression; assess sedation using a sedation scale, and decrease the opioid dose if excessive sedation is detected (see Table 3-10). **Safety** QSEN

- The intraspinal routes include the intrathecal (also called *spinal*) and epidural routes of administration. Intrathecal analgesia is given by single injection of opioid (most often) into the subarachnoid space for acute pain or implanted device for chronic pain; epidural analgesia is given by single injection or continuous infusion with or without PCA capability for all types of pain and usually combines an opioid with a local anesthetic.

- Adjuvant analgesics are drugs that have a primary indication other than pain but are analgesic for some painful conditions. The most commonly used are antidepressants, anticonvulsants, and local anesthetics. Examples are listed in Table 3-6.

- Nonpharmacologic therapies may be effective alone for mild pain and are used to complement, not replace, pharmacologic interventions for moderate to severe pain. **Evidence-Based Practice** QSEN

- PAIN can be managed in any setting, including the home. All patients require teaching with regard to their pain management regimen to ensure continuity of care. Patients or family members will require specialized training when infusion therapy is used in the home setting.

- Request referral or consultation with pain specialists and/or pain centers for patients with PAIN that cannot be managed with customary methods. **Teamwork and Collaboration** QSEN

CHAPTER 4

Genetic and Genomic Concepts for Medical-Surgical Nursing

M. Linda Workman

http://evolve.elsevier.com/Iggy/

PRIORITY CONCEPTS

- Ethics
- Collaboration

LEARNING OUTCOMES

Safe and Effective Care Environment

1. Ensure COLLABORATION with health care team members and genetics professionals when providing genetic testing information to patients and families.

Health Promotion and Maintenance

2. Teach the patient and family who are at increased genetic risk for a disease or disorder to implement environmental modifications to reduce the risk when possible.

Psychosocial Integrity

3. Reduce the psychological impact for the patient and family regarding genetic assessment and genetic testing.

Physiological Integrity

4. Incorporate genetic and genomic principles into patient and family assessment techniques.
5. Ensure the use of professional ETHICS when integrating genomic health into medical-surgical nursing practice.

Genomic health is a growing part of today's comprehensive health care. Although the terms *genetics* and *genomics* often are used interchangeably, there are some differences. **Genetics** is concerned with the general mechanisms of heredity and the variation of inherited traits. Thus how genetic traits are transmitted from one generation to the next is part of genetics. The definition of **genomics** is both broader and more specific, focusing on the function of all of the human DNA, including genes and noncoding DNA regions. Thus how a gene is expressed within a person or family constitutes genomics. **Genomic health care** is the application of known genetic variation to enhance health care to individuals and their families.

Many adult-onset health problems have a genetic basis, meaning that variation of gene sequences and expression contributes to a person's risk for disease development. Some of these health problems also demonstrate **heritability,** meaning that the risk for developing the disorder can be transmitted to one's children in a recognizable pattern. Some adult-onset disorders, such as Huntington disease, are unavoidable when a person inherits a specific genetic mutation that causes the disorder. For other health problems, the risk is increased but is not absolute, indicating a *predisposition* or *susceptibility* toward the problem when a specific genetic mutation is inherited, but such a disorder may never occur. For example, certain gene variations increase the risk for type 2 diabetes; however, the disease is more likely to develop only when the person with the genetic variations has a sedentary lifestyle and is overweight. One outcome of genomic health care is to identify personal risk for disease development and assist the person to reduce

the risk by modifying his or her environment (Manuck & McCaffery, 2014).

Specific discoveries regarding each person's genetic differences are being used to assess disease risk, enhance disease prevention strategies, and personalize disease management approaches (Bielinski et al., 2014). As a result, all health care professionals, including registered nurses, are expected to have at least a minimum knowledge of basic genetics to provide the best possible care for patients and families (Calzone et al., 2013). Table 4-1 lists selected genetic competencies important in medical-surgical nursing. Nurses are expected to know enough about basic genetics to recognize when a patient or family has a possible genetic risk for a health problem and to coordinate the attention of health care team members to ensure appropriate care.

GENETIC BIOLOGY REVIEW

Genes are the coded instructions for the making of all the different proteins the human body produces. For every hormone, enzyme, and other proteins the human body makes, it is the specific genes that tell each cell what protein to make, how to make it, when to make it, and how much to make. Think of each gene as a specific "recipe" for making a protein.

Every human somatic cell with a nucleus contains the entire set of human genes, known as the **genome.** The human genome contains between 20,000 and 25,000 genes. For example, all cells have the gene for insulin. However, the only cell type that allows the insulin gene to be **expressed** (turned on, activated) and

TABLE 4-1 Selected Essential Genetic Competencies for Medical-Surgical Nursing Practice

- Use appropriate genetic terminology.
- Recognize that a person/family with an identified genetic variation is a full member of society deserving of the same quality of health care as that provided to all others.
- Differentiate between genetic predisposition to a health problem and the actual expression or diagnosis of the health problem.
- Recognize the genetic and environmental influences on development of common adult-onset health problems.
- Be aware of genetic-based individual variation in responses to drug therapy.
- Consider genetic transmission patterns when performing a detailed patient and family history assessment.
- Ask appropriate questions during assessment to obtain information relevant to potential genetic risk or predisposition to a specific health problem(s).
- Construct a family pedigree, using standard symbols, that encompasses at least three generations.
- Identify patients/families at increased genetic risk for potential disease development.
- Ensure that patients/families identified to be at increased genetic risk for potential disease development are referred to the appropriate level of genetics professional.
- Individualize patient teaching about genetic issues using terminology and language the patient/family understands.
- Inform patients/families about potential risks and potential benefits of genetic testing.
- Advocate for patients with regard to their rights of accurate information, informed consent, competent counseling, refusal of genetic testing, freedom from coercion, and sharing of testing results.
- Assist patients/families to find credible resources regarding a specific genetic issue.
- Maintain patient/family confidentiality regarding any issue related to genetic testing, genetic predisposition, or genetic diagnosis, including whether genetic testing is even being considered.
- Support the patient's/family's decisions regarding any aspect of genetic testing or genetic diagnosis.

Data from competencies identified by American Association of Colleges of Nursing. (2008). *The essentials of baccalaureate education for nursing practice.* Washington, DC: Author; American Nurses Association. (2008). *Essentials of genetic and genomic nursing: Competencies, curricula guidelines, and outcome indicators* (2nd ed.). Silver Springs, MD: Author; Kirk, M., Calzone, K., Arimori, N., & Tonkin, E. (2011). Genetic-genomics competencies and nursing regulation. *Journal of Nursing Scholarship, 43*(2), 107-116.

FIG. 4-1 The various forms of DNA from a loose double helix to coiled tightly into a chromosome. *bp,* Base pair.

make insulin is the beta cell of the pancreas. So, although the insulin gene is present in skin cells, heart cells, brain cells, and other cells, only in the beta cells is this gene selectively expressed when insulin is needed.

Genes are composed of DNA, which is present as 46 separate large chunks within the nucleus (Fig. 4-1). During cell division, each large chunk of DNA replicates and then organizes into a chromosome form to ensure precise delivery of the genetic information to each of the two new daughter cells. Thus DNA, chromosomes, and genes are all the same basic thing; only the structures differ.

Each chromosome has many genes within it. Humans have 23 pairs of chromosomes—46 individual chromosomes. The Y chromosome is small and has fewer than 100 genes. Larger chromosomes, such as the number 1 chromosome, contain thousands of genes.

One way to think of it is to consider all the DNA in any cell's nucleus (genome) to be a giant "cookbook" containing all the recipes needed to make all the proteins, hormones, enzymes, and other substances your body needs. The chromosome pairs are the different book chapters (so the human genome cookbook has 23 chapters), and the genes are the individual recipes contained within the chapters.

There is a specific chromosome location (**locus**) for every gene. For example, the locus of the gene for blood type is on chromosome 9. The location and the exact DNA sequence for many, but not all, genes is now known.

DNA

DNA Structure

In humans, DNA is a linear, double-stranded structure composed of multiple units of four different nitrogenous bases, each attached to a sugar molecule. The bases in each strand are linked together by phosphate groups. These two individual strands are held together loosely. This double-stranded DNA is arranged like a long set of railroad tracks. The "backbones" of the track are the two long steel rails. For DNA, these backbones are the phosphate groups that hold the bases in place. The bases are the individual railroad ties. Think of each tie as having two pieces—one piece attached to the right-hand rail and one piece attached to the left-hand rail.

Fig. 4-2 shows a very small piece of double-stranded DNA on the left (containing only four base pairs) taken from the larger piece of DNA on the right. The phosphate groups that hold the nucleotides together as a strand are in the red box. The green box in the lower left-hand section shows a whole nucleotide (a base with the sugar and the phosphate group) in place

Phosphate "backbone"

One base pair

One nucleotide

Hydrogen bonds

3.4 Å

34 Å

20 Å

FIG. 4-2 The structure of DNA.

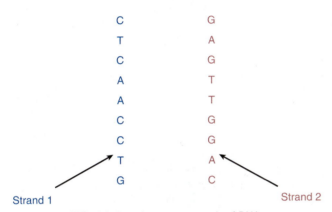

Strand 1	Strand 2
C	G
T	A
C	G
A	T
A	T
C	G
C	G
T	A
G	C

FIG. 4-3 Complementary strands of DNA.

in the left-hand DNA strand. The blue box in the middle of the two strands shows how the base from the left strand lines up with and pairs to a complementary base in the right strand.

Bases are the essential parts of DNA. Many trillions of bases in the DNA are found in the nucleus of just one cell. The four bases in DNA are adenine (A), guanine (G), cytosine (C), and thymine (T). Each base becomes a complete **nucleotide** when a five-sided sugar (known as a *deoxyribose sugar*) and a phosphate group are attached (see Fig. 4-2). Nucleotides form the DNA strands with the phosphate groups holding the bases in place.

Base pairs are the linked bases in the two opposite strands of DNA. The bases always link together across from each other in a very specific way. Thymine always forms a pair with adenine, and cytosine always forms a pair with guanine. Thus the bases of each pair are *complementary* to each other. Because these complementary base pairs in DNA are specific, if the base sequence of one strand of DNA is known, the opposite strand's sequence could be accurately predicted. For example, if the left-hand section of DNA (strand 1 in Fig. 4-3) had the sequence C-T-C-A-A-C-C-T-G, the corresponding (complementary) right-hand section (strand 2 in Fig. 4-3) of DNA would have the sequence G-A-G-T-T-G-G-A-C.

When the two strands of DNA are lined up properly, they twist into a loose helical shape (see Fig. 4-1). In this shape, the DNA is so fine that it can be seen only with electron microscopes. Only when a cell undergoes mitosis does the DNA super-coil tightly into dense pieces called *chromosomes* (Fig. 4-1), which can be seen with standard microscopes.

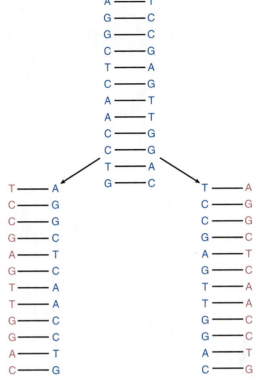

FIG. 4-4 DNA replication. *Blue type,* Original DNA; *red type,* newly replicated DNA.

DNA Replication

DNA must reproduce itself **(replicate)** every time a cell divides (undergoes mitosis). The purpose of mitosis is for one cell to reproduce into two new daughter cells, each of which is identical to the parent cell that started mitosis. For each new cell to have exactly the right amount of DNA and genes, the DNA in the dividing cell must exactly replicate. This process involves having the double strands of DNA separate and then build two new strands that are perfectly complementary to the original strands (Fig. 4-4). The result is two sets of double-stranded DNA. At the time of actual cell division with the separation into two new cells, one set of DNA will move into one of the two new cells made during mitosis and the second set will move into the other new cell. In this way, every new cell ends up with exactly the right amount of DNA with all the genes.

Chromosomes

As shown in Fig. 4-1, a chromosome is a specific large chunk of highly condensed double-stranded DNA, with each chunk containing billions of bases and hundreds (and sometimes thousands) of genes. Each chromosome forms and moves to the center of the cell that is about to divide. Just before the cell splits into two cells, each chromosome is pulled apart so that half of each chromosome goes into one new cell and the other half goes into the other new cell. Thus chromosomes are temporary structures to ensure the precise delivery of DNA to the two new cells. Humans have 46 chromosomes divided into 23 pairs.

Some things about a person can be known by examining his or her chromosomes, but limited information can be obtained by chromosomal analysis because each chromosome is composed of a large chunk of DNA. Only very large deletions, additions, or rearrangements of DNA show up at the level of the

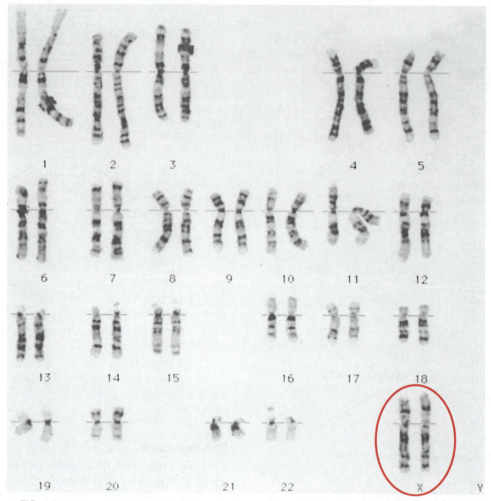

FIG. 4-5 A karyotype of a chromosomally normal female. (The sex chromosomes are *circled in red.*)

chromosome. Losses or gains of even tens of thousands of bases cannot be detected by chromosome analysis.

A **karyotype** is an organized arrangement of all of the chromosomes present in a cell during the metaphase section of mitosis (Fig. 4-5). A picture of the chromosomes is made. Chromosomes are first paired up and then arranged according to size (largest first) and centromere position. This gross organization of DNA can be used to determine missing or extra whole chromosomes and some large structural rearrangements. *A missing gene or a mutated gene would not show up at this level of analysis.* What can be learned about the person from whom the karyotype in Fig. 4-5 was made is that the person is human, female, and **euploid** (has the correct number of chromosome pairs for the species). This person is chromosomally "normal," although she probably has some genes that are different from (variant from or mutated from) the same genes in other people. If the karyotype is abnormal in any way (has more or less than the normal number or has broken chromosomes), the karyotype would be called **aneuploid.**

Autosomes are the 22 pairs of human chromosomes (numbered 1 through 22) that do not code for the sexual differentiation of a person. **Sex chromosomes** are the pair of chromosomes that include the genes for the sexual differentiation of the person. Chromosomally normal males have an X and a Y as the sex chromosomes. Chromosomally normal females have two Xs (XX) as the sex chromosomes (see Fig. 4-5).

Gene Structure and Function

A **gene** is a specific segment(s) of DNA that contains the code (recipe) for a specific protein (see Fig. 4-1). Thus genes are the smallest functional unit of the DNA. Each chromosome is a large segment of DNA that contains hundreds of genes.

For many human traits, one gene controls the expression of that trait in any person. Such traits are known as "single gene traits" *(monogenic traits)*. For each single gene, we have two alleles. An **allele** (pronounced "ah-**lee**-el") is an alternate form (or variation) of a gene. For example, there is one gene for blood type but there are three possible gene alleles (A, B, and O). Each person has only two of the three specific gene alleles for blood type. One of these alleles is on one chromosome 9 of the pair; the other allele is located on the other number 9 chromosome. Because each person only has two number 9 chromosomes, he or she can have only two of the three possible alleles for blood type. One gene allele was inherited from the person's mother, and the other gene allele was inherited from the person's father. *Some traits have even more than three possible alleles, but each person has only two.* Which blood type gene alleles are inherited from a person's parents determines which blood type he or she expresses.

If a person has inherited a blood type A allele from his or her mother and a blood type B allele from his or her father, he or she has the A and B alleles; the blood type expressed when

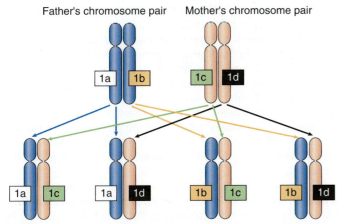

Father's chromosome pair   Mother's chromosome pair

1a 1b   1c 1d

1a 1c   1a 1d   1b 1c   1b 1d

FIG. 4-6 Inheritance of four possible alleles for the single gene trait 1. (Any one person can have only two alleles for a single gene trait.)

the blood bank determines type is type AB. Fig. 4-6 shows this concept. In Fig. 4-6, two people are about to become pregnant. What are the possibilities for this baby to have a specific type of ear shape (pointy, rounded, square, triangular)? The gene for ear shape is trait 1, and it (for the purposes of this explanation) is on chromosome number 6.

Each of the father's sperm contains only one number 6 chromosome and each of the mother's eggs contains only one number 6 chromosome (so that when the sperm fertilizes the egg, the resulting person conceived will have only one pair of chromosome number 6 instead of two pairs of chromosome number 6).

Half the father's sperm have the 1a allele for ear shape, and the other half have allele 1b for ear shape. Half the mother's eggs have 1c for ear shape, and the other half have 1d. The resulting baby can inherit only either a 1a or a 1b from the father, not both; and this same baby can inherit only a 1c or a 1d from the mother—again, not both. The lower portion of Fig. 4-6 shows all the combinations possible for each ear shape gene alleles for any child these two people have.

If a person has two identical alleles for a single gene trait, that person is said to be *homozygous* for that trait. So if a person has an A blood-type gene allele on one number 9 chromosome and an A blood-type gene allele on the other number 9 chromosome, he or she is homozygous for that trait and will express the A blood type.

If a person has two different alleles for a single gene trait, he or she is *heterozygous* for that trait. So if a person has an A blood-type gene allele on one number 9 chromosome and a B blood-type gene allele on the other number 9 chromosome, that person is heterozygous for that trait and will express the AB blood type. Because the A and B alleles are equally dominant (*co-dominant*), they will both be expressed in the actual blood type.

There are differences in expression of the alleles for a trait depending on whether an allele is dominant or is recessive. If a person has an A blood-type gene allele on one number 9 chromosome and an O blood-type gene allele on the other number 9 chromosome, that person is heterozygous for that trait and expresses only the A blood type. Because the A allele is dominant and the O allele is recessive, they will not both be expressed in the actual blood type. Only the dominant allele is expressed, and the recessive allele is "silent." More information about

dominant, recessive, and co-dominant expression is presented later in the Patterns of Inheritance section on p. 56.

Phenotype

The **phenotype** of any gene for a person is what characteristic can actually be observed or, in some cases, determined by a laboratory test. For example, the person who has the AO gene alleles for blood type has the phenotype of type A blood. A person with curly hair has a curly hair phenotype regardless of whether he or she has two alleles for curly hair or one allele for curly hair and one allele for straight hair.

Genotype

The **genotype** for a person's single gene trait is what the actual alleles are for that trait—not just what can be observed. A person with a phenotype of type A blood could have either an AA genotype or an AO genotype. The person who has type O blood would have an OO genotype. When a person has homozygous alleles for a trait, we would expect the genotype and phenotype to be the same. When a person has heterozygous alleles for a trait, the phenotype and the genotype are not always the same. *Recessive traits are expressed only when the person is homozygous for the alleles.* Thus for expressed recessive traits, phenotype and genotype are the same. Dominant traits are expressed whether the person is homozygous for the gene alleles or heterozygous for the gene alleles. Thus for dominant traits, phenotype and genotype can be the same but do not have to be the same.

Gene Expression

The purpose of a gene is to code for the making of a specific protein. For example, the hormone *insulin* is a protein. When a person's blood glucose level starts to rise, the beta cells of the pancreas rapidly make insulin to maintain the person's blood glucose homeostasis.

To continue the cookbook analogy, each gene is the recipe needed to make a specific protein. All the "stuff" that a human body makes—every hormone, every enzyme, every growth factor, every chemical needed to keep the person functioning—is a protein. These proteins are *gene products* because they are produced when the right gene is *expressed*. Just a few examples of gene products are insulin, hemoglobin, erythropoietin, angiotensin, and estrogen.

Protein Synthesis

Protein synthesis is the process by which genes are used to make the proteins needed for physiologic function. Proteins are made up of individual amino acids hooked together like beads on a string. There are 22 different amino acids. Every protein has a specific number of each of the amino acids and a specific order in which they are placed. *If even one amino acid is out of order or completely deleted from the sequence, the protein may be less functional or, perhaps, nonfunctional and unable to perform its job in the body.*

For example, the hormone *insulin* is a protein that contains 51 amino acids in a specific sequence. If some of the amino acids are missing or are in the wrong position, the protein made would be different from real insulin and could not reduce blood glucose levels. *Thus the actual order of the amino acids is critical for the final function of any protein.*

Within the DNA there is a three-nucleotide (base) code for each amino acid. A gene for a specific protein contains all the

FIG. 4-7 A sample protein composed of seven amino acids.

amino acid codes in exactly the right order for that protein. For example, the final active form of the protein *insulin* has 51 amino acids. Thus the minimum number of bases needed in the gene for insulin would be 153 (3 bases per amino acid × 51 amino acids). Fig. 4-7 shows an example of a short protein made up of only 7 amino acids.

The key for making a functional protein is accurate placement of all the amino acids in the order specified by the gene. When problems exist in the base sequence of a gene, its expression may not result in a functional protein. In addition, the process of protein synthesis involves many complex steps and a problem at any step could result in the failure to produce a functional protein.

Mutations

Many human genes have been sequenced, meaning that their base sequence is known and so is the sequence of their amino acids in the expressed proteins. Most people have the same base sequence for a specific gene, like the gene for insulin. When this sequence is the most common one found in a large population of humans, it is referred to as the *wild-type* gene sequence. Think of the term *wild-type* as meaning "normal" or "expected." When a person has a different sequence for a gene compared with the known wild-type sequence, the gene has a variation or mutation. Mutations as small variations in gene sequences occur more often in very large genes, and the significance of some of these changes is not known. It is these differences or variations in the sequences of some genes from the wild-type that are now being examined more closely in health care. Some of these variations can reduce the function of the protein produced, some can eliminate the function of the protein produced, and a few variations have been found that enhance the function of the produced protein compared with the function of the wild-type protein.

Mutations are DNA changes that are passed from one generation to another and thus are *inherited*. An inherited mutation does not have to mean that the mutation is passed from one human generation to another. It can mean that the mutation is passed from one *cell* generation to another and may affect only certain tissues within a person rather than be a problem within a family. These mutations occur in general body cells (somatic cells) and are known as *somatic mutations*. Because these mutations occur in a person's cells after conception, the person cannot pass a somatic mutation on to his or her children. One possible outcome of somatic mutations is an increased risk for cancer in cells with such mutations.

When mutations occur in sex cells, they are called *germline mutations*. A germline mutation *can* be passed on to a person's children, and each of that child's cells, including his or her somatic cells and sex cells, will contain the mutated DNA.

When mutations resulting in sequence variation occur in a gene area of the DNA, the change can alter the expression of that gene and an incorrect gene product (protein) might result. Mutations can have serious results, although some mutations may be beneficial. Gene mutations that increase the risk for a disorder are known as *susceptibility* genes. Gene mutations that

decrease the risk for a disorder are known as *protective* or *resistance* genes (Beery & Workman, 2012).

As stated earlier, the gene sequences for most proteins are generally the same in all people. Sometimes a base in one person's gene for a specific protein is not the same as that in the wild-type. Either this difference can be a variation known as a *single nucleotide polymorphism*, or *SNP* ("snip"), or it can be a mutation. When a base difference allows the protein to be made but there are differences in how well the protein works, the difference is called a *gene variation* or a polymorphism. When a base difference causes a loss of protein function, it is called a mutation.

Clinically, many SNPs exist within different people in the genes of a large family of enzymes involved in drug metabolism. These enzymes are the cytochrome P-450 family, coded for by at least ten separate extremely large genes, with as many as 100 subsets of genes. Cytochrome p is abbreviated as CYP (pronounced "sip"). SNPs in these genes can make the resulting enzyme less active than normal or more active than normal. Either way, a change in activity of any one of these enzymes can affect a person's response to drug therapy. For example, the drug *warfarin* (Coumadin) is metabolized for elimination primarily by two enzymes from this system, CYP2CP and CYP2C19. About 17% to 37% of white people have a SNP variation in CYP2CP that slows the metabolism of warfarin. This means that warfarin remains in the person's system longer, greatly increasing the risk for bleeding and other side effects. For people who have this gene mutation, warfarin doses need to be much lower than those for the general population (Cheek, 2013).

⊕ CULTURAL CONSIDERATIONS

Patient-Centered Care QSEN

Most people of Asian heritage have a SNP in the *CYP2C19* gene that results in low activity of the enzyme produced. This mutation greatly reduces the metabolism of warfarin, leading to a longer warfarin half-life and increased bleeding risks along with other serious side effects. Any person of Asian heritage who needs anticoagulation therapy should be started on very low dosages of warfarin and have his or her international normalized ratio (INR) monitored more frequently than people who do not have a variation of the *CYP2C19* gene.

The most devastating gene mutations are the ones that change the amino acid codes so that a proper protein is not made. Other changes may alter how often or how well a group of cells divides. Gene mutations or variations may cause one person to have a greater-than-normal risk for developing a disease. A different variation in the same gene may cause another person to have a smaller-than-normal risk for developing the same disease.

PATTERNS OF INHERITANCE

For every single gene trait, a person inherits one allele for that gene from his or her mother and one allele from his or her father. How these traits are expressed depends on whether one or both alleles are "dominant" or "recessive." Expression also depends on whether the gene for the trait is located on an autosome or on a sex chromosome.

It is possible to determine how the gene for a specific trait is passed from one human generation to the next (*transmitted*). By looking at how that trait is expressed through several generations of a family, patterns emerge that indicate whether the gene for the trait is dominant or recessive and whether it is located on an autosomal chromosome or on one of the sex chromosomes. This information can be determined through *pedigree analysis.* Determining inheritance patterns for a specific trait makes it possible to predict the relative risk for any one person to have a trait or transmit that trait to his or her children.

Pedigree

A pedigree is a graph of a family history for a specific trait or health problem over several generations. Fig. 4-8 shows common symbols used when creating a pedigree. Fig. 4-9 shows a typical three-generation pedigree. Although the term *pedigree* is the correct genetic term, it can offend some patients. Use the term *family tree* in place of pedigree when talking with patients. Construct a pedigree that includes at least three generations when taking the family history. When analyzing a pedigree, note the answers to these:

- Is any pattern of inheritance recognized, or does the trait appear sporadic?
- Is the trait expressed equally among male and female family members or unequally?
- Is the trait present in every generation, or does it skip one or more generations?
- Do only affected people have children who are affected with the trait, or do unaffected people also have children who express the trait?

The four types of inheritance patterns associated with single gene–controlled traits are autosomal dominant, autosomal recessive, sex-linked dominant, and sex-linked recessive. Each inheritance pattern has specific defining criteria. Table 4-2 lists the patterns of inheritance for some disorders that occur in adults or may be identified in children who live to adulthood.

Autosomal Dominant Pattern of Inheritance

Autosomal dominant (AD) single gene traits require that the gene alleles controlling the trait be located on an autosomal chromosome. A dominant gene allele is usually expressed even

Normal female

Normal male

Gender unknown

Single bar indicates mating

I   Normal parents and normal offspring, two girls and a boy, in birth order indicated by the numbers; I and II
II indicate generations
    1   2   3

Single parent as presented means partner is normal or of no significance to the analysis

Double bar indicates a consanguineous mating (mating between close relatives)

Fraternal twins (not identical)

Identical twins

FIG. 4-8 Standard pedigree symbols.

FIG. 4-9 A three-generation pedigree showing an autosomal dominant pattern of inheritance.

TABLE 4-2	Patterns of Inheritance for Genetic Disorders Among Adults	
PATTERN OF INHERITANCE	**DISORDER**
Autosomal dominant	Breast cancer* (mutation of *BRCA1* or *BRCA2* genes)
	Diabetes mellitus type 2*
	Familial adenomatous polyposis
	Familial melanoma
	Familial hypercholesterolemia
	Hereditary nonpolyposis colon cancer (HNPCC)
	Huntington disease
	Long QT syndrome and sudden cardiac death
	Malignant hyperthermia (MH)
	Marfan syndrome
	Myotonic dystrophy
	Neurofibromatosis (types 1 and 2)
	Ovarian cancer* (mutation of *BRCA1* genes)
	Polycystic kidney disease† (types 1 and 2)
	Retinitis pigmentosa†
	von Willebrand's disease
Autosomal recessive	Albinism
	Alpha$_1$-antitrypsin deficiency
	Beta thalassemia
	Bloom syndrome
	Cystic fibrosis
	Hereditary hemochromatosis
	Sickle cell disease
	Xeroderma pigmentosum
Sex-linked recessive	Glucose-6-phosphate dehydrogenase deficiency
	Hemophilia
	Red-green color blindness
Complex disorders/ Familial clustering	Alzheimer's disease
	Autoimmune disorders
	Bipolar disorder
	Parkinson disease
	Schizophrenia
	Hypertension
	Rheumatoid arthritis

*Some disorders have both a genetic and nongenetic form.
†Some disorders have more than one genetic form and can also be autosomal recessive.

when only one allele of the pair is dominant. Other criteria for AD inheritance include:

- The trait appears in every generation with no skipping.
- The risk for an affected person to pass the trait to a child is 50% with each pregnancy.
- Unaffected people do not have affected children; therefore their risk is essentially 0%.
- The trait is found about equally in males and females.

An example of an AD trait is blood type A. If a person is homozygous for the blood type A allele, he or she will express type A blood (with genotype being identical to the phenotype). If a person is heterozygous for the blood type A allele with the other allele being type O (which is a recessive trait), he or she will also express type A blood. In this case, however, the phenotype is not identical to the genotype. *When a dominant allele is paired with a recessive allele, only the dominant allele is expressed.* The blood type B allele is a dominant allele. When a B allele is paired with an O allele, B blood type is expressed. When a person has one blood type A allele and a blood type B allele, however, both alleles are expressed because they are equally dominant (co-dominant) and the person has type AB blood.

Some health problems inherited as autosomal dominant (AD) single gene traits are not apparent at birth but develop as the person ages (see Table 4-2). Two factors that affect the expression of some AD single gene traits are penetrance and expressivity.

Penetrance

Penetrance is how often or how well, within a population, a gene is expressed when it is present. Some genes are more penetrant than others. For example, the gene for Huntington disease (HD) has an autosomal dominant pattern of transmission. This gene is "highly penetrant" (sometimes called "fully penetrant"). This means that if a person has the HD gene allele, his or her risk for expressing the gene and developing the disease is about 99.99%. Therefore a person who has one HD allele is at high risk for developing HD.

Some dominant gene alleles have "reduced" penetrance. So a person who has the gene mutation has a lower risk for this gene being expressed and actually developing the disorder.

Penetrance has been calculated by examining a population of people known to have the gene mutation and assessing the percentage that go on to express the gene by developing the disorder. For example, the *BRCA2* gene mutation increases a person's risk for breast cancer. This gene is not fully penetrant, so some women (and men) who have the gene do not develop breast cancer. The penetrance rate for this gene mutation is calculated to be between 60% and 80%, meaning that a person who has the gene mutation has a 60% to 80% risk for developing breast cancer. Although this risk is far higher than among people who do not have the mutated gene, the risk is not 100%. Having the gene mutation does not absolutely predict that the person will develop breast cancer—just that the risk is high. However, the person with the mutation can pass on this genetic mutation to his or her children, who will then have an increased risk for breast cancer development.

Expressivity

Expressivity is the degree of expression a person has when a dominant gene is present. So it is a personal issue, not a population issue. The gene is *always* expressed, but some people have more severe problems than do other people. For example, the

FIG. 4-10 A typical pedigree showing an autosomal recessive pattern of inheritance.

gene mutation for one form of neurofibromatosis (*NF1*) is dominant. Some people with this gene mutation have only a few light brown skin tone areas known as *café au lait spots*. Other people with the same gene mutation develop hundreds of tumors (neurofibromas) that protrude through the skin. Expressivity accounts for some variation in genetic disease severity.

Autosomal Recessive Pattern of Inheritance

Autosomal recessive (AR) single gene traits require that the gene controlling the trait be located on an autosomal chromosome. Normally, the trait can be expressed *only* when both alleles are present. Table 4-2 lists some AR adult disorders. Fig. 4-10 shows a typical pedigree for an AR disorder. Criteria for AR patterns of inheritance include:

- The trait may not appear in all generations of any one branch of a family.
- The trait often first appears only in siblings rather than in parents and children.
- About 25% of a family will be affected and express the trait.
- The children of two affected parents will *always* be affected (risk is 100%).
- Unaffected people who are carriers (heterozygous for the trait) and do not express the trait themselves *can* transmit the trait to their children if their partner either is also a carrier or is affected.
- The trait is found about equally in male and female members of the same family.

An example of an AR trait is type O blood. The blood-type O allele is recessive, and both alleles must be type O (homozygous) for the person to express type O blood. If only one allele is a type O allele and the other allele is either type A or type B, the dominant allele will be expressed and the O allele, although present, is not expressed. For AR single gene traits, phenotype and genotype are always the same.

A person who has one mutated allele for a recessive genetic disorder is a **carrier**. A carrier, even though he or she may have one mutated allele, may not have any manifestations of the disorder but can pass this mutated allele on to his or her children. For some autosomal recessive disorders, a carrier may have mild manifestations. One example is sickle cell trait. A person with two sickle cell alleles has the disease and has many associated health problems. A carrier with one sickle cell allele (has "sickle cell trait") may be healthy most of the time and have manifestations only under conditions of severe hypoxia.

Sex-Linked Recessive Pattern of Inheritance

Some genes are present only on the sex chromosomes. The Y chromosome has only a few genes that are not also present on the X chromosome. These genes are important for male sexual

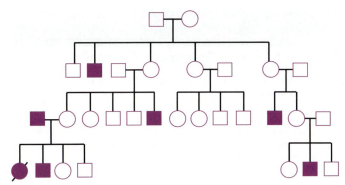

FIG. 4-11 A typical pedigree showing a sex-linked (X-linked) recessive pattern of inheritance.

TABLE 4-3 Purposes of Genetic Testing for Adults	
PURPOSE/TYPE	**DEFINITION**
Carrier testing	Determining whether a patient without symptoms has an allele for a recessive disorder that could be transmitted to his or her children. Disorders for which carrier testing is common include sickle cell disease, hemophilia, hereditary hemochromatosis, cystic fibrosis, beta thalassemia, and Tay-Sachs disease.
Diagnostic testing	Determining whether a patient has or does not have a mutation that increases the risk for a specific disorder.
Symptomatic	Patient has clinical manifestations; test results confirm a diagnosis.
Presymptomatic	Patient has no clinical manifestations but is at high risk for inheriting a specific genetic disorder for which there is no known prevention or treatment. A disorder for which presymptomatic testing is commonly performed is Huntington disease.
Predisposition	Family history or genetic testing indicates risk is high for a known genetic disorder. The patient does not have any manifestations but wants to know whether he or she has the specific mutation and what the chances are that it will be expressed. Disorders for which predisposition testing is often performed include hereditary breast/ovarian cancer and hereditary colorectal cancers. The advantage of predisposition testing is that the patient can then engage in heightened screening activities or medical and surgical interventions that reduce risk.

development. The X chromosome has many single genes that are not present on the Y or elsewhere in the genome. Some of these genes are specific for female sexual development, but there are also several hundred genes on the X chromosome that code for other functions. Few disorders have X-linked dominant expression and are not discussed in this chapter.

Because the number of X chromosomes in males and females is not the same (1:2), the number of X-linked chromosome genes in the two genders is also unequal. Males have only one X chromosome. As a result, X-linked recessive genes have dominant expression in males and recessive expression in females. This difference in expression is because males do not have a second X chromosome to balance the presence of a recessive gene on the first X chromosome.

Sex-linked (X-linked) recessive single gene traits require that the gene allele be present on both of the X chromosomes for the trait to be expressed in females (homozygous) and on only one X chromosome for the trait to be expressed in males. Fig. 4-11 shows a typical pedigree for a sex-linked recessive disorder. Features of a sex-linked recessive pattern of inheritance are:

- The incidence of the trait is much higher among males in a family than among females.
- The trait cannot be passed down (transmitted) from father to son.
- Transmission of the trait is from father to all daughters (who will be carriers).
- Female carriers have a 50% risk (with each pregnancy) of passing the gene to their children.

Complex Inheritance and Familial Clustering

Some health problems appear in families at a rate higher than normal and greater than can be accounted for by chance alone; however, no specific pattern occurs within a family. Although clusters suggest a genetic influence, it is likely that additional factors, such as gender and the environment, also influence disease development or disease severity. Such disorders include Alzheimer's disease, type 1 diabetes, and many others. These disorders are often called *complex* and *multifactorial*, because although an increased genetic risk may be present, the risk is changed by diet, lifestyle, exposure to toxins, infectious agents, and other factors.

GENETIC TESTING

Purpose of Genetic Testing

Many people are eager to have genetic testing but also are fearful of genetic testing. The lay public often believe that a single genetic test can "tell everything about a person." Although genetic testing has the potential to be that informative, this is not currently the case. *It is important to remember that no single person is genetically perfect.*

Genetic testing can be performed with many different techniques. Some genetic tests are specific for a disorder. Others may show a gene variation but the significance of the variation may not be known. Unexpected information can be found during genetic testing. Some ordinary tests, such as blood typing and tissue typing, provide genetic information. Tests that measure the amount of an enzyme or protein also provide genetic information.

Testing for the purpose of assessing genetic information can be performed at many levels. Cellular or biochemical tests provide information about gene products made by a cell, tissue, or organ. Chromosomes and chromosome segments can be assessed for missing, extra, broken, or rearranged chromosomes. The sequence of a gene can be examined to determine variation or mutation. At present, not all genes can be analyzed and the analysis of even one gene is limited by expense and availability. Specific base pairs can be evaluated for mutations (Conley et al., 2013). Many tests are expensive, and the results may not be conclusive. Table 4-3 lists purposes of genetic testing for adults.

Benefits and Risks of Genetic Testing

Genetic testing is different from any other type of testing. Informed consent is required before genetic testing is performed. The person tested is the one who gives consent, even though genetic testing *always* gives information about family members—not just the patient (Badzek et al., 2013).

Benefits of genetic testing include the ability to confirm a diagnosis or to test people who are at risk for a health problem but do not as yet have any manifestations (presymptomatic testing). The information can help a person, family, and their health care provider develop a specific plan of care or early detection. For example, in the case of a strong genetic predisposition for colon cancer, identifying a patient before symptoms appear allows interventions to prevent the disease or to diagnosis it earlier, when cure is more likely.

Risks are associated with genetic testing that are not associated with other types of tests. Genetic testing results do not change. Thus a positive test result cannot be "taken back." Other risks may include psychological or social risks, as well as a risk for family disruption. Often genetic tests are expensive and may not be covered by insurance. Some genetic tests have limited value for predicting future risk. Testing may identify a patient at great risk for the future development of a serious health problem that cannot be prevented or managed. Such a disorder is Huntington disease (HD), which currently has no treatment. Knowing positive test results in this case can lead to depression, blame, and guilt.

Another risk of genetic testing is that positive results may be used to discriminate against a person or a family. Some protection is in place to prevent health insurance companies from failing to insure a person or dropping the coverage of a person who is at high risk for developing a serious illness (e.g., breast or ovarian cancer). However, there are no protections against rate hikes or exclusions of specific treatments. Patients often fear workplace discrimination and personal discrimination if positive test results become known.

Genetic Counseling

Genetic testing is not a standard test that any person should have performed without knowing the benefits and risks. Counseling patients before, during, and after testing is critical and is required by the professional ETHICS governing genetic medicine. Entire families may be a part of the genetic evaluation and follow-up. For example, a 45-year-old woman has breast cancer. In her family, her mother, grandmother, brother, and one sister have all had breast cancer. Genetic testing indicates that she has a *BRCA1* gene mutation. This woman's older daughter wonders whether she has a gene mutation for breast cancer and asks to be tested. When she and her younger sister are tested, the older daughter does not have the mutation but the younger sister does.

Genetic counseling is a process—not a single session or a single recommendation. This process should begin when the patient or family is first identified as potentially having a genetic problem. The process continues through actual testing if the decision to test is made, and it continues through interpretation of results and follow-up. Chart 4-1 lists the steps in the process.

As a nurse and patient advocate, it is your professional duty to determine whether the patient understands the consequences of testing. Often a patient may request genetic testing even when there is no indication of an increased risk for a genetic disorder. Counseling and evaluation can help patients understand whether any useful information could be obtained from testing.

CHART 4-1 Best Practice for Patient Safety & Quality Care QSEN

Steps for Genetic Testing and Counseling

Pretesting Assessment and Patient Education (May Take Multiple Sessions)
- Determining patient understanding and why testing or counseling is being sought
- Determining whether testing is reasonable (considering cost of the test, specificity, probable risk, accuracy of testing)
- Establishing a trusting professional relationship
- Ensuring privacy and confidentiality
- Reviewing informed consent procedures
- Assessing the patient's ability to communicate accurately (including language issues, cognitive function, sensory perception)
- Assessing the patient's psychosocial status and availability of social support
- Taking a detailed patient health history (including drugs, diet, exercise, hormonal history, lifestyle issues)
- Obtaining physical assessment data relevant to the at-risk disorder
- Taking a detailed family history and constructing a three-generation pedigree (minimum)
- Obtaining and verifying information obtained from:
  - Patient
  - Family members
  - Medical records
  - Pathology reports
  - Death certificates
- Interpreting the family history
- Discussing the consequences of testing
- Discussing patient rights and obligations regarding disclosure of information
- Discussing testing options
- Assessing to determine whether coercion is occurring
- Obtaining material to be tested (usually blood)

Test Result Presentation
- Re-assessing the patient's wish to know or not know the test results
- Respecting the patient's decision to not know the test results
- Ensuring privacy and confidentiality
- Presenting the test results
- Interpreting the test results
- Assessing the patient's perception of the test results

Follow-Up
- Supporting the patient's decision to disclose or not disclose the information to other family members
- Discussing the potential risks for other family members
- Ensuring privacy and confidentiality
- Addressing the patient's concerns
- Discussing prevention, early detection, and treatment options
- Discussing family concerns
- Addressing psychosocial issues
- Discussing available resources for information, support, and further counseling
- Providing summary of results and consultation to the patient

Adapted from Beery, T., & Workman, M.L. (2012). *Genetics and genomics in nursing and health care.* Philadelphia: F.A. Davis.

Counseling should be a COLLABORATION performed by a professional or a team who have defined expertise in interpretation of genetic testing results. Such professionals include advanced practice nurses with specialization in genetics, certified genetic counselors, clinical geneticists, and medical geneticists. Each profession has a different level of preparation in genetics and different skills or roles in the counseling process. For example, an advanced practice nurse may counsel a patient about the Huntington disease gene mutation because this test is not ambiguous and the gene is highly penetrant. When a genetic test shows a variation or mutation in an unusual gene region or when penetrance is reduced, the patient may best be served by counseling from a certified genetic counselor or a clinical or medical geneticist.

No matter which professional is involved in genetic counseling, a key feature of this counseling is to be "nondirective." When using a nondirective approach, the counselor provides as much information as possible about the risks and benefits but does not influence the patient's decision to test or not to test. Once the patient has made the decision, the counselor supports the patient and the decision.

Ethical Issues

ETHICS and ethical issues are involved at every level of genetic testing. Some of the most important issues focus on the patient's right to know versus the right not to know his or her gene status, confidentiality, coercion, and sharing of information.

The right to know genetic risk versus the right to not know is the individual patient's choice. Sometimes a patient's right to know has an impact on the right of another family member to not know.

Confidentiality is crucial to the genetic counseling process. *The results of a genetic test must remain confidential to the patient. The results cannot be given to a family member, other health care provider, or insurance carrier without the patient's permission.*

Coercion is possible by other family members and by health care professionals. *The final decision to have genetic testing or to not have testing rests with the patient.* Other people may believe it is important for the patient to have the test; however, the patient must make the decision without such pressures. As a patient advocate, professional ETHICS require you to assess whether the patient is freely making the decision to have genetic testing or whether someone else is urging the patient to test. This important issue can be difficult to assess. Ask the patient who else in his or her family wants to know the results of testing.

Sharing of test result information, negative or positive, can be stressful. The patient makes the final decision whether to share the information with family members. Some patients choose not to share this information even when other family members may also be at risk. This can be difficult for the health care provider who knows the patient has a positive test result for a serious inherited condition and the patient chooses not to tell other family members who may be at risk (Berkman & Hull, 2014). For example, hereditary nonpolyposis colon cancer (HNPCC) has an autosomal dominant inheritance pattern and each child of the patient has a 50% risk for having the gene. If the patient chooses not to tell his or her grown children, they then do not have the opportunity for increased screening to find the cancer at an early stage when cure is possible. An ethical dilemma arises when the health care provider wants to inform the children of their risk.

THE ROLE OF THE MEDICAL-SURGICAL NURSE IN GENETIC COUNSELING

Medical-surgical nurses help patients during the assessing, testing, and counseling processes, although they do not provide in-depth genetic counseling. Patients often feel most comfortable sharing information with nurses and asking nurses to clarify information.

CLINICAL JUDGMENT CHALLENGE
Ethical/Legal

A 22-year-old man has a maternal grandfather with Huntington disease (HD). His father, mother, and paternal grandfather are all healthy and free of HD manifestations. He wants to know whether he also has the HD gene and arranges to be tested. His mother does not want to know whether she has the gene mutation. The man is tested and is found to be positive for the gene mutation that causes HD.
1. Why could a positive test affect this man's mother?
2. Does the mother's right to not know her HD status override the son's right to know his status? Explain your reasoning.
3. Review the ethical principles in Chapter 1. Which principle(s) would be violated if the son informs his mother of his positive test results?

Nurses may be the first health care professionals to identify a patient at specific genetic risk. Some of the "red flags" that a patient may have a genetic risk for a disease or disorder are:
- The disease or disorder occurs at a higher incidence within the family compared with the general population.
- The patient or close family members have another identified genetic problem.
- The incidence of a specific disease or disorder occurs in the patient or in family members at an unusually early age.
- A rare disease is present in two or more family members.
- More than one type of cancer is present in any one person.
- The specific manifestation is associated with one or more genetic disorders (e.g., unusual freckling or skin pigmentation, bicuspid aortic valve, deafness).

The nurse may be the health care professional who first verifies information to bring a genetic problem to light. For example, during an assessment, a patient reveals that her mother died of bone cancer when she was 40 years old. Bone cancer is quite rare among adults; thus the nurse might then ask, "Did your mother ever have any other type of cancer?" Often the patient may then reveal that her mother had breast cancer some years before ("bone cancer" was actually breast cancer that had spread to the bones). Breast cancer at an early age can indicate a genetic predisposition.

Patients may ask questions that indicate they have an interest in genetic testing. These are examples of questions that may be cues that the patient has genetic concerns:
- Will my children get this disease?
- Because my sister has this problem, what are the chances I might also develop it?
- Is there a way to test and see whether my chances of getting this disease or problem are high or low?

Areas of responsibility for any medical-surgical nurse in working with a patient who is considering or having genetic testing include communication, privacy and confidentiality, information accuracy, patient advocacy, and support.

Communication

In congruence with professional ETHICS, act as a patient advocate by ensuring that communication between the patient and whoever is providing the genetic information is clear. First, assess the patient's ability to receive and process information. Can the patient see and hear clearly, or are assistive devices needed? Does the patient understand English, or will an interpreter be needed? Does the patient have adequate cognition at the time of meeting with the genetics professional, or is it impaired by medication, disease, anxiety, or fear?

If the patient appears not to understand terms or jargon during a discussion between him or her and a genetics professional, ask the professional to use common terms and examples for the patient. Verify with the patient that he or she understands or does not understand.

After any discussion about genetic risk or genetic testing, assess the patient's understanding of what was said. Ask the patient to explain, in his or her own words, what the issue means and what his or her expectations are.

Privacy and Confidentiality

Professional ETHICS require that all conversations regarding potential diagnoses or genetic testing need to occur in a private environment. The patient has the right to determine who may be a part of the discussion and can decide to exclude the primary physician and any family member from the discussion with a genetics professional. It is important that health care professionals who may be present during such discussion do not disclose information, formally or informally, without the patient's permission. It is the nurse's ethical duty and responsibility to protect this information from improper disclosure to family members, other health care professionals, other patients, insurance providers, or anyone not specified by the patient.

Information Accuracy

Correct myths about genetic disorders, and teach patients about the nature of genetic testing. In addition, help patients find accurate and helpful resource materials or websites. Medical-surgical nurses are not genetics experts and would not be expected to be the final source of definitive information; however, with COLLABORATION they can help ensure that the patient is referred to the correct level of genetic counseling. If you are present during the patient's discussions with a genetics professional, assess whether the patient understands the issues regarding the health problem.

Patient Advocacy and Support

Ensure that the patient's rights are not neglected or ignored. Ask the patient privately what his or her wishes are regarding genetic testing. Ask whether another person or agency is insisting on the testing. Remind the patient that he or she does not have to agree to be tested. Verify that he or she has signed an informed consent statement for the test.

Considering or having genetic testing is a stressful experience. The patient and family require support and may need help with coping. Ethically, genetic testing should be performed only after genetic counseling has occurred and should be followed with more counseling.

Patients may feel anger, depression, guilt, or hopelessness. Patients who have positive results (results that indicate a specific mutation is present) from genetic testing may have issues of risk for early death or disability and the possibility of having passed the risk for a health problem on to their children. Patients who have an ambiguous test result or one of unknown significance may feel that they have agonized over a decision, spent money, and still have no clear answer. Even patients who have negative genetic test results (results that indicate a specific mutation is not present) need counseling and support. Some patients may have an unrealistic view of what a negative result means for their general health. Others may feel guilty that they were "spared" when other family members were not.

Assess the patient's response to genetic test results. Determine what coping methods were used successfully in the past. If the patient has disclosed information to family members, assess whether they can help provide support or need support themselves. Assess whether the information about positive test results has strained family relationships. Refer the patient to appropriate support groups and general counseling services.

For some positive genetic test results, such as having a *BRCA1* gene mutation, the risk for developing breast cancer is high but is not a certainty. With high risk, the patient needs a plan for prevention and risk reduction. One form of prevention is early detection. Thus a patient who tests positive for a *BRCA1* mutation should have at least yearly mammograms and ovarian ultrasounds to detect cancer at an early stage when it is more easily cured. Teach the patient who has positive test results that indicate an increased risk for a specific health problem about the types of screening procedures that are available and how often screening should occur. For example, some patients at known high genetic risk for breast cancer and ovarian cancer choose the primary prevention methods of bilateral prophylactic mastectomies (surgical removal of the breasts) and oophorectomies (surgical removal of the ovaries). Although these strategies are severe, they are effective and the patient should be informed about their availability.

Teach patients at known high risk for a specific disorder how to modify the environment to reduce risk. For example, a patient who has a specific mutation in the *a1AT* (alpha$_1$-antitrypsin) gene is at increased risk for early-onset emphysema. The onset of emphysema is even earlier when the patient smokes or is chronically exposed to inhalation irritants. By modifying his or her environment, the disease can be delayed or the manifestations reduced.

? NCLEX EXAMINATION CHALLENGE

Psychosocial Integrity

The client who has been found to have a mutation in a gene allele that greatly increases her risk for chronic obstructive lung disease asks the staff nurse to be present when she discloses the test results to her family. What is the nurse's role in this situation?
A. Primary health care provider
B. Genetic counselor
C. Patient advocate
D. Patient support

GET READY FOR THE NCLEX® EXAMINATION!

KEY POINTS

Review these Key Points for each NCLEX Examination Client Needs Category.

Safe and Effective Care Environment

- Ensure that a person or family with indications of an increased genetic risk for a disease or disorder is referred to an appropriate genetics professional. **Teamwork and Collaboration** QSEN
- Advocate for the patient with regard to whether or not to have genetic testing, informed consent before testing, and sharing of test results. **Patient-Centered Care** QSEN
- Ensure that confidentiality of genetic test results is maintained by all health care team members. **Safety** QSEN
- Determine whether an informed consent statement was obtained before any genetic test is performed.
- Keep all patient and family information regarding genetic testing confidential.

Health Promotion and Maintenance

- Identify patients and families at increased genetic risk for disease or disorder.
- Teach patients and families at known increased genetic risk for disease or disorder what types of screening procedures and schedules are most appropriate (check specific disorder chapters for the appropriate screening guidelines). **Evidence-Based Practice** QSEN
- Teach patients and families at known increased genetic risk for disease or disorder what types of environmental modifications can reduce risk, delay disease onset, or reduce symptom severity (check specific disorder chapters for appropriate modifications). **Evidence-Based Practice** QSEN

Psychosocial Integrity

- Assess patients who have received results of genetic testing for responses such as anger, guilt, or depression.

- Allow the patient and family who have been identified as being at increased genetic risk for serious health problems to express concerns and feelings.
- Ensure that the patient who undergoes genetic testing is appropriately counseled before testing, while waiting for test results, and after test results are obtained. **Teamwork and Collaboration** QSEN
- Support the decision of the patient and family to have or not to have genetic counseling or testing.

Physiological Integrity

- Be aware that mutations or variations in gene sequences can change the activity of a protein and have adverse effects on health.
- Keep in mind that many common adult diseases or disorders have a genetic basis (hypertension, diabetes, cancer) although some of these diseases also may occur among people with no genetic risk.
- Remind the patient that having a gene variation that increases the risk for a disorder does not necessarily mean that the disorder will ever develop.
- Ensure that patients understand that genetic testing reveals information about their family members, as well as about themselves.
- Construct a three-generation pedigree from data obtained during the family history section of patient assessment.
- Remind patients that the results of genetic testing cannot be "taken back."
- Be prepared to assume the accepted roles of the medical-surgical nurse in genetic counseling, which include examining assessment data for indications of genetic risk, acting as a patient advocate, correcting myths about genetic disorders and genetic testing, protecting the patient's privacy and rights, and helping to ensure that the patient and/or family at increased genetic risk are referred to a genetics professional.

Evidence-Based Practice in Medical-Surgical Nursing

Rona F. Levin and Fay Wright

http://evolve.elsevier.com/Iggy/

PRIORITY CONCEPTS

- EVIDENCE-BASED PRACTICE
- TEAMWORK AND COLLABORATION
- SAFETY
- QUALITY IMPROVEMENT

LEARNING OUTCOMES

Safe and Effective Care Environment

1. Describe EVIDENCE-BASED PRACTICE (EBP) to include the components of research evidence, clinical expertise, and patient/family values.
2. Explain the role of evidence in making clinical decisions and determining best clinical practice.
3. Explain how to use an EBP approach to identifying a clinical problem, issue, or challenge.
4. Differentiate clinical opinion from research and evidence summaries.
5. Formulate a focused clinical question about clinical practice.
6. List the steps of how to perform a systematic literature review to answer clinical questions.
7. Briefly describe two models of EBP for changing processes of care.
8. Explain the steps of the evidence-based practice improvement (EBPI) model.
9. Discuss how the EBPI model can be used to guide a clinical practice improvement project.

OVERVIEW

All health care professionals need to understand and use an evidence-based practice (EBP) approach to practice. In 2003, the Institute of Medicine (IOM) published a report entitled *Health Professions Education: A Bridge to Quality*. That report contained this mandate: "All health professionals should be educated to deliver patient-centered care as members of an interdisciplinary team, emphasizing EVIDENCE-BASED PRAC-TICE, QUALITY IMPROVEMENT approaches and informatics" (IOM, 2003, p. 3). Since that report was published, EBP to improve the quality of patient care has been a consistent theme in the IOM's publications, with more than 24 reports found on their website to guide implementation of EBP (http://www.iom.edu/Reports.aspx).

In 2010, the IOM in partnership with the Robert Wood Johnson Foundation published *The Future of Nursing: Leading Change, Advancing Health* (IOM, 2010). Key among the four major recommendations is: "Nurses should be full partners, with physicians and other health care professionals, in redesigning health care in the United States" (p. 3). The specifics of this recommendation include the need for nurses to be prepared to be COLLABORATORS in health care improvement efforts and sometimes lead those projects. Aspects of this role include "taking responsibility for identifying problems and areas of system waste, devising and developing improvement plans,

[and] tracking improvement over time ..." (p. 3). Thus all nurses need to be equipped with the knowledge and skill that are required to be a full partner in making positive change in health care. This chapter provides the foundation to begin that preparation.

Definitions of Evidence-Based Practice

According to several nursing experts and the Quality and Safety Education for Nurses (QSEN) movement, EBP incorporates the best current evidence with the expertise of the clinician and the patient's values and preferences to make a decision about health care (Cronenwett et al., 2007; Levin et al., 2013; Melnyk & Fineout-Overholt, 2011). This definition was based on the work of Sackett et al. (2000), who had proposed three components of EBP—best evidence, clinical expertise, and patient values and preferences—as part of the definition of evidence-based medicine.

Ervin (2002) proposed this definition of EBP for nursing: "Evidence-based nursing practice is practice in which nurses make clinical decisions using the best available research and other evidence that is reflected in approved policies, procedures, and clinical guidelines in a particular healthcare agency" (Ervin, 2002, p. 12). DiCenso et al. (2005) further extended this definition to include information about the patient's clinical state and the setting or circumstances in which health care is being provided.

The EBP process is COLLABORATIVE and involves all members of the health care team, including the patient and family. This model is shared by many health care professions and is not unique to nursing. Therefore, although other professions might refer to the model as evidence-based medicine (EBM) or evidence-based social work similar to how DiCenso et al. (2005) specified the practice of nursing, the authors of this text refer to the model as EBP.

Steps of the Evidence-Based Practice Process

The process of EBP is systematic and includes several steps as presented by Sackett et al. (2000) in the context of practicing and teaching medicine.

1. Asking "burning" clinical questions
2. Finding the very best evidence to try to answer those questions
3. Critically appraising and synthesizing the relevant evidence
4. Making recommendations for practice improvement
5. Implementing accepted recommendations
6. Evaluating outcomes

Important to note is that the original approach to EBP developed in the medical community was intended to be used by physicians to solve individual patient problems for which physicians did not have ready answers. The adoption of EBP by nursing and other health care disciplines, however, required a different perspective that incorporated organizational data, goals, and priorities. Most nurses work within a health care agency, not in an independent practice setting. Nurses must COLLABORATE with those in other disciplines who are involved in practice changes within a health care agency. An example of how EBP works within a hospital system is provided later in this chapter.

Asking "Burning" Clinical Questions

Clinical questions are derived when clinicians do not have all the information they need to make the best possible decisions about patient care. A "burning" clinical question is one that usually arises in daily practice or when attending a class or reading a professional journal on a specific topic. The question may arise in relation to an individual patient, a group or population of patients, or a patient care unit or larger organizational area. An example of an *individual* patient question that a nurse might ask is: "My older hospitalized patient who has been placed on fall precautions fell in the bathroom. What else could I have done to prevent this patient from falling, and what can I do to prevent her from falling in the future?" At a *group or population* level, the nurse might ask: "What are current best practices for assessing hospital patients' risk for falls, and/or what are best practices for fall prevention in patients who are at risk for falls? At a *unit or organizational* level, the question might be: "Is the current policy and procedure for assessing patients' risk for falls and for implementing preventive practices based on the best available evidence?"

Once you critically think about and pose a question about clinical practice, you will need to find out at what level the question needs to be answered (i.e., at the individual patient level, patient population level, or organizational level). If the latter two levels are where the problem exists, then begin to gather background information from the literature and internal evidence from your organization to describe the problem more fully (Levin et al., 2010).

One way you can begin to use EBP in your practice is to review the policy and procedure for a specific nursing practice in your clinical setting and determine what type of evidence was used as the basis for that policy and procedure. Does the protocol list references? What types of references are cited?

Once you have described the clinical practice problem and can focus on exactly what concerns you have, ask yourself whether the question is a *background* or a *foreground* question. A *background* question usually asks for a fact, a statement on which most authorities or experts would agree. For example: What is the etiology of congestive heart failure? What are the most frequently prescribed analgesics for the management of postoperative pain? The answers to these types of questions can usually be found in a textbook and are not controversial. A *foreground* question, on the other hand, usually asks a question of relationship and may be controversial. An example of this type of question is: What are the most effective interventions for treating venous leg ulcers?

Qualitative Versus Quantitative Questions. If you are asking a foreground question, develop a more specific, detailed clinical question to guide your search for evidence. Clinical questions may be qualitative or quantitative. A **qualitative question** focuses on the meanings and interpretations of human phenomena or experiences of people and usually analyzes the content of what a person says during an interview or what a researcher observes. Examples of qualitative questions are:

- What is the experience of having cancer like for young adults?
- How do older women respond to a residential move to assisted-living facilities?
- What are the differences in nurses' work culture between acute care and home care agencies?

A **quantitative question** asks about the relationship between or among defined, measurable phenomena and includes a more objective approach to both data collection and data analysis. Answers to quantitative questions necessitate statistical analysis of information that is collected to answer a question. Examples of quantitative questions are:

- What is the effect of using a new assessment tool to predict the likelihood of falling to frequency and severity of falls in patients undergoing hip replacement?
- What is the effect of hydrocolloid dressings compared with silver-impregnated dressings on the rate of wound healing in patients with postsurgical incision wounds?

PICO(T) Format. Nursing authors suggest framing clinical questions in a PICO (Fleming, 2008; Levin, 2013) or PICO(T) format (Fineout-Overholt & Stillwell, 2011). The PICO(T) format is outlined in Table 5-1. The major components of a focused clinical question are the **p**opulation, **i**ntervention, **c**omparison, and **o**utcome, with an added **t**ime component when appropriate.

The *population* indicates the specific group of patients to whom the question applies. This component is important because evidence that may support an intervention with one group of patients may not apply to another group of patients. For example, a fall prevention program for older adults who live at home may be very different from a fall prevention program for patients who attend a rehabilitation program. Be sure to think about the age, gender, ethnicity/race, and specific health problems to narrow your population of interest.

The *intervention* component may pertain to (1) a new therapy that has been supported by best evidence, (2) exposure to disease

TABLE 5-1	Examples of Components of PICO(T) Questions in Relation to Type of Question					
	THERAPY	ETIOLOGY	DIAGNOSIS	PREVENTION	PROGNOSIS	MEANING
Population						
Intervention						
Comparison						
Outcome						
Time						

or harm, (3) a prognostic factor, or (4) a risk behavior or factor—for example, the need for toileting to help prevent falls (Melnyk & Fineout-Overholt, 2011). In terms of a new therapy, one might compare the use of guided imagery to decrease nausea and vomiting among patients receiving chemotherapy with similar patients who receive the current drug therapy for nausea and vomiting, and then evaluate patient outcomes.

The *comparison* component of the clinical question may be either the standard or current treatment as in the above example or may be another intervention with which the innovative practice is compared. In the case of prognostic questions, the comparison may consider another factor or potential influence that could affect the outcome of the patient's health. A preventive question might examine the absence of the risk factor as the comparison—for example, the need for toileting compared with no need for toileting to prevent falls.

The *outcome* component specifies the measurable and desired outcomes of your practice innovation, which may be focused on improving how you assess patients to make a nursing diagnosis or on a prevention or therapeutic intervention. Outcomes must include measures of the results of introducing an innovation to determine whether it was successful. For example, for an intervention outcome, measures might include patients' perception of pain, number of days spent in a hospital, or need for rehabilitative services. Or when testing a way to improve diagnostic accuracy, your outcome might focus on the sensitivity and specificity of a diagnostic test or nursing assessment tool (e.g., What is the best tool for assessing the risk for patient falls on an orthopedic unit?).

Fineout-Overholt and Stillwell (2011) advocated adding a *time* component or time frame to the focused clinical question. The question may include specifying within what time period one would expect the outcome(s) to occur. An example of a completed PICO(T) question is: What is the effect of adding hourly rounding to the standard falls protocol for the geriatric unit (patients 65 years or older) in hospital Y on the process of care provision (to be more specifically defined) and the outcomes of rate of falls, fall morbidity, and clinician satisfaction within a 3-month period?

Arriving at the focused clinical question is not an easy task, even for seasoned clinicians. Clearly identifying each component of the PICO(T) question focuses the clinical question for the next step in the EBP process: finding the best evidence to improve the practice problem.

Finding the Best Evidence

Finding the best available evidence to answer a focused clinical question has been a challenge for clinicians and health care agencies. The major barrier that prevents nurses from engaging in evidence-based practice is lack of time (Pravikoff et al., 2005). Other barriers include:

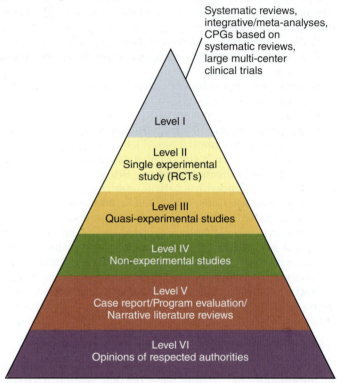

FIG. 5-1 Pyramid of evidence for questions of therapy. *CPGs,* Clinical practice guidelines; *RCTs,* randomized controlled trials.

- Lack of value for research in practice
- Lack of understanding of organization or structure of electronic databases
- Difficulty accessing research materials
- Lack of computer skills
- Difficulty understanding research articles

The health care system is addressing these challenges in many settings to improve the safety and quality of patient care. Many hospitals and community health care agencies are involved in promoting evidence-based practices and projects to reach national safety goals. An example of how staff nurses are essential contributors and collaborators on such projects is presented at the end of this chapter in the Application of the EBPI Model to Clinical Practice section.

Level of evidence (LOE) refers to the status or rank of evidence. Most evidence hierarchies are pyramids with the highest level of evidence at the top (Fig. 5-1). The type of evidence needed depends on the nature of the clinical question—is the question quantitative or qualitative? For example, if you are asking about the effectiveness of different types of compression bandages on healing of venous leg ulcers, you would want to *measure* the change in size of the ulcer as one indication of healing *(quantitative)*. On the other hand, you might be interested in what the experience of having a chronic venous ulcer is like for women *(qualitative)*. Each type of question requires different types and sources of evidence to find an answer. Table 5-2 provides an internationally accepted hierarchy for qualitative levels of evidence. The Evidence-Based Practice boxes in this text identify each study's LOE.

A preliminary evidence search entails identifying whether quality clinical practice guidelines (CPGs) exist to answer the clinical question. A **clinical practice guideline** is an "official recommendation" based on evidence to diagnose and/or manage a health problem (e.g., pain management). If these guidelines are of high quality and they contain the answer to your question, the search may be complete (Levin & Jacobs, 2012). The importance of CPGs is reinforced with the IOM's consensus report on the use and effectiveness of quality clinical practice guidelines for the implementation of EBP (IOM, 2011).

If the guidelines do not provide a sufficient answer to your question and/or they are not based on high-quality evidence, you need to search the "Fantastic Four" databases:

- Cochrane Library of Systematic Reviews
- Joanna Briggs Institute (JBI) systematic reviews
- Medline (or PubMed)
- Cumulative Index to Nursing and Allied Health Literature (CINAHL)

Other databases may also contain a wealth of information depending on the nature of the question. For example, if you are asking a psychological question about the best way to help patients deal with anxiety, then PsycINFO would be a good source. The instructional or health sciences librarian at the local college/university or clinical agency can assist in finding the best current evidence to answer your question. In some cases, you may need to revise the search if the original terms used did not access relevant citations. Table 5-3 provides a template that you can use for any evidence search that you undertake.

If a continued literature search is needed for *quantitative* clinical questions, start with looking for the top level of evidence (i.e., systematic reviews, which are meta-analyses, clinical practice guidelines based on top level evidence, and/or multi-site randomized clinical trials) (see Fig. 5-1). If searching for answers to *qualitative* questions, look first for meta-syntheses. The major purpose of providing systematic reviews of evidence on a topic for both qualitative and quantitative questions is so that busy clinicians will not have to spend many hours finding original single studies and then reviewing, critiquing, and synthesizing each study's evidence. In some cases, evidence summaries are available (Table 5-4). Fig. 5-2 provides a guide for conducting a systematic evidence search.

Critically Appraising and Synthesizing Evidence

The key to this step is a collaborative team effort. One effective strategy is to have each member of an EBP team take responsibility for summarizing and critically appraising a select number of articles (depending, of course, on the number of relevant articles your search revealed) and then presenting a written summary and review to all team members. This allows collegial critique of the evidence, helps clarify areas of uncertainty, and facilitates team consensus on what the best evidence is to answer the clinical question. In addition, summarizing and critically appraising each piece of relevant evidence and entering the results of this activity into a table of evidence makes it easier to synthesize all the relevant evidence succinctly. This evidence synthesis will tell you if there is sufficient evidence to guide practice related to your clinical question.

Making Recommendations to Improve Practice

Once you have reviewed, critically appraised, and synthesized all the relevant evidence, you are ready to make practice recommendations in a written report to whoever needs to review them for potential approval. The clinical application at the end of the chapter illustrates this process.

Implementing Recommendations

This step is perhaps the most exciting and energizing component of an EBP project. After all the hard work of focusing the practice problem, developing a PICO question, retrieving and critically appraising the evidence, and getting practice recommendations approved, the protocol and implementation plan can be developed. This plan should improve practice, patient outcomes, and the desired outcomes of the system (e.g., cost savings). Approaches to implementation are varied. Examples of models to guide EBP projects from the beginning to the end are presented in the next section of this chapter.

TABLE 5-2 JBI Levels of Qualitative Evidence for Meaningfulness*

LEVEL OF EVIDENCE	MEANINGFULNESS M (1-4)
1	Meta-synthesis of research with unequivocal synthesized findings
2	Meta-synthesis of research with credible synthesized findings
3	a. Meta-synthesis of text/opinion with credible synthesized findings b. One or more single research studies of high quality
4	Expert opinion

*From Joanna Briggs Institute. (2008). *Reviewer's manual*. Adelaide, Australia: Author. *JBI*, Joanna Briggs Institute.

TABLE 5-3 Example of a Search Strategy Table with Hypothetical Data

DATABASE	KEY WORDS	DATE RANGE	PEER REVIEWED	# OF CITATIONS	# RETRIEVED	# USED
Medline (PubMed)	Pain Postoperative Behavioral Assessment Scale	2002-2010	All	5	3	0
CINAHL	Pain Postoperative Behavioral Pain Scales	2000-2010	All	25	5	2

CINAHL, Cumulative Index to Nursing and Allied Health Literature.

Keep in mind that the process of implementation needs to be systematic, shared, and consistent. That is, the implementation protocol has to be followed strictly so that any outcomes that are achieved are actually based on the new EBP innovation being implemented. Therefore complete buy-in from the people who will be involved in implementing the new practice is essential.

Evaluating Outcomes

Evaluating outcomes requires valid and reliable measurement tools. For example, if the clinical question is evaluating the effect of music therapy on reducing postoperative abdominal pain, then a tool to measure pain intensity and quality would be used. Many of these tools are cited in the literature and can be used without permission. Others require that permission be

obtained in writing. Be sure to determine whether permission is needed before you use any measurement tool.

MODELS AND FRAMEWORKS FOR IMPLEMENTING EVIDENCE-BASED PRACTICE

Several authors have attempted to develop models or conceptual frameworks to facilitate an understanding of the complex process of introducing evidence-based improvement efforts (Rycroft-Malone & Bucknall, 2010). Each model highlights factors or processes that need to be considered when attempting to implement practice change.

Iowa Model

The major purpose of the Iowa model of EBP is to help health care professionals use evidence to improve patient outcomes. Originally developed as a model for research utilization, Titler revised and enhanced the model in 2010 to incorporate the elements of EBP. Important aspects of the current model include the (Titler, 2010):

- Triggers that lead to clinical questions
- Assessment of whether these questions are priorities for the health care organization
- Focus on forming a team to develop an EBP initiative
- General overview or steps for deciding about whether to implement and then adopt a change in practice

TABLE 5-4	Sources for Pre-Appraised Evidence Guidelines/Summaries
PUBLISHER	**WEBSITE**
BMJ Clinical Evidence	www.clinicalevidence.com
DynaMed	www.ebscohost.com/dynamed
USPSTF Guidelines	www.ahrq.gov/clinic/prevenix.htm
AHRQ Evidence Reports	www.ahrq.gov/clinic/epcix.htm

AHRQ, Agency for Healthcare Research and Quality; *BMJ,* British Medical Journal; *USPSTF,* U.S. Preventive Services Task Force.

FIG. 5-2 Algorithm for systematic review of the published evidence. *CINAHL,* Cumulative Index to Nursing and Allied Health Literature.

CLINICAL JUDGMENT CHALLENGE

Evidence-Based Practice; Quality Improvement; Safety **QSEN**

An 82-year-old alert and oriented woman was admitted with a diagnosis of congestive heart failure. She also has urinary frequency. You notice on her chart that she is a "high falls risk." Over 70% of patients on your unit are also at high risk for falls. The written policy and procedure for fall prevention at your hospital states that patients at risk for falling should have:

- Their health care record flagged with a yellow flower
- A yellow flower placed on their room or bed
- A bed alarm installed
- Their siderails up at all times, except when a visitor, nurse, or nursing assistant is present

The patient felt the urge to urinate and pressed her call light. Someone on the intercom told her that she would assist her shortly. After 15 minutes, the patient had to make a decision to either urinate in bed or climb over the siderails to go to the bathroom. She decided to climb over the siderails and fell. The bed alarm went off after she left the bed.

1. Considering that over 70% of patients admitted to your unit are flagged as "at risk for falls," how do you think the nurses decide that a patient is at risk for falling? Are they using valid, reliable, sensitive, and specific assessment tools to make this determination?
2. In a population of inpatient older adults, what factors can predict patient falls with a high degree of accuracy?
3. Does the best available evidence support the use of bed alarms as an intervention that prevents falls in inpatient adults of any age?
4. In a population of adult inpatients, what are the factors that have been shown by research to be the most predictive of falls?
5. What interventions have been shown to decrease the fall rates in acute care institutions with this population? (Also see Chapter 3.)

Reavy and Tavernier Model

Reavy and Tavernier (2008) developed a model and process to implement EBP that uses concepts from previously developed models (e.g., Stetler model, Iowa model) and builds upon them. The emphasis of the Reavy and Tavernier model is on the crucial role of the direct caregiver (e.g., the staff nurse) in making changes to enhance clinical practice. The authors of the model view the staff nurse as the clinical expert. Given that the staff nurse may not have expertise in research and/or practice improvement, they believe that the expertise of a nurse researcher is needed to facilitate the EBP process. The nurse researcher serves as a role model and supports nursing staff in identifying areas for improvement, assists staff with literature reviews and synthesis of evidence, and helps with the implementation and evaluation of EBP projects. Reavy and Tavernier suggest that if a nurse researcher is not available in the practice setting, then a clinical nurse specialist, advanced practice nurse, or nurse manager might provide the needed support to staff nurses. Also included in this model is an emphasis on patient and family preferences and values; however, there is little explanation of the crucial role of patient as stakeholder in any practice improvement efforts. See Table 5-5 for a more detailed description of this model.

ARCC Model

The Advancing Research and Clinical Practice through Close Collaboration (ARCC) model of evidence-based practice was originally developed by Bernadette Melnyk in 1999 and was enhanced by Melnyk and Fineout-Overholt over a 10-year period (Melnyk & Fineout-Overholt, 2010). The current version of the model consists of several components and how they relate to each other. The major components of the model are:

TABLE 5-5 Processes Used for Implementation of the Reavy and Tavernier Evidence-Based Practice Model for Staff Nurses

	PATIENT VALUES AND PREFERENCES	STAFF NURSE/CLINICAL EXPERT	NURSE RESEARCHER/BEST AVAILABLE EVIDENCE
Assessment	Give verbal and nonverbal communication	Receive verbal and nonverbal messages (collect data)	
Identification and evaluation of problem		1. Identify problem(s) 2. Discuss potential interventions and outcome 3. Conduct literature search	Assist with literature search as needed
Analysis and synthesis of best available evidence		1. Analyze and critique best available evidence 2. Synthesize evidence	Assist with analysis, and critique as needed
Planning		1. Assess feasibility of change 2. Define proposed change 3. Identify resources 4. Define desired outcome	
Implementation and evaluation	Receive nursing care based on best evidence	1. Design and implement peer teaching strategies 2. Implement change 3. Conduct pilot study 4. Evaluate findings 5. Decide to adopt or reject change 6. Communicate findings	1. Provide assistance with pilot study 2. Receive communication related to ideas for research
Integration and maintenance	Receive nursing care based on best evidence	1. Integrate into policies 2. Monitor process 3. Monitor outcomes 4. Communicate updates	Receive communication related to ideas for research

Reprinted with permission from SLACK, Incorporated. From Reavy, K., & Tavernier, S. (2008). Nurses reclaiming ownership of their practice: Implementation of an evidence-based practice model and process. *Journal of Continuing Education in Nursing, 39*(4), 166-172.

- Organizational assessment and readiness to implement EBP
- Identification of strengths and barriers to EBP implementation
- Development and use of EBP mentors
- Implementation of EBP
- Measurement of nurse, system, and patient outcomes

Key to this model is the development and use of EBP mentors who teach, guide, and facilitate agency staff in the implementation and evaluation of evidence-based practices (Melnyk & Fineout-Overholt, 2010).

EVIDENCE-BASED PRACTICE IMPROVEMENT (EBPI) MODEL

The EBPI model developed by Levin et al. under the auspices of the Visiting Nurse Service of New York (Levin et al., 2010) combines the best of the EBP and PI/QI (process/QUALITY IMPROVEMENT) systems into one approach for implementing practice improvement.

Steps of the EBPI Model

The model is prescriptive and easy for guiding health care practitioners from any discipline and setting to achieve positive change. As depicted in Fig. 5-3, the model includes:

- Describing the practice problem
- Formulating a focused clinical question (in PICO format)
- Searching for evidence to answer the question

FIG. 5-3 The Evidence-Based Practice Improvement (EBPI) model.

- Appraising and synthesizing relevant evidence
- Developing an aim statement or project goal
- Developing, implementing, and evaluating the protocol for practice improvement
- Using small tests of change or **p**lan, **d**o, **s**tudy, **a**ct (PDSA) cycles to test methods
- Disseminating best practices

Adopted from the process improvement approach is the idea of PDSA cycles or small tests of change (Langley et al., 2009). Many professionals in health care, business, and other fields implement what they believe is a good idea for an improvement on too-large a scale before they have perfected the new practice or even assessed how successful it may or may not be in their setting with their populations (patients or consumers). One of the most important benefits of small tests of change is that you have a chance to perfect the process or practice that you want to implement before disseminating and using the practice on a wide scale. Small tests of change for EBPI projects in health care are conducted with a small group of people (e.g., patients or staff) for a short period and may be repeated several times until the implementation protocol is perfected (Levin, 2009).

During small tests of change, it is helpful to use the concept of **PDSA** cycles to guide the activities.

- "**P**" stands for "plan" and is the first step in introducing a practice change. During this phase, a project team develops a protocol for implementation, which includes not only the protocol or procedure for the practice innovation but also a total plan for the exact process that will be followed for implementing the project. It includes who will be administering the new practice, how it will be implemented, the time frame for implementation, and how the particular processes implemented for each small test of change will be evaluated.
- "**D**" stands for "do" and is the action-oriented phase of the process. The new innovation or a portion of it is tested according to the plan.
- "**S**" stands for "study" and refers to the review and analysis of data collected during the "do" phase of the cycle.
- "**A**" stands for "act" and is the evaluation of results from the small test to guide decisions about how to proceed with the EBP project.

Decisions then need to be made about how to revise or refine the practice protocol and institute another small test of change to try out the refined protocol and then decide whether the plan is worth continuing.

Application of the EBPI Model to Clinical Practice: A Case Study

Describe the Practice Problem

On an adult general surgical unit in a community hospital, the nursing staff identified that assessing patients' postoperative pain with the current practice of using a numeric 10-point rating scale did not seem to be an effective assessment tool when the patient was lying quietly or appeared to be asleep. The nurses thought that to ask the restful patient to scale his or her pain refocused the patient on the pain and was not supportive of patient relaxation and pain relief. When this type of clinical observational pain assessment was performed, the nurse often did not chart the assessment in the medical record—how could the nurse label the level of pain on the scale when patient behaviors were used to assess pain? To document pain assessment and management in the patient's health record, the nurse would make up a pain rating score. A nurse's note could have been added to the medical record to describe pain behaviors the nurse identified as indicators that pain appeared to be decreasing and pain medication was working. However, the nurses on the unit did not write notes until the end of the shift. Thus the health record appeared as if no re-assessment had taken place and that the nurses were not following hospital policy. Pain assessment and management is a key quality measure for hospital accreditation making EBP quality improvement not only a clinical priority but also an important hospital initiative (The Joint Commission, 2010).

The nurses on the unit identified that pain assessment needed to be improved for quality patient care. A small team of staff nurses who understand the EBP process was formed to lead the project to address the clinical concerns. The staff identified that the main focus of the problem was assessment of patients who were asleep or appeared asleep. Was there a reliable and valid method to assess pain by observing behaviors without disturbing the patient? The nurses identified that the numeric rating scale worked for most postoperative patients after the second postoperative day. The clinical concern was assessing and re-evaluating pain management within the first 24 hours after surgery when patients were tired and often asleep because of the remnants of anesthetic and being heavily medicated for pain.

A chart audit confirmed that the nursing staff consistently assessed and re-evaluated pain with the numeric rating scale on the second postoperative day. Pain was assessed according to standards 95% of the time. On the first day after surgery, the pain scale was documented only 12% of the time. Nurses' notes to describe the patients' pain were written only 60% of the time during the first postoperative day. Clearly, there was a problem documenting pain assessment on the first postoperative day.

No one doubted that the nurses assessed pain frequently and provided pain relief; however, only the administration of pain medication was documented. Pain assessments were not consistently charted and, from a legal standpoint, the pain assessment was not done. When the numeric pain scale was used, the nurses consistently met hospital standards for pain assessment and evaluation of pain relief. The chart audit showed that a new, easy-to-use tool that assessed pain behaviors was needed to improve the documentation of pain assessment.

Formulate a Focused Clinical Question

After conducting the chart audit, the EBP team defined the clinical problem and framed a PICO question to focus the literature search for evidence-based strategies to improve pain assessment. The PICO question developed was: In the adult hospitalized patient (**P**), does the implementation of a behavioral pain scale (**I**) compared with the use of a visual analog scale (**C**) improve the assessment and management of pain in patients on the first postoperative day (**O**)?

Search for Evidence

To start their search, the EBP team began at the Cochrane Library to try to find the highest level of evidence, a clinical practice guideline to answer their question. The Cochrane Library search revealed eight clinical practice guidelines related to pain assessment but none discussed nonverbal/behavioral assessment tools (www.thecochranelibrary.com). The EBP team then went to the hospital library and accessed the CINAHL database. The initial search term used was "Pain Assessment."

This search provided 11,501 article results for the years 1966 to 2013 (www.EBSCOHOST.com). No matter how many nurses worked on the project, it would be impossible to read and evaluate over 11,000 articles. The team then remembered to use the PICO template as a guide to focus the search. Limits to narrow the search were added to the request, and only articles for pain assessment or measurement in adults ages 19 years and older were accessed. Just limiting the articles by the age of the patient reduced the number of articles to 4,836 (www.EBSCOHOST.com). This was a more manageable number of articles but still a huge number to review from a practical standpoint. So the search was further limited to the last 10 years, yielding, 3379 articles, still an insurmountable number of articles to read (www.EBSCOHOST.com). Further limiting the search using the term "inpatient" reduced the number of articles to 237—a much more manageable number, yet still overwhelming (www.EBSCOHOST.com)! Articles from 2013 appeared on the first page of the search screen. The titles revealed many interesting yet varied article topics. The search retrieved articles that addressed pain assessment with culture and pain assessment methods for specific medical diagnoses. Articles that specifically addressed behavioral pain assessment tools in the acute care setting were not immediately apparent in a list of articles.

The team realized that using the PICO question keywords might help narrow the search to the specific topic of interest and to a manageable number of articles to review. Using the search options of "postoperative pain" and "clinical assessment tools," the search engine revealed 89 articles for review (www.EBSCOHOST.com). The nurses then saved the complete search so that they could refer to the list and read other articles as they explored solutions to the PICO question.

The EBP team reviewed the search results and identified five articles that appeared to address the clinical question specifically. One article discussed the use of three evidence-based practices for postoperative pain assessment (Carlson, 2009). The nurses were intrigued by the title of this article—is it possible that the authors have already evaluated three different methods that address their specific clinical question and that it can be read in one article? Another article examined abdominal surgery patients' pain management from the postanesthesia care unit (PACU) to the surgical unit (Wilding et al., 2009). Because PACU-to-unit transition takes place during the early postoperative period, the time that pain assessment using current practice is a concern, this article seemed to address the PICO question. Two articles complemented each other with one reporting the feasibility of using a nonverbal pain assessment tool in the critical care unit (Gélinas, 2010) and another reporting the same tool's reliability (Keane, 2012).

The fifth article also focused on pain assessment tools in the critical care unit (Hall, 2007). This article evaluated three pain assessment tools. Thus the nurses chose to review these three articles in postoperative critical care patients to see if any of the tools discussed could be used on the general surgical floor.

Appraise and Synthesize the Evidence

The team read the articles and completed tables of evidence (TOEs) so the information from the articles could be organized and discussed. The TOEs also helped the nurses systematically organize what they read in a consistent format for group discussion and analysis (Table 5-6). These tables were used as the group discussed their individual review of the articles, which

TABLE 5-6 Sample Entry for a Table of Evidence

NURSING SERVICES TABLE OF EVIDENCE

PROJECT TITLE: PAIN ASSESSMENT
DATE OF REVIEW: FEBRUARY 2013
REVIEWER: F. WRIGHT

ARTICLE INFORMATION: AUTHORS, TITLE, DATE PUBLISHED, JOURNAL	SAMPLE CHARACTERISTICS AND SIZE	STUDY DESIGN, PATIENT SELECTION, EVIDENCE LEVEL/ QUALITY RATING	INTERVENTION	AUTHORS' CONCLUSIONS	REVIEWER'S COMMENTS (STRENGTHS, LIMITATIONS, POTENTIAL PRACTICE CHANGE?)
Keane, K.M. (2012). Validity and reliability of the critical care pain observation tool: a replication study. *Pain Management Nursing, 14*(4), e216-225.	21 postoperative patients assessed for pain at rest, and after repositioning 3 times on postoperative day 1. Mean age of 64 yrs. 67% male patients.	Prospective comparison to determine if there were differences in observed pain behaviors between 2 separate nurse observers and videotaped behaviors to test the reliability and validity of the CPOT instrument. **Level III: quasi-experimental design**	Patients' pain assessed using the CPOT. The CPOT was used to assess pain and compare the results with observations and self-reports of pain when the patient could report pain levels verbally.	Initial CPOT instrument testing: strong discriminant validity ($t = 5.75$, $p > 0.001$). Good face validity; 93% inter-rater reliability; Kappa statistic was 0.36 to 0.72 ($p = 05$). The cognitively and non–cognitively impaired groups' CNPI scores did not differ significantly in total scores. The cognitively impaired group had more pain behaviors identified at rest than the non–cognitively impaired group.	This was a replication of the initial testing (Gélinas, 2010) of the CPOT to assess pain in nonverbal critically ill patients. It seems to be reliable and simple to use. The CPOT seems to be most effective in patients when not intubated and so may be useful on the acute care floor during immediate postoperative assessments.

CNPI, Checklist of nonverbal pain indicators; *CPOT*, Critical-Care Pain Observation Tool.

included a summary of the evidence contained in the article, the strengths and limitations of the evidence, and potential application to their specific PICO question. As the nurses critically appraised the evidence, the group referred to the quantitative evidence pyramid in Fig. 5-1 to identify the level of evidence of each article. The colorful pyramid was posted during the discussion for ease of reference. Through dialog about each article, the authors' methods, outcomes, and the limitations of the different tools to measure pain, the group rated the quality of the articles. This process was used to make an informed decision about the strength of the evidence before any practice recommendations could be made. The staff wanted to use the highest level of evidence possible to inform the practice change. One of the critical care articles was identified as a level III quasi-experimental study and presented a description of a tool that was reported as "easy to use" and reliable for nonverbal patients (Keane, 2012). The staff returned to the literature search to find more information on one of the behavioral pain tools discussed in the same article.

Develop the Aim Statement

After reviewing the evidence to answer the focused clinical question, the nurses developed this aim statement: Improve the frequency of nurses' assessment of first-day postoperative pain from 12% to 70% after 2 weeks of introducing a new behavioral pain assessment tool.

Implement the PDSA Cycles

After the second search for evidence to answer the clinical question and additional review of the new evidence, the team of nurses planned to make a practice change (**Plan**). A small test of the utility of the tool needed to be performed to see if the nurses could accurately assess pain using the behavioral assessment tool and to determine its practicality for use. To evaluate the inter-rater reliability of the tool to determine if the nurses could consistently assess a patient's pain in the same way with the same tool, three of the nurses used the tool simultaneously to assess pain in 10 postoperative patients (**Do**). The assessment results were compared and evaluated to identify whether the nurses were using the tool consistently (**Study**). This small test of change resulted in positive feedback from nurses as to the practicality of the tool, and inter-rater reliability was high (i.e., different nurses observing patients and assessing their pain at the same time using the new tool came up with consistently similar ratings of these patients' pain).

The next step was to perform another small test of change (**Act**) to evaluate if nurses on the EBP team could use the pain assessment tool effectively in the clinical unit to improve patient pain assessment. The team used the tool for 1 week on all first-day postoperative patients. Patient records were monitored daily by the nurse educator and unit manager to evaluate the frequency of pain assessment. Because the team had the initial chart audit data, collecting the same data with the new tool in use would help identify if the behavioral scale for assessment of pain was completed and documented more consistently than before the new scale was introduced. In addition, the EBP nurse team was able to develop a step-by-step process for use of the tool.

The next step in the EBPI implementation process was for the project team to educate the rest of the unit staff on all shifts about the evidence-based intervention—the behavioral pain assessment tool and the process for its use. The TOEs were summarized and discussed to provide the staff with concrete information about the new tool. The EBP nurse team demonstrated how the tool was used. A member of the project team pretended to be asleep in a bed as a patient so that the nurses could role-play how to perform the pain assessment with the proposed tool. Informational posters were placed on the unit and multiple copies were made of the tool for use during the small test of change. The unit secretaries were involved in the education since they were responsible for providing the tools and collecting them when they were completed.

For 2 weeks, the nursing staff used the new tool to assess the pain of first-day postoperative patients. The team reviewed patient charts daily and answered questions about the use of the tool and the documentation of the pain assessment. At the completion of this third small test of change, the team reviewed the chart audits and found that the unit nurses had appropriately documented pain assessment on the first postoperative day 85% of the time—a huge improvement! A short questionnaire was distributed to the nursing staff to determine their feedback about the use and effectiveness of the tool. All unit staff found the new tool easy to use and expressed positive beliefs in its value. They also were very proud to have achieved an outcome that exceeded their outcome in the aim statement.

Disseminate Best Practices

Given the success the nurses achieved on this one postoperative unit with their small tests of change using PDSA cycles, they recommended the introduction of the new behavioral pain assessment tool to the Hospital Standards of Practice Committee. The Committee, consisting of an interdisciplinary team of nurses, physicians, pharmacists, and other health care professionals, was excited about the evidence-based practice improvement effort. They decided to pilot the new tool on all surgical units for 1 month to see if the same results could be achieved with wider dissemination. If the initial benchmark of 70% was achieved in the pilot, then the new protocol for assessment of pain on the first postoperative day would be instituted hospital-wide as the standard of practice. At completion of the pilot, the benchmark of 70% was achieved and the Committee voted to incorporate the new policy and procedure as standard practice.

All nurses who worked on surgical units, the operating suites, and PACU were educated about the new hospital standards for pain assessment. The plan for evaluation of the new practice was to conduct random patient record audits each month for 6 months to determine whether the improvement effort continued after initial implementation. The nurse educator and the EBP mentor worked with the initial EBP nurse team (three staff nurses) to submit an abstract for presentation at an EBP conference. The Vice President of Patient Care Services agreed to pay all expenses for the five nurses who led the project to attend the conference if the abstract was accepted for presentation.

GET READY FOR THE NCLEX® EXAMINATION!

KEY POINTS

Review these Key Points for each NCLEX Examination Client Needs Category.

Safe and Effective Care Environment

- Describe EVIDENCE-BASED PRACTICE (EBP) to include the components of research evidence, clinical expertise, and patient/family values: EBP is a strategy for making clinical decisions about how we practice nursing and other health care professions.
- Describe EBP to include the components of research evidence, clinical expertise, and patient/family values: EBP incorporates the expertise of the clinician and the patient's values and preferences to make decisions about health care. **Evidence-Based Practice** QSEN
- Explain how to use an EBP approach to identifying a clinical problem, issue, or challenge, and formulate a focused clinical question about clinical practice: The first step of the EBP process is to ask a clinical "burning" question using the PICO(T) format (see Table 5-1).
- Recall that quantitative questions focus on the relationship among measurable phenomena and include statistical analysis of information.
- Remember that qualitative questions focus on the meanings and interpretations of human phenomena or experiences of people using interview or observation.

- Explain the roles of levels of evidence by reviewing Fig. 5-1 and Table 5-2, which refer to the status or rank of evidence.
- Briefly describe two models of EBP for changing processes of care: Examples of models of EBP include the Iowa model, the Reavy and Tavernier model (see Table 5-5), and the evidence-based practice improvement (EBPI) model. **Evidence-Based Practice** QSEN
- Differentiate clinical opinion from research and evidence summaries: When performing a literature search on current evidence to answer the clinical question, organize the data into a table of evidence like the one shown in Table 5-6.
- Discuss how the EBPI model can be used to guide a clinical practice QUALITY IMPROVEMENT project: When making changes based on findings from the literature, use PDSA cycles to test the changes on a small scale.
- Discuss how the EBPI model can be used to guide a clinical practice improvement project: Recall that PDSA stands for "Plan," "Do," "Study," and "Act." **Quality Improvement** QSEN
- List the steps of how to perform a systematic literature review to answer clinical questions using the steps in Table 5-5. Recall these steps include searching for clinical practice guidelines, summarizing and appraising research, making recommendations for change, implementing the change, and evaluating the outcomes.

Rehabilitation Concepts for Chronic and Disabling Health Problems

Donna D. Ignatavicius

ⓔ http://evolve.elsevier.com/Iggy/

A **chronic health problem** is one that has existed for at least 3 months. A **disabling health problem** is any physical or mental health/behavioral health problem that can cause disability. This text focuses primarily on physical health problems; mental health/behavioral health problems are discussed in more detail in textbooks on mental health/behavioral health nursing.

Patients with chronic and disabling health problems often participate in rehabilitation programs to prevent further disability, maintain functional ability, and restore as much function as possible. The rehabilitation nurse collaborates with the nursing and health care team and coordinates the patient's interdisciplinary care.

OVERVIEW

Chronic and Disabling Health Problems

Chronic and disabling illnesses are a major health problem in the United States, with almost half of the population having one or more chronic health problems. Complications of chronic disease account for the majority of all deaths, and associated medical costs account for over two thirds of the nation's health care cost. The rate of chronic and disabling conditions is expected to increase as more "baby boomers" approach late adulthood. Some people with chronic and disabling problems are in inpatient settings like rehabilitation centers and skilled nursing facilities, whereas others are managed at home.

Stroke, coronary artery disease, cancer, chronic obstructive pulmonary disease (COPD), asthma, and arthritis are common chronic diseases that can result in varying degrees of disability. Most occur in people older than 65 years. Younger adults are also living longer with potentially disabling genetic disorders that, in the past, would have shortened life expectancy. These specific health problems are discussed throughout this text.

Chronic and disabling conditions are not always illnesses (e.g., heart disease); they may also result from accidents. Accidents are a leading cause of trauma and death among young and middle-aged adults. Increasing numbers of people survive accidents with severe injuries because of advances in medical technology and safety equipment such as motor vehicle airbags. As a result, they are often faced with chronic, disabling neurologic conditions, such as traumatic brain injuries (TBIs) and spinal cord injuries (SCIs).

These health problems are also common among military men and women survivors who served in Iraq and Afghanistan. The most common complications of these wars are TBI and single or multiple limb amputations. These disabilities require months to years of follow-up health care after returning to the community. Because of people living longer with chronic and disabling health problems, the need for rehabilitation is on the rise.

Rehabilitation Settings

Rehabilitation is the continuous process of learning to live with and manage chronic and disabling conditions. The desired outcome of rehabilitation is that the patient will return to the best possible physical, mental, social, vocational, and economic capacity. Rehabilitation is not limited to the return of function in post-traumatic situations. It also includes education and therapy for any chronic illness characterized by a change in a body system function or body structure. Rehabilitation programs related to respiratory, cardiac, and musculoskeletal health problems are common examples that do not involve trauma.

Rehabilitation ("rehab") can occur in a number of settings. This process starts in the acute care hospital (sometimes called *acute* or *short-term rehabilitation*) and continues after discharge from the hospital. The nurse coordinates care from acute care through community-based care to ensure successful rehabilitation.

For continuing rehabilitation services, the most common **inpatient rehabilitation facilities (IRFs)** are freestanding rehabilitation hospitals, rehabilitation or skilled units within hospitals (e.g., transitional care units [TCUs]), and skilled nursing facilities to which the patient is typically admitted for 1 to 3 weeks or longer. **Skilled nursing facilities (SNFs)** are part of either a hospital or long-term care (nursing home) setting (Fig. 6-1). Skilled rehabilitation and nursing services for older residents admitted to SNFs are reimbursed through Medicare A for the first 21 days after admission. After that time, reimbursement is a combination of Medicare and other payer sources for a specified number of days.

Patients in nursing homes or skilled nursing units in hospitals are called *residents*. The term **resident** implies that the person lives in the inpatient facility and has all the rights of anyone living in his or her home. Residents wear street clothes rather than hospital gowns and have choices in what they eat and how they plan each day.

Ambulatory care rehabilitation departments and home rehabilitation programs may be needed for continuing less-intensive services. Eighty percent (80%) of rehabilitation services are paid

FIG. 6-1 Patient (resident) in a skilled nursing facility rehabilitation unit.

for by Medicare B for older adults for a specified period of time if they have this benefit. Some agencies have specialized clinics focused on rehabilitation of patients with specific health problems, such as those that care for patients with strokes; amputations; and large, chronic, and/or nonhealing wounds. After disabled patients become more confident and independent, they may choose to live at home or in a group home. Group homes are facilities in which patients live independently together with other disabled adults. Each patient or group of patients has a care provider, such as a personal care aide, to assist with ADLs and daily decisions requiring accurate judgments. The patients may or may not be actively employed. In some cases, the care home offers employment opportunities to the residents. The purpose of these homes is to provide independent living arrangements outside an institution, especially for younger patients with TBI or SCI.

The Rehabilitation Team

Successful rehabilitation depends on the coordinated effort of a group of the patient, family, and health care professionals in planning, implementing, and evaluating patient-centered care. The focus of the rehabilitation team is to restore and maintain the patient's function to the greatest extent possible.

In addition to the patient, family, and/or significant others, members of the interdisciplinary health care team in the rehabilitation setting may include:

- Physicians, nurse practitioners, and clinical nurse specialists
- Nurses and nursing assistants
- Physical therapists and assistants
- Occupational therapists and assistants
- Speech-language pathologists and assistants
- Rehabilitation assistants/restorative aides
- Recreational or activity therapists
- Cognitive therapists or neuropsychologists
- Social workers or case managers
- Clinical psychologists
- Vocational counselors

- Spiritual care counselors
- Registered dietitians (RDs)
- Pharmacists
- Biomedical technicians

Not all settings that offer rehabilitation services have all of these members on their team. Not all patients require the services of all health care team members.

A physician who specializes in rehabilitative medicine is called a **physiatrist**. Most inpatient rehabilitation settings employ physiatrists. A primary care physician or nurse practitioner may also oversee care for the patient's medical problems.

Rehabilitation nurses in the inpatient setting coordinate the efforts of health care team members and therefore function as the patient's case manager. Nurses also create a rehabilitation milieu, which includes (Pryor, 2010):

- Allowing time for patients to practice self-management skills
- Encouraging patients and providing emotional support
- Protecting patients from embarrassment (e.g., bowel training)
- Making the inpatient unit a more homelike environment

Table 6-1 summarizes the nurse's role as part of the rehabilitation team. Because of an increase in the need for older adult rehabilitation, some nurses specialize in gerontologic rehabilitation (Association of Rehabilitation Nurses [ARN], 2008b). Nurses and other health care professionals may be designated as **rehabilitation case managers** in the home or in acute care settings.

As their name implies, **nursing assistants** or **nursing technicians** assist in the care of patients. These members of the rehabilitation team are under the direct supervision of the registered nurse (RN) or licensed practical or vocational nurse (LPN or LVN).

Physical therapists (PTs), also called **physiotherapists**, intervene to help the patient achieve self-management by focusing on gross MOBILITY skills (e.g., by facilitating ambulation and teaching the patient to use a walker) (Fig. 6-2). They may also teach techniques for performing certain ADLs, such as transferring (e.g., moving into and out of bed), ambulating, and toileting, and can assist with cognitive retraining (often for

patients with TBI). In some settings, PTs play a major role in providing wound care. Physical therapy assistants (PTAs) may be employed to help the PT.

Occupational therapists (OTs) work to develop the patient's fine motor skills used for ADL self-management, such as those required for eating, hygiene, and dressing. OTs also teach patients how to perform independent living skills, such as cooking and shopping. Many inpatient rehabilitation facilities have fully furnished and equipped apartments where patients can practice independent living skills in a mock setting under supervision. To accomplish these outcomes, OTs teach skills related to coordination (e.g., hand movements) and cognitive retraining (Fig. 6-3). Occupational therapy assistants (OTAs) may be available to help the OT.

FIG. 6-2 A physical therapist helping a patient ambulate with a walker.

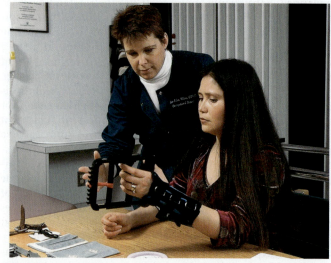

FIG. 6-3 A registered occupational therapist working with a patient on improving hand strength.

TABLE 6-1	Nurse's Role in the Rehabilitation Team

- Advocates for the patient and family
- Creates a therapeutic rehabilitation milieu
- Provides and coordinates holistic patient care in a variety of health care settings, including the home
- Collaborates with the rehabilitation team to establish expected patient outcomes to develop a plan of care
- Coordinates rehabilitation team activities to ensure implementation of the plan of care
- Acts as a resource to the rehabilitation team having specialized knowledge and clinical skills needed to care for patient with chronic and disabling health problems
- Communicates effectively with all members of the rehabilitation team, including the patient and family
- Plans continuity of care when the patient is discharged from the health care facility
- Evaluates the effectiveness of the interdisciplinary plan of care for the patient and family

Adapted from Association of Rehabilitation Nurses. (2008). *Standards and scope of rehabilitation nursing practice*, Glenview, IL: Author.

Speech-language pathologists (SLPs) evaluate and retrain patients with speech, language, or swallowing problems. *Speech* is the ability to say words, and *language* is the ability to understand and put words together in a meaningful way. Some patients, especially those who have experienced a head injury or stroke, have difficulty with both speech and language. Those who have had a stroke also may have dysphagia (difficulty with swallowing). SLPs provide screening and testing for dysphagia. If the patient has this problem, the SLP recommends appropriate foods and feeding techniques. Speech-language pathology assistants (SLPAs) may be employed to help the SLP.

PTs, OTs, and SLPs are collectively referred to as *rehabilitation therapists*. Assistants to PTs, OTs, and SLPs are called *rehabilitation assistants*. Restorative aides, usually in the nursing department, continue the rehabilitation therapy plan of care when therapists are not available. This model of care is common in long-term care settings, such as nursing homes.

Recreational or activity therapists work to help patients continue or develop hobbies or interests. These therapists often coordinate their efforts with those of the OT.

Cognitive therapists, usually neuropsychologists, work primarily with patients who have experienced head injuries with cognitive impairments. These therapists often use computers to assist with cognitive retraining.

Various counselors are helpful in promoting community reintegration of the patient and acceptance of the disability or chronic illness. Social workers help patients identify support services and resources, including financial assistance, and coordinate transfers to or discharges from the rehabilitation setting. Clinical psychologists also counsel patients and families on their psychological problems and on strategies to cope with disability. They may also perform a battery of assessments for COGNITION. Spiritual counselors, usually members of the clergy, specialize in spiritual assessments and care.

Vocational counselors assist with job placement, training, or further education. Work-related skills are taught if the patient needs to change careers because of the disability. If the patient has not yet completed high school, tutors may help with completion of the requirements for graduation.

Registered dietitians (RDs) may be needed to ensure that patients meet their needs for NUTRITION. For example, for patients who need weight reduction, a restricted calorie diet can be planned. For patients who need additional calories or other nutrients, including vitamins, dietitians can plan a patient-specific diet.

Pharmacists collaborate with the other members of the health care team to ensure that the patient receives the most appropriate drug therapy to meet the patient's needs. They oversee the prescription and preparation of medications and provide the health care team with essential information regarding drug safety.

Biomedical technicians maintain the safety of adaptive and electronic devices by monitoring their function and making repairs as needed.

Depending on the patient's health care needs, additional team members may be included in the rehabilitation program, such as the geriatrician, respiratory therapist, and prosthetist. Interdisciplinary team conferences for planning care and evaluating the patient's progress are held regularly with the patient, family members and significant others, and health care providers. The interdisciplinary patient record is shared and read by all team members.

❖ PATIENT-CENTERED COLLABORATIVE CARE

◆ Assessment

History. Collect the history of the patient's present condition, any current drug therapy, and any treatment programs in progress. Begin by obtaining general background data about the patient and family. This information includes cultural practices and the patient's home situation. In collaboration with the occupational therapist, the nurse or case manager addresses the layout of the home. Together they discuss whether the physical layout at home, such as stairs or the width of doorways, will present a problem to the patient after discharge.

Assess the patient's usual daily schedule and habits of everyday living. These include hygiene practices, NUTRITION, ELIMINATION, sexual activity, and sleep. Ask about the patient's preferred method and time of bathing and hygiene activity. In assessing dietary patterns, note food likes and dislikes. Also, obtain information about bowel and bladder function and the normal pattern of elimination.

In assessing sexuality patterns, ask about changes in sexual function since the onset of the disability. The patient's current and previous sleep habits, patterns, usual number of hours of sleep, and use of hypnotics are also assessed. Question whether the patient feels well rested after sleep. Sleep patterns have a significant impact on activity patterns. The assessment of activity patterns focuses on work, exercise, and recreational activities.

CONSIDERATIONS FOR OLDER ADULTS
Patient-Centered Care QSEN

Older adults who need rehabilitation often have other chronic diseases that need to be managed, including diabetes mellitus, coronary artery disease, osteoporosis, and arthritis. These health problems added to the normal physiologic changes associated with aging predispose the older adult to falls, pressure ulcers, and pneumonia. When discharged from a hospital setting, some older patients are undernourished, which causes weakness and fatigue. The longer the hospital stay, the more debilitated the older adult can become.

Health teaching may be challenging because some older patients may have beginning changes in cognition, including short-term memory loss. Sensory losses, like vision and hearing, may also affect their ability to give an accurate history or grasp new information.

Physical Assessment/Clinical Manifestations. Upon admission for baseline and at least daily (depending on agency policy and type of setting), collect physical assessment data systematically according to major body systems (Table 6-2). The primary focus of the assessment related to rehabilitation and chronic disease is the *functional* abilities of the patient.

Cardiovascular and Respiratory Assessment. An alteration in cardiac status may affect the patient's cardiac output or cause activity intolerance. Assess associated signs and symptoms of decreased cardiac output (e.g., chest pain, fatigue). If present, determine when the patient experiences these symptoms and what relieves them. The health care provider may prescribe a change in drug therapy or may prescribe a prophylactic dose of nitroglycerin to be taken before the patient resumes activities. Collaborate with the health care provider and appropriate therapists to determine whether activities need to be modified.

TABLE 6-2   Assessment of Patients in Rehabilitation Settings

BODY SYSTEM	RELEVANT DATA
Cardiovascular system	Chest pain Fatigue Fear of heart failure
Respiratory system	Shortness of breath or dyspnea Activity tolerance Fear of inability to breathe
Gastrointestinal system and nutrition	Oral intake, eating pattern Anorexia, nausea, and vomiting Dysphagia Laboratory data (e.g., serum prealbumin level) Weight loss or gain Bowel elimination pattern or habits Change in stool (constipation or diarrhea) Ability to get to toilet
Renal-urinary system	Urinary pattern Fluid intake Urinary incontinence or retention Urine culture and urinalysis
Neurologic system	Motor function Sensation Perceptual ability Cognitive abilities
Musculoskeletal system	Functional ability Range of motion Endurance Muscle strength
Integumentary system	Risk for skin breakdown Presence of skin lesions

For the patient showing fatigue, the nurse and patient plan methods for using limited energy resources. For instance, frequent rest periods can be taken throughout the day, especially before performing activities. Major tasks could be performed in the morning because most people have the most energy at that time.

A hindrance to rehabilitation for patients with cardiac disorders is fear, particularly for older adults. These patients may have survived a life-threatening experience (e.g., myocardial infarction) and may be so afraid of recurrence or death that they are unable or unwilling to resume any activity. They usually benefit from participation in a structured cardiac rehabilitation program. (See Chapter 38 for a complete description of cardiac rehabilitation.)

Ask the patient whether he or she has shortness of breath, chest pain, or severe weakness and fatigue during or after activity. *Determine the level of activity that can be accomplished without these symptoms.* For example, can the patient climb one flight of stairs without shortness of breath or does shortness of breath occur after climbing only two steps?

Gastrointestinal and Nutritional Assessment. Monitor the patient's oral intake and pattern of eating. Also, assess for the presence of anorexia, dysphagia, nausea, vomiting, or discomfort that may interfere with oral intake. Determine whether the patient wears dentures and, if so, whether they fit. Review the patient's height, weight, hemoglobin and hematocrit levels, serum prealbumin, and blood glucose levels. (See Chapter 60 for discussion of how to perform a screening for NUTRITION

status.) Weight loss or weight gain is particularly significant and may be related to an associated disease or to the illness that caused the disability.

Bowel ELIMINATION habits vary from person to person. They are often related to daily job or activity schedules, dietary patterns, age, and family or cultural background. Elimination habits may be difficult to assess, because many nurses are hesitant to request (and many patients are afraid to volunteer) information pertaining to elimination. Ask about usual bowel patterns before the injury or the illness.

Note any changes in the patient's bowel routine or stool consistency. The most common problem for rehabilitation patients is constipation. In their classic best practice guidelines, the Association of Rehabilitation Nurses (ARN) (2002) defines constipation as the passage of hard, dry stool fewer than 3 times a week or significant change in the patient's usual habits for more than 3 months. Examples of significant changes include abdominal fullness and bloating and straining when having a bowel movement.

If the patient reports any alteration in ELIMINATION pattern, try to determine whether it is due to a change in diet, activity pattern, or medication use. Always assess bowel habits on what is normal for that person.

Ask whether the patient can manage bowel function independently. Independence in bowel elimination requires COGNITION, manual dexterity, sensation, muscle control, and MOBILITY. If the patient requires help, determine whether someone is available at home to provide the assistance. Also assess the patient's and family's ability to cope with any dependency in bowel elimination.

Renal and Urinary Assessment. Ask about the patient's baseline urinary ELIMINATION patterns, including the number of times he or she usually voids. Determine whether he or she routinely awakens during the night to empty the bladder (nocturia) or sleeps through the night. Record fluid intake patterns and volume, including the type of fluids ingested and the time they were consumed.

Question whether the patient has ever had any problems with urinary incontinence or retention. Also, monitor laboratory reports, especially the results of the urinalysis and culture and sensitivity, if needed. *Urinary tract infections (UTIs) among older adults are often missed because acute confusion may be the only indicator of the infection.* Many health care professionals expect older patients to be confused and may not detect this problem. If untreated, UTIs can lead to kidney infection and possible failure.

Neurologic and Musculoskeletal Assessment. The neurologic assessment includes motor function (MOBILITY), sensation, and COGNITION. Assess the patient's pre-existing problems, general physical condition, and communication abilities. Patients may have dysphasia (slurred speech) because of facial muscle weakness or may have aphasia (inability to speak or comprehend), usually the result of a cerebral stroke or traumatic brain injury (TBI). These communication problems are discussed in detail in the chapters on problems of the nervous system.

Determine if the patient has paresis (weakness) or paralysis (absence of movement). Observe the patient's gait. Identify sensory-perceptual changes, such as visual acuity, that could contribute to the patient's risk for injury. Assess his or her response to light touch, hot or cold temperature, and position change in each extremity and on the trunk. Identify levels of decreased sensation. For a perceptual assessment, the nurse evaluates the patient's ability to receive and understand what is heard and seen and the ability to express appropriate motor and verbal responses. During this portion of the assessment, begin to assess short-term and long-term memory.

Assess the patient's cognitive abilities, especially if there is a head injury or stroke. Several tools are available to evaluate COGNITION. One of the most commonly used tools in rehabilitation and long-term care settings is the Brief Interview for Mental Status (BIMS), which is described in detail in Chapter 41. The Confusion Assessment Method (CAM) is used to determine if the patient had delirium, an acute confusional state. (See Table 2-3 in Chapter 2 for description of the CAM tool.)

As with other body systems, nursing assessment of the musculoskeletal system focuses on function. Assess the patient's musculoskeletal status, response to the impairment, and demands of the home, work, or school environment. Determine the patient's endurance level, and measure active and passive joint range of motion (ROM). Review the results of manual muscle testing by physical therapy, which identifies the patient's ROM and resistance against gravity. In this procedure, the therapist determines the degree of muscle strength present in each body segment.

Skin Assessment. Identify actual or potential interruptions in skin and TISSUE INTEGRITY. To maintain healthy skin, the body must have adequate food, water, and oxygen intake; intact waste-removal mechanisms; sensation; and functional MOBILITY. Changes in any of these variables can lead to rapid and extensive skin breakdown. If the patient cannot protect or maintain the skin, assess and plan for his or her needs.

> ### ! NURSING SAFETY PRIORITY (QSEN)
> #### Action Alert
>
> Be sure to remind unlicensed assistive personnel to report changes in the patient's skin promptly, including any new onset of redness. Assess the patient frequently to determine the risk for skin breakdown <u>before</u> it occurs! Older adults are at a very high risk for heel and sacral pressure ulcers, which can occur within 24 hours after admission.

Most rehabilitation settings use special skin assessment tools to identify patients at risk for skin breakdown. For example, the classic Braden Scale for Predicting Pressure Ulcer Risk (see Chapter 25) assesses several areas: sensory perception, skin moisture, activity level, nutritional status, and potential for friction and shear.

Other skin risk assessment tools are available. Some tools also include additional indicators of nutritional status, such as the serum prealbumin. When these levels are low, the patient is at high risk for pressure ulcers. Some tools include incontinence and altered mental state as risk factors.

If a pressure ulcer or other change in skin integrity develops, accurately assess the problem and its possible causes. Inspect the skin every 2 hours until the patient learns to inspect his or her own skin several times a day. Measure the depth and diameter of any open skin areas in inches or centimeters, depending on the policy of the facility. Assess the area around the open lesion to determine the presence of cellulitis or other tissue damage. Chapter 25 includes several widely used classification systems for assessing skin breakdown. Determine the patient's knowledge about the cause and treatment of skin breakdown,

as well as his or her ability to inspect the skin and participate in maintaining TISSUE INTEGRITY.

In most health care agencies, the skin assessment is documented on a special form or part of the electronic health record to keep track of each area of skin breakdown. A baseline assessment is conducted on admission to the agency and updated periodically depending on the agency's policy and the nurse's judgment. In most long-term care, acute care, and rehabilitation settings and with the patient's (or family's if the patient cannot communicate) permission, photographs of the skin are taken on admission and at various intervals for documentation.

> ### ? NCLEX EXAMINATION CHALLENGE
> #### Physiological Integrity
>
> An older adult is admitted for rehabilitation after a total hip replacement. Which statement by the nursing assistant will require follow-up by the nurse?
> A. "The client has an abduction pillow between her legs."
> B. "The client reports being tired after her physical therapy session."
> C. "The client is resting in bed after she had her pain pill."
> D. "The client's sacrum is reddened and uncomfortable."

Functional Assessment. *Functional ability* refers to the ability to perform **activities of daily living (ADLs),** such as bathing, dressing, feeding, and ambulating, and **independent living skills,** including using the telephone, shopping, preparing food, and housekeeping. These latter skills are sometimes referred to as **instrumental activities of daily living (IADLs).** Functional assessment tools are used to assess a patient's abilities. Rehabilitation nurses, physiatrists, or rehabilitation therapists complete one or more of these assessment tools based on the patient's abilities and the policy of the health care setting.

One classic uniform data system still used for outcome data collection across the United States is the Functional Independence Measure (FIM) developed by Granger and Gresham (1984). As a basic indicator of the severity of a disability, the FIM attempts to quantify what the person actually does, whatever the diagnosis or impairment. It does not measure what a person should do or how the person would perform under a different set of circumstances. To eliminate the bias of a particular discipline, the assessment may be performed by trained clinicians. The entire assessment may be performed by one person, or certain categories may be completed by various professionals.

Categories for assessment are self-care, sphincter control, MOBILITY and locomotion, communication, and COGNITION. Scoring is done with numbers that use predetermined criteria for measurement. The patient is evaluated when he or she is admitted to and discharged from a rehabilitation institution and at other specified times to determine progress. The FIM system has also been adapted for use in other health care settings, including acute care and home care, and is available in multiple languages.

In U.S. long-term care settings, the interdisciplinary **Minimum Data Set (MDS) 3.0** is required by the U.S. Centers for Medicare and Medicaid (CMS) to assess patients (residents) in nursing homes. The resident's MOBILITY, sensation, and COGNITION are evaluated, as well as the overall health status. A list

Data from Centers for Medicare and Medicaid Services (CMS). MDS 3.0 for nursing homes and swing bed providers, 2013. Retrieved September 2014 from http://www.cms.gov/Medicare/Quality-Initiatives-Patient-Assessment-Instruments/NursingHomeQualityInits/NHQIMDS30.html.

TABLE 6-3 **Assessment Components of the Minimum Data Set (MDS) 3.0**

- Hearing, Speech and Vision
- Cognitive Patterns
- Mood
- Behavior
- Preferences for Customary Routines and Activities
- Functional Status
- Bowel and Bladder
- Active Disease Diagnoses
- Health Conditions (e.g., pain, fall history)
- Swallowing and Nutritional Status
- Oral/Dental Status
- Skin Condition
- Medications
- Special Treatments and Procedures
- Restraints
- Participation in Assessment and Goal Setting
- Supplemental Therapies

of assessment components for the MDS 3.0 is presented in Table 6-3. Similar to the FIM, all health care team members involved in the resident's care record their assessments on the MDS and the RN coordinates the comprehensive assessment.

Psychosocial Assessment. In addition to determining cognitive function, assess the patient's body image and self-esteem through verbal indicators and descriptions of self-care. Encourage the family to allow the patient to perform as many functions as possible independently to build feelings of self-worth.

Assess the patient's use of defense mechanisms and manifestations of anxiety. To assess the patient's response to loss, ask him or her to describe feelings concerning the loss of a body part or function. Assess for the presence of any stress-related physical problem. Some patients have symptoms of depression, such as fatigue, a change in appetite, or feelings of powerlessness. See Chapter 7 for a thorough discussion of loss and grieving and Chapter 2 for a brief description of depression among the older adult population.

Determine the availability of support systems for the patient. The major support system is typically the family or significant others. Patients who do not have these support systems are more likely to develop depression. Identify the patient's spiritual and/or religious needs, and refer to an appropriate health care team member as needed. Assess sexuality and intimacy needs, and document findings in the electronic health record (EHR).

Vocational Assessment. To assist patients in maximizing functional status, encourage them to resume usual activities. Vocational counselors can help patients find meaningful training, education, or employment after discharge from the rehabilitation setting, if needed.

Patients in the United States should be informed about the Americans with Disabilities Act, which was passed by Congress in 1991 to prevent employer discrimination against disabled people. The employer must offer *reasonable* assistance to a disabled employee to allow him or her to perform the job. For example, if an employee has a severe hearing loss, the employer may need to hire an interpreter for sign language. Workers have a right to ask for special adaptations based on their disabilities.

The rehabilitation team assesses the cognitive and physical demands of the patient's job to determine whether he or she can return to the former job or whether retraining in another field is necessary. The physical demands of jobs range from light in sedentary occupations (0 to 10 lbs often lifted) to heavy

(more than 100 lbs often lifted). The nurse must also consider other aspects of the job, such as mobility or senses required (e.g., hearing).

Job analysis also involves assessing the work environment of the patient's former job. Collaborate with the vocational counselor to determine whether the environment is conducive to the patient's return. Job modifications may be needed to accommodate the patient at work. If an injured worker requires vocational rehabilitation, refer him or her to vocational rehabilitation personnel to evaluate present skills and learn new skills for employment if needed. In most states, Workers' Compensation insurance helps support vocational rehabilitation.

◆ **Analysis**

Regardless of age or specific disability, these priority patient problems are common. Additional problems depend on the patient's specific chronic illness or disability. The priority NANDA-I nursing diagnoses and collaborative problems for patients with chronic and disabling health problems include:

1. Impaired Physical Mobility related to neuromuscular impairment, sensory-perceptual impairment, and/or chronic pain (NANDA-I)
2. Decreased functional ability related to neuromuscular impairment and/or impairment in perception or cognition
3. Risk for Impaired Skin Integrity related to altered sensation and/or altered nutritional state (NANDA-I)
4. Urinary incontinence or Urinary Retention related to neurologic dysfunction and/or trauma or disease affecting spinal cord nerves (NANDA-I)
5. Constipation related to neurologic impairment, inadequate nutrition, or decreased mobility (NANDA-I)

◆ **Planning and Implementation**

Improving Physical Mobility

Planning: Expected Outcomes. The patient with chronic illness or disability is expected to reach a level of physical MOBILITY that allows him or her to function independently with or without assistive devices. In addition, the patient is expected to be free of complications of immobility.

Interventions. Most problems requiring rehabilitation relate to decreased physical MOBILITY. For example, patients with neurologic disease or injury, amputations, arthritis, and cardiopulmonary disease usually experience some degree of immobility. Coordinate care with physical and occupational therapists as the key rehabilitation team members in helping patients meet their mobility outcomes. Patients initially spend 5 to 6 hours a day for at least 5 days a week in rehabilitation therapy departments to regain MOBILITY and self-management skills.

Safe Patient Handling Practices. Before they learn to become independent, patients with decreased MOBILITY in any health care setting or at home often need assistance with positioning in bed and transfers, such as from a bed to a chair, commode, or wheelchair. Patients may not be able to bear full weight, may have inadequate balance, and/or may be very obese. For many years, nurses relied on "body mechanics" to prevent staff injury when moving patients or assisting them to move. This traditional, but outdated, approach was based on the belief that correct body positioning by staff members would protect them from the force of lifting and moving. For example, if the patient could not bear weight or did not have sufficient balance (e.g., quadriplegic spinal cord injury), nurses and therapists used a "bear hug" technique to lift the patient from bed to chair or back again. Obese patients were also lifted with multiple staff assistance.

Heavy lifting and dependent transfers by staff members have resulted in a very high incidence of **work-related musculoskeletal disorders (MSDs)**, most often chronic back injuries, which can be prevented. As a response to this costly problem, the National Institute for Occupational Safety and Health (NIOSH) established evidence-based guidelines for safe patient handling. Based on this document, the American Nurses Association, in partnership with NIOSH and the Veterans Health Administration, developed a curriculum for all nursing students and practicing nurses on how to safely handle and move patients in any health care setting or home environment (American Nurses Association, 2012). In collaboration with other health care team members, nurses assess patient MOBILITY and use best practices for safe patient handling (SPH).

Because each patient has unique needs and characteristics, assess the patient's MOBILITY level using a standardized tool to plan interventions for SPH. An example of an appropriate assessment tool for this purpose is shown in Fig. 6-4. Before moving the patient, assess his or her environment for potential hazards that could cause injury, such as a slippery or uneven floor.

Use these general SPH practices, and teach to staff members:
- Maintain a wide, stable base with your feet.
- Put the bed at the correct height—waist level while providing direct care and hip level when moving patients.
- Try to keep the patient or work directly in front of you to prevent your spine from rotating.
- Keep the patient as close to your body as possible to prevent reaching.

The Veterans Health Administration and many other health care systems follow a no-lift or limited-lift policy for all of their facilities due in large part to technology. That means that nurses and therapists either rely on the patient to independently move and transfer or use a powered, mechanical full-body lift that is either ceiling- or wall-mounted or portable (mobile) (Fig. 6-5). Most lifts use slings that are comfortable, safe, and easy to apply. Electric-powered, portable sit-to-stand devices are also available.

Instead of a no-lift policy, though, some long-term care facilities limit lifting to 35 pounds (15.9 kg). These changes involve intensive staff training and compliance to prevent staff injury. Mechanical lifts are also available for home use.

For patients who are learning to become independent in transfer or bed MOBILITY skills, the physical or occupational therapist usually specifies the procedure for these maneuvers. For example, a quadriplegic patient may use a sliding board for transfer, whereas a paraplegic patient may need a wheelchair with removable arms. A patient still in bed may be taught to turn independently using the siderails. In any case, for safety, always plan or teach the patient to plan the transfer technique before initiating it. The desired outcome is that the patient will eventually be able to transfer independently *and* safely.

If the patient has problems maintaining blood pressure while out of bed, the physical therapist may start him or her on a tilt table to gradually increase tolerance. A low blood pressure is a particularly common problem for patients who are quadriplegic because they have a delayed blood flow to the brain and upper part of the body.

! NURSING SAFETY PRIORITY (QSEN)
Critical Rescue

Before any transfer, carefully observe for potential problems. Orthostatic, or postural, hypotension is a common problem in rehabilitation settings and contributes to falls, which are common for any patient with impaired mobility. If the patient moves from a lying to a sitting or standing position too quickly, his or her blood pressure drops; as a result, he or she becomes dizzy or faints. This problem is worsened by antihypertensive drugs, especially in older adults. To prevent this situation, help the patient change positions slowly, with frequent rest periods to allow the blood pressure to stabilize. If needed, measure blood pressure with the patient in the lying, sitting, and standing positions to examine the differences. **Orthostatic hypotension** is indicated by a drop of more than 20 mm Hg in systolic pressure or 10 mm Hg in diastolic pressure between positions. Notify the health care provider and the therapists about this change.

Weight gain is another potential problem when rehabilitation patients have impaired MOBILITY. Excessive weight hinders transfers both for the nurse or the therapist who is assisting and for the patient who is learning to transfer independently. Weight is usually checked every week to monitor gains or losses. If needed, collaborate with the dietitian to plan a weight-reduction diet for the patient.

Gait Training. The physical therapist works with patients for gait training if they are able to ambulate. While regaining the ability to ambulate, patients may need to use assistive devices, such as a variety of canes or walkers (Fig. 6-6). The specific device selected for each patient depends on the amount of weight bearing that is allowed or tolerated. For example, a stroke patient who has problems with maintaining balance or a steady gait when walking might need a walker. Some patients use walkers with rollers made of tennis ball materials; others who fatigue easily may need a walker with a built-in seat to rest at intervals. A patient who had a total hip replacement 6 weeks ago may be able to use a straight (also called *single-point*) cane.

When working with patients who are using these devices, also known as **ambulatory aids,** the physical therapist ensures that there is a level surface on which to walk. The patient wears a transfer (gait) belt for safety so that the therapist or nurse can guide him or her during ambulation to help prevent falls. Use of transfer belts is recommended as one of the best practices for safe patient handling (Waters & Rockefeller, 2010).

Reinforce the physical therapist's instructions and encourage practice, with the outcome being to walk independently with or without an assistive device. Older patients typically use a walker, with or without rollers, for a broader base of support. Younger or minimally impaired patients often progress to the use of a hemi-cane or straight cane. Chart 6-1 outlines best practices for patient safety when teaching patients how to use ambulatory aids.

Some patients never regain the ability to walk because of their impairment, such as advanced multiple sclerosis or complete high spinal cord injury. They may become wheelchair dependent and need to learn wheelchair or motorized scooter mobility skills. With the help of physical and occupational therapy, most patients can learn to move anywhere in a wheelchair or scooter. For example, quadriplegic patients often use motorized wheelchairs that can be directed and propelled by moving their head or blowing into a device. Patients with multiple sclerosis often use scooters to get around.

Assessment Tool and Care Plan for Safe Patient Handling and Movement

I. Patient's Level of Assistance
_____Independent—Patient performs task safely, with or without staff assistance, with or without assistive devices.
_____Partial Assist—Patient requires no more help than standby, cueing, or coaxing, or caregiver is required to lift no more than 35 lbs of a patient's weight.
_____Dependent—Patient requires nurse to lift more than 35 lbs of the patient's weight, or patient is unpredictable in the amount of assistance offered. In this case, assistive devices should be used.

An assessment should be made before each task if the patient has a varying level of ability to assist because of medical reasons, fatigue, medications, etc. When in doubt, assume the patient cannot assist with the transfer/repositioning.

II. Weight-Bearing Capability
_____Full
_____Partial
_____None

III. Bilateral Upper-Extremity Strength
_____Yes
_____No

IV. Patient's Level of Cooperation and Comprehension
_____Cooperative—May need prompting; able to follow simple commands.
_____Unpredictable or variable (patient whose behavior changes frequently should be considered unpredictable)—Not cooperative or unable to follow simple commands.

V. Weight_____ Height_____

Body Mass Index (BMI) (needed if patient's weight is over 300 lbs)*
If BMI exceeds 50, institute Bariatric Algorithms.

The presence of the following conditions is likely to affect the transfer/repositioning process and should be considered when identifying equipment and techniques needed to move the patient.

VI. Check Applicable Conditions Likely to Affect Transfer/Repositioning Techniques
_____Hip/knee/shoulder replacements
_____History of falls
_____Paralysis/paresis
_____Unstable spine
_____Severe edema
_____Very fragile skin

_____Respiratory/cardiac compromise
_____Wounds affecting transfer/positioning
_____Amputation
_____Urinary/fecal stoma
_____Contractures/spasms
_____Tubes (IV, chest, etc.)

_____Fractures
_____Splints/traction
_____Severe osteoporosis
_____Severe pain/discomfort
_____Postural hypotension

Comments: _____
_____
_____
_____
_____

VII. Appropriate Lift/Transfer Devices Needed
Vertical Lift:
Horizontal Lift:
Other Patient-Handling Devices Needed:

Sling Type
_____Seated
_____Supine

_____Seated (Amputee)
_____Ambulation

_____Standing
_____Limb Support

Sling Size _____

Signature _____ Date _____

*If patient weighs more than 300 lbs, the BMI is needed. For online BMI table and calculator, see http://www.nhlbi.nih.gov/guidelines/obesity/bmi_tbl.htm.

FIG. 6-4 Example of a tool to assess physical mobility.

FIG. 6-5 Example of powered, mechanical full-body lift.

FIG. 6-6 Assistive devices for ambulation. Assistive devices vary in the amount of support they provide. A straight (single-point) cane provides less support than a walker (**A**) or quadripod cane (**B**).

CHART 6-1 Best Practice for Patient Safety & Quality Care (QSEN)

Gait Training with Selected Ambulatory Aids

Walker Assisted
- Apply a transfer belt around the patient's waist.
- Guide the patient to a standing position.
- Remind the patient to place both hands on the walker.
- Ensure that the patient is well balanced.
- Teach the patient repeatedly to perform this sequence:
  - Lift the walker.
  - Move the walker about 2 feet forward, and set it down on all legs.
  - While resting on the walker, take small steps.
  - Check balance.
  - Repeat the sequence.

Cane Assisted
- Apply a transfer belt around the patient's waist.
- Guide the patient to a standing position.
- Be sure the cane is at the height of the patient's wrist when the arm is placed at his or her side. (Many canes can be adjusted to the required height.)
- Remind the patient to place his or her strong hand on the cane.
- Ensure that the patient is well balanced.
- Teach the patient to perform this sequence repeatedly:
  - Move the cane and weaker leg forward at the same time.
  - Move the stronger leg one step forward.
  - Check balance and repeat the sequence.

During the rehabilitation phase, patients are at risk for complications of immobility. Table 6-4 lists some of the common complications and strategies the nurse can use to help prevent each complication. Implementing range-of-motion (ROM) routines, adhering to schedules for turning and repositioning, and maintaining skin care are constant components of rehabilitation nursing care to prevent complications of immobility.

One way to increase MOBILITY, even with patients who are bedridden, is through ROM exercises. ROM techniques are beneficial for any patient with decreased mobility. Although simple ROM techniques are presented in basic nursing textbooks, a few key principles are pertinent to rehabilitation nursing care:
- The human body contains more joints than simply the knees, hips, elbows, and shoulders. For ROM techniques

TABLE 6-4 Prevention of the Common Complications of Immobility

BODY SYSTEM	COMPLICATIONS	PREVENTION
Musculoskeletal	Contractures Footdrop Osteoporosis Susceptibility to fractures Muscular atrophy	Foot support while in bed, range-of-motion exercises, high-top tennis shoes Ambulation if possible (walking) Other weight-bearing exercises
Gastrointestinal	Constipation	Sitting in an upright position Increased activity level Increased fluid and fiber intake
Cardiovascular	Decreased cardiac output Increased venous stasis Thrombus formation Embolism	Range-of-motion exercises Exercise Antiembolism stockings Avoidance of leg massage Low–molecular-weight heparin or other anticoagulant
Neurologic	Disorientation	Sleep-wake schedule in accord with light-dark pattern Reorientation (to person, place, time) Control of sensory stimulation
Renal/urinary	Calculi Infection	Decreased dietary calcium level, if needed Increased fluid intake Ensuring low post-void residuals Intermittent catheterization instead of indwelling if possible
Respiratory	Pneumonia	Frequent oral hygiene Frequent repositioning in wheelchair or bed Breathing exercises
Integumentary (Skin)	Pressure ulcers	Frequent repositioning in wheelchair or bed Pressure reduction or relief devices (in bed and wheelchair) Meticulous skin care Adequate nutrition Frequent skin assessments

to be effective in preventing musculoskeletal contractures, the patient must exercise all joints, including each joint of the fingers, hands, toes, and so forth.

- In performing ROM activities, the nurse or patient performs full-range movement of each joint at least five times and completes the entire process at least three times daily.
- The nurse or PT does not move the joints beyond the point at which the patient expresses pain or beyond the point at which resistance occurs.

Patients with decreased MOBILITY who are able to follow directions are taught by the nurse and the physical therapist to perform active or active-assisted ROM exercises.

Increasing Functional Ability

Planning: Expected Outcomes. The patient with chronic illness or disability is expected to increase functional ability in self-care and other self-management skills with or without assistive/adaptive devices.

Interventions. ADLs, or self-care activities, include eating, bathing, dressing, grooming, and toileting. Encourage the patient to perform as much self-care as possible. Be patient because he or she often takes more time to complete a task than healthy adults do. Collaborate with the occupational therapist (OT) to identify ways in which self-care activities can be modified so the patient can perform them independently and with minimal frustration if possible. For example, the OT teaches a hemiplegic patient to put on a shirt by first placing the affected arm in the sleeve and then putting the unaffected arm in the appropriate sleeve. Slip-on shoes or shoes with Velcro straps may be recommended for some patients. Encourage patients to practice, and allow them time to try to be independent in ADLs.

In long-term care (LTC) settings, federal regulations require that residents not lose their functional skills while they are in the facility. Therefore most facilities have developed *restorative nursing* programs and have coordinated these programs with rehabilitation therapy and activity therapy. The focus of this coordinated effort includes:

- Bed mobility
- Walking
- Transfers
- Dressing
- Grooming
- Active range of motion
- Communication

A variety of devices are available for patients with chronic illness and disability for *assisting with self-care*. An **assistive/adaptive device,** or self-care support device, is any item that enables the patient to perform all or part of an activity independently and safely. Examples include long-handled shoehorns and reachers to prevent bending and losing one's balance. Table 6-5 identifies common devices and describes their use.

Many medical equipment stores and large pharmacies carry clothing and assistive/adaptive devices designed for patients with disabilities. The occupational therapist determines specific patient needs for this equipment. Collaborate with the occupational therapist to look for creative and inexpensive alternatives to meeting these needs. For example, barbecue tongs may be used as "reachers" for pulling up pants or obtaining items on high shelves. A foam curler with the plastic insert removed may be placed over a pencil or eating utensil to make a built-up

TABLE 6-5   Examples and Uses of Common Assistive/Adaptive Devices

DEVICE	USE
Buttonhook	Threaded through the buttonhole to enable patients with weak finger mobility to button shirts Alternative uses include serving as pencil holder or cigarette holder
Extended shoehorn	Assists in the application of shoes for patients with decreased mobility Alternative uses include turning light switches off or on while patient is in a wheelchair
Plate guard and spork (spoon and fork in one utensil)	Applied to a plate to assist patients with weak hand and arm mobility to feed themselves; spork allows one utensil to serve two purposes
Gel pad	Placed under a plate or a glass to prevent dishes from slipping and moving Alternative uses include placement under bathing and grooming items to prevent them from moving
Foam buildups	Applied to eating utensils to assist patients with weak hand grasps to feed themselves Alternative uses include application to pens and pencils to assist with writing or over a buttonhook to assist with grasping the device
Hook and loop fastener (Velcro) straps	Applied to utensils, a buttonhook, or a pencil to slip over the hand and provide a method of stabilizing the device when the patient's hand grasp is weak
Long-handled reacher	Assists in obtaining items located on high shelves or at ground level for patients who are unable to change positions easily
Elastic shoelaces or Velcro shoe closure	Eliminates the need for tying shoes

device. The patient might use an extended shoehorn to operate light switches from wheelchair height. Hook-and-loop fasteners (Velcro) sewn on clothes can prevent the frustrations caused by buttons and zippers.

Assistive technology has further increased the ability for disabled patients to care for themselves using electronic equipment. For example, telephones and computer keyboards can be operated by voice-activation devices. **Robotic technology** provides mechanical parts for the extremities when they are not functional or have been amputated. The cost of these aids has prevented their widespread use (Stein, 2012).

Fatigue often occurs with chronic and disabling conditions. Therefore collaborate with the OT to assess the patient's self-care abilities and to determine possible ways of *conserving energy.* Coordinate with the therapist to develop strategies for energy conservation after evaluating the patient's self-care routines. Preparation for ADLs can help reduce effort and energy expenditure (e.g., gathering all necessary equipment before starting grooming routines). If a patient has high energy levels in the morning, he or she can be taught to schedule energy-intensive activities in the morning rather than later in the day or evening. Spacing activities is also helpful for conserving energy. In addition, allowing time to rest before and after eating and toileting decreases the strain on energy level.

A 61-year-old widower is admitted to an inpatient facility for rehabilitation after a right knee replacement for severe osteoarthritis that resulted from his carpentry job. He lives alone in a one-story house and has two daughters nearby who visit every week. After his wife died 10 years ago, the patient was diagnosed with diabetes mellitus type 2 and hypertension. His serum cholesterol is elevated, and he is overweight. His favorite foods are fried chicken, mashed potatoes and gravy, and homemade buttermilk biscuits, which his daughters frequently prepare for him. As his nurse, you complete his admission assessment.

1. What are this patient's priority problems?
2. With what health care team members will you need to collaborate?
3. What safe patient handling practices would you need to use?
4. What type of ambulatory assistive device would be most appropriate for him at this time?
5. What health teaching does the patient need regarding his mobility and nutrition?

Maintaining Skin Integrity

Planning: Expected Outcomes. The patient with chronic illness or disability is expected to have intact skin and TISSUE INTEGRITY.

Interventions. *The best intervention to prevent skin breakdown and maintain tissue integrity is frequent position changes in combination with adequate skin care and sufficient nutritional intake.* Teach staff to *turn and reposition all patients at least every 2 hours* if they are unable to perform this activity. This time frame may not be sufficient for people who are frail and have thin skin, especially older adults. To determine the best turning schedule, assess the patient's skin condition during each turning and repositioning. For example, if the patient has been sleeping for 2 hours and the nursing assistant decides to postpone turning for 1 hour, reddened areas over the bony prominences may be present. If reddened areas do not fade within 30 minutes after pressure relief or do not blanch, they may be classified as pre-ulcer areas, or stage I pressure areas (see Chapter 25).

Patients who sit for prolonged periods in a wheelchair need to be repositioned at least every 1 to 2 hours. Each patient is evaluated by the physical or occupational therapist for the best seating pad or cushion that is comfortable yet reduces pressure on bony prominences. Patients who are able are taught to perform "wheelchair push-ups" by using their arms to lift their buttocks off the wheelchair seat for 10 seconds or longer every hour, or more often if needed. The PT helps them strengthen their arm muscles in preparation for performing wheelchair push-ups.

If the patient wears high-top tennis shoes for foot positioning to prevent footdrop, remove the shoes and assess for pressure areas every 2 hours. Many patients with neurologic problems have decreased or absent sensation and may not be able to feel the discomfort of increased pressure. Also, check patients who are sitting in wheelchairs for signs of pressure, especially on the lower legs where the leg of the wheelchair could rub against the skin.

Adequate skin care is an essential component of prevention. Perform or assist patients in completing skin care each time they are turned, repositioned, or bathed. Delegate and supervise skin care to unlicensed assistive personnel (UAP), including cleaning soiled areas, drying carefully, and applying a moisturizer. If a patient is incontinent, use topical barrier creams or ointments to help protect the skin from moisture, which can contribute to skin breakdown. *To prevent damage to the already fragile capillary system, teach UAP to avoid rubbing reddened areas.* Instead, carefully observe the areas for further breakdown and relieve pressure on the areas as much as possible. Bed pillows are often good pressure-relieving devices. (See Chapter 25 for a complete discussion of skin care interventions.)

Sufficient NUTRITION is needed both to repair wounds and to prevent pressure ulcers. Collaborate with the dietitian to assess the patient's food selection and ensure that it contains adequate protein and carbohydrates. Both the nurse and the dietitian closely monitor the patient's weight and serum prealbumin levels. If either of these indices decreases significantly, the patient may need high-protein, high-carbohydrate food supplements (e.g., milkshakes) or commercial preparations. Chapter 60 describes nutritional supplementation in detail.

Pressure-relieving or pressure-reducing devices include waterbeds, gel mattresses or pads, air mattresses, low–air loss overlays or beds, and air-fluidized beds. Mattress overlays, such as air and gel types, and replacement mattresses are often effective in reducing pressure. *The use of any mechanical device (except air-fluidized beds) does not eliminate the need for turning and repositioning.*

Specialty beds are categorized as either "low air loss" or "air fluidized." Air-fluidized therapy (e.g., Clinitron Rite Hite® bed) provides the most effective pressure relief by distributing the patient's weight to prevent pressure in any one area. These beds are not often used to *prevent* skin breakdown because insurers may not reimburse the agency for the use of the bed. Therefore these special beds are reserved for *severe skin problems* that have not healed with the use of a conventional bed or other mechanical device. The primary disadvantage of this therapy is its expense, which may exceed several hundred dollars for each day of use. Patients also report discomfort from the heat generated by the bed. Although air-fluidized beds are heavy to move, lighter and more portable versions are available for home use. The cost of air-fluidized therapy is reimbursed by some health insurance providers if the bed is deemed medically necessary to treat the patient's skin problem.

Establishing Urinary Continence

Planning: Expected Outcomes. Most patients with chronic illness or disability are expected to have normal patterns of urinary ELIMINATION without retention, infection, or incontinence.

Interventions. Neurologic disabilities often interfere with successful bladder control in a patient undergoing rehabilitation. These disabilities result in two basic functional types of neurogenic bladder: overactive (e.g., reflex or spastic bladder) and underactive (e.g., hypotonic or flaccid bladder).

An overactive **spastic** (upper motor neuron) **bladder** causes incontinence with sudden, gushing voids. The bladder does not usually empty completely, and the patient is at risk for urinary tract infection. Neurologic problems affecting the upper motor neuron typically occur in patients with strokes or with high-level spinal cord injuries (cervical) or those above the midthoracic region. These injuries result in a failure of impulse transmission from the lower spinal cord areas to the cortex of the brain. Therefore when the bladder fills and transmits impulses to the spinal cord, the patient cannot perceive the sensation. Because there is no injury to the *lower* spinal cord and the voiding reflex arc is intact, the efferent (motor) impulse from a distended bladder is relayed and the bladder contracts.

Experimental technology using sacral neuromodulation is being tested with complete spinal cord–injury patients. The results have been positive in preventing urinary incontinence in patients with spastic bladders (Sievert et al., 2010).

Nonpharmacologic Management. An underactive **flaccid** or **areflexic** (lower motor neuron) **bladder** results in urinary retention and overflow (dribbling). Injuries that damage the lower motor neuron at the spinal cord level of S2-4 (e.g., multiple sclerosis, spinal cord injury or tumor below T12) may directly interfere with the reflex arc or may result in inaccurate interpretation of impulses to the brain. The bladder fills, and afferent (sensory) impulses conduct the message via the spinal cord to the brain cortex. Because of the injury, the impulse is not interpreted correctly by the brain's bladder center and there is a failure to respond with a message for the bladder to contract.

Patients who cannot completely empty their bladder are at risk for post-void residual urine and subsequent possible urinary tract infection. **Post-void residual (PVR)** is the amount of urine remaining in the bladder within 20 minutes after voiding. PVR assessments using a noninvasive ultrasound device called the *BladderScan* are performed by nurses at the bedside. The residual amount measured is accurate if the device is used correctly. It is not accurate when used for morbidly obese patients. The outcome of bladder ultrasonography is to prevent the use of an indwelling urinary catheter. Long-term urinary catheters cause urinary tract infections that are often chronic. A picture of the BladderScan device is in Chapter 65 (see Fig. 65-10).

The nurse can teach a variety of techniques to assist the patient in retraining or repatterning voiding, including (Table 6-6):
- Facilitating, or triggering, techniques
- Intermittent catheterization
- Consistent scheduling of toileting routines; "timed void"

These techniques may not be as effective in patients with physiologic changes associated with aging, including stress incontinence in women with weak pelvic floor muscles and overflow incontinence in men with enlarged prostate glands.

Facilitating (triggering) techniques are used to stimulate voiding. If there is an upper motor neuron problem but the reflex arc is intact (reflex bladder pattern), the voiding response can be initiated by any stimulus that sends the message to the spinal cord level S2-4 that the bladder might be full. Such techniques include stroking the medial aspect of the thigh, pinching the area above the groin, massaging the penoscrotal area, pinching the posterior aspect of the glans penis, and providing digital anal stimulation.

When the patient has a lower motor neuron problem, the voiding reflex arc is not intact (flaccid bladder pattern) and additional stimulation may be needed to initiate voiding. Two techniques used to facilitate voiding are the Valsalva maneuver and the Credé maneuver. For the Valsalva maneuver, teach the patient to hold his or her breath and bear down as if trying to defecate. This technique should not be used by spinal cord–injured patients who are at risk for bradycardia due to loss of vagus nerve control. Assist the patient in performing the **Credé maneuver** by placing the patient's hand in a cupped position directly over the bladder area and instructing him or her to push inward and downward gently as if massaging the bladder to empty.

Intermittent catheterization may be needed for a flaccid or spastic bladder. Initially, a urinary catheter is inserted to drain urine every few hours—after the patient has attempted voiding and has used the Valsalva and Credé maneuvers. If less than 100 to 150 mL of post-void residual is obtained, the nurse typically increases the interval between catheterizations. *The patient should not go beyond 8 hours between catheterizations.* If intermittent self-catheterization is needed at home after discharge from the rehabilitation facility, the patient may use a specialized appliance to help perform the procedure, especially if he or she has problems with manual dexterity. For patients who cannot catheterize themselves, a family member or significant other may need to be taught how to perform the procedure.

Most patients who need intermittent catheterization have chronic bacteriuria (bacteria in the urine with a positive culture), especially those with spinal cord injury (SCI). Unless the patient has symptoms of a urinary tract infection (UTI), such as fever or burning when voiding, the infection is not treated.

! **NURSING SAFETY PRIORITY** (QSEN)
Action Alert

To *prevent* UTI, teach patients and their caregivers to wash their hands thoroughly before and after catheterization and clean the genital area well. Remind the patient to drink at least 8 to 10 glasses of fluid (two quarts) every day by dinnertime and avoid carbonated beverages. If patients have indwelling urinary catheters, remind them to drink 15 glasses of fluid (three quarts) each day before dinner and avoid carbonated beverages.

TABLE 6-6	**Management of Neurogenic Bladder**		
FUNCTIONAL TYPE	**NEUROLOGIC DISABILITY**	**DYSFUNCTION**	**RE-ESTABLISHING VOIDING PATTERNS**
Reflex (spastic)	Upper motor neuron spinal cord injury above T12	Urinary frequency, incontinence but may not empty completely	Triggering or facilitating techniques Drug therapy, as appropriate Bedside bladder ultrasound Intermittent catheterization Consistent toileting schedule Indwelling urinary catheter (as last resort) Increased fluids
Flaccid	Lower motor neuron spinal cord injury below T12 (affects S2-4 reflex arc)	Urinary retention, overflow	Valsalva and Credé maneuvers Increased fluids Intermittent or indwelling urinary catheterization

The Natural Medicines Comprehensive Database states that cranberry juice or extract may be effective to help *prevent* UTI (U.S. National Library of Medicine [NIH], 2011). It is not effective for *treating* urinary infection.

Consistent toileting routines may be the best way to re-establish voiding continence when the patient has an overactive bladder. Assess the patient's previous voiding pattern, and determine his or her daily routine. At a minimum, the nurse or nursing staff assists the patient with voiding after awakening in the morning, before and after meals, before and after physical activity, and at bedtime. *Remind the staff to toilet the patient every 2 hours during the day and every 3 to 4 hours at night.*

Consider the patient's bladder capacity, which may range from 100 to 500 mL, as well as MOBILITY limitations and restrictive clothing. Bladder capacity is determined by measuring urine output. Ensure that the patient is aware of nearby bathrooms at all times or has a call system to contact the nurse or unlicensed assistive personnel for assistance. Chapter 66 also describes methods of achieving bladder control.

Drug Therapy. Drugs are not commonly used for urinary ELIMINATION problems. Mild overactive bladder problems may be treated with antispasmodics, such as oxybutynin (Ditropan XL, Apo-Oxybutynin ✦), solifenacin (VESIcare), or tolterodine (Detrol LA), to prevent incontinence on a short-term basis.

CONSIDERATIONS FOR OLDER ADULTS
Patient-Centered Care (QSEN)

When urinary antispasmodic drugs are used in older adults, observe for, document, and report hallucinations, delirium, or other acute cognitive changes due to the anticholinergic effects of the drugs.

Patients with symptomatic UTIs are managed with short-term antibiotics, such as trimethoprim (Trimpex) or trimethoprim/sulfamethoxazole (Septra, Bactrim). Patients who have frequent UTIs may be placed on pulse antibiotic therapy in which they alternate one week of antibiotic therapy with 3 weeks without antibiotics. Report the patient's progress in bladder training to the rehabilitation team so that the best decision regarding drug therapy can be made.

Establishing Bowel Continence
Planning: Expected Outcomes. The patient with chronic illness or disability is expected to have regular evacuation of stool without constipation. If possible, patients will control their bowel ELIMINATION schedule.

Interventions. Neurologic problems often affect the patient's bowel pattern by causing a reflex (spastic) bowel, a flaccid bowel, or an uninhibited bowel. Bowel retraining programs are designed for each patient to best meet the expected outcomes (Table 6-7). Pardee et al. (2012) found that establishing a successful bowel program can also enhance the quality of life for patients, especially those who have a spinal cord injury (SCI).

Upper motor neuron diseases and injuries, such as a cervical or mid-level spinal cord injury, may result in a reflex (spastic) bowel pattern, with defecation occurring suddenly and without warning. With a reflex pattern, any facilitating or triggering mechanism may lead to defecation if the lower colon contains stool. An example of facilitating or triggering techniques is digital stimulation. For this technique, use a lubricated glove or finger cot and massage the anus in a circular motion for no less than 1 full minute.

⚠ NURSING SAFETY PRIORITY (QSEN)
Critical Rescue

Do not use digital stimulation for patients with cardiac disease because of the risk for inducing a vagal nerve response. This response causes a rapid decrease in heart rate (bradycardia).

Lower motor neuron diseases and injuries interfere with transmission of the nervous impulse across the reflex arc and may result in a flaccid bowel pattern, with defecation occurring infrequently and in small amounts. The use of manual disimpaction may get the best results. Some patients also need oral laxatives and/or stool softeners (Coggrave & Norton, 2010) (see the Evidence-Based Practice box).

Neurologic injuries that affect the brain may cause an uninhibited bowel pattern, with frequent defecation, urgency, and reports of hard stool. Patients may manage uninhibited bowel patterns through a consistent toileting schedule, a high-fiber diet, and the use of stool softeners.

In some cases, patients are not able to regain their previous level of control over their bowel function. The rehabilitation team assists in designing a bowel ELIMINATION program that accommodates the disability.

TABLE 6-7	**Management of Neurogenic Bowel**		
FUNCTIONAL TYPE	**NEUROLOGIC DISABILITY**	**DYSFUNCTION**	**RE-ESTABLISHING DEFECATION PATTERNS**
Reflex (spastic)	Upper motor neuron spinal cord injury above T12	Defecation without warning, but may not empty completely	Triggering mechanisms Facilitation techniques High-fiber diet Increased fluids Laxative use (for some patients) Consistent toileting schedule Manual disimpaction
Flaccid	Lower motor neuron spinal cord injury below T12 (affects S2-4 reflex arc)	Usually absent stools for patients with complete lesions	Triggering or facilitating techniques Increased fluids High-fiber diet Suppository use Consistent toileting schedule Manual disimpaction

EVIDENCE-BASED PRACTICE (QSEN)

Manual Bowel Disimpaction in Patients with Spinal Cord Injury

Coggrave, M.J., & Norton, C. (2010). The need for manual evacuation and oral laxatives in the management of neurogenic bowel dysfunction after spinal cord injury: A randomized controlled trial of a stepwise protocol. *Spinal Cord, 48*(6), 504-510.

The researchers used a randomized controlled design to test interventions needed to maintain bowel continence among patients who had spinal cord injuries for many years. The 68 volunteers were randomized into an intervention group of 35 and a control group of 33. The control group used their usual bowel management program. The intervention group used oral laxatives and manual disimpaction in a stepwise protocol and in combination. All study participants kept bowel diaries for 6 weeks.

Findings from the study showed that manual disimpaction significantly improved bowel continence more than oral laxatives or other bowel management programs. Some patients needed both laxatives and disimpaction to maintain bowel continence.

Level of Evidence: 1

This study used a randomized controlled design to compare bowel management interventions between a control group and an experimental group that used two specific bowel management interventions—manual disimpaction and oral laxatives.

Commentary: Implications for Practice and Research

This research added to the evidence for planning the best bowel management protocol for spinal cord–injured patients. Nurses can use this information to teach patients how to maintain bowel continence. Bowel control is a sensitive and embarrassing patient problem, and nurses can be instrumental in teaching patients about which methods achieve the best outcome.

Collaborate with patients to schedule bowel ELIMINATION as close as possible to their previous routine. For example, a patient who had stools at noon every other day before the illness or injury should have the bowel program scheduled in the same way. An exception is the patient who prefers another time that best fits into his or her daily routine. If the patient is employed during the day, a time-consuming bowel elimination program in the morning may not work. The bowel protocol can then be changed to the evening when there is more time.

Bowel retraining programs for patients with neurologic problems are often designed to include a combination of methods. Although drug therapy should not be a first choice when formulating a bowel training program, consider the need for a suppository if the patient does not re-establish defecation habits through a consistent toileting schedule, dietary modification, anal stimulation, and disimpaction.

Bisacodyl (Dulcolax), a commonly used laxative, may be prescribed either rectally or orally as part of a bowel training program. Suppositories must be placed against the bowel wall to stimulate the sacral reflex arc and promote rectal emptying. Results occur in 15 to 30 minutes. Administer the suppository when the patient expects to defecate, for example, after a meal to coincide with the gastrocolic reflex. Using the suppository every second or third day is usually effective in re-establishing defecation patterns.

Many rehabilitation patients are at high risk for constipation, especially older adults. Encourage fluids (at least 8 glasses a day) and 20 to 35 g of fiber in the diet. Teach patients to eat 2 to 3 daily servings of whole grains, legumes, and bran cereals and 5 daily servings of fruits and vegetables. Do not offer a bedpan when toileting. Instead, be sure that the patient sits upright on a bedside commode or bathroom toilet to facilitate defecation.

? NCLEX EXAMINATION CHALLENGE

Physiological Integrity

Which statement by a quadriplegic client indicates a need for the nurse to provide further teaching about bowel retraining?
A. "I'll eat low-fiber foods each day to prevent diarrhea."
B. "I'll drink at least a quart of water or other liquids every day."
C. "I'll do my daily bowel training routine after I eat breakfast."
D. "I'll use a suppository to help empty my rectum."

Community-Based Care

Discharge planning begins at the time of the patient's admission. If the patient is transferred from a hospital to a rehabilitation unit or long-term care facility, orient him or her to the change in routine and emphasize the importance of self-care. When the patient is admitted, a nurse, case manager, and/or OT assess his or her current living situation at home. Together with the patient and family members or significant others, they determine the adequacy of the current situation and the potential needs after discharge to home. The patient with chronic illness and disability may require home care, assistance with ADLs, nursing care, or physical or occupational therapy after discharge.

Other health care professionals may be necessary to meet the unique needs of special populations. For example, patients with brain injury may benefit from life planning—a process that examines and plans to meet lifelong needs. External case managers specializing in life planning may be part of the interdisciplinary rehabilitation team.

Home Care Management. Before the patient returns home, the nurse assesses his or her readiness for discharge from the rehabilitation facility or hospital. The home may be assessed in multiple ways and points in time.

Predischarge Assessment. Before discharge, the case manager or OT may visit the home to assess its layout and accessibility. These professionals may be employed by the health care agency or by a third-party payer, such as a health maintenance organization. Because of the stress of hospitalization, a patient with a fractured hip who is ambulating well with a walker may neglect to explain to the nurse that the bathroom in the home is accessible by stairway only. The patient may not consider it important to mention that throw rugs, which can cause falls, are scattered throughout the apartment. Fall prevention strategies in the home environment for older adults are discussed in Chapter 2.

During a predischarge visit to the home, the accessibility of bathrooms, bedrooms, and kitchen is assessed. If the patient will be wheelchair dependent after discharge from the facility, home modifications may be needed, such as ramps to replace steps. Doorways should be checked for adequate width. A doorway width of 36 to 38 inches (slightly less than 1 meter [m]) is usually sufficient for a standard-size wheelchair. Obese patients require bariatric wheelchairs and furniture and therefore need a wider door opening. Any room that the patient needs to use is assessed. The bedroom should have sufficient space for the patient to maneuver transfers to and from the wheelchair and the bed, if needed. The bathroom may need a raised toilet seat to at least 17 inches (43 cm).

Space requirements depend on the patient's need to use a wheelchair, walker, or cane. In the bathroom, grab bars may need to be installed before the patient comes home. Bathtub benches can provide support for the patient who has difficulty with mobility and, when used in combination with a handheld showerhead, can provide easily accessible bathing facilities. Assessment of the kitchen may or may not be critical, depending on whether the patient has help with cooking and preparing meals. If the patient will be cooking after discharge, the kitchen may need to be assessed for wheelchair or walker accessibility, appliance accessibility, and the need for adaptive equipment.

Leave-of-Absence Visit. A second method of assessing the patient's home is through a brief home visit, also called a *leave-of-absence (LOA) visit*, before discharge. Explain the need for the trial home visit, and assess the patient's comfort level with this idea. The patient who has been hospitalized for a lengthy period may feel intense anxiety about returning home. The nurse may allay such anxieties with careful preparation. Before the visit, the rehabilitation nurse meets with the patient and family members or significant others to set goals for the visit and to identify specific tasks to be attempted while at home. After the home visit, interview the patient to determine the success of the visit and to assess additional education or training needs before final discharge.

Going home may not be an option for everyone. Some patients may not have a support network of family members or significant others. For example, many older adults have no spouse or close friends living nearby. Children may live far away, which can make home care difficult. If no caregiver is available, the family must decide whether care can be provided in the home by an outside resource. The patient may need to be admitted to a 24-hour supervised health care setting, such as a nursing home. Continued rehabilitation services are available in most long-term care settings (skilled nursing facilities) at least 5 days a week if it is medically necessary.

Self-Management Education. The OT and PT teach the patient to perform ADLs and IADLs independently. The patient's learning potential and cognitive capacity are assessed. The patient is asked to perform or direct each skill or technique independently to verify understanding. Written material explaining the steps in the procedure is provided to the patient and family members to reinforce learning and to provide support with the technique after discharge. Before distributing written material, the rehabilitation team assesses the reading level of the material and determines whether it is appropriate for the patient's reading ability and language skills.

Any chronic illness or disability necessitates changes in lifestyle and body image. Assist the patient in dealing with such changes by encouraging verbalization of feelings and emotions. A focus on existing capabilities instead of disabilities is emphasized.

The patient may fail to relate psychologically to the disability during hospitalization. For example, he or she may display anger or frustration in attempting to perform self-care routines before discharge from the rehabilitation facility. Encourage the patient to be open about such feelings and to talk about ways to prevent worries from becoming realities after discharge. If needed, refer the patient to a mental health care professional to help with adjustment and coping strategies.

The LOA home visit assists the patient and family members or significant others in psychosocial preparation for discharge. It allows the experience of the home situation while being able to return to the hospital environment after a few hours. Often the patient finds new problems in the home that must be addressed before discharge. Review this information with the patient in preparation for discharge to the home.

Health Care Resources. After discharge to the home, various health care resources (e.g., physical therapy, home care nursing, vocational counseling) are available to the patient with chronic illness and disability. Assess the need for additional care and support throughout the hospitalization, and coordinate with the case manager and physician in arranging for home services. A newer process using technology called *tele-health*, or *tele-rehabilitation* allows for care coordination in the home setting. Through the use of various electronic devices, phone, or computer software, a health care team member can monitor the patient's vital signs, weight, and other assessment data. Other programs, such as Rehab@Home, allow patients to perform therapeutic exercises at home using Wii, a webcam, and a computer.

◆ Evaluation: Outcomes

The patient and rehabilitation team evaluate the effectiveness of interdisciplinary interventions based on the common patient problems. Expected outcomes may include that the patient will:

- Reach a level of physical mobility that allows him or her to function independently with or without assistive devices
- Prevent complications of decreased physical mobility
- Perform self-care and other self-management skills independently or with minimal assistance, possibly using assistive/adaptive devices
- Have intact skin and underlying tissues
- Establish urinary continence without infection or retention
- Have regular evacuation of stool without constipation

GET READY FOR THE NCLEX® EXAMINATION!

KEY POINTS

Review these Key Points for each NCLEX Examination Client Needs Category.

Safe and Effective Care Environment

- Recall that rehabilitation is the process of learning to live with chronic and disabling conditions; the role of the rehabilitation nurse is outlined in Table 6-1.
- Collaborate with members of the interdisciplinary rehabilitation team, including physicians, nurse practitioners, physiotherapists, occupational therapists, dietitians, and speech/language pathologists; the patient and family are also members of the team. **Teamwork and Collaboration** QSEN
- Know that acute (short-term) rehabilitation care occurs in a variety of settings, including inpatient rehabilitation facilities (IRFs) and skilled nursing facilities (SNFs) in either a nursing home or hospital.
- Delegate and supervise selected nursing tasks, such as reporting reddened skin areas, as part of quality care for the rehabilitation patient.
- After assessing the home environment, the case manager, OT, and/or rehabilitation nurse make recommendations to the patient and family about home modifications.
- Use evidence-based safe patient handling practices, such as using mechanical lifts and working with other team members, when assessing and moving patients to prevent injury and improve MOBILITY. **Evidence-Based Practice** QSEN
- Recall that the rehabilitation therapists teach patients transfer, bed MOBILITY, and gait training techniques (see Chart 6-1).
- Encourage the patient to be as independent as possible when performing ADLs and safe MOBILITY skills.

Health Promotion and Maintenance

- In coordination with the PT and OT, assess the patient's ability to perform ADLs and MOBILITY skills using a functional assessment process. **Teamwork and Collaboration** QSEN
- Prevent complications of immobility for patients, and teach them how to prevent complications by using interventions listed in Table 6-4. Examples include pressure ulcers, urinary calculi, constipation, and venous thromboembolism. **Evidence-Based Practice** QSEN

Psychosocial Integrity

- Assess the patient's self-esteem and changes in body image caused by chronic or disabling health problems.
- Assess the patient's COGNITION to screen for depression, delirium, and dementia using tools such as the Confusion Assessment Method (CAM), especially for older adults.
- Assess the patient's and family's response to chronic and disabling conditions, including feelings of loss and grief.
- Assist patients in coping with their loss, and assess the availability of patient support systems, especially for older adults. **Patient-Centered Care** QSEN

Physiological Integrity

- Assess rehabilitation patients as outlined in Table 6-2 to help plan appropriate collaborative care.
- Review the Functional Independence Measure (FIM) system as one assessment tool used to assess functional ability of the patient in rehabilitation, including the need for assistive/adaptive devices.
- Recognize that the Minimum Data Set (MDS) 3.0 is the comprehensive assessment tool required by the Centers for Medicare and Medicaid Services that is used in long-term care/nursing home settings (see Table 6-3).
- Assess patients in rehabilitation for risk factors that make them likely to develop skin breakdown; interventions to prevent skin problems include repositioning and adequate NUTRITION. **Quality Improvement** QSEN
- Patients with neurogenic bladder and bowel problems are managed by training programs; overactive (spastic or reflex) and underactive (hypotonic or flaccid) elimination problems are managed differently (see Tables 6-6 and 6-7).
- In collaboration with the rehabilitation therapists, evaluate the ability of patients to use assistive/adaptive devices to promote independence. **Teamwork and Collaboration** QSEN
- Determine patient and family needs regarding discharge to home or other community-based setting.

End-of-Life Care

Mary K. Kazanowski

PRIORTY CONCEPTS

- PALLIATION
- PAIN
- COGNITION
- PERFUSION

LEARNING OUTCOMES

Safe and Effective Care Environment
1. Describe the importance of collaborating with members of the interdisciplinary team when caring for the dying patient and family or other caregivers.
2. Discuss the ethical and legal obligations of the nurse with regard to end-of-life care.

Health Promotion and Maintenance
3. Explain to patients and their families the purpose and procedure for advance directives.

Psychosocial Integrity
4. Assess the patient's and family's ability to cope with the dying process.
5. Assess and plan interventions to meet the dying patient's spiritual needs.

6. Incorporate the patient's cultural practices and beliefs when providing care during the dying process and death.
7. Identify the need for providing psychosocial support to the family or other caregivers during the patient's dying process.

Physiological Integrity
8. Describe the pathophysiology of death.
9. Compare the concepts of hospice and PALLIATION.
10. Assess patients for signs and symptoms related to the end of life.
11. Explain how to provide evidence-based end-of-life care to the dying patient, including symptom management.
12. Explain best practice guidelines for performing postmortem care.

OVERVIEW OF DEATH AND DYING

Although dying is part of the normal life cycle, it is often feared as a time of PAIN and suffering. For the family, death of a member is a life-altering loss that can cause significant and prolonged suffering. As sad and difficult as the death may be, the experience of dying need not be physically painful for the patient or emotionally agonizing for the family. The dying process is an opportunity to change a potentially difficult situation into one that is tolerable, peaceful, and meaningful for the patient and the family left behind.

Because nurses spend more time with patients than do any other health care providers, it is the nurse who often has the greatest impact on a person's experience with death. A nurse can affect the dying process to prevent death without dignity (bad death) from occurring while striving to promote a peaceful and meaningful death (good death). To accomplish this desired outcome, nurses need to have knowledge of end-of-life care, compassion, advocacy, and therapeutic communication skills (Clabots, 2012).

A good death is one that is free from avoidable distress and suffering for patients, families, and caregivers; in agreement with patients' and families' wishes; and consistent with clinical practice standards. Persistent PAIN, not having one's wishes followed at the end of one's life, isolation, abandonment, and agonizing about losses associated with death are characteristics of a bad death.

Death in the United States

Table 7-1 lists the most common causes of death in the United States. Of all people who die, only a small percentage of them die suddenly and unexpectedly. Most people die after a long period of illness (e.g., cardiac, renal, respiratory disease), with gradual deterioration until an active dying phase before the death. Most people who die are older than 65 years.

The U.S. health care system is based on the acute care model, which is focused on prevention, early detection, and cure of disease. This focus and the advances in survival rates for once deadly diseases have made it difficult for many patients and

TABLE 7-1   Leading Causes of Death in the United States
1. Diseases of the heart
2. Malignant neoplasms (cancer)
3. Chronic lower respiratory diseases (e.g., chronic obstructive pulmonary disease [COPD])
4. Cerebrovascular diseases
5. Accidents (unintentional injuries)
6. Alzheimer's disease
7. Diabetes mellitus
8. Influenza and pneumonia
9. Nephritis, nephritic syndrome, and nephrosis
10. Intentional self-harm (suicide)
11. Septicemia
12. Chronic liver disease and cirrhosis
13. Essential hypertension and hypertensive renal disease
14. Parkinson disease
15. Pneumonitis caused by aspiration of solids and liquids

Data from Hoyert, D.L., & Xu, J. (2011). Deaths: Preliminary data for 2011. *National Vital Statistics Reports, 61*(6), 1-52. National Center for Health Statistics. Retrieved December 2013 from www.cdc.gov/nchs/data/nvsr61/nvsr61_06.pdf.

CONSIDERATIONS FOR OLDER ADULTS
Patient-Centered Care QSEN

Older adults in the United States are estimated to account for 75% of deaths each year. Older adults are also more likely than younger adults to think about their needs and preferences related to end of life (EOL). Data suggest that older adults want early discussions with their health care provider in preparation for death (Gillick, 2010). Despite this desire, understanding of preferences and needs related to end of life is lacking.

health care providers to accept death as an outcome of disease. Many view death as a failure.

These negative views have led to a major deficiency in the quality of care provided to many people at the end of life. In 1995, a landmark study highlighted the poor quality of dying experienced by hospitalized patients. The Study to Understand Prognoses and Preferences for Outcomes and Risks of Treatment (SUPPORT) showed that more than 50% of a sample of 9105 hospitalized patients with a life-threatening disease had moderate to severe pain during the last days of their lives. In addition, they did not have their wishes met, even when their wishes were known.

Pathophysiology of Dying

Death is defined as the cessation of integrated tissue and organ function, manifested by lack of heartbeat, absence of spontaneous respirations, or irreversible brain dysfunction. It generally occurs as a result of an illness or trauma that overwhelms the compensatory mechanisms of the body, eventually leading to cardiopulmonary failure/arrest. Direct causes of death include:

- Heart failure secondary to cardiac dysrhythmias, myocardial infarction, or cardiogenic shock
- Respiratory failure secondary to pulmonary embolism, heart failure, pneumonia, lung disease, or respiratory arrest caused by increased intracranial pressure
- Shock secondary to infection, blood loss, or organ dysfunction, which leads to lack of blood flow (i.e., PERFUSION) to vital organs

Inadequate PERFUSION to body tissues deprives cells of their source of oxygen, which leads to anaerobic metabolism with acidosis, hyperkalemia, and tissue ischemia. Dramatic changes in vital organs lead to the release of toxic metabolites and destructive enzymes, referred to as *multiple organ dysfunction syndrome (MODS)*. As illness or organ damage progresses, the syndrome occurs with renal and liver failure. Renal or liver failure can also *start* the dying process.

When the body is hypoxic and acidotic, a lethal dysrhythmia such as ventricular fibrillation or asystole can occur, which ultimately leads to the lack of cardiac output and PERFUSION. Shortly after cardiac arrest, respiratory arrest occurs. When respiratory arrest occurs first, cardiac arrest follows within minutes.

Planning for End-of-Life and Advance Directives

In 1991, the U.S. Congress passed the Patient Self-determination Act (PSDA), which granted people the right to determine the medical care they wanted provided (or not provided) if they became incapacitated. Documentation of this self-determination is accomplished by completing an **advance directive (AD)**. The PSDA requires that a representative in every health care agency ask patients when admitted if they have written advance directives. Patients who do not have ADs should be provided with information on the value of having an AD in place and given the opportunity to complete the state-required forms. Ideally, advance directives should be completed long before a medical crisis.

Advance directives vary from state to state but are readily available through Caring Connections, an online program of the National Hospice and Palliative Care Organization (www.caringinfo.org). Anyone can complete the advance directive forms without legal consultation. Exact titles for each AD form vary from state to state. Generally speaking, most ADs have a section where one names a **durable power of attorney for health care (DPOAHC)**. The DPOAHC is not the same as DPOA for financial affairs. Most legal representatives recommend that the person who is the durable power of attorney be different from the person who is the durable power of attorney for one's finances.

The DPOAHC is the designation for the person or persons appointed to make one's decisions related to health care in the event the person loses decision-making capacity (Fig. 7-1). The DPOAHC, often referred to as a *health care proxy, health care agent,* or *surrogate decision maker,* does not make health care decisions until a physician states that the person loses or lacks the capacity to make his or her own health care decisions because of impairment in COGNITION.

To have decision-making ability, a person must be able to perform three tasks:

- Receive information (but not necessarily oriented × 4)
- Evaluate, deliberate, and mentally manipulate information
- Communicate a treatment preference

By definition, the comatose patient does not have decisional ability.

The second part of the Advance Directive is a **living will** (LW), which identifies what one would (or would not) want if he or she were near death. Treatments that are discussed include cardiopulmonary resuscitation (CPR), artificial ventilation, and artificial nutrition or hydration. The third type of advance directive is a do-not-resuscitate (DNR) form. A **DNR** is an actual order from a physician or other authorized health care provider who instructs that CPR not be attempted in the event

NEW HAMPSHIRE DURABLE POWER OF ATTORNEY FOR HEALTH CARE

INSTRUCTIONS

PRINT YOUR NAME

PRINT THE NAME AND
ADDRESS OF YOUR
AGENT

INSTRUCTION
STATEMENTS

CIRCLE AND INITIAL THE
RESPONSES THAT
REFLECT YOUR WISHES

TERMINAL ILLNESS

PERMANENTLY
UNCONSCIOUS

ARTIFICIAL NUTRITION
AND HYDRATION

ADD PERSONAL
INSTRUCTIONS (IF ANY)

ALTERNATE AGENT

PRINT THE NAME AND
ADDRESS OF YOUR
ALTERNATE AGENT

LOCATION OF THE
ORIGINAL AND COPIES

DATE AND SIGN THE
DOCUMENT HERE

WITNESSING PROCEDURE

WITNESSES MUST SIGN
AND PRINT THEIR
ADDRESSES

AND A NOTARY PUBLIC
OR JUSTICE OF THE
PEACE MUST COMPLETE
THIS SECTION

©2005 National Hospice and
Palliative Care Organization
2006 Revised

I,_____, hereby appoint _____
          (name)   (name of agent)
of _____
                                              (address)

as my agent to make any and all health care decisions for me, except to the extent I state otherwise in this document or as prohibited by law. This durable power of attorney for health care shall take effect in the event I become unable to make my own health care decisions.

STATEMENT OF DESIRES, SPECIAL PROVISIONS, AND LIMITATIONS REGARDING HEALTH CARE DECISIONS.

For your convenience in expressing your wishes, some general statements concerning the withholding or removal of life-sustaining treatment are set forth below. (Life-sustaining treatment is defined as procedures without which a person would die, such as but not limited to the following: cardiopulmonary resuscitation, mechanical respiration, kidney dialysis or the use of other external mechanical and technological devices, drugs to maintain blood pressure, blood transfusions, and antibiotics.) There is also a section that allows you to set forth specific directions for these or other matters. If you wish, you may indicate your agreement or disagreement with any of the following statements and give your agent power to act in those specific circumstances.

1. If I become permanently incompetent to make health care decisions, and if I am also suffering from a terminal illness, I authorize my agent to direct that life-sustaining treatment be discontinued.
   YES   NO (Circle your choice and initial beneath it.)

2. Whether terminally ill or not, if I become permanently unconscious I authorize my agent to direct that life-sustaining treatment be discontinued.
   YES   NO (Circle your choice and initial beneath it.)

3. I realize that situations could arise in which the only way to allow me to die would be to discontinue artificial feeding (artificial nutrition and hydration). In carrying out any instructions I have given above in #1 or #2 or any instructions I may write in #4 below, I authorize my agent to direct that (circle your choice of [a] or [b] and initial beside it):

   (a) artificial nutrition and hydration not be started or, if started, be discontinued,

   —OR—

   (b) although all other forms of life-sustaining treatment be withdrawn, artificial nutrition and hydration continue to be given to me.

   If you do not complete item 3, your agent will not have the power to direct the withdrawal of artificial nutrition and hydration.

4. Here you may include any specific desires or limitations you deem appropriate, such as when or what life-sustaining treatment you would want used or withheld, or instructions about refusing any specific types of treatment that are inconsistent with your religious beliefs or unacceptable to you for any other reason. You may leave this question blank if you desire.

(attach additional pages as necessary)

In the event the person I appoint above is unable, unwilling or unavailable, or ineligible to act as my health care agent, I hereby appoint

_____ of _____
          (name of alternate agent)   (address of alternate agent)
as alternate agent.

I hereby acknowledge that I have been provided with a disclosure statement explaining the effect of this document. I have read and understand the information contained in the disclosure statement.

The original of this document will be kept at _____ and the following persons and institutions will have signed copies:
In witness, whereof, I have hereunto signed my name this _____ day of _____, 20 _____.
                                                          (day)   (month)   (year)

_____
                                                                        (signature)

I declare that the principal appears to be of sound mind and free from duress at the time the durable power of attorney for health care is signed and that the principal has affirmed that he or she is aware of the nature of the document and is signing it freely and voluntarily.

Witness: _____   Address: _____
Witness: _____   Address: _____

STATE OF NEW HAMPSHIRE, COUNTY OF _____
The foregoing instrument was acknowledged before me this _____ day of _____ , 20 ___, by _____.

_____
Notary Public/Justice of the Peace
My commission expires:

FIG. 7-1 An example of a durable power of attorney for health care (DPOAHC).

of cardiac or respiratory arrest. DNR directives are intended for people with known life-limiting conditions, such as terminal cancer. Depending on the state of residence, people who have made the decision not to be resuscitated may have portable DNR documents and or bracelets to identify themselves as having orders not to resuscitate. Some states also have directives referred to as *POLST* (physician orders for life-sustaining treatment), which document additional treatments in case of cardiac or pulmonary arrest. Like portable DNRs, POLST follow the patient across health care settings.

By law, all health care providers must initiate CPR for a person who is not breathing or is pulseless unless that person has a DNR order. The problem with performing CPR is that it can be a violent, likely painful intervention, which prevents a peaceful death. CPR is also likely to be unsuccessful when performed on a patient with advanced disease and comorbidities, especially when the patient is older than 65 years. Many patients and families, however, do not understand the limitations of CPR and do not realize it was never intended to be performed on patients with end-stage disease (Peberdy et al., 2008).

Hospice and Palliative Care

The concept of hospice in the United States came about from a grassroots effort in response to the unmet needs of terminally ill people. As both a philosophy and a system of care, hospice uses an interdisciplinary approach to assess and address the holistic needs of patients and families to facilitate quality of life and a peaceful death. This holistic approach neither hastens nor postpones death but provides relief of symptoms. Hospice systems of care are provided in a variety of settings. They are often affiliated with home care agencies, providing services to patients at home or in a long-term care or assisted-living facility. Some communities also have hospice houses, which provide care to patients in the terminal phase of their lives.

The *Medicare Hospice Benefit* serves as a guide for hospice care in the United States. This benefit pays for hospice services for Medicare recipients who have a prognosis of 6 months or less to live and who agree to forego curative treatment for their terminal illness. Historically, those with terminal cancer made up the majority of patients receiving hospice care. The proportion of patients with terminal cancer, however, has recently decreased, with increases in numbers of patients with other terminal illnesses, (e.g., dementia, end-stage chronic obstructive pulmonary disease [COPD], cardiac disease, or neurologic disease).

Guidelines are available to assist health care providers and families in identifying who is entitled to hospice care under Medicare. Patients who do not qualify for Medicare may have benefits through private insurance or government medical assistance programs (e.g., Medicaid).

CONSIDERATIONS FOR OLDER ADULTS

Patient-Centered Care QSEN

Although twice as many older adults died in hospice care as in a hospital or nursing home compared with a decade ago, hospice is often treated as a last resort after aggressive critical care (see the Evidence-Based Practice box). Earlier referrals to hospice care by physicians in collaboration with the health care team would increase its benefit for older adults and families.

EVIDENCE-BASED PRACTICE QSEN

When Do Medicare Patients Use Hospice Services?

Kelley, A.S., Deb, P., Du, Q., Aldridge Carlson, M.D., & Morrison, R.S. (2013). Hospice enrollment saves money for Medicare and improves care quality across a number of different lengths-of-stay. *Health Affairs, 32(3)*, 552-561.

Despite the demonstrated potential to improve quality of care and lower costs, the Medicare Hospice Benefit has been found to produce savings only for patients enrolled 53 to 105 days before death. The researchers for this study reviewed data from the Health and Retirement Study data (2002-2008) for the most common hospice enrollment periods, which are: 1 to 7 days, 8 to 14 days, 15 to 30 days, and 53 to 105 days before death. Patients enrolling in these periods in hospice were compared with matched, non-hospice controls.

Within all enrollment periods, hospice patients had significantly lower rates of hospital and critical care use, hospital readmissions, and in-hospital death when compared with the matched non-hospice patients.

Level of Evidence: 1

This was a large systematic study that overcame limitations of previous research.

Commentary: Implications for Practice and Research

This study indicates that hospice is the best model of care for people near death, saves health care costs, and addresses quality of care at the end of life. Nurses should provide information to patients at end of life about the value of hospice to ensure a peaceful, dignified death.

Because benefits and care generally require a prognosis of 6 months or less, its use is limited. Many people with chronic, serious illness whose prognosis may be longer than 6 months often do not have access to the support services that work so well within the hospice model. In an effort to address this need, palliative care has evolved.

Palliative care is a philosophy of care for people with life-threatening disease that assists patients and families in identifying their goals of care, assists them with informed decision making, and facilitates quality symptom management. Unlike hospice, PALLIATION is provided by a physician, nurse practitioner, or team of providers, as a consultation visit, with one or more follow-up visits. Palliative care consults are provided in a large number of hospitals and on an ambulatory care basis in some communities. Table 7-2 compares palliative care to hospice care.

Because of their proximity to patients, nurses are often in the position of assisting patients in exploring their wishes for end-of-life care. To elicit this information, the nurse could ask these questions (Steed, 2012):

- Do you have advance directives?
- Have you thought who you would want to speak for you about your medical care, if you were not able to speak for yourself?
- What are your goals for end-of-life care?
- Have you discussed resuscitation with your health care provider?
- Do you want to be at home at the end of your life?
- Do you currently have any distressing symptoms that are not being controlled?
- Do you feel that your spiritual needs are being met? If not, how can we help meet them?

TABLE 7-2	Comparison of Hospice and Palliative Care	
HOSPICE CARE	**PALLIATIVE CARE**	
Patients have a prognosis of six (6) months or less to live.	Patients can be in any stage of serious illness.	
Care is provided when curative treatment, such as chemotherapy, has been stopped.	A consult is provided that is concurrent with curative therapies or therapies that prolong life.	
Care is provided in 60- and 90-day periods with an opportunity to continue if eligibility criteria are met.	Care is not limited by specific time periods.	
Ongoing care is provided by RNs, social workers, chaplains, and volunteers.	Care is in the form of a consult visit by a physician or advanced practice nurse who makes recommendations; follow-up visits may be provided.	

When developing a plan of care for people nearing the end of their lives, consideration should be given for where the person wants to die. A large percentage of Americans would like to die at home. If this is the patient's preference, work with the patient, family, and health care provider to determine if this goal is possible. Providers trained in end-of-life care are available through hospice agencies who can meet with the patient and family to evaluate their needs and assist them in the discharge plan.

? CLINICAL JUDGMENT CHALLENGE

Patient-Centered Care QSEN

A 77-year-old female with stage IV heart failure has had two hospitalizations for congestive heart failure (CHF) exacerbations in the past month. The patient lives alone and has no durable power of attorney for health care or living will. She tells you she does not need an advance directive because she "can just come back to the hospital and they will take care of me."
1. How would you respond to the patient at this time?
2. What types of referral might you make for her? How would you do this?
3. Is the patient a candidate for hospice at this time? Why or why not?
4. What symptoms of distress do you anticipate?
5. How do you feel about the patient wanting re-hospitalization for heart failure?

❖ PATIENT-CENTERED COLLABORATIVE CARE

◆ Assessment

Obtain information about the patient's diagnosis, past medical history, and recent state of health to identify the risks for symptoms of distress at end of life. People with lung cancer, heart failure, or chronic respiratory disease are at high risk for respiratory distress and dyspnea as they decline. Those with brain tumors are at risk for seizure activity. Patients with tumors near major arteries (e.g., head and neck cancer) are at risk for hemorrhage. Those who have been experiencing PAIN often continue to have pain at the end of life, which may increase, decrease, or remain at the same level of intensity.

Physical Assessment/Clinical Manifestations. As death nears, patients often have signs and symptoms of decline in physical function, manifested as weakness, anorexia, and changes in cardiovascular function, breathing patterns, and GI and genitourinary function. As death nears, peripheral circulation decreases and the patient's skin is often cold, mottled, and cyanotic because of poor tissue PERFUSION. Blood pressure decreases and often is only palpable. The dying person's heart rate may increase, become irregular, and gradually decrease before stopping. Changes in breathing pattern are common, with breaths becoming very shallow and rapid. Periods of apnea and Cheyne-Stokes respirations (apnea alternating with periods of rapid breathing) are also common. Death occurs when respirations and heartbeat stop.

Although these signs and symptoms of physical decline are often disturbing to patients and families, they generally do not cause physical discomfort to the patient. However, symptoms that cause suffering can occur in patients with cancer and non-cancer diagnoses.

Near the end of life, the patient often becomes weak and drowsy, often sleeping 23 or more hours of the day. Eventually he or she can become unresponsive. As the patient's ability to speak diminishes, it is difficult to assess his or her perception of symptoms. When caring for those who are unable to communicate their distress or needs, identify alternative ways to assess symptoms of distress. Teach family caregivers to watch closely for objective signs of discomfort (e.g., restlessness, grimacing, moaning) and identify when these symptoms occur in relation to positioning, movement, medication, or other external stimuli. Teach them how to perform interventions that can help relieve discomfort and stress as described in Chart 7-1.

Although the patient's point of view is the most valid indicator of comfort or distress, the family's perception of symptoms is also important. Family caregivers, health care providers, and dying patients may differ in their perceptions of symptoms in terms of intensity, significance, and meaning. Whereas health care providers are often able to identify symptoms of distress, families are often more knowledgeable about the patient's habits and preferences. Incorporate all pertinent information into the plan for symptom management, and work with patients and families toward a common outcome.

Assess any symptom of distress in terms of intensity, frequency, duration, quality, exacerbating (worsening) and relieving factors, and effect on the patient's comfort when awake or asleep. A method for rating the intensity of symptoms should be used to facilitate ongoing assessments and evaluate treatment response. A rating scale of 0 to 10 is commonly used, with 0 indicating no distress and 10 indicating the worst possible distress. The intensity of the symptom before and after an intervention (e.g., medication) is documented by the nurse or the family caregiver and is used daily to evaluate the patient's overall comfort.

Psychosocial Assessment. People facing death may have fear and/or anxiety about their impending death and experience

🌐 CULTURAL CONSIDERATIONS

Patient-Centered Care QSEN

Be aware that patients differ in their needs at end of life depending on their gender and ethnicity. For example, families may not want to know about the terminal conditions of their loved ones. In some cultures, this decision is based on respect for older family members. Ask the family what they want to know and if they desire the assistance of a language interpreter (Clabots, 2012).

CHART 7-1   Patient and Family Education: Preparing for Self-Management

Common Physical Signs and Symptoms of Approaching Death with Recommended Comfort Measures

Coolness of Extremities
Circulation to the extremities is decreased; the skin may become mottled or discolored.
- Cover the person with a blanket.
- Do not use an electric blanket, hot water bottle, electric heating pad, or hair dryer to warm the person.

Increased Sleeping
Metabolism is decreased.
- Spend time sitting quietly with the person.
- Do not force the person to stay awake.
- Talk to the person as you normally would, even if he or she does not respond.

Fluid and Food Decrease
Metabolic needs have decreased.
- Do not force the person to eat or drink.
- Offer small sips of liquids or ice chips at frequent intervals if the person is alert and able to swallow.
- Use moist swabs to keep the mouth and lips moist and comfortable.
- Coat the lips with lip balm.

Incontinence
The perineal muscles relax.
- Keep the perineal area clean and dry. Use disposable underpads (Chux) and disposable undergarments.
- If the person would be more comfortable, consider a Foley catheter.

Congestion and Gurgling
The person is unable to cough up secretions effectively.
- Position the patient on his or her side.
- Administer medications to decrease the production of secretions.

Breathing Pattern Change
Slowed circulation to the brain may cause the breathing pattern to become irregular, with brief periods of no breathing or shallow breathing.
- Elevate the person's head.
- Position the person on his or her side.

Disorientation
Decreased metabolism and slowed circulation to the brain may occur.
- Identify yourself whenever you communicate with the person.
- Reorient the patient as needed.
- Speak softly, clearly, and truthfully.

Restlessness
Decreased metabolism and slowed circulation to the brain may occur.
- Play soothing music, and use aromatherapy.
- Do not restrain the person.
- Massage the person's forehead.
- Reduce the number of people in the room.
- Talk quietly.
- Keep the room dimly lit.
- Keep the noise level to a minimum.
- Consider sedation if other methods do not work.

Adapted from the Hospice of North Central Florida, Inc.

CHART 7-2   Patient and Family Education: Preparing for Self-Management

Common Emotional Signs of Approaching Death

Withdrawal
The person is preparing to "let go" from surroundings and relationships.

Vision-like Experiences
The person may talk to people you cannot see or hear and see objects and places not visible to you. These are not hallucinations or drug reactions.
- Do not deny or argue with what the person claims.
- Affirm the experience.

Letting Go
The person may become agitated or continue to perform repetitive tasks. Often this indicates that something is unresolved or is preventing the person from letting go. As difficult as it may be to do or say, the dying person takes on a more peaceful demeanor when loved ones are able to say things such as, "It's okay to go. We'll be alright."

Saying Goodbye
When the person is ready to die and you are ready to let go, saying "goodbye" is important for both of you. Touching, hugging, crying, and saying "I love you," "Thank you," "I'm sorry," or "I'll miss you so much" are all natural expressions of sadness and loss. Verbalizing these sentiments can bring comfort both to the dying person and to those left behind.

Adapted from the Hospice of North Central Florida, Inc.

difficulty coping. Assess cultural considerations, values, and religious beliefs of the patient and family for their influence on the dying experience, control of symptoms, and family bereavement.

Families of people near death often manifest fear, anxiety, and knowledge deficits regarding the process of death and their role in providing care. Assess the patient and family for fear and anxiety and their expectations of the death experience. Ask them if they want to talk to a **bereavement** (grief) counselor or want guidance from clergy. Explain the common emotional signs of approaching death as described in Chart 7-2.

◆ **Interventions**

The desired outcomes for a patient near the end of life (EOL) are that the patient will have:
- Needs and preferences met
- Control of symptoms of distress
- Meaningful interactions with family
- A peaceful death

Interventions are planned to meet the physical, psychological, social, and spiritual needs of patients using an interdisciplinary approach. The coordinated, interdisciplinary care of hospice is the most successful approach to end-of-life care to date. *Although the perception of hospice is that it provides care for the dying, the major focus of hospice care is on quality of life.* Drug therapy is a major component of hospice care to provide symptom relief. Commonly used drugs are summarized in Chart 7-3.

Interventions to relieve symptoms of distress include positioning, administration of medications, and a variety of complementary and alternative therapies. When medications are used, they are often scheduled around the clock to maintain comfort and prevent reoccurrence of the symptom. The most

CHART 7-3 Best Practice for Patient Safety & Quality Care (QSEN)

Symptom Relief Kit for Patients in Home Hospice

- For unrelieved pain: Morphine solution (20 mg/1 mL solution) 0.25 to 0.5 mL orally or sublingually every 2 to 3 hours as needed.
- For unrelieved dyspnea: Morphine solution (20 mg/1 mL solution) 0.25 to 0.5 mL orally or sublingually every 2 hours as needed.
- For nausea or vomiting: Prochlorperazine 25-mg suppository rectally or 10-mg tablet orally every 6 hours as needed.
- For severe agitation and restlessness:
  - Determine if patient is in pain; treat accordingly.
  - Determine if patient is experiencing urinary retention; insert straight or Foley catheter.
  - Haloperidol 0.5 to 1 mg orally or sublingually every 6 hours.
  - Lorazepam 0.5 to 1 mg elixir or tablet dissolved in 0.5 mL water, administered against buccal mucosa every 4 hours to keep patient comfortable. If patient becomes more agitated after lorazepam, discontinue and contact hospice.
- For oral secretions or loud, wet respirations:
  - Atropine sulfate ophthalmic drops 1%, (2 drops orally or sublingually) every 4 hours as needed; or hyoscyamine drops (Levsin) (0.125-0.25 mg orally every 6 hours).
  - Scopolamine 1 to 3 transdermal patches every 72 hours.
- For unrelieved pain, dyspnea, nausea, vomiting, agitation, or secretions, call hospice.

common end-of-life symptoms that can cause the patient distress are:

- PAIN
- Weakness
- Breathlessness/dyspnea
- Nausea and vomiting
- Restlessness and agitation
- Seizures

Pain Management. *Pain is the most distressing symptom that dying patients fear the most.* Diseases such as cancer often cause tumor pain as a result of the infiltration of cancer cells into organs, nerves, and bones. Other causes of PAIN in dying patients include osteoarthritis, muscle spasms, and stiff joints secondary to immobility.

Patients who have had their PAIN controlled with either short-acting or long-acting opioids should continue their scheduled doses to prevent reoccurrence of the pain. As patients get closer to death, however, they often lose the ability to swallow. Long-acting oral opioids generally cannot be crushed, and rotation to rectal, transdermal, intravenous, or a subcutaneous route may be necessary. Short-acting opioids such as morphine sulfate, oxycodone, or hydromorphone elixir can be given sublingually, via the buccal mucosa, or rectally. They are quick-acting, effective, and safe to administer, even to comatose patients.

CONSIDERATIONS FOR OLDER ADULTS

Patient-Centered Care (QSEN)

Pain relief is often the priority need of older adults receiving PALLIATION. But PAIN is often underreported and undertreated. Do not withhold opioid drugs from older adults. Instead, reduce starting doses, make dose increases slowly, and monitor for changes in mental status or excessive sedation.

Some experts in symptom management at end of life (EOL) recommend discontinuing routine doses of opioids such as morphine when patients become oliguric or anuric. The rationale for this decision is to decrease the risk for delirium that may occur as the result of a failing kidney's inability to excrete morphine metabolites from the body. If delirium is interfering with the patient's ability to achieve a quality end of life, changing the opioid to fentanyl IV is an option. Fentanyl does not have active metabolites, and the delirium may improve. For patients with known renal failure, fentanyl should ideally be used from the start of opioid administration. In cases where it cannot be easily obtained (i.e., when not available by sublingual route or IV route), oxycodone is a better choice over morphine. Chapter 3 describes in detail the management of chronic PAIN.

Complementary and Alternative Therapies. Nonpharmacologic interventions are often integrated into the pain management plan. Some common approaches are presented here, as well as in Chapter 3.

Massage may decrease pain in people with cancer and is one of the most popular complementary interventions used for patients at EOL. This technique involves manipulating the patient's muscles and soft tissue, which improves circulation and promotes relaxation. Patients who are severely weak, are arthritic, or have advanced age may not tolerate extensive massage but may benefit from a short treatment to sites of their choice. In working with patients with cancer, use light pressure and avoid deep or intense pressure. Massage should not be done over the site of tissue damage (e.g., open wounds, tissue undergoing radiation therapy), in patients with bleeding disorders, and in those who are uncomfortable with touch.

Music therapy is another complementary therapy used by people near end of life that has been shown to decrease PAIN by promoting relaxation. Select music based on patient preferences and values.

Therapeutic Touch involves moving one's hands through the patient's energy field to relieve PAIN. Reiki therapy is another type of energy therapy being evaluated for its role in pain and symptom management. Use of Reiki requires a Reiki practitioner who is trained in the method.

Aromatherapy can be used in conjunction with other treatments to relieve pain near EOL. It is thought to decrease PAIN by promoting relaxation and reducing anxiety. Lavender, capsicum, bergamot, chamomile, rose, ginger, rosemary, lemongrass, sage, and camphor have been used in end-of-life care.

❓ NCLEX EXAMINATION CHALLENGE

Physiological Integrity

A client with metastasis to the bone is receiving IV antibiotics for pneumonia but has declined further treatment for his disease. He is experiencing severe back pain rated as a 9 on a 0-to-10 scale. What interventions are the most appropriate for the nurse to implement for this client? **Select all that apply.**
A. Provide both non-opioid and opioid analgesics.
B. Offer music therapy to help the client relax and decrease anxiety.
C. Obtain an order for physical therapy to encourage ambulation.
D. Help the client assume the best position of comfort.
E. Offer Reiki therapy, if available.

Weakness Management. Patients commonly experience weakness and fatigue as death nears. Weakness combined with decreased neurologic function may impair the ability to swallow (dysphagia). Once the patient has difficulty swallowing, oral intake should be limited to soft foods and sips of liquids, only if the patient wants. Teach families about the risk for aspiration, and reassure them that anorexia is normal at this stage. Families often have difficulty accepting that their loved ones are not being fed and may request that IV fluids be started. With great sensitivity, reinforce that stopping food and liquid intake is a natural process. Inform families that giving fluids can actually increase discomfort in a person with multisystem slowdown (Buck, 2012). Discomfort from fluid replacement could lead to respiratory secretions (and distress), increased GI secretions, nausea, vomiting, edema, and ascites. Most experts believe that dehydration in the last hours of life (i.e., terminal dehydration) does not cause distress and may stimulate endorphin release that promotes the patient's sense of well-being. To avoid a dry mouth and lips, moisten them with soft applicators and apply an emollient to soften the lips.

> ⚠️ **NURSING SAFETY PRIORITY** (QSEN)
>
> **Action Alert**
>
> Dysphagia near death presents a problem for oral drug therapy. Although some tablets may be crushed, drugs such as sustained-release capsules should not be taken apart. Reassess the need for each medication. Collaborate with the prescriber about discontinuing drugs that are not needed to control PAIN, dyspnea, agitation, nausea, vomiting, cardiac workload, or seizures. In collaboration with a pharmacist experienced in PALLIATION, identify alternative routes and/or alternative drugs to maintain control of symptoms. Choose the least invasive route such as oral, buccal mucosa (inside cheek), transdermal (via the skin), or rectal. Some oral drugs can be given rectally. Depending on the patient needs, the subcutaneous or IV routes may be used if access is available. The IM route is almost never used at the end of life because it is considered painful and drug distribution varies among patients.

Breathlessness/Dyspnea Management. Dyspnea is a subjective experience in which the patient has an uncomfortable feeling of breathlessness, often described as terrifying. It is a common symptom of distress near the end of life, especially among older adults because of decreased oxygen reserves associated with aging. Patients, families, and health care providers often consider it the major cause of suffering at end of life. Dyspnea can be:

- Directly related to the primary diagnosis (e.g., lung cancer, breast cancer, coronary artery disease)
- Secondary to the primary diagnosis (e.g., pleural effusion)
- Related to treatment of the primary disease (e.g., heart failure caused by chemotherapy, pneumonitis or constrictive pericarditis caused by radiation therapy, anemia related to chemotherapy)
- Unrelated to the primary disease (e.g., pneumonia or congestive heart failure [CHF]).

Depending on the cause, the pathophysiology of dyspnea can involve:

- Obstructive, restrictive, or vascular disturbances in the airways with tumor or lymph node involvement
- Pulmonary congestion secondary to fluid overload and/or cardiac dysfunction

- Bronchoconstriction and bronchospasm as seen with respiratory infection, chronic obstructive pulmonary disease (COPD), or airway blockage by a tumor
- Decreased hemoglobin-carrying capacity as with anemia
- Hyperventilation secondary to neuromuscular disease with limited movement of the diaphragm

Perform a thorough assessment of the patient's dyspnea. Include onset, severity (e.g., 0-to-10 scale), and precipitating factors. Precipitating factors may include time of day, position, anxiety, PAIN, cough, or emotional distress.

Pharmacologic interventions should begin early in the course of dyspnea near death. Nonpharmacologic interventions can be used in conjunction with but not in place of drug therapy.

Opioids such as morphine sulfate are the standard treatment for dyspnea near death. They work by (1) altering the perception of air hunger, reducing anxiety and associated oxygen consumption and (2) reducing pulmonary congestion by dilating pulmonary blood vessels. Patients who have not been receiving opioids are given starting doses of morphine 5 to 6 mg (or less for patients of advanced age) orally every 4 hours during the day and 10 mg at bedtime. If dyspnea occurs only with activity, give morphine before the activity up to every 2 hours. Those who are taking morphine or other opioids for pain may need higher doses for breathlessness, at times up to 50% more than their usual dose.

If a patient is having severe respiratory distress and poor oxygenation, morphine by mouth may need to be repeated as often as every 30 minutes and an IV or subcutaneous route may need to be established. Subcutaneous or intravenous doses of 1 to 2 mg of morphine may be given every 5 to 10 minutes until dyspnea is relieved.

Oxygen therapy for dyspnea near death has not been established as a standard of care for all patients. However, those who do not respond promptly to morphine or other drugs should be tried on oxygen (2 to 6 L by nasal cannula) to assess its effect. Patients often feel more comfortable when the oxygen saturation is greater than 90%. If possible, provide oxygen by nasal cannula (NC) because masks can be frightening. If oxygen is not effective, discontinue it.

> ⚠️ **NURSING SAFETY PRIORITY** (QSEN)
>
> **Action Alert**
>
> Offer oxygen to any patient with dyspnea near death, regardless of his or her oxygen saturation, because comfort is the desired outcome. If the patient is feeling dyspneic even though the oxygen saturation is above 90%, be sure that he or she receives oxygen to relieve respiratory distress. In addition, offer a fan directed toward the patient's face. Some patients find the circulating air more comfortable than oxygen therapy.

Bronchodilators, such as albuterol (Proventil) or ipratropium bromide (Atrovent, Apo-Ipravent ✦) via a metered dose inhaler (MDI) or nebulizer, may be given for symptoms of bronchospasm (heard as wheezes). *Corticosteroids,* such as prednisone (Deltasone, Winpred ✦), may also be given for bronchospasm and inflammatory problems within and outside the lung. Superior vena cava syndrome and cancer-related lymphangitis causing dyspnea may also respond to corticosteroids (also see Chapter 22).

People who have fluid overload with dyspnea, crackles on auscultation, peripheral edema, and other signs of CHF may be given a *diuretic* such as furosemide (Lasix, Uritol ♣) to decrease blood volume, reduce vascular congestion, and reduce the workload of the heart. Furosemide can be administered by mouth, IV, or subcutaneously. IV push administration, which is effective within minutes, may be preferred for heart failure and pulmonary edema.

Antibiotics may be indicated for dyspnea from a respiratory infection. A thorough workup for a respiratory infection is not appropriate when death is imminent. However, if signs or symptoms of a respiratory infection occur with dyspnea, a trial of an appropriate antibiotic may be considered to make the patient comfortable.

Secretions in the respiratory tract and oral cavity may also contribute to dyspnea near death. Loud, wet respirations (referred to as death rattle) are disturbing to family and caregivers even when they do not seem to cause dyspnea or respiratory distress. Reposition the patient onto one side to reduce gurgling, and place a small towel under his or her mouth to collect secretions. *Anticholinergics,* such as atropine (ophthalmic) solution 1% given sublingually every 4 hours as needed or hyoscyamine (Levsin) every 6 hours, are commonly given to dry up secretions. Scopolamine may also be given transdermally to reduce secretion production. Oropharyngeal suctioning is not recommended for loud secretions in the bronchi or oropharynx because it is often not effective and may only agitate the patient.

Fear and anxiety may be components of respiratory distress at end of life. For this reason, benzodiazepines are commonly given when morphine does not fully control the person's dyspnea. Low-dose lorazepam (Ativan) is administered orally, sublingually, or IV every 4 hours as needed or around the clock.

Nonpharmacologic interventions include:
- Applying wet cloths on the patient's face
- Positioning the patient with the head of the bed up either in a hospital bed or a reclining chair to increase chest expansion
- Encouraging imagery and deep breathing

Insertion of a urinary (Foley) catheter to avoid the need for exertion with voiding may be a comfort measure if the patient or family agrees. Risk for infection should not be a consideration when a person is near death.

? NCLEX EXAMINATION CHALLENGE

Physiological Integrity

The nurse is caring for a client who has severe dyspnea because of end-stage chronic obstructive pulmonary disease. Which interventions are the most appropriate to help improve his breathing? **Select all that apply.**
A. Administer morphine sulfate on an around-the-clock schedule.
B. Teach the client and family to keep him in a sitting position.
C. Use a large electric fan to circulate the air.
D. Keep the room temperature warm to prevent respiratory infection.
E. Teach the client and family that he should use bronchodilators as prescribed.

Nausea and Vomiting Management. Although not as common a problem as PAIN or dyspnea, nausea and vomiting occur frequently among terminally ill patients during the last week of life. It is particularly common in patients with acquired immune deficiency syndrome (AIDS) and with breast, stomach, or gynecologic cancers.

Other causes of nausea and vomiting at the end of life include:
- Uremia (increased serum urea nitrogen)
- Hypercalcemia
- Increased intracranial pressure
- Constipation or impaction
- Bowel obstruction

If constipation is identified as the cause of nausea and vomiting, give the patient a biphosphate enema (e.g., Fleet) to remove stool quickly. If stool in the rectum cannot be evacuated, a mineral oil enema followed by gentle disimpaction may relieve the patient's distress. Nausea and vomiting related to other causes can be controlled by one or more antiemetic agents such as prochlorperazine (Compazine), ondansetron (Zofran), dexamethasone (Decadron, Deronil♣, Dexasone♣), or metoclopramide (Reglan, Maxeran♣). Based on a patient's response, one or more of these drugs may be combined and compounded into rectal suppositories or oral troches. In addition to providing medications, be sure to remove sources of odors and keep the room temperature at a level that the patient desires.

Complementary and Alternative Therapies. Aromatherapy using chamomile, camphor, fennel, lavender, peppermint, and rose may reduce or relieve vomiting. Some patients, however, may have worse nausea with aroma. Ask the patient and family about their preferences, and respect culturally established practices.

Agitation and Delirium Management. Agitation at the end of life first requires assessing for PAIN or urinary retention, constipation, or another reversible cause. If constipation is ruled out as the cause and if analgesia and catheterization do not relieve restlessness, delirium (acute confusion) is suspected. Delirium *is a neuropsychiatric syndrome manifested by an acute change in the level of arousal. Clinical manifestations include altered sleep/wake cycle, mumbling speech, disturbance of memory and attention, and perceptual disturbances with delusions and hallucinations. Delirium can be hyperactive or hypoactive. Hypoactive (quiet) delirium is probably not uncomfortable for patients. Agitated (noisy) delirium with emotional and behavioral symptoms (e.g., yelling, hallucinations) can be uncomfortable, especially for family. Chapter 2 discusses delirium in more detail.

When delirium occurs in the week or two before death, it is referred to as *terminal delirium*. Possible causes include the adverse effects of opioids, benzodiazepines, anticholinergics, or steroids. If drugs are suspected causes, they may be decreased or discontinued, particularly if recently started.

! NURSING SAFETY PRIORITY (QSEN)

Drug Alert

Do not give the patient more than one antipsychotic drug at a time because of the risk for adverse drug events (ADEs). A neuroleptic such as a low dose of haloperidol (Haldol, Peridol ♣) 0.5-2 mg orally, IV, subcutaneously, or rectally is commonly used at end of life. Although haloperidol has the potential to cause extrapyramidal symptoms or adverse cardiovascular events and death in older adults with dementia, the benefits of treating delirium usually outweigh the risks.

Benzodiazepines are not generally used as a first choice for older adults with agitation because of their risk for causing delirium. Development of increased agitation after receiving a benzodiazepine could represent a paradoxical reaction—the opposite of what is expected.

Complementary and Alternative Therapies. Music therapy may produce relaxation by quieting the mind and promoting a restful state. Aromatherapy with chamomile may also help overcome anxiety, anger, tension, stress, and insomnia in dying patients.

Seizure Management. Seizures are not common at end of life but may occur in patients with brain tumors, advanced AIDS, and pre-existing seizure disorders. Around-the-clock drug therapy is needed to maintain a high seizure threshold for patients who can no longer swallow antiepileptic drugs (AEDs) and are at risk for seizures. Benzodiazepines, such as diazepam (Valium) and lorazepam (Ativan), are the drugs of choice. For home use, rectal diazepam gel or sublingual lorazepam oral solution (2 mg/mL) may be preferred. As a second choice, barbiturates such as phenobarbital may be given rectally or IV.

Management of the Refractory Symptoms of Distress. Patients receiving opioids for pain or dyspnea and other drugs such as antiemetics or antianxiety agents may experience mild sedation as a side effect to therapy. Depending on the patient and how soon death is expected, this side effect may decrease with time. What is important to understand is that drug therapy for symptoms of distress at end of life are guided by protocols, using medications believed to be safe, with the intent of alleviating suffering. *There is no evidence that administering medications for symptoms of distress using established protocols hastens deaths.* The ethical responsibility of the nurse in caring for patients near death is to follow guidelines for drug use to manage symptoms and to facilitate prompt and effective symptom management until death (Arnstein & Robinson, 2011).

A small percentage of patients have refractory symptoms of distress that do not respond to treatment near the end of life. These patients may be candidates for **proportionate palliative sedation**—a care management approach involving the administration of drugs such as benzodiazepines (e.g., midazolam [Versed]), neuroleptics, barbiturates, or anesthetic agents (e.g., propofol [Diprivan]) for the purpose of "lowering of patient consciousness." *The intent of palliative sedation to promote comfort and not hasten death distinguishes it from euthanasia (discussed later in this chapter).* The use of palliative sedation for refractory symptoms of distress is supported by a consensus of experts in palliative care as a comfort therapy of last resort (Arnstein & Robinson, 2011).

Psychosocial Management. The personal experience of dying or of losing a loved one through death is life altering. Unexpected deaths, particularly in young people, tend to be most traumatic. When a person has a chronic life-threatening disease, he or she and the family may have some knowledge of the expected outcome. Others, however, may have never considered their illness to be potentially terminal. It is important to first assess what patients and family understand about their illness and then help them identify the desired outcomes for care in the context of the illness.

Whereas death is the termination of life, dying is a process. People facing death may demonstrate emotional signs and symptoms of their response to the dying process through behaviors that equate to saying goodbye or through actual withdrawal. Some patients attempt to make families feel better by reassuring them that everything will be fine. Teach families that such behaviors are normal to the process of dying (see Chart 7-2).

Assisting Patients During the Grieving Process. Grief is the emotional feeling related to the perception of the loss. Patients who are dying suffer not only from the anticipated death but

---

TABLE 7-3 **Basic Beliefs Regarding Care at End of Life and Death Rituals for Selected Religions**

Christianity
- There are many Christian denominations, which have variations in beliefs regarding medical care near end of life.
- Roman Catholic tradition encourages people to receive Sacrament of the Sick, administered by a priest at any point during an illness. This sacrament may be administered more than once. Not receiving this sacrament will NOT prohibit them from entering heaven after death.
- People may be baptized as Roman Catholics in an emergency situation (e.g., person is dying) by a layperson. Otherwise, they are baptized by a priest.
- Christians believe in an afterlife of heaven or hell once the soul has left the body after death.

Judaism
- The dying person is encouraged to recite the confessional or the affirmation of faith, called the *Shema*.
- According to Jewish law, a person who is extremely ill and dying should not be left alone.
- The body, which was the vessel and vehicle to the soul, deserves reverence and respect.
- The body should not be left unattended until the funeral, which should take place as soon as possible (preferably within 24 hours).
- Autopsies are not allowed by Orthodox Jews, except under special circumstances.
- The body should not be embalmed, displayed, or cremated.

Islam
- Based on belief in one God Allah and his prophet Muhammad. Qur'an is the scripture of Islam, composed of Muhammad's revelations of the Word of God (Allah).
- Death is seen as the beginning of a new and better life.
- God has prescribed an appointed time of death for everyone.
- Qur'an encourages humans to seek treatment and not to refuse treatment. Belief is that only Allah cures but that Allah cures through the work of humans.
- Upon death, the eyelids are to be closed and the body should be covered. Before moving and handling the body, contact someone from the person's mosque to perform rituals of bathing and wrapping body in cloth.

Data from Giger, J.N. (2013). *Transcultural nursing: Assessment and intervention* (6th ed.). St. Louis: Mosby.

---

also from the loss of the ability to engage with others and in the world. **Mourning** is the outward social expression of the loss. Interventions to assist patients and families in grieving and mourning are based on cultural beliefs, values, and practices. Some patients and their families express their grief openly and loudly, whereas others are quiet and reserved. Table 7-3 lists basic beliefs regarding death, dying, and afterlife for some of the major religions.

Nursing interventions are aimed at providing appropriate emotional support to allow patients and their families to verbalize their fears and concerns. Support includes keeping the patient and family involved in health care decisions and emphasizing that the goal is to keep the patient as comfortable as possible until death. Interventions for providing psychosocial support are summarized in Chart 7-4.

Intervene with those grieving an impending death by "being with" as opposed to "being there." "Being with" implies that you are physically and psychologically with the grieving patient, empathizing to provide emotional support. Listening and acknowledging the legitimacy of the patient's and/or family's

CHART 7-4 Best Practice for Patient Safety & Quality Care (QSEN)

Psychosocial Interventions for Care of the Dying Patient and the Family

- Offer physical and emotional support by "being with" the patient.
- Respect cultural preferences.
- Be realistic.
- Encourage reminiscence.
- Promote spirituality.
- Avoid explanations of the loss.
- Communicate with the patient.
- Provide referrals to bereavement specialists.
- Teach about the physical signs of death (see Chart 9-1).
- Ensure that the patient is receiving palliative care, with an emphasis on symptom management.

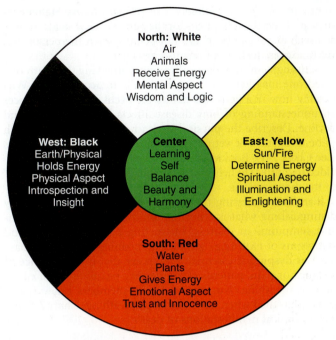

FIG. 7-2 An example of a medicine wheel used by indigenous people to provide harmony and balance in life and transition into the spirit worlds after death.

impending loss are often more therapeutic than speaking; this concept is often referred to as **presence**. Nurses facilitate the expression of grief by giving the person who is mourning permission to express himself or herself. Your manner and words show that these expressions of grief are acceptable and expected. An example of therapeutic communication might be "This must be very difficult for you" or "I'm sorry this is happening."

Do not minimize a patient's or family member's pain of loss. Avoid trite assurances such as "Things will be fine. Don't cry," "Don't be upset. She wouldn't want it that way," or "In a year you will have forgotten." Such comments can be barriers to demonstrating care and concern. Accept whatever the grieving person says about the situation. Remain present, be ready to listen attentively, and guide gently. In this way, you can help the bereaved family and significant others prepare for the necessary reminiscence and integration of the loss.

Storytelling through reminiscence and life review can be an important activity for patients who are dying. **Life review** is a structured process of reflecting on one's life, which is often facilitated by an interviewer. **Reminiscence** is the process of randomly reflecting on memories of events in one's life. The benefits of storytelling through either method provide the ability to attain perspective and enhance meaning. Suggest that the patient and family record autobiographic stories (print or video), write memories in a journal, or develop a scrapbook. Young dying parents often write letters for their children to read when they are older. If the patient does not have enough energy for these activities, familiar objects such as photographs and favorite jewelry can be used to spark ideas for stories.

Meeting Spiritual Needs. **Spirituality** is whatever or whoever gives ultimate meaning and purpose in one's life that invites particular ways of being in the world in relation to others, oneself, and the universe. A person's spirituality may or may not include belief in God. **Religions** are formal belief systems that provide a framework for making sense of life, death, and suffering and responding to universal spiritual questions. Religions often have beliefs, rituals, texts, and other practices that are shared by a community. For some patients, spirituality and religion can help them cope with the thought of death, contributing to quality of life during the dying process.

Perform a spiritual assessment to identify the patient's spiritual needs and to facilitate open expression of his or her beliefs and needs. A spiritual assessment could start with questions such as "What is important to you?" or "What gives you meaning or purpose in your life?"

🌐 CULTURAL CONSIDERATIONS

Patient-Centered Care (QSEN)

When assessing the spiritual needs of the dying patient, consider end-of-life preferences based on ethnic beliefs and practices. For example, the medicine wheel represents the spiritual journey to find one's own path for indigenous people in many countries, including American Indians (e.g., Cherokee, Navajo, Lakota) and Aboriginal people (e.g., Inuit, First Nations) in Canada and Alaska (also known as *Alaska Natives*). The medicine wheel helps people in these groups maintain balance and harmony within four life dimensions (Clarke & Holtslander, 2010) (Fig. 7-2). Depending on specific tribal practices and beliefs, the dimensions may be represented by colors, seasons, or directions.

As part of the dying process, certain tribal ceremonies must take place for patients to have a peaceful transition into the Spirit World and experience a "good death." One special ceremony involves smudging: Selected tribal medicines are burned, and the smoke is passed over the patient's body to cleanse it.

Be aware that supporting patients and their families within their cultural framework is essential as part of the dying process for all patients. Respect all practices, and allow for privacy during ceremonies and ritual practices.

Regardless of whether a person has had an affiliation with a religion or a belief in God or other Supreme Being, he or she can experience what is referred to as *spiritual* or *existential distress*. Existential distress is brought about by the actual or perceived threat to one's continued existence. Terminal illness and facing death can pose a profound threat to one's personhood. The main task for a person at EOL is coming to terms with one's losses, which may include loss of meaning and loss of relationships and facing the unknown. Acknowledge the patient's spiritual pain, and encourage verbalization. Use a family tree to discuss relationships, fears, hopes, and unfinished business. If the patient or family prefers, arrange for counseling with chaplains or others trained in end-of-life care. *Do not try to explain the loss in philosophic or religious terms.* Statements such as "Everything happens for the best" or "God sends us only as much as we can bear" are not helpful when the person has yet to express feelings of anguish or anger.

Although emotionally challenging, witnessing the death of a loved one may help facilitate the family to accept death. Witnessing how ill a person is makes the event real and enhances an understanding of how disease affects bodily function and decline. Describe the physical signs in detail—realistic enough to be unmistakable yet not so graphic as to alarm the listeners (see Chart 7-1). Booklets with this information should be provided to families to help them see what is expected and "normal" to the dying process.

Families witnessing the dying process often have difficulty distinguishing what is a normal finding of decline from signs and symptoms of distress. Instructing families on signs and symptoms of PAIN (e.g., grimacing, moaning, guarding behaviors) or dyspnea is essential. Emphasize that in the absence of dyspnea or pain, patients often die very peacefully with cessation of breathing. Nurses and family members know that a person has died when he or she stops breathing. Chart 7-5 lists other physical manifestations of death.

POSTMORTEM CARE

If the death was in the home and expected, emergency assistance should not be notified. If the person was a patient in a hospice program, the family calls hospice. If a death is unexpected or suspicious, the medical examiner is notified. Otherwise, the nurse or physician performs the pronouncement and completes a death certificate (Chart 7-6). Most states allow nurses to pronounce death in nursing homes and other long-term care facilities, but only a few states permit nurses to pronounce in acute care facilities such as hospitals. Be sure to check your health care agency's policies for who can pronounce death and the specific procedure to follow.

After the patient dies, ask the family or other caregivers if they would like to spend time with the patient to assist them in coping with what has happened and say their good-byes. Even if the death has been anticipated, no one knows how he or she will feel until it occurs. It may take hours to days to weeks or months for each person to realize the full effect of the event. Some family members may find it therapeutic to bathe and prepare the person's body for transfer to the funeral home or the hospital morgue. Offer families this opportunity if it is culturally acceptable.

Before preparing the body for transfer, ask the physician whether an autopsy will be required. When the death is expected, an autopsy is not likely. An autopsy is generally performed only when the cause of death is not known. Some religions do not allow autopsies, such as Orthodox Jews.

After the family or significant others view the body, follow agency procedure for preparing the patient for transfer to either the morgue or a funeral home. In the hospital, a postmortem kit is generally used with a shroud and identification tags. Chart 7-7 describes best practice guidelines for postmortem care.

CHART 7-6 Best Practice for Patient Safety & Quality Care QSEN

Pronouncement of Death

- Note time of death that the family or staff reported the cessation of respirations.
- Identify the patient by the hospital identification (ID) tag; note the general appearance of the body.
- Ascertain that the patient does not rouse to verbal or tactile stimuli. Avoid overtly painful stimuli, especially if family members are present.
- Auscultate for the absence of heart sounds; palpate for the absence of carotid pulse.
- Look and listen for the absence of spontaneous respirations.
- Record the time at which your assessment was completed.
- Document the time of pronouncement and all notifications in the medical record (i.e., to attending physician). Document if the medical examiner needs to be notified (may be required for unexpected or suspicious death). Document if an autopsy is planned per the attending physician and family.
- If your state and agency policy allows an RN to pronounce death, document as indicated on the death certificate.

CHART 7-7 Best Practice for Patient Safety & Quality Care QSEN

Postmortem Care

- Provide all care with respect to communicate that the person was important and valued.
- Ask the family or significant others if they wish to help wash the patient or comb his or her hair; respect and follow their cultural practices for body preparation.
- If no autopsy is planned, remove or cut all tubes and lines according to agency policy.
- Close the patient's eyes unless the cultural/religious practice is for a family member or other person to close the eyes.
- Insert dentures if the patient wore them.
- Straighten the patient, and lower the bed to a flat position.
- Place a pillow under the patient's head.
- Wash the patient as needed, and comb and arrange the patient's hair unless the family desires to perform bathing and body preparation.
- Place waterproof pads under the patient's hips and around the perineum to absorb any excrement.
- Clean the patient's room or unit.
- Allow the family or significant others to see the patient in private and to perform any religious or cultural customs they wish (e.g., prayer).
- Assess that all who need to see the patient have done so, before transferring to the funeral home or morgue.
- Notify the hospital chaplain or appropriate religious leader if requested by the family or significant others.
- Ensure that the nurse or physician has completed and signed the death certificate.
- Prepare the patient for transfer to either a morgue or funeral home; wrap the patient in a shroud (unless the family has a special shroud to use), and attach identification tags per agency policy.

CHART 7-5 Patient and Family Education: Preparing for Self-Management

Signs That Death Has Occurred

- Breathing stops.
- Heart stops beating.
- Pupils become fixed and dilated.
- Body color becomes pale and waxen.
- Body temperature drops.
- Muscles and sphincters relax.
- Urine and stool may be released.
- Eyes may remain open, and there is no blinking.
- The jaw may fall open.
- Observers may hear trickling of fluids internally.

TABLE 7-4 Definitions of Ethical Concepts Related to Issues at End of Life

Withdrawing or withholding life-sustaining therapy (formerly called *passive euthanasia*) An act of omission (e.g., withholding or withdrawing treatment) that might prolong the life of a person who cannot be cured by the treatment. In this situation, the withdrawal of the intervention does not directly cause the patient's death.

Principle of double effect Involves taking an action intended to have a good effect, which also has a known harmful effect. This is not active euthanasia.

Voluntary active euthanasia An act by which the causative agent or treatment in the death of a patient is administered directly by another.

Involuntary active euthanasia The action to end the patient's life is taken without the patient's consent.

Physician-assisted suicide A practice whereby a physician provides a means (e.g., medication) to a patient with the knowledge that the patient will use the means to commit suicide.

THE CONCEPT OF EUTHANASIA

Nurses are usually in the best and most immediate position to discuss end-of-life issues. This includes assisting in the decision-making process regarding immediate or future needs. To do this, nurses must be knowledgeable about terminology and ethical issues related to death and dying (Table 7-4).

Much confusion exists regarding the concept of euthanasia. **Withdrawing or withholding life-sustaining therapy,** formerly called **passive euthanasia,** involves discontinuing one or more therapies that might prolong the life of a person who cannot be cured by the therapy. Another phrase sometimes used is "letting the person die naturally" or "allowing natural death (AND)," as discussed earlier in this chapter. *In this situation, the withdrawal of the intervention does not directly cause the patient's death.* The progression of the patient's disease or poor health status is the cause of death. Professional organizations (e.g., American Nurses Association, American Medical Association) and religious communities (e.g., the Catholic church) support the right of patients and their surrogate decision makers to refuse or stop treatment (e.g., mechanical ventilation, antibiotics, IV fluids) when patients are close to death and interventions are considered medically futile and/or capable of causing harm. The U.S. court system also supports withdrawal of aggressive treatment and the rights of surrogate decision makers to refuse or stop treatment.

By contrast, **active euthanasia** requires that health care providers take action (e.g., give medication or treatment) that purposefully and directly causes the patient's death. *Active euthanasia is not supported by most professional organizations, including the American Nurses Association.* In the states of Oregon, Washington, and Vermont, physician-assisted suicide is legal in certain situations. Nurses should not be involved in active euthanasia or physician-assisted euthanasia. They do, however, play a major role in end-of-life care by advocating for patients' wishes and ensuring quality symptom management and support at the end of life.

GET READY FOR THE NCLEX® EXAMINATION!

KEY POINTS

Review these Key Points for each NCLEX Examination Client Needs Category.

Safe and Effective Care Environment

- Hospice care uses an interdisciplinary approach to assess and address the holistic needs of patients who have a 6-month prognosis or less; examples of health care team members include the social worker, case manager, pharmacist, and physician. **Teamwork and Collaboration** QSEN
- Assess the patient and family to determine if they have written advance directives, such as a durable power of attorney for health care (DPOAHC), a living will, or portable DNR.
- The decision by DPOAHC to withdraw or withhold life-sustaining therapy is supported by the U.S. Supreme Court and other professional/religious organizations.
- Be aware that active euthanasia involves giving a patient a treatment or agent that causes death (see Table 7-4) and is legal only in Oregon, Washington State, and Vermont under certain circumstances.
- Be aware that nurses have an ethical obligation to provide timely information about expected care outcomes so that patients and families can make the best EOL decisions.

Health Promotion and Maintenance

- Stress the importance of having a DPOAHC to inform health care providers of your wishes if you lack capacity.

- Teach the patient and family that an advance directive is a written document that specifies what, if any, extraordinary actions the patient would want if he or she could no longer make decisions about care.

Psychosocial Integrity

- Assess the patient's emotional signs of impending death; assess coping ability of the patient and family or other caregiver (see Chart 7-2).
- Incorporate the patient's personal cultural practices and spiritual beliefs regarding death and dying (see Table 7-3). **Patient-Centered Care** QSEN
- Be aware that people facing death may experience fear and anxiety about their impending death and experience difficulty coping.
- Provide psychosocial interventions to support the patient and family during the dying process, as listed in Chart 7-4.

Physiological Integrity

- Death is defined as the cessation of integrated tissue and organ function, manifested by cessation of heartbeat, absence of spontaneous respirations, or irreversible brain dysfunction.
- Hospice and palliative care are different, as described in Table 7-2.

- Assess the patient for pain, dyspnea, agitation, nausea, and vomiting, which are common problems at the end of life. **Evidence-Based Practice** **QSEN**
- Recognize that older adults are often undertreated for pain or other symptoms at EOL.
- Assess for the common physical signs of approaching death, as listed in Chart 7-1.
- Medications are frequently given to control dyspnea, pain, nausea, vomiting, and agitation in patients near death (see Chart 7-3).
- Because of the risk for delirium, particularly in older adults, providers may avoid use of benzodiazepines for treatment of anxiety, even at end of life. Development of increased agitation after receiving benzodiazepine could represent a paradoxical reaction. **Safety** **QSEN**

- Terminal delirium may occur in a week or two before death. Haloperidol given orally or IV is the drug of choice.
- Assessment of oxygen saturation for patients at end of life is not necessary. Oxygen should be provided based on comfort. **Evidence-Based Practice** **QSEN**
- Common complementary and alternative therapies used for symptom management at end of life include aromatherapy, music therapy, and energy therapies, such as Therapeutic Touch.
- Follow Chart 7-7 for best practice guidelines for performing postmortem care; incorporate the patient's cultural and religious beliefs in body preparation and burial (see Table 7-3). **Patient-Centered Care** **QSEN**

CHAPTER | 8

Concepts of Emergency and Trauma Nursing

Linda Laskowski-Jones and Karen L. Toulson

e http://evolve.elsevier.com/Iggy/

PRIORITY CONCEPTS

- SAFETY
- TEAMWORK AND COLLABORATION
- COMMUNICATION

LEARNING OUTCOMES

Safe and Effective Care Environment

1. Describe the emergency department (ED) environment, including vulnerable populations and interdisciplinary team members.
2. Engage in COLLABORATION with members of the interdisciplinary health care team members in the ED.
3. Plan and implement best practices to maintain staff and patient SAFETY in the ED.
4. Explain selected core competencies that nurses need to function in the ED.
5. Triage patients in the ED to prioritize the order of care delivery.

6. Prioritize resuscitation interventions based on the primary survey of the injured patient.

Psychosocial Integrity

7. Describe the role of the ED nurse in providing support for families after the death of a loved one.

Physiological Integrity

8. Describe the general process of admission through disposition of a patient in the ED.
9. Prevent or reduce common risk factors in the ED that contribute to adverse events in older adults.

The demand for emergency care in the United States is growing rapidly. Emergency departments (EDs) function as safety nets for communities of all sizes by providing services to both insured and uninsured patients seeking medical care. They are also responsible for SAFETY through public health surveillance and emergency disaster preparedness. Some hospital-based emergency departments also provide observation, procedural care, and employee or occupational health services. Other hospital-based emergency departments have interdisciplinary specialty teams who take part in COLLABORATION to provide first-line care for patients with stroke and cardiac problems (Alberts et al., 2011). The role of the ED is so vital that the Centers for Medicare and Medicaid Services (2013) has a process for designating small rural facilities of 25 inpatient beds or fewer as critical access hospitals if they provide around-the-clock emergency care services 7 days a week. Critical access hospitals are considered *necessary providers of health care* to

community residents that are not close to other hospitals in a given region.

Because of the multi-specialty nature of the environment, EDs play a unique role within the U.S. health care system. More than 119 million people visit the ED each year (Centers for Disease Control and Prevention [CDC], 2010). The demand for emergency care has greatly increased over the past 15 years, and the health care consumer has higher expectations. However, the capacity to provide necessary resources has not kept pace in most systems. Emergency department crowding occurs when the need for care exceeds available resources in the department, hospital, or both (Howard, 2009). The Joint Commission has established a set of metrics (Core Measure Sets) based on ED length of stay (LOS) that hospitals are required to submit. The longer the ED length of stay for admitted patients, the more overcrowded the ED becomes. That, in turn, limits access to other patients who are in need of ED beds for emergency care.

A prolonged LOS also indicates problems with inpatient bed availability and poor overall hospital throughput.

Health care reform initiatives stemming from the Affordable Care Act will certainly impact emergency services; the full spectrum of that impact is currently evolving. The widespread availability of health insurance may produce an increase in the number of patients who use the emergency department because they now have greater access to the necessary financial resources. Emergency department use may actually decrease for some types of patients as hospitals and providers partner in Accountable Care Organization models. This will better control costs by managing patient outcomes through primary care networks and disease management programs. Emergency departments may also experience a shift in focus from admitting the majority of acutely ill patients to the hospital for care to COLLABORATING more with home care services and establishing better access to resources in the community to enable patients to be safely discharged home from the ED when possible.

THE EMERGENCY DEPARTMENT ENVIRONMENT OF CARE

In the emergency care environment, rapid change is the rule. The typical ED is fast paced and, at the height of activity, might even appear chaotic. Patients seek treatment for a number of physical, psychological, spiritual, and social reasons. In general, nurses work in this environment because they dislike routines and thrive in challenging, stimulating work settings. Although most EDs have treatment areas that are designated for certain populations such as patients with trauma or cardiac, psychiatric, or gynecologic problems, care can actually take place almost anywhere. In a crowded ED, patients may receive initial treatment outside of the usual treatment rooms, including the waiting room and hallways.

The ED is typically alive with activity and noise, although the pace decreases at times because arrivals are random. Emergency nurses can expect background sounds that include ringing telephones, monitor alarms, vocal patients, crying children, and radio transmissions between staff and incoming ambulance or helicopter personnel. Interruptions and distractions are the norm, and the nurse must ensure these events do not impact patient SAFETY.

Demographic Data and Vulnerable Populations

Staff members in the ED provide care for people across the life span with a broad spectrum of issues, illnesses, and injuries—as well as various cultural and religious values. Especially vulnerable populations who visit the ED include the homeless, the poor, and older adults. During a given shift, for example, the emergency nurse may function as a cardiac nurse, a geriatric nurse, a psychiatric nurse, a pediatric nurse, and a trauma nurse. Patient acuity ranges from life-threatening emergencies to minor symptoms that could be addressed in a primary care office or community clinic. Some of the most common reasons that people seek ED care are:
- Abdominal pain
- Chest pain
- Breathing difficulties
- Injuries (especially falls in older adults)
- Headache
- Fever
- Pain (the most common symptom)

CONSIDERATIONS FOR OLDER ADULTS
Patient-Centered Care QSEN

Older adults usually visit the ED because of worsening of an existing chronic condition or because the condition affects their ability to perform ADLs. Older adults are also sometimes admitted from nursing homes or assisted-living facilities for procedures (e.g., insertion of a percutaneous endoscopic gastrostomy [PEG] tube or peripherally inserted central catheter [PICC]) or for treatments (e.g., blood transfusions). Some hospitals plan direct admission of the patient to same-day surgery or hold a bed for the procedure or treatment to bypass the ED. This arrangement decreases the patient's wait time and therefore decreases the risks for adverse events, such as pressure ulcer development or hospital-acquired infection. Incorporating family members of older adults into the ED care process can aid in overall patient evaluation, decision making, and satisfaction with the ED experience (Nikki et al., 2013).

Special Nursing Teams

Many EDs have specialized nursing teams that deal with high-risk populations of patients. One example is the forensic nurse examiner team. **Forensic nurse examiners (RN-FNEs)** are educated to obtain patient histories, collect forensic evidence, and offer counseling and follow-up care for victims of rape, child abuse, and domestic violence—also known as *intimate partner violence (IPV)* (Desy, 2010). They are trained to recognize evidence of abuse and to intervene on the patient's behalf. Forensic nurses who specialize in helping victims of sexual assault are called *sexual assault nurse examiners (SANEs)* or *sexual assault forensic examiners (SAFEs)*.

Interventions performed by forensic nurses may include providing information about developing a SAFETY plan or how to escape a violent relationship. Forensic nurse examiners document injuries and collect physical and photographic evidence. They may also provide testimony in court as to what was observed during the examination and information about the type of care provided.

The **psychiatric crisis nurse team** is another example of an ED specialty team. Many patients who visit the ED for their acute problems also have chronic mental health disorders. The availability of mental health nurses can improve the quality of care delivered to these patients who require specialized interventions in the ED and can offer valuable expertise to the emergency health care staff. For example, the team evaluates patients with emotional behaviors or mental illness and facilitates the follow-up treatment plan, including possible admission to an appropriate psychiatric facility. These nurses also interact with patients and families when sudden illness, serious injury, or death of a loved one may have caused a crisis. On-site interventions can help patients and families cope with these unexpected changes in their lives.

Interdisciplinary Team Collaboration

The emergency nurse is one member of the large interdisciplinary team who provides care for patients in the ED. A team approach to emergency care using COLLABORATION is considered a standard of practice (Fig. 8-1). In this setting, the nurse coordinates care with all levels of health care team providers, from prehospital emergency medical services (EMS) personnel to physicians, hospital technicians, and professional and ancillary support staff.

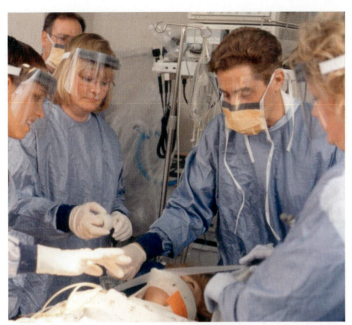

FIG. 8-1 The ability to work as part of an interdisciplinary team is crucial to positive outcomes for emergency department (ED) patients.

FIG. 8-2 Advanced life support helicopter arriving at emergency department landing zone. Helicopters are used to rapidly transport critically ill and injured patients to the hospital for emergent care.

FIG. 8-3 Prehospital providers take a patient from the ambulance to be brought into the emergency department.

Prehospital care providers are typically the first caregivers that patients see before transport to the ED by an ambulance or helicopter (Fig. 8-2). Local protocols define the skill level of the EMS responders dispatched to provide assistance. **Emergency medical technicians (EMTs)** offer basic life support (BLS) interventions such as oxygen, basic wound care, splinting, spinal immobilization, and monitoring of vital signs. Some units carry automatic external defibrillators (AEDs) and may be authorized to administer selected drugs such as an EpiPen or nitroglycerin based on established medical protocols. For patients who require care that exceeds BLS resources, paramedics are usually dispatched. **Paramedics** are advanced life support (ALS) providers who can perform advanced techniques, which may include cardiac monitoring, advanced airway management and intubation, establishing IV access, and administering drugs en route to the ED (Fig. 8-3).

The prehospital provider is a key source for valuable patient data. Emergency nurses rely on these providers to be the "eyes and ears" of the health care team in the prehospital setting and to ensure COMMUNICATION of this information to other staff members for continuity of care.

Another integral member of the emergency health care team is the **emergency medicine physician**. These medical professionals receive specialized education and training in emergency patient management. As emergency care has become increasingly complex and specialized, emergency medicine is a recognized physician specialty practice.

The emergency nurse interacts with a number of staff and community physicians involved in patient care but is involved in close COLLABORATION with emergency medicine physicians. Even though other physician specialists may be involved in ED patient treatment, the emergency medicine physician typically directs the overall care in the department. Many EDs also employ nurse practitioners (NPs) and physician assistants (PAs) to assume designated roles in patient assessment and treatment. Teaching hospitals also have resident physicians who train in the ED. They act in collaboration with or under the supervision of the emergency medicine physician to assist with emergency care delivery.

The emergency nurse interacts and regularly takes part in COLLABORATION with *professional and ancillary staff* who function in support roles. These personnel include radiology and ultrasound technicians, respiratory therapists, laboratory technicians, social workers, case managers, nursing assistants, and clerical staff. Each support staff member is essential to the success of the emergency health care team. The ED nurse is accountable for communicating pertinent staff considerations, patient needs, and restrictions to support staff (e.g., physical limitations, Transmission-Based Precautions) to ensure that ongoing patient and staff safety issues are addressed. For example, the respiratory therapist can assist the nurse to troubleshoot mechanical ventilator issues. Laboratory technicians can offer advice regarding best practice techniques for specimen collection. During the discharge planning process, social workers or case managers can be tremendous patient advocates in locating community resources, including temporary housing, durable medical equipment (DME), drug and alcohol counseling, health insurance information, and prescription services.

The emergency nurse's interactions extend beyond the walls of the ED. COMMUNICATION with nurses from the inpatient units is necessary to ensure continuity of patient care. Providing a concise but comprehensive report of the patient's ED experience is essential for the *hand-off communication* process and patient SAFETY (Blouin, 2011). Information should include the patient's:

- Situation (reason for being in the ED)
- Brief medical history
- Assessment and diagnostic findings
- Transmission-Based Precautions if needed
- Interventions
- Response to those interventions

The Joint Commission's National Patient Safety Goals (NPSGs) (The Joint Commission [TJC], 2013) advocate that hospitals and other health care agencies use a standardized approach to hand-off communications to prevent errors caused by poor or inadequate communication. Many agencies use the SBAR method (**s**ituation, **b**ackground, **a**ssessment, **r**esponse) or some variation of that method to ensure complete and clearly understood COMMUNICATION. Chapter 1 discusses the SBAR technique in more detail.

Both emergency nurses and nurses on inpatient units need to understand the unique aspects of their two practice environments to prevent conflicts. For example, nurses on inpatient units may be critical of the push to move patients out of the ED setting quickly, particularly when the unit activity is high. Similarly, the emergency nurse may be critical of the inpatient unit's lack of understanding or enthusiasm for accepting admissions rapidly. Effective interpersonal communication skills and respectful negotiation can optimize teamwork and COLLABORA-TION between the emergency nurse and the inpatient unit nurse. For instance, when ED patient volume or acuity is overwhelming, the unit nurse can volunteer to assist the ED nurse by moving a monitored patient to the hospital bed. Whenever possible, the emergency nurse may decide to delay sending admitted patients to inpatient units during change of shift or crisis periods such as a cardiac arrest on the unit.

STAFF AND PATIENT SAFETY CONSIDERATIONS

In the emergency department (ED) setting, staff and patient SAFETY are major concerns (Chart 8-1).

Staff Safety

Staff safety concerns center on the potential for transmission of disease and on personal safety when dealing with aggressive, agitated, or violent patients and visitors. The emergency nurse uses Standard Precautions at all times when a potential for contamination by blood or other body fluids exists. Patients with tuberculosis or other airborne pathogens are preferentially

> **! NURSING SAFETY PRIORITY (QSEN)**
> ### Action Alert
>
> Hostile patient and visitor behaviors also pose injury risks to staff members. Be alert for volatile situations or people who demonstrate aggressive or violent tendencies through verbal abuse or acting out. Be sure to follow the hospital's security plan, including looking for an escape route, attempting de-escalation strategies before harm can occur, and notifying security staff as well as supervisory staff of the situation. Emergency visits resulting from gang or domestic violence can produce particularly hazardous conditions. Report all episodes of assaultive or violent behaviors through the hospital's event documentation process so that hospital leaders and risk managers are aware of the scope of the problem and can plan safety strategies, including staff education, accordingly (Harding, 2011).

placed in a negative pressure room if available. The nurse wears a powered air-purifying respirator (PAPR) or a specially fitted facemask before engaging in any close interaction with these patients (see Chapter 23).

EDs employ several methods of ensuring SAFETY. Many EDs have at least one security guard present at all times for immediate assistance with these situations. Metal detectors may be used as a screening device for patients and visitors who are suspected of having weapons. Strategically located panic buttons and remote door access controls allow staff to get help and secure major ED or hospital entrances. The triage reception area—a particularly vulnerable access point into the ED—is often designed to serve as a security barrier with bullet-proof glass and staff-controlled door entry into the treatment area. Hospitals may even employ canine units made up of specially trained officers and dogs to patrol high-risk areas and respond to handle threatening situations (Johnson & Parker, 2009).

Patient Safety

In addition to concerns about staff safety, some of the most common *patient SAFETY* issues are:

- Patient identification
- Fall risk
- Skin breakdown in vulnerable populations
- High risk for medical errors or adverse events

Hospital emergency departments have unique factors that can affect patient SAFETY. These factors include the provision of

---

CHART 8-1　**Best Practice for Patient Safety & Quality Care (QSEN)**

Maintaining Patient and Staff Safety in the Emergency Department

SAFETY CONSIDERATION	INTERVENTIONS TO MINIMIZE RISK
Patient identification	Provide an identification (ID) bracelet for each patient. Use two unique identifiers (e.g., name, date of birth). If patient identity is unknown, use a special identification system.
Injury prevention for patients	Keep rails up on stretcher. Keep stretcher in lowest position. Remind the patient to use call light for assistance. Reorient confused patient frequently. If patient is confused, ask a family member or significant other to remain with him or her. Implement measures to protect skin integrity for patients at risk for skin breakdown.
Risk for errors and adverse events	Obtain a thorough patient and family history. Check the patient for a medical alert bracelet or necklace. Search the patient's belongings for weapons or other harmful devices when he or she has altered mental status.
Injury prevention for staff	Use Standard Precautions at all times. Anticipate hostile, violent patient, family, and/or visitor behavior. Plan options if violence occurs, including assistance from the security department.

complex emergency care, constant interruptions, and the need to interact with the many providers involved in caring for one patient.

Correct *patient identification* is critical in any health care setting. All patients are issued an identification bracelet at their point of entry in the ED—generally at the triage registration desk or at the bedside if emergent needs exist. For patients with an unknown identity and those with emergent conditions that prevent the proper identification process (e.g., unconscious patient without identification, emergent trauma patient), hospitals commonly use a "Jane/John Doe" or another identification system. Whatever method is used, always verify the patient's identity using two unique identifiers before each intervention and before medication administration per The Joint Commission's 2013 National Patient Safety Goals. Examples of appropriate identifiers include the patient's name, birth date, agency identification number, home telephone number or address, and/or Social Security number.

Fall prevention starts with identifying people at risk for falls and then applying appropriate fall precautions and SAFETY measures. Patients can enter the ED without apparent fall risk factors, but because of interventions such as pain medication, sedation, or lower extremity cast application, they can develop a risk for falls. Falls can also occur in patients with medical conditions or drugs that cause syncope ("blackouts"). Many older adults also experience orthostatic (postural) hypotension as a side effect of cardiovascular drugs. In this case, patients become dizzy when changing from a lying or sitting position (see Chapter 2).

! NURSING SAFETY PRIORITY (QSEN)
Action Alert

Help patients move slowly from a supine to an upright position and when ambulating, if needed. Also, confirm that siderails are up and locked on stretchers, that the call light is within reach, and that a patient's fall risk is communicated clearly to visitors and staff members who may assume responsibility for care.

Older adults who are on beds or stretchers should *always* have all siderails up and the bed or stretcher in the lowest position. Access to a call light is especially important; instruct the patient to call for the nurse if assistance is needed rather than attempt independent ambulation. Many older adults have difficulty adjusting to the noise and pace of the ED and/or have illnesses or injuries that cause delirium, an acute confusional state. Reorient the patient frequently, and re-assess mental status. Undiagnosed delirium increases the risk for mortality for older adults who are admitted to the hospital. Assess the need for a family member, significant other, or sitter to stay with the patient to prevent falls and assist with reorientation. Additional safety strategies are listed in Chart 8-1.

Some patients spend a lengthy time on stretchers while awaiting unit bed availability—possibly as long as 1 to 2 days in some hospitals, especially during high census periods as often occurs in flu season. During that time, basic health needs require attention, including providing nutrition, hygiene, SAFETY, and privacy for all ED patients. Waiting in the ED can cause increased pain in patients with back pain or arthritis.

Protecting skin integrity also begins in the ED. Emergency nurses need to assess the skin frequently and implement preventive interventions into the ED plan of care, especially when caring for older adults or those of any age who are immobilized. Interventions that promote clean, dry skin for incontinent patients, mobility techniques that decrease shearing forces when moving the immobile patient, and routine turning help prevent skin breakdown. Chapter 25 describes additional nursing interventions for preventing skin breakdown.

A significant SAFETY risk for all patients who enter the emergency care environment is the *potential for medical errors or adverse events*, especially those associated with medication administration. The episodic and often chaotic nature of emergency management in an environment with frequent interruptions can easily lead to errors.

To reduce error potential, the emergency nurse makes every attempt to obtain essential and accurate medical history information from the patient, family, or reliable significant others as necessary. When dealing with patients who arrive with an altered mental status, a quick survey to determine whether the person is wearing a medical alert bracelet or necklace is important to gain medical information. In addition, a two-person search of patient belongings may yield medication containers; the name of a physician, pharmacy, or family contact person; or a medication list. In this case, the nurse serves as a detective to find clues, which may not only promote SAFETY but also help determine the diagnosis and influence the overall emergency treatment plan. Automated electronic tracking systems are also available in some EDs to assist staff in identifying the location of patients at any given time and in monitoring the progress of care delivery during the visit. These valuable safety measures are especially important in large or busy EDs with a high population of older adults (Laskowski-Jones, 2008).

In addition to falls and pressure ulcer development, another adverse event that can result from a prolonged stay in the ED is a *hospital-acquired infection*. Older adults, in particular, are at risk for urinary tract or respiratory infections. Patients who are immune suppressed, especially those on chronic steroid therapy or immune modulators, are also at a high risk. Nurses and other ED personnel need to wash their hands frequently and thoroughly or use hand sanitizers to help prevent pathogen transmission.

? CLINICAL JUDGMENT CHALLENGE
Safety (QSEN)

The emergency department manager has created a task force to decrease the rate of adverse incidents in patients who have increased safety needs during their stay in the department. At their meeting, each person discussed a specific safety need and actions that can be taken to reduce that risk.

1. What populations are at highest risk for safety compromise while in the emergency department?
2. What specific procedures can the unit implement to decrease medication errors?
3. What actions can be delegated to unlicensed personnel in these areas: medication administration, skin protection, and fall risk?
4. How can the staff reduce hazard risk for patients who are confused (either as a chronic condition or as the result of medication side effects) or who have delirium?

SCOPE OF EMERGENCY NURSING PRACTICE

The scope of emergency nursing practice encompasses management of patients across the life span—from birth through death—and all health conditions that prompt a person of any age to seek emergency care.

Core Competencies

Emergency nursing practice requires that nurses be skilled in patient assessment, priority setting and clinical decision making, multitasking, and COMMUNICATION. A sound knowledge base is also essential. Flexibility and adaptability are vital traits because situations within the ED, as well as individual patients, can change rapidly.

Like that of any nurse in practice, the foundation of the emergency nurse's skill base is *assessment*. He or she must be able to rapidly and accurately interpret assessment findings according to acuity and age. For example, mottling of the extremities may be a normal finding in a newborn but it may indicate poor peripheral perfusion and a shock state in an adult.

CONSIDERATIONS FOR OLDER ADULTS
Patient-Centered Care QSEN

Some older adults may not be able to provide an accurate history because of memory loss or acute delirium. If possible, review their prior hospitalization records to obtain complete histories, or ask a family member or friend for pertinent information. Older adults usually have many pre-existing diseases (comorbidities) that must be considered as part of the assessment. *Knowing the history is vital because these conditions might adversely affect or complicate the cause for the ED visit.* For example, a patient who has rib fractures but has a history of chronic obstructive pulmonary disease (COPD) may not be able to maintain adequate oxygenation without endotracheal intubation and mechanical ventilatory support in the ED.

Another consideration for older adult assessment is that the presenting symptoms of older adults are often different or less specific than those of younger adults. For example, increasing weakness, fatigue, and confusion may be the only admission concerns. These vague symptoms can be caused by serious illnesses, such as an acute myocardial infarction (MI), urinary tract infection, or pneumonia. Diagnosing older adults often keeps them in the ED for extended periods, which can lead to patient safety concerns as discussed on p. 108.

Another skill for the emergency nurse is *priority setting*, which is essential in the triage process. Priority setting depends on accurate assessment, as well as good critical thinking and clinical decision-making skills. These skills are generally gained through hands-on clinical experience in the ED. However, discussion of case studies and the use of human patient simulation and simulation software and aids can help prepare nurses to acquire this skill base in a nonthreatening environment and then apply it in the actual clinical situation (Kisner & Johnson-Anderson, 2010).

The knowledge base for emergency nurses is broad and ranges from critical care emergencies to less common problems, such as snakebites and hazardous materials contamination (see Chapters 9 and 10). ED nurses also learn to recognize and manage the legal implications of societal problems such as domestic violence, elder abuse, and sexual assault.

Although most EDs have physicians available around the clock who are physically located within the ED, the nurse often initiates COLLABORATIVE interdisciplinary protocols for lifesaving interventions such as cardiac monitoring, oxygen therapy, insertion of IV catheters, and infusion of appropriate parenteral solutions. In many EDs, nurses function under clearly defined medical protocols that allow them to initiate drug therapy for emergent conditions such as anaphylactic shock and cardiac arrest. Emergency care principles extend to knowing what essential laboratory and diagnostic tests may be needed and, when necessary, obtaining them.

The emergency nurse must be proficient in performing a variety of technical skills (multitasking), sometimes in a stressful, high-pressure environment such as a cardiac or trauma resuscitation. In addition to basic skills, he or she may also need to be proficient with critical care equipment, such as invasive pressure monitoring devices and mechanical ventilators. This type of equipment is commonly found in EDs that are part of Level I and Level II trauma centers.

The nurse also COLLABORATES with and assists the physician with a number of procedures. Knowledge and skills related to procedural setup, patient preparation, teaching, and postprocedure care are key aspects of emergency nursing practice. Common ED procedures include:
- Simple and complex suturing for wound closure
- Foreign body removal
- Central line insertion
- Endotracheal intubation and initiation of mechanical ventilation
- Transvenous pacemaker insertion
- Lumbar puncture
- Pelvic examination
- Chest tube insertion
- Paracentesis
- Fracture management

More than one nurse may be necessary to assist with some procedures. For example, if moderate sedation is used to produce amnesia and relaxation during fracture reduction, one nurse assists the physician with the actual procedure while the other nurse monitors the patient before, during, and after the moderate sedation medications are administered.

Finally, an essential aspect of the emergency nurse's skill base is COMMUNICATION. The ED environment is complex; therefore multiple barriers to effective communication are likely. One common barrier is the patient's cultural beliefs and practices, especially if they differ from those of the health care team. Assess each patient as an individual, and be careful not to

⊕ CULTURAL CONSIDERATIONS
Patient-Centered Care QSEN

Be aware of the various cultural and religious values of patients that may influence care. Many people have distinct beliefs that must be respected in the health care setting. For example, some Mexican Americans are modest and do not like to have their bodies exposed. They often tend to be very family-oriented and affectionate toward each other.

Patients with language barriers can present a challenge. The population of non-English-speaking people is rapidly increasing in the United States. When a patient who is not proficient in English arrives to the ED seeking care, access available resources such as telephone language lines and dedicated interpreters contracted by the hospital to ensure an understanding of all aspects of care.

A religious belief system can also affect the delivery of care. For example, Jehovah's Witness patients do not accept blood transfusions and may not accept certain medications that are derived from human blood components.

Be aware that not all patients identify themselves as male or female. Some patients may be in the process of changing their gender identity from male to female or female to male (transgender people). Ask the patient what pronoun (he, she, or other term) that the person prefers to be called. Demonstrate professional behaviors that promote trust. Chapter 73 discusses the special care for this population in detail.

stereotype anyone based on his or her ethnicity, socioeconomic status, gender identity, or religion.

ED crowding and insufficient nursing personnel to meet the demand for services also create difficulties with COMMUNICATION of pertinent patient information and quality of written documentation. The high-stress ED environment can negatively affect effective interpersonal behaviors, particularly when nurses must deal with angry, violent, or demanding patients.

Training and Certification

Two general types of certification are referred to in emergency nursing practice: the "certification" that marks successful completion of a particular course of study; and emergency nursing specialty certification (Table 8-1). As part of the orientation and employment requirements for staff nurses in most U.S. EDs, successful completion of the Basic Life Support (BLS) for Healthcare Providers and Advanced Cardiac Life Support (ACLS) and Pediatric Advanced Life Support (PALS) provider courses through the American Heart Association is necessary. These courses provide instruction in fundamental, evidence-based management theory and techniques for cardiopulmonary resuscitation (CPR). Course participants include physicians, nurses, and prehospital personnel. The ACLS course builds on the BLS content to include:

- Advanced concepts in cardiac monitoring
- Invasive airway management skills
- Pharmacologic and electrical therapies
- Intravascular access techniques
- Special resuscitation situations
- Post-resuscitation management considerations

Additional certification may be required through successful completion of trauma continuing education courses.

EMERGENCY NURSING PRINCIPLES

Triage

ED triage is an organized system for sorting or classifying patients into priority levels depending on illness or injury severity. The organization of emergency care and the ED is structured through triage principles. The key concept is that patients who present to the ED with the highest acuity needs receive the quickest evaluation, treatment, and prioritized resource utilization such as x-rays, laboratory work, and computed tomography (CT) scans. These patients also have priority for hospital service areas, such as the operating room or cardiac catheterization laboratory. A person with a lower acuity problem may wait

longer in the ED because the higher acuity patient is moved to the "head of the line." The staff may need to COMMUNICATE information about this system to the patient and family who may not understand why other patients are treated first.

The triage nurse is the gatekeeper in the emergency care system. When patients present to the ED, regulatory standards dictate that a registered nurse (RN), physician, or physician assistant (PA) perform a rapid assessment to determine triage priority. However, the RN is typically the person assigned to perform the triage function in most hospitals. The triage nurse requires appropriate training and experience in both emergency nursing and triage decision-making concepts to develop an expert knowledge base, as well as ongoing mentoring and quality improvement feedback (Dateo, 2013). In some instances, the triage nurse may seek the input of an emergency physician, advanced practice nurse (e.g., nurse practitioner [NP]), or PA to help establish the acuity level if the patient's presentation is highly unusual.

Based on the triage priority, patients may be rushed into a treatment room, directed to a lower acuity area within the ED, or asked to sit in the waiting room. Variations on this theme include:

- Triage nurse–initiated protocols for laboratory work or diagnostic studies that may be performed before the patient is actually evaluated by a physician
- Initiation of care while the patient is on a stretcher in the hallway of a crowded ED

These protocols are especially beneficial for certain populations who require rapid diagnosis and COLLABORATIVE treatment within a defined time frame from ED arrival to meet established standards of care. Examples are patients with chest pain or those with a clinical presentation indicative of stroke, sepsis, or pneumonia.

Emergent, Urgent, and Nonurgent Categories

Many triage systems can be used by a hospital ED. Any system must be applied consistently by triage nursing staff and endorsed by the emergency medicine physician staff. Based on the severity of the patient's condition, a well-known triage scheme used in the United States is the three-tiered model of "emergent, urgent, and nonurgent" (Table 8-2). In this system, for example,

---

TABLE 8-1   Descriptions of Training and Certifications for Emergency Nursing

CERTIFICATION	DESCRIPTION
Basic Life Support (BLS) (required)	Noninvasive assessment and management skills for airway maintenance and cardiopulmonary resuscitation (CPR)
Advanced Cardiac Life Support (ACLS) (usually required)	Invasive airway management skills, pharmacology, and electrical therapies, special resuscitation
Pediatric Advanced Life Support (PALS) (may be required)	Neonatal and pediatric resuscitation
Certified Emergency Nurse (CEN) (optional)	Validates core emergency nursing knowledge base

---

TABLE 8-2   Three-Tiered Triage System and Examples of Patients Triaged in Each Tier

TIER LEVEL	EXAMPLES OF PATIENTS TRIAGED IN EACH TIER
Emergent (life threatening)	Respiratory distress Chest pain with diaphoresis Stroke Active hemorrhage Unstable vital signs
Urgent (needs quick treatment, but not immediately life threatening)	Severe abdominal pain Renal colic Displaced or multiple fractures Complex or multiple soft tissue injuries New-onset respiratory infection, especially pneumonia in older adults
Nonurgent (could wait several hours if needed without fear of deterioration)	Skin rash Strains and sprains "Colds" Simple fracture

a patient experiencing crushing substernal chest pain, shortness of breath, and diaphoresis would be classified as emergent and triaged immediately to a treatment room within the ED. Similarly, a critically injured trauma patient or a person with an active hemorrhage would also be prioritized as emergent. The emergent triage category implies that a condition exists that poses an immediate threat to life or limb.

The urgent triage category indicates that the patient should be treated quickly but that an immediate threat to life does not exist at the moment. Reassessment is needed if a physician cannot evaluate the patient in a timely manner. In people with evidence of clinical deterioration, triage priority may be upgraded from urgent to emergent. Examples of patients who typically fall into the urgent category are those with a new onset of pneumonia (as long as respiratory failure does not appear imminent), renal colic, complex lacerations not associated with major hemorrhage, displaced fractures or dislocations, and temperature greater than 101° F (38.3° C). Those categorized as nonurgent can generally tolerate waiting several hours for health care services without a significant risk for clinical deterioration. Conditions within this classification include patients with sprains and strains, simple fractures, "cold" symptoms, and skin rashes.

Other Multi-Tiered Models

To further sort patient conditions within an acuity classification or triage priority system, four- and five-tier triage models also exist. Such models are based either on comprehensive lists of conditions that indicate the particular triage priority to which a patient should be assigned or on the nature of resources that a patient will use in the ED setting. A patient situation may generate various triage classifications in different hospitals depending on the triage priority system used at that particular institution. Some schemes may even take into account the presence of pre-existing conditions such as a history of anticoagulant use, diabetes, heart disease, and organ transplantation.

It is surprising that there is no universally accepted triage system recognized in the United States. Thus there is no standardization of triage acuity data to compare patient acuity among hospitals. Medical providers, health insurance companies, and patients often disagree on the definition of an emergent versus a nonurgent ED visit, making it essential to use a practical triage system to maintain department efficiency and allocation of resources (Aacharya et al., 2011). The Emergency Nurses Association in COLLABORATION with the American College of Emergency Physicians studied the available research literature on acuity scales and concluded that two standardized five-level systems, the Emergency Severity Index (ESI) and the Canadian Triage Acuity Scale (CTAS), are the most reliable (Shelton, 2010). The ESI model uses an algorithm that fosters rapid, reliable, and clinically pertinent categorization of patients into five groups, from level 1 (emergent) to level 5 (nonurgent). The CTAS model differs from ESI in that lists of descriptors are used to establish the triage level.

Whatever triage model is used, triage nurses must employ a systematic approach, apply solid clinical decision-making skills, and maintain a caring ethic. Compassion fatigue, or burn-out, can hinder objectivity in dealing with patients who present to the ED. A biased approach threatens the ED nurse's ability to triage patients accurately. Mistriage is a patient SAFETY risk that can be the "root cause" of delayed or inadequate treatment with potentially deadly consequences.

 NCLEX EXAMINATION CHALLENGE

Safe and Effective Care Environment

The emergency department nurse is assigned to five clients waiting for orders to be implemented. Which client does the nurse assess first?

A. 60-year-old waiting for transport to the operating room for an emergency appendectomy
B. 25-year-old with a closed femur fracture who received pain medication 10 minutes ago
C. 30-year-old with nausea and vomiting who has IV fluids infusing and is now sleeping
D. 28-year-old construction worker with a laceration to the arm that is waiting to be sutured

Disposition

At the conclusion of the assessment, the physician must make a decision regarding patient disposition (i.e., where the patient should go after being discharged from the ED). Should the patient be admitted to the hospital, transferred to a specialty care center, or be discharged to home with instructions for continued care and follow-up? Usually, the answer is straightforward. A patient who has an evolving myocardial infarction, stroke, or acute surgical need is admitted.

Sometimes, though, the ED disposition decision is less clear. Often the physician discusses this decision in COLLABORATION with the emergency nurse. The nurse may have a greater sense of how well a patient will manage in a home setting depending on whether other family members or friends are available to assist and are reliable. For example, in the event a patient with a minor head injury has suffered a loss of consciousness, someone is typically expected to remain with that person for

CONSIDERATIONS FOR OLDER ADULTS

Patient-Centered Care QSEN

If discharge from the ED to home is possible, ensure that safety issues are considered. For example, collaborate with the emergency department physician to evaluate the patient's prescription and over-the-counter medications to determine if the drug regimen should be continued. Involve the ED-based pharmacist if one is available for consultation when necessary. If the medication regimen needs to be changed, be sure that the patient and family member or significant other has the new information in writing and that it is explained verbally. If needed, assess whether the patient has someone who can dispense medications into a "medi-set" to ensure accuracy and prevent adverse drug events. Consider a social services or case management referral for those patients in need of financial resources to obtain prescribed medications.

To prevent future ED visits, screen older adults per agency policy for functional assessment, cognitive assessment, and risk for falls. Depression screening is also important because suicide rates are two times higher among older adults when compared with younger adults. White men older than 85 years are at the highest risk (Touhy & Jett, 2012).

More than half of all older patients are admitted to the hospital directly from the ED (Nolan, 2009). If hospitalization is needed, determine if the patient has advance directives or is able to make decisions about advance directives before admission. If the patient was admitted from a nursing home, contact the facility to let them know the patient's status. If the patient was receiving home health care services, notify the agency about the hospital admission. Contact the patient's primary physician and designated family member if he or she is not present with the patient.

the first 12 to 24 hours to be sure that he or she does not show any evidence of neurologic deterioration. Another common scenario involves the potential risk to the patient in cases of actual or suspected domestic violence. If discharge to home is not deemed safe, the patient may be admitted to the hospital in an observation status until resources can be organized to provide for a safe environment. Coordinate the discharge plan and continuing care with the social worker or case manager.

Case Management

Some EDs employ registered nurse case managers who screen ED patients and intervene when necessary to arrange appropriate referral and follow-up. This is an evolving role in the ED setting that can be beneficial in providing comprehensive care and as a strategy to avoid inappropriate use of resources.

ED case managers, supported by electronic information systems, can review the ED census on both a "real-time" and a retrospective basis to determine which patients have visited the ED frequently in a given period. The case manager can then determine the reasons they sought emergency services, such as lack of a primary health care provider, exacerbation ("flare-up") of a chronic condition, a lack of health education, or lack of the financial resources necessary to manage the health condition. COLLABORATIVE case management interventions include facilitating referrals to primary care providers or to subsidized community-based health clinics for patients or families in need of routine services.

For those with needs related to chronic conditions, the case manager can arrange referral into appropriate disease management programs in the community if available. Disease management programs are specific to a particular condition such as asthma, COPD, diabetes, hypertension, heart failure, and renal failure. They help patients learn how to manage their condition on a day-to-day basis to prevent exacerbations or clinical deterioration. The desired outcome is to keep the person out of the hospital as long as possible. Health teaching is a key component of these programs. For other health teaching needs, the ED case manager directs the patient to the appropriate educational resources such as a health educator, registered dietitian, or community organization (e.g., the American Cancer Society, the American Heart Association).

Other functions of the ED case manager might include working in COLLABORATION with staff to plan disposition for homeless people, locating a safe environment for victims of domestic violence or elder abuse, or providing information on resources for low-cost or free prescriptions. Homeless adults often have multiple chronic medical illnesses for which they visit emergency departments frequently. A large study of homeless adults with chronic medical illnesses demonstrated a decrease in ED visits and hospital admissions as a result of an organized follow-up system for housing and ongoing case management support. (See the Quality Improvement box.)

Patient and Family Education

A key role of the emergency nurse is health teaching. At the most basic level, nurses review discharge instructions with the patient and family before signing them out of the department.

In addition to discharge instructions, the ED environment and community-at-large present many opportunities for health education. Emergency nurses are in an ideal position to educate the public about wellness and injury-prevention strategies. If

Improving the Flow of Stable Patients Through an Emergency Department

Popovich, M.A., Boyd, C., Dachenhaus, T., & Kusler, D. (2012). Improving stable patient flow through the emergency department by utilizing evidence-based practice: One hospital's journey. *Journal of Emergency Nursing, 38*(5), 474-478.

Many nonemergent patients use emergency departments (EDs) for medical care, resulting in overcrowding, lengthy wait times, patient dissatisfaction, and increasing numbers of patients who leave without being seen (LWBS). Increased length of wait has been correlated with poorer outcomes. A project was designed in the country's fifth-largest pediatric emergency department to investigate whether an evidence-based, volume-driven protocol would increase rapid treatment of stable patients. The protocol included a volume-based driver, unlike other tools used in EDs to manage patient flow, staffing, and resource allocation, such as the Emergency Severity Index (ESI), which is a 5-level decision-making tool used in triage. The protocol was designed to determine when to open the satellite unit for stable patients.

A participating hospital contained a 68-bed Level I trauma center and a nearby 8-bed satellite unit. A benchmark of 120 minutes for total length of stay (TLOS) was established as the quality indicator. After reviewing ED statistics, a tool was developed that considered total patient census and the number of ESI 4 and 5 patients in the unit. The triggers were a total census of 55 and/or 11 to 16 ESI level 4 patients and/or 5 to 7 ESI level 5 patients in the department. Other considerations included more than two people in the triage line, more than three people in the lobby waiting to be seen, and whether the urgent care section was full. Training was conducted to ensure consistency among the nurses in categorizing level 4 and level 5 patients. Use of the tool increased the number of days the satellite was open and decreased the number of patients who LWBS by 29%. The 120-minute benchmark was not met, but only by 7.5 minutes.

Commentary: Implications for Practice and Research

This demonstrated that patient satisfaction and outcomes were diminished as waiting times for ED services increased. EDs using an evidence-based tool can eliminate personal opinions when considering whether to use additional resources to expedite the flow of stable patients through the department. Specifying triggers for activating these resources can allow for better use of ED services. Research should continue on fine-tuning the tool to meet the needs of individual EDs, correlating use of the tool and patient outcomes, and should investigate patient satisfaction with the resulting (it is hoped decreased) wait times.

CULTURAL CONSIDERATIONS

Patient-Centered Care (QSEN)

Most discharge instructions are either preprinted or computer generated and can be customized to address the patient's needs. Consider his or her reading level, primary language, and visual acuity. Educational materials and instructions should be available at no higher than the 6th-grade reading level. For patients who have English as a second language, many hospitals have educational materials available in Spanish and other regional languages. However, interpreters may be necessary to assist the health care provider customize the information appropriately. For older adults and others with vision deficits, large-print materials may be helpful.

the patient presented after a motor vehicle crash, for instance, the nurse can reinforce the need to wear seat belts or use child safety seats correctly. ED visits that result from mishaps in the home provide an excellent opportunity to discuss home SAFETY issues (e.g., the need for smoke detectors and carbon monoxide detectors) and fall prevention tips (e.g., the need for proper lighting, removal of throw rugs). Injury is not the only topic that affords a teaching opportunity. A new onset or an exacerbation of a medical condition also allows for education, such as how to measure blood glucose and ways to control blood pressure or reduce the risk for heart disease.

Death in the Emergency Department

Not all critically ill or injured patients who come to the ED can be saved. Sometimes a patient's death is expected by family members, typically when they have dealt with a loved one's terminal condition or age-related decline. Usually, however, a death in the ED is a sudden and unexpected event that produces a state of crisis and chaos for family and significant others. Emergency department staff members need to address the needs of the family members in this overwhelming time.

If resuscitation efforts are still underway when the family arrives, one or two family members may be given the opportunity to be present during lifesaving procedures. Family presence during resuscitation is gaining wider acceptance in the health care community; however, a significant number of hospitals still have not devised clear policies or guidelines to facilitate family-witnessed resuscitation (Feagan & Fisher, 2011).

If the patient dies before family members arrive, ED staff members try to prepare the body and the room for viewing by the family. However, certain types of ED deaths may require forensic investigation or become medical examiner's cases. Therefore ED staff may not be able to remove IV lines and indwelling tubes or clean the patient's skin if these actions could potentially damage evidence. Trauma deaths, suspected homicide, or abuse cases always fall into this category. In these situations, cover the body with a sheet or blanket while leaving the patient's face exposed, and dim the lights before family viewing.

When dealing with family members in crisis, simple and concrete COMMUNICATION is best. Words such as *death* or *died,* although seemingly harsh, create less confusion than terms such as *expired* or *passed away.* Demonstrate caring, compassion, and empathy during all interactions, even in periods of heightened emotions. Intense grief can provoke a range of family reactions from silence to violence. If available, coordinate with crisis staff (social workers or psychiatric nurses) to assist families and maintain SAFETY during this time. Offer the family the option of speaking with clergy or calling someone of their choice for additional support. A family member may need to be admitted to the ED to be treated for anxiety or physical manifestations of stress such as chest pain, difficulty breathing, or severe headache.

Dealing with death is often difficult for ED personnel, especially during busy periods when the ability to console family members may be limited. In response, some emergency departments have developed bereavement committees that focus on meeting the needs of grieving families. Actions such as sending sympathy cards, attending funerals, making follow-up phone calls, and creating memory boxes are common. These actions help COMMUNICATE caring and compassion after the moment of crisis.

THE IMPACT OF HOMELESSNESS

Homelessness affected 636,000 people in 2011, an increase of 1% from the prior year (National Alliance to End Homelessness, 2012). The homeless population is made up of both adults and children who live from day to day in a state of fear, chaos,

and confusion (Gerber, 2013). People become homeless as a result of a crisis or persistent poverty (Gerber, 2013). They have a high incidence of acute and chronic health conditions, psychiatric illnesses, physical disabilities or limitations, and problems with substance abuse (Gerber, 2013). They are vulnerable to physical trauma, weather exposure, sexually transmitted diseases, infestation, and infectious diseases such as tuberculosis and influenza.

Homeless patients often seek ED care for a variety of reasons. Because the ED is open 24 hours per day and is mandated by federal law to perform an emergency medical screening examination on all of their patients, patients who are homeless know that they will gain entry despite their inability to pay for services. The ED represents a safe place to go for shelter in poor weather and for food, medical care, pain relief, and human interaction. Some homeless patients simply seek a temporary respite from their current living conditions, which may be a park, homeless shelter, car, abandoned building, or cardboard box. Those people who have been persistently homeless may assimilate into the homeless culture, learn to take great pride in their survival skills, and fiercely protect their few belongings as well as their living space. They may develop a distrust of outsiders, including members of the health care profession, and are especially sensitive to any perceived bias or stereotyping (Gerber, 2013).

Patients who are homeless bring special challenges to their ED evaluation, treatment, and disposition. Some visit the ED frequently and do not adhere to treatment recommendations or follow-up with community referrals. Those with mental illness or substance abuse may act out or become disruptive, posing a SAFETY risk to staff and patients.

To best care for homeless patients in the ED setting, nurses must first maintain their situational awareness and attend to their own needs for personal safety. These include not only anticipating the potential for violent behavior but also using Standard Precautions and assessing the need to isolate the patient in a negative pressure room if airborne disease such as tuberculosis (TB) is a concern. The key nursing action is to demonstrate behaviors that promote trust. These include making eye contact (if culturally appropriate), speaking calmly, avoiding any prejudicial or stereotypical remarks, being patient, showing genuine care and concern by listening, following through on promises, and exercising caution when there is a need to enter into the patient's personal space (Gerber, 2013). Clear professional boundaries must be stated if the patient becomes disruptive, profane, or sexually inappropriate. While collaborating with the emergency care provider to ensure that the patient's emergency medical needs are identified and treated, consult a social worker or case manager to work with the patient in identifying safety needs, referral options, and community resources. It is also important to develop an individual care plan with the interdisciplinary health care team if the patient uses the ED frequently. This type of care plan is extremely beneficial in establishing a consistent approach to patient management, especially when the patient has complex conditions or exhibits drug-seeking and disruptive behavior.

TRAUMA NURSING PRINCIPLES

The general public tends to use the term *trauma* to mean any type of crisis ranging from a heart attack to psychological stress. Among health care professionals, though, trauma refers to bodily injury. More than 180,000 people in the United States die each year as a result of injuries, and nearly 2 million are hospitalized, often with permanent and disabling consequences (National Center for Injury Prevention and Control [NCIPC], 2012). Injuries can be categorized as either intentional (i.e., assault, homicide, suicide) or unintentional (i.e., accidents). *Unintentional injury,* such as a motor vehicle crash, is the leading cause of death for Americans younger than 35 years and is one of today's most significant public health problems (NCIPC, 2012).

Injury management is a key component of emergency department services. About 30 million people in the United States visit the ED each year to receive treatment for injuries (NCIPC, 2012). Therefore an important part of emergency nursing practice is a core competency in general trauma care. For emergency nurses who work in accredited trauma centers, opportunities typically exist to further develop expertise in trauma nursing through ongoing clinical practice, specialty training programs, and continuing education. Trauma nursing is a field that encompasses the continuum of care from injury prevention and prehospital services to acute care, rehabilitation, and, ultimately, community reintegration.

Trauma Centers and Trauma Systems

Trauma centers have their roots in military medicine. Injured soldiers who received rapid transport from the battlefield and treatment from skilled health care personnel had a survival advantage in the mobile army surgical hospital (MASH) units first deployed in the Korean and Vietnam wars. Consequently, the MASH unit became the original model for the development of civilian trauma centers. Today's **trauma center** in the United States is a specialty care facility that provides competent and timely trauma services to patients, depending on its designated level of capability.

Trauma Centers

Not all EDs that offer around-the-clock emergency services are trauma centers. The American College of Surgeons Committee on Trauma (2006) has set forth national standards for trauma center accreditation and categorizes the resource requirements necessary for the highest capability trauma center (Level I) to the lowest (Level IV) (Table 8-3).

A *Level I trauma center* is a regional resource facility that is capable of providing leadership and total COLLABORATIVE care for every aspect of injury, from prevention through rehabilitation. These centers also have a responsibility to offer professional and community education programs, conduct research, and participate in system planning. Because a significant resource and experience commitment is required to maintain strict accreditation standards, Level I trauma centers are usually located in large teaching hospitals and serve dense population areas (Fig. 8-4).

Level II trauma centers are usually located in community hospitals and are capable of providing care to the vast majority of injured patients. However, a Level II trauma center may not be able to meet the resource needs of patients who require very complex injury management, such as those in need of advanced surgical care. These people are generally transferred to a Level I trauma center for specialty care. In communities without a Level I trauma center, Level II centers play a significant leadership role in injury management, education, prevention, and emergency preparedness planning.

A *Level III trauma center* is a critical link to higher capability trauma centers in communities that do not have ready access to Level I or Level II centers. The primary focus is initial injury

LEVELS OF TRAUMA CENTER	FUNCTIONS OF TRAUMA CENTER
Level I	Usually located in large teaching hospital systems in densely populated areas
	Provides a full continuum of trauma services for all patients
	Conducting research is a requirement for designation
Level II and Level III	Both typically located in community hospitals
	Level II
	Provides care to most injured patients
	Transports patient if needs exceed resource capabilities
	Level III
	Stabilizes patients with major injuries
	Transports patient if needs exceed resource capabilities
Level IV	Usually located in rural and remote areas
	Provides basic trauma patient stabilization and advanced life support within resource capabilities
	Arranges transport to higher trauma center levels as necessary

TABLE 8-3 Levels and Functions of Trauma Centers

FIG. 8-4 A trauma team participates in a realistic trauma resuscitation simulation. This type of training ensures staff remain proficient in skills and able to care for any situation that might present to the emergency department (ED).

stabilization and patient transfer. Level III trauma centers are usually found in smaller, rural hospitals and serve areas with low population density. Because Level III trauma centers have general surgeons and orthopedic surgeons immediately available, patients with some major injuries may be admitted for care. However, if the injuries are severe or critical, transfer to a Level I or II trauma center occurs after ED assessment, resuscitation, and stabilization—sometimes after emergent, lifesaving surgery. Patients are typically transported out in either an advanced life support ambulance or helicopter with critical care transport personnel in attendance.

The function of a *Level IV trauma center* is to offer advanced life support care in rural or remote settings that do not have ready access to a higher-level trauma center, such as a ski area. Patients are stabilized to the best degree possible before transfer, using available personnel such as advanced practice nurses, physician assistants, nurses, and paramedics. Resources, including the consistent availability of a physician, may be extremely limited. Transport time to the final care center can be prolonged because of both distance and bad weather conditions that may prevent transfer by air.

Level III and Level IV trauma centers establish close COL-LABORATIVE relationships with Level I and Level II trauma centers. Based on accreditation standards, care providers at Levels I and II trauma centers have a responsibility to readily accept injured patients in transfer. They provide timely feedback to trauma personnel at referring hospitals and share expertise by offering educational opportunities to advance trauma care delivery in the region. In addition, personnel from all levels of trauma centers participate in focused system improvement and patient safety initiatives that enhance quality of care and solve identified problems.

Trauma Systems

Trauma centers save lives—but a trauma center is only as good as the overall trauma system that supports it. A **trauma system** is an organized and integrated approach to trauma care designed to ensure that all critical elements of trauma care delivery are aligned to meet the injured patient's needs. These elements include (Cooper & Laskowski-Jones, 2006):

- Access to care through COMMUNICATION technology (e.g., an enhanced 911 service)
- Timely availability of prehospital emergency medical care
- Rapid transport to a qualified trauma center
- Early provision of rehabilitation services
- System-wide injury prevention, research, and education initiatives

The overall desired outcome of an organized trauma system is to enable an injured patient not only to recover from trauma but also to return to a productive role in society.

A well-functioning trauma system is also essential to general public health and SAFETY. It provides the structure necessary for disaster readiness and community emergency preparedness (see Chapter 10). Although most states now have at least some basic elements of a trauma system in place, significant gaps still exist in many regions.

Mechanism of Injury

The **mechanism of injury (MOI)** describes how the patient's traumatic event occurred, such as a high-speed motor vehicle crash, a fall from a standing height, or a gunshot wound to the torso. Knowing key details about the MOI can provide insight into the energy forces involved and may help trauma care providers predict injury types and, in some cases, patient outcomes. Prehospital care providers report the MOI as a COMMUNICA-TION standard when handing off care to ED and trauma personnel. Similarly, patients who present to the ED for medical care will often relate the MOI by describing the particular chain of events that caused their injuries.

Two of the most common injury-producing mechanisms are blunt trauma and penetrating trauma. **Blunt trauma** results from impact forces like those sustained in a motor vehicle crash, a fall, and an assault with fists, kicks, or a baseball bat. **Blast effect** from an exploding bomb also causes blunt trauma. The energy transmitted from a blunt trauma mechanism, particularly the rapid **acceleration-deceleration** forces involved in high-speed crashes or falls from a great height, produces injury

by tearing, shearing, and compressing anatomic structures. Trauma to bones, blood vessels, and soft tissues occurs.

Penetrating trauma is caused by injury from sharp objects and projectiles. Examples are wounds from knives, ice picks, and other comparable implements, as well as bullets (gunshot wounds [GSWs]) or pellets. Fragments of metal, glass, or other materials that become airborne in an explosion (shrapnel) can also produce penetrating trauma. Each mechanism has the risk for specific injury patterns and severity that the trauma team considers when planning diagnostic evaluation and management strategies. Certain injury mechanisms, such as a gunshot wound to the chest or abdomen or a stab wound to the neck, are so highly associated with life-threatening consequences that they automatically require trauma team intervention for a rapid and coordinated resuscitation response.

Primary Survey and Resuscitation Interventions

A basic tenet of emergency care in any environment is scene SAFETY. In the prehospital setting, emergency care providers must ensure that they are aware of any hazards that might pose a threat to rescuers and take actions to decrease or eliminate the risk. This same concept applies to the hospital ED setting. Before engaging in trauma resuscitation as a nurse member of the trauma team, keep in mind that there is a high risk for contamination with blood and body fluids. For this reason, use Standard Precautions in *all* resuscitation situations and at other times when exposure to blood and body fluids is likely. Proper attire consists of an impervious cover gown, gloves, eye protection, a facemask, and surgical cap, as well as shoe covers (if *significant* blood loss is anticipated, such as during an ED procedure).

The initial assessment of the trauma patient is called the **primary survey,** which is an organized system to rapidly identify and effectively manage immediate threats to life. The primary survey is based on a standard "ABC" mnemonic plus a "D" and "E" for trauma patients: airway/cervical spine (**A**); breathing (**B**); circulation (**C**); disability (**D**); and exposure (**E**). Resuscitation efforts occur simultaneously with each element of the primary survey (American College of Surgeons Committee on Trauma, 2008; Laskowski-Jones, 2009). Even though the resuscitation team may encounter multiple clinical problems or injuries, issues identified in the primary survey are managed before the team engages in interventions of lower priority, such as splinting fractures and dressing wounds.

A: Airway/Cervical Spine

Like for any patient, the highest priority intervention is to establish a patent airway. Even minutes without an adequate oxygen supply can lead to brain injury that can progress to anoxic brain death.

In general, a non-rebreather mask is best for the spontaneously breathing patient. Bag-valve-mask (BVM) ventilation with the appropriate airway adjunct and a 100% oxygen source is indicated for the person who needs ventilatory assistance during resuscitation. A patient with significantly impaired consciousness requires an endotracheal tube and mechanical ventilation (American College of Surgeons Committee on Trauma, 2008).

B: Breathing

After the airway is successfully secured, breathing becomes the next priority in the primary survey. *This assessment determines*

Critical Rescue

> Clear the airway of any secretions or debris either with a suction catheter or manually if necessary. Protect the cervical spine in any trauma patient with the potential for spinal injury by manually aligning the neck in a neutral, in-line position and using a jaw-thrust maneuver when establishing an airway. Provide supplemental oxygen for all patients who require resuscitation.

whether or not ventilatory efforts are effective—not only whether or not the patient is breathing. Listen to breath sounds and evaluate chest expansion, respiratory effort, and any evidence of chest wall trauma or physical abnormalities. Both apneic patients and those with poor ventilatory effort need BVM ventilation for support until endotracheal intubation is performed and a mechanical ventilator is used. If cardiopulmonary resuscitation (CPR) becomes necessary, the mechanical ventilator is disconnected and the patient is manually ventilated with a BVM device. Lung compliance can be assessed through sensing the degree of difficulty in ventilating the patient with the BVM.

C: Circulation

When effective ventilation is ensured, the priority shifts to circulation. The adequacy of heart rate, blood pressure, and overall perfusion becomes the focus of the assessment. Common threats to circulation include cardiac arrest, myocardial dysfunction, and hemorrhage leading to a shock state. Interventions are targeted at restoring effective circulation through cardiopulmonary resuscitation, hemorrhage control, IV vascular access with fluid and blood administration as necessary, and drug therapy. *External* hemorrhage is usually quite obvious and best controlled with firm, direct pressure on the bleeding site with thick, dry dressing material. This method is effective in decreasing blood flow for most wounds. *Tourniquets that occlude arterial blood flow distal to the injury may be considered to manage severe bleeding from extremity trauma when direct pressure fails to achieve hemorrhage control; hemostatic dressings (e.g., dressings impregnated with substances that speed the formation of a blood clot) are another essential tool to manage life-threatening hemorrhage* (Strickler, 2010). *Internal* hemorrhage is a more hidden complication that must be suspected in injured patients or those who present in a shock state.

In a resuscitation situation, blood pressure can be quickly and easily estimated before a manual cuff pressure can be obtained by palpating for the presence or absence of peripheral and central pulses:

- Presence of a radial pulse: BP at least 80 mm Hg systolic
- Presence of a femoral pulse: BP at least 70 mm Hg systolic
- Presence of a carotid pulse: BP at least 60 mm Hg systolic

By the time hypotension occurs, compensatory mechanisms used by the body in an attempt to maintain vital signs in a shock state have been exhausted. Timely, effective intervention is critical to preserve life and vital organ function.

IV access is best achieved initially with insertion of large-bore (16-gauge) peripheral IV lines in the antecubital area (inside bend of the elbow). Additional access can be obtained via central veins in the femoral, subclavian, or jugular sites using large-bore (8.5 Fr) central venous catheters. Intraosseous access is an excellent initial approach for critically ill patients when

veins cannot be rapidly accessed by the resuscitation team (see Chapter 13 for discussion of intraosseous infusion therapy). Ringer's lactate and 0.9% normal saline (NS) are the crystalloid solutions of choice for resuscitation; hypertonic saline may also be prescribed in some situations, particularly in the case of head trauma. Fluids and blood products should be warmed before administration to prevent hypothermia. Anticipate the need for rapid blood component administration in a hemorrhagic shock state using packed red blood cells, fresh frozen plasma, and platelets to both replace blood loss and prevent coagulopathy when significant hypotension persists after infusion of 2 L of solution (Davis et al., 2012). However, the priority intervention is to stop the bleeding.

D: Disability

The disability examination provides a rapid baseline assessment of neurologic status. A simple method to evaluate level of consciousness is the "AVPU" mnemonic:

- A: **A**lert
- V: Responsive to **v**oice
- P: Responsive to **p**ain
- U: **U**nresponsive

Another common way of determining and documenting level of consciousness is the **Glasgow Coma Scale (GCS),** an assessment that scores eye opening, verbal response, and motor response. The lowest score is 3, which indicates a totally unresponsive patient; a normal GCS score is 15. Metabolic abnormalities (e.g., severe hypoglycemia), hypoxia, neurologic injury, and illicit drugs or alcohol can impair level of consciousness. Frequent reassessment is needed for rapid intervention in the event of neurologic compromise or deterioration.

E: Exposure

The final component of the primary survey is **exposure.**

Action Alert

> Remove all clothing to allow for thorough assessment. Always *cut away* clothing with scissors:
> - During resuscitation when rapid access to the patient's body is critical
> - When manipulating a patient's limbs to remove clothing could cause further injury
> - When thermal or chemical burns have caused fabrics to melt into the patient's skin

If evidence preservation is an issue, handle items per institutional policy. Evidence may include articles of clothing, impaled objects, weapons, drugs, and bullets. Emergency nurses are often called upon to provide testimony in court regarding their recall of the presentation and treatment of patients in the ED. Examples of types of cases in which evidence collection is vital are rape, elder abuse, domestic violence, homicide, suicide, drug overdose, and assault.

Once clothing is removed, hypothermia (body temperature less than or equal to 97° F [36° C]) poses a risk to injured patients, especially those with burns and traumatic shock states (Moore, 2011). Hypothermia is discussed in detail in Chapter 9.

Table 8-4 highlights the primary survey and associated resuscitation interventions.

TABLE 8-4 The Primary Survey and Resuscitation Interventions

PRIORITIES OF THE PRIMARY SURVEY	EXAMPLES OF SPECIFIC INTERVENTIONS
A: Airway/cervical spine	Establish a patent airway by positioning, suctioning, and oxygen as needed. Protect the cervical spine by maintaining alignment; use a jaw-thrust maneuver if there is a risk for spinal injury. If the Glasgow Coma Scale (GCS) score is 8 or less or the patient is at risk for airway compromise, prepare for endotracheal intubation and mechanical ventilation.
B: Breathing	Assess breath sounds and respiratory effort. Observe for chest wall trauma or other physical abnormality. Prepare for chest decompression if needed. Prepare to assist ventilations if needed.
C: Circulation	Monitor vital signs, especially blood pressure and pulse. Maintain vascular access using a large-bore catheter. Use direct pressure for external bleeding; anticipate need for a tourniquet for severe, uncontrollable extremity hemorrhage and use of a hemostatic dressing.
D: Disability	Evaluate the patient's level of consciousness (LOC) using the GCS. Re-evaluate the patient's LOC frequently.
E: Exposure	Remove all clothing for a complete physical assessment. Prevent hypothermia (e.g., cover the patient with blankets, use heating devices, infuse warm solutions).

NCLEX EXAMINATION CHALLENGE
Safe and Effective Care Environment

A trauma client has been brought to the emergency department after a motor vehicle crash. The client has severe injuries. What action does the nurse perform first?
A. Start 2 large-bore IVs and run normal saline.
B. Apply oxygen and an oximeter probe to the client.
C. Stabilize the cervical spine and assess the airway.
D. Place pressure on a large bleeding wound to the forehead.

The Secondary Survey and Resuscitation Interventions

After the ED resuscitation team addresses the immediate life threats, other activities that the emergency nurse can anticipate include insertion of a gastric tube for decompression of the GI tract to prevent vomiting and aspiration, insertion of a urinary catheter to allow careful measure of urine output, and preparation for diagnostic studies. The resuscitation team also performs a more comprehensive head-to-toe assessment, known as the secondary survey, to identify other injuries or medical issues that need to be managed or that might affect the course of treatment.

Disposition

The patient may be transported immediately to the operating room or interventional radiology suite directly from the ED, depending on the nature of the injury. When no immediate procedural intervention is indicated, patients are admitted to inpatient units for management and nursing care based on the nature and severity of their injuries, as well as any other pre-existing medical conditions that could complicate trauma care. However, if the facility does not have the resource capabilities to manage the injured patient, the physician arranges for transfer to a higher level of care.

Work in COLLABORATION with the interdisciplinary team to address the trauma patient's complex health care needs, including early consultation with social services and the rehabilitation team. Coordinate with other support services as necessary, such as pastoral care, nutrition support, psychiatry, behavioral health specialists, and substance abuse counselors. Trauma centers are required to incorporate systems to identify patients with high-risk alcohol use (American College of Surgeons Committee on Trauma, 2006). An effective strategy is to implement an SBIRT (**s**creening, **b**rief **i**ntervention, and **r**eferral to **t**reatment) program in which interdisciplinary trauma team members, including emergency and trauma nurses, are educated to assess patients for problem drinking. The typical interaction involves a brief, respectful conversation that offers feedback, advice, and motivation to reduce alcohol consumption (Desy et al., 2010).

Consider the needs of family members in crisis and address them when planning nursing care. A trauma advanced practice nurse, if available, can help coordinate trauma care by offering clinical expertise, facilitating COMMUNICATION among caregivers, and serving as an educator for the patient, staff, and family (Mower-Wade & Pirrung, 2010). They can organize family meetings with the interdisciplinary team and arrange for necessary resources. If this resource is not available, a case manager or specially educated direct care nurse may perform these functions.

GET READY FOR THE NCLEX® EXAMINATION!

KEY POINTS

Review these Key Points for each NCLEX Examination Client Needs Category.

Safe and Effective Care Environment
- Understand that emergency departments (EDs) are fast-paced, often crowded environments where care occurs for patients across the life span with a variety of health problems.
- Recognize that some vulnerable populations who present to the ED include patients who are uninsured (poor), homeless, and older adults. **Patient-Centered Care** QSEN
- Anticipate that some of the most common reasons that patients seek ED care are chest pain, abdominal pain, difficulty breathing, injury, headache, fever, and pain.
- COLLABORATE with members of the interdisciplinary health care team in the ED, which includes prehospital providers,

physicians, nurses, specialty teams, and support staff. **Teamwork and Collaboration** [QSEN]

- Review Chart 8-1 to plan and implement best practices to maintain staff and patient SAFETY in the ED. **Safety** [QSEN]
- Explain the core competencies needed for nurses to function in the ED, including assessment, priority setting, knowledge, technical skills, and COMMUNICATION.
- Understand that the three-level triage model categorizes patients as emergent, urgent, and nonurgent (see Table 8-2). The Emergency Severity Index is a five-tier triage system that uses both acuity and the prediction of necessary resources to rapidly categorize the priority of patients.
- Recall that trauma centers are categorized as Levels I through IV, based on their resource capabilities as listed in Table 8-3.
- Remember that the mechanism of injury describes the manner in which the traumatic event occurred.
- Recall that the two most common injury-producing mechanisms are blunt trauma and penetrating trauma.
- Prioritize resuscitation interventions based on the primary survey of the injured patient by implementing the steps of the primary survey and trauma resuscitation as outlined in Table 8-4.
- Recall that patient education as part of the discharge plan is an important part of ED nursing practice.

Psychosocial Integrity

- Provide support by working in COLLABORATION with the psychiatric crisis team as needed.

Physiological Integrity

- Remember the general process of admission through discharge in the ED. Patients managed in the ED are treated and stabilized before discharge. Patients may be discharged to their homes or be admitted for observation or inpatient care.
- Recall that about half of all older adults who visit the ED are admitted to the hospital. **Patient-Centered Care** [QSEN]
- Understand that ED nurses are accountable for preventing or reducing risks such as falls, medication errors, pressure ulcers, and hospital-acquired infections. COMMUNICATION with the older adult may be challenging if he or she has memory loss or develops acute delirium while in the ED. **Safety** [QSEN]

Care of Patients with Common Environmental Emergencies

Linda Laskowski-Jones

 http://evolve.elsevier.com/Iggy/

PRIORITY CONCEPTS

- PAIN
- THERMOREGULATION

- TISSUE INTEGRITY

LEARNING OUTCOMES

Safe and Effective Care Environment

1. Collaborate with the interdisciplinary health care team when providing care for patients with common environmental emergencies.

Health Promotion and Maintenance

2. Teach people at risk how to prevent heat-related and cold-related injuries, especially older adults.
3. Teach people at risk how to prevent arthropod bites and stings and snakebites.

Physiological Integrity

4. Assess patients at high risk for environmental emergencies.
5. Prioritize first aid/prehospital interventions for patients who have THERMOREGULATION problems.

6. Prioritize first aid/prehospital interventions for patients who have arthropod bites affecting TISSUE INTEGRITY.
7. Prioritize first aid/emergency care interventions for patients who have venomous snakebites.
8. Apply knowledge of pathophysiology to identify best practices for care of patients with environmental emergencies.
9. Develop an evidence-based plan of care for a patient who is allergic to bees and is stung.
10. Prioritize care for patients who have been struck by lightning.
11. Prioritize care for patients who survive a drowning incident.
12. Explain best practices for patients who are at risk for or experience altitude-related illnesses.

Recreational activities, as well as home and work responsibilities, inspire people of all ages to leave their homes and go outdoors. However, seemingly harmless outside activities can have associated environmental risks, especially for older adults. Some risks, such as insect bites or stings, reptile bites, and environmental conditions, may also pose threats indoors. This chapter provides an overview of selected environmental emergencies, their initial emergency management (first aid), and acute care interventions. Illness and injury prevention strategies for nurses to incorporate into their own lifestyle and health teaching opportunities are also discussed.

HEAT-RELATED ILLNESSES

High environmental temperature (above 95°F [35°C]) and high humidity (above 80%) are the most common environmental factors causing heat-related illnesses. These THERMOREGULATION-related illnesses include heat exhaustion and heat stroke. Some of the most vulnerable, at-risk populations for these problems are:

- Older adults
- People with mental health conditions
- People who work outside, such as construction and agricultural workers (more men than women)
- Homeless people
- Illicit drug users (especially cocaine users)
- Outdoor athletes (recreational and professional)
- Members of the military who are stationed in countries with hot climates (e.g., Iraq, Afghanistan)

Older adults have less body fluid volume and can easily become dehydrated when exposed to excessive heat and humidity. Wearing heavy clothing, inadequate acclimatization to hot weather, and social disadvantage (e.g., poor housing, lack of air-conditioning) are also significant contributing factors.

A patient's health status can also increase the risk for heat-related illness, especially obesity, heart disease, fever, infection, strenuous exercise, seizures, mental health disorders, and all degrees of burns (even sunburn). In addition, the use of certain prescribed drugs such as lithium, neuroleptics, beta-adrenergic blockers, anticholinergics, angiotensin-converting

CHART 9-1 **Nursing Focus on the Older Adult**

Heat-Related Illness Prevention

- Avoid alcohol and caffeine.
- Prevent overexposure to the sun; use a sunscreen with an SPF of at least 30 with UVA and UVB protection.
- Rest frequently, and take breaks from being in a hot environment. Plan to limit activity at the hottest time of day.
- Wear clothing suited to the environment. Lightweight, light-colored, and loose-fitting clothing is best.
- Pay attention to your personal physical limitations; modify activities accordingly.
- Take cool baths or showers to help reduce body temperature.
- Stay indoors in air-conditioned buildings, if possible.
- Ask a neighbor, friend, or family member to check on the older adult at least twice a day during a heat wave.

SPF, Sun protection factor; *UVA,* ultraviolet A; *UVB,* ultraviolet B.

enzyme (ACE) inhibitors, and diuretics increases the risk for heat-related illness (Cusack et al., 2011).

HEALTH PROMOTION AND MAINTENANCE

Teach older adults before participating in any hot weather activity how to consider their risks and to take steps to eliminate or minimize them whenever possible. Ask them to have a family member, friend, or neighbor check on them several times each day to ensure that there are no signs of heat-related illness. Chart 9-1 lists other essential heat-related illness prevention strategies for older adults, many of which apply to adults of any age.

HEAT EXHAUSTION

❖ PATHOPHYSIOLOGY

Heat exhaustion is a syndrome resulting primarily from dehydration. It is caused by heavy perspiration, as well as inadequate fluid and electrolyte intake during heat exposure over hours to days. Patients feel ill, and their clinical manifestations resemble the flu. Profuse diaphoresis can lead to profound, even fatal, dehydration and hyponatremia caused by excessive sodium lost in perspiration. *If untreated, heat exhaustion can lead to heat stroke, which is a true emergency condition that has a very high mortality rate.*

❖ PATIENT-CENTERED COLLABORATIVE CARE

In heat exhaustion, patients usually have flu-like symptoms with headache, weakness, nausea, and/or vomiting. Body temperature is not significantly elevated in this condition. The patient may continue to perspire despite dehydration.

❗ NURSING SAFETY PRIORITY (QSEN)

Action Alert

Assess the patient for orthostatic hypotension and tachycardia, especially the older adult who is predisposed to rapid dehydration. Older adults who are already dehydrated often experience acute confusion and are at risk for falls.

Ask the person experiencing heat exhaustion to immediately stop physical activity; move him or her to a cool place, and use cooling measures. Effective cooling measures include placing cold packs on the neck, chest, abdomen, and groin; soaking the person in cool water; or fanning him or her while spraying water on the skin. Remove any constrictive clothing. Provide an oral rehydrating solution such as a sports drink or an oral rehydration therapy solution. Mistakenly drinking plain water can worsen the sodium deficit. *Do not give salt tablets*—they can cause stomach irritation, nausea, and vomiting. If these signs and symptoms persist, call an ambulance to transport the patient to the hospital.

In the clinical setting, monitor vital signs. Rehydrate the patient with IV 0.9% saline solution if nausea or vomiting persists. Draw blood for serum electrolyte analysis. Hospital admission is indicated only for patients who have other health problems that are worsened by the heat-related illness or for those with severe dehydration. The management of hypovolemic dehydration is discussed in more detail in Chapter 11.

HEAT STROKE

❖ PATHOPHYSIOLOGY

Heat stroke is a *true medical emergency* in which body temperature may exceed 104° F (40° C). It has a high mortality rate if not treated in a timely manner. The victim's THERMOREGULATION mechanisms fail and cannot adjust for a critical elevation in body temperature (Laskowski-Jones, 2010). If the condition is not treated or the patient does not respond to treatment, organ dysfunction and death can result. In their cohort study of 16 emergency departments, Hausfater et al. (2010b) found that nine factors help predict mortality in patients admitted to emergency departments with non-exertional heat stroke (see the Evidence-Based Practice box).

The two major types of heat stroke are exertional and classic. **Exertional heat stroke** has a sudden onset and is often the result of strenuous physical activity in hot, humid conditions. Not being used to hot weather and wearing clothing too heavy for the environment are common contributing factors. **Classic heat stroke,** also referred to as *non-exertional heat stroke,* occurs over a period of time as a result of chronic exposure to a hot, humid environment, such as a home without air-conditioning in the high heat of the summer. It generally affects ill and older adults and causes several hundred deaths in the United States every year. The risk factors for heat stroke are similar to those for heat exhaustion.

❖ PATIENT-CENTERED COLLABORATIVE CARE

◆ Assessment

Victims of heat stroke have a profoundly elevated body temperature (above 104° F [40° C]). *Although the patient's skin is hot and dry, the presence of sweating does not rule out heat stroke—people with heat stroke may continue to perspire.*

Mental status changes occur as a result of thermal injury to the brain. Manifestations can include confusion, bizarre behavior, seizures, or even coma (Chart 9-2). Vital sign abnormalities may include hypotension, tachycardia, and tachypnea. Recent research demonstrates that cardiac troponin I (cTnI) is frequently elevated during non-exertional heat-related illnesses. A severe increase (>1.5 ng/mL) indicates severe myocardial damage and decreases the chance of patient survival 1 year after the event (Hausfater et al., 2010a).

Complications of THERMOREGULATION failure due to classic heat stroke include multiple organ dysfunction syndrome (MODS), renal impairment, electrolyte and acid-base

EVIDENCE-BASED PRACTICE QSEN

What Factors Predict Who Will Develop Non-exertional Heat Stroke?

Hausfater, P., Megarbane, B., Dautheville, S., Patzak, A., Andronikof, M., Andre, S., et al. (2010). Prognostic factors in non-exertional heatstroke. *Intensive Care Medicine, 36*, 272-280.

Heat-related illnesses are often medical emergencies that can lead to death. The authors presented findings of a large multi-center observational cohort study of 1456 patients who were admitted to 16 emergency departments (EDs) in teaching hospitals during heat waves. The mean age of the sample was 79 years, and 391 of them were critically ill on admission. All of the study patients had an elevated core body temperature. The survival rate for the study sample was only 57% at 1 year after diagnosis.

On retrospective review of the patients' charts, it was found that nine factors negatively influenced survival rates. They included an age older than 80 years, body temperature of over 104°F (40°C), systolic blood pressure less than 100 mm Hg, Glasgow Coma Scale score of less than 12, presence of cancer and/or cardiac disease, previous treatment with diuretics, living in an institution, and transported to the ED by ambulance.

Level of Evidence: 4

This study is a nonexperimental or descriptive cohort study, but it used a large sample size in multiple emergency departments. Random assignment or comparison of two groups was not appropriate for answering the research question.

Commentary: Implications for Practice and Research

The results of this study indicate that older, institutionalized patients with cardiac disease or cancer and heat stroke have a high risk for not surviving a year after the heat-related illness. The major nursing implication from this study is that more emphasis on preventing heat-related illnesses in institutionalized patients is needed, particularly if they are older than 80 years. Strengths of the study included the large sample size collected from multiple emergency departments. A weakness might be the level of evidence (Level 4: nonexperimental or descriptive cohort study), but this is probably outweighed by the sampling method and the fact that an experimental design was not appropriate to answer the research question. Nurses are in a key position to advocate for these patients and to implement interventions that can help prevent heat stroke. Early detection and treatment also are needed. Chart 9-1 lists best practices for decreasing the risk for heat-related illnesses in older adults.

CHART 9-2   Key Features
Heat Stroke

- Body temperature more than 104°F (40°C)
- Hot and dry skin; may or may not perspire
- Mental status changes, such as:
  - Acute confusion
  - Bizarre behavior
  - Anxiety
  - Loss of coordination
  - Hallucinations
  - Agitation
  - Seizures
  - Coma
- Vital sign changes, including:
  - Hypotension
  - Tachycardia
  - Tachypnea (increased respiratory rate)
- Electrolyte imbalances, especially sodium and potassium
- Decreased renal function (oliguria)
- Coagulopathy (abnormal clotting)
- Pulmonary edema (crackles)

! NURSING SAFETY PRIORITY QSEN
Critical Rescue

After ensuring that the patient has a patent airway, effective breathing, and adequate circulation, use rapid cooling as the first priority for care. Methods for rapidly cooling include:
- Removing clothing
- Placing ice packs on the neck, axillae, chest, and groin
- Immersing the victim in cold water
- Wetting the patient's body with cold water and then fanning rapidly to aid in cooling by evaporation

Drenching the victim with large amounts of icy water may be the fastest, most effective means to reduce core body temperature (O'Brien et al., 2012).

---

indwelling urinary catheter. Continue aggressive interventions to cool the patient until the rectal temperature is 102°F (38.9°C) (O'Brien et al., 2012). External continuous cooling methods include using cooling blankets and applying ice packs in the axillae and groin and on the neck and head. Internal cooling methods may include iced gastric and bladder lavage. Use a continuous core temperature–monitoring device (e.g., rectal or esophageal probe) or a temperature-monitoring urinary bladder catheter to prevent hypothermia.

If shivering occurs during the cooling process, give a parenteral benzodiazepine such as diazepam (Valium). Lorazepam (Ativan) is an alternative agent. Seizure activity can further elevate body temperature and is also treated with an IV benzodiazepine. Once the patient is stabilized, admission to a critical care unit is warranted to monitor for complications such as multi-system organ dysfunction syndrome and severe electrolyte imbalances; these problems increase mortality risk.

---

disturbances, coagulopathy (abnormal clotting), pulmonary edema, and cerebral edema (O'Brien et al., 2012). Any of these problems can lead to death and are described in detail elsewhere in this book.

◆ Interventions

Coordinate care with the health care team to recognize and treat immediately and aggressively to achieve optimal patient outcomes. Chart 9-3 lists evidence-based emergency care of patients with heat stroke.

First Aid/Prehospital Care. Do not give food or liquid by mouth because vomiting and aspiration are risks in patients with neurologic impairment. Immediate medical care using advanced life support is essential.

Hospital Care. *The first priority for collaborative care is to monitor and support the patient's airway, breathing, and circulatory status.* Provide high-concentration oxygen therapy, start several IV lines with 0.9% saline solution, and insert an

---

? NCLEX EXAMINATION CHALLENGE
Physiological Integrity

An older client with heat exhaustion is being cooled with cool water spray and fanning. What assessment indicates to the nurse that the client needs hospitalization?
A. The client is alert and oriented.
B. The client's mucous membranes are dry and sticky.
C. The client reports weakness and nausea.
D. The client continues to sweat while being cooled.

Emergency Care of the Patient with Heat Stroke: Restoring Thermoregulation

At the Scene
- Ensure a patent airway.
- Remove the patient from the hot environment (into air-conditioning or into the shade).
- Remove the patient's clothing.
- Pour or spray cold water on the patient's body and scalp.
- Fan the patient (not only the person providing care, but all surrounding people should fan the patient with newspapers or whatever is available).
- If ice is available, place ice in cloth or bags and position the packs on the patient's scalp, in the groin area, behind the neck, and in the armpits.
- Contact emergency medical services to transport the patient to the emergency department.

At the Hospital
- Give oxygen by mask or nasal cannula; be prepared for endotracheal intubation.
- Start at least one IV with a large-bore needle or cannula.
- Administer normal saline (0.9% sodium chloride) as prescribed, using cooled solutions if available.
- Use a cooling blanket.
- Do not give aspirin or any other antipyretics.
- Insert a rectal probe to measure core body temperature continuously, or use a rectal thermometer and assess temperature every 15 minutes.
- Insert an indwelling urinary drainage catheter.
- Monitor vital signs frequently as clinically indicated.
- Obtain baseline laboratory tests as quickly as possible: serum electrolytes, cardiac enzymes, liver enzymes, and complete blood count (CBC).
- Assess arterial blood gases.
- Administer muscle relaxants (benzodiazepines) if the patient begins to shiver.
- Measure urine output and specific gravity to determine fluid needs.
- Stop cooling interventions when core body temperature is reduced to 102°F (39°C).
- Obtain urinalysis, and monitor urine output.

FIG. 9-1 Southern copperhead *(Agkistrodon contortrix)* has markings that make it almost invisible when lying in leaf litter.

FIG. 9-2 Cottonmouth water moccasin *(Agkistrodon piscivorus)*. The open-mouthed threat gesture is characteristic of this semiaquatic pit viper.

Snakebite Prevention

- Do not keep venomous snakes as pets.
- Be extremely careful in locations where snakes may hide, such as tall grass, rock piles, ledges and crevices, woodpiles, brush, boxes, and cabinets. Snakes are most active on warm nights.
- Don protective attire such as boots, heavy pants, and leather gloves. When walking or hiking, use a walking stick or trekking poles.
- Inspect suspicious areas before placing hands and feet in them.
- Do not harass any snakes you may encounter. Striking distance can be up to two-thirds the length of the snake. Even young snakes pose a threat; they are capable of envenomation from birth.
- Be aware that newly dead or decapitated snakes can inflict a bite for up to an hour after death because of persistence of the bite reflex.
- Do not transport the snake with the victim to the medical facility for identification purposes; instead, take a digital photo of the snake at a safe distance if possible.

SNAKEBITES

Although most snake species are nonvenomous (nonpoisonous) and harmless, there are two families of poisonous snakes in North America: pit vipers *(Crotalidae)* and coral snakes *(Elapidae)*.

Pit vipers are named for the characteristic depression between each eye and nostril that serves as a heat-sensitive organ for locating warm-blooded prey. They include various species of rattlesnakes, copperheads, and cottonmouths and account for the majority of the poisonous snakebites in the United States (Figs. 9-1 and 9-2).

Coral snakes are found from North Carolina to Florida and in the Gulf states through Texas and the southwestern United States. They have broad bands of red and black rings, separated by yellow or cream rings. These nonaggressive snakes have short, fixed fangs and inject highly neurotoxic venom into prey.

Most snakes fear humans and attempt to avoid contact with them. Sudden, unexpected confrontations at close range often lead to defensive strikes. Awareness is the key to snakebite prevention.

HEALTH PROMOTION AND MAINTENANCE

Chart 9-4 provides common-sense actions to avoid being bitten by a poisonous snake. Teach people who own snakes to follow these precautions. Remind them that snakebites can be life threatening.

NORTH AMERICAN PIT VIPERS

North American pit vipers can be differentiated from harmless snakes by these key anatomic features:
- A heat-sensing "pit"
- A triangular head that indicates the presence of venom glands and elliptical pupils

- Two retractable, curved fangs that have canals for venom flow
- Up to three sets of developing "replacement" fangs behind the primary fangs

Unlike copperheads and cottonmouths, rattlesnakes also have interlocking horny rings in their tails that vibrate and serve as a characteristic warning signal. Pit vipers can regulate the amount of venom flow through their fangs, depending, in part, on the size of the prey. The amount of venom injected in bites to humans varies. A bite might actually be "dry," meaning there is no envenomation (venom injection), yet there are distinctive fang marks on the patient. In contrast, "harmless" snakes do not have venom glands or fangs but can bite and leave skin marks.

❖ PATHOPHYSIOLOGY

When providing emergency care to a victim of snakebite, assess for evidence that venom has been injected into the body. The primary functions of venom are to immobilize, kill, and aid in digestion of prey. Therefore venom causes local and systemic toxic effects. The enzymes in venom break down human tissue proteins, alter membrane integrity, and impair blood clotting. The pathophysiologic effects of pit viper envenomation can lead to impaired TISSUE INTEGRITY from local tissue necrosis and massive tissue swelling, intravascular fluid shifts and hypovolemic shock, pulmonary edema, renal failure, hemorrhagic complications from disseminated intravascular coagulation (DIC), and death. These complications are discussed elsewhere in this book.

❖ PATIENT-CENTERED COLLABORATIVE CARE

◆ Assessment

The clinical manifestations of venom release are based on the type and amount of venom injected; the bite location; and the age, size, and health status of the victim. Puncture wounds in the skin are a key local sign of pit viper envenomation. One or more puncture wounds may be present, depending on how many fangs the snake has and how many times the snake struck the patient. Severe PAIN, swelling, and redness or ecchymosis (bruising) in the area around the bite are common. Hours later, vesicles or hemorrhagic bullae may form. Systemic responses to venom must be distinguished from the effects of anxiety and panic related to being bitten by a snake. Common reports by the victim include a minty, rubbery, or metallic taste in the mouth and tingling or paresthesias of the scalp, face, and lips. Other effects include muscle fasciculations (twitching) and weakness, nausea, vomiting, hypotension, seizures, and coagulopathy (clotting abnormalities) or DIC. If the bite site does not show evidence of local tissue swelling or redness within 8 hours, systemic effects are less likely to develop.

◆ Interventions

First Aid/Prehospital Care. First aid interventions for snakebite should begin in the field and can improve the victim's outcome.

Immobilizing the affected extremity in a position of function with a splint may help limit the spread of the venom. Maintain the extremity at the level of the heart. Keep the person warm, and provide calm reassurance. Do not offer any alcohol because it can cause the venom to spread through vasodilation (Bledsoe et al., 2009). *Do not incise or suck the wound, apply ice to it, or*

> **⚠ NURSING SAFETY PRIORITY** (QSEN)
> *Critical Rescue*
>
> The first priority is to move the person to a safe area away from the snake and encourage rest to decrease venom circulation. Next, remove jewelry and constricting clothing before swelling worsens. Call for immediate emergency assistance. Do not attempt to capture or kill the snake, but do take digital photographs at a safe distance if possible to aid in snake identification.

use a tourniquet—these actions are ineffective and can worsen the patient's outcome (Norris et al., 2012).

Hospital Care. *Acute care in a hospital is required as soon as possible because envenomation is a medical emergency.* Supportive care includes supplemental oxygen, two large-bore IV lines, and infusion of crystalloid fluids such as normal saline solution or Ringer's lactate solution. Apply continuous cardiac and blood pressure monitoring equipment to quickly detect clinical deterioration. Because venom can cause severe PAIN at the bite site, opioids are indicated. Provide tetanus prophylaxis and wound care as part of the collaborative plan of care.

Severe pit viper bites cause coagulopathy and promote hemorrhage and tissue destruction. Along with typical baseline laboratory studies, anticipate obtaining specimens for a coagulation profile, complete blood count (CBC), creatine kinase (CK), type and crossmatch for possible blood transfusion, and urinalysis. An electrocardiogram (ECG) is necessary to detect evidence of myocardial ischemia or other cardiac abnormalities.

Obtain pertinent patient history related to the event, including a full description of the snake's appearance, the time the bite occurred, prehospital interventions, and any past incidence of snakebite or antivenom use. To accurately assess the development of tissue edema at the bite site, measure and record the circumference of the bitten extremity every 15 to 30 minutes. Delineate the border of skin discoloration or edema with a skin marker to better track the progression of venom effects.

Venom potency varies. Not all snakebite victims need antivenom administration. The decision whether or not to give antivenom is based on the severity of the snakebite. Table 9-1 classifies envenomation severity. *Contact the regional poison*

TABLE 9-1	**Grades of Pit Viper Envenomation**
ENVENOMATION	**CHARACTERISTICS**
None	Fang marks, but no local or systemic reactions
Minimal	Fang marks, local swelling and pain, but no systemic reactions
Moderate	Fang marks and swelling progressing beyond the site of the bite; systemic signs and symptoms, such as nausea, vomiting, paresthesias, and hypotension
Severe	Fang marks present with marked swelling of the extremity, subcutaneous ecchymosis, severe symptoms, including manifestations of coagulopathy

From Auerbach, P.S., Donner, H.J., & Weiss, E.A. (2013). *Field guide to wilderness medicine* (4th ed.). St. Louis: Mosby.

control center so that toxicologists can provide specific advice for antivenom dosing and medical management.

The newest and safest antivenom for pit viper bites is Crotalidae Polyvalent Immune Fab (CroFab), which is derived from sheep (ovine). This drug consists of specific antibody fragments of immunoglobulin G (IgG) that bind and neutralize toxins in pit viper venom to counteract its effects on the body (Norris et al., 2012). Unlike the older antivenoms that were derived from horse serum, serum sickness rarely occurs after IV CroFab administration. **Serum sickness** is a type III hypersensitivity reaction that develops within 3 to 21 days, first as a skin rash with progression to fever, joint PAIN, and **pruritus** (itching). Although mild to moderate allergic reactions such as pruritus and **urticaria** (hives) can occur, anaphylaxis is rare. If the patient has a known hypersensitivity to papain or papaya, which is used during the manufacturing process, CroFab is contraindicated unless the benefits are believed to outweigh the risks (Fougera Pharmaceuticals, Inc., 2008). Give CroFab cautiously to patients who have:

- A previous allergic reaction to antivenom therapy
- A hypersensitivity to bromelain (a pineapple-derived enzyme) or sheep protein
- Prior CroFab therapy for a past envenomation (patients can become sensitized to the foreign sheep protein)
- Pregnancy
- Sensitivity to mercury-containing products (the antivenom contains mercury)

CroFab should be given to patients as soon as possible, with the optimal timing within 6 hours of the bite (Fougera Pharmaceuticals, Inc., 2008). The recommended initial IV dose is 4 to 6 vials infused over 60 minutes. During the first 10 minutes, the infusion should be slow (25-50 mL/hr). Monitor the patient closely for an allergic reaction (e.g., hives, rash, difficulty breathing). If symptoms are not effectively controlled with the first dose, an additional 4 to 6 vials are recommended. Once the symptoms are under control, 2 more vials of CroFab are administered every 6 hours for a total of 18 hours of administration (Fougera Pharmaceuticals, Inc., 2008).

CORAL SNAKES

❖ PATHOPHYSIOLOGY

North American coral snakes are found in the southeastern and southwestern United States (Fig. 9-3). These snakes burrow into the ground and are nonaggressive. Coral snakes account for fewer than 1% of venomous snakebites in the United States (Norris, 2011). Their ability to inject venom is less efficient than that of the pit vipers. Their maxillary fangs are small and fixed in an upright position. Most bites occur when people attempt to handle the snake. Coral snake venom has two toxins: a nerve toxin and a muscle toxin. The amount of venom in an adult coral snake is enough to kill an adult.

Coral snakes can be recognized by bands of black, red, and yellow that circle around the body of the snake. Several harmless snake species closely resemble the coral snake. If a black band lies between the red and yellow bands, the snake is usually nonvenomous. If the red band touches the yellow band, the snake is venomous. A helpful memory aid for identifying coral snakes is "red on yellow can kill a fellow" and "red on black, venom lack." *Be aware that this saying applies only to coral snakes found in the United States!*

❖ PATIENT-CENTERED COLLABORATIVE CARE
◆ Assessment

Manifestations of coral snake envenomation are the result of its neurotoxic properties. The physiologic effect is to block neurotransmission, which produces weakness, cranial nerve deficits (ptosis, diplopia, swallowing difficulty), an altered level of consciousness, and, ultimately, respiratory paralysis (Norris, 2011). Unlike the PAIN from pit viper bites, pain at the coral snakebite site may be only mild and transient. The venom is spread via the lymphatic system, but swelling, if present, is typically mild. Fang marks may be difficult to find because of the coral snake's small teeth. The toxic effects of coral snake venom also may be delayed up to 13 hours after a bite but then produce rapid clinical deterioration (Norris et al., 2012). Early signs and symptoms include nausea, vomiting, headache, pallor, and abdominal pain. Assess for neurologic manifestations, such as paresthesias (painful tingling), numbness, muscle fasciculations, and mental status changes, as well as cranial nerve and peripheral nerve deficits. Total flaccid paralysis may occur later, and the patient may have difficulty speaking, swallowing, and breathing. Clotting disorders do not occur.

Respiratory problems and cardiovascular collapse can occur in severe cases (Norris, 2011). Arterial blood gas analysis reveals respiratory insufficiency. The muscle toxin in the venom can cause an elevation in creatine kinase (CK) levels from muscle breakdown and produce **myoglobinuria** (release of muscle myoglobulin into the urine). Despite these clinical effects, death is rare if the patient receives timely management.

◆ Interventions

First Aid/Prehospital Care. Because several varieties of harmless snakes resemble the coral snake, the first priority, if possible, is to identify the snake as a coral snake. *However, if the snake cannot be positively identified, the victim should be treated as if venom has been injected.* Because coral snake venom does not destroy tissue, the field treatment to limit the spread of venom includes the use of pressure immobilization techniques (Norris et al., 2012). The affected extremity is encircled snugly with an elastic bandage or roller gauze dressing to impede lymphatic flow; it is then splinted. *This compression bandage must not be so tight that it impairs arterial flow. It should not be removed until the victim is managed at an acute care facility* (Norris et al., 2012).

FIG. 9-3 Sonoran coral snake *(Micruroides euryxanthus)* is also known as the *Arizona coral snake.* No documented fatality has followed a bite by this species.

Hospital Care. Once in an acute care setting, patients who have had an actual or potential coral snake envenomation will have continuous cardiac, blood pressure, and pulse oximetry monitoring and are admitted to a critical care unit. Prepare to provide aggressive airway management via endotracheal intubation if respiratory insufficiency or severe neurologic impairment occurs. Aspiration of secretions is a significant risk for this patient.

Coral snake antivenom is no longer manufactured in the United States. Until another drug manufacturer takes over production, supportive care is recommended as the primary patient management strategy (Norris, 2011). A patient can survive a coral snake bite without antivenom but may require prolonged mechanical ventilation; the effects of severe bites can persist for many days (Norris, 2011). *Contact the regional poison control center immediately for specific advice on patient management.*

! NURSING SAFETY PRIORITY (QSEN)

Critical Rescue

The most significant risk to the victim is airway compromise and respiratory failure. Therefore ensure that the patient's IV lines are patent and that resuscitation equipment is immediately available.

ARTHROPOD BITES AND STINGS

Arthropods include spiders, scorpions, bees, and wasps. Unlike snakes, almost all species of spiders are venomous to some degree—most are not harmful to humans either because their mouth is too small to pierce human skin or the quantity or quality of their venom is inadequate to produce major health problems. Brown recluse and black widow spiders, scorpions, bees, and wasps are examples of venomous arthropods that can cause toxic reactions in humans. Chart 9-5 lists actions that help prevent arthropod bites and stings.

CHART 9-5   Patient and Family Education: Preparing for Self-Management

Arthropod Bite/Sting Prevention

- Wear protective clothing, including gloves and shoes, when working in areas known to harbor venomous arthropods, such as spiders, scorpions, bees, and wasps.
- Cover garbage cans. Bees and wasps are attracted to uncovered garbage.
- Use screens in windows and doors to prevent flying insects from entering buildings.
- Inspect clothing, shoes, and gear for insects before putting on these items.
- Shake out clothing and gear that have been on the ground to prevent arthropod "stowaways" and inadvertent bites and stings.
- Consult an exterminator to control arthropod populations in and around the home. Eliminating insects that are part of the arthropod's food source may also limit their presence.
- Identify nesting areas such as yard debris and rock piles; remove them whenever possible.
- Do not place unprotected hands where the eyes cannot see.
- Avoid handling insects or keeping them as "pets."
- Do not swat insects, wasps, and Africanized bees because they can send chemical signals that alert others to attack.
- Carry a prescription epinephrine autoinjector and antihistamines if known to be allergic to bee and wasp stings. Ensure at least one family member is also able to use the autoinjector.

FIG. 9-4 Brown recluse spider *(Loxosceles reclusa).*

BROWN RECLUSE SPIDER

❖ PATHOPHYSIOLOGY

Brown recluse spiders are known for producing bites that result in skin ulcers. Also known as "fiddlebacks" or "violin spiders," they are medium-size spiders that are light brown and have a dark brown, fiddle-shaped mark that extends from their eyes down their back (Fig. 9-4). Like their name implies, brown recluse spiders are shy and hide in areas that are dark and secluded, such as boxes, closets, basements, sheds, and garages. Most indoor bites occur when people are sleeping, reaching into boxes or closets, or donning clothing that contains the spider. Few people ever see the spider that bit them. The only evidence may be impaired TISSUE INTEGRITY from a skin lesion or a necrotic wound or, less often, systemic effects from the injected toxin, commonly referred to as **loxoscelism**. Note that it is also common for patients to mistake a skin lesion for a spider bite; the lesion may actually be due to a skin infection, an insect bite, or even the manifestation of a health condition (Suchard, 2011).

❖ PATIENT-CENTERED COLLABORATIVE CARE

◆ Assessment

Brown recluse spider venom causes cell damage. The bite may be described as painless or stinging to sharp and painful. Some victims are unaware that they were bitten until intense local aching and pruritus develop over minutes to hours. The central bite site may demonstrate impaired TISSUE INTEGRITY appearing as a bleb or vesicle surrounded by edema and erythema, which may expand over the course of hours as the toxin spreads to surrounding tissues. The center of the bite becomes bluish purple. Some people have few or no tissue changes and therefore do not require medical attention.

For other people who are bitten, over the next 1 to 3 days the central part of the wound becomes dark and necrotic (Fig. 9-5). **Eschar** (a necrotic, leathery covering over the wound) eventually forms. The combination of these tissue changes is often referred to as the classic "red, white, and blue sign" that is associated with severe brown recluse spider bites.

When the eschar sloughs, TISSUE INTEGRITY is impaired by an open wound or ulcer that can remain for weeks to months. In rare cases, some patients may also have manifestations of systemic toxicity to brown recluse spider bites. These can include a rash, fever, chills, nausea, vomiting, malaise, and joint PAIN. In the worst cases, hemolytic reactions, renal failure, pulmonary edema, cardiovascular collapse, and death can occur.

FIG. 9-5 Brown recluse spider bite after 24 hours, with central ischemia and rapidly advancing cellulitis.

◆ Interventions

First Aid/Prehospital Care. The basic first aid for a brown recluse spider bite is to apply cold compresses over the site intermittently until there is no further progression of the wound (Arnold, 2012). Cold helps decrease the enzyme activity of the venom and may limit tissue swelling and necrosis. *Do not use heat because it increases the enzyme activity and potentially worsens the wound.* Recommended actions include elevation of the affected extremity, local wound care, and rest.

Hospital Care. Supportive care and ongoing monitoring for complications meet the needs of most patients with a brown recluse spider bite. For patients with wounds that appear infected, topical antiseptic and sterile dressings are necessary. Wound cultures and antibiotics may also be indicated. Tetanus prophylaxis is recommended.

A surgeon evaluates patients whose wounds require interventions beyond conservative management. Débridement (removal of necrotic tissue) and skin grafting may be required to promote TISSUE INTEGRITY and healing in severe wounds. Where available, collaborate with a wound specialist nurse.

A small number of patients experience severe systemic complications (loxoscelism). Manifestations include:

- Fever and chills
- Nausea and vomiting
- Renal failure
- Hemolytic anemia (anemia caused by destruction of red blood cells)
- Thrombocytopenia (decreased platelets)
- Disseminated intravascular coagulation (DIC)
- Death

These problems are discussed elsewhere in this text. Critical care management, including aggressive hydration, blood transfusions, hemodialysis, and supportive therapies, is required to prevent further deterioration and promote recovery.

BLACK WIDOW SPIDER

❖ PATHOPHYSIOLOGY

Black widow spiders can be found in every state in the United States except Alaska. They can inflict deadly bites and are found in cool, damp environments like outdoor log piles, vegetation, and rocks. They also commonly inhabit barns, sheds, and garages. The female spider is best identified by her shiny black color and the red hourglass pattern on her abdomen. Male spiders are smaller in size and lighter in color with white and gray markings. The hourglass pattern is faint in males. Black widow spiders carry neurotoxic venom. Bites to humans are usually defensive when the spider is at risk for being crushed.

The initial bite of a black widow spider ranges from nearly painless to sharply painful. Typically, the person notices a tiny papule or small, red punctate mark. Some people have intense PAIN, which seems out of proportion to the lesion. In many cases, the symptoms do not progress beyond a local reaction in the area of the bite site. If systemic signs and symptoms do occur, they generally develop within 1 hour and involve the neuromuscular system.

❖ PATIENT-CENTERED COLLABORATIVE CARE

◆ Assessment

Black widow spider venom produces a syndrome known as **latrodectism**, in which the venom causes neurotransmitter release from nerve terminals. Severe abdominal PAIN, muscle rigidity and spasm, hypertension, and nausea and vomiting are common. The problem may be incorrectly diagnosed as an acute abdomen, and surgical consultation may be considered because of the clinical features similar to peritonitis (Boyer et al., 2012). Muscle spasms involve the large muscles of the abdomen, back, and limbs. Other problems include facial edema, **ptosis** (eyelid drooping), diaphoresis, weakness, increased salivation, respiratory difficulty from excessive secretions, fasciculations (twitching), and **paresthesias** (painful tingling or numbness). The effects of the bite are self-limited and generally resolve in a few days. *However, older adults with other health problems like cardiovascular disease are at much higher risk for complications.*

◆ Interventions

First Aid/Prehospital Care

> **! NURSING SAFETY PRIORITY** (QSEN)
>
> **Action Alert**
>
> The priority intervention for a black widow spider bite in the prehospital setting is to apply an ice pack because cold application decreases the action of the neurotoxin.

Monitor the person for evidence of systemic toxicity as described in the previous Assessment section. If this problem occurs, support the patient's airway, breathing, and circulation. Patients should be transported to a medical facility as soon as possible for advanced life support care.

Hospital Care. In the emergency department, closely monitor vital signs, with special attention to blood pressure and respiratory function. Supportive therapy in the hospital includes administration of opioid pain medication and muscle relaxants such as diazepam (Valium) or other benzodiazepines. Provide tetanus prophylaxis as needed. Observe the patient for seizures related to a rapidly rising blood pressure (Boyer et al., 2012). For some patients, antihypertensive agents are needed. Although relapses may occur, the patient usually recovers within a week.

Less often, pulmonary edema, uncontrollable hypertension, seizures, respiratory arrest, and shock occur. These patients require critical care management. Antivenom is available for black widow spider bites. Although it can cause anaphylaxis and serum sickness, antivenom is considered effective in treating severe reactions (Boyer et al., 2012). The drug is also given to pregnant women because they may have uterine contractions from a black widow spider bite that can lead to a premature delivery (Boyer et al., 2012). The regional poison control center provides information about antivenom dosing and management for women who are pregnant.

SCORPIONS

❖ PATHOPHYSIOLOGY

Scorpions are found in many states within the United States although not typically in the Midwest or New England. However, stings are always possible when people keep scorpions as pets or when scorpions are accidentally transported in baggage and packaging. Unlike spiders that envenom their prey by inflicting a bite, scorpions inject venom through a stinging apparatus on their tail. Most scorpion stings produce a mild reaction characterized by local PAIN, inflammation, and mild systemic symptoms. These effects are usually self-limiting and best treated by analgesics, supportive management, and basic wound care.

One species of scorpion found in the southwestern United States that can inflict a sting associated with a potentially fatal systemic response is the bark scorpion (Fig. 9-6). It is often found in trees and woodpiles and around debris. Humans are usually stung when the scorpion gets into clothing, shoes, blankets, and personal items left on the ground.

❖ PATIENT-CENTERED COLLABORATIVE CARE

◆ Assessment

Because bark scorpion venom is neurotoxic, clinical manifestations result from cranial nerve and/or skeletal muscle involvement. The sting site may or may not show evidence of the venom release. There may be no redness or other obvious sign of inflammation. Gentle tapping at the potential sting site causing increased PAIN is associated with a bark scorpion sting (Suchard, 2012). The severity of the reaction varies from local pain to severe systemic manifestations, such as excessive salivation, hyperactivity, high fever, hypertension, GI disorders, tachycardia, cardiac dysfunction, pulmonary edema, and nervous system involvement. In rare cases, death can occur.

Symptoms usually begin immediately after the sting and can reach a crisis level within 12 hours. Recovery occurs gradually. PAIN and paresthesias can remain for up to 2 weeks (Suchard, 2012).

FIG. 9-6 The bark scorpion of Arizona *(Centruroides sculpturatus).*

◆ Interventions

Hospital Care. The first priority of patient management is vital sign assessment and continuous monitoring for several hours in a hospital emergency department or critical care unit. As symptoms worsen, the patient may develop respiratory failure and need intubation and mechanical ventilation.

Provide supplemental oxygen and IV fluid replacement immediately. Apply an ice pack to the sting site to control pain. Give analgesic and sedative agents with caution in the non-intubated, spontaneously breathing patient. Potent opioids, benzodiazepines, and barbiturates can cause loss of airway reflexes and precipitate respiratory failure. Fever is treated with acetaminophen (Tylenol) and application of a cooling blanket as needed. Because scorpion stings produce a puncture wound impairing TISSUE INTEGRITY, provide tetanus prophylaxis and basic wound care with an antiseptic agent. *Contact the poison control center as soon as possible to assist with patient management, particularly in regard to use of pharmacologic agents for scorpion stings.*

BEES AND WASPS

❖ PATHOPHYSIOLOGY

Bees and wasps are also venomous arthropods. Stings can produce a wide range of reactions from discomfort at the sting site to severe PAIN, multi-system problems, and life-threatening anaphylaxis in allergic people. Bumblebees, hornets, and wasps are capable of stinging repeatedly when disturbed. They have a smooth stinger that may or may not become lodged in the victim. Only honeybees can sting just once. When a honeybee stings a person, the stinger and venom sac pull away from the bee. The bee dies, but venom injection continues because the stinger and sac remain in the victim.

"Africanized" bees, also called "killer bees," are a very aggressive species that are found in the southwestern states. They are known to attack in groups and can remain agitated for several hours. People under attack should attempt to outrun the bees, if possible, and keep their mouth and eyes protected from the swarm. A person should never go into a body of water because the bees will attack when he or she comes up for air. When a person sustains multiple stings, reactions are more severe and may be fatal because multiple venom doses have cumulative toxic effects.

Health Promotion and Maintenance

Chart 9-5 lists actions that may help prevent arthropod bites and stings.

❖ PATIENT-CENTERED COLLABORATIVE CARE

◆ Assessment

The person who is stung by a bee or wasp first has a local reaction of immediate PAIN and a wheal-and-flare skin reaction. For some people, swelling can be extensive and involve an entire limb or body area. Systemic effects can then develop based on the venom load and the person's sensitivity to the venom. These effects may include generalized edema, nausea, vomiting, and diarrhea and are reactions to the toxic effects of the venom itself, not necessarily an allergic reaction. Other toxic venom effects include destruction of red and white blood cells and platelets, damage to the blood vessel walls, acute kidney injury, renal failure, liver injury, and cardiac complications; multi-system organ failure can develop (Lin et al., 2011).

If the patient has an *allergy to the venom*, then urticaria (hives), pruritus (itching), and swelling of the lips and tongue may occur. An allergic response can rapidly progress to an anaphylactic reaction in highly sensitive patients. Anaphylaxis is a life-threatening allergic response and is evidenced by respiratory distress with bronchospasm and laryngeal edema, hypotension, deterioration in mental status, and cardiac dysrhythmias. *This type of reaction constitutes a true medical emergency that is imminently life threatening and may lead to cardiac arrest.* Initially it may be impossible to distinguish an allergic reaction from a toxic venom reaction because they both can cause the same types of early signs and symptoms.

◆ **Interventions**

First Aid/Prehospital Care. Basic emergency care for bee and wasp stings includes quick removal of the stinger (if present) and application of an ice pack (Laskowski-Jones, 2010). Tweezers formerly were avoided for stinger removal because it was believed that pinching the stinger would cause additional venom to be injected. However, this concern appears to be unfounded (Auerbach, 2009). The stinger is best removed with tweezers or by gently scraping or brushing it off with the edge of a knife blade, credit card, or needle. The method used to remove the stinger is not as important as the speed of removal (Auerbach, 2009).

Advanced prehospital emergency care interventions are prioritized to ensure that airway, breathing, and circulation are maintained. First, determine whether the patient has a history of allergic reactions to bee stings. If the patient has a severe allergic reaction with wheezing, facial swelling, and respiratory distress, epinephrine must be given immediately. Allergic adult patients typically carry an epinephrine autoinjector (e.g., EpiPen®, Auvi-Q™. This device administers a quick and simple single dose of epinephrine in an emergency with just a click of a button. The injection is given via the IM route, typically in the mid-portion of the outer thigh. (See Chapter 20 for further discussion of epinephrine administration for anaphylaxis management.)

After epinephrine administration, an antihistamine such as diphenhydramine (Benadryl, Allerdryl ✤) or chlorpheniramine (Chlor-Trimeton, Novo-Pheniram ✤) is also given. In the field setting, oral liquid diphenhydramine (available over the counter) may be easier for the victim to swallow than the tablet form if there is tongue or pharyngeal edema. *Call 911 to transport the patient to a medical facility as soon as possible, since epinephrine administration may need to be repeated in 15 minutes if symptoms persist.*

Hospital Care. Once in a clinical setting, patients who sustain serious reactions to bee or wasp stings need oxygen administration and continuous cardiac and blood pressure monitoring. Establish an IV infusion with normal saline solution to support blood pressure. Advanced life support drugs and resuscitation equipment should be made immediately available. If epinephrine IM fails to relieve the life-threatening reaction, a different epinephrine formulation may be requested as a very slow IV bolus.

Bronchospasm can be treated with albuterol (Proventil, Novo-Salmol ✤) via inhalation or a similar bronchodilating agent. Parenteral antihistamines, such as diphenhydramine (Benadryl, Allerdryl ✤), and corticosteroids are also commonly

---

> **! NURSING SAFETY PRIORITY** (QSEN)
> **Drug Alert**
>
> IV epinephrine administration has much greater risk for adverse cardiovascular effects than IM epinephrine. Use the IV form of epinephrine with extreme caution, especially in older adults with cardiovascular disease, because it can dramatically increase pulse rate and blood pressure. Monitor the patient's vital signs frequently—at least every 10 to 15 minutes for 1 hour after IV administration.

prescribed to decrease the immune response. The toxin in the bee and wasp venom may outlast the effects of the initial doses of epinephrine and antihistamines and cause a recurrence of the allergic reaction over time. Therefore doses may need to be repeated for hours or days. Corticosteroids in tapered doses are often given to manage or prevent delayed allergic effects, termed a *biphasic reaction*, which generally occurs within 4 to 6 hours of the sting; however, the evidence regarding the effectiveness of corticosteroid administration is unclear (Choo et al., 2013).

All patients who have sustained multiple stings (particularly more than 50) are observed in an emergency care setting for several hours to monitor for the development of toxic venom effects. A critical care admission may be needed.

> **! NURSING SAFETY PRIORITY** (QSEN)
> **Action Alert**
>
> Teach anyone who develops an allergic reaction to bee or wasp stings to always carry a prescription epinephrine autoinjector and wear a medical alert tag or bracelet.

LIGHTNING INJURIES

❖ PATHOPHYSIOLOGY

Lightning is a year-round force of nature responsible for multiple injuries and deaths each year. It is caused by an electric charge generated within thunderclouds that may become cloud-to-ground lightning—the most dangerous form to people and structures. Young adult males account for the majority of lightning-related deaths. Most lightning-related injuries occur in the summer months during the afternoon and early evening because of increased thunderstorm activity and greater numbers of people spending time outside. Anyone without adequate shelter, including golfers, hikers, campers, beach-goers, and swimmers, is at risk.

Lightning has an enormous magnitude of energy and a different current flow than a typical high-voltage electric shock. The duration of contact is nearly instantaneous, resulting in a flashover phenomenon—an effect that may account for the relatively low overall mortality rate. Because water is a conductor of electricity and current takes the path of least resistance to the ground, any wetness on the body increases the flashover effect of a lightning strike. Lightning flashover produces an explosive force that can injure victims directly, as well as cause them to fall or to be thrown. The clothing and shoes of victims may be damaged or blown off in the process.

Lightning produces injury by directly striking a victim, by splashing off a nearby object, or by traveling through the ground. Although few people die after a lightning strike, many survivors are left with permanent disabilities.

Health Promotion and Maintenance

Injuries caused by lightning strike are highly preventable. Teach people to stay indoors during an electrical storm. Chart 9-6 lists common prevention strategies. For more information, the Wilderness Medical Society (http://wms.org) also offers evidence-based practice guidelines for the prevention and treatment of lightning injuries (Davis et al., 2012).

❖ PATIENT-CENTERED COLLABORATIVE CARE

◆ Assessment

Both the cardiopulmonary and the central nervous systems are profoundly affected by lightning injuries. *The most lethal initial effect of massive electrical current discharge on the cardiopulmonary system is cardiac arrest.* Because cardiac cells are autorhythmic, an effective cardiac rhythm may return spontaneously. However, prolonged respiratory arrest from impairment of the medullary respiratory center can produce hypoxia and, subsequently, a second cardiac arrest. Therefore, when attempting to manage multiple victims of a lightning strike, provide care to those who are in cardiopulmonary arrest first. Initiate resuscitation measures with immediate airway and ventilatory management, chest compressions, and other appropriate life-support interventions.

People who survive the immediate lightning strike may be treated in a less emergent fashion. However, these victims can have serious myocardial injury, which may be manifested by ECG and myocardial perfusion abnormalities, such as angina and dysrhythmias. The initial appearance of mottled skin and decreased to absent peripheral pulses usually arises from arterial vasospasm and typically resolves spontaneously in several hours.

Central nervous system (CNS) injury is common in lightning strike victims. A classic finding is an immediate but temporary paralysis that affects the lower limbs to a greater extent than the upper limbs. This condition usually resolves within hours, but the patient must be evaluated for spinal injury. Other clinical manifestations and complications resulting from lightning strikes include cataracts, tympanic membrane rupture, cerebral hemorrhage, depression, and post-traumatic stress disorder. Lightning strikes also cause skin burns. Most burns are superficial and heal without incident. Patients may have full-thickness burns, charring, and contact burns from overlying metal objects. An uncommon but characteristic skin manifestation of lightning is the appearance of branching or ferning marks on the skin called Lichtenberg figures.

◆ Interventions

First Aid/Prehospital Care. Because of lightning's powerful impact to the body, patients are at great risk for multi-system trauma. The full extent of injury may not be known until thorough monitoring and diagnostic evaluation can be performed in the hospital. Initial care includes spinal immobilization with priority attention to stabilization of airway, breathing, and circulation through standard basic and advanced life support measures. Cardiopulmonary resuscitation (CPR) is performed immediately when a person is in cardiac arrest. If cardiopulmonary or CNS injury is present, skin burns are *not* an initial priority. However, if time and resources permit, a sterile dressing may be applied to cover the sites. *Victims of lightning strike are not electrically charged; the rescuer is in no danger from physical contact.* Nonetheless, the storm can present a continued threat to everyone in the vicinity who lacks adequate shelter. Contrary to popular belief, lightning can and does strike in the same place more than once.

Hospital Care. Once in the acute care hospital setting, the focus of care is advanced life support management, including cardiac monitoring to detect cardiac dysrhythmias and a 12-lead ECG. The patient may require mechanical ventilation until spontaneous breathing returns. Collaborate with the health care team to perform a thorough physical and diagnostic evaluation

---

CHART 9-6 Patient and Family Education: Preparing for Self-Management

Lightning Strike Prevention

- Observe weather forecasts when planning to be outside.
- Seek shelter when you hear thunder. Safe choices include going inside the nearest building or an enclosed vehicle. Isolated sheds and the entrances to caves are dangerous, however. Do not stand under an isolated tall tree or structure (e.g., ski lift, flagpole, boat mast, power line) in an open area such as a field, ridge, or hilltop; lightning seeks the highest point. A stand of dense trees offers better protection.
- Leave the water immediately (including an indoor shower or bathtub), and move away from any open bodies of water.
- Avoid metal objects like chairs or bleachers; put down tools, fishing rods, garden equipment, golf clubs, and umbrellas; stand clear of fences, exposed pipes, motorcycles, bicycles, tractors, and golf carts.
- If camping in a tent, stay away from the metal tent poles and wet walls.
- Once inside a building, stay away from open doors, windows, fireplaces, metal fixtures, and plumbing.
- Turn off electrical equipment including computers, televisions, and stereos.
- Stay off the telephone. Lightning can enter through the telephone line and produce head and neck trauma, including cataracts and tympanic membrane disruption. Death can result.
- If you are caught out in the open and cannot seek shelter, attempt to move to lower ground such as a ravine or valley; stay away from any tall trees or objects that could result in a lightning strike splashing over to you; place insulating material between you and the ground (e.g., sleeping pad, rain parka, life jacket). A lightning strike is imminent if your hair stands on end, you see blue halos around objects, and hear high-pitched or crackling noises. If you cannot move away from the area immediately, crouch on the balls of your feet and tuck your head down to minimize the target size; do not lie down on the ground or have hand contact with the ground.

Data from Auerbach, P.S., Donner, H.J., & Weiss, E.A. (2013). *Field guide to wilderness medicine* (4th ed.). St. Louis: Mosby.

❓ CLINICAL JUDGMENT CHALLENGE

Patient-Centered Care QSEN

A nurse is working at a day camp for church leaders when a sudden severe thunderstorm occurs. Several adults participating in outdoor activities appear to have been hit by lightning. The nurse arrives on scene and finds four injured people. One person appears to be unconscious, one has ferning marks and burns on his skin, and the other two are sitting up against the wall of a building and reporting severe weakness of their lower extremities.

1. What risk factors did these people have for lightning injury?
2. Which person should the nurse assess first and what is the priority of care of this patient?
3. What potential complication does the nurse plan to address in the immediate rescue period?
4. What direction should the nurse give the large crowd of campers and camp staff?

to identify obvious and occult (hidden) traumatic injuries because the patient may have suffered a fall or blast effect during the strike. A computed tomography (CT) scan of the head may be performed to identify intracranial hemorrhage. A creatine kinase (CK) measurement may be requested to detect skeletal muscle damage resulting from the lightning strike. In severe cases, rhabdomyolysis (circulation of by-products of skeletal muscle destruction) can lead to renal failure. Burn wounds are assessed and treated according to standard burn care protocols. Tetanus prophylaxis is necessary for burns or any break in skin integrity. Some institutions transfer these victims to a burn center for follow-up management.

COLD-RELATED INJURIES

Two common cold-related injuries are hypothermia and frostbite. Both types of injury can be prevented by implementing protection from the cold. Teach patients at risk ways to prevent these injuries through methods to maintain THERMOREGULATION, which can range from mild discomfort to major systemic complications.

HEALTH PROMOTION AND MAINTENANCE

When participating in cold weather activities, clothing choices are critical to the prevention of hypothermia and frostbite. Teach the importance of wearing synthetic clothing because it moves moisture away from the body and dries fast. Cotton clothing, especially as an undergarment, holds moisture, becomes wet, and contributes to the development of hypothermia. Cotton clothing should be strictly avoided in a cold outdoor environment; this rule applies to gloves and socks as well. Wet socks and gloves promote frostbite in the toes and fingers. Wearing too many pairs of socks can decrease circulation and lead to frostbite.

Clothing should be layered so that it can be easily added or removed as the temperature changes. The inner layers, such as polyester fleece, provide warmth and insulation. The outer layer's purpose is to block the wind and provide moisture protection. This layer is best made of a windproof, waterproof, breathable fabric. A hat is an essential clothing item that significantly decreases body heat loss through the head. Face protection with a facemask should be used on particularly cold days when wind chill poses a risk. Sunscreen (minimum sun protection factor [SPF] 30) and sunglasses are also important to protect skin and eyes from the sun's harmful rays.

Teach people to keep water, extra clothing, and food in their car when driving in winter in case the vehicle becomes stranded. Maintaining personal fitness and conditioning is also an important consideration to prevent hypothermia and frostbite. People should not diet or restrict food or fluid intake when participating in winter outdoor activities. Malnutrition and dehydration contribute to cold-related illnesses and injuries. Finally, it is important for people to know their physical limits and to come in out of the cold when these limits have been reached.

HYPOTHERMIA

❖ PATHOPHYSIOLOGY

Hypothermia is a core body temperature below 95°F (35°C). Common predisposing conditions that promote hypothermia include:

- Cold water immersion
- Acute illness (e.g., sepsis)
- Traumatic injury
- Shock states
- Immobilization
- Cold weather (especially for the homeless and people working outdoors)
- Advanced age
- Selected medications (e.g., phenothiazines, barbiturates)
- Alcohol intoxication and substance abuse
- Malnutrition
- Hypothyroidism
- Inadequate clothing or shelter (e.g., the homeless population)

An environmental temperature below 82°F (28°C) can produce impaired THERMOREGULATION and hypothermia in any susceptible person. *Therefore people, especially older adults, are actually at risk on a year-round basis in most areas of the world.* Wind chill is a significant factor: heat loss increases as wind speed rises. Wet conditions further increase heat loss through evaporation. Weather is the most common cause of hypothermia for outdoor sports enthusiasts and for those with inadequate clothing or shelter. It is also a problem for the older adult, the homeless, and the poor who cannot afford heating.

❖ PATIENT-CENTERED COLLABORATIVE CARE

◆ Assessment

Hypothermia is commonly divided into three categories by severity: *mild* (90° to 95°F [32° to 35°C]); *moderate* (82.4° to 90°F [28° to 32°C]); and *severe* (below 82.4°F [28°C]). Treatment decisions are based on the severity of hypothermia. Chart 9-7 summarizes by category the common key features for the patient who is hypothermic.

◆ Interventions

First Aid/Prehospital Care. For treatment of *mild hypothermia*, the person needs to be sheltered from the cold environment, have all wet clothing removed, and undergo passive or active external rewarming. Passive methods involve applying

---

CHART 9-7 Key Features
Hypothermia

Mild
- Shivering
- Dysarthria (slurred speech)
- Decreased muscle coordination
- Impaired cognition ("mental slowness")
- Diuresis (caused by shunting of blood to major organs)

Moderate
- Muscle weakness
- Increased loss of coordination
- Acute confusion
- Apathy
- Incoherence
- Possible stupor
- Decreased clotting (caused by impaired platelet aggregation and thrombocytopenia)

Severe
- Bradycardia
- Severe hypotension
- Decreased respiratory rate
- Cardiac dysrhythmias, including possible ventricular fibrillation or asystole
- Decreased neurologic reflexes
- Decreased pain responsiveness
- Acid-base imbalance

warm clothing or blankets. Active methods incorporate heating blankets, warm packs, and convective air heaters or warmers to speed rewarming. If a heating blanket is used, monitor the patient's skin at least every 15 to 30 minutes to reduce the risk for burn injury.

In the case of mild, uncomplicated hypothermia as the only health problem, having the victim drink warm high-carbohydrate liquids that do not contain alcohol or caffeine can aid in rewarming. Alcohol is a peripheral vasodilator; both alcohol and caffeine are diuretics. These effects can potentially worsen dehydration and hypothermia.

Hospital Care. General management principles apply to both *moderate* and *severe* hypothermia. Protect patients from further heat loss and handle them gently to prevent ventricular fibrillation. Positioning the patient in the supine position prevents orthostatic changes in blood pressure from cardiovascular instability. Follow standard resuscitation efforts with special attention to maintenance of airway, breathing, and circulation as recommended by the American Heart Association (2011):

- Administer drugs with caution and/or spaced at longer intervals because metabolism is unpredictable in hypothermic conditions.
- Remember that drugs can accumulate without obvious therapeutic effect while the patient is cold but may become active and potentially lead to drug toxicity as effective rewarming is underway.
- Consider withholding IV drugs, except vasopressors, until the core temperature is above 86°F (30°C).
- Initiate CPR for patients without spontaneous circulation.
- For a hypothermic patient in ventricular fibrillation or pulseless ventricular tachycardia, one defibrillation attempt is appropriate. Be aware that defibrillation attempts may be ineffective until the core temperature is above 86°F (30°C).

Treatment of *moderate* hypothermia may involve both active external and core (internal) rewarming methods. Applying external heat with heating blankets can promote core temperature "after-drop" by producing peripheral vasodilation. **"After-drop"** is the continued decrease in core body temperature after the victim is removed from the cold environment; it is caused by the return of cold blood from the periphery to the central circulation. Therefore the patient's trunk should be actively rewarmed before the extremities. Core rewarming methods for moderate hypothermia include administration of warm IV fluids, heated oxygen or inspired gas to prevent further heat loss via the respiratory tract, and heated peritoneal, pleural, gastric, or bladder lavage.

> ## ! NURSING SAFETY PRIORITY (QSEN)
> ### *Critical Rescue*
>
> Patients who are *severely* hypothermic are at high risk for cardiac arrest. Avoid using active *external* rewarming with heating devices because it is dangerous and contraindicated in this population due to rapid vasodilation.

The treatment of choice for *severe* hypothermia is to use *extracorporeal* rewarming methods such as cardiopulmonary bypass or hemodialysis (Leikin et al., 2012). Cardiopulmonary bypass is the fastest core rewarming technique. However, this device is not available in all hospitals. It also requires specialized

personnel and resources to operate it properly. Monitor for early signs of complications that can occur after rewarming, such as fluid, electrolyte, and metabolic abnormalities; acute respiratory distress syndrome (ARDS); acute renal failure; and pneumonia.

A long-standing principle in the treatment of patients with hypothermic cardiac arrest is that "no one is dead until they are warm and dead." There is a factual basis to this statement when considering the number of survivors who have suffered a prolonged hypothermic cardiac arrest. Prolonged resuscitation efforts may not be reasonable in cases in which survival appears highly unlikely, such as in an anoxic event followed by a hypothermic cardiac arrest.

FROSTBITE

❖ PATHOPHYSIOLOGY

Another significant cold-related injury that may or may not be associated with hypothermia is frostbite. The main risk factor is inadequate insulation against cold weather; that is, either the skin is exposed to the cold or the person's clothing offers insufficient protection, leading to injury. Wet clothing, in particular, is a poor insulator and facilitates the development of frostbite. Fatigue, dehydration, and poor nutrition are other contributing factors. People who smoke, consume alcohol, or have impaired peripheral circulation have a higher incidence of frostbite. Any previous history of frostbite further increases a person's susceptibility.

> ## 💡 NCLEX EXAMINATION CHALLENGE
> ### *Health Promotion and Maintenance*
>
> An occupational health nurse is teaching a safety class to city employees who work outdoors year round. What does the nurse teach are risk factors for developing frostbite? **Select all that apply.**
> A. Excessive fatigue
> B. Prior episodes of frostbite
> C. Diabetes or other peripheral vascular disease
> D. Dehydration
> E. Smoking
> F. Wearing polyester socks

❖ PATIENT-CENTERED COLLABORATIVE CARE

◆ Assessment

Frostbite occurs when body tissue freezes and causes damage. Like burns, frostbite injuries can be superficial, partial, or full thickness. By contrast, **frostnip** is a type of superficial cold injury that may produce pain, numbness, and pallor of the affected area but is easily relieved by applying warmth; it does not cause tissue damage (impaired TISSUE INTEGRITY). Frostnip typically develops on skin areas such as the face, nose, finger, or toes. Untreated, it is a precursor to more severe forms of frostbite.

First-degree frostbite, the least severe type of frostbite, involves **hyperemia** (increased blood flow) of the involved area and edema formation. In *second-degree frostbite,* large fluid-filled blisters develop with partial-thickness skin necrosis (Fig. 9-7). *Third-degree frostbite* appears as small blisters that contain dark fluid and an affected body part that is cool, numb, blue, or red and does not blanch. Full-thickness and subcutaneous tissue

FIG. 9-7 Edema and blister formation 24 hours after frostbite injury occurring in an area covered by a tightly fitted boot.

necrosis occurs and requires débridement. In *fourth-degree frostbite*, the most severe form, there are no blisters or edema; the part is numb, cold, and bloodless. The full-thickness necrosis extends into the muscle and bone. At this stage, gangrene develops, which may require amputation of the affected part.

◆ **Interventions**

First Aid/Prehospital Care. Recognition of frostbite is essential to early, effective intervention and prevention of further tissue damage. Asking a partner to frequently observe for early signs of frostbite such as a white, waxy appearance to exposed skin, especially on the nose, cheeks, and ears, is an effective strategy to identify the problem before it worsens. In persons with dark skin, skin becomes paler, waxy, and somewhat gray. In this case, the best remedy is to have the person seek shelter from the wind and cold and to attend to the affected body part. Superficial frostbite is easily managed using body heat to warm the affected area. Teach patients to place their warm hands over the affected areas on their face or to place cold hands under the arms.

Hospital Care. Patients with more severe and deeper forms of frostbite need aggressive management. For all degrees of partial-thickness to full-thickness frostbite, rapid rewarming in a water bath at a temperature range of 104° to 108°F (40° to 42°C) is indicated to thaw the frozen part (Auerbach et al., 2010). Because patients experience severe PAIN during the rewarming process, this intervention is best accomplished in a medical facility; however, it may be done in another setting if no other options exist for prompt transport or rescue. Administer analgesics, especially IV opiates, and IV rehydration.

> ! **NURSING SAFETY PRIORITY** QSEN
>
> **Critical Rescue**
>
> Do not apply dry heat or massage the frostbitten areas as part of the warming process. These actions can produce further tissue injury.

When the rewarming process is complete, handle the injured areas gently and elevate them above heart level if possible to decrease tissue edema. Sometimes splints are used to immobilize extremities during the healing process. Assess the person at least hourly for the development of compartment syndrome—a limb-threatening complication caused by severe neurovascular impairment. Observe for early manifestations, which include increasing pain (even after analgesics are given) and paresthesias (painful tingling and numbness). Compare the affected extremity with the unaffected one to assess for pallor. Assess for pulses and muscle weakness. Management of compartment syndrome is discussed in detail in Chapter 51.

Frostbite destroys tissue and produces a deep tetanus-prone wound; the patient should be immunized to prevent tetanus.

Apply only loose, nonadherent sterile dressings to the damaged areas. Avoid compression of the injured tissues. Both topical and systemic antibiotics may be used. Once a patient's frozen part has thawed, do not allow it to refreeze, which worsens the injury. Antiprostaglandin therapy with ibuprofen may be used because it may decrease tissue damage for some patients (Auerbach et al., 2010).

In cases of severe, deep frostbite, débridement of necrotic tissue may be needed to evaluate tissue viability and provide wound management. Amputation may be indicated for patients with severe injuries or for those who develop gangrene or severe compartment syndrome.

ALTITUDE-RELATED ILLNESSES

❖ **PATHOPHYSIOLOGY**

High altitude illnesses, also known as **high altitude disease (HAD)** or *altitude sickness,* cause pathophysiologic responses in the body as a result of exposure to low partial pressure of oxygen at high elevations. Although most consider high altitude to be an elevation over 5000 feet, millions of people worldwide who ascend to or live at altitudes above 2500 feet are at risk for acute and chronic mountain sickness.

As altitude increases, atmospheric (barometric) pressure decreases. Oxygen makes up 21% of the pressure. Therefore, as this pressure falls, the partial pressure of oxygen in the air decreases, resulting in less available oxygen to humans. The pathophysiologic consequence is hypoxia. Hypoxia is more pronounced as elevation increases. Elevations higher than 18,000 feet are extreme altitudes. Supplemental oxygen is necessary at these levels in non-acclimatized people to prevent altitude-related illnesses, including death, from occurring during abrupt ascent.

The cause of HAD is an interaction of environmental and genetic factors (Guoen et al., 2009). Those who are obese or have chronic illnesses, especially cardiovascular problems, are more at risk than those who are thinner and healthier. Dehydration and central nervous system depressants, such as alcohol, also increase the risk. The age of the person does not seem to be a factor in altitude-related illnesses.

> 🧬 **GENETIC/GENOMIC CONSIDERATIONS**
>
> **Patient-Centered Care** QSEN
>
> Genetic differences among certain ethnic groups who live in high altitude areas have been studied. For example, chronic mountain sickness is less common in Tibetans and Sherpas than in Andeans, Hans, or Peruvian Quechuas (Guoen et al., 2009).
>
> In addition, the pathogenesis of mountain sickness is associated with unidentified variations in hypoxia-related genes and the genes responsible for the human leukocyte antigen (HLA) system. Examples of genes with variants that may contribute to the development of HAD include:
> - *EPO* (erythropoietin), which regulates red blood cell production
> - *HIF1A* (hypoxia inducible factor), which mediates the effects of hypoxia on body cells
> - *EDN1* (endothelin), which causes vasoconstriction and thus increases blood pressure
> - *NOS3* (endothelial nitric oxide synthase), which makes nitric acid in vascular tissue to maintain vessel tone and altitude adaptation
>
> At this time, no clinical genetic testing to determine a person's risk for altitude sickness is available; however, further research is being conducted to identify specific gene variations that contribute to altitude-related illnesses.

The process of adapting to high altitude is called *acclimatization*. **Acclimatization** involves physiologic changes that help the body adapt to less available oxygen in the atmosphere. As the carotid bodies sense a decline in Pao_2 at about 5000 feet, they increase the respiratory rate to improve oxygen delivery. This mechanism is called the "hypoxic-ventilatory response." Increased respiratory rate causes **hypocapnia** (decreased carbon dioxide) and respiratory alkalosis, which limit further increases in respiratory rate. Rapid eye movement (REM) sleep is impaired. Hypoxia can occur from periods of apnea. Within 24 to 48 hours of being at high altitude, the kidneys excrete the excess bicarbonate, which helps the pH to return to normal and ventilatory rate to again increase.

Increased sympathetic nervous system activity increases heart rate, blood pressure, and cardiac output. Pulmonary artery pressure rises as an effect of generalized hypoxia-induced pulmonary vasoconstriction. Cerebral blood flow increases to maintain cerebral oxygen delivery. Hypoxia also induces red blood cell production by stimulating the release of erythropoietin. The result is an increase in red blood cells and hemoglobin concentration. Over time, polycythemia can develop in people who remain in a high altitude environment.

People who plan to climb to high altitudes are advised to ascend slowly, over the course of days or even weeks, depending on the degree of elevation. Ascending too rapidly is the primary cause of altitude-related illnesses. They are much more common in people who sleep at elevations above 8000 feet.

The three most common clinical conditions that are considered high altitude illnesses are acute mountain sickness (AMS), high altitude cerebral edema (HACE), and high altitude pulmonary edema (HAPE). AMS may occur with HACE and/or HAPE; the underlying pathophysiology is hypoxia. Chronic mountain sickness can occur in people who live at high elevations. Although each syndrome has several unique manifestations, the basic assessment and management approach are the same.

❖ **PATIENT-CENTERED COLLABORATIVE CARE**

◆ **Assessment**

Assessment findings for the typical patient with AMS include reports of throbbing headache, anorexia, nausea, and vomiting. Feeling chilled, irritable, and apathetic is also associated with AMS. The syndrome produces effects similar to an alcohol-induced hangover. The patient may relate a feeling of extreme illness. Vital signs are variable: the patient can be tachycardic or bradycardic, have normal blood pressure, or have postural hypotension. He or she may experience dyspnea both on exertion and at rest. Exertional dyspnea is expected as a person adjusts to high altitude. However, dyspnea at rest is abnormal and may signal the onset of HAPE.

If AMS progresses to *high altitude cerebral edema (HACE)*, the extreme form of this disorder, the patient cannot perform ADLs and has extreme apathy. A key sign of HACE is the development of ataxia (defective muscular coordination). The patient also has a change in mental status with confusion and impaired judgment. Cranial nerve dysfunction and seizures may occur. If untreated, a further decline in the patient's level of consciousness results. Stupor, coma, and death can result from brain swelling and the subsequent damage caused by increased intracranial pressure over the course of 1 to 3 days.

High altitude pulmonary edema (HAPE) often appears in conjunction with HACE but may occur during the progression of AMS within the first 2 to 4 days of a rapid ascent to high altitude, commonly on the second night. It is the most common cause of death associated with high altitude. Patients notice poor exercise tolerance and a prolonged recovery time after exertion. Fatigue and weakness, as well as other signs and symptoms of AMS, are present. Important clinical indicators of HAPE include a persistent dry cough and cyanosis of the lips and nail beds. Tachycardia and tachypnea occur at rest. Crackles may be auscultated in one or both lungs. Pink, frothy sputum is a late sign of HAPE. A chest x-ray demonstrates pulmonary infiltrates and pulmonary edema. Arterial blood gas analysis shows respiratory alkalosis and hypoxemia (decreased oxygen). Pneumonia also may be present. Pulmonary artery pressure is usually very elevated because of pulmonary edema.

◆ **Interventions**

First Aid/Prehospital Care. The most important intervention to manage serious altitude-related illnesses is descent to a lower altitude. Patients must be monitored carefully for any evidence of symptom progression. With mild AMS, the victim should be allowed to rest and acclimate at the current altitude. The person is instructed not to ascend to a higher altitude, especially for sleep, until symptoms lessen. If symptoms persist or worsen, he or she should be moved to a lower altitude as soon as possible. Even a descent of about 1600 feet may improve the patient's condition and reverse altitude-related pathologic effects. Oxygen should also be administered if available to effectively treat symptoms of AMS.

Prevention and Treatment. The oral drug *acetazolamide* (Diamox, Apo-Acetazolamide ✦) is commonly used to both prevent and treat AMS (Hackett & Roach, 2012). Acetazolamide is a carbonic anhydrase inhibitor. It acts by causing a bicarbonate diuresis, which rids the body of excess fluid, and induces metabolic acidosis. The acidotic state increases respiratory rate and decreases the occurrence of periodic respiration during sleep at night. In this way, it helps patients acclimate faster to a high altitude. For best results, the drug should be taken 24 hours before ascent and be continued for the first 2 days of the trip.

> ❗ **NURSING SAFETY PRIORITY** (QSEN)
>
> **Drug Alert**
>
> Because acetazolamide is a sulfa drug, ask about an allergy to sulfa before the patient takes the drug because it may cause hypersensitivity reactions in those who are sulfa-sensitive.

Another drug that is indicated in the treatment of moderate to severe AMS is dexamethasone (Decadron, Deronil ✦). This drug's mechanism of action is unclear for AMS treatment, but it reduces cerebral edema by acting as an anti-inflammatory in the central nervous system. It does not speed acclimatization like acetazolamide does, but it does relieve the symptoms of AMS. Symptoms may recur when the drug is stopped, an effect termed the "rebound phenomenon" (Hackett & Roach, 2012).

For the treatment of HACE, early recognition of ataxia or a change in level of consciousness should prompt a rapid descent by rescuers or companions to a lower altitude. While undergoing descent, the patient can be given supplemental oxygen and dexamethasone. If mental status is severely impaired and the patient's airway is at risk, all drugs should be given parenterally. Ultimately, the patient with HACE must be admitted to the hospital. Critical care management may be necessary.

Like HACE, early recognition of HAPE is essential to improve the patient's chance for survival. Phosphodiesterase inhibitors such as tadalafil (Cialis) and sildenafil (Viagra) may be used to prevent HAPE because of their pulmonary vasodilatory effects (Hackett & Roach, 2012). When it occurs, HAPE is a serious condition that requires quick evacuation to a lower altitude, oxygen administration, and bedrest to save the patient's life. If descent must be delayed because of weather conditions or other factors, oxygen administration is essential as soon as possible. Keep the patient warm at all times. Drugs are not substitutes for descent and oxygen. However, the treatment of HAPE may include the calcium channel blocker *nifedipine* (Procardia, Adalat PA ✦, Apo-Nifed ✦) to decrease pulmonary vascular resistance (Hackett & Roach, 2012). Hospital admission is required. In uncomplicated cases of HAPE, recovery occurs quickly but effects such as weakness and fatigue may persist for 2 weeks.

Chart 9-8 summarizes best practices for preventing, recognizing, and treating altitude-related illnesses.

🔲 NCLEX EXAMINATION CHALLENGE

Physiological Integrity

A client on a climbing expedition reports a headache and nausea. The client rests 1 day at the current altitude and then climbs further the following day. The third day, other members of the climbing team note that the client has developed gross motor coordination difficulties. What action by the team nurse takes priority?
A. Administering acetazolamide (Diamox)
B. Providing 100% oxygen by facemask
C. Having the client descend to a lower altitude
D. Ensuring that the client stays warm at all times

CHART 9-8 Best Practice for Patient Safety & Quality Care (QSEN)

Preventing, Recognizing, and Treating Altitude-Related Illnesses

- Plan a slow ascent to allow for acclimatization.
- Learn to recognize clinical manifestations of altitude-related illnesses.
- Avoid overexertion and overexposure to cold; rest at present altitude before ascending further.
- Ensure adequate hydration and nutrition.
- Avoid alcohol and sleeping pills when at high altitude.
- For progressive or advanced acute mountain sickness (AMS), recognize symptoms and implement an immediate descent; provide oxygen at high concentration.
- To prevent the occurrence of AMS, discuss the use of acetazolamide (Diamox) and other agents as indicated with your health care provider.
- Protect skin and eyes from the sun's harmful ultraviolet rays at high altitude. Wear sunscreen (at least SPF 30) and high-quality wraparound sunglasses or goggles.

SPF, Sun protection factor.

DROWNING

❖ PATHOPHYSIOLOGY

Drowning is a leading cause of accidental death in the United States. It occurs when a person suffers primary respiratory impairment from submersion or immersion in a liquid medium (usually water) (Szpilman et al., 2012). Near-drowning was previously defined as recovery after submersion; however, this term is no longer used because language that describes drowning incidents has been standardized. Today the drowning process is considered a continuum with outcomes that range from survival to death.

Health Promotion and Maintenance

Prevention is the key to avoiding drowning incidents. When providing health teaching, include these points:
- Constantly observe people who cannot swim and are in or around water.
- Do not swim alone.
- Test the water depth before diving in head first; never dive into shallow water.
- Avoid alcoholic beverages when swimming and boating and while in proximity to water.
- Ensure that water rescue equipment, such as life jackets, flotation devices, and rope, is immediately available when around water.

❖ PATIENT-CENTERED COLLABORATIVE CARE

◆ Assessment

When water is aspirated into the lungs, the quantity and the makeup of the water are key factors in the pathophysiology of the drowning event. Aspiration of both fresh water and salt water causes surfactant to wash out of the lungs. Surfactant reduces surface tension within the alveoli, increases lung compliance and alveolar radius, and decreases the work of breathing. Loss of surfactant destabilizes the alveoli and leads to increased airway resistance. Salt water—a hypertonic fluid—also creates an osmotic gradient that draws protein-rich fluid from the vascular space into the alveoli. In both cases, pulmonary edema results. Salt water and fresh water aspiration cause similar degrees of lung injury (Szpilman et al., 2012). Another concern is water quality; the victim's outcome may be negatively affected by contaminants in the water such as chemicals, algae, microbes, sand, and mud. These substances can worsen lung injury and cause a lung infection.

The duration and severity of hypoxia are the two most important factors that determine outcomes for victims of drowning. Very cold water seems to have a protective effect. Successful resuscitations have been reported even after prolonged arrest intervals. Hypothermia might offer some protection to the hypoxic brain by reducing cerebral metabolic rate. The diving reflex is a physiologic response to asphyxia, which produces bradycardia, a reduction in cardiac output, and vasoconstriction of vessels in the intestine, skeletal muscles, and kidneys. These physiologic effects are thought to reduce myocardial oxygen use and enhance blood flow to the heart and cerebral tissues. Survival may be linked to some combination of the effects of hypothermia and the diving reflex.

The cause of the drowning should also be determined, if possible. The patient may have suffered a medical condition or injury that caused the drowning event such as a seizure, myocardial infarction, stroke, or spinal cord injury while in the water. Injuries sustained from diving into shallow water or body surfing, such as cervical spine trauma, can also increase the difficulty of rescue and resuscitation efforts.

◆ **Interventions**

First Aid/Emergency Care. Immediate emergency care focuses on a safe rescue of the victim. Potential rescuers must consider their own swimming abilities and limitations, as well as any natural or human-made hazards, before attempting to save the victim; failure to do so could place additional lives in jeopardy. *Once rescuers gain access to the victim, the priority is safe removal from the water.* Spine stabilization with a board or flotation device should be considered only for those victims who are at high risk for spine trauma (e.g., history of diving, use of a water slide, signs of injury or alcohol intoxication), as opposed to all drowning victims (Szpilman et al., 2012). Time is of the essence; efforts directed toward a rapid rescue have the most potential benefit. Initiate airway clearance and ventilatory support measures, including delivering rescue breaths while the patient is still in the water, as soon as possible (Szpilman et al., 2012). If hypothermia is a concern, handle the victim gently to prevent ventricular fibrillation.

> ⚠ **NURSING SAFETY PRIORITY** (QSEN)
>
> **Critical Rescue**
>
> Do not attempt to get the water out of the victim's lungs; deliver abdominal or chest thrusts only if airway obstruction is suspected.

Hospital Care. Once the person is safely removed from the water, airway and cardiopulmonary support interventions begin, including oxygen administration, endotracheal intubation, CPR, and defibrillation, if necessary. In the clinical setting, gastric decompression with a nasogastric or orogastric tube is needed to prevent aspiration of gastric contents and improve ventilatory function. After a period of artificial ventilation by mask, the victim typically has a distended abdomen, which impairs movement of the diaphragm and decreases lung ventilation. Patients who experience drowning require complex care to support their major body systems. The full spectrum of critical care technology may be needed to manage the pathophysiologic complications of drowning, including pulmonary edema, infection, acute respiratory distress syndrome (ARDS), and CNS impairment. These complications are discussed elsewhere in this text.

> ❓ **CLINICAL JUDGMENT CHALLENGE**
>
> **Patient-Centered Care** (QSEN)
>
> Emergency Medical Services (EMS) brought a drowning victim to the emergency department (ED). The patient is mildly hypothermic, bradycardic, and hypotensive.
> 1. What further information will the nurse need to obtain from the paramedics?
> 2. How does the nurse explain the major pathophysiologic event of drowning to the nursing student observing in the ED?
> 3. The paramedics state that the patient was submerged in a polluted, fresh water pond. How does that environment affect the patient?
> 4. What action does the nurse take to prevent a complication from CPR in this patient and why?

NURSING CONCEPTS AND CLINICAL JUDGMENT REVIEW

What might you NOTICE if the patient has impaired THERMO-REGULATION as a result of a cold-related injury?
- Body temperature below 95°F (35°C) (hypothermia)
- Shivering (hypothermia)
- Possible ventricular fibrillation (hypothermia)
- Cold, pale extremities (frostnip)
- Patient reports numbness or pain (frostnip)
- Hyperemia and edema (1st-degree frostbite)
- Fluid-filled blisters and deep skin necrosis (2nd-degree frostbite)
- Small blisters containing dark fluid, pale or red cool skin that does not blanch, patient reports numbness (3rd-degree frostbite)
- Numb, cold, bloodless body part that eventually develops necrosis (4th-degree frostbite)

What should you INTERPRET and how should you RESPOND to the patient with impaired THERMOREGULATION as a result of a cold-related injury?

Perform focused physical assessment findings and interpret their relationship to impaired thermoregulation, including:
- Temperature
- Skin integrity
- Reports of pain or numbness
- Other vital signs
- Cardiac assessment
- Neurologic assessment
- Fluid status

Respond by:
- *Providing rewarming measures:* Remove patient from the environment; remove wet, cold clothing; initiate passive external rewarming, active external rewarming, or internal rewarming measures as appropriate for hypothermia; thaw frozen body parts in a warm water bath and handle gently; handle hypothermic patients gently to prevent ventricular fibrillation
- Providing pain control measures
- Applying loose, dry dressings
- Administering tetanus prophylaxis and possible antibiotics for open wounds
- Preparing patient for possible débridement
- Using caution when administering drugs because of unpredictable metabolism; alternatively consider withholding drugs except vasopressors until core temperature is at least 86°F (30°C)

- Initiating CPR if needed; one defibrillation attempt is appropriate but may be ineffective if core temperature is lower than 86° F (30° C)
- Providing hydration

On what should you REFLECT?
- Monitor the patient's response to pain medication and rewarming techniques.
- Monitor for further injury from rewarming techniques.
- Evaluate the patient's and family's knowledge about the injury and treatment plans.
- Educate the patient and family on ways to prevent future cold-related injury.
- Monitor the patient's nutrition and hydration status.

GET READY FOR THE NCLEX® EXAMINATION!

KEY POINTS

Review these Key Points for each NCLEX Examination Client Needs Category.

Safe and Effective Care Environment
- Collaborate with the health care team to assess high-risk patients, especially older adults, for their knowledge of safety precautions to prevent THERMOREGULATION alterations such as heat-related and cold-related injuries. **Evidence-Based Practice** QSEN
- Assess high-risk patients, including those who do not know how to swim, for their knowledge of safety precautions to avoid drowning.

Health Promotion and Maintenance
- Teach people how to prevent heat-related illnesses as outlined in Chart 9-1.
- Educate people how to prepare for cold environments, including proper clothing (no cotton) and avoidance of wind and wet weather.
- Instruct people how to prevent arthropod bites and stings as described in Chart 9-5.
- Teach people how to avoid getting bitten by a snake as listed in Chart 9-4.

Physiological Integrity
- Recall that heat-related injuries can be mild (heat exhaustion) to severe (heat stroke).
- Recall that the priority for first aid for heat stroke, after a patent airway is established, is to cool the patient as quickly as possible (see Chart 9-3). **Patient-Centered Care** QSEN
- Remember that North American pit vipers can be identified by their triangular-shaped head and retractable fangs; non-poisonous snakes do not have these features.
- Recall that the management of a patient who has a snakebite depends on the severity of envenomation (venom injection) (see Table 9-1); both local and systemic manifestations can occur.
- Remember that the priority for first aid/prehospital care when a patient has a snakebite is to decrease the venom circulation. **Patient-Centered Care** QSEN
- Administer antivenom drugs that are available for most types of poisonous snakebites; monitor for an allergic response when these medications are given.

- Recall that the bite of a brown recluse spider can cause tissue necrosis; in rare cases, systemic manifestations can occur, including death.
- Remember that cold applications, such as ice, should be used as first aid/prehospital care for poisonous spider bites.
- Understand that the effect of the bark scorpion venom is neurotoxic; monitor the patient for signs of respiratory failure that may require mechanical ventilation.
- Recall that single bee and wasp stings cause only local reactions unless the person is allergic to them.
- Remember that epinephrine is the drug of choice for bee and wasp sting allergic reactions, followed by an antihistamine drug. **Patient-Centered Care** QSEN
- Teach people that the best way to prevent lightning injury is to avoid places where lightning is likely to strike (see Chart 9-6).
- Recall that lightning causes central nervous system and cardiovascular complications, as well as skin burns.
- Instruct people that two common cold injuries are hypothermia and frostbite; both may be prevented by selecting appropriate layered clothing; cotton should not be worn.
- Teach patients that in moderate to severe cases of hypothermia, coagulopathy (abnormal clotting) or cardiac failure can occur.
- Remember that the priority for care of a patient with a cold injury is warming; alcohol should be avoided. **Patient-Centered Care** QSEN
- Recall that frostbite causes various degrees of impaired TISSUE INTEGRITY and is classified as mild (frostnip) to serious (fourth degree); severe frostbite can result in amputation due to compartment syndrome or gangrene.
- Know that high altitude can cause a range of physiologic consequences in the body, primarily due to hypoxia.
- Teach people that the priority for care of the patient with illness related to high altitude is descent to a lower altitude.
- Recall that acetazolamide (Diamox, Apo-Acetazolamide ♣) is the drug of choice for prevention and treatment of mild altitude-related illness.
- Review Chart 9-8, which outlines best practice strategies for preventing, recognizing, and treating altitude-related illnesses.
- Remember that drowning victims often require cardiopulmonary support, including CPR.
- Recall that a drowning victim is at risk for pulmonary infection, ARDS, and central nervous system impairment.

Concepts of Emergency and Disaster Preparedness

Linda Laskowski-Jones

http://evolve.elsevier.com/Iggy/

PRIORITY CONCEPTS

- COMMUNICATION
- SAFETY
- TEAMWORK AND COLLABORATION

LEARNING OUTCOMES

Safe and Effective Care Environment

1. Apply principles of triage to prioritize care delivery in a disaster situation.
2. Identify the roles of the nurse in emergency preparedness and response.
3. Compare the key personnel roles in an emergency preparedness and response plan.
4. Describe the components of an emergency preparedness and response plan.
5. Develop a personal emergency preparedness plan.
6. Identify which patients to recommend for hospital discharge in a disaster situation.

Psychosocial Integrity

7. Assess survivors for ability to adapt to the effects of disaster changes or traumatic events.
8. Provide support to the person and/or family in coping with life changes resulting from a disaster.

Physiological Integrity

9. Explain how to maintain physical SAFETY when responding to disaster and mass casualty situations.

A **disaster** is commonly defined as an event in which illness or injuries exceed resource capabilities of a health care facility or community because of destruction and devastation. The disaster can be either *internal* to a health care facility or *external* from situations that create casualties in the community. Both internal and external disasters can occur simultaneously.

TYPES OF DISASTERS

An *internal* disaster is any event inside a health care facility or campus that could endanger the SAFETY of patients or staff. The event creates a need for evacuation or relocation. It often requires extra personnel and the activation of the facility's emergency preparedness and response plan (also called an *emergency management plan*). Examples of potential internal disasters include fire, explosion, loss of critical utilities (e.g., electricity, water, and communications capabilities), and violence. Each health care organization develops policies and procedures for preventing these events through organized facility and security management plans. The most important outcome for any internal disaster is to maintain patient, staff, and visitor safety.

An *external* disaster is any event outside the health care facility or campus, somewhere in the community, which requires the activation of the facility's emergency management plan. The number of facility staff and resources may not be adequate for the incoming emergency department (ED) patients. External disasters can be either natural, such as a hurricane, earthquake or tornado, or technologic, such as an act of terrorism with explosive devices or a malfunction of a nuclear reactor with radiation exposure. Recent external disasters include the Boston Marathon bombing on April 15, 2013, and the West, Texas, fertilizer plant explosion 2 days later. St. John's Regional Medical Center in Joplin, Missouri, had an internal disaster compounding an external disaster on May 2011 when it was directly hit by an EF-5 tornado that destroyed a large part of the town. Of the 142 dead, only 6 people inside the hospital died (Letner, 2011) (Fig. 10-1).

Both internal and external disasters can result in many casualties, including death. Multi-casualty and mass casualty (disaster) events are not the same. The main difference is based on the scope and scale of the incident, considering the number and severity of victims or casualties involved. Both require specific response plans to activate necessary resources. In general, a **multi-casualty event** can be managed by a hospital using local resources; a **mass casualty event** overwhelms local medical capabilities and may require the COLLABORATION of multiple agencies and health care facilities to handle the crisis (Smith,

FIG. 10-1 St. John's Regional Medical Center in Joplin, Missouri, after a powerful tornado struck in May 2011.

Nurse's Role in Responding to Health Care Facility Fires

- Remove any patient or staff from immediate danger of the fire or smoke.
- Discontinue oxygen for all patients who can breathe without it.
- For patients on life support, maintain their respiratory status manually until removed from the fire area.
- Direct ambulatory patients to walk to a safe location.
- If possible, ask ambulatory patients to help push wheelchair patients out of danger.
- Move bedridden patients from the fire area in bed, by stretcher, or in a wheelchair; if needed, have one or two staff members move patients on blankets or carry them.
- After everyone is out of danger, seek to contain the fire by closing doors and windows and using an ABC extinguisher (can put out any type of fire), if possible.
- Do not risk injury to you or staff members while moving patients or attempting to extinguish the fire.

2010). State, regional, and/or national resources may be needed to support the areas affected by the event. Trauma centers have a special role in all emergency preparedness activities because they provide a critical level of expertise and specialized resources for complex injury management.

To maintain ongoing disaster preparedness, hospital personnel participate in emergency training and drills regularly. In the United States, The Joint Commission (2008) mandates that hospitals have an emergency preparedness plan that is tested through drills or actual participation in a real event at least twice yearly. One of the drills or events must involve community-wide resources and an influx of actual or simulated patients to assess the ability of collaborative efforts and command structures. In addition, accredited health care organizations are required to take an "all-hazards approach" to disaster planning. Using this approach, preparedness activities must address *all credible threats* to the SAFETY of the community that could result in a disaster situation. Disaster drills, then, are ideally planned based on a risk assessment or vulnerability analysis that identifies the events most likely to occur in a particular community. For example, a flood is more likely in the Gulf of Mexico and an avalanche is more likely in ski areas of the Rocky Mountains. It is essential that staff actively participate in these drills and take them seriously to enable their ongoing competency. The importance of training was emphasized in all the recent disasters and is credited with saving lives (Caramenico, 2013).

Hospitals are not the only health care agencies that are required to practice disaster drills. Nursing homes and other long-term care (LTC) facilities are also mandated to have annual drills to prepare for mass casualty events. Part of the response plan must include a method for evacuation of residents from the facility in a timely and safe manner as was demonstrated in the West, Texas, nursing home evacuation.

An evacuation plan is also part of fire prevention and preparedness plans for health care facilities. The Life Safety Code® published by the National Fire Protection Association (2013) provides guidelines for building construction, design, maintenance, and evacuation. The Centers for Medicare and Medicaid Services (CMS) (2012) requires every health care facility to practice at least one fire drill or actual fire response once a year. Patient evacuation is not required if the event is a drill. All facility personnel are mandated to have training on fire prevention and responsiveness each year. Chart 10-1 lists general guidelines for fire responsiveness and building evacuation to ensure SAFETY.

IMPACT OF EXTERNAL DISASTERS

The events of September 11, 2001, substantially changed hospital and community disaster planning efforts (Wielawski, 2006). With the shocking terrorist attacks on the Twin Towers of the World Trade Center and the Pentagon and the actual and perceived threat of domestic terrorism, including the anthrax exposure that followed, hospital emergency preparedness concepts became much more fully integrated into the daily operations of emergency departments (EDs) by necessity. Weapons of mass destruction (WMD) rapidly became a focus of public health risk.

The term "NBC" was coined to describe **n**uclear, **b**iologic, and **c**hemical threats. In response, emergency medical services (EMS) agencies and hospitals improved SAFETY by upgrading their decontamination facilities, equipment, and all levels of personal protective equipment to better protect staff. ED physician and nursing staff now routinely undergo hazardous materials (HAZMAT) training and learn how to recognize patterns of illness in patients who present for treatment that potentially indicate biologic terrorism agents, such as anthrax or smallpox (Fig. 10-2). Protocols for the pharmacologic treatment of infectious disease agents, as well as stockpiles of antibiotics and nerve agent antidotes, are readily available.

The most immediate outcome of improving emergency preparedness after September 11 is that the ability to competently handle the more typical multi-casualty or mass casualty incident such as a bus crash, tornado, or building collapse has been greatly improved in many communities. However, disaster situations can still exceed the scope of usual day-to-day crisis operations, pointing to the necessity of well-defined regional and national emergency preparedness plans and the need for ongoing drills.

In 2005, Hurricane Katrina made landfall in Louisiana and other Gulf states as a category 4 storm and caused more than 1000 deaths and devastating environmental and property damage. Volunteers from all over the United States, as well as

FIG. 10-2 Hazardous materials (HAZMAT) training to decontaminate people exposed to toxic agents in an outdoor decontamination area.

FIG. 10-3 Temporary shelter set up for homeless victims of Hurricane Katrina in New Orleans.

local, regional, and federal agencies, took part in the large-scale disaster evacuation, rescue, and relief effort that severely challenged available resources and established disaster plans. Critical systems failed and were eventually re-established through COLLABORATION with multiple agencies to ensure that the most basic human needs were met (Fig. 10-3). Hurricane Katrina overwhelmed the existing emergency care system and caused the mobilization of a national mutual aid response on a level that had not been experienced in recent U.S. history.

Many health care facilities still have not made structural changes that would offer SAFETY and protection from flooding and utilities failures. A case in point is the devastation brought by "Superstorm Sandy" that made landfall on New York City in October 2012. Though it was downgraded from a category 1 hurricane, the flooding that occurred destroyed critical equipment, including emergency power generators, in the lower levels of several health care facilities, causing the loss of utilities and crippling hospital operations. Hospitals that were severely impacted had to evacuate patients to other facilities, many of which were already overwhelmed by an influx of patients from the storm's damage in the community. Staff worked for several days in harsh conditions, evacuating critical patients via stairwells since elevators were nonfunctional, carrying glow sticks and flashlights and wearing headlamps (Evans, 2012).

Lessons learned from Hurricane Katrina and other natural disasters, as well as worldwide incidents such as Superstorm Sandy, the earthquakes in Japan and Haiti, tsunamis, and terrorist attacks, enable improved facility design, staff preparation, and coordination of efforts that are beneficial for future disasters. These insights also can be applied to health care facility and community agency plans for pandemic infections, including influenza.

A pandemic (an infection or disease that occurs throughout the population of a country or the world) leads a vast number of people to seek medical care, even the "worried well." Though not yet ill, the "worried well" want evaluation, preventive treatment, or reassurance from a health care provider. A pandemic influenza outbreak, such as the 2009-2010 swine flu outbreak caused by the H1N1 virus, raised significant concerns that the resource capabilities of the entire health care system could be overwhelmed and that community systems and critical supply chains could be severely damaged. Worker illness, absenteeism, and personal choices to remain quarantined to avoid being exposed to the illness negatively affect the number of health care staff available to care for patients. Fortunately, because of widespread vaccination programs and public information campaigns, the swine flu pandemic of 2009-2010 was well managed. Concern remains that avian influenza A strain (H5N1), also known as "bird flu," could pose a global pandemic threat if a gene mutation occurs to allow easy human-to-human spread. Because of the mass casualty nature of pandemic influenza, emergency preparedness planners must COLLABORATE to incorporate strategies for handling an influx of ill patients into the system as part of ongoing disaster readiness. Quarantine of selected nursing units or the entire hospital could become necessary, prompting closure until the risk has passed.

Common to all mass casualty events, the goal of emergency preparedness is to effectively meet the extraordinary need for resources such as hospital beds, staff, drugs, personal protective equipment (PPE), supplies, and medical devices, such as mechanical ventilators. The U.S. government stockpiles critical equipment and supplies in case they are needed for a pandemic influenza outbreak and organizes large-scale vaccination programs (see Chapter 23 for more information on emerging infections). Each state has its own specific emergency preparedness plan for pandemic influenza, including who would receive vaccines in a mass casualty event.

EMERGENCY PREPAREDNESS AND RESPONSE

Mass Casualty Triage

A key process in any multi-casualty or mass casualty response is effective triage to rapidly sort ill or injured patients into priority categories based on their acuity and survival potential.

Triage functions may be performed by EMS providers in the field, such as:
- Emergency medical technicians (EMTs) and paramedics
- Nurse and physician field teams who are called from the hospital to a disaster scene to assist EMS providers
- Nurse and physician hospital teams to assess and reassess incoming patients

Triage concepts in a mass casualty incident differ from the "civilian triage" methods discussed in Chapter 8 that are practiced during usual emergency department operations (Table 10-1). Although disaster triage practices can vary widely based

TABLE 10-1 Comparison of Triage Under Usual Versus Mass Casualty Conditions

TRIAGE UNDER USUAL CONDITIONS	TRIAGE UNDER MASS CASUALTY CONDITIONS
Emergent (immediate threat to life)	Emergent or class I (red tag) (immediate threat to life)
Urgent (major injuries that require immediate treatment)	Urgent or class II (yellow tag) (major injuries that require treatment)
Nonurgent (minor injuries that do not require immediate treatment)	Nonurgent or class III (green tag) (minor injuries that do not require immediate treatment)
Does not apply	Expectant or class IV (black tag) (expected and allowed to die)

on local EMS protocols, some concepts are fairly universal. Most mass casualty response teams both in the field (at the disaster site) and in the hospital setting use a **disaster triage tag system** that categorizes triage priority by color and number (Smith, 2010):

- Emergent (class I) patients are identified with a red tag.
- Patients who can wait a short time for care (class II) are marked with a yellow tag.
- Nonurgent or "walking wounded" (class III) patients are given a green tag.
- Patients who are expected to die or are dead are issued a black tag (class IV).

> **! NURSING SAFETY PRIORITY** (QSEN)
> ### *Action Alert*
>
> In mass casualty or disaster situations, implement a military form of triage with the overall desired outcome of doing the greatest good for the greatest number of people (Smith, 2010). This means that patients who are critically ill or injured and might otherwise receive attempted resuscitation during usual operations may be triaged into an "expectant" or "black-tagged" category and allowed to die or not be treated until others received care.
>
> Typical examples of black-tagged patients are those with massive head trauma, extensive full-thickness body burns, and high cervical spinal cord injury requiring mechanical ventilation. The rationale for this seemingly heartless decision is that limited resources must be dedicated to saving the most lives rather than expending valuable resources to save one life at the possible expense of many others.

In general, *red-tagged* patients have immediate threats to life, such as airway obstruction or shock, and require immediate attention. *Yellow-tagged* patients have major injuries, such as open fractures with a distal pulse and large wounds that need treatment within 30 minutes to 2 hours. *Green-tagged* patients have minor injuries that can be managed in a delayed fashion, generally more than 2 hours. Examples of green-tag injuries include closed fractures, sprains, strains, abrasions, and contusions.

Green-tagged patients are often referred to as the "walking wounded" because they may actually evacuate themselves from the mass casualty scene and go to the hospital in a private vehicle. Green-tagged patients usually make up the greatest number in most large-scale multi-casualty situations. Therefore they can overwhelm the system if provisions are not made to handle them as part of the disaster plan. Also, because they

often come to the hospital on their own, the hospital may not be able to determine how many actual casualties will arrive. A related concern is that green-tagged patients who self-transport may unknowingly carry contaminants from a nuclear, biologic, or chemical incident into the hospital environment with potentially disastrous consequences. ED staff must anticipate these issues and COLLABORATE to devise emergency response plans accordingly, including appropriate decontamination measures.

> **? NCLEX EXAMINATION CHALLENGE**
> ### *Physiological Integrity*
>
> The nurse is triaging clients arriving at the hospital after a large scale disaster. Which of these clients is correctly classified?
> A. Young adult with closed fractures of her right leg and arm: Yellow tag
> B. Older adult with severe abdominal pain who is dazed and confused: Black tag
> C. Middle-aged adult with third-degree burns over 90% of his body: Red tag
> D. Young adult with bruises and superficial lacerations: Green tag

Once patients are in the triage area of the hospital, they typically receive a special bracelet with a disaster number. Preprinted labels with this number can be applied to the patients' chart forms and personal belongings. Digital photos may be used as part of the identification process in some systems. The standard hospital registration process and identification band can be applied after the patient's identity is confirmed.

Automated tracking systems using infrared and radiofrequency technology (RFT) are available in some emergency departments to track a patient's triage priority upon arrival, location, and process of care. The interactions the patient has with caregivers can also be tracked, an important SAFETY strategy if the patient is later found to have contaminants or a disease that could pose a risk to staff members who had close contact and require decontamination or prophylaxis (Laskowski-Jones, 2008). These systems are valuable components of the hospital's emergency preparedness infrastructure because they can rapidly portray the overall census and acuity of patients. They also enable ED leaders to determine how many casualties of a particular acuity level a hospital can safely accept from the incident scene.

Notification and Activation of Emergency Preparedness/Management Plans

When the number of casualties exceeds the usual resource capabilities, a disaster situation exists. What may be a routine day in the emergency department of a large urban trauma center could be defined as a disaster for a small rural community hospital if the same number of patients were to arrive. Each facility, then, decides when criteria are met to declare a disaster. Flexibility is needed because resources may change by time of day and by day of the week. For instance, hospitals typically have the fewest staff available after midnight on the weekend. An incident that occurs in this time frame may require activation of the emergency preparedness plan to bring extra resources into the hospital. The same incident during weekday business hours might be handled with on-site personnel alone without the need for activation of the plan.

Notification that a multi-casualty or mass casualty situation exists usually occurs by radio, cellular, or electronic COMMUNI-CATION between the ED and EMS providers at the scene. A state or regional emergency management agency may also notify the ED of the event. Each hospital has its own policy that specifies *who* has the authority to activate and *how* to activate the disaster or emergency preparedness plan. Group paging systems, telephone trees, and instant computer-based alert messages are the most common means of notifying essential personnel of a mass casualty incident or disaster.

A catastrophic event, such as a major earthquake or tornado, or a terrorist incident involving weapons of mass destruction (WMD) also requires the COLLABORATION of volunteers from all levels of health care providers in the region. In this case, the media may be contacted to broadcast messages to the health care community-at-large via television, radio, and electronic announcements. For such incidents, the National Guard, the American Red Cross, the public health department, various military units, a Medical Reserve Corps (MRC), or a Disaster Medical Assistance Team (DMAT) can be activated by state and federal government authorities.

- An MRC is made up of a group of volunteer medical and public health care professionals, including physicians and nurses. They offer their services to health care facilities or to the community in a supportive or supplemental capacity during times of need such as a disaster or pandemic disease outbreak. This group may help staff hospitals or community health settings that face personnel shortages and establish first aid stations or special-needs shelters. As a means to alleviate emergency department and hospital overcrowding, the MRC may also set up an acute care center (ACC) in the community for patients who need acute care (but not intensive care) for days to weeks.
- A DMAT is a medical relief team made up of civilian medical, paraprofessional, and support personnel that is deployed to a disaster area with enough medical equipment and supplies to sustain operations for 72 hours (U.S. Department of Health & Human Services, 2013). DMATs are part of the National Disaster Medical System (NDMS) in the United States. They provide relief services ranging from primary health care and triage to evacuation and staffing to assist health care facilities that have become overwhelmed with casualties (Merchant et al., 2010). *Because licensed health care providers such as nurses act as federal employees when they are deployed, their professional licenses are recognized and valid in all states.* Additional examples of services provided by the NDMS include:
  - Disaster Mortuary Operational Response Teams (DMORTs) to manage mass fatalities
  - National Veterinary Response Teams (NVRTs) for emergency animal care
  - International Medical Surgical Response Teams (IMSuRTs) to establish fully functional field surgical facilities wherever they are needed in the world

Nurses can join these teams, complete the required training, and offer their expertise as part of a coordinated federal response team in times of critical need (U.S. Department of Health & Human Services, 2013).

Before going to the incident in the field, nurses, physicians, and support staff must have adequate training to prepare them to recognize the risks in an unstable environment

(Laskowski-Jones, 2010; Olchin & Krutz, 2012; Yin et al., 2012). Such risks can include the potential for structural collapse, becoming the secondary target of a terrorist attack, interpersonal violence in unsecured locales, and working in an environment in which contagious diseases and natural hazards are common (e.g., poisonous snake bites and mosquito-borne illnesses). Disaster workers must take measures such as obtaining prophylactic medications and vaccinations, having a personal evacuation plan, and ensuring access to necessary supplies and protective equipment so that they do not become victims as well.

The National Disaster Life Support Foundation, Inc. (2013) offers Core, Basic, and Advanced Disaster Life Support training courses that include all essential aspects of disaster response and management. They include the core competencies of disaster management to all levels of health care professionals. In addition, the Federal Emergency Management Agency (FEMA) (2013) provides numerous online resources, including Community Emergency Response Team (CERT) training so that people are better prepared for disasters and are able to respond more self-sufficiently to incidents and hazard situations in their own communities. These courses include mass casualty triage education.

Hospital Emergency Preparedness: Personnel Roles and Responsibilities

Nurses play a major role in the emergency preparedness or emergency management plan. In the event of a disaster, the Hospital Incident Command System is established for organization and structure.

Hospital Incident Command System

The facility-level organizational model for disaster management is the **Hospital Incident Command System (HICS)**, which is a part of the National Incident Management System (NIMS) implemented by the Department of Homeland Security and FEMA to standardize disaster operations. In this system, roles are formally structured under the hospital or long-term care facility incident commander with clear lines of authority and accountability for specific resources (FEMA, 2013). Officers are named to oversee essential emergency preparedness functions such as public information, safety and security, and medical command. Chiefs are appointed to manage logistics, planning, finance, and operations as appropriate to the type and scale of the event. In turn, chiefs delegate specific duties to other departmental officers and unit leaders. The idea is to achieve a manageable span of control over the personnel or resources allocated to achieve efficiency. FEMA offers free courses on the NIMS model and HICS structure through their website (www.training.fema.gov/IS/).

Because mass casualty events typically involve large numbers of people and can create a chaotic work environment, many EMS agencies and health care facilities use brightly colored vests with large lettering to help identify key leadership positions. Specific job action sheets are distributed to all personnel with leadership roles in HICS that pre-define reporting relationships and list prioritized tasks and responsibilities. The HICS personnel also establish an **emergency operations center (EOC)** or **command center** in a designated location with accessible communication technology. They then use their collective expertise to manage the overall incident. All internal requests for additional personnel and resources, as well as COMMUNICATION with

TABLE 10-2 Summary of Key Personnel Roles and Functions for Emergency Preparedness and Response Plan

PERSONNEL ROLE	PERSONNEL FUNCTION
Hospital incident commander	Physician or administrator who assumes overall leadership for implementing the emergency plan
Medical command physician	Physician who decides the number, acuity, and resource needs of patients
Triage officer	Physician or nurse who rapidly evaluates each patient to determine priorities for treatment
Community relations or public information officer	Person who serves as a liaison between the health care facility and the media

field teams and external agencies, should be coordinated through the EOC to maintain unity of command.

The roles and responsibilities of health care personnel in a mass casualty event or disaster are defined within the institution's emergency response or preparedness plan (Table 10-2). Each plan can be as individual as the particular facility's operations. However, virtually all plans identify certain key functions. For example, one of the primary roles in a hospital to be established at the onset of an incident is that of a **hospital incident commander** who assumes overall leadership for implementing the institutional plan. This person is usually either a physician in the ED or a hospital administrator who has the authority to activate resources. The role can also be fulfilled by a nursing supervisor functioning as the on-site hospital administrator after usual business hours. The hospital incident commander's role is to take a global view of the entire situation and facilitate patient movement through the system. The commander brings in both personnel and supply resources to meet patient needs. For example, a hospital incident commander might dictate that all patients due to be discharged from an inpatient unit be moved to a lounge area immediately to free up hospital beds for mass casualty victims. He or she could also direct departments such as physical therapy or a surgical clinic to cancel their usual operations to convert the space into a minor treatment area. The incident commander assists in the organization of hospital-wide services to rapidly expand hospital capacity, recruit paid or volunteer staff, and ensure the availability of medical supplies.

Another typical role defined in hospital or other health care emergency preparedness plans is that of the **medical command physician**. He or she focuses on determining the number, acuity, and medical resource needs of victims arriving from the incident scene to the hospital and organizing the emergency health care team response to the injured or ill patients. Responsibilities include identifying the need for and calling in specialty-trained providers such as:

- Trauma surgeons
- Neurosurgeons
- Orthopedic surgeons
- Pulmonologists
- Plastic surgeons
- Burn surgeons
- Infectious disease physicians
- Industrial hygienists
- Radiation safety personnel

In smaller hospitals with limited specialty resources, the medical command physician might also help determine which patients should be transported out of the facility to a higher level of care or to a specialty hospital (e.g., burn center).

Closely affiliated with the medical command physician is the **triage officer**. This person is generally a physician in a large hospital who is assisted by triage nurses. When physician resources are limited, an experienced nurse may assume this role. The triage officer rapidly evaluates each person who presents to the hospital, even those who come in with triage tags in place. Patient acuity is re-evaluated for appropriate disposition to the area within the ED or hospital best suited to meet the patient's medical needs.

Many other roles and responsibilities can be defined within the institutional emergency response plan and may include the supply officer, the COMMUNICATIONS officer, the infection control officer, and the community relations/public information officer, to name a few. The community relations or public information officer is an especially important role to delineate in advance. Mass casualty incidents tend to attract a large amount of media attention. This staff member can draw media away from the clinical areas so that essential hospital operations are not hindered. He or she can also serve as the liaison between hospital administration and the media to release only appropriate and accurate information.

Role of Nursing in Health Care Facility Emergency Preparedness and Response

Nurses play key roles before, during, and after a disaster. Before an event, they contribute to developing internal and external emergency response plans, including defining specific nursing roles. Nurses take into account the security needs, COMMUNICATION methods, training, alternative treatment areas, staffing for high-demand or surge situations, and requirements for resources, equipment, and supplies. They then test the plans by actively participating in disaster drills and evaluating the outcomes.

During an actual disaster, the ED charge nurse, trauma program manager, and other ED nursing leadership personnel act in COLLABORATION with the medical command physician and triage officer to organize nursing and ancillary services to meet patient needs. Telephone trees may be activated to call in ED nurses who are not working or are not scheduled to work. ED areas are identified and prepared to stage, triage, resuscitate, and treat the disaster victims. Efforts are made to quickly discharge or admit other ED patients as appropriate to make room for the new arrivals. ED nurses apply principles of triage as disaster victims enter the system to prioritize care delivery and direct patients to the designated areas best suited to meet their needs.

Nursing roles in a disaster extend to all areas within a health care facility. The level of involvement is determined by the scope and scale of the disaster. In any mass casualty event, nurses from medical-surgical nursing units may be asked, in COLLABORATION with the health care provider, to recommend patients for discharge to free up inpatient beds for disaster victims. Patients who are the most medically stable may be discharged early, including those who:

- Were admitted for observation and are not bedridden
- Are having diagnostic evaluations and are not bedridden
- Are soon scheduled to be discharged or could be cared for at home with support from family or home health care services

- Have had no critical change in condition for the past 3 days
- Could be cared for in another health care facility, such as rehabilitation or long-term care

💡 NCLEX EXAMINATION CHALLENGE

Safe and Effective Care Environment

The ED charge nurse is assigning duties to nurses who have been floated to the ED or who have volunteered to help staff the ED during a mass casualty situation. Which assignments are most appropriate? **Select all that apply.**

A. GI laboratory nurse assigned to orthopedic clients having sedation procedures

B. Critical care nurse assigned to client, not related to the mass casualty, having chest pain

C. Medical-surgical nurse assigned to accompany clients to radiology

D. Nursing manager from an inpatient unit assigned to monitor clients in the waiting room

E. Liaison nurse from the operating room assigned to work with families

General staff nurses also may be recruited to COLLABORATE in providing care for stable ED patients, thus allowing ED nurses to focus their efforts on aiding the mass casualty victims. Critical care unit nurses need to identify patients who can be transferred out of the unit to rapidly expand critical care bed capacity. In addition, they can supplement ED nurses in the resuscitation setting or assist in monitored care and transport to critical care units. Hospital and ED nurse leaders also typically direct the ancillary departments to deliver supplies, instrument trays, medications, food, and personnel to meet service demands.

Hospital staff of all levels may be required to alter their routine operations to accommodate a high volume of patients, including those with special needs such as decontamination, burn management, or quarantine. Emergency plans dictate specific actions by staff members, such as who should be called when the plan is activated, who should report, where to report, what supplies or equipment carts should be brought to a pre-designated location, and what type of paperwork or system should be implemented for patient identification in a large-scale event. Some staff may even have their roles changed completely. For example, nurses from the performance improvement department or case management may be reassigned to fulfill a clinical responsibility for a nursing unit. The key concept is that staff members are expected to remain flexible in a mass casualty situation and perform at their highest level to address the needs of both the health care system and the patients. The greatest good for the greatest number of people is still the organizing principle when considering roles and responsibilities in mass casualty events—not necessarily individual staff preferences. However, the SAFETY of all patients is vital.

Creativity and flexibility of nursing leaders and nursing staff are essential to provide the staffing coverage necessary for a large-scale or extended incident. The willingness of staff to show up for work is directly impacted by their concerns for their home and family in a disaster; inadequate staffing can jeopardize a facility's ability to provide care. A **personal emergency preparedness plan** developed by each nurse can help in such situations. It should outline the preplanned specific

TABLE 10-3 Basic Supplies for Personal Preparedness (3-Day Supply)

- Backpack
- Clean clothing, sturdy footwear
- Potable water—at least 1 gallon per person per day for at least 3 days
- Food—non-perishable, no cooking required
- Headlamp or flashlight—battery powered; extra batteries and/or chemical light sticks (**NOTE**: a headlamp is superior because it allows hands-free operation)
- Pocket knife or multi-tool
- Personal identification (ID) with emergency contacts and phone numbers, allergies, and medical information; lists of credit card numbers and bank accounts (keep in watertight container)
- Towel and washcloth; towelettes, soap, hand sanitizer
- Paper, pens, and pencils; regional maps
- Cell phone and charger
- Sunglasses/protective and/or corrective eyewear
- Emergency blanket and/or sleeping bag and pillow
- Work gloves
- Personal first aid kit with over-the-counter (OTC) and prescription medications/vitamins
- Rain gear
- Roll of duct tape and plastic sheeting
- Radio—battery powered or hand-crank generator
- Toiletries (toothbrush and toothpaste, comb, brush, razor, shaving cream, mirror, feminine supplies, deodorant, shampoo, lip balm, sunscreen, insect repellent, toilet paper)
- Plastic garbage bags and ties, resealable plastic bags
- Matches in a waterproof container
- Whistle
- Household liquid bleach for disinfection

arrangements that are to be made for childcare, pet care, and older adult care if the need arises, especially if the event prevents returning home for an extended period.

❗ NURSING SAFETY PRIORITY (QSEN)

Action Alert

Include emergency contact names, addresses, and telephone numbers to use in a crisis as part of a personal emergency preparedness plan. In addition, pre-assemble **personal readiness supplies** or **"go bag"** (disaster supply kit) for the home and automobile with clothing and basic survival supplies, which allows for a rapid response for disaster staffing coverage (Table 10-3). "Go bags" are needed for all members of the family, including pets, in the event the disaster requires evacuation of the community or people to take shelter in their own homes.

When called to respond to work during a mass casualty event, some nurses may experience ethical and moral conflict between their family obligations and professional responsibilities (Chaffee, 2006). The American Nurses Association's (ANA's) *Code of Ethics for Nurses with Interpretive Statements* (2001) does not offer clear guidance in this situation. Each person has to make a choice about whether to be involved in helping during the emergency or when to become involved.

EVENT RESOLUTION AND DEBRIEFING

When the last major casualties have been treated and no more are expected to arrive in numbers that could overwhelm the health care system, the incident commander considers "standing down" or deactivating the emergency response plan.

However, although the casualties may have left the ED, other areas in the hospital may still be under stress and need the support of the supplemental resources provided by emergency plan activation. Before terminating the response, it is essential to ensure that the needs of the other hospital departments have been met and all are in agreement to resume normal operations.

A vital consideration in event resolution is staff and supply availability to meet ongoing operational needs. If nursing staff and other personnel were called in from home during their off hours or if they worked well beyond their scheduled shifts to meet patient and departmental needs, provision for adequate rest periods should be made. Exhaustion poses a risk not only to patient safety but also to the nurse when he or she must drive home. Sleeping quarters at the hospital might be necessary in this case, especially if the disaster event contributed to treacherous travel conditions.

Severe shortages of supplies also pose a threat to usual operations at the conclusion of a mass casualty incident. Taking inventory and restocking the ED are high priority assignments. COLLABORATION between the ED and the central supply department is essential to resolving stock availability problems. Instrument trays must be washed, packaged, and re-sterilized. Critical supplies that have been depleted from hospital stores must be reordered and delivered to the hospital quickly. Contracts with key vendors outlining emergency re-supply expectations and arrangements should be a part of the hospital's overall emergency preparedness plan.

Two general types of **debriefing**, or formal systematic review and analysis, occur after a mass casualty incident or disaster. The first type entails bringing in critical incident stress debriefing (CISD) teams to provide sessions for small groups of staff to promote effective coping strategies. The second type of debriefing involves an administrative review of staff and system performance during the event to determine whether opportunities for improvement in the emergency management plan exist.

Critical Incident Stress Debriefing

CISD is only one component of a much broader critical incident stress management (CISM) program. CISM programming addresses pre-crisis through post-crisis interventions for small to large groups, including communities. After working through the turmoil and the emotional impact of the incident as well as the aftermath, the staff may find it difficult to "get back to normal." Without intervention during *and* after the emergency, they may develop post-traumatic stress disorder (PTSD). PTSD can lead to multiple characteristic psychological and physical effects, including flashbacks, avoidance, less interest in previously enjoyable events, and detachment, as well as rapid heart rate and insomnia. People suffering from PTSD can have great difficulty relating in their usual way to family and friends. Ultimately, professional "burnout" can stem from the inability to cope with the stress effectively. A resource for CISM is the International Critical Incident Stress Foundation, Inc. (2013); their mission is "to provide leadership, education, training, consultation, and support services in comprehensive crisis intervention and disaster behavioral health services to the emergency response professions, other organizations, and communities worldwide" (www.icisf.org/who-we-are). Chart 10-2 lists recommendations proposed by several national organizations to help prevent PTSD during the emergency situation.

CHART 10-2 **Best Practice for Patient Safety & Quality Care** (QSEN)

Preventing Staff Post-Traumatic Stress Disorder (PTSD) During a Mass Casualty Event

- Use available counseling.
- Encourage and support co-workers.
- Monitor each other's stress level and performance.
- Take breaks when needed.
- Talk about feelings with staff and managers.
- Drink plenty of water, and eat healthy snacks for energy.
- Keep in touch with family, friends, and significant others.
- Do not work for more than 12 hours per day.

Adapted from Papp, E. (2005). Preparing for disasters: Helping yourself as you help others. *AJN*, *105*(5), 112.

A CISD team comprises two or three specially trained people who come together quickly when called to deal with the emotional needs of health care team members after a particularly devastating or disturbing incident. The team leader typically has background in a mental health/behavioral health field. The co-leader is ideally a peer of the group being debriefed. Thus, if nurses are debriefed, then a nurse member of the CISD team is generally assigned to the session. CISD-trained physicians, police, firefighters, EMTs, and paramedics may also be used, depending on the needs of the group. The third member of the team is known as the "doorkeeper." This person is responsible for keeping inappropriate people out (e.g., media, spectators) and talking with anyone who leaves the session early in an effort to have him or her return or accept follow-up. Staff involved in the incident need protected time to undergo stress debriefing, which generally lasts from 1 to 3 hours per session.

Typical "ground rules" for stress debriefing include strict confidentiality of information shared during the session and unconditional acceptance of the thoughts and feelings expressed by people within the group. The usual arrangement for the most effective group interaction is a circular configuration of chairs in a private setting. Food should be available so that hunger is not a distraction. CISD group leaders encourage group discussion through asking a series of questions designed to get everyone involved to tell his or her own story about the incident and explain the personal impact. The group leaders enable participants to place the incident into perspective and dispel any feelings of blame or guilt. They also educate participants about self-care concepts and coping strategies to use immediately. People who require more than a CISD session may need referral for mental health/behavioral health counseling.

Administrative Review

The second type of debriefing is an administrative evaluation directed at analyzing the hospital or agency response to an event while it is still in the forefront of the minds of everyone who participated in it. The goal of this type of debriefing is to discern what went right and what went wrong during activation and implementation of the emergency preparedness plan so that needed changes can be made. Typically, representatives from all groups that were involved in the incident come together soon after plan activation has been discontinued. They each are given an opportunity to hear and express both positive and negative comments related to their experiences with the event. Then, in the days after the plan activation, written critique forms are also solicited to gain additional information after participants have had time to consider their overall impressions of the response as well as the impact it had on their respective departments or clinical areas.

Although drills are important, implementing the emergency preparedness plan during an actual mass casualty event is the most effective means of "reality testing" the plan's utility. Feedback provided by participants can be used to modify or revise the plan and create new processes in preparation for future events.

ROLE OF NURSING IN COMMUNITY EMERGENCY PREPAREDNESS AND RESPONSE

During a community disaster, nurses and other emergency personnel may be needed for triage, first aid/emergency care, and shelter assistance. The first action of first-responders in a disaster is to remove people from danger, both the injured and uninjured. This job is typically managed by firefighters and other disaster-trained emergency personnel; unless they have had specific search and rescue training, nurses are not usually involved in this process. In all cases, developing and maintaining accurate *situational awareness* is critical for appropriate priority setting and SAFETY in a rapidly changing environment (Busby & Witucki-Brown, 2011).

After removal from danger, victims are triaged by health care personnel as described earlier in this chapter. After triage, nurses often provide on-site first aid and emergency care. They may also be involved in teaching and supervising volunteers. The American Red Cross sets up shelters for people who have lost their homes or have been evacuated from their homes.

Nurses may also need to teach those living temporarily in shelters about procedures that will be needed for SAFETY when they return home. For example, clean drinking water may not be available for several days or longer. Community residents may need to boil their water before drinking. If electricity and gas are not available, an outdoor grill or camp stove can be used. As alternative procedures, commercial water purification filters, sterilizing ultraviolet pens, or tablets or 10 to 20 drops of chlorine bleach added to a gallon of water will make the water safe to drink.

Human waste management creates another challenge if toilets do not flush. If not managed safely, enteric pathogens spread disease. A toilet bowl or bucket lined with a plastic bag can be used for human waste. To sanitize it and provide odor control, chlorine bleach can be added and the bag tied and sealed. Portable toilet chemicals or chlorinated lime may be used as alternatives. To prevent a toxic gas reaction, remind residents not to mix any chemicals. Treated human waste bags can be buried in the ground. In an austere environment, a pit can be dug in the ground as an improvised toilet. In all cases, emphasize the importance of handwashing with soap and water or using a hand sanitizer to prevent disease transmission.

PSYCHOSOCIAL RESPONSE OF SURVIVORS TO MASS CASUALTY EVENTS

One of the most important roles of the nurse after a community disaster is health assessment, including psychosocial health. Experiencing a disaster can produce both immediate and long-lasting psychosocial effects in people personally affected by the event. Depending on the nature and magnitude of the incident, survivors experience the tragic loss of loved ones, property, and valued possessions. They and their family members may have suffered injuries or illnesses brought about by the catastrophe. Lifestyles, roles, and routines are drastically altered, preventing people from achieving any sense of normalcy in the hours, the days, and perhaps even the weeks and months that follow a disaster. Coping abilities in survivors are severely stressed, leading to many individual responses that can range from functional and adaptive behaviors to maladaptive coping.

Survivors have to confront feelings of vulnerability resulting from the devastating event, knowing that it could occur again—a particularly relevant issue for people who live in areas prone to acts of terrorism or to natural disasters. The decision—be it voluntary or involuntary—to abandon a family home or geographic region and then relocate to a "safe" area either temporarily or permanently results in a further sense of loss and grief. Some people may feel guilty about living through an event that caused so many others to die. The range of intense emotions can appear as physical illness, as well as psychological and social dysfunction.

When helping people in crisis after a mass casualty event, be calm and reassuring. Establish rapport through active listening and honest COMMUNICATION. Survivors benefit from talking about their experiences and being helped as they work to problem-solve. Offer choices whenever possible to help survivors gain a sense of personal control. Help survivors adapt to their new surroundings and routines through simple, concrete explanations. Convey caring behaviors, and provide a sense of safety and security to the best extent possible. If available, request that crisis counselors respond and assist in providing compassionate support to victims and their families (Kallman & Feury, 2011).

A disaster may cause some survivors to develop posttraumatic stress disorder (PTSD), which can potentially last for a lifetime. People who are unable to sleep, are easily startled, have "flashbacks" to relive the disaster, or report "feeling numb" 2 weeks or more after a disaster or traumatic event are at risk for PTSD (Hyer & Brown, 2008).

❓ CLINICAL JUDGMENT CHALLENGE

Patient-Centered Care QSEN

An ED nurse has gone on an emergent medical mission trip to a Third World country after an earthquake with multiple building collapses in a remote rural area. Hundreds are reported missing, and even more are injured. Medical resources in this country are scarce.

1. What challenges does this nurse face in terms of his or her own safety and health?
2. How can the nurse manage basic hygiene and meet basic needs?
3. Some local residents are so distraught that they are unable to function and are not eating or sleeping. What assistance can the nurse provide?
4. After returning from the mission trip, the nurse feels apathetic, disengaged with regular employment, and is often short tempered with co-workers and staff. What resources exist for the nurse?

Nurses caring for survivors with these manifestations should perform further assessment. One tool that can be used to assess survivor response to a disaster is the Impact of Event Scale—

Revised (IES-R). The IES-R is a 22-item self-administered questionnaire including several subscales, such as avoidance. Before giving the tool, determine the patient's reading level because it is written at a 10th-grade reading level. The tool should not be used for patients with short-term memory loss. For that reason, many older survivors are often not adequately assessed for post-disaster PTSD (Hyer & Brown, 2008). However, assess all older survivors of a disaster for this complication when possible.

> **! NURSING SAFETY PRIORITY** (QSEN)
>
> **Action Alert**
>
> A high score on any IES-R subscale indicates a need for further evaluation and counseling. Refer the patient to a social worker or qualified mental health counselor. A high score on all subscales requires referral to a psychiatrist or clinical psychologist to evaluate the possibility of current or past trauma, such as abuse or neglect.

GET READY FOR THE NCLEX® EXAMINATION!

KEY POINTS

Review these Key Points for each NCLEX Examination Client Needs Category.

Safe and Effective Care Environment
- Describe the hospital emergency preparedness and response team that all hospitals are required to have in case of mass casualty (disaster). **Teamwork and Collaboration** (QSEN)
- Use the guidelines in Chart 10-1 to respond to a fire in any facility. **Safety** (QSEN)
- Apply principles of triage by using the typical triage system for a mass casualty situation, which includes an additional category for those patients allowed to die (black-tagged) (see Table 10-1).
- Describe the special roles that are assigned in a mass casualty incident as identified in Table 10-2.
- Understand how to assist in determining the need for initiating the emergency preparedness plan based on available resources, including staffing. **Teamwork and Collaboration** (QSEN)
- Be prepared for an emergency by developing a personal emergency preparedness plan, including a plan for child, pet, and older adult care; have a "go bag," or disaster supply kit, packed for both the automobile and the home (see Table 10-3).
- Compare key personnel roles in an emergency preparedness and response plan, including those involved in the two types of debriefing that occur after a mass casualty event or period—critical incident stress debriefing and an administrative review or evaluation. **Teamwork and Collaboration** (QSEN)

- Identify the important roles of nurses in preparing for, managing, and debriefing after internal health care facility and community disasters.
- Recall that nurses play a major role in triage, first aid and emergency care, and shelter assistance in external community disasters.
- Understand how to identify which patients to recommend for hospital discharge in a disaster situation. **Patient-Centered Care** (QSEN)

Psychosocial Integrity
- Assess survivors and families for their ability to adapt to the effects of disaster changes or traumatic events, including post-traumatic stress disorder (PTSD). **Patient-Centered Care** (QSEN)
- Provide emotional support to the person and/or family in coping with life changes resulting from a disaster by encouraging relaxation, listening to survivor feelings, and referring for appropriate counseling. **Patient-Centered Care** (QSEN)
- Be honest with victims and their families, and help them adapt to their changed or new surroundings.
- Provide support by taking precautions to prevent staff from developing PTSD as outlined in Chart 10-2.

Physiological Integrity
- Take precautions for meeting basic needs in a mass casualty situation; know your own limitations, and develop situational awareness when responding. **Safety** (QSEN)

11 | CHAPTER

Assessment and Care of Patients with Fluid and Electrolyte Imbalances

M. Linda Workman

 http://evolve.elsevier.com/Iggy/

PRIORITY CONCEPTS

- FLUID AND ELECTROLYTE IMBALANCE

LEARNING OUTCOMES

Safe and Effective Care Environment

1. Protect the patient with a change in FLUID AND ELECTROLYTE BALANCE.

Health Promotion and Maintenance

2. Teach people how to prevent, recognize, and manage a change in FLUID AND ELECTROLYTE BALANCE.

Psychosocial Integrity

3. Reduce the psychological impact for the patient experiencing a change in FLUID AND ELECTROLYTE BALANCE.

Physiological Integrity

4. Use knowledge from anatomy and physiology to assess the patient's FLUID AND ELECTROLYTE BALANCE.
5. Use laboratory data and clinical manifestations to determine the effectiveness of interventions to restore FLUID AND ELECTROLYTE BALANCE.
6. Prioritize interventions for a patient who has a change in FLUID AND ELECTROLYTE BALANCE.

HOMEOSTASIS

The body works best when FLUID AND ELECTROLYTE BALANCE is kept within a narrow range of normal. For example, no body system works well if 2 liters of blood volume are gained or lost. To keep conditions as close to normal as possible (known as **homeostasis**), the body has many control actions (known as **homeostatic mechanisms**) to prevent dangerous changes.

Homeostasis requires that the body's volume and composition of FLUIDS remain within normal limits. Water (fluid) is the most common substance in the body, making up about 55% to 60% of total weight for healthy younger adults and 50% to 55% of total weight for healthy older adults. This water is divided into two main compartments (spaces)—the fluid outside the cells (**extracellular fluid [ECF]**); and the fluid inside the cells (**intracellular fluid [ICF]**). The ECF space is about one third (about 15 L) of the total body water. The ECF includes **interstitial fluid** (fluid between cells, sometimes called the "third space"); blood, lymph, bone, and connective tissue water; and the transcellular FLUIDS. **Transcellular fluids** are in special body spaces and include cerebrospinal fluid, synovial fluid, peritoneal fluid, and pleural fluid. ICF is about two thirds (about 25 L) of total body water. Fig. 11-1 shows normal total body water distribution.

Water is needed to deliver dissolved nutrients, ELECTROLYTES, and other substances to all organs, tissues, and cells. In health, the volume of water in the fluid compartments remains within the normal range although the water moves constantly between compartments. Changes in either the amount of water or the amount of electrolytes in body FLUIDS can affect the functioning of all cells, tissues, and organs. *For proper function, the volume of all body fluids and the types and amount of dissolved substances must be carefully balanced.*

PHYSIOLOGIC INFLUENCES ON FLUID AND ELECTROLYTE BALANCE

Body fluids are composed of water and particles dissolved or suspended in water. The **solvent** is the water portion of fluids. **Solutes** are the particles dissolved or suspended in the water.

Solutes vary in type and amount from one fluid space to another. When solutes express an overall electrical charge, they are known as *electrolytes*. Body function depends on keeping the correct FLUID AND ELECTROLYTE BALANCE within each body fluid space (compartment).

Three processes control FLUID AND ELECTROLYTE BALANCE so the internal environment remains stable even when the external environment changes. These processes—filtration, diffusion, and osmosis—determine how, when, and where fluids and particles move across cell membranes.

FILTRATION

Physiologic Action

Filtration is the movement of FLUID (water) through a cell or blood vessel membrane because of water pressure **(hydrostatic pressure)** differences on both sides of the membrane. Water pressure is related to water volume pressing against confining membranes.

Fluid weight in a space is related to the amount of FLUID present in that area. Water molecules in a confined space constantly press outward against the membranes, creating hydrostatic pressure. This is a "water-pushing" pressure, because it is the force that pushes water outward from a confined space through a membrane (Fig. 11-2).

The amount (volume) of water in any body fluid space determines the hydrostatic pressure of that space. Blood, which is "thicker" than water (more *viscous*), is confined within the blood vessels. Blood has hydrostatic pressure because of its weight and volume. Another factor that affects blood hydrostatic pressure in arteries is the pumping action of the heart.

The hydrostatic pressures of two fluid spaces can be compared whenever a porous **(permeable)** membrane separates the two spaces. If the hydrostatic pressure is the same in both fluid spaces, there is no pressure difference between the two spaces and the hydrostatic pressure is at *equilibrium*. If the hydrostatic pressure is not the same in both spaces, **disequilibrium** exists. This means that the two spaces have a graded difference (*gradient*) for hydrostatic pressure: one space has a higher hydrostatic pressure than the other. *The human body constantly seeks equilibrium.* When a gradient exists, water movement (filtration) occurs until the hydrostatic pressure is the same in both spaces (see Fig. 11-2).

Water moves through the membrane **(filters)** from the space with higher hydrostatic pressure to the space with lower pressure. Filtration continues only as long as the hydrostatic pressure gradient exists. Equilibrium is reached when enough fluid leaves one space and enters the other space to make the hydrostatic pressure in both spaces equal. In equilibrium, water molecules are evenly exchanged between the two spaces but no net further filtration of fluid occurs. Neither space gains or loses water molecules, and the hydrostatic pressure in both spaces remains the same.

Clinical Significance

Blood pressure is an example of a hydrostatic filtering force. It moves whole blood from the heart to capillaries where filtration can occur to exchange water, nutrients, and waste products between the blood and the tissues. The hydrostatic pressure difference between the capillary blood and the interstitial fluid (fluid in the tissue spaces) determines whether water leaves the blood vessels and enters the tissue spaces.

Capillary membranes are only one cell layer thick, making a thin "wall" to hold blood in the capillaries. Large spaces **(pores)** in the capillary membrane help water filter freely when a hydrostatic pressure gradient is present (Fig. 11-3).

Extracellular space   Intracellular space

Plasma volume

Interstitial space

About 25 liters

About 3.5-6 liters

About 10-12 liters

FIG. 11-1 Normal distribution of total body water in adults.

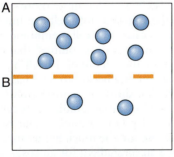

Compartment A has more water molecules and greater hydrostatic pressure than does compartment B.

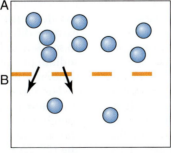

Water molecules move down the hydrostatic pressure gradient from compartment A through the permeable membrane into compartment B, which has a lower hydrostatic pressure.

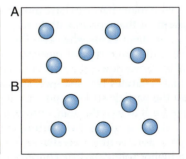

Enough water molecules have moved down the hydrostatic pressure gradient from compartment A into compartment B that both sides now have the same amount of water and the same amount of hydrostatic pressure. An equilibrium of hydrostatic pressure now exists between the two compartments, and no further *net* movement of water will occur.

○ = Water molecule

━ = Permeable membrane

FIG. 11-2 The process of filtration.

Endothelial cells

Intercellular spaces (pores)
through which diffusion, filtration,
and osmosis can occur

FIG. 11-3 The basic structure of a capillary.

Edema (tissue swelling from excess FLUID) forms with changes in hydrostatic pressure differences between the capillary blood and the interstitial fluid, such as in patients with right-sided heart failure. In this condition, the volume of blood in the right side of the heart increases because the right ventricle is too weak to pump blood efficiently into the lung blood vessels. As blood backs up into the venous and capillary systems, the capillary hydrostatic pressure rises until it is higher than the hydrostatic pressure in the interstitial space. Then, excess filtration of fluids from the capillaries into the interstitial tissue space occurs, forming visible edema.

DIFFUSION

Physiologic Action

Diffusion is the movement of particles (solute) across a permeable membrane from an area of higher particle concentration to an area of lower particle concentration (down a *concentration gradient*). Particles in a fluid have totally random movement from the vibration of atoms in the nucleus. This random movement allows molecules to bump into each other within a confined fluid space. Each collision increases the speed of particle movement. The more particles (higher concentration) present in the confined fluid space, the greater the number of collisions.

As a result of the collisions, molecules in a solution spread out evenly through the available space. They move from an area of higher amounts (higher concentration) of molecules to an area of lower amounts until an equal amount is present in all areas. Fluid spaces with many particles have more collisions and faster particle movement than spaces with fewer particles.

A concentration gradient exists when two fluid spaces have different amounts of the same type of particles. Particle collisions cause them to move down the concentration gradient. Any membrane that separates two spaces is struck repeatedly by particles. When the particle strikes a pore in the membrane that is large enough for it to pass through, diffusion occurs (Fig. 11-4). The chance of any single particle hitting the membrane and going through a pore is much greater on the side of the membrane with a higher solute particle concentration.

The speed of diffusion is related to the difference in amount of particles (concentration gradient) between the two sides of the membrane. The degree of difference is the *steepness* of the gradient: the larger the concentration difference between the two sides, the steeper the gradient. Diffusion is more rapid when the gradient is steeper (just as a ball rolls downhill faster when the hill is steep than when the hill is nearly flat). Particles move from the fluid space with a higher concentration of solute particles to the fluid space with a lower concentration of solute particles.

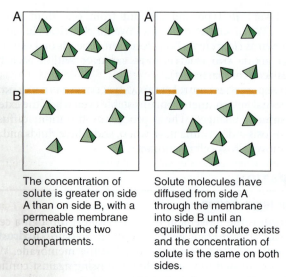

The concentration of solute is greater on side A than on side B, with a permeable membrane separating the two compartments.

Solute molecules have diffused from side A through the membrane into side B until an equilibrium of solute exists and the concentration of solute is the same on both sides.

FIG. 11-4 Diffusion of solute particles through a permeable membrane from an area of higher solute concentration to an area of lower solute concentration until an equilibrium is reached.

Particle diffusion continues as long as a concentration gradient exists between the two sides of the membrane. When the concentration of particles is the same on both sides of the membrane, the particles are in equilibrium and only an equal exchange of particles continues.

Clinical Significance

Diffusion is what transports most ELECTROLYTES and other particles through cell membranes. Unlike capillary membranes, which permit the diffusion of most small-size particles down a gradient, cell membranes are *selective* for which particles can diffuse. They permit diffusion of some particles but not others. Some particles cannot move across a cell membrane, even when a steep "downhill" gradient exists, because the membrane is **impermeable** (closed) to that particle. For these particles, the concentration gradient is maintained across the membrane.

Impermeability and special transport systems cause differences in the amounts of specific particles from one fluid space to another. For example, usually the fluid outside the cell (the extracellular fluid [ECF]) has ten times more sodium ions than the fluid inside the cell (the intracellular fluid [ICF]). This extreme difference is caused by cell membrane impermeability to sodium and by special "sodium pumps" that move any extra sodium present inside the cell out of the cell "uphill" against its concentration gradient and back into the ECF.

For some particles, diffusion cannot occur without help, even down steep concentration gradients, because of selective membrane permeability. One example is glucose. Even though the amount of glucose may be much higher in the ECF than in the ICF (creating a steep gradient for glucose), glucose cannot cross many cell membranes without the help of insulin. When insulin is present, it binds to insulin receptors on cell membranes, which then makes the membranes much more permeable to glucose. As a result, glucose can cross the cell membrane down its concentration gradient until equilibrium of glucose concentration is achieved.

Diffusion across a cell membrane that requires the assistance of a membrane-altering system (e.g., insulin) is called **facilitated diffusion** or **facilitated transport**. This type of movement is still a form of diffusion.

OSMOSIS

Physiologic Action

Osmosis is the movement of water only through a selectively permeable *(semipermeable)* membrane. For osmosis to occur, a membrane must separate two fluid spaces and one space must have particles that cannot move through the membrane. (The membrane is impermeable to this particle.) A concentration gradient of this particle must also exist. Because the membrane is impermeable to these particles, they cannot cross the membrane but water molecules can. (Usually water can *always* move through a cell membrane.)

For the fluid spaces to have equal concentrations of the particle, the water molecules move down their concentration gradient from the side with the higher concentration of water molecules (and thus a lower concentration of particles along with a greater hydrostatic pressure) to the side with the lower concentration of water molecules (and a higher concentration of particles along with a lower hydrostatic pressure). This movement continues until both spaces contain the same proportions of particles to water. Dilute (less concentrated) FLUID has fewer particles and more water molecules than the more concentrated fluid. Thus water moves by osmosis down its hydrostatic pressure gradient from the dilute fluid to the more concentrated fluid until a concentration equilibrium occurs (Fig. 11-5).

At this point, the *concentrations* of particles in the fluid spaces on both sides of the membrane are equal even though the total amounts of particles and volumes of water are different. *The concentration equilibrium occurs by the movement of water molecules rather than the movement of solute particles.*

Particle concentration in body FLUID is the major factor that determines whether and how fast osmosis and diffusion occur. This concentration is expressed in milliequivalents per liter (mEq/L), millimoles per liter (mmol/L), and milliosmoles per liter (mOsm/L). **Osmolarity** is the number of milliosmoles in a *liter* of solution; **osmolality** is the number of milliosmoles in a *kilogram* of solution. The normal osmolarity value for plasma and other body fluids ranges from 270 to about 300 mOsm/L. The body functions best when the osmolarity of all body fluid spaces is close to 300 mOsm/L. When all fluids have this particle concentration, the fluids are **isosmotic** or **isotonic** (also called **normotonic**) to each other.

FLUIDS with osmolarities greater than 300 mOsm/L are **hyperosmotic**, or **hypertonic**, compared with isosmotic fluids. These fluids have a *greater* osmotic pressure than do isosmotic fluids and tend to pull water from the isosmotic fluid space into the hyperosmotic fluid space until an osmotic balance occurs. If a hyperosmotic IV solution (e.g., 3% or 5% saline) were infused into a patient with normal ECF osmolarity, the infusing fluid would make the person's blood hyperosmotic. To balance this situation, the interstitial fluid would be pulled into the circulation in an attempt to dilute the blood osmolarity back to normal. As a result, the interstitial volume would shrink and the plasma volume would expand.

FLUIDS with osmolarities of less than 270 mOsm/L are **hypoosmotic**, or **hypotonic**, compared with isosmotic fluids. Hypoosmolar fluids have a *lower* osmotic pressure than isosmotic fluids, and water is pulled from the hypo-osmotic fluid space into the isosmotic fluid space. An example of a hypotonic IV fluid is 0.45% saline.

Clinical Significance

Osmosis and filtration act together at the capillary membrane to maintain both extracellular fluid (ECF) and intracellular fluid (ICF) volumes within their normal ranges. The thirst mechanism is an example of how osmosis helps maintain homeostasis. The feeling of thirst is caused by the activation of cells in the brain that respond to changes in ECF osmolarity.

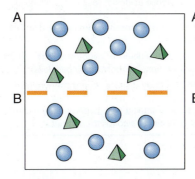

Side A has more solute molecules than does side B, even though the number of water molecules is the same on both sides. Thus side A has a greater osmotic (water pulling) pressure than does side B.

DISEQUILIBRIUM
Side A 1.5:1 ratio of water to solute
Side B 3:1 ratio of water to solute

○ = Water molecule
━ = Permeable membrane
△ = Solute molecule

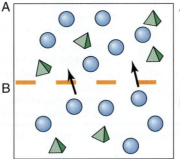

Movement of water occurs by osmosis toward side A because it has greater osmotic pressure. The membrane is *not* permeable to the solute molecules, so the actual number of solute molecules on side A and side B does not change. *Only the water molecules move, because the membrane is not permeable to the solute molecules.*

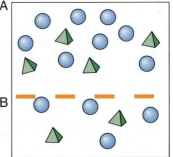

Enough water molecules have moved from side B into side A that the actual concentration of solute is now the same on both sides, with a ratio of water to solute of 2:1. An equilibrium of osmotic pressure now exists between the two compartments, and no further *net* movement of water molecules or solute molecules will occur.

EQUILIBRIUM
Side A 2:1 ratio of water to solute
Side B 2:1 ratio of water to solute

FIG. 11-5 The process of osmosis to generate a concentration equilibrium (but not a volume equilibrium) for a solute particle that cannot move through a cell membrane.

These cells, so very sensitive to changes in ECF osmolarity, are called *osmoreceptors.* When a person loses body water but most of the particles remain, such as through excessive sweating, ECF volume is decreased and osmolarity is increased (is hypertonic). The cells in the thirst center shrink as water moves from the cells into the hypertonic ECF. The shrinking of these cells triggers a person's awareness of thirst and increases the urge to drink. Drinking replaces the amount of water lost through sweating and dilutes the ECF osmolarity, restoring it to normal. The thirst mechanism is less sensitive in older adults, increasing their risk for dehydration.

FLUID BALANCE

BODY FLUIDS

Fluid balance is closely linked to and affected by electrolyte concentrations. Table 11-1 lists the normal ranges of the major serum electrolytes. Chart 11-1 lists the normal electrolyte values for people older than 60 years.

A person's age, gender, and amount of fat affect the amount and distribution of body fluids. An older adult has less total body water than a younger adult. Chart 11-2 discusses age-related changes in fluid balance. An obese person has less total water than a lean person of the same weight because fat cells contain almost no water.

GENDER HEALTH CONSIDERATIONS
Patient-Centered Care QSEN

Women of any age have less total body water than men of similar sizes and ages. This difference is because men tend to have more muscle mass than women and because women have more body fat. (Muscle cells contain mostly water, and fat cells have little water.) This difference in water distribution may be responsible for differences seen in women's and men's responses to drugs.

Body fluids are constantly filtered and replaced as fluid balance is maintained through intake and output. The total amount of water within each fluid space is stable, but individual

TABLE 11-1	Major Serum Electrolyte Concentrations and Significance of Abnormal Values		
ELECTROLYTE	**REFERENCE RANGE**	**INTERNATIONAL RECOMMENDED UNITS**	**SIGNIFICANCE OF ABNORMAL VALUES**
Sodium (Na^+)	136-145 mEq/L	136-145 mmol/L	*Elevated:* Hypernatremia; dehydration; kidney disease; hypercortisolism *Low:* Hyponatremia; fluid overload; liver disease; adrenal insufficiency
Potassium (K^+)	3.5-5.0 mEq/L	3.5-5.0 mmol/L	*Elevated:* Hyperkalemia; dehydration; kidney disease; acidosis; adrenal insufficiency; crush injuries *Low:* Hypokalemia; fluid overload; diuretic therapy; alkalosis; insulin administration; hyperaldosteronism
Calcium (Ca^{2+})	9.0-10.5 mg/dL	2.25-2.62 mmol/L	*Elevated:* Hypercalcemia; hyperthyroidism; hyperparathyroidism *Low:* Hypocalcemia; vitamin D deficiency; hypothyroidism; hypoparathyroidism; kidney disease; excessive intake of phosphorus-containing foods and drinks
Chloride (Cl^-)	98-106 mEq/L	98-106 mmol/L	*Elevated:* Hyperchloremia; metabolic acidosis; respiratory alkalosis; hypercortisolism *Low:* Hypochloremia; fluid overload; excessive vomiting or diarrhea; adrenal insufficiency; diuretic therapy
Magnesium (Mg^{2+})	1.3-2.1 mEq/L	0.65-1.05 mmol/L	*Elevated:* Hypermagnesemia; kidney disease; hypothyroidism; adrenal insufficiency *Low:* Hypomagnesemia; malnutrition; alcoholism; ketoacidosis
Phosphorus (P) (Phosphate [PO_4^{3+}]P)	3.0-4.5 mg/dL	0.97-1.45 mmol/L	*Elevated:* Hyperphosphatemia; kidney disease; hypoparathyroidism; acidosis; hypocalcemia *Low:* Hypophosphatemia; chronic antacid use; hyperparathyroidism; hypercalcemia; vitamin D deficiency; alcoholism; malnutrition

Data from Pagana, K., & Pagana, T. (2014). *Mosby's manual of diagnostic and laboratory tests* (5th ed). St. Louis: Mosby.

CHART 11-1	Nursing Focus on the Older Adult			

Normal Plasma Electrolyte Values for People Older Than 60 Years

	REFERENCE RANGE		INTERNATIONAL RECOMMENDED UNITS	
ELECTROLYTE	**60-90 YEARS**	**>90 YEARS**	**60-90 YEARS**	**>90 YEARS**
Calcium (Ca^{2+})	9.0-10.5 mg/dL	8.2-9.6 mg/dL	2.2-2.62 mmol/L	2.05-2.40 mmol/L
Chloride (Cl^-)	98-106 mEq/L	98-111 mEq/L	98-106 mmol/L	98-111 mmol/L
Magnesium (Mg^{2+})	1.3-2.1 mEq/L	1.3-2.1 mEq/L	0.65-1.05 mmol/L	0.65-1.05 mmol/L
Phosphorus (P)	3.0-4.5 mg/dL	3.0-4.5 mg/dL	0.97-1.45 mmol/L	0.97-1.45 mmol/L
Potassium (K^+)	3.5-5.0 mEq/L	3.5-5.0 mEq/L	3.5-5.0 mmol/L	3.5-5.0 mmol/L
Sodium (Na^+)	136-145 mEq/L	132-146 mEq/L	136-145 mmol/L	132-146 mmol/L

Data for adults 60 to 90 years from Pagana, K., & Pagana, T. (2014). *Mosby's manual of diagnostic and laboratory tests* (5th ed). St. Louis: Mosby.
Data for adults >90 years from Tietz, N.W. (Ed.). (1995). *Clinical guide to laboratory tests* (3rd ed.). Philadelphia: Saunders.

water molecules move continually among all spaces. As a result, water in all spaces is exchanged continually while maintaining constant fluid volume.

Fluid intake is regulated through the thirst drive. FLUID enters the body as liquids and as solid foods, which contain up to 85% water (Table 11-2).

A rising blood osmolarity or a decreasing blood volume triggers the sensation of thirst. Sensations such as mouth dryness or the thought that a person has not had a drink recently also triggers the thirst drive. An adult takes in about 2300 mL of fluid daily from food and liquids.

Fluid loss occurs through several routes (see Table 11-2). The kidney is the most important and the most sensitive water loss route because it is regulated and is adjustable. The volume of urine excreted daily varies depending on the amount of FLUID taken in and the body's need to conserve fluids.

The minimum amount of urine per day needed to excrete toxic waste products is 400 to 600 mL. This minimum volume is called the **obligatory urine output**. If the 24-hour urine output falls below the obligatory output amount, wastes are retained and can cause lethal electrolyte imbalances, acidosis, and a toxic buildup of nitrogen.

The ability of the kidneys to make either concentrated or very dilute urine helps maintain FLUID BALANCE. The kidney works with various hormones to maintain fluid balance when extracellular fluid concentrations, volumes, or pressures change.

Other normal water loss occurs through the skin, the lungs, and the intestinal tract. Water losses also can result from salivation, drainage from fistulas and drains, and GI suction.

Water loss from the skin, lungs, and stool is called **insensible water loss** because there are no mechanisms to control this loss. In a healthy adult, insensible water loss is about 500 to 1000 mL/day. This loss increases greatly during thyroid crisis, trauma, burns, states of extreme stress, and fever. Insensible water loss also increases when the environment is hot and dry. Patients at risk for increased insensible water loss include those being mechanically ventilated, those with rapid respirations (*tachypnea*), and those undergoing continuous GI suctioning. Loss by sweating is variable and can reach a maximum rate of about 2 L/hr. Water loss through stool is normally minimal. However, this loss can increase greatly with severe diarrhea or excessive fistula drainage. If not balanced by intake, insensible loss can lead to severe dehydration and electrolyte imbalances.

HORMONAL REGULATION OF FLUID BALANCE

Three hormones help control FLUID AND ELECTROLYTE BALANCE. These are aldosterone, antidiuretic hormone (ADH), and natriuretic peptide (NP).

Aldosterone is a hormone secreted by the adrenal cortex whenever sodium levels in the extracellular fluid (ECF) are decreased. Aldosterone prevents both water and sodium loss. When aldosterone is secreted, it acts on the kidney nephrons, triggering them to reabsorb sodium and water from the urine back into the blood. This action increases blood osmolarity and blood volume. Aldosterone prevents excessive kidney excretion of sodium. It also helps prevent blood potassium levels from becoming too high.

Antidiuretic hormone (ADH), or vasopressin, is released from the posterior pituitary gland in response to changes in blood osmolarity. The hypothalamus contains the osmoreceptors that are sensitive to changes in blood osmolarity. Increased blood osmolarity, especially an increase in the level of plasma sodium, results in a slight shrinkage of these cells and triggers ADH release from the posterior pituitary gland. Because the action of ADH retains just water, it only indirectly regulates electrolyte retention or excretion.

ADH acts directly on kidney tubules and collecting ducts, making them more permeable to water only. As a result, more water is *reabsorbed* by these tubules and returned to the blood, decreasing blood osmolarity by making it more dilute. When blood osmolarity decreases with low plasma sodium levels, the osmoreceptors swell slightly and inhibit ADH release. Less water is then reabsorbed, and more is lost from the body in the urine. As a result, the amount of water in the extracellular fluid (ECF) decreases, bringing osmolarity up to normal.

Natriuretic peptides (NPs) are hormones secreted by special cells that line the atria of the heart (atrial natriuretic peptide [ANP]) and the ventricles of the heart. (The peptide secreted by the heart ventricular cells is known as *brain natriuretic peptide [BNP]* because it was first discovered in the brain.) These peptides are secreted in response to increased blood volume and blood pressure, which stretch the heart tissue. NP binds to receptors in the nephrons, creating effects that are

CHART 11-2 Nursing Focus on the Older Adult

Impact of Age-Related Changes on Fluid Balance

SYSTEM	CHANGE	RESULT
Skin	Loss of elasticity Decreased turgor Decreased oil production	Skin becomes an unreliable indicator of fluid status, especially the back of the hand Dry, easily damaged skin
Kidney	Decreased glomerular filtration Decreased concentrating capacity	Poor excretion of waste products Increased water loss, increasing the risk for dehydration
Muscular	Decreased muscle mass	Decreased total body water Greater risk for dehydration
Neurologic	Diminished thirst reflex	Decreased fluid intake, increasing the risk for dehydration
Endocrine	Adrenal atrophy	Poor regulation of sodium and potassium, increasing the risk for hyponatremia and hyperkalemia

TABLE 11-2 Routes of Fluid Ingestion and Excretion

INTAKE	OUTPUT
Measurable	
Oral fluids	Urine
Parenteral fluids	Emesis
Enemas*	Feces
Irrigation fluids*	Drainage from body cavities
Not Measurable	
Solid foods	Perspiration
Metabolism	Vaporization through the lungs

*Measured by subtracting the amount returned from the amount instilled.

opposite of aldosterone. Kidney reabsorption of sodium is inhibited at the same time that glomerular filtration is increased, causing increased urine output. The outcome is decreased circulating blood volume and decreased blood osmolarity.

SIGNIFICANCE OF FLUID BALANCE

The Renin-Angiotensin II Pathway

The human body requires FLUID AND ELECTROLYTE BALANCE, as well as a balance of acids and bases, for best function. The most important fluids to keep in balance are the blood volume (plasma volume) and the fluid inside the cells (intracellular fluid). Of these two, the most critical FLUID BALANCE to prevent death is maintaining blood volume at a sufficient level for blood pressure to remain high enough to ensure adequate perfusion and gas exchange of all organs and tissues. Balance of both water and electrolytes is needed for this very vital function.

Because low blood volume and low blood pressure can rapidly lead to death, the body has many specific actions (compensatory mechanisms) that guard against excessive fluid loss from the plasma volume. These actions involve specific hormone levels, kidney function, and blood vessel responses to change how water and sodium are handled to maintain blood pressure.

Because the kidney is a major regulator of water and sodium balance to maintain blood pressure and perfusion to all tissues and organs, the kidneys monitor blood pressure, blood volume, blood oxygen levels, and blood osmolarity (related to sodium concentration). When the kidneys sense that any one of these parameters is getting low, they begin to secrete a substance called *renin* that sets into motion a group of hormonal and blood vessel responses to ensure that blood pressure is raised back up to normal. Fig. 11-6 summarizes these responses.

So, the triggering event is any change in the blood that indicates to the kidney that tissue and organ perfusion are at risk. Low blood pressure is a triggering event because when it gets too low, blood cannot flow through vessels into tissues and organs. Anything that reduces blood volume (e.g., dehydration, hemorrhage) below a critical level *always* lowers blood pressure. Low blood oxygen levels also are triggering events because with too little oxygen in the blood, even if the blood reaches the tissues and organs, it cannot supply the needed oxygen and the tissues and organs could die. A low blood sodium level also is a triggering event because sodium and water are closely linked. Where sodium goes, water follows. So, anything that causes the blood to have too little sodium prevents water from staying in the blood. The result is low blood volume with low blood pressure and poor tissue perfusion.

Once the kidneys sense that tissue and organ perfusion are at risk, special cells in the kidney tubule begin to secrete renin into the blood. Renin then activates some blood proteins, one of which is *angiotensinogen*. Activated angiotensinogen is *angiotensin I*, which is relatively weak and has little action. It is then acted on by another enzyme known as *angiotensin-converting enzyme* or *ACE*, which converts angiotensin I into its most active form, angiotensin II.

Angiotensin II starts several different activities that all work to increase blood volume and blood pressure. First, because angiotensin II is a powerful vasoconstrictor, it causes constriction of small arteries and veins throughout the body. This action increases peripheral resistance and reduces the size of the vascular bed, which raises blood pressure as a compensatory

FIG. 11-6 The role of the renin-angiotensin II pathway in fluid and electrolyte balance and blood pressure regulation.

mechanism without adding more blood volume. At the same time, a second action of angiotensin II is that it constricts the size of the arterioles that feed the kidney nephrons. This action results in a lower glomerular filtration rate and a huge reduction of urine output. Decreasing urine output prevents further loss of water so that more is retained in the blood to help raise blood pressure. The last and slightly slower action of angiotensinogen II is to cause the adrenal glands to secrete the hormone *aldosterone*. Aldosterone is nicknamed the "water-and-sodium-saving hormone" because it causes the kidneys to reabsorb water and sodium, preventing them from being excreted into the urine. This response allows more water and sodium to be returned to the blood, increasing blood pressure and blood volume. All of these actions help maintain perfusion to vital organs.

Clinical Application

The renin-angiotensin II pathway is highly stimulated whenever the patient is in shock or when the stress response occurs. This is why urine output is used as an indicator of perfusion adequacy after surgery or any time the patient has undergone an invasive procedure and is at risk for hemorrhage.

An additional application of this pathway is related to management of *hypertension* (high blood pressure). Patients who have hypertension are often asked to limit their intake of sodium. The reason for this is that a high sodium intake raises the blood level of sodium, causing more water to be retained in the blood volume and raising blood pressure. Drug therapy for hypertension management may include diuretic drugs that increase the excretion of sodium so that less is present in the blood, resulting in a lower blood volume. Another class of drugs often used to manage blood pressure is the "ACE inhibitors." These drugs disrupt the renin-angiotensin II pathway by reducing the amount of angiotensin-converting enzyme (ACE) made so that less angiotensin II is present. With less angiotensin II, there is less vasoconstriction and reduced peripheral resistance, less aldosterone production, and greater excretion of water and sodium in the urine. All of these responses lead to decreased blood volume and blood pressure. Another class of drugs used to manage hypertension is the angiotensin receptor blockers (ARBs). These drugs disrupt the renin-angiotensin II pathway by blocking the receptors that bind with angiotensin II so that the tissues cannot respond to it and blood pressure is lowered.

FLUID IMBALANCES

All patients are at risk for some degree of fluid imbalance because many health problems can disrupt fluid intake or output. Fluid imbalances can occur in any setting.

DEHYDRATION

❖ PATHOPHYSIOLOGY

In **dehydration**, fluid intake or retention is less than what is needed to meet the body's fluid needs, resulting in a Fluid volume deficit, especially a plasma volume deficit. It is a condition rather than a disease and can be caused by many factors (Table 11-3). Dehydration may be an *actual* decrease in total body water caused by either too little intake of fluid or too great a loss of fluid. It also can occur without an actual loss of total body water, such as when water shifts from the plasma into the interstitial space. This condition is called *relative* dehydration.

Dehydration may occur with just water (fluid) loss or with water and electrolyte loss (isotonic dehydration). *Isotonic dehydration is the most common type of fluid loss problem.* Fluid is lost only from the extracellular fluid (ECF) space, including both the plasma and the interstitial spaces. There is no shift of fluids between spaces, so the intracellular fluid (ICF) volume remains normal (Fig. 11-7). Circulating blood volume is decreased (**hypovolemia**) and leads to inadequate tissue perfusion. The body's defenses adapt (compensate) during dehydration to maintain adequate blood flow to vital organs in spite of

---

CONSIDERATIONS FOR OLDER ADULTS
Patient-Centered Care QSEN

Older patients are at high risk for dehydration because they have less total body water than younger adults. In addition, many older adults have decreased thirst sensation and may have difficulty with walking or other motor skills needed for obtaining fluids. They also may take drugs such as diuretics, antihypertensives, and laxatives that increase fluid excretion.

TABLE 11-3	Common Causes of Fluid Imbalances
Dehydration	**Fluid Overload**
• Hemorrhage	• Excessive fluid replacement
• Vomiting	• Kidney failure (late phase)
• Diarrhea	• Heart failure
• Profuse salivation	• Long-term corticosteroid therapy
• Fistulas	• Syndrome of inappropriate
• Ileostomy	antidiuretic hormone (SIADH)
• Profuse diaphoresis	• Psychiatric disorders with
• Burns	polydipsia
• Severe wounds	• Water intoxication
• Long-term NPO status	
• Diuretic therapy	
• GI suction	
• Hyperventilation	
• Diabetes insipidus	
• Difficulty swallowing	
• Impaired thirst	
• Unconsciousness	
• Fever	
• Impaired motor function	

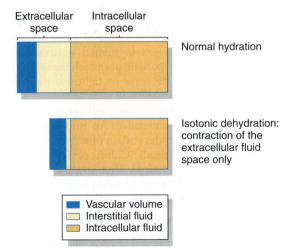

FIG. 11-7 Changes in fluid compartment volumes with dehydration.

hypovolemia. The main defense is increasing vasoconstriction and peripheral resistance to maintain blood pressure and circulation.

Health Promotion and Maintenance

Mild dehydration is very common among healthy adults and is corrected or prevented easily by matching fluid intake with fluid output. Teach all patients to drink more fluids, especially water, whenever they engage in heavy or prolonged physical activity or live in dry climates or at higher altitudes. Beverages with caffeine can increase fluid loss, as can drinks containing alcohol; thus these beverages should not be used to prevent or treat dehydration.

Moderate to severe dehydration is more likely to occur in people who are unable to obtain fluids without help, such as some older adults. Dehydration in older adults in long-term care facilities can be prevented with programs that include routinely offering residents fluids every hour or two during the day and when administering medications.

❖ PATIENT-CENTERED COLLABORATIVE CARE

◆ Assessment

History. The nutrition history can reveal problems that affect FLUID BALANCE. Ask specific questions about food and liquid intake. Also assess the types of fluids and foods ingested to determine amount and osmolarity. Many patients do not know that solid foods contain liquid. Other foods such as ice cream, gelatin, and ices are liquids at body temperature, and these must be included when calculating fluid intake.

Collect specific information about exact intake and output volumes, and obtain serial daily weight measurements. If possible, weigh the patient directly rather than asking what he or she weighs because weight loss is an indication of dehydration. *Because 1 L of water weighs 2.2 pounds (1 kg), changes in daily weights are the best indicators of fluid losses or gains. A weight change of 1 pound corresponds to a fluid volume change of about 500 mL.*

Output includes losses not only as urine but also as sweat, diarrhea, and insensible loss during fevers. Ask specific questions about prescribed and over-the-counter drugs, and check the dosage, the length of time taken, and the patient's adherence with the drug regimen.

Other important areas of the patient history include a sense of thirst or excessive drinking, exposure to hot environments, living at higher altitudes, and the presence of kidney or endocrine diseases. Assess the patient's level of consciousness and mental status, because changes in mental status occur with FLUID imbalance. Ask the patient about changes in ring or shoe tightness. A sudden decrease in tightness may indicate dehydration.

Older adults may use diuretics or laxatives that can lead to FLUID AND ELECTROLYTE imbalance. An important issue for older adults is that they may depend on other people to provide assistance in meeting fluid needs (Collins & Claros, 2011).

Physical Assessment/Clinical Manifestations. Nearly all body systems are affected by dehydration to some degree. The most obvious changes occur in the cardiovascular and integumentary systems.

Cardiovascular changes are good indicators of hydration status because of the relationship between plasma fluid volume and blood pressure. Heart rate increases in an attempt to

maintain blood pressure with less blood volume. Peripheral pulses are weak, difficult to find, and easily blocked with light pressure. The blood pressure also decreases, as does the pulse pressure, with a greater decrease in the systolic blood pressure. Hypotension is more severe with the patient in the standing position than in the sitting or lying position (**orthostatic** or **postural hypotension**). Because the blood pressure with the patient standing may be much lower than in other positions, first measure blood pressure with the patient lying down, then sitting, and finally standing. (These measures are also called "ortho checks" or "ortho changes.") As the blood pressure decreases when changing position, the person may not have sufficient blood flow to the brain, causing the sensations of light-headedness and dizziness. This problem increases the risk for falling, especially among older adults.

Neck veins are normally distended when a patient is in the supine position, and hand veins are distended when lower than the level of the heart. Neck veins normally flatten when the patient moves to a sitting position. With dehydration, neck and hand veins are flat, even when the neck and hands are not raised above the level of the heart.

Respiratory changes include an increased rate because the decreased blood volume reduces perfusion and oxygenation. The increased respiratory rate is a compensatory mechanism that attempts to maintain oxygen delivery when perfusion is decreased.

Skin changes can indicate dehydration. Assess the skin and mucous membranes for color, moisture, and turgor. In older patients, this information is less reliable because of poor skin turgor resulting from the loss of elastic tissue and increased skin dryness from the loss of tissue FLUID with aging. Assess skin turgor by checking:

- How easily the skin over the back of the hand and arm can be gently pinched between the thumb and the forefinger to form a "tent"
- How soon the pinched skin resumes its normal position after release

In dehydration, skin turgor is poor, with the tent remaining for minutes after pinching the skin. The skin is dry and scaly.

CONSIDERATIONS FOR OLDER ADULTS

Patient-Centered Care **QSEN**

Assess skin turgor in an older adult by pinching the skin over the sternum or on the forehead, rather than the back of the hand (Fig. 11-8). With aging, the skin loses elasticity and tents on hands and arms even when the person is well hydrated.

FIG. 11-8 Examining the skin turgor of an older patient.

In dehydration, oral mucous membranes are not moist. They may be covered with a thick, sticky coating and may have cracks and fissures. The surface of the tongue may have deep furrows. This manifestation may not be accurate for assessing dehydration in patients taking drugs that have the side effect of dry mouth.

Neurologic changes with dehydration include changes in mental status and temperature with reduced blood flow in the brain. Confusion is more common among older adults and may be the first indication of a FLUID imbalance. Check to determine whether the patient is alert and oriented. Chapter 41 provides more information about assessment of mental status.

The patient with dehydration often has a low-grade fever, and fever can also cause dehydration. A patient with a temperature higher than 102°F (39°C) for longer than 6 hours is especially at risk because the increased body temperature increases the rate at which FLUID is lost. For every degree (Celsius) increase in body temperature above normal, a minimum of an additional 500 mL of body fluid is lost.

Kidney changes in dehydration affect urine volume and concentration. Monitor urine output, comparing total output with total fluid intake and daily weights. The urine may be concentrated, with a specific gravity greater than 1.030. The color is dark amber and has a strong odor. *Urine output below 500 mL/day for any patient without kidney disease is cause for concern.* Use daily weights to assess fluid loss. Weight loss over a half pound per day is fluid loss.

Laboratory Assessment. No single laboratory test result confirms or rules out dehydration. Instead, dehydration is determined by laboratory findings along with clinical manifestations (see Table 11-1). Usually, laboratory findings with dehydration show elevated levels of hemoglobin, hematocrit, serum osmolarity, glucose, protein, blood urea nitrogen, and various ELECTROLYTES because more water is lost and other substances remain, increasing blood concentration (**hemoconcentration**). Hemoconcentration is not present when dehydration is caused by hemorrhage, because loss of all blood and plasma products occurs together.

◆ **Interventions**

The focus of management for the patient with dehydration is to prevent injury, prevent further fluid loss, and increase fluid volumes to normal. Nursing priorities include patient safety, fluid replacement, and drug therapy.

Patient safety issues and strategies are priorities of care before and during other therapies for dehydration. Monitor vital signs, especially heart rate and blood pressure. The patient with dehydration is at risk for falls because of orthostatic hypotension, dysrhythmia, muscle weakness, and possible confusion. Assess his or her muscle strength, gait stability, and level of alertness. Instruct the patient to get up slowly from a lying or sitting position and to immediately sit down if he or she feels light-headed. Implement the falls precautions listed in Chart 2-4 in Chapter 2.

Fluid replacement is key to correcting dehydration and preventing death from reduced perfusion. Best practices for nursing care of the patient with dehydration are listed in Chart 11-3. Mild to moderate dehydration is corrected with oral fluid replacement if the patient is alert enough to swallow and can tolerate oral fluids. Encourage fluid intake, and measure the amount ingested.

Determine whether the patient has any special fluid needs (e.g., sugar-free fluids, thickened fluids). Provide FLUID the

---

CHART 11-3 Best Practice for Patient Safety & Quality Care (QSEN)

The Patient with Dehydration

- When possible, provide oral fluids that meet the patient's dietary restrictions (e.g., sugar-free, low-sodium, thickened).
- Collaborate with other members of the health care team to determine the amount of fluids needed during a 24-hour period.
- Ensure the fluids are offered and ingested on an even schedule at least every 2 hours throughout 24 hours.
- Teach unlicensed assistive personnel to actively participate in the hydration therapy and not to withhold fluids to prevent incontinence.
- Administer prescribed IV fluids at a rate consistent with hydration needs and any known cardiac, pulmonary, or kidney problems.
- Monitor the patient's response to fluid therapy at least every 2 hours for indicators of adequate rehydration or the need for continuing therapy, especially:
  - Pulse quality
  - Urine output
  - Pulse pressure
  - Weight (every 8 hours)
- Monitor for and report indicators of fluid overload, including:
  - Bounding pulse
  - Difficulty breathing
  - Neck vein distention in the upright position
  - Presence of dependent edema
- Assess the IV and the infusion site at least hourly for indications of infiltration, extravasation, or phlebitis (e.g., swelling around the site, pain, cordlike veins, reduced drip rate).
- Administer drugs prescribed to correct the underlying cause of the dehydration (e.g., antiemetics, antidiarrheals, antibiotics, antipyretics).

---

patient enjoys, and time the intake schedule. Dividing the total amount of fluids needed by nursing shifts helps meet fluid needs more evenly over 24 hours with less danger of overload. Offer the conscious patient small volumes of fluids hourly.

Coordinate with unlicensed assistive personnel (UAP) to meet patients' specific fluid needs. Teach UAP to offer 2 to 4 ounces of fluid every hour to patients who are dehydrated or who are at risk for dehydration. If incontinence is a concern, ensure that UAP understand that withholding fluids is not appropriate to prevent the problem. Instruct them to take the time to stay with patients while they drink the fluid and to note the exact amount ingested. Direct UAP to report any difficulties patients may have in swallowing or managing fluids.

Oral rehydration solutions (ORS) for rehydration therapy are an effective way to replace fluids. Specifically formulated solutions containing glucose and ELECTROLYTES are absorbed even when the patient is vomiting or has diarrhea. These are more often used in the home setting, in long-term care, and for patients who have poor veins, making IV therapy difficult. A variety of commercial ORS are available over the counter.

Drug therapy for dehydration is directed at restoring FLUID BALANCE and controlling the causes of dehydration. Whenever possible, fluid is replaced orally. When dehydration is severe or the patient cannot tolerate oral fluids, IV fluid replacement is needed. Calculation of how much fluid to replace is based on the patient's weight loss and clinical manifestations. The rate of fluid replacement depends on the degree of dehydration and the patient's cardiac, pulmonary, or kidney status.

The type of fluid prescribed varies with the patient's cardiovascular status and the osmolarity of the blood. Table 11-4 lists

TABLE 11-4   **Characteristics of Common Intravenous Therapy Solutions**

SOLUTION	OSMOLARITY (mOsm/L)	pH	CALORIES (KCAL) PER LITER	TONICITY
0.9% saline	308	5	0	Isotonic
0.45% saline	154	5	0	Hypotonic
5% dextrose in water (D_5W)	272	3.5-6.5	170	Isotonic*
10% dextrose in water ($D_{10}W$)	500	3.5-6.5	340	Hypertonic*
5% dextrose in 0.9% saline	560	3.5-6.5	170	Hypertonic*
5% dextrose in 0.45% saline	406	4	170	Hypertonic*
5% dextrose in 0.225% saline	321	4	170	Isotonic*
Ringer's lactate	273	6.5	9	Isotonic
5% dextrose in Ringer's lactate	525	4-6.5	179	Hypertonic*

Data from Trissel, L. (2013). *Handbook on injectable drugs* (17th ed.). Bethesda, MD: American Society of Hospital-System Pharmacists.
*Solution tonicity at the time of administration. Within a short time after administration, the dextrose is metabolized and the tonicity of the infused solution decreases in proportion to the osmolarity or tonicity of the non-dextrose components (electrolytes) within the water.

the composition of common IV fluids. The two most important areas to monitor during rehydration are pulse rate and quality and urine output.

Drug therapy may correct some causes of the dehydration. For example, antidiarrheal drugs are prescribed when diarrhea causes dehydration. Antimicrobial therapy may be used in patients with bacterial diarrhea. Antiemetics may be used when vomiting causes dehydration. Antipyretics to reduce fever are helpful when fever makes dehydration worse.

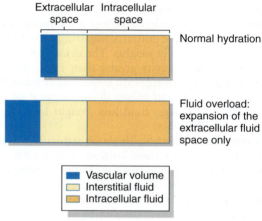

FIG. 11-9 Changes in fluid compartment volumes with fluid overload.

> ### ❓ NCLEX EXAMINATION CHALLENGE
> #### *Safe and Effective Care Environment*
>
> Which assessment finding indicates to the nurse that fluid resuscitation therapy for the client with isotonic dehydration is effective?
> A. Respiratory rate has changed from 16 to 18 breaths/min.
> B. Urine specific gravity has increased from 1.040 to 1.050.
> C. Neck veins are flat when the client moves to a sitting position.
> D. Pulse pressure has changed from 22 mm Hg to 32 mm Hg.

FLUID OVERLOAD

❖ PATHOPHYSIOLOGY

Fluid overload, also called *overhydration,* is an excess of body FLUID. It is not a disease but, rather, a clinical indication of a problem in which fluid intake or retention is greater than the body's fluid needs. The most common type of fluid overload is hypervolemia (Fig. 11-9) because the problems result from excessive fluid in the extracellular fluid (ECF) space. Most problems caused by fluid overload are related to excessive fluid in the vascular space or to dilution of specific electrolytes and blood components. The conditions leading to fluid overload are related to excessive intake or inadequate excretion of fluids. See Table 11-3 for causes of fluid overload. Fig. 11-10 outlines the adaptive changes the body makes in response to mild or moderate fluid overload, especially increased urine output and edema formation. When overload is severe or occurs in a person with poor cardiac or kidney function, it can lead to heart failure and pulmonary edema. Dilution of electrolytes, especially sodium and potassium, can lead to seizures, coma, and death (McGraw, 2012).

❖ PATIENT-CENTERED COLLABORATIVE CARE

◆ Assessment

Patients with fluid overload often have pitting edema (Fig. 11-11). Other manifestations are usually seen in the cardiovascular, respiratory, neuromuscular, integumentary, and GI systems (Chart 11-4).

Fluid overload is diagnosed based on assessment findings and the results of laboratory tests. Usually, serum electrolyte values are normal but decreased hemoglobin, hematocrit, and serum protein levels may result from excessive water in the vascular space (**hemodilution**).

◆ Interventions

The focus of priority nursing interventions for patients with fluid overload is to ensure patient safety, restore normal FLUID BALANCE, provide supportive care until the imbalance is resolved, and prevent future fluid overload. Drug therapy, nutrition therapy, and monitoring are the basis of intervention.

Patient safety is the first priority. Interventions are implemented to prevent fluid overload from becoming worse, leading to pulmonary edema, heart failure, and complications of electrolyte dilution. Any patient with fluid overload, regardless of age, is at risk for these complications. Older adults or those with cardiac problems, kidney problems, pulmonary problems, or liver problems are at greater risk.

FIG. 11-10 Adaptive actions and mechanisms to prevent cardiac and pulmonary complications during fluid overload. (*ADH,* Antidiuretic hormone; *ECF,* extracellular fluid.)

FIG. 11-11 Pitting edema of the left foot and ankle.

Monitor for indicators of increased fluid overload (bounding pulse, increasing neck vein distention, presence of crackles in lungs, increasing peripheral edema, reduced urine output) at least every 2 hours.

! NURSING SAFETY PRIORITY (QSEN)

Critical Rescue

Pulmonary edema can occur very quickly and can lead to death. Notify the health care provider of any change that indicates the fluid overload either is not responding to therapy or is becoming worse.

The patient with fluid overload and edema is at risk for skin breakdown. Use a pressure-reducing or pressure-relieving overlay on the mattress. Assess skin pressure areas daily for signs of redness or open area, especially the coccyx, elbows, hips, and heels. Because many patients with fluid overload may be receiving oxygen by mask or nasal cannula, check the skin integrity around the mask, nares, and ears and under the elastic band. Help the patient change positions every 2 hours, or ensure that unlicensed assistive personnel (UAP) perform this action.

CHART 11-4 Key Features

Fluid Overload

Cardiovascular Changes
- Increased pulse rate
- Bounding pulse quality
- Elevated blood pressure
- Decreased pulse pressure
- Elevated central venous pressure
- Distended neck and hand veins
- Engorged varicose veins
- Weight gain

Respiratory Changes
- Increased respiratory rate
- Shallow respirations
- Shortness of breath
- Moist crackles present on auscultation

Skin and Mucous Membrane Changes
- Pitting edema in dependent areas
- Skin pale and cool to touch

Neuromuscular Changes
- Altered level of consciousness
- Headache
- Visual disturbances
- Skeletal muscle weakness
- Paresthesias

Gastrointestinal Changes
- Increased motility
- Enlarged liver

Drug therapy focuses on removing the excess FLUID. Diuretics are prescribed for fluid overload if kidney failure is not the cause. Prescribed drugs may include high-ceiling (loop) diuretics, such as furosemide (Lasix, Furoside ✦). If there is concern that too much sodium and other ELECTROLYTES would be lost using loop diuretics or if the patient has syndrome of inappropriate antidiuretic hormone (SIADH), conivaptan (Vaprisol) or tolvaptan (Samsca) may be prescribed.

Monitor the patient for response to drug therapy, especially weight loss and increased urine output. Observe for manifestations of electrolyte imbalance, especially changes in electrocardiogram (ECG) patterns. Assess laboratory findings, especially sodium and potassium values, every 8 hours or whenever they are drawn.

Nutrition therapy for the patient with *chronic* fluid overload may involve restrictions of both FLUID and sodium intake. Often sodium restriction involves only "no added salt" to ordinary table foods when fluid overload is mild. For more severe fluid overload, the patient may be restricted to 2 g/day to 4 g/day of sodium. When sodium restriction is ongoing, teach the patient and family how to check food labels for sodium content and how to keep a daily record of sodium ingested. Explain to the patient and family the reason for any fluid restriction and the importance of adhering to the restriction.

Monitoring intake and output and weight provides information on therapy effectiveness. Teach UAP that these measurements need to be accurate, not just estimated, because treatment decisions are based on these findings. Schedule fluid offerings throughout the 24 hours. Teach UAP to check urine for color and character and to report these findings. Check the urine specific gravity (a specific gravity below 1.005 may indicate fluid overload). If the patient is receiving IV therapy, infuse the exact amount prescribed.

Fluid retention may not be visible. Rapid weight gain is the best indicator of fluid retention and overload. Metabolism can account for only a half pound of weight gain in one day. Each pound of weight gained (after the first half pound) equates to about 500 mL of retained FLUID. Weigh the patient at the same time every day (before breakfast), using the same scale. Whenever possible, have the patient wear the same type of clothing for each weigh-in. When in-bed weights are taken, lift tubing and equipment off the bed. Record the number of blankets and pillows on the bed at the initial weigh-in, and ensure ongoing weights always include the same number.

If the patient is discharged to home before the fluid overload has completely resolved or has continuing risk for fluid overload, teach him or her and the family to monitor weight at home. Suggest that a record of these daily weights be kept to show the health care provider at checkups. Patients may choose to use mobile "apps" to record and trend this information. Also, instruct the patient to call his or her health care provider for more than a 3-pound gain in a week or more than a 2-pound gain in 24 hours.

ELECTROLYTE BALANCE AND IMBALANCES

Electrolytes, or **ions**, are substances dissolved in body FLUID that carry an electrical charge. **Cations** have positive charges; **anions** have negative charges. Body fluids are electrically neutral, which means that the number of positive ions is balanced by an equal number of negative ions. However, the

distribution of ions differs in the extracellular fluid (ECF) and the intracellular fluid (ICF) (Fig. 11-12).

Most ELECTROLYTES have different concentrations in the ICF and ECF. This concentration difference helps maintain membrane excitability and allows nerve impulse transmission. The normal ranges of electrolyte concentration are very narrow. So, even small changes in these levels can cause major problems.

Electrolyte imbalances can occur in healthy people as a result of changes in fluid intake and output. These imbalances are usually mild and are easily corrected. Severe electrolyte imbalances with actual losses or retention of specific electrolytes are life threatening and can occur in any setting. People at greatest risk for severe imbalances are older patients, patients with chronic kidney or endocrine disorders, and those who are taking drugs that alter FLUID AND ELECTROLYTE BALANCE. *All ill people are at some risk for electrolyte imbalances.*

Table 11-1 lists the normal serum levels of the major electrolytes. Most ELECTROLYTES enter the body in ingested food. The normal concentration of blood electrolytes changes slightly with the aging process. Chart 11-1 lists the normal electrolyte values for people older than 60 years.

ELECTROLYTE BALANCE occurs by matching the dietary intake of electrolytes with the kidney excretion or reabsorption of

Plasma volume	Interstitial fluid	Intracellular fluid
Volume 3.5-5.5 L	Volume ~10 L	Volume 25-30 L
Osmolarity 270-300 mOsm	Osmolarity 270-300 mOsm	Osmolarity 270-300 mOsm
Sodium 136-145 mEq/L	Sodium 135-145 mEq/L	Sodium 14 mEq/L
Potassium 3.5-5.0 mEq/L	Potassium 3.5-5.0 mEq/L	Potassium 140 mEq/L
Chloride 96-109 mEq/L	Chloride ~118 mEq/L	Chloride ~4-6 mEq/L
Calcium 9.0-10.5 mg/dL	Calcium 7.0-9.0 mg/dL	Calcium 1.0-8.0 mg/dL
Magnesium 1.3-2.1 mEq/L	Magnesium ~1.3 mEq/L	Magnesium 6-30 mEq/L
Protein 7-8 g/L	Protein ~2 g/L	Protein 16 g/L

FIG. 11-12 The electrolyte composition of various body fluids.

electrolytes. For example, the plasma level of potassium is maintained between 3.5 and 5.0 mEq/L (mmol/L). The high potassium level in foods such as meat and citrus fruit could increase the ECF potassium level and lead to major problems. In health, this does not occur because kidney excretion of potassium keeps pace with potassium intake and prevents major changes in the blood potassium level.

CONSIDERATIONS FOR OLDER ADULTS
Patient-Centered Care QSEN

> Older adults are at risk for electrolyte imbalances as a result of age-related organ changes, especially reduced kidney function. They are more likely to be taking drugs that affect fluid or electrolyte balance.

SODIUM

Sodium (Na^+), a mineral, is the major *cation* (positively charged particle) in the extracellular fluid (ECF) and maintains ECF osmolarity. Sodium levels of the ECF are high (136 to 145 mEq/L [mmol/L]), and the intracellular fluid (ICF) sodium levels are low (about 14 mEq/L [mmol/L]). Keeping this difference in sodium levels is vital for skeletal muscle contraction, cardiac contraction, and nerve impulse transmission. Sodium levels and movement influence water balance because "where sodium goes, water follows." The ECF sodium level determines whether water is retained, excreted, or moved from one fluid space to another.

To maintain electrical balance, the sodium (a cation) level within body FLUIDS must be matched by an equal number of anions (negatively charged substances). When this balance is present, the fluid is electrically neutral. Changes in plasma sodium levels seriously change fluid volume and the distribution of other ELECTROLYTES.

Sodium enters the body through the ingestion of many foods and fluids. Foods with the highest sodium levels are those that are processed or preserved, such as smoked or pickled foods, snack foods, and many condiments. Foods lowest in sodium include fresh fish and poultry and most fresh vegetables and fruit.

Despite variation in sodium intake from one day to the next, the blood sodium level usually remains within the normal range. Serum sodium balance is regulated by the kidney under the influences of aldosterone, antidiuretic hormone (ADH), and natriuretic peptide (NP), as described on p. 153.

Low serum sodium levels inhibit the secretion of ADH and NP and trigger aldosterone secretion. Together these compensatory actions increase serum sodium levels by increasing kidney reabsorption of sodium and enhancing kidney loss of water.

High serum sodium levels inhibit aldosterone secretion and directly stimulate secretion of ADH and NP. Together these hormones increase kidney excretion of sodium and kidney reabsorption of water.

HYPONATREMIA
❖ PATHOPHYSIOLOGY

Hyponatremia is an ELECTROLYTE imbalance in which the serum sodium (Na^+) level is below 136 mEq/L (mmol/L). Sodium imbalances often occur with a fluid imbalance because the same hormones regulate both sodium and water balance. The problems caused by hyponatremia occur from two

TABLE 11-5	Common Causes of Hyponatremia

Actual Sodium Deficits
- Excessive diaphoresis
- Diuretics (high-ceiling diuretics)
- Wound drainage (especially gastrointestinal)
- Decreased secretion of aldosterone
- Hyperlipidemia
- Kidney disease (scarred distal convoluted tubule)
- Nothing by mouth
- Low-salt diet
- Cerebral salt-wasting syndrome
- Hyperglycemia

Relative Sodium Deficits (Dilution)
- Excessive ingestion of hypotonic fluids
- Psychogenic polydipsia
- Freshwater submersion accident
- Kidney failure (nephrotic syndrome)
- Irrigation with hypotonic fluids
- Syndrome of inappropriate antidiuretic hormone secretion
- Heart failure

changes—reduced excitable membrane depolarization and cellular swelling.

Excitable cell membrane depolarization depends on high extracellular fluid (ECF) levels of sodium being available to cross cell membranes and move into cells in response to a stimulus. Hyponatremia makes depolarization slower so that excitable membranes are less excitable.

With hyponatremia, the osmolarity of the ECF is lower than that of the intracellular fluid (ICF). As a result, water moves into the cell, causing swelling. Even a small amount of swelling can reduce cell function. Larger amounts of swelling can make the cell burst (*lysis*) and die.

Many conditions and drugs can lead to hyponatremia (Table 11-5). A common cause of low sodium levels is the prolonged use and overuse of diuretics, especially in older adults. When these drugs are used to manage FLUID overload, sodium is lost along with the extra water. Hyponatremia can result from the loss of total body sodium, the movement of sodium from the blood to other fluid spaces, or the dilution of serum sodium from excessive water in the plasma.

❖ PATIENT-CENTERED COLLABORATIVE CARE
◆ Assessment

The manifestations of hyponatremia are caused by its effects on excitable cellular activity. The cells especially affected are those involved in cerebral, neuromuscular, intestinal smooth muscle, and cardiovascular functions.

Cerebral changes are the most obvious problems of hyponatremia. Behavioral changes result from cerebral edema and increased intracranial pressure. Closely observe and document the patient's behavior, level of consciousness, and mental status. A sudden onset of acute confusion or increased confusion is often seen in older adults who have low serum sodium levels. When sodium levels become very low, seizures, coma, and death may occur (McGraw, 2012).

Neuromuscular changes are seen as general muscle weakness. Assess the patient's neuromuscular status during each nursing shift for changes from baseline. Deep tendon reflexes diminish, and muscle weakness is worse in the legs and arms. Test arm muscle strength by having the patient squeeze your hand.

Another way to test arm muscle strength is to have the patient flex his or her arms against the chest and keep them flexed while you attempt to pull them away from the chest. Test leg muscle strength by having the patient push both feet against a flat surface (like a box or a board) while you apply resistance to the opposite side of the flat surface.

> **⚠ NURSING SAFETY PRIORITY** (QSEN)
> **Action Alert**
>
> If muscle weakness is present, immediately check respiratory effectiveness because ventilation depends on adequate strength of respiratory muscles.

Intestinal changes include increased motility, causing nausea, diarrhea, and abdominal cramping. Assess the GI system by listening to bowel sounds and observing stools. Bowel sounds are hyperactive, with rushes and gurgles over the splenic flexure and in the lower left quadrant. Bowel movements are frequent and watery.

Cardiovascular changes are seen as changes in cardiac output. The cardiac responses to hyponatremia with **hypovolemia** (decreased plasma volume) include a rapid, weak, thready pulse. Peripheral pulses are difficult to palpate and are easily blocked with light pressure. Blood pressure is decreased, and the patient may have severe orthostatic hypotension, leading to light-headedness or dizziness. The central venous pressure is low. When hyponatremia occurs with **hypervolemia** (FLUID overload), cardiac changes include a full or bounding pulse with normal or high blood pressure. Peripheral pulses are full and difficult to block; however, they may not be palpable if edema is present.

◆ **Interventions**

The specific cause of the low sodium level is determined to plan the most appropriate management. Interventions with drug therapy and nutrition therapy are used to restore serum sodium levels to normal and prevent complications from FLUID overload or a too-rapid change in serum sodium level. *The priorities for nursing care of the patient with hyponatremia are monitoring the patient's response to therapy and preventing hypernatremia and fluid overload.*

Drug therapy involves reducing the doses of any drugs that increase sodium loss, such as most diuretics. Other regimens vary depending on whether a FLUID imbalance occurs with hyponatremia. When hyponatremia occurs with a fluid deficit, IV saline infusions are prescribed to restore both sodium and fluid volume. Severe hyponatremia may be treated with small-volume infusions of hypertonic saline, most often 3% saline (Schreiber, 2013b) although 5% saline can be used for extreme hyponatremia. These infusions are delivered using a controller to prevent accidental increases in infusion rate. Monitor the infusion rate and the patient's response.

When hyponatremia occurs with FLUID excess, drug therapy includes giving drugs that promote the excretion of water rather than sodium, such as conivaptan (Vaprisol) or tolvaptan (Samsca). Drug therapy for hyponatremia caused by inappropriate secretion of antidiuretic hormone (ADH) may include lithium and demeclocycline (Declomycin). Assess hourly for signs of excessive fluid loss, potassium loss, and increased sodium levels.

Nutrition therapy can help restore sodium balance in mild hyponatremia. Collaborate with the registered dietitian (RD) to teach the patient about which foods to increase in the diet. Therapy involves increasing oral sodium intake and restricting oral fluid intake. Fluid restriction may be needed long-term when FLUID overload is the cause of the hyponatremia or when kidney fluid excretion is impaired. Nursing actions for patient safety, skin protection, monitoring, and patient and family teaching are the same as those for fluid overload on pp. 161-162.

HYPERNATREMIA

❖ *PATHOPHYSIOLOGY*

Hypernatremia is an ELECTROLYTE imbalance in which the serum sodium level is over 145 mEq/L (mmol/L). It can be caused by or can cause changes in FLUID volume. Table 11-6 lists causes of hypernatremia.

As serum sodium level rises, a larger difference in sodium levels occurs between the extracellular fluid (ECF) and the intracellular fluid (ICF). More sodium is present to move rapidly across cell membranes during depolarization, making excitable tissues more easily excited. This condition is called **irritability,** and excitable tissues over-respond to stimuli. In addition, water moves from the cells into the ECF to dilute the hyperosmolar ECF. So, when serum sodium levels are high, severe cellular dehydration with cellular shrinkage occurs. Eventually the dehydrated excitable tissues may no longer be able to respond to stimuli.

❖ *PATIENT-CENTERED COLLABORATIVE CARE*

◆ *Assessment*

The manifestations of hypernatremia vary with the severity of sodium imbalance and whether a FLUID imbalance is also present. Changes are first seen in excitable membrane activity, especially nerve, skeletal muscle, and cardiac function.

Nervous system changes start with altered cerebral function. Assess the patient's mental status for attention span and cognitive function. In hypernatremia with normal or decreased FLUID volumes, the patient may have a short attention span and be agitated or confused. When hypernatremia occurs with fluid overload, the patient may be lethargic, drowsy, stuporous, and even comatose.

Skeletal muscle changes vary with the degree of sodium increases. Mild rises cause muscle twitching and irregular muscle contractions. As hypernatremia worsens, the muscles and nerves are less able to respond to a stimulus and muscles become progressively weaker. Late, the deep tendon reflexes are reduced or absent. Muscle weakness occurs bilaterally and has

TABLE 11-6 **Common Causes of Hypernatremia**	
Actual Sodium Excesses	**Relative Sodium Excesses**
• Hyperaldosteronism	• Nothing by mouth
• Kidney failure	• Increased rate of metabolism
• Corticosteroids	• Fever
• Cushing's syndrome or disease	• Hyperventilation
• Excessive oral sodium ingestion	• Infection
• Excessive administration of sodium-containing IV fluids	• Excessive diaphoresis
	• Watery diarrhea
	• Dehydration

no specific pattern. Observe for twitching in muscle groups. Assess muscle strength by having the patient perform handgrip and arm flexion against resistance as described on pp. 161-162. Assess deep tendon reflexes by lightly tapping the patellar (knee) tendons and Achilles (heel) tendons with a reflex hammer and measuring the movement.

Cardiovascular changes include decreased contractility because high sodium levels slow the movement of calcium into the heart cells. Measure blood pressure and the rate and quality of the apical and peripheral pulses. Pulse rate and blood pressure may be normal, above normal, or below normal, depending on the FLUID volume and how rapidly the imbalance occurred.

Pulse rate is increased in patients with hypernatremia and hypovolemia. Peripheral pulses are difficult to palpate and are easily blocked. Hypotension and severe orthostatic (postural) hypotension are present, and pulse pressure is reduced.

Patients with hypernatremia and hypervolemia have slow to normal bounding pulses. Peripheral pulses are full and difficult to block. Neck veins are distended, even with the patient in the upright position. Blood pressure, especially diastolic blood pressure, is increased.

◆ *Interventions*

Drug and nutrition therapies are used to prevent further sodium increases and to decrease high serum sodium levels. Interventions used when sodium levels become life threatening include hemodialysis. *Priorities for nursing care of the patient with hypernatremia include monitoring his or her response to therapy and ensuring patient safety by preventing hyponatremia and dehydration.*

Drug therapy is used to restore FLUID balance when hypernatremia is caused by fluid loss. Isotonic saline (0.9%) and dextrose 5% in 0.45% sodium chloride are most often prescribed (Schreiber, 2013a). Although the dextrose 5% in 0.45% sodium chloride is hypertonic in the IV bag, once it is infused, the glucose is rapidly metabolized and the fluid is really hypotonic. Hypernatremia caused by poor kidney excretion of sodium requires drug therapy with diuretics that promote sodium loss, such as furosemide (Lasix, Furoside✦) or bumetanide (Bumex). Assess the patient hourly for symptoms of excessive losses of fluid, sodium, or potassium.

Nutrition therapy to prevent or correct mild hypernatremia involves ensuring adequate water intake, especially among older adults. Dietary sodium restriction may be needed to prevent sodium excess when kidney problems are present. Collaborate with the dietitian to teach the patient how to determine the sodium content of foods, beverages, and drugs. Nursing actions for patient safety, skin protection, monitoring, and patient and family teaching are similar to those for fluid overload on pp. 158-160.

? NCLEX EXAMINATION CHALLENGE

Physiological Integrity

Which condition or manifestation in the client with a serum sodium level of 149 mEq/L indicates to the nurse that this electrolyte imbalance may be caused by excessive fluid loss?
A. The client has twitching muscle contractions in the lower extremities.
B. The client's skin is cool and clammy.
C. The urine specific gravity is increased.
D. The hematocrit is 52%.

POTASSIUM

Potassium (K^+) is the major cation of the intracellular fluid (ICF). The normal plasma potassium level ranges from 3.5 to 5.0 mEq/L (mmol/L) (see Table 11-1). The normal ICF potassium level is about 140 mEq/L (mmol/L). Because of its high levels inside cells, potassium has some control over intracellular osmolarity and volume. Keeping this large difference in potassium concentration between the ICF and the extracellular fluid (ECF) is critical for excitable tissues to depolarize and generate action potentials.

Because potassium levels in the blood and interstitial fluid are so low, any change seriously affects physiologic activities. For example, a decrease in blood potassium of only 1 mEq/L (from 4 mEq/L to 3 mEq/L) is a 25% difference in total ECF potassium concentration. In contrast, a 1 mEq/L decrease in blood sodium level (from 130 mEq/L to 129 mEq/L) is, overall, a much smaller change (less than 1%) in total ECF sodium concentration.

Almost all foods contain potassium. It is highest in meat, fish, and many (but not all) vegetables and fruits. It is lowest in eggs, bread, and cereal grains. Typical potassium intake is about 2 to 20 g/day. Despite heavy potassium intake, the healthy adult keeps plasma potassium levels within the narrow range of normal values.

The main controller of ECF potassium level is the sodium-potassium pump within the membranes of all body cells. This pump moves extra sodium ions from the ICF and moves extra potassium ions from the ECF back into the cell. In this way, the serum potassium level remains low and the cellular potassium remains high. At the same time, this action also helps the serum sodium level remain high and the cellular sodium level remain low.

About 80% of potassium is removed from the body by the kidney. Kidney excretion of potassium is enhanced by aldosterone.

HYPOKALEMIA

❖ *PATHOPHYSIOLOGY*

Because 98% of total body potassium (K^+) is inside cells, minor changes in extracellular potassium levels cause major changes in cell membrane excitability. Hypokalemia is an ELECTROLYTE imbalance in which the serum potassium level is below 3.5 mEq/L (mmol/L). *It can be life threatening because every body system is affected.*

Low serum potassium levels increase the difference in the amount of potassium between the fluid inside the cells (ICF) and the fluid outside the cells (ECF). This increased difference reduces the excitability of cells. As a result, the cell membranes of all excitable tissues, such as nerve and muscle, are less responsive to normal stimuli. Gradual potassium loss may have no manifestations until the loss is extreme. Rapid reduction of serum potassium levels causes dramatic changes in function. Table 11-7 lists causes of hypokalemia.

Actual potassium depletion occurs when potassium loss is excessive or when potassium intake is not adequate to match normal potassium loss. Relative hypokalemia occurs when total body potassium levels are normal but the potassium distribution between fluid spaces is abnormal or it is diluted by excess water.

TABLE 11-7   Common Causes of Hypokalemia

Actual Potassium Deficits

- Inappropriate or excessive use of drugs:
  - Diuretics
  - Digitalis
  - Corticosteroids
- Increased secretion of aldosterone
- Cushing's syndrome
- Diarrhea
- Vomiting
- Wound drainage (especially gastrointestinal)
- Prolonged nasogastric suction
- Heat-induced excessive diaphoresis
- Kidney disease impairing reabsorption of potassium
- Nothing by mouth

Relative Potassium Deficits

- Alkalosis
- Hyperinsulinism
- Hyperalimentation
- Total parenteral nutrition
- Water intoxication
- IV therapy with potassium-poor solutions

❖ **PATIENT-CENTERED COLLABORATIVE CARE**

◆ **Assessment**

Age is important because urine concentrating ability decreases with aging, which increases potassium loss. Older adults are more likely to use drugs that lead to potassium loss.

Drugs, especially diuretics, corticosteroids, and beta-adrenergic agonists or antagonists, can increase potassium loss through the kidneys. Ask about prescription and over-the-counter drug use. In patients taking digoxin (Lanoxin, Novo-Digoxin ✦), hypokalemia increases the sensitivity of the cardiac muscle to the drug and may result in digoxin toxicity, even when the digoxin level is within the therapeutic range. Ask whether the patient takes a potassium supplement, such as potassium chloride (KCl), or eats foods that have high concentrations of potassium, such as bananas, citrus juices, raisins, and meat. The patient may not be taking the supplement as prescribed because of its unpleasant taste.

Disease can lead to potassium loss. Ask about chronic disorders, recent illnesses, and medical or surgical interventions. A thorough nutrition history, including a typical day's food and beverage intake, helps identify patients at risk for hypokalemia.

Respiratory changes occur because of respiratory muscle weakness resulting in shallow respirations. *Thus respiratory status should be assessed first in any patient who might have hypokalemia.* Assess the patient's breath sounds, ease of respiratory effort, color of nail beds and mucous membranes, and rate and depth of respiration.

!   **NURSING SAFETY PRIORITY**   (QSEN)

Action Alert

Assess the respiratory status of a patient who has hypokalemia at least every 2 hours because respiratory insufficiency is a major cause of death for these patients.

Musculoskeletal changes include skeletal muscle weakness. A stronger stimulus is needed to begin muscle contraction. A patient may be too weak to stand. Hand grasps are weak, and deep tendon reflexes may be reduced (hyporeflexia). Severe hypokalemia causes flaccid paralysis. Assess for muscle weakness and the patient's ability to perform ADLs.

Cardiovascular changes are assessed by palpating the peripheral pulses. In hypokalemia, the pulse is usually thready and weak. Palpation is difficult, and the pulse is easily blocked with light pressure. The pulse rate can range from very slow to very rapid, and an irregular heartbeat (dysrhythmia) may be present. Measure blood pressure with the patient in the lying, sitting, and standing positions, because orthostatic (postural) hypotension occurs with hypokalemia.

Neurologic changes from hypokalemia include altered mental status. The patient may have short-term irritability and anxiety followed by lethargy that progresses to acute confusion and coma as hypokalemia worsens.

Behavioral changes caused by hypokalemia can occur quickly. The patient may be lethargic and unable to perform simple problem-solving tasks such as counting by threes. As hypokalemia progresses, confusion increases and coma may develop.

Intestinal changes occur with hypokalemia because GI smooth muscle contractions are decreased, which leads to decreased peristalsis. Bowel sounds are hypoactive, and nausea, vomiting, constipation, and abdominal distention are common. Measure abdominal girth, and auscultate for bowel sounds in all four abdominal quadrants. *Severe hypokalemia can cause the absence of peristalsis (paralytic ileus).*

Laboratory data confirm hypokalemia (serum potassium value below 3.5 mEq/L [mmol/L]). Hypokalemia causes ECG changes in the heart, including ST-segment depression, flat or inverted T waves, and increased U waves. *Dysrhythmias can lead to death, particularly in older adults who are taking digoxin.*

◆ **Interventions**

Interventions for hypokalemia focus on preventing potassium loss, increasing serum potassium levels, and ensuring patient safety. Drug and nutrition therapies help restore normal serum potassium levels. *The priorities for nursing care of the patient with hypokalemia are (1) ensuring adequate oxygenation, patient safety for falls prevention, and prevention of injury from potassium administration and (2) monitoring the patient's response to therapy.* Chart 11-5 highlights best practice activities when caring for a patient with hypokalemia.

Drug therapy for management and prevention of hypokalemia includes additional potassium and drugs to prevent potassium loss (Scotto et al., 2014). Most potassium supplements are potassium chloride, potassium gluconate, or potassium citrate. The amount and the route of potassium replacement depend on the degree of loss.

Potassium is given IV for severe hypokalemia. The drug is available in different concentrations, and this drug carries a high alert warning as a concentrated electrolyte solution. The Joint Commission's National Patient Safety Goals has mandated that concentrated potassium be diluted and added to IV solutions only in the pharmacy by a registered pharmacist and that vials of concentrated potassium not be available in patient care areas. *Before infusing any IV solution containing potassium chloride (KCl), check and recheck the dilution of the drug in the IV solution container.*

NURSING SAFETY PRIORITY QSEN

CHART 11-5 Best Practice for Patient Safety & Quality Care QSEN

The Patient with Hypokalemia

- Question the continued use of drugs that increase excretion of potassium (e.g., thiazide and loop diuretics).
- Administer prescribed oral potassium supplement, well diluted and with a meal or just after a meal or snack to prevent nausea and vomiting.
- Prevent accidental overdose of IV potassium by checking and re-checking the concentration of potassium in the IV solution, ensuring that the maximum concentration is no greater than 1 mEq/10 mL of solution.
- Establish an IV access in a large vein with a high volume of flow, avoiding the hand.
- Assess the IV access for placement and an adequate blood return *before* administering potassium-containing solutions.
- Use a controller for solution delivery, maintaining an infusion rate not faster than 5 to 10 mEq of potassium per hour.
- Assess the IV site hourly.
- Stop the infusion immediately if the patient reports pain or burning or if any manifestation of infiltration occurs.
- If possible, monitor electrocardiography (ECG) continuously.
- Monitor patient responses every 1 to 2 hours to determine therapy effectiveness and the potential for hyperkalemia.
  - Indications of therapy effectiveness:
    - Respiratory rate is greater than 12 breaths per minute
    - Oxygen saturation is at least 95% (or has returned to the patient's normal baseline)
    - The patient can cough effectively
    - Hand grasp strength increases
    - Deep tendon reflexes are present
    - Bowel sounds are present and active
    - Pulse is easily palpated and regular
    - Systolic blood pressure when standing remains within 20 mm Hg of the systolic pressure obtained when the patient is sitting or lying down
    - ST segment returns to the isoelectric line
    - T waves increase in size and are positive
    - U waves decrease or disappear
    - Patient's cognition resembles his or her prehypokalemic state
    - Serum potassium level is between 3.5 and 5.0 mEq/L
  - Indications of hyperkalemia:
    - Heart rate is less than 60 beats per minute
    - P waves are absent
    - T waves are tall
    - PR intervals are prolonged
    - QRS complexes are wide
    - Deep tendon reflexes are hyperactive
    - Bowel sounds are hyperactive
    - Numbness or tingling is present in the hands and feet and around the mouth
    - The patient is anxious
    - Serum potassium level is above 5.0 mEq/L
- Keep patient on bedrest until hypokalemia resolves, or provide assistance when out of bed to prevent falls.

NURSING SAFETY PRIORITY QSEN

Drug Alert

A dilution no greater than 1 mEq of potassium to 10 mL of solution is recommended for IV administration. The maximum recommended infusion rate is 5 to 10 mEq/hr; this rate is never to exceed 20 mEq/hr under any circumstances. In accordance with National Patient Safety Goals (NPSGs), potassium is not given by IV push to avoid causing cardiac arrest.

Potassium is a severe tissue irritant and is never given by IM or subcutaneous injection. Tissues damaged by potassium can become necrotic, causing loss of function and requiring surgery. IV potassium solutions irritate veins and cause phlebitis. Check the prescription carefully to ensure that the patient receives the correct amount of potassium. Assess the IV site hourly, and ask the patient whether he or she feels burning or pain at the site.

NURSING SAFETY PRIORITY QSEN

Action Alert

If infiltration of solution containing potassium occurs, stop the IV solution immediately, remove the venous access, and notify the health care provider or Rapid Response Team. Document these actions along with a complete description of the IV site.

Oral potassium preparations may be taken as liquids or solids. Potassium has a strong, unpleasant taste that is difficult to mask, although it can be mixed with many liquids. Because potassium chloride can cause nausea and vomiting, give the drug during or after a meal and advise patients using the drug at home not to take it on an empty stomach.

Diuretics that increase the kidney excretion of potassium can cause hypokalemia, especially high-ceiling (loop) diuretics (e.g., furosemide [Lasix, Furoside ✦] and bumetanide [Bumex]) and the thiazide diuretics. These drugs are avoided in patients with hypokalemia. A potassium-sparing diuretic may be prescribed to increase urine output without increasing potassium loss. Potassium-sparing diuretics include spironolactone (Aldactone, Novospiron ✦), triamterene (Dyrenium), and amiloride (Midamor).

Nutrition therapy involves collaboration with a dietitian to teach the patient how to increase dietary potassium intake. Eating foods that are naturally rich in potassium helps prevent further loss, but supplementation is needed to restore normal potassium levels.

Implement safety measures with a patient who has muscle weakness from hypokalemia, including the falls precautions listed in Chart 2-4 in Chapter 2. Be sure to have the patient wear a gait belt when ambulating with assistance.

Respiratory monitoring is performed at least hourly for severe hypokalemia, especially checking for increasing rate and decreasing depth. Also check oxygen saturation by pulse oximetry to determine breathing effectiveness. Assess respiratory muscle effectiveness by checking the patient's ability to cough. Examine the face, oral mucosa, and nail beds for pallor or cyanosis. Evaluate arterial blood gas values (when available) for decreased blood oxygen levels (**hypoxemia**) and increased arterial carbon dioxide levels (**hypercapnia**), which indicate inadequate breathing effectiveness.

NCLEX EXAMINATION CHALLENGE

Physiological Integrity

Which question is most important for the nurse to ask the client who has a serum potassium level of 2.9 mEq/L?
A. "Do you use sugar substitutes?"
B. "Do you use diuretics or laxatives?"
C. "Have you had any muscle twitches or cramps, especially at night?
D. "Have you or any member of your family ever been diagnosed with lung disease?"

HYPERKALEMIA

❖ PATHOPHYSIOLOGY

Hyperkalemia is an ELECTROLYTE imbalance in which the serum potassium level is higher than 5.0 mEq/L (mmol/L). Even small increases above normal values can affect excitable tissues, especially the heart.

A high serum potassium increases cell excitability; as a result, most excitable tissues respond to less intense stimuli and may even discharge spontaneously. The heart is very sensitive to serum potassium increases, and hyperkalemia interferes with electrical conduction, leading to heart block and ventricular fibrillation.

The problems that occur with hyperkalemia are related to how rapidly ECF potassium levels increase. Sudden potassium rises cause severe problems at serum levels between 6 and 7 mEq/L. When serum potassium rises slowly, problems may not occur until potassium levels reach 8 mEq/L or higher.

Hyperkalemia is rare in people with normal kidney function. Most cases of hyperkalemia occur in hospitalized patients and in those undergoing medical treatment. Those at greatest risk are chronically ill patients, debilitated patients, and older adults (Table 11-8).

❖ PATIENT-CENTERED COLLABORATIVE CARE

◆ Assessment

Age is important because kidney function decreases with aging. Ask about kidney disease, diabetes mellitus, recent medical or surgical treatment, and urine output, including frequency and amount of voidings. Ask about drug use, particularly potassium-sparing diuretics and angiotensin-converting enzyme (ACE) inhibitors. Obtain a nutrition history to determine the intake of potassium-rich foods and the use of salt substitutes (which contain potassium).

Collect specific information about manifestations related to hyperkalemia. Ask whether the patient has had palpitations, skipped heartbeats, other cardiac irregularities, muscle twitching, leg weakness, or unusual tingling or numbness in the hands, feet, or face. Ask about recent changes in bowel habits, especially diarrhea.

Cardiovascular changes are the most severe problems from hyperkalemia and are the most common cause of death in patients

---

TABLE 11-8 Common Causes of Hyperkalemia

Actual Potassium Excesses
- Overingestion of potassium-containing foods or medications:
  - Salt substitutes
  - Potassium chloride
  - Rapid infusion of potassium-containing IV solution
  - Bolus IV potassium injections
- Transfusions of whole blood or packed cells
- Adrenal insufficiency
- Kidney failure
- Potassium-sparing diuretics
- Angiotensin-converting enzyme inhibitors (ACEIs)

Relative Potassium Excesses
- Tissue damage
- Acidosis
- Hyperuricemia
- Uncontrolled diabetes mellitus

---

with hyperkalemia. Cardiac manifestations include bradycardia, hypotension, and ECG changes of tall, peaked T waves, prolonged PR intervals, flat or absent P waves, and wide QRS complexes. As serum potassium levels rise, ectopic beats may appear. Complete heart block, asystole, and ventricular fibrillation are life-threatening complications of severe hyperkalemia.

Neuromuscular changes with hyperkalemia have two phases. Skeletal muscles twitch in the early stages of hyperkalemia, and the patient may be aware of tingling and burning sensations followed by numbness in the hands and feet and around the mouth (**paresthesia**). As hyperkalemia worsens, muscle weakness occurs followed by flaccid paralysis. The weakness moves up from the hands and feet and first affects the muscles of the arms and legs. Respiratory muscles are not affected until serum potassium levels reach lethal levels.

Intestinal changes include increased motility with diarrhea and hyperactive bowel sounds. Bowel movements are frequent and watery.

Laboratory data confirm hyperkalemia (potassium level over 5.0 mEq/L). If it is caused by dehydration, levels of other ELECTROLYTES, hematocrit, and hemoglobin also are elevated. Hyperkalemia caused by kidney failure occurs with elevated serum creatinine and blood urea nitrogen, decreased blood pH, and normal or low hematocrit and hemoglobin levels.

◆ Interventions

Interventions for hyperkalemia focus on reducing the serum potassium level, preventing recurrences, and ensuring patient safety. Drug therapy is key. *The priorities for nursing care of the patient with hyperkalemia are assessing for cardiac complications, patient safety for falls prevention, monitoring the patient's response to therapy, and health teaching.*

Drug therapy can restore normal potassium balance by enhancing potassium excretion and promoting the movement of potassium from the extracellular fluid (ECF) into the cells.

Stop potassium-containing infusions, and keep the IV access open. Withhold oral potassium supplements, and provide a potassium-restricted diet.

Increasing potassium excretion helps reduce hyperkalemia if kidney function is normal. Potassium-excreting diuretics, such as furosemide, are prescribed. When kidney problems exist, drug therapy to increase potassium excretion includes cation exchange resins that promote intestinal sodium absorption and potassium excretion, such as sodium polystyrene sulfonate (Kayexalate). However, this therapy may take hours to reduce potassium levels. If potassium levels are dangerously high, additional measures, such as dialysis, are needed.

Movement of potassium from the extracellular fluid (ECF) to the intracellular fluid (ICF) can help reduce serum potassium levels temporarily. Potassium movement into the cells is enhanced by insulin. Insulin increases the activity of the sodium-potassium pumps, which move potassium from the ECF into the cell. IV fluids containing glucose and insulin are prescribed to help decrease serum potassium levels (usually 100 mL of 10% to 20% glucose with 10 to 20 units of regular insulin) (Cottrell, 2012). These IV solutions are hypertonic and are infused through a central line or in a vein with a high blood flow to avoid local vein inflammation. Observe the patient for manifestations of hypokalemia and hypoglycemia during this therapy.

CHART 11-6 Patient and Family Education: Preparing for Self-Management

Nutritional Management of Hyperkalemia

You Should Avoid	You May Eat
• Meats, especially organ meat and preserved meat	• Eggs
• Dairy products	• Breads
• Dried fruit	• Butter
• Fruits high in potassium:	• Cereals
■ Bananas	• Sugar
■ Cantaloupe	• Fruits low in potassium (fresh, frozen, or canned):
■ Kiwi	■ Apples
■ Oranges	■ Apricots
• Vegetables high in potassium:	■ Berries
■ Avocados	■ Cherries
■ Broccoli	■ Cranberries
■ Dried beans or peas	■ Grapefruit
■ Lima beans	■ Peaches
■ Mushrooms	■ Pineapple
■ Potatoes (white or sweet)	• Vegetables low in potassium:
■ Seaweed	■ Alfalfa sprouts
■ Soybeans	■ Cabbage
■ Spinach	■ Carrots
	■ Cauliflower
	■ Celery
	■ Eggplant
	■ Green beans
	■ Lettuce
	■ Onions
	■ Peas
	■ Peppers
	■ Squash

Data from Pennington, J.A., & Spungen, J.S. (2010). *Bowes and Church's food values of portions commonly used* (19th ed.). Philadelphia: Lippincott Williams & Wilkins.

Cardiac monitoring allows for the early recognition of dysrhythmias and other manifestations of hyperkalemia on cardiac muscle. Compare recent ECG tracings with the tracings obtained when the patient's serum potassium level was close to normal.

! NURSING SAFETY PRIORITY (QSEN)

Critical Rescue

Notify the health care provider or Rapid Response Team if the patient's heart rate falls below 60 beats per minute or if the T waves become spiked, both of which accompany hyperkalemia.

Health teaching is key to the prevention of hyperkalemia and the early detection of complications. The teaching plan includes diet, drugs, and recognition of the manifestations of hyperkalemia. Collaborate with the dietitian to teach the patient and family about which foods to avoid (those high in potassium). Foods that are low in potassium are listed in Chart 11-6. Instruct the patient and family to read the labels on drug and food packages to determine the potassium content. Warn them to avoid salt substitutes, which contain potassium.

CALCIUM

Calcium (Ca^{2+}) is a mineral with functions closely related to those of phosphorus and magnesium. It is an ion having two positive charges *(divalent cation)* that exists in the body in a bound form and an ionized (unbound or free) form.

Bound calcium is usually attached to serum proteins, especially albumin. Ionized calcium is present in the blood and other extracellular fluid (ECF) as free calcium. Free calcium is the active form and must be kept within a narrow range in the ECF. The body functions best when blood calcium levels are maintained between 9.0 and 10.5 mg/dL, or between 2.25 and 2.62 mmol/L (see Table 11-1). Calcium has a steep gradient between ECF and intracellular fluid (ICF) because the amount of calcium in the ICF is very low. This mineral is important for maintaining bone strength and density, activating enzymes, allowing skeletal and cardiac muscle contraction, controlling nerve impulse transmission, and allowing blood clotting.

Calcium enters the body by dietary intake and absorption through the intestinal tract. Dairy products are common foods high in calcium. Absorption of dietary calcium requires the active form of vitamin D. Calcium is stored in the bones. When more calcium is needed, parathyroid hormone (PTH) is released from the parathyroid glands. PTH increases serum calcium levels by:

- Releasing free calcium from bone storage sites (bone *resorption* of calcium)
- Stimulating vitamin D activation to help increase intestinal *absorption* of dietary calcium
- Inhibiting kidney calcium excretion
- Stimulating kidney calcium *reabsorption*

When excess calcium is present in plasma, PTH secretion is inhibited and the secretion of *thyrocalcitonin (TCT)*, a hormone secreted by the thyroid gland, is increased. TCT causes the plasma calcium level to decrease by inhibiting bone resorption of calcium, inhibiting vitamin D–associated intestinal uptake of calcium, and increasing kidney excretion of calcium in the urine.

HYPOCALCEMIA

❖ PATHOPHYSIOLOGY

Hypocalcemia is an ELECTROLYTE imbalance in which a total serum calcium (Ca^{2+}) level is below 9.0 mg/dL or 2.25 mmol/L. Calcium is stored in bone, with only a small amount of total body calcium present in extracellular fluid (ECF). Because the normal blood level of calcium is so low, any change in calcium levels has major effects on function.

Calcium is an excitable membrane stabilizer, regulating depolarization and the generation of action potentials. It decreases sodium movement across excitable membranes, slowing the rate of depolarization. Low serum calcium levels increase sodium movement across excitable membranes, allowing depolarization to occur more easily and at inappropriate times.

Hypocalcemia is caused by many chronic and acute conditions, as well as medical or surgical treatments. Table 11-9 lists causes of hypocalcemia. Acute hypocalcemia results in the rapid onset of life-threatening manifestations. Chronic hypocalcemia occurs slowly over time, and excitable membrane manifestations may not be severe because the body has adjusted to the gradual reduction of serum calcium levels.

Actual calcium loss (a reduction in total body calcium) occurs when the absorption of calcium from the GI tract slows or when calcium is lost from the body. Relative calcium loss causes total body calcium amounts to remain normal while serum calcium levels are low. This problem occurs when the

TABLE 11-9 Common Causes of Hypocalcemia

Actual Calcium Deficits

- Inadequate oral intake of calcium
- Lactose intolerance
- Malabsorption syndromes:
  - Celiac sprue
  - Crohn's disease
- Inadequate intake of vitamin D
- End-stage kidney disease
- Diarrhea
- Steatorrhea
- Wound drainage (especially gastrointestinal)

Relative Calcium Deficits

- Hyperproteinemia
- Alkalosis
- Calcium chelators or binders
  - Citrate
  - Mithramycin
  - Penicillamine
  - Sodium cellulose phosphate (Calcibind)
  - Aredia
- Acute pancreatitis
- Hyperphosphatemia
- Immobility
- Removal or destruction of parathyroid glands

GENDER HEALTH CONSIDERATIONS
Patient-Centered Care QSEN

Postmenopausal women are at risk for chronic calcium loss. This problem is related to reduced weight-bearing activities and a decrease in estrogen levels. As they age, many women decrease weight-bearing activities such as running and walking, which allows osteoporosis to occur at a more rapid rate. Also, the estrogen secretion that protects against osteoporosis diminishes. (See Chapter 50 for a complete discussion of osteoporosis.)

FIG. 11-13 Palmar flexion indicating a positive Trousseau's sign in hypocalcemia.

FIG. 11-14 Facial muscle response indicating a positive Chvostek's sign in hypocalcemia.

unbound calcium in the body is reduced or when parathyroid gland function is decreased.

❖ PATIENT-CENTERED COLLABORATIVE CARE
◆ Assessment

Assess the nutrition history for the risk for hypocalcemia. Ask the patient about his or her intake of dairy products and whether he or she takes a calcium supplement regularly.

One indicator of hypocalcemia is a report of frequent, painful muscle spasms ("charley horses") in the calf or foot during rest or sleep. Ask about a history of recent orthopedic surgery or bone healing. Endocrine disturbances and treatments are risk factors for hypocalcemia. A history of thyroid surgery, therapeutic irradiation of the upper middle chest and neck area, or a recent anterior neck injury increases the risk for hypocalcemia. Most manifestations of acute hypocalcemia are caused by overstimulation of the nerves and muscles.

Neuromuscular changes often occur first in the hands and feet. Paresthesias occur at first, with sensations of tingling and numbness. If hypocalcemia continues or worsens, muscle twitching or painful cramps and spasms occur. Tingling

may also affect the lips, nose, and ears. These problems may signal the onset of neuromuscular overstimulation and tetany (Crawford & Harris, 2012).

Assess for hypocalcemia by testing for Trousseau's and Chvostek's signs. To test for Trousseau's sign, place a blood pressure cuff around the upper arm, inflate the cuff to greater than the patient's systolic pressure, and keep the cuff inflated for 1 to 4 minutes. Under these hypoxic conditions, a positive Trousseau's sign occurs when the hand and fingers go into spasm in palmar flexion (Fig. 11-13). To test for Chvostek's sign, tap the face just below and in front of the ear (over the facial nerve) to trigger facial twitching of one side of the mouth, nose, and cheek (Fig. 11-14).

Cardiovascular changes involve heart rate and ECG changes. The heart rate may be slower or slightly faster than normal, with a weak, thready pulse. Severe hypocalcemia causes severe hypotension and ECG changes of a prolonged ST interval and a prolonged QT interval.

Intestinal changes include increased peristaltic activity. Auscultate the abdomen for hyperactive bowel sounds. The patient may report painful abdominal cramping and diarrhea.

Skeletal changes are common with chronic hypocalcemia. Calcium leaves bone storage sites, causing a loss of bone density (osteoporosis). The bones are less dense, more brittle, and fragile and may break easily with slight trauma. Vertebrae become more compact and may bend forward, leading to an overall loss of height. See Chapter 50 for discussion of osteoporosis.

Ask about changes in height and any unexplained bone pain. Observe for spinal curvatures and any unusual bumps or protrusions in bones that may indicate old fractures.

◆ Interventions

Interventions focus on restoring normal calcium levels and preventing complications. These include drug therapy, nutrition therapy, reducing environmental stimuli, and preventing injury. Patient safety during restoration of serum calcium levels is a nursing care priority.

Drug therapy for hypocalcemia includes direct calcium replacement (oral and IV) and drugs that enhance the absorption of calcium, such as vitamin D. When hypocalcemia is a result of hyperphosphatemia, aluminum hydroxide may help raise serum calcium levels. When neuromuscular manifestations are troublesome, drugs that decrease nerve and muscle responses also may be used.

Nutrition therapy involves a high-calcium diet for patients with mild hypocalcemia and for those who are at continuing risk for hypocalcemia. Collaborate with the dietitian to assist the patient in selecting calcium-rich foods.

Environmental management for safety is needed because the excitable membranes of the nervous system and the skeletal system are overstimulated in hypocalcemia. Reduce stimulation by keeping the room quiet, limiting visitors, adjusting the lighting, and using a soft voice.

Use seizure precautions for the patient with hypocalcemia (see Chapter 42). Keep emergency equipment (e.g., oxygen, suction) at the bedside.

Injury prevention strategies are needed because the patient with long-standing calcium loss may have brittle, fragile bones that fracture easily and cause little pain. When lifting or moving a patient with fragile bones, use a lift sheet rather than pulling the patient. Observe for normal range of joint motion and for any unusual surface bumps or depressions over bony areas that may indicate bone fracture.

HYPERCALCEMIA
❖ PATHOPHYSIOLOGY

Hypercalcemia is an ELECTROLYTE imbalance in which the total serum calcium level is above 10.5 mg/dL or 2.62 mmol/L. Even small increases above normal have severe effects. Although the effects of hypercalcemia occur first in excitable tissues, all systems are affected.

Hypercalcemia means either that the amount of serum calcium is so great that the normal calcium-controlling actions cannot keep pace or that a control action is not functioning properly (Table 11-10). Hypercalcemia causes excitable tissues to be less sensitive to normal stimuli, thus requiring a stronger stimulus to function. The excitable tissues affected most by hypercalcemia are the heart, skeletal muscles, nerves, and intestinal smooth muscles.

TABLE 11-10 Common Causes of Hypercalcemia	
Actual Calcium Excesses	**Relative Calcium Excesses**
• Excessive oral intake of calcium	• Hyperparathyroidism
• Excessive oral intake of vitamin D	• Malignancy
• Kidney failure	• Hyperthyroidism
• Use of thiazide diuretics	• Immobility
	• Use of glucocorticoids
	• Dehydration

❖ PATIENT-CENTERED COLLABORATIVE CARE
◆ Assessment

The manifestations of hypercalcemia are related to its severity and how quickly the imbalance occurred. The patient with a mild but rapidly occurring calcium excess often has more severe problems than the patient whose imbalance is severe but has developed slowly.

Cardiovascular changes are the most serious and life-threatening problems of hypercalcemia. Mild hypercalcemia at first causes increased heart rate and blood pressure. Severe or prolonged calcium imbalance depresses electrical conduction, slowing heart rate.

Measure pulse rate and blood pressure, and observe for indications of poor tissue blood flow, such as cyanosis and pallor. Examine ECG tracings for dysrhythmias, especially a shortened QT interval.

Hypercalcemia allows blood clots to form more easily whenever blood flow is poor. Blood clotting is more likely in the lower legs, the pelvic region, areas where blood flow is blocked by internal or external constrictions, and areas where venous obstruction occurs.

Assess for slowed or impaired blood flow. Measure and record calf circumferences with a soft tape measure. Assess the feet for temperature, color, and capillary refill to determine the blood flow to and from the area.

Neuromuscular changes include severe muscle weakness and decreased deep tendon reflexes without paresthesia. The patient may be confused and lethargic.

Intestinal changes are first reflected as decreased peristalsis. Constipation, anorexia, nausea, vomiting, and abdominal distention and pain are common. Bowel sounds are hypoactive or absent. Assess abdominal size by measuring abdominal girth with a soft tape measure in a line circling the abdomen at the umbilicus.

◆ Interventions

Interventions for hypercalcemia focus on reducing serum calcium levels through drug therapy, rehydration, and, depending on the cause and severity, dialysis. Cardiac monitoring is also important.

Drug therapy involves preventing increases in calcium, as well as drugs to lower calcium levels. IV solutions containing calcium (e.g., Ringer's lactate) are stopped. Oral drugs containing calcium or vitamin D (e.g., calcium-based antacids) are discontinued.

FLUID volume replacement can help restore normal serum calcium levels. IV normal saline (0.9% sodium chloride) is usually given because sodium increases kidney excretion of calcium.

Thiazide diuretics are discontinued and are replaced with diuretics that enhance the excretion of calcium, such as furosemide (Lasix, Furoside ♣). Calcium chelators (calcium binders) help lower serum calcium levels. Such drugs include plicamycin (Mithracin) and penicillamine (Cuprimine, Pendramine ♣).

Drugs to prevent hypercalcemia include agents that inhibit calcium resorption from bone, such as phosphorus, calcitonin (Calcimar), bisphosphonates (etidronate), and prostaglandin synthesis inhibitors (aspirin, NSAIDs).

Cardiac monitoring of patients with hypercalcemia is needed to identify dysrhythmias and decreased cardiac output. Compare recent ECG tracings with the patient's baseline tracings. Especially look for changes in the T waves and the QT interval and changes in rate and rhythm.

? NCLEX EXAMINATION CHALLENGE

Health Promotion and Maintenance

Which intervention is most important for the nurse to teach the client who is at continuing risk for hypercalcemia and has normal kidney function?

A. "Report a weight gain of 1 lb or more a day to your health care provider immediately."
B. "Keep track of the number of bowel movements you have each day."
C. "Avoid taking aspirin or any aspirin-containing products."
D. "Be sure to drink at least 2 liters of fluids each day."

PHOSPHORUS

Normal serum levels of phosphorus range from 3.0 to 4.5 mg/dL, or 0.97 to 1.45 mmol/L (see Table 11-1). Most phosphorus (80%) can be found in the bones. It is the major anion in the ICF, and its levels inside cells are much higher than in the ECF. Phosphorus is needed for activating vitamins and enzymes, forming energy supplies, and assisting in cell growth and metabolism. It also functions in acid-base balance and calcium homeostasis.

Phosphorus balance and calcium balance are intertwined. Plasma levels of calcium and phosphorus exist in a balanced, reciprocal relationship, which means that when you multiply the two values, the product remains constant. Therefore a change in the level of serum phosphorus results in an equal and opposite change in the level of serum calcium (and vice versa).

The regulation of ECF phosphorus occurs through the activity of parathyroid hormone (PTH). Increased PTH levels cause a net loss of phosphorus. Reduced PTH levels enhance kidney reabsorption of phosphorus, resulting in increased plasma levels of phosphorus.

HYPOPHOSPHATEMIA
❖ PATHOPHYSIOLOGY

Hypophosphatemia is an electrolyte imbalance in which the serum phosphorus level is below 3.0 mg/dL. Body functions are not usually impaired with rapid changes in serum phosphorus levels. Reduced function occurs more often with chronic hypophosphatemia. Table 11-11 lists causes of phosphorus imbalance.

Most effects of hypophosphatemia are related to decreased energy metabolism, as well as to other FLUID AND ELECTROLYTE imbalances. Because phosphorus and calcium are inter-related,

---

TABLE 11-11   **Common Causes of Phosphorus Imbalance**
Hypophosphatemia
• Malnutrition
• Starvation
• Use of aluminum hydroxide–based antacids
• Use of magnesium-based antacids
• Hyperparathyroidism
• Hypercalcemia
• Kidney failure
• Malignancy
• Hyperglycemia
• Hyperalimentation
• Respiratory alkalosis
• Uncontrolled diabetes mellitus
• Alcohol abuse
Hyperphosphatemia
• Decreased kidney excretion resulting from kidney disease
• Tumor lysis syndrome
• Increased intake of phosphorus
• Hypoparathyroidism

decreases in serum phosphorus levels cause *increases* in serum calcium levels.

❖ PATIENT-CENTERED COLLABORATIVE CARE

◆ Assessment

Manifestations of hypophosphatemia are most apparent in the cardiac, musculoskeletal, hematologic, and central nervous systems. Cardiac changes include weak contractility, decreased stroke volume, and decreased cardiac output. Peripheral pulses are slow, difficult to find, and easy to block. Prolonged hypophosphatemia causes progressive but reversible cardiac muscle damage.

Musculoskeletal changes include weak skeletal muscles that may progress to acute muscle breakdown (**rhabdomyolysis**). With profound muscle weakness, respiratory efforts are ineffective, leading to respiratory failure. Assess for muscle strength, and observe respiratory effort.

The manifestations of *chronic* hypophosphatemia are most evident in the skeletal system. Bone density is decreased, which leads to fractures. Assess the patient for unusual lumps or depressions over bony areas that indicate bone fractures.

Central nervous system changes are not apparent until hypophosphatemia is severe. These first appear as irritability and may progress to seizure activity followed by coma.

◆ Interventions

Drugs that promote phosphorous loss (e.g., antacids, osmotic diuretics, calcium supplements) are discontinued. Oral replacement of phosphorus along with a vitamin D supplement may correct moderate hypophosphatemia. IV phosphorus is given only when serum phosphorus levels fall below 1 mg/dL and the patient has serious manifestations. Infuse IV phosphorus slowly because the problems caused by hyperphosphatemia are equally serious.

Nutrition therapy involves increasing the intake of phosphorus-rich foods while decreasing the intake of calcium-rich foods. Collaborate with the dietitian to teach the patient and family which foods to eat and which to avoid.

HYPERPHOSPHATEMIA

Hyperphosphatemia is an electrolyte imbalance in which the serum phosphorus level is above 4.5 mg/dL. High levels are well tolerated by most body systems. Causes of increased serum phosphorus levels include kidney disease, certain cancer treatments, increased phosphorus intake, and hypoparathyroidism. Table 11-11 lists common causes of hyperphosphatemia.

The problems caused by hyperphosphatemia center on the hypocalcemia that results when serum phosphorus levels increase. These problems include increased membrane excitability and can cause life-threatening side effects (see p. 168). Thus the management of hyperphosphatemia entails the management of hypocalcemia (see p. 169).

MAGNESIUM

Magnesium (Mg^{2+}) is a mineral that forms a cation when dissolved in water. Most magnesium is stored in bones and cartilage. Little magnesium is present in the extracellular fluid (ECF). Plasma levels of free magnesium range from 1.3 to 2.1 mEq/L, or 0.65 to 1.05 mmol/L (see Table 11-1). The intracellular fluid (ICF) has more magnesium and it has more functions inside the cells than in the blood. It is important for skeletal muscle contraction, carbohydrate metabolism, generation of energy stores, vitamin activation, blood coagulation, and cell growth. Magnesium regulation occurs through the kidney and the intestinal tract although the exact mechanisms are not known. When blood magnesium levels are low, ingested magnesium is rapidly absorbed and kidney excretion of magnesium stops. When blood magnesium levels are high, little magnesium is absorbed from food and kidney magnesium excretion increases.

HYPOMAGNESEMIA

Hypomagnesemia is an electrolyte imbalance in which the serum magnesium (Mg^{2+}) level is below 1.3 mEq/L. It is most often caused by decreased absorption of dietary magnesium or increased kidney magnesium excretion. Table 11-12 lists the specific causes of hypomagnesemia.

The effects of hypomagnesemia are caused by increased membrane excitability and the accompanying serum calcium

---

TABLE 11-12 Common Causes of Magnesium Imbalance

Hypomagnesemia
- Malnutrition
- Starvation
- Diarrhea
- Steatorrhea
- Celiac disease
- Crohn's disease
- Drugs (diuretics, aminoglycoside antibiotics, cisplatin, amphotericin B, cyclosporine)
- Citrate (blood products)
- Ethanol ingestion

Hypermagnesemia
- Increased magnesium intake:
  - Magnesium-containing antacids and laxatives
  - IV magnesium replacement
- Decreased kidney excretion of magnesium resulting from kidney disease

---

and potassium imbalances. Excitable membranes, especially nerve cell membranes, may depolarize spontaneously.

Neuromuscular changes are caused by increased nerve impulse transmission. Normally, magnesium inhibits nerve impulse transmission at synapse areas. Decreased levels increase impulse transmission from nerve to nerve or from nerve to skeletal muscle. The patient has hyperactive deep tendon reflexes, numbness and tingling, and painful muscle contractions. Positive Chvostek's and Trousseau's signs may be present because hypomagnesemia may occur with hypocalcemia (see the earlier discussion of these assessment signs of neuromuscular changes on p. 168 in the Hypocalcemia section). The patient may have tetany and seizures as hypomagnesemia worsens.

Intestinal changes are from decreased intestinal smooth muscle contraction. Reduced motility, anorexia, nausea, constipation, and abdominal distention are common. A paralytic ileus may occur when hypomagnesemia is severe.

Interventions for hypomagnesemia aim to correct the imbalance and manage the specific problem that caused it. In addition, because hypocalcemia often occurs with hypomagnesemia, interventions also aim to restore normal serum calcium levels.

Drugs that promote magnesium loss, such as high-ceiling (loop) diuretics, osmotic diuretics, aminoglycoside antibiotics, and drugs containing phosphorus, are discontinued. Magnesium is replaced intravenously with magnesium sulfate (MgSO$_4$) when hypomagnesemia is severe. Assess deep tendon reflexes at least hourly in the patient receiving IV magnesium to monitor effectiveness and prevent hypermagnesemia. If hypocalcemia is also present, drug therapy to increase serum calcium levels is prescribed.

HYPERMAGNESEMIA

Hypermagnesemia is an ELECTROLYTE imbalance in which the serum magnesium level is above 2.1 mEq/L. Table 11-12 lists the specific causes of hypermagnesemia.

Magnesium is a membrane stabilizer. Most manifestations of hypermagnesemia occur as a result of reduced membrane excitability. They usually are not apparent until serum magnesium levels exceed 4 mEq/L.

Cardiac changes include bradycardia, peripheral vasodilation, and hypotension. These problems become more severe as serum magnesium levels increase. ECG changes show a prolonged PR interval with a widened QRS complex. Bradycardia can be severe, and cardiac arrest is possible. Hypotension is also severe, with a diastolic pressure lower than normal. *Patients with severe hypermagnesemia are in grave danger of cardiac arrest.*

Central nervous system changes result from depressed nerve impulse transmission. Patients may be drowsy or lethargic. Coma may occur if the imbalance is prolonged or severe.

Neuromuscular changes include reduced or absent deep tendon reflexes. Voluntary skeletal muscle contractions become progressively weaker and finally stop.

Hypermagnesemia has no direct effect on the lungs; however, when the respiratory muscles are weak, respiratory insufficiency can lead to respiratory failure and death.

Interventions for hypermagnesemia focus on reducing the serum level and correcting the underlying problem that caused the imbalance. All oral and parenteral magnesium is discontinued. When kidney failure is not present, giving magnesium-free IV fluids can reduce serum magnesium levels. High-ceiling (loop) diuretics such as furosemide (Lasix, Furoside ✦) can further reduce serum magnesium levels. When cardiac problems are severe, giving calcium may reverse the cardiac effects of hypermagnesemia.

CHLORIDE

Chloride (Cl^-) is the major anion of the extracellular fluid (ECF) and works with sodium to maintain ECF osmotic pressure. The normal plasma concentration of chloride ranges from 98 to 106 mEq/L or mmol/L (see Table 11-1). It enters the body through dietary intake and is important in the formation of hydrochloric acid in the stomach.

Only a small amount of chloride is present inside the cells because negative charges on the cell membrane repel chloride and prevent it from crossing the membrane. However, extracellular chloride can enter cells when exchanged for another anion that is leaving the cell. This situation, called a *chloride shift*, decreases plasma chloride without a net body loss of chloride. Bicarbonate (HCO_3^-) is the anion most commonly exchanged for chloride.

Imbalances of chloride usually occur as a result of other electrolyte imbalances. An exception is chloride loss from excessive vomiting or prolonged gastric suction. Imbalances of chloride are usually corrected by interventions for correcting other electrolyte or acid-base problems.

❓ CLINICAL JUDGMENT CHALLENGE
Patient-Centered Care; Safety QSEN

The patient is a 29-year-old woman admitted 20 hours ago for an acute exacerbation of Crohn's disease with intense abdominal pain. She is NPO and receiving normal saline intravenously at 175 mL per minute. She was last given hydromorphone (Dilaudid) 4 mg IV 30 minutes ago. Because she did have an episode of hypotension earlier after Dilaudid, you now take her vital signs. On inflating the blood pressure cuff, she develops palmar flexion. The flexion remains after the cuff is deflated.
1. What is most likely the cause of this problem?
2. What electrolytes are most likely to be out of balance and why?
3. What is your best first action?
4. Should the Rapid Response Team be called? Why or why not?
5. What additional assessment data are most important to collect? Explain your selection.

NURSING CONCEPTS AND CLINICAL JUDGMENT REVIEW

What might you NOTICE in a patient who has adequate FLUID AND ELECTROLYTE BALANCE?

Vital signs:
- Heart rate and rhythm within usual range for the patient
- Respiratory rate and depth within usual range for the patient

Physical assessment:
- Skin turgor normal, no tenting, no edema
- Skin color normal (no cyanosis or pallor)
- Oral mucous membrane and nail beds pink with rapid capillary refill

- Strong and equal peripheral pulses
- Deep tendon reflexes present and normal
- Muscle strength consistent with what is normal for the patient
- Urine output about equal to fluid intake

Psychological assessment:
- Oriented and not confused
- Easily aroused from sleep

Laboratory assessment:
- Serum electrolyte values within normal limits
- Normal electrocardiogram

GET READY FOR THE NCLEX® EXAMINATION!

KEY POINTS

Review these Key Points for each NCLEX Examination Client Needs Category.

Safe and Effective Care Environment
- Assess any patient with a problem of FLUID AND ELECTROLYTE BALANCE for falls risk.
- Ensure access to adequate fluids for patients who cannot talk or who have limited mobility.
- Supervise the oral fluid therapy and intake and output measurement aspects of care delegated to unlicensed assistive personnel.
- Use a pump or controller to deliver IV fluids to patients with fluid overload. **Safety** QSEN
- Do not give IV potassium at a rate greater than 20 mEq/hr.
- Never give potassium supplements by the IM, subcutaneous, or IV push routes. **Safety** QSEN

- Use a pump or controller when giving IV potassium-containing solutions. **Safety** QSEN
- Use a gait belt when assisting a patient with muscle weakness to walk or transfer. **Safety** QSEN
- Collaborate with the dietitian to teach patients about diets that are restricted in potassium, sodium, or calcium.
- Use a lift sheet to move or reposition a patient with chronic hypocalcemia. **Safety** QSEN

Health Promotion and Maintenance
- Encourage all patients to maintain an adequate fluid intake (minimum of 2 L per day) unless another condition requires fluid restriction.
- Teach all people to increase fluid intake when exercising, when in hot or dry environments, or during conditions that increase metabolism (e.g., fever).

- Instruct patients at risk for FLUID imbalance to weigh themselves on the same scale daily, close to the same time each day, and with about the same amount of clothing on each time and to monitor these daily weights for changes or trends. **Patient-Centered Care** QSEN
- Instruct patients who exercise heavily (athletes) to take scheduled fluid replacement breaks.
- Instruct caregivers of older adults who have cognitive impairments or mobility problems to schedule offerings of fluids at regular intervals throughout the day. **Patient-Centered Care** QSEN
- Teach patients how to determine electrolyte content of processed foods by reading labels.
- Teach patients who are prescribed to take diuretics to take the drugs as prescribed.
- Teach patients who are taking digoxin to measure their pulse for rate, rhythm, and quality.
- Teach patients who are taking diuretics to measure their pulse for rate, rhythm, and quality.

Psychosocial Integrity

- Explain the purpose of fluid restriction to the patient and the family to ensure cooperation and prevent any misunderstandings.
- Assess patients who have a sudden change in cognition for a change in FLUID AND ELECTROLYTE BALANCE. **Safety** QSEN
- Determine the patient's food preferences and dislikes when planning an electrolyte-restricted diet.

Physiological Integrity

- Assess skin turgor on the forehead or the sternum of older patients.
- Use daily weights to determine fluid gains or losses. **Evidence-Based Practice** QSEN
- Ask patients about the use of drugs such as diuretics, laxatives, salt substitutes, and antihypertensives that may alter FLUID AND ELECTROLYTE BALANCE.
- Correctly interpret laboratory electrolyte values.
- Do not give oral fluids to an unconscious patient.
- Monitor the cardiac and pulmonary status at least every hour when patients with dehydration are receiving IV fluid replacement therapy.
- Offer or ensure that oral care is performed at least every 4 hours for patients with dehydration.
- Assess the IV site hourly of a person receiving IV solutions containing potassium, and document its condition. **Safety** QSEN
- Immediately stop the infusion of potassium-containing solutions if infiltration is suspected.
- Assess all patients with hyperkalemia for cardiac dysrhythmias and ECG abnormalities, especially tall T waves, conduction delays, and heart block.
- Assess the respiratory status of all patients with hypokalemia.
- Assess the bowel sounds; heart rate, rhythm and quality; and muscle strength to evaluate the patient's responses to therapy for an ELECTROLYTE imbalance.

Assessment and Care of Patients with Acid-Base Imbalances

M. Linda Workman

 http://evolve.elsevier.com/Iggy/

PRIORITY CONCEPTS

- ACID-BASE BALANCE

LEARNING OUTCOMES

Safe and Effective Care Environment

1. Identify patients at risk for falls as a result of problems with ACID-BASE BALANCE, especially older adults.

Health Promotion and Maintenance

2. Teach patients measures to take to maintain ACID-BASE BALANCE and avoid imbalances.

Psychosocial Integrity

3. Reduce the psychological impact for the patient experiencing a problem with ACID-BASE BALANCE.

Physiological Integrity

4. Apply knowledge of anatomy and physiology to explain regulation of ACID-BASE BALANCE.
5. Assess the patient for ACID-BASE BALANCE status, using laboratory data and clinical manifestations.
6. Prioritize nursing care for the patient with a problem affecting ACID-BASE BALANCE.

ACID-BASE BALANCE occurs through control of hydrogen ion (H^+) production and elimination. Body fluid **pH** is a measure of the body fluid's free hydrogen ion level. *This value has the narrowest range of normal and the tightest control mechanisms of all the electrolytes.* The level of free hydrogen ions, formed from acids, must be rigidly controlled. Even small changes in the free hydrogen ion level (pH) of body fluids can cause major problems in function. Keeping the pH within the normal range involves balancing acids and bases in body fluids. Normal pH ranges from 7.35 to 7.45 for arterial blood and from 7.31 to 7.41 for venous blood.

The normal free hydrogen ion level of blood and other body fluids is quite low (less than 0.0001 mEq/L) compared with other electrolytes (see Chapter 11). Because it is so low, the hydrogen ion concentration is not measured directly but, instead, is calculated in negative logarithm units. The value of pH is *inversely* related (negatively related) to the level of free hydrogen ions. Thus the *lower* the pH value of a fluid, the *higher* the level of free hydrogen ions in that fluid. The pH of a solution may range from 1 (as acidic as possible) to 14 (as alkaline as possible), with 7 being neutral. *A change of 1 pH unit actually represents a tenfold change in free hydrogen ion level.* Therefore any pH unit change (e.g., a change from 7.4 to 7.3) represents a large increase in the free hydrogen ion level.

Keeping the pH of the blood within the normal range by regulating ACID-BASE BALANCE is important because changes from normal interfere with many functions. These include:

- Changing the shape and reducing the function of hormones and enzymes
- Changing the distribution of other electrolytes, causing fluid and electrolyte imbalances
- Changing excitable membranes, making the heart, nerves, muscles, and GI tract either less or more active than normal
- Decreasing the effectiveness of many drugs

ACID-BASE BALANCE

Most body fluids have a pH value between 7.35 and 7.45 even though they contain acidic substances and basic substances. This value is slightly alkaline rather than strictly neutral (7.0 is neutral). Normal body fluid pH remains at this near-neutral value when the acids and bases are nearly balanced, limiting the total number of free or unbalanced hydrogen ions. ACID-BASE BALANCE occurs by matching the rate of hydrogen ion production (which is a continuous normal process) with hydrogen ion loss.

Acid-Base Chemistry

Acids

Acids are substances that release hydrogen ions when dissolved in water (H_2O), *increasing* the amount of free hydrogen ions in that solution. The strength of an acid is measured by how easily it releases a hydrogen ion in solution. A strong acid, such as hydrochloric acid (HCl), separates completely in water and releases *all* of its hydrogen ions, as shown in Fig. 12-1.

A weak acid releases only *some*, not all, of its hydrogen ions. In the following example, each molecule of acetic acid (CH_3COOH), a weak acid, contains a total of four hydrogen molecules. When acetic acid combines with water, as shown in Fig. 12-2, it releases only one of its four hydrogen molecules, keeping the other three hydrogen molecules bound to the molecule (CH_3COO^-).

Bases

A base binds free hydrogen ions in solution and *lowers* the amount of free hydrogen ions in solution. Strong bases bind hydrogen ions easily. Examples are sodium hydroxide (NaOH) and ammonia (NH_3).

Weak bases bind hydrogen ions less readily. An example of a weak base is bicarbonate (HCO_3^-). Although a weak base, the many bicarbonate ions in the body are critical in preventing major changes in body fluid pH.

Buffers

Buffers are critical in keeping body fluid pH at normal levels because they can react either as an acid (releasing a hydrogen ion) or as a base (binding a hydrogen ion). How a buffer reacts depends on the existing ACID-BASE BALANCE of that fluid. Buffers always try to bring the fluid as close as possible to the normal body fluid pH of 7.35 to 7.45. If the fluid is basic (with few free hydrogen ions), the buffer *releases hydrogen ions* into the fluid (Fig. 12-3). If the fluid is acidic (with many free hydrogen ions), the buffer *binds some of the excess hydrogen ions*. In this way, buffers act like hydrogen ion "sponges," soaking up hydrogen ions when too many are present and squeezing out hydrogen ions when too few are present. This flexibility allows buffers to keep body fluid pH in the normal range.

Liquids with a pH of 7.0 are neutral by having a free hydrogen ion level in which the amount and strength of acids and bases are equal. Fig. 12-4 shows the concept of neutral pH in which the combined *strength* and *amount* of all acids are equal to the combined *strength* and *amount* of all bases in a given solution. With human acid-base homeostasis, the relative

$$HCl + H_2O \leftrightarrow H^+ + Cl^- + H_2O$$

Hydrochloric acid · Water · Hydrogen ion · Chloride ion · Water

FIG. 12-1 Release of hydrogen ions by a strong acid (hydrochloric acid) in which the strong acid completely dissociates in water.

$$CH_3COOH + H_2O \leftrightarrow H^+ + CH_3COO^- + H_2O$$

Acetic acid (not ionized) · Water · Hydrogen ion · Acetic acid (ionized) · Water

FIG. 12-2 Release of hydrogen ions by a weak acid (acetic acid) in which the weak acid only partially dissociates in water and most of its hydrogen ions remain bound.

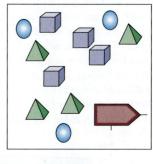

Fluid pH 7.38 (normal). The number and strength of acid components are equal to the number and strength of base components. Hydrogen ion concentration is limited and constant.

Fluid pH 7.51 (alkaline). The number and strength of base components are greater than the number and strength of acid components. Hydrogen ion concentration is below normal.

Buffer is added to the alkaline fluid.

The buffer acts as an acid, releasing a hydrogen ion.

△ Acid component ▢ Base component ◯ Hydrogen ion ⬡ Buffer

FIG. 12-3 Action of buffer in solution.

AAABBB	AAAABBB	AAABB
AAABBB	AAAABBB	AAABB
AAABBB	AAAABBB	AAABB
Neutral or acid-base balance	Acidic (acid excess) (actual acidosis)	Acidic (base deficit) (relative acidosis)

FIG. 12-4 Concept of acidic versus normal pH. (A = acid; B = base.)

AAABBB	AAABBBB	AABBB
AAABBB	AAABBBB	AABBB
AAABBB	AAABBBB	AABBB
Neutral	Alkaline (base excess)	Alkaline (acid deficit)

FIG. 12-5 Concept of alkaline versus normal pH. (A = acid; B = base.)

amounts and strengths of acids and bases are nearly equal and, normally, hydrogen ion production is balanced with hydrogen ion loss so that the overall free hydrogen ion levels remain constant.

Liquids with a pH ranging from 1.0 to 6.99 have more or stronger (or both) acids compared with bases. These liquids are *acidic* (see Fig. 12-4), with more free hydrogen ions released than bound, increasing the amount of free hydrogen ions in the liquid.

Liquids with a pH ranging from 7.01 to 14.0 have more or stronger (or both) bases compared with acids. These liquids are *basic,* in which more hydrogen ions are being bound than released, decreasing the amount of free hydrogen ions (Fig. 12-5).

Body Fluid Chemistry

Bicarbonate Ions

Body fluids contain different types of acids and bases. The most common base in human body fluid is bicarbonate (HCO_3^-); the most common acid is carbonic acid (H_2CO_3). In health, the body keeps these substances at a constant ratio of 1 molecule of carbonic acid to 20 free bicarbonate ions (1:20) (Fig. 12-6). To maintain this ratio, both carbonic acid and bicarbonate must be carefully controlled. This constant ratio is related to balancing the production and elimination of carbon dioxide (CO_2) and hydrogen ions (H^+).

Relationship Between Carbon Dioxide and Hydrogen Ions

A key process in understanding ACID-BASE BALANCE is the carbonic anhydrase equation. This equation, driven by the enzyme *carbonic anhydrase,* shows how hydrogen ion levels and carbon dioxide levels are directly related to one another, so that an increase in one causes an equal increase in the other (Fig. 12-7).

Carbon dioxide is a gas that forms carbonic acid when combined with water, making carbon dioxide a part of carbonic acid. Carbonic acid is not stable, and the body needs to keep a 1:20 ratio of carbonic acid to bicarbonate. When carbonic acid is formed from water and carbon dioxide, it begins to separate into free hydrogen ions and bicarbonate ions. *Therefore the carbon dioxide content of a fluid is directly related to the amount of hydrogen ions in that fluid. Whenever conditions cause carbon dioxide to increase, more free hydrogen ions are created. Likewise,* *whenever free hydrogen ion production increases, more carbon dioxide is produced.*

When excess carbon dioxide is produced, the equation shifts to the *right,* causing an *increase* in hydrogen ions (and a *decrease* in pH), as shown in Fig. 12-8. When very little carbon dioxide is produced, no free hydrogen ions are created by this equation.

When excess hydrogen ions are present, the carbonic anhydrase equation shifts to the *left,* causing the creation of more carbon dioxide, as shown in Fig. 12-9. When the amount of free hydrogen ions in body fluids is low, no extra carbon dioxide is produced.

How is the relationship between free hydrogen ions and carbon dioxide helpful? Carbon dioxide is a gas that can be eliminated during exhalation, and this action is important for ACID-BASE BALANCE. When any condition causes the hydrogen ion concentration of body fluids to increase, extra CO_2 is produced in the same proportion. This extra CO_2 is eliminated during exhalation, helping to bring the hydrogen ion concentration down to normal. Whenever the CO_2 level changes, the pH changes to the same degree, in the opposite direction. Thus when the CO_2 level of a liquid increases, the pH drops, indicating more free hydrogen ions (more acidic). Likewise, when the CO_2 level of a liquid decreases, the pH rises, indicating fewer free hydrogen ions (more alkaline).

An increase in bicarbonate causes the amount of hydrogen ions to decrease and the pH to increase, or become more alkaline (basic). Likewise, a decrease in bicarbonate causes the free hydrogen ion level to increase and the pH to decrease, or become more acidic.

Because the kidneys control bicarbonate levels and the lungs control CO_2 levels in the healthy person, pH is also described as the function of the kidneys divided by the function of the lungs (Fig. 12-10).

Sources of Acids and Bicarbonate

When acids are present in body fluids, free hydrogen ions are released and must be controlled for pH balance. Acids and hydrogen ions are produced continuously through normal body physiologic work and metabolism.

Normal metabolism of carbohydrate, protein, and fat creates natural waste products. Carbohydrate metabolism forms carbon dioxide (CO_2). Carbon dioxide is exhaled by the lungs during breathing. One factor that determines blood pH is how much CO_2 is produced by body cells during metabolism versus how rapidly that CO_2 is removed by breathing. Protein breakdown forms sulfuric acid. Fat breakdown forms fatty acids and ketoacids.

Incomplete breakdown of glucose, which occurs whenever cells metabolize under **anaerobic** (no oxygen) conditions, forms lactic acid. Anaerobic conditions occur with hypoxia, sepsis, and shock. Incomplete breakdown of fatty acids, occurring when large amounts of fatty acids are being metabolized, forms ketoacids.

Cell destruction allows cell contents to be released, including the structures that contain acids. These released acids in the extracellular fluid (ECF) increase free hydrogen ion levels.

FIG. 12-6 Normal ratio of carbonic acid to bicarbonate is 1:20.

$$CO_2 + H_2O \leftrightarrow H_2CO_3 \leftrightarrow HCO_3^- + H^+$$

FIG. 12-7 The carbonic anhydrase equation showing that the concentration of carbon dioxide is directly related to the concentration of hydrogen ions.

$$CO_2 + H_2O \rightarrow H_2CO_3 \rightarrow HCO_3^- + H^+$$

FIG. 12-8 Increased carbon dioxide levels force the equation to the right and increase the concentration of hydrogen ions proportionately.

$$CO_2 + H_2O \leftarrow H_2CO_3 \leftarrow HCO_3^- + H^+$$

FIG. 12-9 Increased hydrogen ion levels force the equation to the left and increase the concentration of carbon dioxide levels proportionately.

(Slow but powerful response)

$$pH = \frac{\text{Kidney function} = \text{Bicarbonate levels}}{\text{Lung function} = \text{Carbon dioxide levels}}$$

(Rapid but limited response)

FIG. 12-10 Contribution of pH balance by kidney and lung function.

CHART 12-1	**Laboratory Profile**

Acid-Base Assessment

TEST	NORMAL RANGE FOR ADULTS ARTERIAL	VENOUS	SIGNIFICANCE OF ABNORMAL FINDINGS
pH Adult <90 yr >90 yr	7.35-7.45 7.25-7.45	7.31-7.41 7.31-7.41	Increased: metabolic alkalosis, loss of gastric fluids, decreased potassium intake, diuretic therapy, fever, salicylate toxicity, respiratory alkalosis, hyperventilation Decreased: metabolic or respiratory acidosis, ketosis, renal failure, starvation, diarrhea, hyperthyroidism
PaO₂ Adult <90 yr >90 yr	80-100 mm Hg 70-90 mm Hg		Increased: increased ventilation, oxygen therapy, exercise Decreased: respiratory depression, high altitude, carbon monoxide poisoning, decreased cardiac output
PaCO₂	35-45 mm Hg	40-50 mm Hg	Increased: respiratory acidosis, emphysema, pneumonia, cardiac failure, respiratory depression Decreased: respiratory alkalosis, excessive ventilation, diarrhea
Bicarbonate	21-28 mEq/L	24-29 mEq/L	Increased: metabolic alkalosis, bicarbonate therapy Decreased: metabolic acidosis, diarrhea, pancreatitis
Lactate	3-7 mg/dL 0.3-0.8 mmol/L	5-20 mg/dL 0.6-2.2 mmol/L	Increased: hypoxia, exercise, insulin infusion, alcoholism, pregnancy Decreased: fluid overload

Data from Pagana, K., & Pagana, T. (2014). *Mosby's manual of diagnostic and laboratory tests* (5th ed). St. Louis: Mosby.
PaCO₂, Partial pressure of arterial carbon dioxide; *PaO₂,* partial pressure of arterial oxygen.

Bicarbonate, a weak base, is the main buffer of the ECF. It comes from the GI absorption of ingested bicarbonate, pancreatic production of bicarbonate, movement of cellular bicarbonate into the ECF, kidney reabsorption of filtered bicarbonate, and the breakdown of carbonic acid. Once bicarbonate is in the ECF, it is kept at a level 20 times greater than that of carbonic acid.

Acid-Base Regulatory Actions and Mechanisms

As long as body cells are healthy, they continuously produce acids, carbon dioxide, and free hydrogen ions. Despite this production, hydrogen ion, bicarbonate, oxygen, and carbon dioxide levels are kept within normal limits when ACID-BASE BALANCE controlling actions are normal. Chart 12-1 lists their normal values in arterial and venous blood. This homeostasis depends on:

- Hydrogen ion production being consistent and not excessive
- CO₂ loss from the body through breathing keeping pace with all forms of hydrogen ion production

To keep the free hydrogen ion level (pH) of the ECF within the narrow normal range, the body has chemical, respiratory, and kidney actions (mechanisms) for acid-base balance (Table 12-1).

Chemical Acid-Base Control Actions and Mechanisms

Buffers are the first line of defense against changes in free hydrogen ion levels. These buffers are always present in body fluids and act fast to reduce or raise the amount of free hydrogen ions to normal. By acting as hydrogen ion "sponges," buffers can bind hydrogen ions when too many are present or release hydrogen ions when not enough are present.

Buffers are composed of chemicals or proteins. The two most common chemical buffers are bicarbonate (which is active in both the extracellular fluid [ECF] and intracellular fluid [ICF]) and phosphate (which is active in the ICF). Protein buffers are the most common buffers. Extracellular protein buffers are albumin and globulins. A major intracellular protein buffer is hemoglobin. When the amount of free hydrogen ions in the blood increases, some of the excess hydrogen ions cross the membranes of red blood cells and bind to the large numbers of hemoglobin molecules in each red blood cell. This binding of hydrogen ions to hemoglobin results in fewer hydrogen ions remaining in the blood, bringing blood pH back up toward normal.

Respiratory Acid-Base Control Actions and Mechanisms

When chemical buffers alone cannot prevent changes in blood pH, the respiratory system is the second line of defense against changes. Breathing controls the amount of free hydrogen ions by controlling the amount of carbon dioxide (CO₂) in arterial blood. Because CO₂ is converted into hydrogen ions with the carbonic anhydrase reaction, the CO₂ level is *directly* related to the hydrogen ion level. Breathing rids the body of any excess CO₂.

The CO₂ level in venous blood increases with metabolism. This CO₂ moves into lung capillary blood. Because the amount (pressure) of CO₂ is far higher in lung capillary blood than it is

TABLE 12-1 Acid-Base Regulatory Mechanisms

MECHANISM TYPE	KEY CHARACTERISTICS
Chemical	
Protein buffers (albumin, globulins, hemoglobin)	Very rapid response
Chemical buffers (bicarbonate, phosphate)	Provide immediate response to changing conditions
	Can handle relatively small fluctuations in hydrogen ion production during normal metabolic and health conditions
Respiratory	
Increased hydrogen ions or increased carbon dioxide:	Primarily assist buffering systems when the fluctuation of hydrogen ion
Triggers the brain to increase the rate and depth of breathing, causing more carbon dioxide to be lost and decreasing the hydrogen ion concentration	concentration is acute
Decreased hydrogen ions or decreased carbon dioxide:	
Inhibits brain stimulation, leading to decreased rate and depth of breathing, causing carbon dioxide to be retained and increasing the hydrogen ion concentration	
Kidney	
Actions to decrease pH:	The most powerful regulator of acid-base balance
Increased kidney excretion of bicarbonate	Respond to large or chronic fluctuations in hydrogen ion production or
Increased kidney reabsorption of hydrogen ions	elimination
Actions to increase pH:	Slowest response (hours to days)
Decreased kidney excretion of bicarbonate	Longest duration
Decreased kidney reabsorption of hydrogen ions	

FIG. 12-11 Neural regulation of respiration and hydrogen ion concentration. (*H+*, Hydrogen ion, *Paco2*, partial pressure of arterial carbon dioxide.)

in the air in the alveoli, CO_2 diffuses freely from the blood into the alveolar air. Once in the alveoli, CO_2 is exhaled during breathing and is lost from the body. Because the amount (pressure) of CO_2 in room air is nearly zero, CO_2 can continue to be exhaled even when breathing is impaired.

Respiratory regulation of ACID-BASE BALANCE is under the control of the central nervous system (Fig. 12-11). Special receptors in the respiratory areas of the brain are sensitive to changes in the amount of CO_2 in brain tissues. As the amount of CO_2 begins to rise above normal in brain blood and tissues, these central receptors trigger neurons to increase the rate and depth of breathing (**hyperventilation**). As a result, more

CO_2 is exhaled ("blown off") from the lungs and the CO_2 level in the ECF decreases. When the arterial CO_2 level returns back down to normal, the rate and depth of breathing return to levels that are normal for the person.

If the amount of ECF free hydrogen ions is too low, then the CO_2 level also is too low. Central receptors sense these low CO_2 levels and stop or slow the neuron activity in the respiratory centers of the brain, decreasing the rate and depth of breathing (**hypoventilation**). As a result, less CO_2 is lost through the lungs and more CO_2 is retained in arterial blood. This retention of already-formed CO_2, together with the normal production of CO_2 from metabolism, results in a rapid return of the arterial CO_2 levels (and hydrogen ion levels) back up to normal. When these levels are normal, the rate and depth of breathing also return to normal levels.

The respiratory system's response in acid-base balance is rapid. Changes in the rate and depth of breathing occur within minutes after changes in the hydrogen ion level or CO_2 level of the ECF occur.

Kidney Acid-Base Control Actions and Mechanisms

The kidneys are the third line of defense against wide changes in body fluid pH. Kidney actions are stronger for regulating ACID-BASE BALANCE but take 24 to 48 hours to completely respond. When blood pH changes are persistent, kidney actions to increase excretion and reabsorption rates of acids or bases (depending on which way pH changes) start. These actions are kidney movement of bicarbonate, formation of acids, and formation of ammonium.

Kidney movement of bicarbonate is the first kidney pH control action. It occurs in the kidney tubules in two ways: (1) kidney movement of bicarbonate produced elsewhere in the body and (2) kidney movement of bicarbonate produced in the kidneys. Much of the bicarbonate made in other body areas is excreted in the urine. When blood hydrogen ion levels are high, this bicarbonate is reabsorbed from the kidneys back into circulation, where it can help buffer excess hydrogen ions. The kidney tubules also can make additional bicarbonate and reabsorb it to increase the buffer effect. When blood hydrogen ion levels are low, the bicarbonate stays in the urine and is excreted.

Formation of acids occurs through the phosphate-buffering system inside the cells of the kidney tubules. When the newly created bicarbonate made in kidney cells is reabsorbed into the blood, the urine has an excess of anions, including phosphate (HPO_4^{2-}). This negatively charged fluid draws hydrogen ions (which have a positive charge) into the urine. Once in the urine, the hydrogen ion binds to phosphate ions, forming an acid (H_2PO_4) that is then excreted in the urine.

Formation of ammonium converts the ammonia (NH_3), which is formed during normal protein breakdown, into ammonium (NH_4^+) in the urine. The ammonium "traps" the hydrogen ions and then allows them to be excreted in the urine. The result is a loss of hydrogen ions and an increase in blood pH.

Compensation

In the process of *compensation,* the body adapts to attempt to correct changes in blood pH and maintain ACID-BASE BALANCE. A pH below 6.9 or above 7.8 is usually fatal. The normal pH range for human extracellular fluid (ECF) is 7.35 to 7.45. Both the kidneys and the lungs can compensate for acid-base imbalances, but they are not equal in their final responses. The respiratory system is much more sensitive to acid-base changes and can begin compensation efforts within seconds to minutes after a change in pH. However, these efforts are limited and can be overwhelmed easily. The kidney compensatory actions are much more powerful and result in rapid changes in ECF composition. However, these more powerful actions are not fully triggered unless the acid-base imbalance continues for several hours to several days.

Respiratory compensation occurs through the lungs, usually to correct for acid-base imbalances from metabolic problems. For example, when prolonged running causes buildup of lactic acid, hydrogen ion levels in the ECF increase and the pH drops. To bring the pH back to normal, breathing is triggered in response to increased carbon dioxide levels. Both the rate and depth of respiration increase. These respiratory efforts cause the blood to lose carbon dioxide with each exhalation, so ECF levels of carbon dioxide and free hydrogen ions gradually decrease. When the lungs can *fully compensate,* the pH returns to normal.

Kidney compensation results when a healthy kidney works to correct for changes in blood pH that occur when the respiratory system either is overwhelmed or is not healthy. For example, in a person with chronic obstructive pulmonary disease (COPD), the respiratory system cannot exchange gases adequately. Carbon dioxide is retained continuously, hydrogen ion levels increase, and the blood pH falls (becomes more acidic). To oppose this process, the kidney excretes more hydrogen ions and increases the reabsorption of bicarbonate back into the blood. As a result, the blood pH remains either within or closer to the normal range. When these backup actions are completely effective, acid-base problems are *fully compensated* and the pH of the blood returns to normal even though the levels of oxygen and bicarbonate may be abnormal (Blevins, 2014).

Sometimes, however, the respiratory problem causing the acid-base imbalance is so severe that kidney actions can only *partially compensate* and the pH is not quite normal. Partial compensation helps because it prevents the acid-base imbalance from becoming severe (Blevins, 2014).

ACID-BASE IMBALANCES

Acid-base imbalances are problems of ACID-BASE BALANCE resulting from changes in the blood hydrogen ion level or pH. These changes are caused by problems with the acid-base regulatory actions or by exposure to dangerous conditions. Imbalances in which blood pH is below normal reflect **acidosis**, and imbalances in which blood pH is above normal reflect **alkalosis**. Acid-base imbalances impair the function of many organs and can be life threatening.

ACIDOSIS
❖ *PATHOPHYSIOLOGY*

In acidosis, the acid-base balance of the blood and other extracellular fluid (ECF) is upset by an excess of hydrogen ions (H^+). This is seen as an arterial blood pH below 7.35. The amount of acids present is greater than normal compared with the amount or strength of bases.

Acidosis is not a disease; it is a condition caused by a disorder or pathologic process. It can be caused by metabolic problems, respiratory problems, or both. Patients at greatest risk for acute acidosis are those with problems that impair breathing. Older adults with chronic health problems are at greater risk for developing acidosis (Chart 12-2).

Acidosis can result from an actual or relative increase in the amount or strength of acids. An *actual acid excess* results in acidosis by either overproducing acids (and release of hydrogen ions) or undereliminating normally produced acids (retention of hydrogen ions). Either way, more hydrogen ions are present than should be. Problems that increase acid production include diabetic ketoacidosis and seizures. Problems that decrease acid

---

CHART 12-2 **Nursing Focus on the Older Adult**

The Older Patient Experiencing Acid-Base Imbalance

When Obtaining a Patient's History
- Assess risk factors for acid-base imbalance, including drugs, chronic health problems (especially kidney disease, pulmonary disease), and acute health problems.
- Ask the patient to list all prescribed and over-the-counter drugs (especially diuretics and antacids). If the patient is unable to provide this information, ask the family to bring the drugs in from home.
- Ask the patient to recall what liquids were taken in the past 24 hours and whether urination amounts have changed.

When Assessing the Patient
- Compare the patient's mental status with what the family, significant other, or health record states is the patient's baseline.
- Observe the rate and depth of respiration.
  - Determine whether the patient can complete a sentence without stopping for breath.
- Examine the color of nail beds and mucous membranes.
- Obtain a urine specimen, and observe for color and character. Test for specific gravity and pH.
- Examine skin turgor for dehydration. Attempt to pinch the skin to form a tent over the sternum and on the forehead. If a tent forms, record how long it remains.
- Measure the rate and quality of the pulse.
- Monitor clinical responses and laboratory values while the acid-base imbalance is being corrected.
- Administer IV therapy by pump or controller.

elimination include respiratory impairment and kidney impairment.

In *relative* acidosis, the amount of acids does not increase. Instead, the amount or strength of the bases decreases (to create a *base deficit*), which makes the fluid relatively more acidic than basic. A relative acidosis *(base deficit)* is caused by either overeliminating or underproducing bicarbonate ions (HCO_3^-) (see Fig. 12-4). Problems that underproduce bases include pancreatitis and dehydration. A condition that overeliminates bases is diarrhea.

Regardless of its cause, acidosis causes major changes in body function. The main problems occur because hydrogen ions are positively charged ions. An increase in hydrogen ions creates imbalances of other positively charged electrolytes, especially potassium. The changes in potassium levels because of excess hydrogen ions is described in the Laboratory Assessment section for acidosis. These electrolyte imbalances then disrupt the functions of nerves, cardiac muscle, and skeletal muscle. Manifestations of acidosis first appear in the musculoskeletal, cardiac, respiratory, and central nervous systems. Even slight increases in blood hydrogen ion levels reduce the activity of many hormones and enzymes, leading to death.

Acidosis can be caused by metabolic problems, respiratory problems, or combined metabolic and respiratory problems. Specific causes of acidosis are listed in Table 12-2.

Metabolic Acidosis

Four processes can result in metabolic acidosis: overproduction of hydrogen ions, underelimination of hydrogen ions, underproduction of bicarbonate ions, and overelimination of bicarbonate ions.

TABLE 12-2   Common Causes of Acidosis

PATHOLOGY	CONDITION
Metabolic Acidosis	
Overproduction of hydrogen ions	Excessive oxidation of fatty acids: Diabetic ketoacidosis Starvation Hypermetabolism: Heavy exercise Seizure activity Fever Hypoxia, ischemia Excessive ingestion of acids: Ethanol or methanol intoxication Salicylate intoxication
Underelimination of hydrogen ions	Kidney failure
Underproduction of bicarbonate	Kidney failure Pancreatitis Liver failure Dehydration
Overelimination of bicarbonate	Diarrhea
Respiratory Acidosis	
Underelimination of hydrogen ions	Respiratory depression: Anesthetics Drugs (especially opioids) Electrolyte imbalance Inadequate chest expansion: Muscle weakness Airway obstruction Alveolar-capillary block

Overproduction of hydrogen ions can occur with excessive breakdown of fatty acids, anaerobic glucose breakdown *(lactic acidosis)*, and excessive intake of acids. Excessive breakdown of fatty acids occurs with diabetic ketoacidosis or starvation. When insufficient glucose is available for fuel, the body breaks down fats (lipids). The products of excessive fatty acid breakdown are strong acids *(ketoacids)*, which release large amounts of hydrogen ions.

Lactic acidosis occurs when cells use glucose without adequate oxygen *(anaerobic metabolism)*; glucose then is incompletely broken down and forms lactic acid. This acid releases hydrogen ions, causing acidosis. Lactic acidosis occurs whenever the body has too little oxygen to meet metabolic oxygen demands (e.g., heavy exercise, seizure activity, reduced oxygen).

Excessive intake of acids floods the body with hydrogen ions. Agents that cause acidosis when ingested in excess include ethyl alcohol, methyl alcohol, and acetylsalicylic acid (aspirin).

Underelimination of hydrogen ions leads to acidosis when hydrogen ions are produced at the normal rate but are not removed at the same rate they are produced. Most hydrogen ion loss occurs through the lungs and the kidneys. Kidney failure causes acidosis when the kidney tubules cannot secrete hydrogen ions into the urine and they are retained. Severe lung problems also can result in retention of CO_2 with a corresponding retention of hydrogen ions.

Underproduction of bicarbonate ions (base deficit) leads to acidosis when hydrogen ion production and removal are normal but too few bicarbonate ions are present to balance the hydrogen ions. Because bicarbonate is made in the kidneys and in the pancreas, kidney failure and impaired liver or pancreatic function can cause a base-deficit acidosis.

Overelimination of bicarbonate ions (base deficit) leads to acidosis when hydrogen ion production and removal are normal but too many bicarbonate ions have been lost. One cause of base deficit acidosis is diarrhea.

Respiratory Acidosis

Respiratory acidosis results when respiratory function is impaired and the exchange of oxygen (O_2) and carbon dioxide (CO_2) is reduced. This problem causes CO_2 retention, which leads to the same increase in hydrogen ion levels and acidosis. (See the carbonic anhydrase equation in Fig. 12-7.)

Unlike metabolic acidosis, respiratory acidosis results from only one cause—retention of CO_2, causing increased production of free hydrogen ions. Table 12-2 lists the four types of respiratory problems and their possible causes.

Respiratory depression results from depressed function of the brainstem neurons that trigger breathing movements. This lowered rate and depth of breathing leads to poor gas exchange and retention of carbon dioxide. Common causes include anesthetic agents, opioids, and poisons. Physical respiratory depression occurs when respiratory neurons are damaged or destroyed by trauma or when problems in the brain increase the intracranial pressure. Problems causing cerebral edema and respiratory depression include brain tumors, cerebral aneurysm, stroke, and overhydration.

Inadequate chest expansion reduces gas exchange and leads to acidosis. Chest expansion can be restricted by skeletal trauma or deformities, respiratory muscle weakness, or external constriction. Respiratory muscle weakness, caused by electrolyte imbalances, fatigue, muscular dystrophy, muscle damage, or muscle breakdown, reduces chest movement. External conditions, such as casts, tight scar tissue around the chest, obesity, and ascites, can restrict chest movement.

Airway obstruction prevents air movement into and out from the lungs *(ventilation)* and leads to poor gas exchange, CO_2 retention, and acidosis. External obstruction can be caused by clothing, neck edema, and local lymph node enlargement. Internal obstruction can be caused by aspiration of foreign objects, bronchoconstriction, mucus, and edema.

Reduced alveolar-capillary diffusion causes poor gas exchange and leads to CO_2 retention and acidosis. Disorders that reduce diffusion include pneumonia, pneumonitis, tuberculosis, emphysema, acute respiratory distress syndrome, chest trauma, pulmonary emboli, pulmonary edema, and drowning.

Combined Metabolic and Respiratory Acidosis

Metabolic and respiratory acidosis can occur at the same time. Uncorrected acute respiratory acidosis always leads to poor oxygenation and lactic acidosis (McCance et al., 2014). For example, a person who has diabetic ketoacidosis and chronic obstructive pulmonary disease has a combined metabolic and respiratory acidosis. Combined acidosis is more severe than either metabolic acidosis or respiratory acidosis alone.

❖ PATIENT-CENTERED COLLABORATIVE CARE

◆ Assessment

History. Collect data about risk factors related to the development of acidosis. Information about age, nutrition, and current manifestations are especially important.

Older adults are more at risk for problems leading to acid-base imbalance, including cardiac, kidney, or pulmonary impairment. Also, older adults may be taking drugs that disrupt ACID-BASE BALANCE, especially diuretics and aspirin. Ask about specific risk factors, such as any type of breathing problem, kidney failure, diabetes mellitus, diarrhea, pancreatitis, and fever.

Obtain a detailed nutrition history to determine total caloric intake and the proportions of carbohydrates, fats, and proteins ingested. Ask whether the patient has fasted or followed a strict diet within the past week.

Ask about headaches, behavior changes, increased drowsiness, reduced alertness, reduced attention span, lethargy, anorexia, abdominal distention, nausea or vomiting, muscle weakness, or increased fatigue. Ask the patient to relate activities of the previous 24 hours to identify activity intolerance, behavior changes, and fatigue. Because the central nervous system is often depressed in acidosis, you may need to obtain this information from the patient's family.

Physical Assessment/Clinical Manifestations. Manifestations of acidosis are similar whether the cause is metabolic or respiratory (Chart 12-3). Acidosis reduces the ability of excitable membranes to respond appropriately, especially in cardiovascular tissue, neurons, skeletal muscle, and GI smooth muscle.

Cardiovascular changes are first seen with mild acidosis and are more severe as the condition worsens. Early changes include increased heart rate and cardiac output. With worsening acidosis or with acidosis and hyperkalemia (elevated blood potassium levels), heart rate decreases, T waves become tall and peaked, and QRS complexes are widened. Peripheral pulses may be hard to find and are easily blocked. Hypotension occurs with vasodilation.

CHART 12-3 Key Features

Acidosis

Cardiovascular Manifestations
- Delayed electrical conduction:
  - Ranges from bradycardia to heart block
  - Tall T waves
  - Widened QRS complex
  - Prolonged PR interval
- Hypotension
- Thready peripheral pulses

Central Nervous System Manifestations
- Depressed activity (lethargy, confusion, stupor, coma)

Neuromuscular Manifestations
- Hyporeflexia
- Skeletal muscle weakness
- Flaccid paralysis

Respiratory Manifestations
- Kussmaul respirations (in metabolic acidosis with respiratory compensation)
- Variable respirations (generally ineffective in respiratory acidosis)

Integumentary Manifestations
- Warm, flushed, dry skin in metabolic acidosis
- Pale to cyanotic and dry skin in respiratory acidosis

! NURSING SAFETY PRIORITY (QSEN)

Critical Rescue

Assess the cardiovascular system first in any patient at risk for acidosis, because acidosis can lead to cardiac arrest from the accompanying hyperkalemia.

Central nervous system (CNS) changes include depression of CNS function. Problems may range from lethargy to confusion, especially in older patients. As acidosis worsens, the patient may become unresponsive. Assess the patient's mental status (see Chapter 41).

Neuromuscular changes include reduced muscle tone and deep tendon reflexes as a result of the accompanying hyperkalemia. Assess arm muscle strength and leg muscle strength. Test arm muscle strength by having the patient squeeze your hand. Test leg muscle strength by having the patient push both feet against a flat surface (like a box or a board) while you apply resistance to the opposite side of the flat surface. Muscle weakness is bilateral and can progress to paralysis.

Respiratory changes may cause the acidosis and can be caused by the acidosis. Assess the patient's rate, depth, and ease of breathing. Use pulse oximetry to determine how well oxygen is delivered to the peripheral tissues.

If acidosis is metabolic in origin, the rate and depth of breathing increase as the hydrogen ion level rises. Breaths are deep and rapid and not under voluntary control, a pattern called Kussmaul respiration.

If acidosis is caused by respiratory problems, breathing efforts are reduced. Respirations are usually shallow and rapid. Muscle weakness makes this problem worse.

Skin changes occur with metabolic or respiratory acidosis. With metabolic acidosis, breathing is unimpaired and the rate is increased and CO_2 is lost. This causes vasodilation and makes the skin and mucous membranes warm, dry, and pink. With respiratory acidosis, breathing is ineffective and skin and mucous membranes are pale to cyanotic.

Psychosocial Assessment. Behavioral changes may be the first manifestations of acidosis. Observe and document the patient's behavior by description (objectively) rather than by interpretation (subjectively). Ask family members if the patient's behavior is typical for him or her, and establish a baseline for comparison with later assessment findings.

Laboratory Assessment. Arterial blood pH is the laboratory value used to confirm acidosis. Acidosis is present when arterial blood pH is less than 7.35. However, this test alone does not indicate what is causing the acidosis. Manifestations of metabolic acidosis and respiratory acidosis are similar, but their treatments are different. *Therefore it is critical to obtain and interpret other laboratory data, such as arterial blood gas (ABG) values and blood levels of electrolytes* (Chart 12-4).

Metabolic acidosis is reflected by several changes in ABG values. The pH is low (<7.35) because buffering and respiratory compensation are not adequate to keep the amount of free hydrogen ions at a normal level. The bicarbonate level is low (<21 mEq/L). It is low because (1) bicarbonate has been lost, causing a base-deficit acidosis; (2) bicarbonate production is inadequate,

causing a base-deficit acidosis; or (3) bicarbonate may be bound to other substances. The partial pressure of arterial oxygen (Pao_2) is normal because gas exchange is not impaired. The partial pressure of arterial carbon dioxide ($Paco_2$) is normal or even slightly decreased because gas exchange is adequate and carbon dioxide retention is not a factor (Jones, 2010).

The serum potassium level is often high in acidosis as the body attempts to maintain electroneutrality during buffering. Fig. 12-12 shows the movement of potassium ions as serum pH changes. As the blood hydrogen ion level rises, some of the excess hydrogen ions enter red blood cells for intracellular buffering. The movement of hydrogen ions into the cells creates an excess of positive ions inside the cells. To balance these extra positive charges, an equal number of potassium ions (that also have a positive charge) move from the cells into the blood. This increases the blood potassium level, causing hyperkalemia.

Respiratory acidosis is reflected by several changes in ABG values. The pH is low (<7.35) because of the increased amount of free hydrogen ions in the blood. Buffering and kidney compensation are not adequate to keep the amount of free hydrogen ions at a normal level. If the kidneys partially compensate for this acidosis, pH is low but not as abnormal as could be expected with the degree of CO_2 retention.

CHART 12-4   Laboratory Profile

Acid-Base Imbalances (Uncompensated)

IMBALANCE	LABORATORY VALUE CHANGES						
	pH	HCO_3^-	Pao_2	$Paco_2$	K^+	Ca^{2+}	Cl^-
Metabolic acidosis	↓	↓	Ø	Ø and ↓	↑	Ø	Ø and ↑
Respiratory acidosis	↓	Ø	↓	↑	↑	Ø	↑↓
Combined acidosis	↓	↓↑	↓	↑	↑	Ø	↑
Metabolic alkalosis	↑	↑	Ø	Ø and ↑	↓	↓	↓
Respiratory alkalosis	↑	Ø	Ø	↓↓	↓	↓	↑
Combined alkalosis	↑	↑	Ø	↓	↓	↓	↓

↑, Above normal; ↓, below normal; ↑↓, value can increase or decrease depending on other factors; Ø, normal; Ca^{2+}, calcium ions; Cl^-, chloride ions; $Paco_2$, partial pressure of arterial carbon dioxide; Pao_2, partial pressure of arterial oxygen; HCO_3^-, bicarbonate ions; K^+, potassium ions.

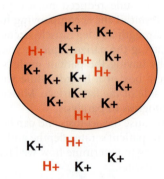

Under normal conditions, the intracellular potassium content is much greater than that of the extracellular fluid. The concentration of hydrogen ions is low in both compartments.

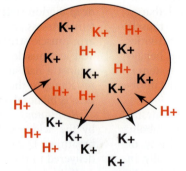

In acidosis, the extracellular hydrogen ion content increases and the hydrogen ions move into the intracellular fluid. To keep the intracellular fluid electrically neutral, an equal number of potassium ions leave the cell, creating a relative hyperkalemia.

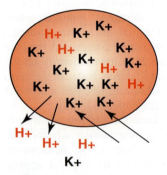

In alkalosis, more hydrogen ions are present in the intracellular fluid than in the extracellular fluid. Hydrogen ions move from the intracellular fluid into the extracellular fluid. To keep the intracellular fluid electrically neutral, potassium ions move from the extracellular fluid into the intracellular fluid, creating a relative hypokalemia.

FIG. 12-12 Movement of potassium (K^+) in response to changes in the extracellular fluid hydrogen ion (H^+) concentration.

The partial pressure of arterial oxygen (Pao_2) is low and the partial pressure of arterial carbon dioxide ($Paco_2$) is high because the pulmonary problem impairs gas exchange, causing poor oxygenation and CO_2 retention. *(The hallmarks of respiratory acidosis are a decreasing Pao_2 coupled with a rising $Paco_2$.)* Because carbon dioxide diffuses more easily across the alveolar membrane than oxygen, a decreased Pao_2 usually occurs before an increased $Paco_2$.

The serum bicarbonate level is variable. A patient with rapid onset of respiratory acidosis often has a normal bicarbonate level because kidney compensation has not started. When the acidosis persists for 24 hours or longer, kidney compensation increases the levels of bicarbonate. Chronic respiratory acidosis is indicated by an elevated bicarbonate level and increased $Paco_2$.

Serum potassium levels are elevated in acute respiratory acidosis. They are normal or low in chronic respiratory acidosis when kidney compensation is present.

Priority Patient Problems. Priority problems for the patient experiencing acidosis are associated with the decreased function of excitable membranes. These problems include hypotension and decreased perfusion, impaired memory and cognition, and increased risk for falls.

◆ **Interventions**

Interventions for acidosis focus on correcting the underlying problem and monitoring for changes. To ensure appropriate interventions, first identify the specific type of acidosis present.

Metabolic Acidosis. Interventions for metabolic acidosis include hydration and drugs or treatments to control the problem causing the acidosis. For example, if the acidosis is a result of diabetic ketoacidosis, insulin is given to correct the hyperglycemia and halt the production of ketone bodies. Rehydration and antidiarrheal drugs are given if the acidosis is a result of prolonged diarrhea. *Bicarbonate is administered only if serum bicarbonate levels are low.*

Nursing priorities include continuously monitoring the patient for changes that indicate either he or she is responding to the treatment or the acidosis is becoming worse. The cardiovascular system and the skeletal muscle system are sensitive to acidosis and are the most important systems to monitor. Interpreting ABG results is an important part of monitoring.

Respiratory Acidosis. Priority interventions for respiratory acidosis are focused on improving ventilation and oxygenation and maintaining a patent airway. These include drug therapy, oxygen therapy, pulmonary hygiene (positioning and breathing techniques), ventilatory support, and prevention of complications. (See Chapter 30 for disorders causing respiratory acidosis.)

Drug therapy is focused on improving ventilation and oxygenation rather than directly on altering pH. Drug categories useful for respiratory acidosis include bronchodilators, anti-inflammatories, and mucolytics.

Oxygen therapy helps promote gas exchange for patients with respiratory acidosis. Carefully monitor oxygen saturation to ensure that the lowest flow of oxygen that prevents hypoxemia is used to avoid oxygen-induced tissue damage.

Ventilation support with mechanical ventilation may be needed for patients who cannot keep their oxygen saturation at 90% or who have respiratory muscle fatigue. Chapter 32 discusses the nursing care needs of patients who are being mechanically ventilated.

Preventing complications is a nursing priority when caring for a patient with respiratory acidosis. Monitoring breathing status hourly and intervening when changes occur are critical in preventing complications. Listen to breath sounds, and assess how easily air moves into and out of the lungs. Check for any muscle retractions, the use of accessory muscles (especially the neck muscles [sternocleidomastoids]), and whether breathing produces a grunt or wheeze that can be heard without a stethoscope. Assess nail beds and oral membranes for cyanosis (a late finding).

> **? NCLEX EXAMINATION CHALLENGE**
> *Physiological Integrity*
>
> What type of acid-base problem does the nurse expect in a client who is being insufficiently mechanically ventilated and whose most recent arterial blood gas results include a pH of 7.29?
> A. Metabolic acidosis with an acid excess
> B. Metabolic acidosis with a base deficit
> C. Respiratory acidosis with an acid excess
> D. Respiratory acidosis with a base deficit

ALKALOSIS
❖ PATHOPHYSIOLOGY

In patients with alkalosis, the ACID-BASE BALANCE of the blood is disturbed and has an excess of bases, especially bicarbonate (HCO_3^-). The amount or strength of the bases is greater than normal compared with the amount of the acids. Alkalosis is a *decrease* in the free hydrogen ion level of the blood and is reflected by an arterial blood pH *above* 7.45. Like acidosis, alkalosis is not a disease but, rather, is a manifestation of a problem. It can be caused by metabolic problems, respiratory problems, or both (Table 12-3).

Alkalosis can result from an actual or relative increase in the amount or strength (or both) of bases. In an actual base excess, alkalosis occurs when base (usually bicarbonate) is either overproduced or undereliminated.

TABLE 12-3	Common Causes of Alkalosis
PATHOLOGY	**CONDITION**
Metabolic Alkalosis	
Increase of base components	Oral ingestion of bases: Antacids Parenteral base administration: Blood transfusion Sodium bicarbonate Total parenteral nutrition
Decrease of acid components	Prolonged vomiting Nasogastric suctioning Hypercortisolism Hyperaldosteronism Thiazide diuretics
Respiratory Alkalosis	
Excessive loss of carbon dioxide	Hyperventilation, fear, anxiety Mechanical ventilation Salicylate toxicity High altitudes Shock Early-stage acute pulmonary problems

AAABBB   AAABBBB   AABBB
AAABBB   AAABBBB   AABBB
AAABBB   AAABBBB   AABBB

| Acid-base balance | Actual alkalosis (base excess) | Relative alkalosis (acid deficit) |

FIG. 12-13 Concepts of actual and relative alkalosis. (A = acid; B = base.)

In *relative* alkalosis, the actual amount or strength of bases does not increase but the amount of the acids decreases, creating an *acid deficit*. A relative base-excess alkalosis (actual acid deficit) results from an overelimination or underproduction of acids (Fig. 12-13).

The problems of alkalosis are serious and can be life threatening. Management focuses on correcting the cause after identifying whether the alkalosis origin is respiratory or metabolic.

Whether metabolic, respiratory, or both, alkalosis affects specific functions. The pathologic effects are caused by the electrolyte imbalances that occur in response to decreased blood cation (positively charged particles) levels. Most problems of alkalosis are related to increased stimulation of the nervous, neuromuscular, and cardiac systems.

Metabolic alkalosis is an acid-base imbalance caused by either an increase of bases (base excess) or a decrease of acids (acid deficit). Base excesses are caused by excessive intake of bicarbonates, carbonates, acetates, and citrates. Excessive use of bicarbonate-containing antacids can cause a metabolic alkalosis. Other base excesses can occur during medical treatments, such as citrate excesses during massive blood transfusions and IV sodium bicarbonate given to correct acidosis. The hallmark of a base-excess acidosis is an ABG result with an elevated pH and an elevated bicarbonate level along with normal oxygen and carbon dioxide levels.

Acid deficits can be caused by disease processes or medical treatment. Disorders causing acid deficits include prolonged vomiting, excess cortisol, and hyperaldosteronism. Treatments that promote acid loss causing metabolic alkalosis include thiazide diuretics and prolonged gastric suctioning.

Respiratory alkalosis is usually caused by an excessive loss of CO_2 through hyperventilation (rapid respirations). Patients may hyperventilate in response to anxiety, fear, or improper settings on mechanical ventilators. Hyperventilation can also result from direct stimulation of central respiratory centers because of fever, central nervous system lesions, and salicylates. The hallmark of respiratory alkalosis is an ABG result with an elevated pH coupled with a low carbon dioxide level. Usually, the oxygen and bicarbonate levels are normal.

❖ PATIENT-CENTERED COLLABORATIVE CARE

◆ Assessment

Manifestations of problems with ACID-BASE BALANCE are the same for metabolic and respiratory alkalosis. Many symptoms are the result of the low calcium levels (**hypocalcemia**) and low potassium levels (**hypokalemia**) that usually occur with alkalosis (see Fig. 12-12). These problems change the function of the nervous, neuromuscular, cardiac, and respiratory systems (Chart 12-5).

Central nervous system (CNS) changes are caused by overexcitement of the nervous systems. Patients have dizziness, agitation, confusion, and hyperreflexia, which may progress to

---

CHART 12-5   Key Features

Alkalosis

Central Nervous System Manifestations
- Increased activity
- Anxiety, irritability, tetany, seizures
- Positive Chvostek's sign
- Positive Trousseau's sign
- Paresthesias

Neuromuscular Manifestations
- Hyperreflexia
- Muscle cramping and twitching
- Skeletal muscle weakness

Cardiovascular Manifestations
- Increased heart rate
- Normal or low blood pressure
- Increased digitalis toxicity

Respiratory Manifestations
- Increased rate and depth of ventilation in respiratory alkalosis
- Decreased respiratory effort associated with skeletal muscle weakness in metabolic alkalosis

---

seizures. Tingling or numbness may occur around the mouth and in the toes. Other indicators of alkalosis with hypocalcemia are positive Chvostek's and Trousseau's signs (see Chapter 11).

Neuromuscular changes are related to the hypocalcemia and hypokalemia that occur with alkalosis. Nervous system activity increases, causing muscle cramps, twitches, and "charley horses." Deep tendon reflexes are hyperactive. **Tetany** (continuous contractions) of muscle groups also may be present. Tetany is painful and indicates a rapidly worsening condition.

Skeletal muscles may contract as a result of nerve stimulation, but they become weaker because of the hypokalemia. Handgrip strength decreases, and the patient may be unable to stand or walk. Respiratory efforts become less effective as the respiratory muscles weaken.

Cardiovascular changes occur because alkalosis increases myocardial irritability, especially when accompanied by hypokalemia. Heart rate increases, and the pulse is thready. When decreased blood volume is also present, the patient may have severe hypotension. The hypokalemia increases heart sensitivity to digoxin, which increases the risk for digoxin toxicity.

Respiratory changes, especially increases in the rate of breathing, are the main causes of respiratory alkalosis. Although the volume of air inhaled and exhaled with each breath is nearly normal, the total volume of air inhaled and exhaled each minute rises with the increased respiratory rate. The increased minute volume may be caused by anxiety or physiologic changes.

Arterial blood pH greater than 7.45 confirms alkalosis, but this test alone does not identify its cause. Because the manifestations of metabolic alkalosis and respiratory alkalosis are similar, it is critical to obtain additional laboratory data, especially arterial blood gas (ABG) values and specific serum electrolyte levels (see Chart 12-4) (Blevins, 2014).

◆ Interventions

Interventions are planned to prevent further losses of hydrogen, potassium, calcium, and chloride ions; to restore fluid balance; to monitor changes; and to provide for *patient safety*. Treatments that may have caused alkalosis (e.g., prolonged gastric suctioning, excessive infusion of certain IV solutions, drugs that promote hydrogen ion excretion) are modified or stopped. Drug therapy is prescribed to resolve the causes of alkalosis and to restore normal fluid, electrolyte, and acid-base balance. For example, the patient with metabolic alkalosis caused by diuretic therapy receives fluid and electrolyte replacement, and the diuretic therapy is adjusted or stopped. Antiemetic drugs are prescribed for vomiting. Monitor the patient's progress, and adjust fluid and electrolyte therapy. Monitor electrolytes daily until they return to near normal.

During correction of alkalosis, a nursing care priority is prevention of injury from falls. The patient with alkalosis has hypotension and muscle weakness, which increase the risk for falls, especially among older adults. Implement the general falls prevention nursing interventions and the high-risk falls prevention nursing interventions outlined in Chart 2-4 in Chapter 2.

> ## ? CLINICAL JUDGMENT CHALLENGE
> ### *Patient-Centered Care; Safety* QSEN
>
> The patient is a 21-year-old college student brought to the emergency department by his friends when he was found unconscious during a fraternity party. He was seen drinking heavily at the party and had not eaten for 2 days before the event. He takes no prescription drugs, and his current vital signs are: T = 97.8° F; P = 48, slightly irregular and thready; R = 28, deep and regular; BP = 88/50. His current arterial blood gas results are: pH = 7.31; $HCO_3^- = 25$ mEq/L; $PaCO_2 = 28$ mm Hg; $PaO_2 = 99$ mm Hg.
> 1. What specific type of acid-base problem does this patient have? Explain your choice.
> 2. What is the most probable origin of the acid-base imbalance?
> 3. Should oxygen be applied? Why or why not?
> 4. What nursing interventions for safety are most appropriate for this patient?
> 5. What additional laboratory and assessment data should be performed? Provide a rationale for your selections.

NURSING CONCEPTS AND CLINICAL JUDGMENT REVIEW

What might you NOTICE in a patient with appropriate ACID-BASE BALANCE?

Vital signs:
- Respiratory rate and depth within usual range for the patient
- Heart rate and rhythm within usual range for the patient
- Oxygen saturation of 95% or higher

Physical assessment:
- Able to speak a sentence of 12 words without stopping for breath
- Able to walk and talk without stopping for breath
- Skin color normal (no cyanosis or pallor)
- Oral mucous membrane and nail beds pink with rapid capillary refill

- Breathing quiet
- Muscle strength consistent with what is normal for the patient
- Urine output about equal to fluid intake

Psychological assessment:
- Oriented and not confused
- Energy level good; can engage in desired work, recreational, and personal activities

Laboratory assessment:
- Arterial blood gas values within normal limits
- Serum electrolyte values, especially potassium and calcium, within normal limits

GET READY FOR THE NCLEX® EXAMINATION!

KEY POINTS

Review these Key Points for each NCLEX Examination Client Needs Category.

Safe and Effective Care Environment
- Assess the ACID-BASE BALANCE of any patient with new-onset muscle weakness.
- Use fall precautions for any patient with a problem in ACID-BASE BALANCE. **Safety** QSEN

Health Promotion and Maintenance
- Teach patients to take drugs as prescribed, especially diuretics, antihypertensives, and cardiac drugs.
- Instruct patients at continuing risk for respiratory acidosis to stop smoking.

Psychosocial Integrity
- Assess the oxygenation status of any patient with acute confusion.

- Monitor the neurologic status at least every 2 hours in patients being treated for a problem with ACID-BASE BALANCE.
- Assist patients who have anxiety-induced respiratory alkalosis to identify causes of anxiety.

Physiological Integrity
- Be aware of how the following principles, processes, and mechanisms influence the regulation of ACID-BASE BALANCE:
  - The normal pH of the body's extracellular fluids (including blood) is 7.35 to 7.45.
  - The more hydrogen ions present, the more acidic the fluid; the fewer hydrogen ions present, the more alkaline the fluid.
  - pH values below 7.35 indicate acidosis; pH values above 7.45 indicate alkalosis.
  - Anything that increases the CO_2 level in the blood increases the hydrogen ion content and lowers the pH.

- Acids are normally formed in the body as a result of metabolism.
- Chemical blood buffers are the immediate way that acid-base imbalances are corrected.
- The lungs control the amount of CO_2 that is retained or exhaled.
- The kidneys regulate the amount of hydrogen and bicarbonate ions that are retained or excreted by the body.
- If a lung problem causes retention of carbon dioxide, the healthy kidney compensates by increasing the amount of bicarbonate that is produced and retained.
- Acidosis reduces the excitability of cardiovascular muscle, neurons, skeletal muscle, and GI smooth muscle.
- Alkalosis increases the sensitivity of excitable tissues, allowing them to over-respond to normal stimuli and respond even without stimulation.

- Check the serum potassium level for any patient who has acidosis. **Evidence-Based Practice** **QSEN**
- Assess the cardiovascular system first in any patient at risk for acidosis because acidosis can lead to cardiac arrest from the accompanying hyperkalemia. **Evidence-Based Practice** **QSEN**
- Assess the airway of any patient who has acute respiratory acidosis.
- Assess heart rate and rhythm at least every 2 hours for any patient with an acid-base imbalance.
- Monitor arterial blood gas (ABG) values to evaluate the effectiveness of therapy for acid-base imbalances. **Evidence-Based Practice** **QSEN**

CHAPTER 13

Infusion Therapy*

Cheryl J. Dumont

ℰ http://evolve.elsevier.com/Iggy/

PRIORITY CONCEPTS

- FLUID AND ELECTROLYTE BALANCE
- TISSUE INTEGRITY
- INFECTION
- PERFUSION

LEARNING OUTCOMES

Safe and Effective Care Environment

1. Prevent IV administration errors by following best practices that ensure patient and staff safety.
2. Describe the benefits and limitations of selected safety-enhancing technologies used for infusion therapy.
3. Identify the evidence-based guidelines for prevention of intravenous (IV) catheter–related bloodstream INFECTION (CR-BSI).

Health Promotion and Maintenance

4. Describe the special needs and care for older adults receiving IV therapy.
5. Teach the patient and family about the type and care related to the patient's infusion therapy.

Physiological Integrity

6. Explain how to check the accuracy of prescriptions for IV fluids and drug therapy.
7. Identify the appropriate veins for peripheral IV catheter insertion.
8. Differentiate types of vascular access devices (VADs) used for peripheral and central IV therapy.
9. Outline best practice for inserting peripheral VADs.
10. Assess the patient's infusion site frequently for local complications, such as phlebitis and infiltration.
11. Prioritize nursing interventions for maintaining an infusion system.
12. Assess, prevent, and manage systemic complications related to infusion therapy and VADs.
13. Describe nursing care associated with intra-arterial, intraperitoneal, subcutaneous, intraosseous, and intraspinal infusion therapy.

Infusion therapy is the delivery of medications in solution and fluids by parenteral (piercing of skin or mucous membranes) route through a wide variety of catheter types and locations using multiple procedures. IV therapy is the most common route for infusion therapy. It delivers solutions directly into the veins of the vascular system. This chapter focuses on access for and administration of all types of infusion therapy.

OVERVIEW

Infusion therapy is delivered in all health care settings, including hospitals, home care, ambulatory care clinics, physicians' offices, and long-term care facilities. The most common reasons for using infusion therapy are to:

- Maintain FLUID BALANCE or correct fluid imbalance
- Maintain ELECTROLYTE or acid-base BALANCE or correct electrolyte or acid-base imbalance
- Administer medications
- Replace blood or blood products

IV therapy is the most common invasive therapy administered to hospitalized patients. Advances in medicine and technology have made it possible for people with chronic diseases such as diabetes mellitus, chronic kidney disease, and malabsorption syndromes to live long and productive lives. These patients often depend on long-term infusion therapy of some kind. They often have very poor vascular integrity and, therefore, accessing their peripheral veins takes a high level of skill.

Having a specialized team of infusion nurses to initiate and maintain infusion therapy has been recommended as best practice by the Centers for Disease Control and Prevention (CDC) to reduce complications of infusion therapy (O'Grady et al., 2011). These teams have demonstrated value in cost savings, patient satisfaction, and patient outcomes.

*With recognition given to the Winchester Medical Center Vascular Access Team: Meredith Baker, Tammy Brannon, Cathy Dalton, Ronee Fertig, Ozlem Getz, Debbie Knippenberg, Paula McCarren, Sheri Miller, and Nancy Stoop.

Infusion nurses may perform any or all of these activities:

- Develop evidence-based policies and procedures
- Insert and maintain various types of peripheral and central venous catheters
- Monitor patient outcomes of infusion therapy
- Educate staff, patients, and families regarding infusion therapy
- Consult on product selection and purchasing decisions
- Provide therapies such as blood withdrawal, therapeutic phlebotomy, hypodermoclysis, intraosseous infusions, and administration of medications including chemotherapy

The registered nurse (RN) generalist is taught to insert peripheral IVs; most institutions have a process for credentialing this skill. Depending on the state's nurse practice act, licensed practical/vocational nurses (LPNs/LVNs) and technicians may be trained and credentialed to perform the skill of peripheral IV insertion and assist with infusions. *The RN is ultimately accountable for all aspects of infusion therapy and delegation of associated tasks (Infusion Nurses Society [INS], 2011).* You have a strategic role in selection of the correct device and managing the patient requiring infusion therapy (Santolim et al., 2012).

The Infusion Nurses Society (INS) publishes guidelines and standards of practice for policy and procedure development in all health care settings. These standards establish the criteria for all nurses delivering infusion therapy. The Infusion Nurses Certification Corporation (INCC) offers a written certifying examination. Nurses who successfully complete this examination have mastered an advanced body of knowledge in this specialty and may use the initials *CRNI*, which stand for *certified registered nurse infusion*.

Types of Infusion Therapy Fluids

Many types of parenteral fluids are used for infusion therapy. These fluids are IV solutions, including parenteral nutrition, blood and blood components, and drug therapy.

Intravenous Solutions

More than 200 IV fluids (solutions) are available that meet the requirements established by the United States Pharmacopeia (USP). Each solution is classified by its tonicity (concentration) and pH. Tonicity is typically categorized by comparison with normal blood plasma as osmolarity (mOsm/L). As discussed in Chapter 11, normal serum osmolarity for adults is between 270 and 300 mOsm/L. Parenteral solutions within that normal range are isotonic; those fluids greater than 300 mOsm/L are hypertonic; and those fluids less than 270 mOsm/L are hypotonic.

When an *isotonic infusate* (solution that is infused into the body) is used, water does not move into or out of the body's cells. Therefore patients receiving isotonic solutions are at risk for fluid overload, especially older adults (see Chapter 11). *Hypertonic* solutions are used to correct FLUID AND ELECTROLYTE and acid-base imbalances by moving water out of the body's cells and into the bloodstream. Electrolytes and other particles also move across cell membranes across a concentration gradient (from higher concentration to lower concentration). Parenteral nutrition solutions are hypertonic (see Chapter 60). Instead of moving water out of cells, *hypotonic* infusates move water into cells to expand them. Patients receiving either hypertonic or hypotonic fluids are at risk for phlebitis and infiltration. Phlebitis is the inflammation of a vein caused by

mechanical, chemical, or bacterial irritation. Infiltration occurs when IV solution leaks into the tissues around the vein.

The pH of IV solutions is a measure of the acidity or alkalinity and usually ranges from 3.5 to 6.2. Extremes of both osmolarity and pH can cause vein damage leading to phlebitis and thrombosis (blood clot in the vein). Thus FLUIDS and medications with a pH value less than 5 and more than 9 and with an osmolarity more than 600 mOsm/L are best infused in the central circulation where greater blood flow provides adequate hemodilution (Perucca, 2010). For example, total parenteral nutrition (TPN) solutions have an osmolarity greater than 1400 mOsm/L. TPN should not be infused in peripheral circulation because it can damage blood cells and the endothelial lining of the veins and decrease PERFUSION.

> **! NURSING SAFETY PRIORITY** (QSEN)
> **Drug Alert**
>
> Drugs such as amiodarone (Cordarone), vancomycin (Vancocin), and ciprofloxacin (Cipro I.V.) are venous irritants that have a pH less than 5. Phlebitis occurs when patients require long-term infusion of these drugs in peripheral circulation. Drugs with vasoconstrictive action (e.g., dopamine or chemotherapeutic agents [e.g., vinblastine]) are vesicants (chemicals that damage body tissue on direct contact) that can cause extravasation. Extravasation results in severe TISSUE INTEGRITY impairment as manifested by blistering, tissue sloughing, or necrosis from infiltration into the surrounding tissues. (See Complications of Intravenous Therapy section on p. 204 for further explanation and Chapter 22 for more detail.) Monitor the IV insertion site carefully for early manifestations of infiltration, including swelling, coolness, or redness. If any of these symptoms are present, discontinue the drug immediately and notify the infusion therapy team, if available. If an infusion specialist is not available, plan to remove the IV catheter and consider central line placement.

Blood and Blood Components

Blood transfusion is given by using packed red blood cells, created by removing a large portion of the plasma from whole blood. Other available blood components include platelets, fresh frozen plasma, albumin, and several specific clotting factors. Each component has detailed requirements for blood-type compatibility and infusion techniques. For patient safety, The Joint Commission's (TJC) 2014 National Patient Safety Goals (NPSGs) require agencies to ensure that blood components are properly ordered, handled and dispensed, and administered and that patients are appropriately monitored. Positive patient identification using two patient identifiers and requiring two qualified health care professionals is essential before any blood or blood component is administered.

Most organizations use the International Society of Blood Transfusion (ISBT) universal bar-coding system to ensure the right blood for the right patient (Fig. 13-1). The ISBT system includes four components that must be present on the blood label both in bar code and in eye-readable format. These four components are (1) a unique facility identifier, (2) the lot number relating to the donor, (3) the product code, and (4) the ABO group and Rh type of the donor.

An acute hemolytic transfusion reaction caused by an incompatible blood transfusion is a "sentinel event." The Joint Commission defines a sentinel event as an unexpected occurrence involving serious physical or psychological injury or

FIG. 13-1 Unit of blood showing the International Society of Blood Transfusion (ISBT) universal bar code for blood transfusions.

the risk thereof and requiring an intense analysis of the contributing factors and corrective action. As a measure to improve the quality of health care, The Joint Commission reviews organizations' activities in response to sentinel events. Established policies and procedures must be rigidly followed to ensure a safe transfusion and reduce the risk for complications. (See Chapter 40 for a complete discussion of blood transfusion administration.)

Drug Therapy

IV drugs provide a rapid therapeutic effect but can lead to immediate serious reactions, called **adverse drug events (ADEs)**. Hundreds of drugs are available for infusion by a variety of techniques. As with all drug administration, nurses must be knowledgeable about drug indications, proper dosage, contraindications, and precautions. IV administration also requires knowledge of appropriate dilution, rate of infusion, pH and osmolarity, compatibility with other IV medications, appropriate infusion site (peripheral versus central circulation), potential for vesicant/irritant effects, and specific aspects of patient monitoring because of its immediate effect. *Regardless of familiarity with the drug, never assume that IV administration is the same as giving that drug by other routes.* New information is continuously being published, and new drugs are rapidly being introduced.

Medication safety is extremely important in all health care settings today. The Joint Commission's 2014 NPSGs include as a major goal improving the safety of high-alert drugs. An example of these drugs is concentrated electrolyte solutions (e.g., potassium chloride), which require restricted access, prominent warnings about the concentration, and storage in a secured location.

Procedures must be established to prevent errors resulting from look-alike, sound-alike drugs such as Celebrex IV (celecoxib) and Cerebyx (fosphenytoin). Other strategies to reduce errors include limiting available concentrations of drugs and dispensing all drugs, including catheter flush solutions, in single-dose containers. Smart pumps with drug libraries (see Infusion Systems section), in combination with computer provider (physician, nurse practitioner, physician assistant) order

entry (CPOE) and bar code medication administration (BCMA) systems, use recent technology to help reduce adverse drug events (ADEs). Electronic medication administration records (MARs) and multiple checks by pharmacists, as required by The Joint Commission's NPSGs, also help reduce errors.

Prescribing Infusion Therapy

A prescription for infusion therapy written by an authorized provider (physician, nurse practitioner, or physician assistant) is necessary before IV therapy begins. To be complete, the prescription for infusion fluids should include:

- Specific type of fluid
- Rate of administration written in milliliters per hour (mL/hr) or the total amount of fluid and the total number of hours for infusion (e.g., 125 mL/hr or 1000 mL/8 hr)
- Drugs and the specific dose to be added to the solution, such as electrolytes or vitamins

A drug prescription should include:

- Drug name, preferably by generic name
- Specific dose and route
- Frequency of administration
- Time of administration
- Length of time for infusion
- Purpose (required in some health care agencies, especially nursing homes)

Some continuously infused drugs, such as those for pain management, are prescribed as milligrams per hour. The type and volume of dilution for infusion medications may be included in the prescription or calculated by the infusion pharmacist.

❗ NURSING SAFETY PRIORITY (QSEN)

Action Alert

Determine that the IV prescription is appropriate for the patient and clarify any questions with the health care provider before administration. Be sure to check for the accuracy and completeness of the treatment prescription. An example of an incomplete one is "5% dextrose in water to keep the vein open" (TKO or KVO). This statement does not specify the rate of infusion and is not considered complete.

Vascular Access Devices

An infusion catheter, also known as a **vascular access device (VAD)**, is a plastic tube placed in a blood vessel to deliver fluids and medications. This catheter should not be confused with the ventricular assist device also called a VAD. In this chapter, VAD refers to vascular access devices. The specific type and purpose of the therapy determine whether the infusion can be given safely through peripheral veins or if the large central veins of the chest are needed. Advances in catheter materials and insertion techniques have radically expanded the types of VADs currently used. This discussion includes the description of each type of catheter used for peripheral and central IV therapy. Seven major types are described:

- Short peripheral catheters
- Midline catheters
- Peripherally inserted central catheters (PICC)
- Nontunneled percutaneous central venous catheters (CVCs)
- Tunneled catheters
- Implanted ports
- Hemodialysis catheters

Assess the patient's needs for vascular access, and choose the device that has the best chance of infusing the prescribed therapy for the required length of time. Depending on the patient and type of VAD to be inserted, a topical anesthetic agent or intradermal lidocaine HCl 1% may be helpful to decrease patient discomfort. Obtain a health care provider's order and check for patient allergies before administering any anesthetic.

💡 NCLEX EXAMINATION CHALLENGE
Safe and Effective Care Environment

A client receiving ciprofloxacin intravenously reports that the peripheral IV insertion site has become painful and reddened. In what order will the nurse perform the needed actions to manage this problem?
A. Report the patient's problem to the health care provider.
B. Document findings and actions in the electronic health record.
C. Change the IV insertion site to a new location.
D. Stop the infusion of the drug immediately.

PERIPHERAL INTRAVENOUS THERAPY

Short infusion catheters are the most commonly used vascular access devices (VADs) for **peripheral IV therapy**. They are usually placed in the veins of the arm. Another catheter used for peripheral IV therapy is a midline catheter.

Short Peripheral Catheters

Short peripheral catheters are composed of a plastic cannula built around a sharp stylet extending slightly beyond the cannula (Fig. 13-2). The stylet (sharp) allows for the venipuncture, and the cannula is advanced into the vein. Once the cannula is advanced into the vein, the stylet is withdrawn. These catheters are designed with a safety mechanism to cover the sharp end of the stylet after it is removed from the patient. The stylet is a hollow-bore, blood-filled needle that carries a high risk for exposure to bloodborne pathogens if needle stick injury occurs. A federal law enacted in 2000 amended the Bloodborne Pathogen Standards from the Occupational Safety and Health Administration (OSHA) requiring the use of catheters with an engineered safety mechanism to prevent needle sticks.

Insertion and Placement Methods

Short peripheral catheters are most often inserted into superficial veins of the forearm using sterile technique. In emergent situations, these catheters can be used also in the external jugular vein of the neck. *Avoid the use of veins in the lower extremities of adults, if possible, because of an increased risk for deep vein thrombosis and infiltration.*

Short catheters range in length from ¾ inch to 1¼ inch with gauge sizes from 26 gauge (the smallest) to 14 gauge (large

bore). *Choose the smallest gauge catheter capable of delivering the prescribed therapy.* Current design improves the fluid flow through the catheter while using a smaller gauge and thereby decreases the possibility of vein irritation from a large catheter. For example, a thin-walled 24-gauge Insyte catheter has about the same flow-rate ability as a 22-gauge non–thin-walled Angiocath. Larger gauge sizes allow for faster flow rates but also cause phlebitis more often. Table 13-1 lists each gauge size and its common uses.

The current recommendations for dwell (stay in) time of short peripheral catheters do not include a specific time frame. The recommendations from both the CDC and the INS are that the catheter should be removed and/or rotated to a different site based on clinical indications (e.g., signs of phlebitis [warmth, tenderness, erythema or palpable venous cord], infection, or malfunction) (CDC, 2011; INS, 2011). This process requires conscientious and frequent assessment of the site. However, if the patient's therapy is expected to be longer than 6 days, a midline catheter or PICC should be chosen (O'Grady et al., 2011). When selecting the site for insertion of a peripheral catheter, consider the patient's age, history, and diagnosis; the type and duration of the prescribed therapy; and, whenever possible, the patient's preference. Chart 13-1 lists the major criteria for the placement of peripheral VADs.

Vein transilluminators and ultrasound devices are now available as tools to assist in IV line placement. Several different types of portable *vein transilluminators* are available, such as VeinViewer, Veinlite LED, and AccuVein AV 300 (Fig. 13-3). Although they may have different mechanisms of action (some use infrared light and some use laser), these devices penetrate only up to about 10 mm and are limited to finding superficial veins.

FIG. 13-2 BD Insyte Autoguard IV catheter. With the push of a button, the needle instantly retracts, reducing the risk for accidental needle stick injuries.

TABLE 13-1	Choosing the Gauge Size for Peripheral Catheters	
CATHETER GAUGE	**INDICATIONS**	**APPROXIMATE FLOW RATES**
24-26 gauge Smallest, shortest (¾-inch length)	Not ideal for viscous infusions Expect blood transfusion to take longer Preferred for infants and small children	24 mL/min (1440 mL/hr)
22 gauge	Adequate for most therapies; blood can infuse without damage	38 mL/min (2280 mL/hr)
20 gauge (1-1¼-inch length)	Adequate for all therapies Most providers of anesthesia prefer not to use a smaller size than this for surgery cases	65 mL/min (3900 mL/hr)
18 gauge	Preferred size for surgery Vein needs to be large enough to accommodate the catheter	110 mL/min (6600 mL/hr)
14-16 gauge	For trauma and surgical patients requiring rapid fluid resuscitation Needs to be in a vein that can accommodate it	

Ultrasound-guided peripheral IV insertion can allow insertion into deeper veins (White et al., 2010). This technology has been shown to be very valuable in assisting with cannulation of peripheral veins that the nurse cannot access with sight and touch. However, there are risks the nurse must be aware of when using ultrasound guidance. This technology should be used only by nurses who have been trained and whose competencies are maintained. Arteries and nerves lie parallel to deep veins, and training is needed to learn to identify these structures and avoid damaging them. In addition, when deeper veins are accessed, infiltration may go undetected until a significant amount of fluid has collected in the tissues. This complication can be particularly devastating if the solution is an irritant or vesicant.

CHART 13-1   Best Practice for Patient Safety & Quality Care (QSEN)

Placement of Short Peripheral Venous Catheters

- Verify that the prescription for infusion therapy is complete and appropriate for infusion through a short peripheral catheter.
- For adults, choose a site for placement in the upper extremity. DO NOT USE THE WRIST.
- Choose the patient's nondominant arm when possible.
- Choose a distal site, and make all subsequent venipunctures proximal to previous sites.
- Do not use the arm on the side of a mastectomy, lymph node dissection, arteriovenous shunt or fistula, or paralysis.
- Avoid choosing a site in an area of joint flexion.
- Avoid choosing a site in a vein that feels hard or cordlike.
- Avoid choosing a site close to areas of cellulitis, dermatitis, or complications from previous catheter sites.
- Choose a vein of appropriate length and width to fit the size of the catheter required for infusion.

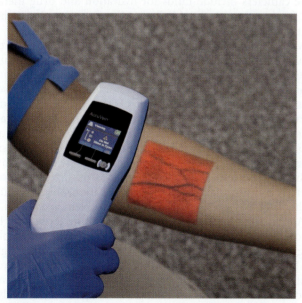

FIG. 13-3 The AccuVein AV300 is a vein illumination device that helps health care professionals locate veins for blood draw, IV infusion, and blood donation by projecting a pattern of light on the patient's skin to reveal the position of underlying veins on the skin's surface. The device uses red and infrared light, which the hemoglobin in blood absorbs to detect the position of the vein.

For patients who need IV access but are at risk for fluid overload or do not need extra IV fluids, the peripheral vascular access device (VAD) can be converted into an intermittent IV lock, also called a *saline lock*. This device allows administration of specific drugs given IV push (e.g., furosemide [Lasix, Furoside ✦]) or on an intermittent basis using a medication administration set. IV antibiotics are frequently given this way. In some cases, the saline lock is placed in case there is a need for emergency drug administration via IV push. The intermittent device is flushed with saline before and after drug administration to ensure patency and prevent occlusion with a blood clot.

Site Selection and Skin Preparation

The most appropriate veins for peripheral catheter placement include the dorsal venous network, basilic, cephalic, and median veins, as well as their branches (Fig. 13-4). *However, cannulation of veins on the hand is not appropriate for older patients with a loss of skin turgor and poor vein condition and for active patients receiving infusion therapy in an ambulatory care clinic or home care. Use of veins on the dorsal surface of the hands should be reserved as a last resort for short-term infusion of non-vesicant and non-irritant solutions in young patients.*

Mastectomy, axillary lymph node dissection, lymphedema, paralysis of the upper extremity, and the presence of dialysis grafts or fistulas alter the normal pattern of blood flow through the arm. Using veins in the extremity affected by these conditions requires a physician's request. Short peripheral catheters are not recommended for obtaining routine blood samples.

⚠ NURSING SAFETY PRIORITY (QSEN)

Critical Rescue

Avoid veins on the palmar side of the wrist because the median nerve is located close to veins in this area, making the venipuncture more painful and difficult to stabilize. The cephalic vein begins above the thumb and extends up the entire length of the arm. This vein is usually large and prominent, appearing as a prime site for catheter insertion. Damage to the nerve from any injury can result in permanent loss of function or complex regional pain syndrome, type 2 (CRPS) (Watts & Kremer, 2011). Reports of tingling, feeling "pins and needles" in the extremity, or numbness during the venipuncture procedure can indicate nerve puncture. If any of these symptoms occur, stop the IV insertion procedure immediately, remove the catheter, and choose a new site.

Winged needles ("butterfly needles") are easy to insert but are associated with a high frequency of infiltration. They are most commonly used for injection of single-dose drugs or for drawing blood samples. Like a short peripheral catheter, winged needles should also have an engineered safety mechanism to house the needle when removed.

Aseptic skin preparation and technique before IV insertion are crucial. Catheter-related bloodstream INFECTION (CR-BSI) can occur from a peripheral IV site. The CDC recommendations include:

- Perform evidence-based hand hygiene before palpating the insertion site.
- Clip hair—do not shave.
- Ensure that skin is clean. If visibly soiled, cleanse with soap and water.
- Wear clean gloves for peripheral IV insertion; do not touch the access site after application of antiseptics.

FIG. 13-4 Common IV sites in the inner arm.

FIG. 13-5 Midline catheter; the tip of this catheter resides in a peripheral vein.

- Prepare clean skin with a skin antiseptic (chlorhexidine 2% with 70% alcohol, 70% isopropyl alcohol, or povidone-iodine) using a back-and-forth motion for 30 seconds, and allow the solution to dry before peripheral venous catheter insertion.

Midline Catheters

Midline catheters can be anywhere from 3 to 8 inches long, 3 to 5 Fr, and double or single lumen. They are inserted through the veins of the upper arm. The median antecubital vein is used most often if insertion is done without the aid of ultrasound guidance. With ultrasound guidance, deeper veins can be accessed and the insertion site can be further above the antecubital fossa. The basilic vein is preferred over the cephalic vein because of its larger diameter and straighter path. It also allows greater hemodilution of the fluids and medications being infused. The catheter tip is located in the upper arm with the tip residing no further into the venous network than the axillary vein (Fig. 13-5). These catheters are used for therapies lasting from 1 to 4 weeks; however, there are no recommendations for the optimal dwell time. In a 2014 study, the average dwell time for midlines was identified as 6.9 days (Dumont, Getz, & Miller, 2014). Because of the extended dwell time, strict sterile technique is used for insertion and dressing changes for a midline catheter. Additional education and skill assessment are required for the nurse to be qualified to insert midline catheters.

Midline catheters have been found to reduce the number of repeated IV cannulations, which reduces patient discomfort, increases patient satisfaction, and contributes to organizational

efficiency (Alexandrou et al., 2011). A midline catheter can be used when skin integrity or limited peripheral veins make it difficult to maintain a short peripheral catheter. Indications for these catheters include fluids for hydration and drug therapy that is given longer than 6 days and up to 4 weeks, such as antibiotics, heparin, steroids, and bronchodilators.

Midline catheters are considered to dwell in the peripheral circulation; the recommendations for infusates (fluids or drugs) are the same as for short peripheral IVs. Fluids and medications infused through a midline catheter should have a pH between 5 and 9 and a final osmolarity of less than 600 mOsm/L (Perucca, 2010). The pH and osmolarity outside these parameters increase the risk for complications like phlebitis and thrombosis. Midline catheters should not be used for infusion of vesicant medications—drugs that cause severe tissue damage if they escape into the subcutaneous tissue (extravasation). There is concern that at a midline tip location, larger amounts of the drug may extravasate before the problem is detected.

All parenteral nutrition formulas, including those with low concentrations of dextrose, and solutions that have an osmolarity greater than 600 mOsm/L should not be infused through a midline catheter. Do not draw blood from these catheters routinely. Midline catheters should not be placed in extremities affected by mastectomy with lymphedema, paralysis, or dialysis grafts and fistulas. When using a double-lumen midline catheter, do not administer incompatible drugs simultaneously through both lumens because the blood flow rate in the axillary vein is not high enough to ensure adequate hemodilution and prevention of drug interaction in the vein.

A new midline, PowerGlide, has been developed by Bard Access Systems. This catheter is approved for power injection of 5 mL/sec for computed tomography (CT) scans (Bard, 2013). There is no evidence in the literature to date on the efficacy of this practice.

CENTRAL INTRAVENOUS THERAPY

In **central IV therapy,** the vascular access device (VAD) is placed in the central circulation, specifically within the superior vena cava (SVC) near its junction with the right atrium, also called the *caval-atrial junction (CAJ).* Blood flow in the SVC is about 2 L/min compared with about 200 mL/min in the axillary vein. Most central vascular access devices require confirmation of tip location at the CAJ by chest radiograph before solutions are infused. However, newer technologies use either a magnet tip locator or identification of the CAJ by electrocardiogram rather than by x-ray. Both the Sherlock 3CG by Bard and the VasoNova/Teleflex systems have received Food and Drug Administration (FDA) approval as an alternative to chest x-ray or fluoroscopy to verify PICC tip location.

A number of types of central vascular access devices (CVADs) are available, depending on the purpose, duration, and insertion site availability. Several recent improvements in catheter materials allow antimicrobial and heparin coatings to reduce INFECTION risk and improve the longevity of the catheter. Not all central line catheters are approved for power injection used in radiologic tests. The catheter can rupture if it is not designed to handle the injection pressure necessary for some tests such as pulmonary CT angiography or CT angiography of the aorta (5 mL/sec and 300 per square inch [psi]). Check with the radiology department and read the indications on the packaging before using them for power injection (Macha et al., 2009).

Peripherally Inserted Central Catheters

A **peripherally inserted central catheter (PICC)** is a long catheter inserted through a vein of the antecubital fossa (inner aspect of the bend of the arm) or the middle of the upper arm. Nurses who insert these CVADs require special training and certification.

In adults, the PICC length ranges from 18 to 29 inches (45-74 cm) with the tip residing in the superior vena cava (SVC) ideally at the caval-atrial junction (CAJ) (Fig. 13-6). Placement of the catheter tip in veins distal to the SVC is avoided. This inappropriate tip location, often called a *mid-clavicular catheter,* is associated with much higher rates of thrombosis than when the tip is located in the SVC at the CAJ. Mid-clavicular tip locations are used only when anatomic or pathophysiologic changes prohibit placing the catheter into the SVC.

PICCs should be inserted early in the course of therapy before veins of the extremity have been damaged from multiple venipunctures and infusions. Insertion methods using

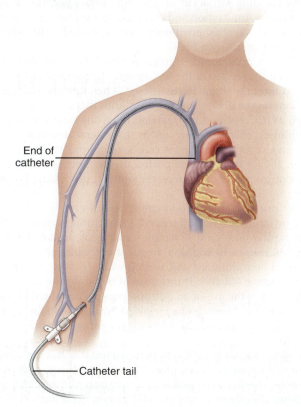

FIG. 13-6 Peripherally inserted central catheter (PICC) is placed peripherally in a vein of the upper arm with the tip resting in the superior vena cava.

guidewires and ultrasound systems greatly improve insertion success. The basilic vein is the preferred site for insertion; the cephalic vein can be used if necessary. Two brachial veins are not recommended because they are more difficult to access; they are deeper in the arm and run close to the brachial artery. *Sterile technique is used for insertion to reduce the risk for catheter-related bloodstream INFECTION (CR-BSI). Before the catheter can be used for infusion, a chest x-ray indicating that the tip resides in the lower SVC is required when the catheter is not placed under fluoroscopy or with the use of the electrocardiogram tip locator technique.*

PICCs are available in single-, dual-, or triple-lumen configurations and are available with both the Groshong valve and the pressure-activated safety valve (PASV). PICCs are also available as "Power PICCs" and can be used for contrast injection at a maximum of 5 mL/sec and a maximum pressure of 300 psi. They can also be connected to transducers and used to monitor central venous pressure (Bard Access Systems, 2011).

The most common complications from PICCs include phlebitis, thrombophlebitis, deep vein thrombosis (DVT), and CR-BSIs. Thrombophlebitis and DVT can be very serious, threaten the integrity of the vein, and decrease PERFUSION. The smallest possible French size should be used to decrease the rate of upper extremity DVT, a potentially life-threatening event.

CR-BSI has been noted to be less common in PICCs than in other central venous catheters (CVCs) because of the insertion site in the upper extremity. The cooler, drier skin of the upper arm has fewer types and numbers of microorganisms, leading to lower rates of INFECTION. Accidental arterial puncture or excessive bleeding can occur on insertion and is controlled by direct pressure. Infiltration and extravasation are rare. Insertion complications such as pneumothorax associated with other CVCs do not occur with PICCs.

PICCs can accommodate infusion of all types of therapy because the tip resides in the SVC where the rapid blood flow quickly dilutes the fluids being infused. Therefore there are no limitations on the pH or osmolality of fluids that can be infused through a PICC. For example, patients requiring lengthy courses of antibiotics, chemotherapy agents, parenteral nutrition formulas, and vasopressor agents can benefit from this type of catheter. PICCs have been reported to dwell successfully for months or even years; however, the optimal dwell time is not known.

PICCs can be used for blood sampling; however, lumen sizes of 4 Fr or larger are recommended. Using lumens with small diameters may not yield a sample capable of producing the needed test results. In addition, frequent entry into any central line should be minimized and treated with strict aseptic technique to prevent CR-BSI. Transfusion of blood through a PICC usually requires the use of an infusion pump. Packed red blood cells are cold and viscous. The length of the catheter adds resistance and may prevent the blood from infusing within the 4-hour limit.

Teach patients with a PICC to perform usual ADLs; however, they should avoid excessive physical activity. Muscle contractions in the arm from physical activity like heavy lifting can lead to catheter dislodgment and possible lumen occlusion. PICCs may be contraindicated in paraplegic patients who rely on their arms for mobility and in patients using crutches that provide support in the axilla.

PICC insertion is commonly performed in the patient's hospital room, an ambulatory care treatment facility, or the imaging department. Regardless of where they are inserted, the same precautions must be taken as with any other central line insertion using the catheter-related bloodstream INFECTION (CR-BSI) prevention bundle. Major components of this prevention bundle include:

- Hand hygiene
- Maximal barrier precautions upon insertion
- Chlorhexidine skin antisepsis
- Optimal catheter site selection and post-placement care with avoidance of the femoral vein for central venous access in adult patients
- Daily review of line necessity with prompt removal of unnecessary lines

Other helpful interventions include use of a check list for sterility during the procedure, a line cart with all equipment, and a stop sign on the door of the room to stop unnecessary traffic through the room during the procedure.

> **! NURSING SAFETY PRIORITY** (QSEN)
>
> ***Action Alert***
>
> The INS recommendation for flushing PICC lines not actively used is 5 mL of heparin (10 units/mL) in a 10-mL syringe at least daily when using a non-valved catheter and at least weekly with a valved catheter. Use 10 mL of sterile saline to flush before and after medication administration; 20 mL of sterile saline is flushed after drawing blood. *Always use 10-mL barrel syringes to flush any central line because the pressure exerted by a smaller barrel poses a risk for rupturing the catheter.*

Nontunneled Percutaneous Central Venous Catheters

Nontunneled percutaneous central venous catheters (CVCs) are inserted by a physician, trained physician assistant, or nurse practitioner through the subclavian vein in the upper chest or the internal jugular veins in the neck using sterile technique. Occasionally the patient's condition may require insertion of the CVC in a femoral vein, but the rate of infection is very high. If the femoral site must be used, it is removed as soon as possible.

CVCs are usually 7 to 10 inches (18 to 25 cm) long and have one to as many as five lumens (Fig. 13-7). These catheters are also available with antimicrobial coatings such as chlorhexidine and silver sulfadiazine. The tip resides in the superior vena cava (SVC) and is confirmed by a chest x-ray. Nontunneled percutaneous CVCs are most commonly used for emergent or trauma situations, critical care, and surgery. There is no recommendation for optimal dwell time. However, these catheters are commonly used for short-term situations and are *not* the catheter of choice for home care or ambulatory clinic settings.

Insertion of these central catheters requires the patient to be placed in the Trendelenburg position, usually with a rolled towel between the shoulder blades. This position may be difficult or contraindicated for patients with respiratory conditions, spinal curvatures, and increased intracranial pressure, especially for older adults. Trauma, surgery, or radiation in the neck or chest prohibits the use of these devices as well. Insertion with ultrasound guidance has been demonstrated to

FIG. 13-7 The Edwards Lifesciences PreSep central venous catheter (CVC); often placed in the subclavian or internal jugular vein with the tip of the catheter resting in the superior vena cava.

improve the safety of insertion in the internal jugular site (Griswold-Theodorson et al., 2009). The presence of a tracheotomy increases the risk for cross-contamination of the insertion site. The warmer, moister skin of the neck and upper chest has more types and higher numbers of microorganisms, resulting in more CR-BSIs with this type of catheter.

Tunneled Central Venous Catheters

Tunneled central venous catheters are VADs that have a portion of the catheter lying in a subcutaneous tunnel, separating the points where the catheter enters the vein from where it exits the skin. This separation is intended to prevent the organisms on the skin from reaching the bloodstream (Fig. 13-8). Today these catheters are usually inserted by physicians in the radiology suite, rather than placed surgically. The catheter has a cuff made of a rough material that is positioned inside the subcutaneous tunnel. These cuffs commonly contain antibiotics, which also reduce the risk for INFECTION. The tissue granulates into the cuff, providing a mechanical barrier to microorganisms and anchoring the catheter in place.

The design of tunneled CVCs requires surgical techniques for insertion and removal. Single-, dual-, and triple-lumens are available. These catheters were originally named for the physicians who designed them, including Broviac, Hickman, and Leonard catheters.

Tunneled catheters are used primarily when the need for infusion therapy is frequent and long-term. Patients needing parenteral nutrition for months, years, or the remainder of their life commonly choose a tunneled catheter. Tunneled catheters are also chosen when several weeks or months of infusion therapy are needed and a PICC is not a good choice. For example, paraplegic patients needing 6 to 8 weeks of antibiotics are not good candidates for a PICC because of the excessive use of the upper extremities for mobility. Some oncology patients may prefer a tunneled catheter instead of an implanted port

because they cannot tolerate the needle sticks required for accessing those devices.

Implanted Ports

Implanted ports are very different from other central vascular access devices (CVADs). This type of device is chosen for patients who are expected to require IV therapy for more than a year (Santolim et al., 2012). This device is typically inserted by a physician in the radiology department or by a surgeon in the operating suite. Implanted ports consist of a portal body, a dense septum over a reservoir, and a catheter. They can be single- or double-lumen and come in various sizes. A subcutaneous pocket is surgically created to house the port body. The catheter is inserted into the vein and attached to the portal body. The septum is made of self-sealing silicone and is located in the center of the port body over the reservoir; the catheter extends from the side of the port body. The incision is closed, and no part of the catheter is visible externally; therefore this device has the least impact on body image (Fig. 13-9).

Some implanted ports are power-injectable and can be used for obtaining contrast-enhanced computed tomography (CECT). These devices can withstand 5 mL/sec at up to 300 psi pressure. The BARD PowerPort can be identified by palpation of three bumps on the top of the septum and a triangular-shaped port. Be careful not to press firmly on the bumps because it can be painful to the patient. Be sure to use a power-injection–rated noncoring needle with this type of port when it is used for this purpose. These needles come with labeling identifying that they are power-injection rated (Fig. 13-10).

Venous ports may be placed on the upper chest or the upper extremity. The venous catheter may enter either the subclavian or internal jugular vein. Although an implanted port is most commonly used in the venous system, the catheter may be placed in arteries, the epidural space, or the peritoneal cavity, with the port pocket located over a bony prominence.

Implanted ports are accessed by using a noncoring needle (a common brand name is *Huber*) that is specially designed with a deflected tip. This design slices through the dense septum

FIG. 13-8 Tunneled catheter. A portion of this catheter lies in a subcutaneous tunnel, separating the point where the catheter enters the vein from where it exits the skin.

FIG. 13-9 Positioning of an implanted port.

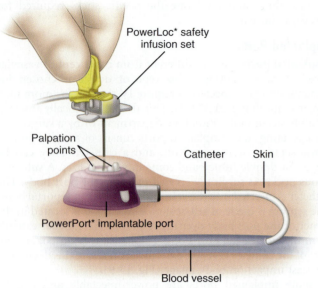

PowerLoc* safety
infusion set

Palpation
points

Catheter   Skin

PowerPort* implantable port

Blood vessel

FIG. 13-10 A noncoring needle for accessing an implanted powerport.

without coring out a small piece of it, thus preserving the integrity of the septum. Port bodies placed in the chest have a larger septum and usually tolerate about 2000 punctures. Port bodies placed in the upper extremity are smaller and are rated to tolerate about 750 punctures.

Port access should be done only by formally trained health care professionals using a mask and aseptic technique. Implanted ports are used most often for patients receiving chemotherapy. These patients are immune-compromised making them highly susceptible to INFECTION. Before puncture, palpate the port to locate the septum. Carefully palpate to feel the shape and depth of the port body to ensure puncture of the septum, not the attached catheter. Some have attached extension sets and wings to stabilize the needle. One important feature is an engineered safety mechanism to contain the needle when it is removed from the septum. Because the dense septum holds tightly to the needle, there can be a rebound when it is pulled from the septum, which can result in needle stick injury to the nurse.

Implanted ports need to be flushed after each use and at least once a month between courses of therapy. This procedure is done to prevent clot formation in the internal chamber of the port and is often referred to as "locking" or "de-accessing." The INS recommendation for locking or de-accessing a port is 5 mL of 100 units heparin/mL (INS, 2011). When the port is not accessed, there is no external catheter requiring a dressing. Puncture of the skin over the port is required to gain access to the port body, causing pain for some patients. Topical anesthetic creams can be used to make the access procedure more tolerable.

> **⚠ NURSING SAFETY PRIORITY** (QSEN)
> ### *Drug Alert*
>
> Before giving a drug through an implanted port, always check for blood return. If there is no blood return, withhold the drug until patency and adequate noncoring needle placement of the port are established. Serious extravasations of vesicant drugs can occur because a fibrin sheath (flap or tail) may occur at the tip of the catheter, clot it, and cause retrograde subcutaneous leakage.

Hemodialysis Catheters

Hemodialysis catheters have very large lumens to accommodate the hemodialysis procedure or a pheresis procedure that harvests specific blood cells. They may be tunneled for long-term needs or nontunneled for short-term needs. A hemodialysis catheter is critical to the management of renal failure and must function well. CR-BSIs and vein thrombosis are common problems; therefore this catheter should not be used for administration of other fluids or drugs except in an emergency.

The concentration of heparin used to lock hemodialysis catheters ranges from 1,000 to 10,000 units/mL. Researchers have demonstrated that using 1,000 units/mL reduces the incidence of postinsertion bleeding but may be associated with an increased need for recombinant tissue plasminogen activator (tPA) to maintain patency. A flush of 1,000 units heparin/mL or a solution of 4% sodium citrate in the amount of the dwell volume of each lumen has been recommended (Moran & Ash, 2008). Heparin is most often used because sodium citrate has not been as commercially available in the preparation needed. To prevent systemic anticoagulation and subsequent bleeding, be sure to aspirate the heparin from the lumens before use.

INFUSION SYSTEMS

Nurses administering infusion therapies need to understand how infusion systems work. This knowledge ensures that the patient can benefit from a particular system's advantages while minimizing any potential complications.

Containers

Infusion containers are made of glass or plastic. *Glass* bottles were the original fluid container to be mass produced. They are easily sterilized, and it is easy to read the amount of fluid remaining in the bottle. Also, glass is inert and so cannot interact with some drugs like plastic can. However, glass bottles are heavy and cannot easily be used in many situations, such as patient transport during emergencies. These containers require an air vent for fluids to flow freely from them. The most common method is to use an administration set with a special filtered vent. Some bottles may have a straw tube open to the room air through the rubber stopper in the bottle and extending to above the level of the fluid. Bottles with a venting straw do not have a barrier to prevent contaminants in the air from entering the fluid.

Plastic containers are considered *closed systems* because they do not rely on outside air to allow the fluid to infuse. Instead, atmospheric pressure pushes against the flexible sides of the container, allowing the fluid to flow by gravity. For this reason, plastic containers do not require vented administration sets. These containers are lightweight, resistant to breaking, easier to store, and easy to use in emergency conditions. Therefore they are used more frequently than glass containers.

All plastic containers were commonly made of polyvinyl chloride (PVC). To increase flexibility and strength, PVC required the addition of a plasticizer, such as di-2-ethylhexylphthalate or DEHP. Concern has been growing in the past few years over the exposure of patients to this chemical because it can leach from the plastic fluid container or tubing and infuse into the patient with the IV fluid or medication. The FDA has determined that there is little to no risk posed to most patients by exposure to the amount of DEHP released from IV bags with infusion of crystalloids or drugs. However, there is concern about the buildup of chemical exposure from many sources over a lifetime and specifically the potential effects of DEHP on the development of the male reproductive system. Therefore many hospitals are using PVC-free and DEHP-free IV bags, especially for high-risk groups.

One disadvantage of removing DEHP from the plastic bags is that the bags are less pliable and more prone to rupture. Some institutions do not allow these bags to be sent through a pneumatic tube system because the pressure exerted has caused the bags to rupture during transport.

A problem with plastic containers is that they are not compatible with insulin, nitroglycerin, lorazepam (Ativan), fat emulsions, and lipid-based drugs. Nitroglycerin and insulin adhere to the walls of the PVC container, making it impossible to know exactly how much medication the patient is receiving. There is evidence that a priming volume of 20 mL of insulin solution is required to minimize the effect of insulin absorption losses to the plastics in IV lines (Thompson et al., 2012).

Another concern with plastic bags is the accuracy of reading the amount of fluid remaining in the container. The middle graduations have been shown to be 10% above or below the actual amount of fluid, but the first and last markings could be inaccurate by as much as 40% (Perucca, 2010).

NURSING SAFETY PRIORITY (QSEN)
Action Alert

Regardless of the type of fluid container being used, check it for cracks or pinholes before use. Always observe the fluid for **turbidity** (cloudiness) or any unusual color that could indicate contamination.

Administration Sets

The administration set is the connection between the catheter and the fluid container. Numerous sets are available in many different configurations. The type and purpose of the infusion determine the type of administration set needed. Some sets are *generic*, meaning that they are appropriate for most infusions. Other sets are used for specific types of infusions, such as blood transfusion. Still others are *dedicated*, meaning that they must be used with a specific manufacturer's infusion controlling device. Information that describes their proper use is provided on the packaging of administration sets.

Secondary Administration Sets

A primary continuous administration set is used to infuse the primary IV fluid by either a gravity infusion or an electronic infusion pump. A short **secondary administration set**, also known as a **piggyback set**, is attached to the primary set at a Y–injection site and is used to deliver intermittent medications (Fig. 13-11). Directions and diagrams for use are typically on the packaging. Once attached, these sets should remain connected together as an infusion system. Primary and secondary continuous infusion administration sets used to infuse fluids other than parenteral nutrition, lipids, blood, or blood products should be changed no more frequently than every 96 hours (INS, 2011).

FIG. 13-11 Secondary IV administration set attached to the primary set at a Y-injection site.

Intermittent Administration Sets

When no primary continuous fluid is being infused, use an intermittent administration set to infuse multiple doses of medications through a catheter that has been capped with a needleless connection device. Remove the medication bag from the previous dose, and attach the new one. Remove the sterile cap covering the distal end of the set, and attach the set to the catheter. Because both ends of the set are being manipulated with each dose, the INS standards of practice state that this set should be changed every 24 hours. When the administration set is used for infusion of parenteral nutrition or lipid solution, change it every 24 hours. Change blood tubing within 4 hours; use new tubing to infuse propofol (Diprivan) every 6 to 12 hours (McGoldrick, 2010).

Administration sets are sterile in the fluid pathway and under the sterile caps on each end of the set. The set is not packaged as a completely sterile product and cannot be added to a sterile field. Careful attention is required to maintain sterility of the spike and the connection end of the tubing to prevent introduction of microorganisms into the catheter and bloodstream.

Add-on Devices

Several other types of add-on devices include short extension sets, injection caps, and filters. Extension sets may be packaged as a sterile product for adding to a sterile field; however, always check the product label for this information.

Administration sets have two ways to connect to the catheter hub: a slip lock or a Luer-Lok. The *slip lock* is a male end that slips into the female catheter hub. A *Luer-Lok* connection has the same male end with a threaded collar that requires twisting onto the corresponding threads of the catheter hub. All connections, including *extension sets*, should have a Luer-Lok design to ensure that the set remains firmly connected. Loose connections lead to fluid leakage and increase the risk for contamination and subsequent bloodstream infection. When using a central venous catheter, a Luer-Lok connection is critical to reduce the risk for air embolism. Tape is not considered an adequate mechanism for securing set connections.

Luer-Lok devices may be purposefully or accidentally disconnected. Patients or visitors may disconnect the system to allow the patient to get out of bed or the chair. Or, the device may become accidentally disconnected when the patient turns or moves. In either case, be sure to reconnect the device by following the proper sequence to reassemble the IV system components. Fatalities have resulted when nurses have accidently reconnected IV tubing to a tracheostomy or other inappropriate port.

Filters may be part of the administration set or may be separate add-on pieces. Their purpose is to remove particulate matter, microorganisms, and air from the infusion system. Filter sizes depend on the pore size, with common sizes being 1.2 microns used to filter lipid-containing parenteral nutrition and 0.2 microns intended to remove all particles and bacteria. Filters should be placed as close to the catheter hub as possible.

Particulate matter in the IV fluid, a primary reason to use filters, comprises undissolved, unintended substances and may include rubber pieces, glass particles, cotton fibers, drug particles, paper, and metal fibers. These particles become trapped in the small circulation of the lungs. A red blood cell is about 5 microns in diameter and is the largest size that can pass through the pulmonary capillary bed; IV fluids may contain particles larger than 5 microns. For patients receiving infusion therapy for long periods, a significant number of particles could block the blood flow through the pulmonary circulation. Microcirculation in the spleen, kidneys, and liver could also be affected. Particulate matter has also been implicated in the development of phlebitis in peripheral veins.

Other concerns with using filters include the possibility for their rupture, their use with certain drugs that bind to the filter surface, using the incorrect size of filter for drugs with large molecules, and choosing a filter that will not tolerate the pressure exerted by infusion pumps. Rupture is most commonly associated with the exertion of high pressure exceeding the limit tolerated by the specific filter. Some drugs cannot be filtered because they are retained inside the filter because of their chemical nature or molecule size. For these reasons, medication filtration during the process of admixing is commonly used today as an alternative to final filtration at the bedside. Drugs of a very small quantity should be administered below the filter.

Filters used on blood administration sets have much larger pore size and are not interchangeable with filters used for fluids and medications. A standard blood filter ranges from 170 to 260 microns and removes microclots and other debris caused by blood collection and storage. Microaggregate filters have a pore size of 20, 40, or 80 microns and are used to remove degenerating platelets, white blood cells, and fibrin strands. Leukocyte-removal filters are used to remove white blood cells that cause febrile and allergic blood transfusion reactions.

Needleless Connection Devices

In July 1992, the Occupational Safety and Health Administration (OSHA) published guidelines entitled *Occupational Exposure to Bloodborne Pathogens, Final Rule.* This document requires health care organizations to initiate engineering controls "that isolate or remove the bloodborne pathogen hazard from the workplace." This standard was amended in 2001 with the passage of the Needlestick Safety and Prevention Act. This regulation requires the use of devices engineered with safety mechanisms and mandates that staff who perform these tasks be directly involved with selecting products. It also requires each employer to maintain a sharps injury log with details of each incident. Many products are designed to minimize health care workers' exposure to contaminated needles. Luer-activated devices are the most common design for needleless systems today.

Although these devices have reduced the incidence of accidental needle sticks for health care professionals, concern remains about a possible increase in the risk for catheter-related bloodstream infections (CR-BSIs) (Jarvis et al., 2009). This concern stems from the crevices created with the diaphragm and Luer-Lok design. Blood and bacteria can be trapped in the crevices, and meticulous cleaning is required with each use.

Various designs are available for connectors that provide positive or negative displacement of fluid when the needleless syringe is removed. Needleless positive-pressure valve (PPV) connectors were developed to prevent backflow of blood into the IV catheter, thereby decreasing chances of thrombus formation and CR-BSI. Several newer connectors are silver-impregnated to reduce bacterial growth (Fig. 13-12). Be sure to check which type of connector valve is used in your facility because the flushing technique differs depending on type. Researchers have found conflicting results about the relationships between these devices and CR-BSI and catheter occlusion (Khalidi et al., 2009; Mitchell et al., 2009; O'Grady et al., 2011).

Conclusive studies are needed to determine the best design for needleless systems. Until then, implement these interventions to reduce infection risk:

- Clean all needleless system connections vigorously with antimicrobial for 30 seconds (usually 70% alcohol or alcohol and 2% chlorhexidine swabs) before connecting infusion sets or syringes, paying special attention to the small ridges in the Luer-Lok device. There are newer caps that are impregnated with alcohol or chlorhexidine that may be used to keep the port aseptic; however, these will increase costs and research is needed to demonstrate the benefit.
- Do not tape connections between tubing sets.
- Use evidence-based hand hygiene guidelines from the CDC and OSHA

Rate-Controlling Infusion Devices

The ability to regulate the rate and volume of infusions is critical to the safe and accurate administration of medications and

FIG. 13-12 Example of a needleless connector.

fluids to patients. Nurses have a choice of numerous devices that can be electronically or mechanically regulated.

Electronic infusion devices (IV pumps) are used universally in acute care institutions. They are also used in long-term care settings and at home. In addition, "smart pumps" provide the latest infusion computer technology to promote patient safety and save nursing time. *Remember that the use of pumps does not decrease your responsibility to carefully monitor the patient's infusion site and the infusion rate.*

In inpatient settings, IV pumps are pole-mounted. As their name implies, these electronic devices with battery backup pump drugs or fluids under pressure. They accurately measure the volume of fluid being infused by using one of three mechanisms:

- A syringe-type mechanism that fills and empties
- A wavelike, peristaltic action that pushes fluid along the tubing
- A series of microchambers that fill and empty

Regardless of the pumping mechanism, these devices require dedicated cassette tubing designed to match the pump.

Syringe pumps use an electronic or battery-powered piston to push the plunger continuously at a selected milliliter-per-hour rate. The use of syringe pumps is limited to small-volume continuous or intermittent infusions and depends on the syringe size. Antibiotics and patient-controlled analgesia are frequently delivered with syringe pumps. Patients requiring fluid restrictions can also benefit from using a syringe pump because smaller yet accurate volumes can be used to dilute medications.

Ambulatory pumps are generally used for home care patients and allow them to return to their usual activities while receiving infusion therapy. These pumps have a wide range of sizes, with some requiring a backpack, but they usually weigh less than 6 pounds. They are typically used to accurately deliver continuous infusions, such as parenteral nutrition, pain medication, and many programmable drug schedules. Frequent battery recharging or replacement is usually necessary.

Electronic infusion devices can be programmed in many different ways and require a thorough knowledge of the specific brand being used. Infusion rate and the volume to be infused are usually entered in single milliliter increments, but some can be programmed as fractions of a milliliter. Some pumps allow the rate to be programmed to taper or ramp up and down at the beginning and ending of the infusion. Secondary syringe infusion, secondary infusion rate, remote site programming, adjustable infusion pressure, and integration into the nurse call system also are possible.

Electronic infusion devices have a variety of alarms, such as air-in-line, upstream and downstream occlusion, infusion complete, and low-battery or power warnings. All devices must have some mechanism to prevent free flow of the infusing fluid or medication. When the cassette or tubing is removed from the pump, this mechanism automatically stops fluid flow until it is properly replaced in the pump. This safety measure prevents accidental rapid infusion of large amounts of fluid or medication, which could lead to serious clinical problems.

In the past few years, **smart pumps** (infusion pumps with dosage calculation software) have been promoted to reduce adverse drug events (ADEs). Incorrect programming of pumps without this feature is one of the most common types of drug errors, especially in hospitals. Multiple libraries of drug information are stored in the pump manufacturer's medical management system. This software allows the facility to pre-program dosing limits, especially for high-alert drugs. Examples of smart pumps are the B. Braun Outlook 400ES and the Baxter Sigma Spectrum infusion system.

The newest development in smart pumps is a wireless network connection. Drug libraries can be updated via a wireless connection, thus eliminating the necessity of manually updating each pump. In addition to preventing drug errors, smart pump systems record potential errors that would have occurred without these safety mechanisms (Breland, 2010).

Dose-track technology is intended to transmit the infusion data to the institution's pharmacy so that the correct patient receives the correct medication. Dose-guard technology alerts the nurse if institution-defined dose limits are exceeded. These newer technologies provide safeguards for patients to keep them safe. However, the "smarter" the pump, the more extensive the programming steps are and the more alarms that the nurse must respond to. In addition, technology and wireless connections can fail. The challenge for nurses is to maintain the skill of manual dose calculation and rate control, to acknowledge and validate all alarms, and to guard against becoming desensitized to alarms.

Mechanically regulated devices can be used to deliver intermittent medications such as antibiotics or continuous pain medications in community-based health or home care settings. In acute care settings, devices called "infusers" may be found in surgical services. They are powered by positive pressure from the collapsing balloon or roller returning to its coiled position.

The systems include elastomeric balloons, spring-coiled syringes and containers, and a multi-chambered fluid container placed in a mechanical roller (Accufuser or On-Q PainBuster) (Fig. 13-13). These small portable devices do not require power sources such as batteries or electricity. They deliver a preset

FIG. 13-13 On-Q PainBuster pump (mechanical infuser).

infusion rate, and fluid volume is determined by the size of the fluid container; however, most hold only 50 to 100 mL.

NURSING CARE FOR PATIENTS RECEIVING INTRAVENOUS THERAPY

Educating the Patient

The current trend in health care demands that we partner with our patients to provide the best patient-centered care. In 2010, The Joint Commission added the requirement that all patients who have central lines placed in the hospital must have education on prevention of catheter-related bloodstream infection (CR-BSI). Before catheter insertion, educate the patient and family about:

- The type of catheter to be used
- Hand hygiene and aseptic technique for care of the catheter
- The therapy required
- Alternatives to the catheter and therapy
- Activity limitations
- Any signs or symptoms of complications that should be reported to a health care professional

Provide written information before placement of a long-term catheter, and continue to assess the patient's knowledge level and provide more information or answers as needed. Most manufacturers of PICCs, tunneled catheters, and implanted ports provide patient information booklets. However, specific information about the chosen procedures and supplies may be required. Conversation and pictures will be helpful for patients who are *literacy challenged* (have a low reading level ability).

Performing the Nursing Assessment

All central VADs require documentation of tip location at the CAJ by either electrocardiogram technology, fluoroscopy, or chest x-ray. The initial verbal and subsequent written report should contain specific information about the catheter tip location in relation to anatomic structures. The nurse's knowledge of accurate tip location is required before beginning infusion through the catheter. Repeating the x-ray during catheter use may be necessary if the patient reports unusual pain or sensation.

Nursing assessment for all infusion systems should be systematic. Begin with the insertion site and work upward, following the tubing. Know the type of catheter your patient has in place. Be sure to find out the length of catheter, the insertion site, and tip location to perform a complete assessment. Assess the insertion site by looking for redness, swelling, hardness, or drainage. Lightly palpate the area over the dressing. When a midline catheter or PICC is used, assess the entire extremity and upper chest for signs of phlebitis and thrombosis. When a tunneled catheter is used, assess the exit site, the entire length of the tunnel, and the point where the catheter enters the vein. For a well-healed catheter, it may not be possible to detect the vein entrance site. On newly inserted catheters, there could be a small puncture site with a suture or other securement device. For implanted ports, assess the incision and surgically created subcutaneous pocket.

Assess the integrity of the dressing, making sure it is clean, dry, and adherent to the skin on all sides. Check all connections on the administration set, and ensure that they are secure. Be sure they are not taped. Check the rate of infusion for all fluids by either counting drops or checking the infusion pump. Assess the amount of fluid that has infused from the container. Is it accurate, or is it infusing too fast or too slow? Adjust the rate to the prescribed flow rate. Check all labels on containers for the patient's name and fluid or medication. *Be sure that the correct solution is being infused!*

! NURSING SAFETY PRIORITY (QSEN)
Action Alert

Remind unlicensed assistive personnel (UAP) to avoid taking blood pressures in an extremity with any type of catheter in place. If a short peripheral catheter is being used for continuous infusion, the compression while taking the blood pressure can increase venous pressure, causing fluid to overflow from the puncture site and infiltration. When a midline catheter or PICC is being used, compression from the blood pressure cuff could increase vein irritation and lead to phlebitis.

Draw blood samples in the extremity opposite from all catheters. Blood should not be drawn from a venipuncture site proximal to (above) an infusing peripheral catheter because the infusing fluid could alter the results of the test to be performed. Venipuncture at or near the insertion site of a midline catheter or PICC could damage the catheter, add to areas of venous inflammation, and decrease PERFUSION.

Securing and Dressing the Catheter

Adequate catheter securement is vital to prevent many complications. Tape, sutures, and specially designed securement devices can be used for this purpose. For a short peripheral catheter, tape strips are most common; however, the tape should be *clean*. Tape strips from a peripheral IV start kit are preferred. Strips of tape should not be taken from rolls of tape moved between patient's rooms, from other procedures, or from uniform pockets. Precutting tape and placing it on the patient's bedrails, your uniform or scrubs, or other object should also be avoided to prevent infection.

Newer *securement devices* are designed for all catheter types and provide an evidence-based method to prevent VAD movement (INS, 2011). Recent studies have shown that these devices, such as the StatLock IV stabilization device, prevent peripheral and central catheters from becoming dislodged (Fig. 13-14) (see the Evidence-Based Practice box). In addition, they prevent complications like phlebitis and infiltration. To prevent skin tears, remove the adhesive on a StatLock with 70% alcohol.

PICCs and nontunneled percutaneous central catheters may be sutured in place; however, this creates additional breaks in the skin that could become infected. If these sutures are loose or broken, notify the health care provider to replace them. IV catheter sutures are being replaced with securement devices and Dermabond glue in some facilities, which can decrease infection and avoid the need to remove sutures after infusion therapy is discontinued.

Tunneled catheters usually have sutures placed near the skin exit site, which are removed after the tunnel has healed. The incision over an implanted port pocket will have sutures until it has healed. After it is healed and when it is not accessed, no dressing is required. When an implanted port is accessed, the sterile occlusive dressing should cover the entire needle and site.

Sterile dressings used over the insertion site protect the skin and puncture site. For a short *peripheral* catheter, the transparent membrane dressings do not require routine changes. Short peripheral lines do not usually dwell longer than a few days, and as long as the dressing is dry, clean, and intact, it does not have

FIG. 13-14 The StatLock provides a standardized method to prevent catheter movement.

EVIDENCE-BASED PRACTICE (QSEN)

What is the Best Method for Securing a Patient's Peripheral IV Line?

Alekseyev, S., Byrne, M., Carpenter, A., Franker, C., Kidd, C., & Hulton, L. (2012). Prolonging the life of a patient's IV: An integrative review of intravenous securement devices. *MEDSURG Nursing, 21*(5), 285-292.

Intravenous catheter stabilization is recognized as an important intervention to maintain peripheral IV therapy. The researchers sought to answer this clinical question: What is the best device or method for securing a patient's IV to preserve its integrity and prevent migration and loss of access? A thorough literature search for available research was performed, and 13 articles were identified as usable for this review. Twelve of the reported studies found that manufactured catheter stabilization devices were preferred over traditional tape and surgical strips methods. Although most studies included use of the StatLock anchoring device, no one securement device was recommended. Studies of the StatLock device showed that it significantly improved peripheral IV survival rates and reduced complication rates. These findings reduced health care costs and staff time.

Level of Evidence: 1

This study used an integrative research review and analysis methodology to determine best practices for use of IV securement devices.

Commentary: Implications for Practice and Research

This research validated the effectiveness of manufactured IV catheter securement and stabilization devices for all patients receiving peripheral infusion therapy. These devices reduce the need for IV restarts, IV complications, and costs associated with IV therapy. Future studies are needed to determine which device(s) are the best to standardize care of patients receiving peripheral infusion therapy.

2011). The initial dressing on a midline catheter or PICC is usually tape and gauze, changed within 24 hours after insertion because some bleeding is likely. Transparent membrane dressings can be used for subsequent dressing. For patients who develop erythema (redness) from Tegaderm, the IV3000 dressing from Smith and Nephew may be used. Document when you change the sterile dressing and your IV site assessments in the appropriate electronic health record according to agency policy.

⚠ NURSING SAFETY PRIORITY (QSEN)

Action Alert

Site protection may be needed for short peripheral catheters or for port access needles. Plastic shields can be placed over the site to prevent accidental bumping or pressure from clothing. Make sure you can easily assess the site frequently. Never place a restraint or opaque dressing over a peripheral IV site, especially when infusing an irritant or vesicant.

When changing the dressing, remove it by pulling laterally from side to side. It can also be removed by holding the external catheter and pulling it off toward the insertion site. *Never pull it off by pulling away from the insertion site because this could dislodge the catheter!*

After removing the dressing from a midline catheter or any central venous catheter, note the external catheter length. Compare this length with the original length at insertion. If the length has changed, the catheter tip location has also changed and may no longer be in a vein appropriate for infusion. Follow agency policy or notify the health care provider about the length change. A chest x-ray may be needed, and careful assessment of the type of therapy and remaining length of therapy will likely be required.

Protect the external catheter, dressing, and all attached tubing from water because it is a source of contamination. *Remind unlicensed assistive personnel (UAP) to cover the extremity where the IV is located when giving the patient a bath.* A plastic bag or wrap can be taped over the extremity to keep the dressing and site dry.

to be changed. Any VAD dressing should be changed when it is loose or soiled.

For central lines and midline catheters, tape and sterile gauze or a transparent membrane dressing may be used. Change tape and gauze dressings every 48 hours; change transparent membrane dressings, such as Tegaderm, every 5 to 7 days (INS,

? CLINICAL JUDGMENT CHALLENGE
Evidence-Based Practice; Safety (QSEN)

A new graduate nurse is being oriented to your medical-surgical nursing unit. Today he is assigned to care for three patients. One patient is an older adult with an infiltrated peripheral IV in her forearm. The second patient has a PICC line for antibiotic therapy, and the third patient has an arterial implanted port for chemotherapy. As his preceptor, you are responsible for teaching him how to assess patients with these devices and prevent and/or monitor for complications. Your unit has several memory checklists for IV care that you plan to review with him.

1. What best clinical practices will you teach the new nurse about how to care for patients who have a PICC line?
2. For what life-threatening complication is the patient with the implanted port most at risk?
3. You observe the new nurse as he prepares to restart the IV for the older adult patient. He chooses a vein in the dorsum of the hand. What is your best response about his IV site selection?
4. What is the value of memory checklists to ensure consistency among nurses caring for patients receiving IV therapy?

Changing Administration Sets and Needleless Connectors

Plan the change of administration sets and fluid containers to occur at the same time, if possible, to minimize the number of times the system is opened. For short peripheral catheters, the administration set and catheter should also be changed at the same time to avoid excessive manipulation of the catheter. Document these changes per agency policy.

Needleless connector devices can be changed when the administration set is changed. If it is being used for intermittent infusions, the device should be changed at least once per week. Fluid leakage from the device indicates the integrity has been compromised, and it should be changed immediately.

Precautions to prevent *air emboli* are required when changing the set or connectors attached to any catheter; however, central venous catheters require special attention. Most catheters have a pinch clamp that can be closed during this procedure. Techniques used to increase the intrathoracic pressure and prevent air embolism during IV set change include:

- Placing the patient in a flat or Trendelenburg position to ensure that the catheter exit site is at or below the level of the heart
- Asking the patient to perform a Valsalva maneuver by holding his or her breath and bearing down
- Timing the IV set change to the expiratory cycle when the patient is spontaneously breathing
- Timing the IV set change to the inspiratory cycle when the patient is receiving positive-pressure mechanical ventilation

Controlling Infusion Pressure

Fluid flow through the infusion system requires that the pressure on the external side be greater than the pressure at the catheter tip. Fluid flow can be slowed or obstructed by many causes. Inside the catheter lumen, resistance is created by the catheter length and diameter or by deposits of fibrin, thrombus, or drug precipitate. Near the catheter tip, resistance to flow comes from the catheter tip impinging on the vein wall, thrombus, or venous spasm.

All catheter manufacturers have warnings about the use of excessive pressure. Gravity and infusion pumps do not exert pressure too high for the catheter to handle; however, excessive pressure from syringes can lead to catheter damage. For this reason, use 10-mL syringes for central venous catheters. Although these larger syringes generate less pressure, it is still possible to reach excessive pressure levels if great force is applied against a syringe attached to a catheter that is partially occluded.

Flushing the Catheter

Catheter flushing prevents contact between incompatible drugs and maintains patency of the lumens. Normal saline alone or normal saline followed by heparinized saline may be used. When using valved catheters and certain positive fluid-displacement needleless devices, normal saline alone is acceptable because these devices have mechanisms that prevent the backflow of blood into the catheter lumen.

! NURSING SAFETY PRIORITY (QSEN)
Critical Rescue

Assess catheter patency carefully before each use. Use sterile technique to flush with normal saline while applying slow, gentle pressure to the syringe plunger. If you feel any resistance, stop the procedure immediately! If you continue, catheter rupture or forcing a blood clot into circulation could result. During the flushing procedure, always aspirate for a brisk blood return from the catheter lumen.

If the catheter will not yield a blood return, further diagnostic studies may be needed to determine the cause of the problems. Thrombolytic agents such as alteplase (Cathflo Activase) may be used to dissolve blood clots in venous catheters (Genentech, 2011).

For short peripheral catheters, usually 3 mL normal saline is adequate to flush the catheter. For all other catheters, 5 to 10 mL of preservative-free normal saline is needed. Bacteriostatic normal saline is limited to no more than 30 mL in a 24-hour period in adults. By using 10 mL before and after each dose of medication, it is easy to exceed this limitation. Check your agency's policy and procedure about specific flushing amounts.

Flush catheters immediately after each use. Delay in disconnecting the intermittent administration set and flushing the catheter could cause lumen occlusion from blood that backflows into the lumen when the infusion pressure is lower than venous pressure.

All fluids used to flush catheters should be obtained from single-dose containers or prefilled syringes. Vials used for multiple doses contribute to medication errors and increase the risk for contamination.

Obtaining Blood Samples from Central Venous Catheters

Short peripheral catheters should not be used routinely for obtaining blood samples. This additional manipulation could lead to vein irritation that requires removal of the catheter. Central venous catheters and midlines can be used for obtaining blood samples after a careful assessment of the risks versus the benefits. If your patient has no peripheral venipuncture sites or is fearful of needles, using the central venous catheter may be appropriate. The risks associated with obtaining blood samples from a central venous catheter are numerous. This procedure requires additional hub manipulation, which is a major cause of CR-BSI. Consider the laboratory tests needed and the types of fluids that have recently been infused. For

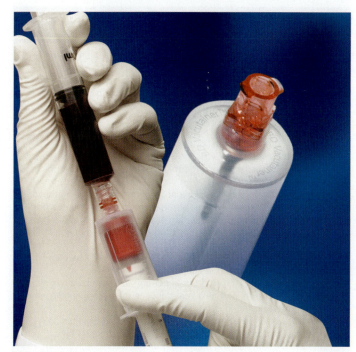

FIG. 13-15 Vacutainer needle holder prevents needle stick injuries when drawing blood.

example, heparin interferes with coagulation studies and electrolytes in the fluid may alter the results of serum electrolytes. Drawing blood from catheters for blood culture should not be done within an hour of completion of antimicrobial infusions (Garcia & Isenberg, 2010).

If blood sampling from a central venous catheter is the best alternative, vigorous cleaning of the connections with 70% alcohol is necessary. Use methods that do not require exposed needles. Vacuum tubes attached via a "vacutainer" to the catheter hub eliminate the need to transfer the blood from a syringe into the tubes. For small-diameter catheters, the vacuum in the tube may cause the catheter to temporarily collapse, preventing the backflow of blood into the tube. In this situation, small syringes should be used because they create less pressure on aspiration, the opposite of what small syringes do on injection. Transfer of the blood from the syringe to the vacuum tube requires the use of a "vacutainer needle holder." This device keeps the needle housed in a plastic case and covered, preventing needle stick injuries (Fig. 13-15). After blood draw from any catheter, a flush of 10 to 20 mL sterile normal saline is necessary to ensure a patent line. Be sure to clear the line and cap of blood to prevent a breeding ground for infection.

Removing the Vascular Access Device

To remove a short peripheral IV, lift opposite sides of the transparent dressing and pull laterally to remove the dressing from the site while stabilizing the catheter. Slowly withdraw the catheter from the skin, and immediately cover the puncture site with dry gauze. Hold pressure on the site until hemostasis is achieved. Assess the catheter tip to make sure it is intact and completely removed. Document the time of catheter removal and the appearance of the IV site.

Removal of midline catheters and PICCs must be performed with the same slow, gentle techniques used to insert the catheter. Veins can develop venospasms when rapid or forceful

techniques are used. After explaining to the patient that this procedure will not be painful, remove the dressing and withdraw the catheter in short segments by pulling from the insertion site. *If you feel resistance, always stop and never apply force to the catheter. Extreme traction or force could cause the catheter to break and embolize (travel) to the heart or pulmonary circulation.*

Simple distraction techniques and deep breathing may be sufficient to relax the patient and remove the catheter. If these fail, replace the dressing and apply heat; allow time for the vein wall to relax. Keeping the extremity warm and dry and asking the patient to drink warm liquids could facilitate removal. Use of medications to relax the vein wall may be required if the catheter cannot be removed after several hours. Imaging studies may also be needed to determine whether the cause is a thrombosis instead of venospasm.

Nontunneled percutaneous central catheters are removed by clipping any sutures and withdrawing the catheter in short segments. Venospasm does not commonly occur when removing these catheters because the vein diameter is large.

To prevent venous air embolism when removing any central venous catheter (including PICCs), position the patient in a flat supine or Trendelenburg position according to agency policy. To ensure the intrathoracic pressure is higher than atmospheric pressure, have the patient hold his or her breath or perform a Valsalva maneuver during removal. If the patient is mechanically ventilated, time the removal to the delivery of an inhalation by the ventilator. Be sure to keep the catheter clamped during this procedure. When a central venous catheter is removed, a tract between the skin and vein may create a conduit that could allow air to be pulled into the vein.

After removal, measure the catheter length and compare it with the length documented on insertion. *If the entire catheter length was not removed, contact the health care provider immediately!* Removal of tunneled catheters and implanted ports is usually performed by nurse practitioners or physicians.

Documenting Intravenous Therapy

Intravenous therapy is risk prone. Nurses can protect themselves from malpractice claims with conscientious assessment, intervention, and documentation. Be sure you document after insertion of a vascular access device (VAD) and throughout the course of the therapy. When inserting a venous catheter, remember to document the:
- Date and time of the VAD insertion
- Name of the nurse (you) who inserted the VAD
- Vein that was used for insertion
- Type of VAD used
- Number of insertion attempts and locations of attempts before successful insertion
- Response of the patient to the VAD insertion process
- Type of dressing applied
- Type of securement device, if used
- Special barrier precautions used, if any
- Patient and family education provided related to IV therapy

During the course of the patient's infusion therapy, be sure to continue documenting in the electronic health record your assessments and any interventions needed as a result of complications. Follow your agency's policies and procedures for additional requirements.

COMPLICATIONS OF INTRAVENOUS THERAPY

Complications from IV therapy can be minor and limited or life threatening. Serious life-altering or life-threatening complications are dramatically increasing in frequency and severity and present a tremendous financial burden to the U.S. health care system. Catheter-related bloodstream INFECTION (CR-BSI) is one of the most serious problems, often resulting in patient death. They are more common in patients with central VADs but can also occur with peripheral catheters.

Catheter-Related Bloodstream Infection

The Institute for Healthcare Improvement identified catheter-related bloodstream INFECTION (CR-BSI) as one of several preventable hospital-acquired infections (HAIs). They report that CR-BSIs are responsible for up to 28,000 deaths per year. As part of their previous *100,000 Lives Campaign*, a number of evidence-based interventions were combined into the CR-BSI prevention bundle. As a nurse, your accountability is to ensure that these interventions are followed (Table 13-2).

Other Complications of Intravenous Therapy

Local complications of IV therapy occur at or near the catheter. A priority for care for patients with IV therapy is to prevent, assess, and detect these complications. In some cases, nurses also manage these problems. Definitions, causes, signs and symptoms, treatment, and prevention of local complications are summarized in Table 13-3. *Systemic complications* of IV therapy involve the entire vascular system or multiple systems.

TABLE 13-2 **The Catheter-Related Bloodstream Infection (CR-BSI) Prevention Bundle**

- Use a *checklist* during insertion to make sure everything is done correctly. Tell anyone who violates the correct steps to stop the procedure immediately.
- *Hand hygiene* before inserting a central line must be thorough (i.e., no quick scrub). Anyone who touches the central line must also perform thorough hand hygiene.
- *Maximal barrier precautions* during line insertion require that the patient be draped from head to toe with a sterile barrier.
- The health care provider who inserts the VAD wears sterile *gloves, gown, and mask.* Anyone in the room during the procedure must also wear a mask.
- *Traffic in and out of the room must be minimized.* Many institutions use a "stop" sign on the door of the room to prevent people from coming in and going out during the procedure and a special "central line cart" to ensure they have everything they need in the room.
- *Chlorhexidine is used for skin disinfection* because it has best outcomes for preventing infection.
- *Use preferred sites.* PICC in the upper arm and subclavian veins are the first choice. The next preference is the internal jugular vein, and the least preferred is the femoral vein.
- *Post-placement care* requires meticulous dressing changes and care of all parts of the IV system, such as keeping ports and stopcocks clean; hanging bags using sterile technique; vigorous scrub of catheter hub with alcohol when used.
- *Review daily the need* for the patient's VAD. The incidence of CR-BSI increases each day the device is in place. As soon as it is determined that the patient no longer needs the IV line, it should be removed.

PICC, Peripherally inserted central catheter; *VAD,* vascular access device.

TABLE 13-3 **Local Complications of Intravenous Therapy**

COMPLICATION	CAUSE	SIGNS AND SYMPTOMS	TREATMENT	PREVENTION
Infiltration				
Leakage of a non-vesicant IV solution or medication into the extravascular tissue	Peripheral catheter has punctured opposite vein wall Obstruction of blood flow causing backflow through original entrance site Inflammatory process causing fluid leakage at the capillary level Fibrin sheath fully encasing a central venous catheter leading to retrograde flow and leakage from venipuncture site Damaged septum of implanted port Dislodged port access needle	IV rate slows Increasing edema around site Patient report of skin tightness; blanching or coolness of skin; burning, tenderness, or general discomfort at the insertion site; fluid leaking from puncture site; absence of a blood return (though this may not be reliable with a short peripheral catheter)	Stop infusion and remove short peripheral catheter immediately after identification of problem. Apply sterile dressing if weeping from tissue occurs. Elevate extremity. Warm or cold compresses may be used according to the solution infiltrated and organizational policy. Warm compresses increase circulation to the area and speed healing. Cool compresses may be used to relieve discomfort and reduce swelling. Insert a new catheter in the opposite extremity. For all central venous catheters, obtain a study to determine the cause of the problem. For implanted port, remove and insert a new port access needle. Rate the infiltration using the INS Infiltration Scale and document (Table 13-7).	Catheter stabilization—use smallest catheter appropriate; avoid area of flexion, or use arm board. Avoid placing restraints at the IV site. Make successive venipunctures proximal to the previous site. Monitor site frequently; educate patient about activities and signs and symptoms. Central venous catheters—obtain a brisk blood return before using the catheter for infusion. Frequently assess proper positioning of port access needle. Stabilize it well, and protect from clothing.

TABLE 13-3 Local Complications of Intravenous Therapy—cont'd

COMPLICATION	CAUSE	SIGNS AND SYMPTOMS	TREATMENT	PREVENTION
Extravasation Leakage of a vesicant IV solution or medication into the extravascular tissue This can occur with both peripheral and central catheters	Same as for infiltration	Same as for infiltration Blistering and tissue sloughing may not appear for a few days and resolves over 1-4 wk with infiltration of some chemotherapeutic agents such as anthracycline and alkylating agents	Stop infusion, and disconnect administration set. Aspirate drug from short peripheral catheter or port access needle. Leave short peripheral catheter or port access needle in place to deliver antidote, if indicated by established policy. If possible, aspirate residual drug from the exit site of a central venous catheter. Administer antidote according to established policy. Apply cold compresses for all drugs EXCEPT vinca alkaloids and epipodophyllotoxins. Photograph site. Monitor at 24 hr, 1 wk, 2 wk, and as needed. Surgical interventions may be required. Provide written instructions to patient and family.	Same as for infiltration. Know the vesicant potential before giving any IV medication. Prevention is key.
Phlebitis Inflammation of the vein Post-infusion phlebitis presents within 48-96 hr after the catheter has been removed	Mechanical cause from insertion technique, catheter size, and lack of catheter securement Chemical cause from extremes of pH and/or osmolarity of the fluid or medication Bacterial cause from a break in aseptic technique, poor securement, and extended dwell time	Patient may report pain at the IV site; nurse may observe that vein appears red and inflamed along the length; vein may become hard and cordlike (Table 13-6)	Remove short peripheral catheter at the first sign of phlebitis; use warm compresses to relieve pain. Monitor frequently. Document using Phlebitis Scale. Insert a new catheter using the opposite extremity. Mechanical phlebitis occurring in the first week after PICC insertion may be treated without catheter removal. Apply continuous heat; rest and elevate the extremity. Significant improvement is seen in 24 hr, and complete resolution is seen within 72 hr. Remove catheter if treatment is unsuccessful.	Choose the smallest-gauge catheter for the required therapy. Avoid sites of joint flexion, or stabilize with an armboard. Avoid infusing fluids or medications with a pH below 5 or above 9 through a peripheral vein. Avoid infusing fluids or medications with a final osmolarity above 500 mOsm/L through a peripheral vein. Rotate sites every 72-96 hr according to established policy. Adequately secure the catheter. Use aseptic technique. For PICCs, teach patient to avoid excessive physical activity with the extremity.
Thrombosis Blood clot inside the vein	Anything that damages the endothelial lining of the intima can initiate clot formation Traumatic venipuncture Multiple venipuncture attempts Use of catheters too large for the chosen vein Hyper-coagulable state and venous stasis	Slowed or stopped infusion rate Swollen extremity Tenderness and redness Engorged peripheral veins of the ipsilateral chest and extremity	Stop infusion and remove short peripheral catheter immediately. Apply cold compresses to decrease blood flow and stabilize the clot. Elevate extremity. Surgical intervention may be required. For central venous catheters, notify the physician and obtain requests for a diagnostic study. Low-dose thrombolytic agents can be used to lyse the clot.	Use evidence-based venipuncture technique. Make only two attempts to perform venipuncture. Choose the smallest-gauge catheter in the largest vein possible. Secure catheter adequately. Use armboards if short peripheral catheters are placed in areas of joint flexion. Ensure adequate hydration to avoid changes in blood composition and flexion of the extremity. Prophylactic low-dose warfarin (Coumadin, Warfilone ♦) may be prescribed for patients with a central venous catheter.

Continued

TABLE 13-3 Local Complications of Intravenous Therapy—cont'd

COMPLICATION	CAUSE	SIGNS AND SYMPTOMS	TREATMENT	PREVENTION
Thrombophlebitis The presence of a blood clot and vein inflammation	Same as for phlebitis and thrombosis	Same as for phlebitis and thrombosis	Same as for phlebitis and thrombosis. Apply cold compresses initially, followed by warm.	Same as for phlebitis and thrombosis.
Ecchymosis and Hematoma Ecchymosis results from infiltration of blood into the surrounding tissue Hematoma results from uncontrolled bleeding	Unskilled or multiple IV insertion attempts Patients with coagulopathy or fragile veins (e.g., older adults and patients on steroids) Accidental laceration of a large vein or artery	Swelling Bruising Pain or tenderness	When removing device, apply light pressure; excessive pressure could cause other fragile veins in the area to rupture. For hematoma, apply direct pressure until bleeding has stopped. Elevate extremity, apply ice for first 24 hours, and then warm compress for comfort.	Avoid veins that cannot be easily seen or palpated. Use extra caution in patients with coagulopathies. Use evidence-based venipuncture technique.
Site Infection Invasion of microorganisms at the insertion site in the absence of simultaneous bloodstream infection Infection localized at the insertion site, the port pocket, or subcutaneous tunnel	Break in aseptic technique during insertion or the handling of sterile equipment Lack of proper hand hygiene and skin antisepsis	Site appears red, swollen, and warm; patient may report tenderness at the site; may observe purulent or malodorous exudates	Clean exit site with alcohol, expressing drainage if present. For short peripheral catheter, midline catheter, or PICC, remove using sterile technique and avoid contact between skin and catheter. Send catheter tip for culture, if requested. Clean site with alcohol, and cover with dry sterile dressing; physician to evaluate for septic phlebitis and need for antimicrobial therapy or surgical intervention.	Use strict aseptic technique when inserting, maintaining, or removing catheters. Practice evidence-based hand hygiene. Ensure dressing remains clean, dry, and adherent to skin at all times.
Venous Spasm A sudden contraction of the vein	A normal response to irritation or injury of the vein wall	Cramping or pain at or above the insertion site Numbness in the area Slowing of the infusion rate Inability to withdraw midline catheter or PICC	Temporarily slow infusion rate. Apply warm compress. Do not immediately remove short peripheral catheter. If occurring during midline catheter or PICC removal, do not apply tension or attempt forceful removal. Reapply a dressing, apply heat, encourage patient to drink warm liquids, and keep extremity covered and dry. 12-24 hr may be required before catheter can be removed.	Allow time for vein diameter to return to normal after tourniquet removal and before advancing catheter. Infuse fluids at room temperature, if possible. For a midline catheter or PICC, gently withdraw the catheter in short segments.
Nerve Damage Inadvertent piercing or complete transection of a nerve	Venipuncture near known nerve locations Unanticipated nerve locations	Reports of tingling or feeling "pins and needles" at or below the insertion site Numbness at or near the insertion site	Immediately stop the insertion procedure if the patient reports extreme pain. Remove the catheter if reports of discomfort do not improve when the catheter is secured.	Avoid using the cephalic vein near the wrist. Avoid using veins on the palm side of the wrist. Adequately secure the catheter, but avoid tape that is too tight. Support areas of joint flexion with an armboard.

INS, Infusion Nurses Society; *PICC,* peripherally inserted central catheter.

TABLE 13-4	**Systemic Complications of Intravenous Therapy**			
COMPLICATION	**CAUSE**	**SIGNS AND SYMPTOMS**	**TREATMENT**	**PREVENTION**
Circulatory Overload Disruption of fluid homeostasis with excess fluid in the circulatory system	Infusion of fluids at a rate greater than the patient's system can accommodate	Patient may report shortness of breath and cough; patient's blood pressure is elevated, and there is puffiness around the eyes and edema in dependent areas; patient's neck veins may be engorged, and nurse may hear moist breath sounds.	Slow the IV rate, and notify physician; raise patient to an upright position; monitor vital signs, and administer oxygen as prescribed; administer diuretics as prescribed.	Monitor intake and output carefully, and notify physician as soon as an imbalance is noticed between the patient's intake and output.
Speed Shock Systemic reaction to the rapid infusion of a substance unfamiliar to the patient's circulatory system	Rapid infusion of drugs or bolus infusion, which causes the drug to reach toxic levels quickly	Patient may report lightheadedness or dizziness and chest tightness; nurse may note that patient has a flushed face and an irregular pulse; without intervention, patient may lose consciousness and go into shock and cardiac arrest.	Immediately discontinue the drug infusion and hang isotonic solution to keep the vein open; monitor vital signs carefully, and notify physician for further treatments.	Be aware of the appropriate infusion rate of medications and adhere to them; use of infusion control devices assists in prevention of speed shock.
Catheter Embolism A shaving or piece of catheter breaks off and floats freely in the vessel	Anything that damages the catheter—during insertion, dressing change, excessive force with flushing or medication administration	Depending on where the catheter embolizes, this could be life threatening. Cardiopulmonary arrest could occur.	Emergently notify the physician. Remove the catheter, and apply a tourniquet high on the limb of the catheter site; inspect catheter to determine how much may have embolized; an x-ray is taken to determine the presence of any catheter piece; surgical intervention may be necessary.	When inserting over-the-needle catheters, never reinsert the needle into the catheter; avoid pulling a through-the-needle catheter back through the needle during insertion. Avoid scissors near the catheter with dressing changes.

Information on common systemic complications can be found in Table 13-4. For central venous catheters (CVCs), complications can occur during the insertion procedure or during the dwell time (Table 13-5). Tables 13-6 and 13-7 are the INS criteria for grading phlebitis and infiltrations. Document all assessments and complications in the patient's electronic health record. Notify the infusion therapy team and/or health care provider per agency policy when complications occur.

IV THERAPY AND CARE OF THE OLDER ADULT

The aging process causes numerous changes in all body functions, and yet aging occurs differently in each person. Nutrition, environment, genetics, social factors, and education are just a few of the factors that influence the older adult's needs. Because all body functions are affected, IV therapy can be affected by these changes.

Skin Care

Aging skin becomes thinner and loses subcutaneous fat, decreasing the skin's ability for thermal regulation. Fewer nerve endings mean the decreased ability to feel pain. Older patients *may* not perceive acute pain from traumatic venipuncture requiring excessive probing or multiple attempts. However, this action increases the risk for fluid leakage and subsequent infiltration or extravasation injury. Inserting and removing a catheter and dressing could tear the skin layers.

Skin antisepsis is extremely important because of the decreased immunity seen as part of the aging process. Lipids are normally found in skin as a protective agent, and alcohol easily dissolves lipids. Although greater numbers of organisms may be killed, the skin can also become excessively dry and cracked. Current recommendations call for using friction when cleaning the skin to penetrate the layers of the epidermis. However, excessive friction may damage fragile skin and cause impaired TISSUE INTEGRITY. Chlorhexidine is the preferred agent, and the product currently available contains alcohol. Check for allergies to iodine before using iodine or iodophors. Iodophors such as povidone-iodine require contact with the skin for a minimum of 2 minutes to be effective. All antiseptic solutions must be thoroughly dry before applying the dressing or tape.

Skin should never be shaved before venipuncture, but excessive amounts of hair should be clipped. Shaving causes microabrasions that can lead to infection. The skin of an older adult may be more delicate and therefore more easily nicked while shaving.

Skin and TISSUE INTEGRITY can easily be compromised by the application of tape or dressings. Use of skin protectant solutions puts a protective barrier between the skin and dressing and improves the adherence of the dressing to the skin. Removal of tape and dressings may require adhesive remover solutions, or an alcohol pad may accomplish the same purpose. Securement devices like the StatLock require the use of a skin

TABLE 13-5 **Complications During the Dwell of Central Venous Catheters**

COMPLICATION	POSSIBLE CAUSES	SIGNS AND SYMPTOMS	TREATMENT	PREVENTION
Catheter Migration Movement of a properly placed catheter tip to another vein No change in the external catheter length	Changes in intrathoracic pressure caused by coughing, vomiting, sneezing, heavy lifting, and congestive heart failure	For migration to the jugular vein: reports of hearing a running stream or gurgling sound on the side of catheter insertion For migration to the azygos vein: back pain between the shoulder blades Neurologic complications if medications are infused	Stop all infusions, and flush catheter. Notify physician. Obtain a chest radiograph, if required, to assess tip location. Spontaneous repositioning back to the SVC is possible. Repositioning by radiology may be required.	Place catheter tip properly in the lower third of the SVC near the junction with the right atrium. Instruct patient to perform usual ADLs but to avoid excessive physical activity.
Catheter Dislodgment Movement of catheter into or out of the insertion site	Inadequate catheter securement Excessive physical activity with a PICC	External catheter length has changed, also changing the internal tip location No other signs or symptoms may be immediately noticed	Stop all infusions, and flush catheter. NEVER re-advance the catheter into the insertion site. Determine the amount of external catheter length, and compare with the length documented on insertion. Notify the physician or nurse inserting the catheter for further assessment.	Use proper catheter securement device. Instruct patient to perform normal ADLs but to avoid excessive physical activity.
Catheter Rupture Catheter is broken, damaged, or separated from hub or port body	Forcefully flushing a catheter with any size syringe against resistance Using scissors to remove a dressing Catheter compression of a subclavian inserted catheter between the clavicle and first rib (also known as *pinch-off syndrome*)	Fluid leaking from insertion site Pain or swelling during infusion Reflux of blood into the catheter extension Inability to aspirate blood from catheter	Repair the damaged segment; depends on the availability of a repair kit designed for the specific brand of catheter being used; repair may be considered a temporary measure instead of a permanent treatment. Remove catheter.	NEVER use excessive force when flushing a catheter, regardless of syringe size. On injection, small syringes generate more pressure than larger syringes. Use of a 10-mL syringe is generally recommended for flushing procedures. Insert catheter through jugular or upper extremity sites instead of subclavian site.
Lumen Occlusion Catheter lumen is partially or totally blocked	Drug or mineral precipitate (calcium, diazepam, and phenytoin are common) Lipid sludge from long-term infusion of fat emulsion Blood clots and fibrin sheath caused by blood reflux into lumen Allowing administration sets to remain connected for extended periods after medication has infused	Infusion stops, or pump alarm sounds Inability or difficulty administering fluids Inability or difficulty drawing blood Increased resistance to flushing of the catheter	Assess history of catheter use. A suddenly developing problem may indicate contact between incompatible medications. A problem that develops over an extended period may indicate a gradual clot formation. For drug precipitate, determine the pH of the precipitated drug. Use hydrochloric acid for acidic drug. Use sodium bicarbonate for alkaline drugs. For blood clot, use thrombolytic enzymes such as alteplase.	Always flush with normal saline between, before, and after each medication given through the catheter. Use positive-pressure flushing techniques when a negative fluid displacement needleless connector is being used. Use a positive fluid displacement needleless connector. Flush catheters immediately when medication infusion is complete.
Catheter-Related Bloodstream Infection (CR-BSI) Pathogenic organisms invade the patient's circulation The CDC has specific criteria to classify these infections	Lack of sterile field during insertion Inadequate skin antiseptic agents and application techniques Manipulation of the catheter hub leading to intraluminal contamination Inadequate hand hygiene Long dwell time	Early symptoms include fever, chills, headache, and general malaise	Change the entire infusion system from solution to IV device; notify physician, obtain cultures, and administer antibiotics as prescribed. If the infusate is the suspected cause, send a specimen to the laboratory for evaluation.	Maintain sterile technique. Use the recommended CR-BSI prevention bundle.

CDC, Centers for Disease Control and Prevention; *PICC*, peripherally inserted central catheter; *SVC*, superior vena cava.

TABLE 13-6   Phlebitis Scale from INS Standards of Practice

GRADE	CLINICAL CRITERIA
0	No symptoms
1	Erythema with or without pain
2	Pain at access site with erythema and/or edema
3	Pain at access site with erythema and/or edema Streak formation Palpable cord
4	Pain at access site with erythema and/or edema Streak formation Palpable venous cord more than 1 inch long Purulent drainage

Data from Infusion Nurses Society (INS). (2011). Infusion nursing standards of practice. *Journal of Infusion Nursing, 34(IS)*, S8.

TABLE 13-7   Infiltration Scale from INS Standards of Practice

GRADE	CLINICAL CRITERIA
0	No symptoms
1	Skin blanched Edema <1 inch in any direction Cool to touch With or without pain
2	Skin blanched Edema 1-6 inches in any direction Cool to touch With or without pain
3	Skin blanched, translucent Gross edema >6 inches in any direction Cool to touch Mild to moderate pain Possible numbness
4	Skin blanched, translucent Skin tight, leaking Skin discolored, bruised, swollen Gross edema >6 inches in any direction Deep pitting tissue edema Circulatory impairment Moderate to severe pain Infiltration of any amount of blood product, irritant, or vesicant

Data from Infusion Nurses Society (INS). (2011). *Standards of Practice*, Norwood, MA.

protectant (e.g., Skin-Prep) before applying the device. The protectant prevents skin tearing when the device is removed.

Vein and Catheter Selection

Vein and catheter selection are of highest importance in older adults. Choose insertion sites carefully after considering the patient's skin integrity, vein condition, and functional ability. The general principle of starting with the most distal sites usually indicates use of hand veins. *However, avoid fragile skin and small, tortuous veins on the back of the hand (dorsum); select the initial IV site higher on the arm.*

Venous distention must be accomplished with a flat tourniquet; however, the veins may require longer to adequately distend. Allowing a tourniquet to remain in place for extended periods causes an overfilling of the vein and can result in a hematoma when the vein is punctured. On extremely fragile skin, the tourniquet application can lead to ecchymotic areas or skin tears. Protect the skin by placing a wash cloth or the patient's gown between the skin and tourniquet. A tourniquet may not be required in veins that are already distended; however, carefully palpate these veins to determine their condition. Avoid hard, cordlike veins. Blood pressure cuffs can also be used for venous distention. Inflate the cuff and release until the pressure is slightly less than diastolic pressure. Other methods to distend veins include:

- Tapping lightly, but avoiding forceful slapping
- Asking the patient to open and close the fist so the muscles can force blood into the veins, making sure the hand is relaxed when the venipuncture is attempted
- Placing the extremity lower than the heart
- Applying warm compresses or a heating pad (be careful not to make it too hot) to the entire extremity for 10 to 20 minutes and removing just before making the venipuncture

As with all patients, venipuncture technique requires adequate skin and vein stabilization during the puncture and complete catheter advancement. Veins of an older adult are more likely to roll away from the needle. Low angles of 10 to 15 degrees between the skin and catheter will improve your success with venipuncture.

As soon as the catheter enters the vein, it may be necessary to release the tourniquet. Release of venous pressure from the puncture can lead to ecchymosis. Allowing the tourniquet to remain in place during the complete catheter advancement could increase this problem.

! NURSING SAFETY PRIORITY (QSEN)

Action Alert

Catheter securement may mean that administration sets are placed out of easy reach of a confused patient. Use flexible netting over the extremity to help prevent the patient from pulling at the dressing or tubing, while allowing easy access to the site. A device such as the I.V. House UltraDressing shown in Fig. 13-16 can also protect the site. Do not use rolled bandages to cover the extremity because they prevent insertion site assessment. Complications may progress to an advanced state before they are noticed.

Choosing a midline catheter or PICC may be best in older patients with poor skin turgor, limited venous sites, or veins that are fragile, tortuous, or hard. These catheters are placed in the upper extremity where venous distention techniques can be used. Inserting nontunneled percutaneous central catheters in older adults can be much more challenging. Venous distention for insertion requires the Trendelenburg position and a well-hydrated patient. FLUID volume deficit prevents adequate distention of the subclavian or jugular veins. Patients with conditions like chronic obstructive pulmonary disease and kyphosis cannot tolerate the Trendelenburg position. Tunneled catheters and implanted ports may be appropriate after considering the surgical techniques required to insert these catheters.

Cardiac and Renal Changes

Because of changes in cardiac and renal status in older adults, the accuracy of infusion volume and flow rate measurements is

FIG. 13-16 I.V. House UltraDressing IV site protector, a safety device used for IV site protection, guards the integrity of the older adult's skin while helping secure the site.

CLINICAL JUDGMENT CHALLENGE

Patient-Centered Care; Teamwork and Collaboration; Informatics QSEN

A 63-year-old obese, diabetic woman is transferred from the hospital to the skilled nursing facility (SNF) where you work as a charge nurse. The resident is being managed with IV cefoxitin 2 g IV piggyback (IVPB) every 8 hours for osteomyelitis resulting from an arterial foot ulcer. On review of her admission orders, you note that she has a newly inserted intermittent saline lock in her right forearm and is prescribed to receive the antibiotic for 4 more weeks.

1. The SNF policy for administration of drugs prescribed every 8 hours is a 6 PM–2 AM–10 AM schedule. Would you schedule her antibiotic at these times? Why or why not?
2. Two days later as you are planning to end your shift, the resident reports that her IV site seems red and swollen. What action will you take at this time? What will you document on the resident's electronic health record?
3. Is a peripheral vascular access device (VAD) the best choice for this resident? Why or why not? With whom will you or the oncoming nurse collaborate to make this decision? What does the evidence say about the type of VAD that would be best to meet this resident's needs? Where would you go to find the answer to this clinical question?
4. Using the SBAR technique, what will you report to the oncoming nurse about the resident's IV complications?

very important in the older adult. The health care provider's prescription for infusion therapy should be assessed for appropriateness for the patient's condition. Older adults are very prone to FLUID overload and resulting congestive heart failure. Electronic controlling devices may be required to ensure the necessary accuracy. Clinical manifestations of fluid overload are described in Chapter 11.

When fluid restrictions are required, medications could be diluted in small quantities and delivered using a syringe pump or a manual IV push. Consult with a pharmacist to determine the smallest amount of diluent required. This alternative may allow the patient to have more fluid to drink. Serum sodium levels should be considered when normal saline is routinely used for dilution in patients with hypertension or cardiac problems.

An increasing number of patients with chronic illness require repeated and frequent IV therapies. Many of these patients are vein depleted and need vein preservation. Subcutaneous and intraosseous routes have demonstrated effectiveness in emergency resuscitation. These procedures may also be beneficial for routine infusion of isotonic, non-irritant, non-vesicant solutions in patients with chronic illness and vein depletion (Aguiar, 2010).

Specific therapies requiring infusion into arteries and peritoneal, epidural, and intrathecal space are also available. These therapies are most commonly used to administer chemotherapy, lytic therapy, or pain medication.

SUBCUTANEOUS INFUSION THERAPY

Subcutaneous infusion therapy has been used for a variety of drug infusions. Most commonly it is used for administration of pain medications and insulin therapy. It is beneficial for palliative care patients who cannot tolerate oral medications, when IM injections are too painful, or when vascular access is not available or is too difficult to obtain.

Hypodermoclysis or "clysis" involves the slow infusion of isotonic FLUIDS into the patient's subcutaneous tissue. Although common in the early twentieth to mid-twentieth century, this method had not been widely used again until the 1990s. The growth of geriatric and palliative health care has helped spur the use of this method of infusion therapy for selected patients (Scales, 2011).

Hypodermoclysis can be used for short-term FLUID volume replacement. The patient must have sufficient sites of intact skin without INFECTION, inflammation, bruising, scarring, or edema. The most common sites are the front and sides of the thighs and hips, the upper abdomen, and the area under the clavicle. Unlike IV therapy, the upper extremities should not be used because fluid is absorbed more readily from sites with larger stores of adipose tissue. Hypodermoclysis is not appropriate for emergency resuscitations and should not be used if the fluid replacement needs exceed 2000 to 3000 mL/day and should not exceed 1500 mL/day at any single infusion site (Scales, 2011).

Hyaluronidase may be ordered by the health care provider and is mixed with each liter of infusion fluid. This substance is an enzyme that improves the absorption of the infusion from the subcutaneous tissue (Connolly et al., 2011; INS, 2011).

A small-gauge (25 to 27) winged infusion or "butterfly" needle, a small-gauge short peripheral catheter, or an infusion set specially designed for subcutaneous infusion can be chosen. The subcutaneous infusion sets have a small needle extending at a right angle from a flat disk that helps stabilize the needle.

When choosing the infusion site, consider the patient's level of activity. The area under the clavicle or the abdomen prevents difficulty with ambulation. Clip excess hair in the area, and clean the chosen site with the antiseptic solution, preferably 2% chlorhexidine gluconate in 70% isopropyl alcohol to prevent infection (Candon et al., 2010). Prime the infusion tubing and the attached subcutaneous infusion set or winged needle. Gently pinch an area of about 2 inches (5 cm), and insert the needle using sterile technique. After securing the needle, cover the site with a transparent dressing. Flow rates for hydration fluids begin at 30 mL/hr. After 1 hour, the rate can be increased if the patient has experienced no discomfort. The maximum rate is usually 2 mL/min or 120 mL/hr. Assess the site every 4 hours while in a hospital setting and at least twice daily while at home. Redness, warmth, leakage, bruising, swelling, and reports of pain indicate tissue irritation and possible impaired tissue integrity. If these symptoms occur, remove the infusion needle. Rotate the site at least once a week. More frequent rotation may be needed depending on TISSUE INTEGRITY (INS, 2011).

Other complications include pooling of the fluid at the insertion site and an uneven fluid drip rate. Both of these problems may be resolved by restarting the infusion in another location. An infusion pump may also be used. Small ambulatory infusion pumps can be used to allow for greater mobility.

INTRAOSSEOUS INFUSION THERAPY

Intraosseous (IO) therapy allows access to the rich vascular network in the red marrow of bones. Although IO has previously been regarded as a pediatric procedure, it is now considered acceptable for use in adults. Victims of trauma, burns, cardiac arrest, diabetic ketoacidosis, and other life-threatening conditions benefit from this therapy because often clinicians cannot access these patients' vascular systems for traditional IV therapy (Aguiar, 2010). Intraosseous catheters may be established in the prehospital setting when IV access cannot be readily obtained in an emergency.

Absorption rates of large-volume parenteral (LVP) infusions and drugs administered via the IO route are similar to those achieved with peripheral or central venous administration. The IO route should be used only during the immediate period of resuscitation and should not be used longer than 24 hours (Aguiar, 2010). After establishing access, efforts should continue to obtain IV access as well.

There are few contraindications for intraosseous infusion. The only absolute contraindication is fracture in the bone to be used as a site. Conditions such as severe osteoporosis, osteogenesis imperfecta, or other conditions that increase the risk for fracture with insertion of the IO needle and skin infection over the site may also be contraindications for some patients. Repeated attempts to access the same site should be avoided (Madigan, 2008).

Any needle could be used to provide therapy and access the medullary space (marrow). However, 15- or 16-gauge needles specifically designed for IO are preferred. New technology using a battery-powered drill has improved the ease of IO insertion. A number of sites can be used, including the proximal tibia (tibial tuberosity), distal femur, medial malleolus (inner ankle), proximal humerus, and iliac crest. The proximal tibia is the most common site accessed for IO therapy (Fig. 13-17).

If IV access cannot be obtained within the first few minutes of resuscitation procedures, IO may be attempted. The leg is restrained, and the site is cleaned with an antiseptic agent such as chlorhexidine. After successful insertion, the needle must be secured to prevent movement out of the bone. The same doses of fluids and medications can be infused IO as IV. An infusion pump may be used for rapid flow rates.

FIG. 13-17 Proximal tibial intraosseous (IO) access.

During the procedure, most patients rate the pain as a 2 or 3 on a scale of 0 to 10. Lidocaine 1% is used to anesthetize the skin, the subcutaneous tissue, and the periosteum to promote comfort (Madigan, 2008). Pain is also reported during the initial infusion. This may be reduced by injecting 0.5 mg/kg of preservative-free lidocaine through the intraosseous port before initiating the infusion (Phillips et al., 2010).

Improper needle placement with infiltration into the surrounding tissue is the most common complication of IO therapy. An accumulation of fluid under the skin at either the insertion site or on the other side of the limb indicates that the needle either is not far enough in to penetrate the bone marrow or is too far into the limb and has protruded through the other side of the shaft. Needle obstruction occurs when the puncture has been accomplished but flushing has been delayed. This delay may cause the needle to become clotted with bone marrow.

Osteomyelitis is an unusual but serious complication of IO therapy. You can help prevent this with meticulous aseptic technique, hand hygiene, and removal of the catheter as soon as it is no longer needed.

Compartment syndrome is a condition in which increased tissue pressure in a confined anatomic space causes decreased

PERFUSION (blood flow to the area). The decreased circulation to the area leads to hypoxia and pain in the area. Although the complication is rare in IO therapy, the nurse should monitor the site carefully and alert the physician promptly if the patient exhibits any signs of decreased circulation to the limb, such as coolness, swelling, mottling, or discoloration. Without improvement in PERFUSION to the limb, the patient could ultimately require amputation of the limb. Nursing assessment and interventions for compartment syndrome are discussed in detail in Chapter 51.

INTRA-ARTERIAL INFUSION THERAPY

Catheters are placed into arteries to obtain repeated arterial blood samples, to monitor various hemodynamic pressures continuously, and to infuse chemotherapy agents or fibrinolytics (intra-arterial infusion therapy). Catheters placed in the radial, brachial, or femoral arteries are used for obtaining blood samples and arterial pressure monitoring. Arterial waveforms and pressures are converted to digital values displayed on attached monitors. Between the catheter and the monitor is a special administration set capable of handling high infusion pressure, a pressurized fluid container, a continuous flush attachment, a three-way stopcock, and a transducer. The transducer is positioned at the level of the patient's atrium and secured to an IV pole to enable correct arterial pressure measurements.

The pulmonary artery is used to monitor pressures in the heart and lungs. This artery is cannulated via the large central venous system and through the right side of the heart. Hemodynamic monitoring and how to interpret these values are described in Chapter 38.

Chemotherapy agents administered arterially allow infusion of a high concentration of drug directly to the tumor site before it is diluted in blood or metabolized by the liver or kidneys. Drug infusion through the same blood supply feeding the tumor optimizes cell destruction at the tumor site while minimizing systemic side effects. The most common arterial sites include the hepatic and celiac arteries for liver tumors, although the carotid artery for tumors of the head, neck, or brain and pelvic arteries for cervical tumors have been used. Arterial catheter insertion can be performed through the skin via a surgical procedure or by an interventional radiologist. Implanted ports are commonly used for extended therapies. For short-term therapy, an external catheter may be used for 3 to 7 days, although the risks for complications increase during dwell time.

> **! NURSING SAFETY PRIORITY** (QSEN)
>
> **Critical Rescue**
>
> Carefully secure all junctions on the administration sets with Luer-Lok devices. Life-threatening hemorrhage can occur if an accidental disconnection occurs! When an infusion pump is used, be sure that it has a pressure high enough to overcome arterial pressure. Closely monitor the arterial insertion site and affected extremity. Assess the extremity for warmth, sensation, capillary refill, and pulse.

When the carotid artery is involved, perform neurologic assessments. When a femoral catheter is used, apply antiembolic stockings or other measures to prevent deep vein thrombosis. Complications from arterial catheters are similar to those from venous catheters, including infection, bleeding from the insertion site, hemorrhage from a catheter disconnection, catheter migration, infiltration, and catheter lumen or arterial occlusion. Specialized training is required to manage patients with arterial catheters.

INTRAPERITONEAL INFUSION THERAPY

Intraperitoneal (IP) infusion therapy is the administration of chemotherapy agents into the peritoneal cavity. IP therapy is used to treat intra-abdominal malignancies such as ovarian and gastrointestinal tumors that have moved into the peritoneum after surgery.

Catheters used for IP therapy may be an implanted port for long-term treatment or an external catheter for temporary use. These catheters, including those attached to an implanted port, have large internal lumens with multiple side-holes along the catheter length to allow for delivery of large quantities of fluid. Administration of IP therapy includes three phases: the instillation phase; the dwell phase, usually 1 to 4 hours; and the drain phase. Because this treatment involves the delivery of biohazardous agents, additional competency is required to handle the infusion properly.

The patient should be in the semi-Fowler's position for the infusion. He or she may experience nausea and vomiting caused by increasing pressure on the internal organs from the infusing fluid. Pressure on the diaphragm may cause respiratory distress. Reducing the flow rate and treatment with antiemetic drugs may be needed. Severe pain may indicate that the catheter has migrated, and an abdominal x-ray is needed to determine its location.

During the dwell and drainage phases, the patient may need assistance in frequently moving from side to side to distribute the fluid evenly around the abdominal cavity. After the fluid has drained, the catheter is flushed with normal saline, although heparinized saline may be used in implanted ports. Catheter lumen occlusion is caused by the formation of fibrous sheaths or fibrin clots or plugs inside the catheter or around the tip.

Exit site INFECTION, indicated by redness, tenderness, and warmth of the tissue around the catheter, can occur. Microbial peritonitis and inflammation of the peritoneal membranes from the invasion of microorganisms are other complications. If peritonitis occurs, the patient may experience a fever and report abdominal pain. Abdominal rigidity and rebound tenderness may be present. This condition is preventable by using strict aseptic technique in the handling of all equipment and infusion supplies. Management includes antimicrobial therapy administered either IV or intraperitoneally.

INTRASPINAL INFUSION THERAPY

The spinal column is covered by three layers: the dura mater, or outermost covering; the arachnoid, or middle layer; and the pia mater, which is closest to the spinal cord. Two spaces used for infusion are the epidural space between the dura mater and vertebrae and the subarachnoid space. The epidural space consists of fat, connective tissue, and blood vessels that protect the spinal cord. Medications infused into the epidural space must diffuse through the dura mater, and there is the possibility that some drug will be absorbed systemically. Intrathecal medications are infused into the subarachnoid space and directly into the cerebral spinal fluid, allowing reduced doses (McHugh et al., 2012). Care of patients with these therapies requires competency training and validation.

Postoperative and chronic pain is the primary indication for epidural infusion (see Chapter 3). Opioids administered epidurally slowly diffuse across the dura mater to the dorsal horn of the spinal cord. They lock onto receptors and block pain impulses from ascending to the brain. The patient receives pain relief from the level of the injection caudally (toward the toes). Local anesthetics administered epidurally work on the sensory nerve roots in the epidural space to block pain impulses. The physician administers the first dose of medication; then, depending on state law, the type of medication, and facility policies, nurses trained in epidural therapy may administer subsequent doses.

Intrathecal infusion of chemotherapy has been used for treating central nervous system (CNS) cancers. The belief was that lower total body doses delivered directly to the tumor would help prevent side effects. However, more recent studies have linked intrathecal infusion of methotrexate with increased neuromuscular impairments in acute lymphoblastic leukemia (ALL) survivors (Ness et al., 2012). Intrathecal infusion has also been used to manage chronic pain and to treat spasticity of neurologic diseases such as cerebral palsy, multiple sclerosis, reflex sympathetic dystrophy, and traumatic and anoxic acquired brain injuries (Hayek et al., 2011; McHugh et al., 2012).

A temporary catheter used for epidural therapy can be a percutaneous catheter that is secured at the site and extends up the back toward the shoulder. These catheters are used for postoperative pain management and usually dwell for only several hours or a few days. Infection and subsequent meningitis and catheter migration are the possible complications.

Epidural catheters used for longer periods include a tunneled catheter and implanted port. Tunneled catheters are tunneled toward the abdomen and have a subcutaneous cuff to act as a barrier to infection. The external catheter exits the skin on the abdomen, so it can be easily reached for use by the patient or caregiver. An epidural implanted port is the same design as an IV implanted port and is accessed with the same noncoring needle. The catheter extends from the lumbar puncture site to the port pocket and is located over a bony prominence on the abdomen through a subcutaneous tunnel. Surgically implanted pumps can also be used to deliver epidural and intrathecal infusion.

Using sterile technique, an intraspinal catheter usually is inserted in the lumbar region. The external portion of a temporary epidural catheter is laid along the back toward the head and usually extends over the shoulder. The entire catheter length is taped for added security. Dressings are usually not routinely changed because they are used only for short periods. If bleeding or fluid leakage requires dressing removal, use extreme care to prevent dislodging the catheter.

For a tunneled catheter or implanted port, the entire subcutaneous tunnel and port pocket should be frequently assessed. Measurement of an external catheter segment could help identify catheter migration.

An in-line filter is used on all intraspinal infusions to block the infusion of particulate matter. Medications commonly contain preservatives such as alcohol, phenols, or sulfites; however, these are toxic to the CNS. All medications used for intraspinal infusion must be free of preservatives. Alcohol and products containing alcohol should not be applied to the insertion site because the solution could track along the catheter and cause nerve damage. Povidone-iodine solutions are preferred for skin antisepsis before insertion and during catheter dwell, including tunneled catheter exit sites and implanted port pockets.

Complications from epidural and intrathecal infusion can be caused by the type of medication being infused or can be related to the catheter. It is important to know the specific location of the intraspinal catheter because the doses of medications are quite different. When used for pain management, doses are usually 10 times greater for epidural than for intrathecal infusion. Assess the patient for response to the drugs being given, level of alertness, respiratory status, and itching.

Catheter-related complications include INFECTION, bleeding, leakage of cerebrospinal fluid (CSF), occlusion of the catheter lumen, and catheter migration. It is important to be aware of coagulopathy and timing of anticoagulant therapy when epidural catheters are inserted. Epidural hematoma can cause neurologic damage if not corrected promptly. Infection in the patient receiving either epidural or intrathecal therapy could be the result of a lack of asepsis when handling the medication or during the administration. Evidence of local infection, such as redness or swelling at the catheter exit site, may be present. The patient may also exhibit neurologic and systemic signs of infection (e.g., meningitis), such as headache, stiff neck, or temperature higher than 101° F (38.3° C). Report any neurologic change to the health care provider immediately!

GET READY FOR THE NCLEX® EXAMINATION!

KEY POINTS

Review these Key Points for each NCLEX Examination Client Needs Category.

Safe and Effective Care Environment

- Check IV administration orders for accuracy and completeness before implementing them. **Safety** QSEN
- Prevent IV administration errors by using smart pumps and other emerging technology-based safety infusion systems; these devices do not replace careful monitoring and assessment of the patient receiving infusion therapy. **Informatics** QSEN
- Devices engineered with safety mechanisms are required by the Occupational Safety and Health Administration (OSHA) to prevent staff injuries from needles, thus preventing bloodborne pathogen hazards. **Safety** QSEN
- Use the evidence-based catheter-related bloodstream infection (CR-BSI) prevention bundle during insertion and care of patients who have central lines, including using a checklist

during insertion, hand hygiene, maximal barrier precautions, and chlorhexidine for skin disinfection (see Table 13-2). **Evidence-Based Practice** **QSEN**

Health Promotion and Maintenance

- Older adults present special challenges when infusion therapy is used; physiologic changes of the skin and cardiac/renal systems must be considered.
- Use small IV catheters for older adults, and insert using a 10- to 15-degree angle to prevent rolling of the vein. **Patient-Centered Care** **QSEN**
- Teach patients and their families about the patient's infusion therapy, including purpose, type, and safety precautions.

Physiological Integrity

- Infusion therapy is the delivery of parenteral medications and fluids through a wide variety of catheters and locations.
- Infusion therapy is used for establishing FLUID AND ELECTROLYTE BALANCE, achieving optimum nutrition, maintaining hemostasis, and treating or preventing illnesses with medications.
- Vascular access devices (VADs) are catheters that are used to deliver fluids and electrolytes and medications into the intravascular space.
- Common types of VADs include short peripheral catheters, midline catheters, peripherally inserted central catheters (PICCs), nontunneled percutaneous and tunneled central catheters, implanted ports, and hemodialysis catheters.
- Use best practice for placement of short peripheral VADs, including avoiding the small veins of the hands (see Chart 13-1). **Evidence-Based Practice** **QSEN**
- Document care for the patient receiving IV therapy, including the type of VAD inserted. **Informatics** **QSEN**
- The type of VAD that is used depends on the reason for infusion therapy, the patient's condition, and the length of therapy.
- Choose the appropriate peripheral catheter gauge size of the VAD depending on its purpose (see Table 13-1).

- PICCs, tunneled central catheters, and implanted ports are commonly used for long-term infusion therapy.
- Infusion controllers and pumps are electronic devices used to regulate the flow of infusion fluids and medications, but be sure to monitor the infusion rate.
- Nursing care for patients receiving all types of infusion therapy includes using sterile technique when starting the therapy and when changing components of the infusion system, changing and securing the site dressing, and assessing the site for local complications (see Table 13-3). **Evidence-Based Practice** **QSEN**
- Assess and document the presence of phlebitis using the INS Phlebitis Scale (see Table 13-6). **Evidence-Based Practice** **QSEN**
- Use normal saline to flush IV catheters on a periodic basis per agency policy.
- Assess, prevent, and manage systemic complications related to IV therapy as outlined in Table 13-4.
- Assess, prevent, and manage complications during the course of central IV therapy as listed in Table 13-5.
- Subcutaneous therapy of fluids (hypodermoclysis) involves a slow infusion for a short time; the thighs, hips, and abdomen are commonly used.
- Intraosseous infusion therapy allows fluids and medications to be absorbed by the rich vascular network of the bones; it is used for both children and adults, particularly in emergency situations.
- Arterial therapy is used primarily for the administration of chemotherapy agents directly into a tumor site; the liver is the most common arterial site for this purpose.
- Intraperitoneal therapy is used for chemotherapy agent administration into the peritoneal cavity, especially for ovarian and gastrointestinal tumors that have metastasized into the peritoneum.
- Epidural and intrathecal administration of medications are the common uses for intraspinal infusion. Epidural infusions are usually for pain management; intrathecal infusions are usually chemotherapy agents used for cancers that cross the blood-brain barrier into the central nervous system.

CHAPTER | 14

Care of Preoperative Patients

Robin Chard

 http://evolve.elsevier.com/Iggy/

PRIORITY CONCEPTS

- INFECTION

LEARNING OUTCOMES

Safe and Effective Care Environment
1. Differentiate among the various types and purposes of surgery.
2. Examine personal factors for each patient for potential threats to safety, especially with older adults.
3. Protect the patient from injury and INFECTION during the perioperative period.

Health Promotion and Maintenance
4. Teach patients about dietary restrictions, preoperative preparations, and interventions to perform after surgery to prevent complications.

Psychosocial Integrity
5. Reduce the psychological impact for the patient and family regarding the preoperative experience.

6. Ensure patient concerns and needs are communicated to other members of the health care team.

Physiological Integrity
7. Use knowledge of physiology and behavioral principles to describe an accurate and complete preoperative assessment.
8. Implement interventions to reduce the risk for perioperative complications.
9. Use laboratory and clinical data to assess for changes that may affect the patient's response to drugs, anesthesia, and surgery.

Patients undergoing surgery have benefitted greatly from advances in surgical techniques, anesthesia, pharmacology, medical devices, and supportive interventions. Research defining best practices has resulted in improved outcomes in all areas of the perioperative experience. New interventions, such as robotics and other types of minimally invasive surgeries (MISs), are continually being developed. Advances in anesthetic agents and techniques have made surgery safer than ever before. Many surgical procedures have moved from the operating room to other departments such as interventional radiology, cardiac catheterization, and endoscopy. Ambulatory care facilities, known as ambulatory surgical centers (ASCs), are being used for many surgical procedures outside acute care hospitals and account for more than 23 million surgical procedures performed annually (Ambulatory Surgery Center Association,

2013). These changes affect the role of the perioperative nurse and have an impact on how patient teaching is performed.

Cost-reduction is a driving force for the management of the surgical patient. Shortened stays and ambulatory surgeries are common. Patient histories may be conducted by telephone or online before surgery rather than in person. Some patients may be observed only after surgery and not admitted as an inpatient. In response to the ongoing health care delivery changes and the use of multiple settings, nurses have modified their interventions, remaining focused on patient care before (**preoperative**), during (**intraoperative**), and after (**postoperative**) surgery. Together, these time periods are known as the **perioperative** experience.

Patient safety throughout the perioperative period is the number-one priority for all personnel. Fig. 14-1 shows an

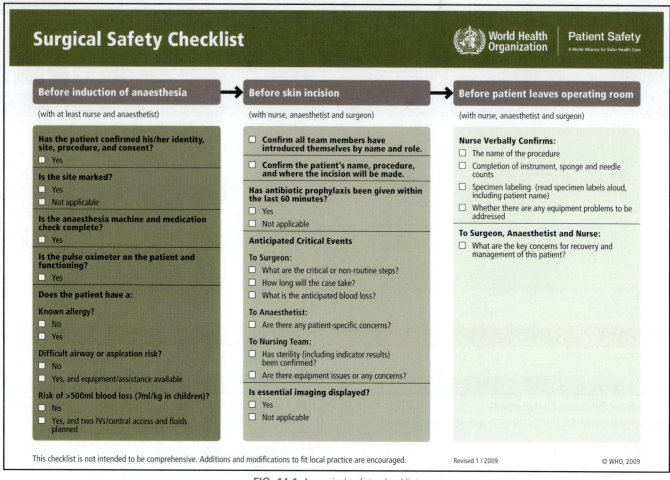

FIG. 14-1 A surgical safety checklist.

overview of a surgical safety checklist as recommended by the World Health Organization (WHO). Quality measures such as wrong-site surgery, patient falls, hospital-acquired pressure ulcers, and vascular catheter–associated INFECTIONS must now be reported to the Centers for Medicare and Medicaid Services (CMS). These data are used for tracking patient outcomes and ensuring patient-centered care and accountability on the part of health care facilities.

Because surgery is invasive and involves exposure to various anesthetic agents and drugs, as well as positioning and other environmental hazards, complications are common. Some complications are predictable and are considered preventable or "never events." As a result, The Joint Commission (TJC) has partnered with other groups and agencies and developed a plan for the reduction and eventual elimination of preventable surgical complications known as the *Surgical Care Improvement Project (SCIP)*. Implementation of these core measures is now mandatory for patient safety. The current plan focuses on INFECTION prevention, prevention of serious cardiac events, and prevention of venous thromboembolism (VTE) (also known as *deep vein thrombosis [DVT]*). Ten specific core measures have been identified as actions required for prevention of these complications in patients identified as at risk. Table 14-1 provides an overview of these core measures areas. (The numbers associated with the core measures are not always chronologic, indicating that some areas are still in development.) The perioperative areas of responsibility for these core measures and their

prevention strategies are highlighted in the appropriate areas of this chapter. In addition, some core measures also are discussed in patient care chapters most associated with the complication.

? NCLEX EXAMINATION CHALLENGE
Safe and Effective Care Environment

Because of an unexpected emergency case, a client scheduled for colon surgery at 8 AM has been rescheduled for 11 AM. What is the nurse's best action related to preoperative prophylactic antibiotic administration according to the Surgical Care Improvement Project (SCIP) guidelines?
A. Administer the preoperative antibiotic at 7 AM as originally prescribed.
B. Administer the antibiotic at the same time as the other prescribed preoperative drugs.
C. Adjust the antibiotic administration time to be within 1 hour before the surgical incision.
D. Hold the preoperative antibiotic until the client is actually in the operating room and has been anesthetized.

OVERVIEW

The preoperative period begins when the patient is scheduled for surgery and ends at the time of transfer to the surgical suite. As a nurse, you will function as an educator, an advocate, and a promoter of health. The surgical environment demands the

TABLE 14-1 Surgical Care Improvement Project (SCIP) Core Measure Overview

CORE MEASURE IDENTIFICATION	MEASUREMENT NAME/DESCRIPTION
SCIP Infection-1 (SCIP Inf-1)	*Prophylactic Antibiotic Received Within One Hour Prior to Surgical Incision* The purpose is to use short-duration antibiotics to establish bactericidal blood and tissue levels by the time the surgical incision is made.
SCIP Infection-2 (SCIP Inf-2)	*Prophylactic Antibiotic Selection for Surgical Patients* The purpose is to ensure that prophylactic antibiotics are used for patients who are at increased risk for surgical site infections. The guidelines for risk and for the exact antibiotic to be used are specific to each type of surgical procedure and follow evidence-based published recommendations.
SCIP Infection-3 (SCIP Inf-3)	*Prophylactic Antibiotics Discontinued Within 24 Hours After Surgery End Time* The purpose is to ensure that prophylactic antibiotic therapy provides benefit without risk. Prolonged prophylactic antibiotic therapy has not been shown to increase benefit and is known to increase the risk for *C. difficile* infection and the development of microorganisms that are resistant to antimicrobial drugs.
SCIP Infection-4 (SCIP Inf-4)	*Cardiac Surgery Patients with Controlled 6 AM Postoperative Blood Glucose* (Applies to cardiac surgery patients only) The purpose is to avoid hyperglycemia (which is defined as blood glucose levels above 200 mg/dL and is associated with increased complications and mortality) in cardiac surgery patients, especially patients undergoing coronary artery bypass graft surgery and patients with diabetes who are having cardiac surgery.
SCIP Infection-6 (SCIP Inf-6)	*Surgery Patients with Appropriate Hair Removal* The purpose is to avoid hair removal procedures, specifically shaving, that cause skin abrasions and increase the risk for surgical site infections. If hair must be removed from the surgical site, removal is performed with electric clippers or chemical depilatories.
SCIP Infection-9 (SCIP Inf-9)	*Urinary Catheter Removed on Postoperative Day 1 (POD 1) or Postoperative Day 2 (POD 2) with Day of Surgery Being Day Zero* The purpose is to avoid urinary catheter–associated urinary tract infections, which increase with longer duration indwelling catheters. It is unacceptable to have an indwelling urinary catheter in place longer than 48 hours after surgery unless there is a documented specific and medically validated reason for it.
SCIP Infection-10 (SCIP Inf-10)	*Surgery Patients with Perioperative Temperature Management* The purpose is to prevent prolonged hypothermia, which is associated with impaired wound healing, serious cardiac complications, altered drug metabolism, coagulation problems, and a higher incidence of surgical site infections. Temperature must be measured within 15 minutes from the end of anesthesia administration. Intentional hypothermia must be documented.
SCIP CARD-2	*Surgery Patients on Beta-Blocker Therapy Prior to Arrival Who Received a Beta-Blocker During the Perioperative Period* The purpose is to ensure that patients with specific medical conditions receive beta-blocker therapy before surgery and continue the therapy in the immediate postoperative period. This evidence-based action has resulted in a significant reduction in coronary events, cardiovascular mortality, and overall mortality.
SCIP Venous thromboembolism-1 (SCIP VTE-1)	*Surgery Patients with Recommended Venous Thromboembolism Prophylaxis Ordered* The purpose is to reduce the complications from postoperative venous thromboembolism (VTE). Surgery is a major risk factor responsible for VTE formation and subsequent pulmonary embolism. Although VTE prophylaxis is effective, it is underused. Specific preoperative and postoperative VTE prophylaxis strategies are recommended on the basis of patient risk, type and duration of surgery, and extent of expected postoperative immobilization.
SCIP Venous thromboembolism-2 (SCIP VTE-2)	*Surgery Patients Who Received Appropriate Venous Thromboembolism Prophylaxis Within 24 Hours Prior to Surgery to 24 Hours After Surgery* The purpose is to reduce the complications from postoperative venous thromboembolism (VTE), particularly among patients undergoing the types of surgeries in which the risk is highest.

Data from The Joint Commission. (2014). *National Patient Safety Goals*. Retrieved April 2014, from www.jointcommission.org/surgical_care_improvement_project/.
C. difficile, Clostridium difficile.

use of knowledge, judgment, and skills based on the principles of nursing science. Perioperative nursing places special emphasis on safety, advocacy, and patient education, although ensuring a "culture of safety" is the responsibility of all health care team members.

The patient's readiness for surgery is critical to the outcome. Preoperative care focuses on preparing the patient for the surgery and ensuring patient safety. This care includes education and any intervention needed before surgery to reduce anxiety and complications and to promote patient cooperation in procedures after surgery. Use adult teaching and learning principles in teaching patients and families before surgery. Validate, clarify, and reinforce information the patient has received

from the surgeon or other members of the surgical team. In addition, during the nursing assessment before surgery, problems may be identified that warrant further patient assessment or intervention before the procedure. As required by The Joint Commission's National Patient Safety Goals (NPSGs), communication and collaboration with the surgical team are essential so that correct actions are taken to achieve the desired outcome.

Categories and Purposes of Surgery

Surgical procedures are categorized by the purpose, body location, extent, and degree of urgency. Table 14-2 explains the categories and gives examples of surgical procedures.

TABLE 14-2	Selected Categories of Surgical Procedures	
CATEGORY	**DESCRIPTION**	**CONDITION OR SURGICAL PROCEDURE**
Reasons for Surgery		
Diagnostic	Performed to determine the origin and cause of a disorder or the cell type for cancer	Breast biopsy Exploratory laparotomy Arthroscopy
Curative	Performed to resolve a health problem by repairing or removing the cause	Cholecystectomy Appendectomy Hysterectomy
Restorative	Performed to improve a patient's functional ability	Total knee replacement Finger reimplantation
Palliative	Performed to relieve symptoms of a disease process, but does not cure	Colostomy Nerve root resection Tumor debulking Ileostomy
Cosmetic	Performed primarily to alter or enhance personal appearance	Liposuction Revision of scars Rhinoplasty Blepharoplasty
Urgency of Surgery		
Elective	Planned for correction of a nonacute problem	Cataract removal Hernia repair Hemorrhoidectomy Total joint replacement
Urgent	Requires prompt intervention; may be life threatening if treatment is delayed more than 24 to 48 hr	Intestinal obstruction Bladder obstruction Kidney or ureteral stones Bone fracture Eye injury Acute cholecystitis
Emergent	Requires immediate intervention because of life-threatening consequences	Gunshot or stab wound Severe bleeding Abdominal aortic aneurysm Compound fracture Appendectomy
Degree of Risk of Surgery		
Minor	Procedure without significant risk; often done with local anesthesia	Incision and drainage (I&D) Implantation of a venous access device (VAD) Muscle biopsy
Major	Procedure of greater risk; usually longer and more extensive than a minor procedure	Mitral valve replacement Pancreas transplant Lymph node dissection
Extent of Surgery		
Simple	Only the most overtly affected areas involved in the surgery	Simple/partial mastectomy
Radical	Extensive surgery beyond the area obviously involved; is directed at finding a root cause	Radical prostatectomy Radical hysterectomy
Minimally invasive surgery (MIS)	Surgery performed in a body cavity or body area through one or more endoscopes; can correct problems, remove organs, take tissue for biopsy, re-route blood vessels and drainage systems; is a fast-growing and ever-changing type of surgery	Arthroscopy Tubal ligation Hysterectomy Lung lobectomy Coronary artery bypass Cholecystectomy

Surgical Settings

The term **inpatient** refers to a patient who is admitted to a hospital. The patient may be admitted the day before or, more often, the day of surgery (often termed *same-day admission [SDA]*), or the patient may already be an inpatient when surgery is needed. The terms **outpatient** and **ambulatory** refer to a patient who goes to the surgical area the day of the surgery and returns home on the same day (i.e., *same-day surgery [SDS]*). Hospital-based ambulatory surgical centers, freestanding surgical centers, physicians' offices, and ambulatory care centers are common. More than half of all surgical procedures in North America are performed in ambulatory centers (Ambulatory Surgery Center Association, 2013).

One advantage of outpatient surgery is that patients are not separated from the comfort and security of their home and family. Same-day surgery, however, places more responsibility on the patient and family, especially for care after surgery. Often a case manager is needed to coordinate post-discharge care for the patient.

❖ PATIENT-CENTERED COLLABORATIVE CARE

◆ Assessment

History. Data collection about the patient before surgery begins in various settings (e.g., the surgeon's office, the preadmission or admission office, the inpatient unit, the telephone, the Internet). Use privacy to increase the patient's comfort with the interview process. Anesthesia and surgery are both physical and emotional stressors. Collect these data:

- Age
- Use of tobacco, alcohol, or illicit substances, including marijuana
- Current drugs
- Use of complementary or alternative practices, such as herbal therapies, folk remedies, or acupuncture
- Medical history
- Prior surgical procedures and how these were tolerated
- Prior experience with anesthesia, pain control, and management of nausea or vomiting
- Autologous or directed blood donations
- Allergies, including sensitivity to latex products
- General health
- Family history
- Type of surgery planned
- Knowledge about and understanding of events during the perioperative period
- Adequacy of the patient's support system

When taking a history, screen the patient for problems that increase the risk for complications during and after surgery. Some problems that increase the surgical risk or increase the risk for complications after surgery are listed in Table 14-3.

Older patients are at increased risk for complications from both anesthesia and surgery (Doerflinger, 2009). The normal aging process decreases immune system functioning and delays wound healing. The frequency of chronic illness increases in older patients. Gas exchange is more profoundly affected by general anesthetic agents and by opioid analgesics. Age-related changes in kidney and liver function may delay the elimination of anesthetic and analgesic agents, increasing the risk for adverse reactions. See Chart 14-1 for other changes in older adults that may alter the operative response or risk.

Drugs and substance use may affect patient responses to surgery. Tobacco use increases the risk for pulmonary complications because of changes to the lungs, blood vessels, and chest cavity. Alcohol and illicit substance use can alter the patient's responses to anesthesia and pain medication. Withdrawal of alcohol before surgery may lead to delirium tremens. Prescription and over-the-counter drugs may also affect how the patient reacts to the operative experience. Adverse effects can occur with the use of some herbs. Thus asking about and documenting past and current use of herbs or botanicals are important.

Medical history is important to obtain because many chronic illnesses increase surgical risks and need to be considered when planning care. For example, a patient with systemic lupus erythematosus may need additional drugs to offset the stress of the surgery. A patient with diabetes may need a more extensive bowel preparation because of decreased intestinal motility. An INFECTION may need to be treated before surgery.

TABLE 14-3 Selected Factors That Increase the Risk for Surgical Complications

Age
- Older than 65 years

Medications
- Antihypertensives
- Tricyclic antidepressants
- Anticoagulants
- Nonsteroidal anti-inflammatory drugs (NSAIDs)

Medical History
- Decreased immunity
- Diabetes
- Pulmonary disease
- Cardiac disease
- Hemodynamic instability
- Multi-system disease
- Coagulation defect or disorder
- Anemia
- Dehydration
- Infection
- Hypertension
- Hypotension
- Any chronic disease

Prior Surgical Experiences
- Less-than-optimal emotional reaction
- Anesthesia reactions or complications
- Postoperative complications

Health History
- Malnutrition or obesity
- Drug, tobacco, alcohol, or illicit substance use or abuse
- Altered coping ability

Family History
- Malignant hyperthermia
- Cancer
- Bleeding disorder

Type of Surgical Procedure Planned
- Neck, oral, or facial procedures (airway complications)
- Chest or high abdominal procedures (pulmonary complications)
- Abdominal surgery (paralytic ileus, venous thromboembolism)

Ask the patient specifically about cardiac problems because complications from anesthesia occur more often in patients with cardiac problems (Johnson, 2011). A patient with a history of rheumatic heart disease may be prescribed antibiotics before surgery. Cardiac problems that increase surgical risks include coronary artery disease, angina, myocardial infarction (MI) within 6 months before surgery, heart failure, hypertension, and dysrhythmias. These problems impair the patient's ability to withstand hemodynamic changes and alter the response to anesthesia. The risk for an MI during surgery is higher in patients who have heart problems. Patients with cardiac disease may require perioperative therapy with beta-blocking drugs, as recommended by core measures for SCIP CARD-2 (see Table 14-1).

Pulmonary complications during or after surgery are more likely to occur in older patients, those with chronic respiratory

CHART 14-1   Nursing Focus on the Older Adult

Age-Related Changes as Surgical Risk Factors

PHYSIOLOGIC CHANGE	NURSING INTERVENTIONS	RATIONALES
Cardiovascular System		
Decreased cardiac output	Determine normal activity levels, and note when the patient tires.	Knowing limits helps prevent fatigue.
Increased blood pressure		
Decreased peripheral circulation	Monitor vital signs, peripheral pulses, and capillary refill.	Having baseline data helps detect deviations.
Respiratory System		
Reduced vital capacity	Teach coughing and deep-breathing exercises.	Pulmonary exercises help prevent pulmonary complications.
Loss of lung elasticity		
Decreased oxygenation of blood	Monitor respirations and breathing effort.	Having baseline data helps detect deviations.
Renal/Urinary System		
Decreased blood flow to kidneys	Monitor intake and output.	Ongoing assessment helps detect fluid and electrolyte imbalances and decreased renal function.
Reduced ability to excrete waste	Assess overall hydration.	
Decline in glomerular filtration rate	Monitor electrolyte status.	
Nocturia common	Assist frequently with toileting needs, especially at night.	Frequent toileting helps prevent incontinence and falls.
Neurologic System		
Sensory deficits	Orient the patient to the surroundings.	An individualized preoperative teaching plan is developed based on the patient's orientation and any neurologic deficits.
Slower reaction time	Allow extra time for teaching the patient.	
Decreased ability to adjust to changes in the surroundings	Provide for the patient's safety.	Safety measures help prevent falls and injury.
Musculoskeletal System		
Increased incidence of deformities related to osteoporosis or arthritis	Assess the patient's mobility.	Interventions help prevent complications of immobility.
	Teach turning and positioning.	
	Encourage ambulation.	
	Place on falls precautions, if indicated.	Safety measures help prevent injury.
Skin		
Dry with less subcutaneous fat makes the skin at greater risk for damage; slower skin healing increases risk for infection	Assess the patient's skin before surgery for lesions, bruises, and areas of decreased circulation.	Having baseline data helps detect changes and evaluate interventions.
	Pad bony prominences.	Padding can protect at-risk areas.
	Use pressure-avoiding or pressure-reducing overlays.	Overlays can prevent pressure ulcer formation by redistributing body weight.
	Avoid applying tape to skin.	Tape removal damages thin skin.
	Teach the patient to change position at least every 2 hours.	Changing position frequently helps prevent reduced blood flow to an area and changes external pressure patterns.

problems, and smokers because of smoking- or age-related lung changes (Doerflinger, 2009). Increased chest rigidity and loss of lung elasticity reduce anesthetic excretion. Smoking increases the blood level of carboxyhemoglobin (carbon monoxide on oxygen-binding sites of the hemoglobin molecule), which decreases oxygen delivery to organs. Action of cilia in pulmonary mucous membranes decreases, which leads to retained secretions and predisposes the patient to INFECTION (pneumonia) and atelectasis (collapse of alveoli). Atelectasis reduces gas exchange and causes intolerance of anesthesia. It is also a common problem after general anesthesia.

Chronic lung problems such as asthma, emphysema, and chronic bronchitis also reduce the elasticity of the lungs, which reduces gas exchange. As a result, patients with these problems have reduced tissue oxygenation.

Previous surgical procedures and anesthesia affect the patient's readiness for surgery. Previous experiences, especially with complications, may increase anxiety about the scheduled surgery. Ask about the patient's experience with anesthesia and all allergies. These data provide information about tolerance of and possible fears about the use of anesthesia. The family medical history and problems with anesthetics may indicate possible reactions to anesthesia, such as malignant hyperthermia (see Chapter 15).

An allergy to certain substances alerts you to a possible reaction to anesthetic agents or to substances that are used before or during surgery. For example, povidone-iodine (e.g., Betadine) used for skin cleansing contains the same allergens found in shellfish. Patients who are allergic to shellfish may have an adverse reaction to povidone-iodine. The patient with an allergy to avocados, bananas, strawberries, and other fruits may also have a latex sensitivity or allergy. Patients who have an egg, peanut, or soy allergy may have a reaction to propofol (Diprivan), which is an anesthetic agent often used in the induction and maintenance of anesthesia (MDConsult, 2012).

Blood donation for surgery can be made by the patient (autologous donations) a few weeks just before the scheduled surgery date. Then, if blood is needed during or after surgery, an autologous blood transfusion can be given. This practice eliminates transfusion reactions and reduces the risk for acquiring bloodborne disease. Specific patient criteria, which may vary by surgical type and patient health problem, must be met to qualify for autologous transfusion.

A special tag is placed on the blood bag when an autologous blood donation has been made. The blood donor center gives the patient a matching tag that he or she wears or brings to the surgical area before surgery as required by The Joint Commission's National Patient Safety Goals (NPSGs). This procedure helps ensure that patients receive only their own donated blood. Patients may wish to have family and friends donate blood exclusively for their use, if needed. This practice (called *directed blood donation*) is possible only if the blood types are compatible and the donor's blood is acceptable. Directed donation is not practiced in all blood donation centers. When directed blood donations are used, a special tag is attached to the blood bag. This tag notes the names of the patient and the donor and bears the patient's signature.

Ask whether autologous or directed blood donations have been made, and document this information in the chart. It is important to know the specific blood collection center where the donation was made and whether the blood has arrived before the patient goes into surgery. The hospital receives and stores the blood units until they are used or are no longer needed. Unused blood is returned to the collection center.

Increased use of "bloodless surgery" and minimally invasive surgery (MIS) provides alternatives for patients with religious or medical restrictions to blood transfusions. These programs reduce the need for transfusion during and after surgery. Some techniques used are limiting blood samples (the number of samples, as well as the volume of blood drawn per sample) before surgery and stimulating the patient's own red blood cell production with epoetin alpha (e.g., Epogen, Procrit). Supplemental iron, folic acid, vitamin B_{12}, and vitamin C may be prescribed to help red blood cell formation. Newer equipment and surgical techniques cause less blood loss than older techniques. Such advances include recycling blood suctioned during surgery and immediately transfusing it back into the patient. Assess, monitor, teach, and support the patient during the bloodless surgery process.

Discharge planning is started before surgery. Assess the patient's home environment, self-care capabilities, and support systems and anticipate postoperative needs before surgery. *All patients, regardless of how minor the procedure or how often they have had surgery, should have discharge planning.* Older patients and dependent adults may need transportation referrals to and from the physician's office or the surgical setting. A home care nurse may be needed to monitor recovery and to provide instructions. Patients with few support systems may need follow-up care at home. Some patients need a planned direct admission to a rehabilitation facility or center for physical therapy after surgery, especially joint replacement surgery. Shortened hospital stays require adequate discharge planning to achieve the desired outcomes after surgery.

Physical Assessment/Clinical Manifestations. The preoperative patient may be any age, with a health status that varies from well to debilitated. Perform a complete assessment before surgery to obtain baseline data. Use this information to identify current health problems, potential complications related to anesthesia, and risk for complications that may occur after surgery.

Begin the assessment by obtaining a complete set of vital signs. You may need to obtain vital signs several times at different time intervals for accurate baseline values. Previous vital signs from another admission (if available) are helpful to compare with current vital signs. Abnormal vital signs may

---

CHART 14-2   Nursing Focus on the Older Adult

Specific Considerations When Planning Care for the Older Preoperative Patient

- Greater incidence of chronic illness
- Greater incidence of malnutrition
- More allergies
- Increased incidence of impaired self-care abilities
- Inadequate support systems
- Decreased ability to withstand the stress of surgery and anesthesia
- Increased risk for cardiopulmonary complications after surgery
- Risk for a change in mental status when admitted (e.g., related to unfamiliar surroundings, change in routine, drugs)
- Increased risk for a fall and resultant injury

---

require postponement of surgery until the problem is treated and the patient's condition is stable. Also assess for anxiety, which could increase blood pressure, pulse, and respiratory rate. Document these findings as part of the overall assessment.

Throughout the assessment, focus on problem areas identified from the patient's history and on all body systems affected by the surgical procedure. The older adult (Chart 14-2; see also Chapter 2) or chronically ill patient is at increased risk for complications during and after surgery. The number of serious problems (**morbidity**) and death (**mortality**) during or after surgery is higher in older and chronically ill patients (Johnson, 2011).

Report any abnormal assessment findings to the surgeon and to anesthesia personnel, as required by The Joint Commission's NPSGs. In this way, you are a proactive patient advocate exercising professional legal responsibility. Often, established protocols or care maps identify what interventions are to be performed before surgery.

Cardiovascular status is critical to assess because cardiac problems are associated with many surgery-related deaths. Check the patient for hypertension, which is common, is often undiagnosed, and can affect the response to surgery. Cardiac assessment includes listening to heart sounds for rate, regularity, and abnormalities. Ask whether the patient has ever had a venous thromboembolism (VTE). Examine the patient's hands and feet for temperature, color, peripheral pulses, capillary refill, and edema. Report any problems (e.g., absent peripheral pulses, pitting edema, cardiac manifestations, chest pain, shortness of breath, and dyspnea) to the surgeon for further assessment and evaluation. (Cardiac assessment is discussed in Chapter 33.)

Respiratory status considers age, smoking history (including exposure to secondhand smoke), and any chronic illness (Doerflinger, 2009). Obese patients may have undiagnosed respiratory problems such as obstructive sleep apnea (OSA), which can lead to complications from anesthesia (Graham et al., 2011). Observe the patient's posture; respiratory rate, rhythm, and depth; overall respiratory effort; and lung expansion. Document any clubbing of the fingertips (swelling at the base of the nail beds caused by a chronic lack of oxygen) or cyanosis. Auscultate the lungs to assess for any abnormal breath sounds (crackles, wheezes, rubs). (More information on respiratory assessment is found in Chapter 27.)

Kidney function affects the excretion of drugs and waste products, including anesthetic and analgesic agents. If kidney function is reduced, fluid and electrolyte balance can be altered, especially in older patients. Ask about problems such as urinary frequency, dysuria (painful urination), nocturia (awakening during nighttime sleep because of a need to void), difficulty starting urine flow, and oliguria (scant amount of urine). Ask the patient about the appearance and odor of the urine. Assess the patient's usual fluid intake and degree of continence. If the patient has kidney or urinary problems, consult with the physician about further workup. (Kidney/urinary assessment is discussed further in Chapter 65.)

Kidney impairment decreases the excretion of drugs and anesthetic agents. As a result, drug responses may be prolonged. Scopolamine (Buscopan ✦), morphine, other opioids, benzodiazepines, and barbiturates often cause confusion, disorientation, apprehension, and restlessness when given to patients with decreased kidney function.

Neurologic status includes the patient's overall mental status, level of consciousness, orientation, and ability to follow commands. This information is needed before planning preoperative teaching and care after surgery. A problem in any of these areas affects the type of care needed during the surgical experience. Determine the patient's baseline neurologic status to be able to identify changes that may occur later. Also assess for any motor or sensory deficits. (See Chapter 41 for complete nervous system assessment.)

The usual neurologic status of a mentally impaired patient may be difficult to assess (Doerflinger, 2009). The patient who has been independent and oriented at home may become disoriented in the hospital setting. Family members can often provide information about what the patient was like at home.

The Joint Commission's NPSGs require that you ensure patient safety by assessing the patient's risk for falling, especially older patients. Evaluate factors such as mental status, muscle strength, steadiness of gait, and sense of independence to determine the patient's risk. Document the patient's ability to ambulate and the steadiness of gait as baseline data.

Musculoskeletal status problems may interfere with positioning during and after surgery. For example, patients with arthritis may be able to assume surgical positions but have discomfort after surgery from prolonged joint immobilization. Other anatomic features, such as the shape and length of the neck and the shape of the chest cavity, may interfere with respiratory and cardiac function or require special positioning during surgery.

> ### ! NURSING SAFETY PRIORITY (QSEN)
>
> #### Action Alert
>
> Ask about a history of joint replacement, and document the exact location of any prostheses. Communicate this information to operating room personnel to ensure that electrocautery pads, which could cause an electrical burn, are not placed on or near the area of the prosthesis. Other areas to avoid electrocautery pad placement include on or near bony prominences, scar tissue, hair, tattoos, weight-bearing surfaces, pressure points, and metal piercings (Spruce & Braswell, 2012).

Nutrition status, especially malnutrition and obesity, can increase surgical risk. Surgery increases metabolic rate and depletes potassium, vitamin C, and B vitamins, all of which are needed for wound healing and blood clotting. In poorly nourished patients, decreased serum protein levels slow recovery. Negative nitrogen balance may result from depleted protein stores. This problem increases the risk for skin breakdown, delayed wound healing, possible dehiscence or evisceration (see Chapter 16), dehydration, and sepsis.

Some older patients may have poor nutrition because of chronic illness, diuretic or laxative use, poor dietary planning or habits, anorexia, lack of motivation, or financial limitations (Touhy & Jett, 2014). Indications of poor fluid or nutrition status include:

- Brittle nails
- Muscle wasting
- Dry or flaky skin, decreased skin turgor, and hair changes (e.g., dull, sparse, dry)
- Orthostatic (postural) hypotension
- Decreased serum protein levels and abnormal serum electrolyte values

The obese patient is often malnourished because of an imbalanced diet. Obesity increases the risk for poor wound healing because of excessive *adipose* (fatty) tissue. Fatty tissue has few blood vessels, little collagen, and decreased nutrients, all of which are needed for wound healing. Obesity stresses the heart and reduces the lung volumes, which can affect the surgery and recovery. Obese patients may need larger drug doses and may retain them longer after surgery.

Skin assessment is important. Many insurers have denied coverage to hospitals for care provided to patients who develop skin breakdown or pressure ulcers during the perioperative period. Assess the patient's skin for signs of breakdown, open sores, or areas that may be exposed to excessive pressure during the surgical procedure, and document these findings. Communicate this information to the circulating nurse so that precautions can be taken to prevent injury.

> ### ? NCLEX EXAMINATION CHALLENGE
>
> #### Safe and Effective Care Environment
>
> An 81-year-old client, scheduled for a long orthopedic procedure, appears to have a low body mass index. In addition to the body mass index value, which additional client information is most important for the nurse to report to the surgeon and perioperative team as indicating an increased risk for skin breakdown?
> A. Negative nitrogen balance
> B. Previous abdominal surgery
> C. Allergy to latex products
> D. Change in mental status upon admission

Psychosocial Assessment. Perform a psychosocial assessment to determine the patient's level of anxiety, coping ability, and support systems. Provide information and offer support as needed.

Most patients have some degree of anxiety or fear before surgery. The extent of these reactions varies according to the type of surgery, the perceived effects of the surgery and its potential outcome, and the patient's personality. Surgery may be seen as a threat to life, body image, self-esteem, self-concept, or lifestyle. Patients may fear death, pain, helplessness, a change in role or work status, a diagnosis of life-threatening conditions, possible disabling or crippling effects, or the unknown.

Anxiety or fear affects the patient's ability to learn, cope, and cooperate with teaching and operative procedures. Anxiety may also influence the amount and type of anesthetic needed and may slow recovery. In some cases, severe preoperative anxiety can increase the degree of pain after surgery. Be aware of potential anxiety when interviewing the patient and planning teaching.

Assess coping mechanisms used by the patient under similar situations or in the past when confronted with a stressful situation. Ask open-ended questions about the patient's feelings about the entire surgical experience. Factors that influence coping include age, previous surgical or sick-role experiences, and physical discomfort. Manifestations of anxiety include anger, crying, restlessness, profuse sweating, increased pulse rate, palpitations, sleeplessness, diarrhea, and urinary frequency.

Laboratory Assessment. Laboratory tests before surgery provide baseline data about the patient's health and help predict potential complications. The patient scheduled for surgery in an ambulatory surgical center or admitted to the hospital on the morning of or day before surgery may have preadmission testing (PAT) performed from 24 hours to 28 days before the scheduled surgery. These test results are usually valid unless there has been a change in the patient's condition that warrants repeated testing or the patient is taking drugs that can alter laboratory values (e.g., warfarin [Coumadin], aspirin, diuretics). Some facilities have time limits for tests, especially pregnancy testing or any other test results that would require altering the surgical plan.

The choice of laboratory testing before surgery varies among facilities and depends on the patient's age, medical history, and type of anesthesia planned (Rothrock, 2011). The most common tests include:

- Urinalysis
- Blood type and screen
- Complete blood count or hemoglobin level and hematocrit
- Clotting studies (prothrombin time [PT], international normalized ratio [INR], activated partial thromboplastin time [aPTT], platelet count)

- Electrolyte levels
- Serum creatinine and blood urea nitrogen levels
- Depending on a female patient's age and the nature of the planned procedure, a pregnancy test may also be needed

Urinalysis is performed to assess for abnormal substances in the urine such as protein, glucose, blood, and bacteria. If kidney disease is suspected or if the patient is older, the physician may request other tests to determine the type and degree of disease present.

Report electrolyte imbalances or other abnormal results to the anesthesia team and the surgeon before surgery. **Hypokalemia** (decreased serum potassium level) increases the risk for toxicity if the patient is taking digoxin, slows recovery from anesthesia, and increases cardiac irritability. **Hyperkalemia** (increased serum potassium level) increases the risk for dysrhythmias, especially with the use of anesthesia.

> **! NURSING SAFETY PRIORITY** (QSEN)
>
> **Critical Rescue**
>
> Any potassium imbalance—hypokalemia or hyperkalemia—must be corrected before surgery.

Other studies may be needed, depending on the patient's medical history. For example, baseline arterial blood gas (ABG) values are assessed before surgery for patients with chronic pulmonary problems. Chart 14-3 lists abnormal laboratory findings and their possible causes.

CHART 14-3 Laboratory Profile

Perioperative Assessment

TEST	NORMAL RANGE FOR ADULTS	SIGNIFICANCE OF ABNORMAL FINDINGS	
		INCREASED IN	**DECREASED IN**
Potassium (K⁺)	3.5-5.0 mEq/L, or 3.5-5.0 mmol/L	Dehydration Kidney impairment Acidosis Cellular/tissue damage Hemolysis of the specimen	NPO status when potassium replacement is inadequate Excessive use of non–potassium-sparing diuretics Vomiting Malnutrition Diarrhea Alkalosis
Sodium (Na⁺)	90 yr or younger: 136-145 mEq/L, or 136-145 mmol/L Older than 90 yr: 132-146 mEq/L, or 132-146 mmol/L	Cardiac failure or kidney impairment Hypertension Excessive amounts of IV fluids containing sodium chloride Edema Dehydration (hemoconcentration)	Nasogastric drainage Vomiting or diarrhea Excessive use of laxatives or diuretics Excessive amounts of IV fluids containing water Syndrome of inappropriate antidiuretic hormone (SIADH)
Chloride (Cl⁻)	90 yr or younger: 98-106 mEq/L, or 98-106 mmol/L Older than 90 yr: 98-111 mEq/L, or 98-111 mmol/L	Respiratory alkalosis Dehydration Kidney impairment Excessive amounts of IV fluids containing sodium chloride (NaCl)	Excessive nasogastric drainage Vomiting Excessive use of diuretics Diarrhea
Carbon dioxide (CO₂)	60 yr or younger: 23-30 mEq/L, or 23-30 mmol/L 60-90 yr: 23-31 mEq/L, or 23-31 mmol/L Older than 90 yr: 20-29 mEq/L, or 20-29 mmol/L	Chronic pulmonary disease Intestinal obstruction Vomiting or nasogastric suctioning Metabolic alkalosis	Hyperventilation Diabetic ketoacidosis Diarrhea Lactic acidosis Renal failure Salicylate toxicity

Continued

CHART 14-3   Laboratory Profile—cont'd

Perioperative Assessment

TEST	NORMAL RANGE FOR ADULTS	SIGNIFICANCE OF ABNORMAL FINDINGS	
		INCREASED IN	DECREASED IN
Glucose (fasting)	60 yr or younger: 70-110 mg/dL, or 4.1-5.9 mmol/L 60-90 yr: 82-115 mg/dL, or 4.6-6.4 mmol/L Older than 90 yr: 75-121 mg/dL, or 4.2-6.7 mmol/L	Hyperglycemia Excessive amounts of IV fluids containing glucose Stress Steroid use Pancreatic or hepatic disease	Hypoglycemia Excess insulin

Creatinine	*Females:*
	    60 yr or younger: 0.5-1.1 mg/dL, or 44-97 μmol/L
	    60-90 yr: 0.6-1.2 mg/dL, or 53-106 μmol/L
	    Older than 90 yr: 0.6-1.3 mg/dL, or 53-115 μmol/L
	Males:
	    60 yr or younger: 0.6-1.2 mg/dL, or 53-106 μmol/L
	    60-90 yr: 0.8-1.3 mg/dL, or 71-115 μmol/L
	    Older than 90 yr: 1.0-1.7 mg/dL, or 88-150 μmol/L
		Kidney damage with destruction of large number of nephrons
		Renal insufficiency
		Acute kidney injury
		Chronic kidney disease
		End-stage kidney disease (ESKD)
			Atrophy of muscle tissue

Blood urea nitrogen (BUN)	Younger than 60 yr: 10-20 mg/dL, or 3.61-7.1 mmol/L 60-90 yr: 8-23 mg/dL, or 2.9-8.2 mmol/L Older than 90 yr: 10-31 mg/dL, or 3.6-11.1 mmol/L	Dehydration Kidney impairment Excessive protein in diet Liver failure	Overhydration Malnutrition
Prothrombin time (pro time, PT)	11-12.5 sec, 85%-100%, or 1:1.1 patient-control ratio	Coagulation defect (bleeding disorder) Vitamin K deficiency	Coagulation (clotting) disorder, such as thrombophlebitis or pulmonary embolus
International normalized ratio (INR)	0.7-1.8	Anticoagulant therapy (aspirin, warfarin)	Extensive cancer
Partial thromboplastin time, activated (aPTT)	30-40 sec	Coagulation defect (bleeding disorder) Anticoagulant therapy (heparin) Liver disease	Coagulation (clotting) disorder, such as thrombophlebitis or pulmonary embolus Extensive cancer
White blood cell (WBC) count (leukocyte count)	Total: 5,000-10,000/mm³	Infection Inflammation Stress Tissue necrosis	Immune disorder Immunosuppressant therapy

Hemoglobin, total	*Females:*
	    18-44 yr: 12-16 g/dL, or 117-155 g/L
	    45-64 yr: 11.7-16.0 g/dL, or 117-160 g/L
	    65-74 yr: 11.7-16.1 g/dL, or 117-161 g/L
	Males:
	    18-44 yr: 14-18 g/dL, or 132-173 g/L
	    45-64 yr: 13.1-17.2 g/dL, or 131-172 g/L
	    65-74 yr: 12.6-17.4 g/dL, or 126-174 g/L
		Dehydration
		Polycythemia
		Chronic pulmonary disease
		Congestive heart failure
			Blood loss
			Anemia
			Renal failure

Hematocrit	*Females:*
	    18-44 yr: 35%-45%
	    45-74 yr: 37%-47%
	Males:
	    18-44 yr: 42%-52%
	    45-64 yr: 39%-50%
	    65-74 yr: 37%-51%
		Dehydration
		Polycythemia
		High altitude
			Blood loss
			Anemia
			Kidney failure

Source: Pagana, K., & Pagana, T. (2014). *Mosby's manual of diagnostic and laboratory tests* (5th ed). St. Louis: Mosby.

Imaging Assessment. A chest x-ray may be requested before surgery. Often, healthy adults are not required to have a chest x-ray. A chest x-ray determines the size and shape of the heart, lungs, and major vessels and provides evidence of the presence of pneumonia or tuberculosis. It also provides baseline data in case of complications. Abnormal x-ray findings alert the surgeon to potential cardiac or pulmonary complications. Heart failure, cardiomyopathy, pneumonia, or infiltrates may cause cancellation or delay of elective surgery. For emergency surgery, x-ray results assist the anesthesia provider in selecting anesthesia type.

Other imaging studies are based on patient need, medical history, and the nature of the surgical procedure. For example, a patient with back pain may have CT scans or MRI examinations before spinal surgery to identify the exact location of the problem.

Other Diagnostic Assessment. An electrocardiogram (ECG) may be required for patients older than a specific age who are to have general anesthesia. The age varies among facilities but is often 40 to 45 years. An ECG may also be required for patients with a history of cardiac disease or those at risk for cardiac complications. It provides baseline information on new or existing cardiac problems, such as an old myocardial infarction (MI). A patient with a known cardiac problem may need a cardiology consultation before surgery. Drugs for problem prevention, such as nitroglycerin, beta blockers, and antibiotics, may be needed throughout the surgical period to reduce or prevent stress on the heart. Abnormal or potentially life-threatening ECG results may cause the cancellation of surgery until the patient's cardiac status is stable.

A focused assessment of the preoperative patient is shown in Chart 14-4.

CHART 14-4 Focused Assessment

The Preoperative Patient

As part of the cardiopulmonary assessment, take and record vital signs; report:
- Hypotension or hypertension
- Heart rate less than 60 or more than 120 beats/min
- Irregular heart rate
- Chest pain
- Shortness of breath or dyspnea
- Tachypnea
- Pulse oximetry reading of less than 94%

Assess for and report any signs or symptoms of infection, including:
- Fever
- Purulent sputum
- Dysuria or cloudy, foul-smelling urine
- Any red, swollen, draining IV or wound site
- Increased white blood cell count

Assess for and report signs or symptoms that could contraindicate surgery, including:
- Increased prothrombin time (PT), international normalized ratio (INR), or activated partial thromboplastin time (aPTT)
- Hypokalemia or hyperkalemia
- Patient report of possible pregnancy or positive pregnancy test

Assess for and report other clinical conditions that may need to be evaluated by a physician or advanced practice nurse before proceeding with the surgical plans, including:
- Change in mental status
- Vomiting
- Rash
- Recent administration of an anticoagulant drug

❓ NCLEX EXAMINATION CHALLENGE

Physiological Integrity

The preoperative admitting nurse notices that the client scheduled for total joint replacement surgery in 2 hours has a smell of alcohol on his breath even though he has just stated that he has fasted completely for the past 10 hours. What is the nurse's best first action?

A. Accept the client's statement and continue the preoperative preparation.

B. Report the discrepancy to the surgeon and anesthesiologist immediately.

C. Tell the client the observation and provide the opportunity for him to explain.

D. Remind the client that alcohol consumption may require changes in anesthesia procedure.

◆ Analysis

The priority NANDA-I nursing diagnoses and collaborative problems for preoperative patients include:

1. Deficient Knowledge related to unfamiliarity with surgical procedures and preparation (NANDA-I)
2. Anxiety related to new or unknown experience, possibility of pain, and possible surgical outcomes (NANDA-I)

◆ Planning and Implementation

As the nurse, your role is to ensure coordination of care for the patient before surgery. This responsibility continues until the patient is transferred to the operating room (OR).

Providing Information

Planning: Expected Outcomes. The patient needs to know what to expect during and after surgery and participate in his or her recovery as indicated by consistently demonstrating these behaviors:

- Explaining in his or her own words the purpose and expected results of the planned surgery
- Asking questions when a term or procedure is not known
- Adhering to the NPO requirements
- Stating an understanding of preoperative preparations (e.g., skin preparation, bowel preparation)

- Demonstrating correct use of exercises and techniques to be used after surgery for the prevention of complications (e.g., splinting the incision, using an incentive spirometer, performing leg exercises, ambulating as early as permitted)

Interventions. Because the surgical experience is foreign to many people, focus on teaching the patient and family members. Teaching may begin in the surgeon's office for planned or elective surgery. Pamphlets, written instructions, approved websites, and video recordings or DVDs may be given or sent to the patient. More teaching may occur when the patient has preadmission testing. Some facilities hold classes before surgery for groups of patients or show videos for those who are having the same or similar surgical procedures. A tour of the operating suite and the postanesthesia care unit (PACU) may be included.

Explore the patient's level of knowledge and understanding. Increased access to information via the Internet may be helpful but is also a concern. Some Internet information may not be accurate or may not apply to a specific patient's plan of care.

The Joint Commission's NPSGs require that you provide information about informed consent, dietary restrictions, specific preparation for surgery (bowel and skin preparations), exercises after surgery, and plans for pain management to promote patients' participation and help achieve the expected outcome. A sample educational checklist is shown in Table 14-4. Because education occurs in a variety of settings, coordination of patient teaching efforts is challenging. When you care for the patient just before surgery (same-day, ambulatory surgery [outpatient] unit, inpatient hospital unit), assess the patient's

TABLE 14-4 Preoperative Teaching Checklist

Consider these items when planning individualized preoperative teaching for patients and families:

- Fears and anxieties
- Surgical procedure
- Preoperative routines (e.g., NPO, blood samples, showering)
- Invasive procedures (e.g., lines, catheters)
- Coughing, turning, deep breathing
- Incentive spirometer
  - How to use
  - How to tell when used correctly
- Lower extremity exercises
- Stockings and pneumatic compression devices
- Early ambulation
- Splinting
- Pain management

and family members' knowledge and provide additional information as needed. If the patient is receiving sedation or general anesthesia, stress the importance of having another person drive the patient home after the procedure. Document in the patient record information about who was involved in teaching, what specifically was taught, and what education materials were given to the patient and family.

Ensuring Informed Consent. Surgery of any type involves invasion of the body and requires informed consent from the patient or legal guardian (Fig. 14-2). The Joint Commission's NPSGs state that patients deserve to be informed and involved in decisions affecting their health care. Consent implies that the patient has sufficient information to understand:

- The nature of and reason for surgery
- Who will be performing the surgery and whether others will be present during the procedure (e.g., students)
- All available options and the risks associated with each option
- The risks associated with the surgical procedure and its potential outcomes
- The risks associated with the use of anesthesia

Informed consent is one way to help ensure patient safety. It helps protect the patient from any unwanted procedures and protects the surgeon and the facility from lawsuit claims related to unauthorized surgery or uninformed patients. Written record of informed consent is documented on a "consent form" but can also be documented in the surgeon's notes. The consent form documents the patient's consent and signature for the procedure listed.

As a competent adult, it is the patient's right to refuse treatment for any reason, even when refusal might lead to death. For example, in the case of Jehovah's Witnesses, some patients will not accept blood transfusions because of their religious convictions.

The surgeon is responsible for having the consent form signed before sedation is given and before surgery is performed. *You, as a nurse, are not responsible for providing detailed information about the surgical procedure. Rather, your role is to clarify facts that have been presented by the surgeon and dispel myths that the patient or family may have about the surgical experience. You verify that the consent form is signed, and you serve as a witness to the signature, not to the fact that the patient is informed* (Rock & Hoebeke, 2014).

! NURSING SAFETY PRIORITY (QSEN)

Action Alert

If you believe that the patient has not been adequately informed, contact the surgeon and request that he or she see the patient for further clarification. Document this action in the medical record.

Patients who cannot write may sign with an X, which must be witnessed by two people. In an emergency, telephone or telegram authorization is acceptable and should be followed up with written consent as soon as possible. The number of witnesses (usually two) and the type of documentation vary according to the facility's policy. For a life-threatening situation in which every effort has been made to contact the person with medical power of attorney, consent is desired but not essential. In place of written or oral consent, written consultation by at least two physicians who are not associated with the case may be requested by the surgeon. This formal consultation legally supports the decision for surgery until the appropriate person can sign a consent form. If the patient is not capable of giving consent and has no family, the court can appoint a legal guardian to represent the patient's best interests.

A blind patient may sign his or her own consent form, which usually needs to be witnessed by two persons. Patients who do not speak the general language of the facility or who are hearing impaired may require a qualified translator and a second witness. Many facilities have consent forms written in more than one language and also have health care professionals who are proficient with American Sign Language. Qualified translators may be health care professionals, other types of hospital employee, or family members. They are required to keep patient information confidential.

Some surgical procedures, such as sterilization and experimental procedures, may require a special permit in addition to the standard consent. National and local governing bodies and the individual facility determine which procedures require a separate permit. Separate consents for anesthesia and blood products may be required.

Surgical procedures that are site-specific, such as left, right, or bilateral, require patient identification before surgery. As required by The Joint Commission's NPSGs, to ensure the correct site is selected and the wrong site is avoided, the site is marked by a licensed independent practitioner and, whenever possible, involves the patient. The surgeon is accountable and should be present during the procedure. The nurse is an important part of this safety measure. Before starting the operative procedure, facilities use a "time-out" procedure to verify the correct site, patient, and procedure. The perioperative nurse is in a position of ensuring these safety measures are implemented immediately before the procedure is started (Association of periOperative Registered Nurses [AORN], 2014c). The "time-out" involves the participation of all members of the procedure team including the surgeon, anesthesia provider, circulating nurse, scrub person, and any other active participants.

! NURSING SAFETY PRIORITY (QSEN)

Critical Rescue

At a minimum, the patient's identity, correct side and site, correct patient position, and agreement on the proposed procedure must be verified by all members of the surgical team.

GENERAL REQUEST AND CONSENT

FOR OFFICE USE ONLY:
Patient Name: _____
Date of Birth: _____
Date of Procedure: _____

I _____ request and give consent to _____
　　　(Type or print patient name)　　　　　　　　　　　　　　　　(Type or print Doctor or Practitioner Name(s))

to perform the following procedure(s) _____
　　　　　　　　　　　　　　　　(Please list site and side if appropriate)

_____

The benefits, risks, complications, and alternatives to the above procedure(s) have been explained to me.

I understand that the procedure(s) will be performed at Christiana Care by and under supervision of my doctor or practitioner. My doctor or practitioner may use the services of other doctors or practitioners, or members of the resident staff as he or she deems necessary or advisable.

I authorize my doctor or practitioner and his or her associates and assistants to perform such additional procedures, which in their judgment are necessary and appropriate to carry out my diagnosis or treatment.

I authorize the hospital to retain, preserve and use for scientific, teaching or transplant purposes, or to make other dispositions of, at their convenience, any specimens, tissues, or parts taken from my body during the course of this operation.

I consent to observers in the operating room in accordance with hospital policy. I consent to photography or video taping of my surgical procedure for educational purposes, provided my identity remains anonymous and confidential.

I agree to being given blood or blood products as deemed advisable during the course of my procedure. The risks, benefits, and alternatives to receiving blood or blood products have been explained to me.

I consent to the administration of sedation or analgesia during my procedure. The risks, benefits, and alternatives to receiving sedation or analgesia have been explained to me.

If anesthesia is required, I consent to the administration of anesthesia by members of the Department of Anesthesiology. I also consent to the use of non-invasive and invasive monitoring techniques as deemed necessary. I understand that anesthesia involves risks that are in addition to those resulting from the operation itself including, but not limited to, dental injury, hoarseness, vocal cord injury, infection, nerve injury, corneal abrasion, seizures, heart attack, stroke and even death.

Please initial one of the following statements (females only):

_____ To the best of my knowledge I am not pregnant.   _____ I believe I am pregnant.

I certify that I have read and understand the above consent statements. In addition, I have been offered the opportunity to ask my doctor or practitioner any questions I have regarding the procedure(s) to be performed and they have been answered to my satisfaction. I acknowledge that I have been given no guarantee or assurance as to the results that may be obtained from the procedure(s).

_____　_____   _____　_____
Signature of Patient or Decision Maker　Date and Time   Doctor or Practitioner Signature　　　Date and Time

_____   _____
Relationship to Patient if Decision Maker   Doctor ID # or Print Name

_____　_____   _____
Witness Signature　　　　　　　　　　Date and Time   Practitioner Print Name/Title

_____
Witness Print Name

Telephone
Consent: _____
　　　　　　　Name of person obtained from/Relationship to Patient

_____　_____   _____　_____
Witness's (es') Signature(s)　　　　　Date and Time   Witness's (es') Signature(s)　　　　　Date and Time

_____   _____
Witness's (es') Print Name(s)   Witness's (es') Print Name(s)

FIG. 14-2 A surgical consent form.

CLINICAL JUDGMENT CHALLENGE

Safety QSEN

The patient states the surgeon discussed the addition of a second procedure to the one indicated on the consent. The patient is visibly upset that the consent he is asked to sign with the surgical resident reflects only one procedure and cannot understand why the nurse and resident do not have the authority to "fix" the consent. In addition, he states he will not take his wedding ring off because it has never left his hand since his wife put it there 30 years ago.

1. How would you address the patient's immediate concern regarding the consent?
2. Under what conditions could the second procedure be performed?
3. What remedy would you propose to prevent such occurrences in the future?
4. How will you respond to the patient's unwillingness to remove his wedding ring?

Patient Self-Determination. Patients receiving medical care have the right to have or to initiate advance directives, such as a living will or durable power of attorney, as mandated by the Patient Self-Determination Act. Advance directives provide legal instructions to the health care providers about the patient's wishes and are to be followed. *Surgery does not provide an exception to a patient's advance directives or living will* (AORN, 2014b). Chapter 7 discusses advance directives in more detail.

Implementing Dietary Restrictions. Regardless of the type of surgery and anesthesia planned, the patient is restricted to NPO status before surgery. **NPO** means no eating, drinking (including water), or smoking (nicotine stimulates gastric secretions). The exact amount of time a patient must be NPO before surgery is controversial. Patients, especially older adults, who fast for 8 or more hours may have imbalances of fluids, electrolytes, and blood glucose levels. The American Society of Anesthesiologists (ASA) recommends a reduced NPO time—6 or more hours for easily digested solid food and 2 hours for clear liquids (Crenshaw, 2011; Sendelbach, 2010). A major problem is that these guidelines for duration of fasting have not been implemented universally.

NPO status ensures that the stomach contains a limited volume of gastric secretions, which decreases the risk for aspiration. Outpatients and patients who are scheduled for admission to the hospital on the same day that surgery is performed must receive written and oral instructions about when to begin NPO status.

NURSING SAFETY PRIORITY QSEN

Action Alert

Emphasize the importance of adhering to the prescribed NPO restriction. Failure to adhere can result in cancellation of surgery or increase the risk for aspiration during or after surgery.

Administering Regularly Scheduled Drugs. On the day of surgery, the patient's usual drug schedule may need to be altered. Consult the medical health care provider and the anesthesia provider for instructions about drugs such as those taken for diabetes, cardiac disease, or glaucoma, as well as regularly scheduled anticonvulsants, antihypertensives, anticoagulants, antidepressants, and corticosteroids. The surgeon may prescribe some drugs, including over-the-counter drugs such as aspirin, other NSAIDs, and herbal supplements, to be stopped until after surgery. Other drugs may be given IV to maintain the drug level in the blood. *Drugs for cardiac disease, respiratory disease, seizures, and hypertension are commonly allowed with a sip of water before surgery.* Some antihypertensive or antidepressant drugs are withheld on the day of surgery to reduce adverse effects on blood pressure during surgery. Even when beta blockers are not part of a patient's usual medications, they may be prescribed for some patients who are at risk for cardiac problems. Check with the health care provider, surgeon, or anesthesia provider to determine whether a specific patient requires perioperative therapy with beta-blocking drugs, as recommended by core measures for SCIP CARD-2 (see Table 14-1).

The patient who takes insulin for diabetes may be given a reduced dose of intermediate- or long-acting insulin based on the blood glucose level or may be given regular (fast-acting) insulin in divided doses on the day of surgery. As an alternative, an IV infusion of 5% dextrose in water may be given with the insulin to prevent low blood sugar during surgery. Because of the many treatment approaches to diabetes, clarify drug and IV prescriptions with the health care provider. (See Chapter 64 for more information about diabetes.)

Intestinal Preparation. Bowel or intestinal preparations are performed to prevent injury to the colon and to reduce the number of intestinal bacteria. Bowel evacuation is needed when a patient is having major abdominal, pelvic, perineal, or perianal surgery. In addition, colonoscopy procedures, routinely performed in outpatient ambulatory care facilities, require the patient to follow a strict preoperative protocol for bowel evacuation. The surgeon's preference and the type of surgical procedure determine the type of bowel preparation. Enemas ordered to be given until return flow is clear is a stressful procedure, especially for the older patient. Repeated enemas can cause electrolyte imbalance, fluid volume imbalances, vagal stimulation, and postural (orthostatic) hypotension. Enemas cause severe anal discomfort in patients with hemorrhoids. Some physicians prescribe potent laxatives instead of enemas, especially for older patients. Bowel preparations can exhaust the patient, and you must take safety precautions to prevent falls.

Skin Preparation. The skin is the body's first line of defense against INFECTION. A break in this barrier increases the risk for infection, especially for older patients. Skin preparation before surgery is the first step to reduce the risk for surgical site infection (AORN, 2014d).

One or two days before the scheduled surgery, the surgeon may ask the patient to shower using an antiseptic solution. Instruct the patient to be especially careful to clean well around the proposed surgical site. If the patient is hospitalized before surgery, showering and cleaning are repeated the night before surgery or in the morning before transfer to the surgical suite. This cleaning reduces contamination of the surgical field and reduces the number of organisms at the site. Remove any soil or debris from the surgical site and surrounding areas.

Factors that predispose to wound contamination and surgical site INFECTION (SSI) include bacteria found in hair follicles, disruption of the normal protective mechanisms of the skin, and nicks in the skin. Shaving of hair creates the potential for infection. Hair clipping with electrical clippers and depilatories are to be used for hair removal as required by The Joint Commission's NPSGs (Tanner et al., 2011). This type of skin preparation is part of the Surgical Care Improvement Project's (SCIP) core measures for SCIP Inf-6 (see Table 14-1).

The Centers for Disease Control and Prevention (CDC) recommends that if shaving is necessary, the hair should be removed using disposable sterile supplies and aseptic principles *immediately* before the start of the surgical procedure. If needed, shaving is performed in the treatment room, the holding area of the operating suite, or the operating room (OR). Fig. 14-3 shows areas of hair removal for various surgical procedures.

Preparing the Patient for Tubes, Drains, and Vascular Access. Prepare the patient for possible placement of tubes, drains, and vascular access devices. Preparation reduces the

FIG. 14-3 Skin preparation of common surgical sites. *Shaded areas* indicate preparation areas.

patient's anxiety and fear and the family's negative reaction. Be careful not to scare the patient while providing information about the purpose of each tube.

Tubes of all sorts are common after surgery. A nasogastric (NG) tube may be inserted before abdominal surgery to decompress or empty the stomach and the upper bowel. Usually the tube is placed after the induction of anesthesia, when insertion is less disturbing to the patient and is easier to perform. The patient may need an indwelling urinary (Foley) catheter before, during, or after surgery to keep the bladder empty and to monitor kidney function.

Drains are often placed during surgery to help remove fluid from the surgical site. Some drains are under the dressing; others are visible and require emptying. Drains come in various shapes and sizes (see Chapter 16). Inform the patient that drains are often used routinely and that generally they are not painful but may cause some discomfort. Discuss the reasons drains should not be kinked or pulled.

Vascular access is placed for patients receiving a general anesthetic and for most patients receiving other types of anesthetics. Access is needed to give drugs and fluids before, during, and after surgery. Patients who are dehydrated or are at risk for dehydration may receive fluids before surgery.

CONSIDERATIONS FOR OLDER ADULTS
Patient-Centered Care [QSEN]

Older adult patients are at greater risk for dehydration because their fluid reserves are lower than those of young or middle-aged adults. Carefully monitor older adult patients and patients with cardiac disease receiving IV fluids. (See Chapter 13 for more information on IV therapy.)

The IV access is usually placed in the arm using a large-bore, short catheter (e.g., 18-gauge, 1-inch catheter) or placed in the back of the hand using a smaller-bore (20-gauge) catheter. A larger vein provides the least resistance to fluid or blood infusion, especially in an emergency when rapid infusions may be needed. Depending on the patient's needs and the facility's policies, the IV access can be placed before surgery when the patient is in the hospital room, in the holding or admission area of the surgical suite, or in the OR.

Postoperative Procedures and Exercises. Teach the patient and family members about exercises and procedures (e.g., checking dressings, obtaining vital signs frequently) to be performed after surgery. Family members can be helpful in reminding patients to perform the exercises. Teaching before surgery reduces apprehension and fear, increases cooperation and participation in care after surgery, and decreases respiratory and vascular complications. When the fear or anxiety level is high, explore the patient's feelings before discussing procedures.

Discussion, demonstration with return demonstration, and practice by the patient aid in the ability to perform various breathing (Chart 14-5) and leg (Chart 14-6) exercises after surgery. Stress the need to begin exercises early in the recovery phase and to continue them, with 5 to 10 repetitions each, every 1 to 2 hours after surgery for at least the first 48 hours. Explain that the patient may need to be awakened for these activities.

Procedures and Exercises to Prevent Respiratory Complications. *Breathing exercises* include deep, or diaphragmatic, breathing to enlarge the chest cavity and expand the lungs. After

---

CHART 14-5 *Patient and Family Education:* **Preparing for Self-Management**

Perioperative Respiratory Care

Deep (Diaphragmatic) Breathing
1. Sit upright on the edge of the bed or in a chair, being sure that your feet are placed firmly on the floor or a stool. (After surgery, deep breathing is done with the patient in Fowler's position or in semi-Fowler's position.)
2. Take a gentle breath through your mouth.
3. Breathe out gently and completely.
4. Then take a deep breath through your nose and mouth, and hold this breath to the count of five.
5. Exhale through your nose and mouth.

Expansion Breathing
1. Find a comfortable upright position, with your knees slightly bent. (Bending the knees decreases tension on the abdominal muscles and decreases respiratory resistance and discomfort.)
2. Place your hands on each side of your lower rib cage, just above your waist.
3. Take a deep breath through your nose, using your shoulder muscles to expand your lower rib cage outward during inhalation.
4. Exhale, concentrating first on moving your chest, then on moving your lower ribs inward, while gently squeezing the rib cage and forcing air out of the base of your lungs.

Splinting of the Surgical Incision
1. Unless coughing is contraindicated, place a pillow, towel, or folded blanket over your surgical incision and hold the item firmly in place.
2. Take three slow, deep breaths to stimulate your cough reflex.
3. Inhale through your nose, and then exhale through your mouth.
4. On your third deep breath, cough to clear secretions from your lungs while firmly holding the pillow, towel, or folded blanket against your incision.

---

you demonstrate and explain the technique, urge the patient to practice deep breathing.

For patients with chronic lung disease or limited chest expansion, as seen in older patients because of the aging process, expansion breathing exercises are useful. For the patient having chest surgery, expansion breathing exercises strengthen accessory muscles and are started before surgery. Expansion breathing after surgery during chest physiotherapy (percussion, vibration, postural drainage) may help loosen secretions and maintain an adequate air exchange.

Incentive spirometry is another way to encourage the patient to take deep breaths. Its purpose is to promote complete lung expansion and to prevent pulmonary problems. Various types of incentive spirometers are available; Fig. 14-4 shows a patient using one type. With all types, the patient must be able to seal the lips tightly around the mouthpiece, inhale spontaneously, and hold his or her breath for 3 to 5 seconds for effective lung expansion. Goals (e.g., attaining specific volumes) can be set according to the patient's ability and the type of incentive spirometer. Seeing a ball move up a column or a bellows expanding reinforces and motivates the patient to continue performance.

Coughing and splinting may be performed along with deep breathing every 1 to 2 hours after surgery. The purposes of coughing are to expel secretions, keep the lungs clear, allow full aeration, and prevent pneumonia and atelectasis. Coughing may be uncomfortable for the patient, but when performed correctly, it should not harm the incision. Splinting (i.e., holding) the incision area provides support, promotes a feeling

Postoperative Leg Exercises

Exercise No. 1

1. Lie in bed with the head of your bed elevated to about 45 degrees.
2. Beginning with your right leg, bend your knee, raise your foot off the bed, and hold this position for a few seconds.
3. Extend your leg by unbending your knee, and lower the leg to the bed.
4. Repeat this sequence four more times with your right leg; then perform this same exercise five times with your left leg.

Exercise No. 2

1. Beginning with your right leg, point your toes toward the bottom of the bed.
2. With the same leg, point your toes up toward your face.
3. Repeat this exercise several times with your right leg; then perform this same exercise with your left leg.

Exercise No. 3

1. Beginning with your right leg, make circles with your ankle, first to the left and then to the right.
2. Repeat this exercise several times with your right leg; then perform this same exercise with your left leg.

Exercise No. 4

1. Beginning with your right leg, bend your knee and *push* the ball of your foot into the bed or floor until you feel your calf and thigh muscles contracting.
2. Repeat this exercise several times with your right leg; then perform this same exercise with your left leg.

FIG. 14-4 A patient using an incentive spirometer.

of security, and reduces pain during coughing. The proper technique for splinting the incision site and coughing is described in Chart 14-5. A folded bath blanket or pillow is helpful to use as a splint. Cardiac surgery patients may receive their own heart-shaped pillow for splint use.

The use of routine coughing exercises after surgery is controversial. Some surgeons believe coughing may harm the surgical wound and that it would be better to use other, safer measures for lung hygiene, such as deep breathing and incentive spirometer exercises. When routine coughing exercises should be avoided for a specific patient, such as after a hernia repair or craniotomy, the surgeon usually writes a "do not cough" prescription.

Procedures and Exercises to Prevent Cardiovascular Complications. Venous stasis and venous thromboembolism (VTE) (a group of vascular disorders that includes deep vein thrombosis [DVT] and pulmonary embolism [PE]) are potential but often avoidable complications of surgery. VTE or DVT can lead to a PE if the blood clot breaks off and travels to the lungs. Patients at greater risk for VTE:

- Are obese
- Are older than 40 years
- Have cancer
- Have decreased mobility or are immobile
- Have a spinal cord injury
- Have a history of VTE, DVT, PE, varicose veins, or edema
- Are taking oral contraceptives

- Smoke
- Have decreased cardiac output
- Have hip fracture or total hip or total knee surgery

Always assess for VTE before surgery. Sudden swelling in one leg is a common physical finding of VTE caused by DVT. A patient may feel a dull ache in the calf area that becomes worse with ambulation. A careful assessment and timely intervention may prevent the potentially fatal complication of pulmonary embolism.

Because surgical-related VTE can be prevented, prophylaxis is required by the Surgical Care Improvement Project (SCIP) core measures (see Table 14-1). All patients should be evaluated for VTE risk based on history, type and duration of surgery, and expected time of immobilization after surgery. VTE prophylaxis may involve devices and drug therapy, depending on a specific patient's evaluated risk. Devices may be used during and after surgery along with leg exercises and early ambulation to promote venous return. Specific interventions depend on the patient's risk factors (Larkin et al., 2012). (See the Evidence-Based Practice box.)

Antiembolism stockings (TED or Jobst stockings) and elastic (Ace) wraps provide graduated compression of the legs, starting at the end of the foot and ankle. Measure the patient's leg length and circumference before ordering the stocking size. Elastic wraps are used when the legs are too large or too small for the stockings. Assist the patient in applying the stockings or wraps, and ensure that they are neither too loose (are ineffective) nor too tight (inhibit blood flow). They need to be worn properly and should be removed 1 to 3 times per day for 30 minutes for skin inspection and skin care.

Pneumatic compression devices enhance venous blood flow by providing intermittent periods of compression on the legs. Measure the patient's legs, and order the correct size. Place the boots on the patient's legs, and then set and check the compression pressures (usually 35-55 mm Hg). *Unless these devices are applied properly, there is no benefit* (Elpern et al., 2013). Fig. 14-5 shows various types of sequential compression devices. Antiembolism stockings may be worn in addition to the boots and may reduce some of the uncomfortable sensations of the boots (e.g., itching, sweating, heat).

Leg exercises also promote venous return. Teach the leg exercises outlined in Chart 14-6, and then urge the patient to practice these exercises before surgery. The exercises are important, even when other devices are used.

FIG. 14-5 An external pneumatic compression device used to promote venous return and prevent deep vein thrombosis (DVT).

Mobility soon after surgery (early ambulation) has many cardiovascular and other benefits. It stimulates intestinal motility, enhances lung expansion, mobilizes secretions, promotes venous return, prevents joint rigidity, and relieves pressure. For most types of surgery, teach the patient to turn at least every 2 hours after surgery while confined to bed. Teach patients how

EVIDENCE-BASED PRACTICE QSEN

VTE Prevention Beyond the Surgical Care Improvement Project (SCIP): What Works?

Larkin, B., Mitchell, K., & Petrie, K. (2012). Translating evidence to practice for mechanical venous thromboembolism prophylaxis. *AORN Journal, 96*(5), 513-527.

Both pharmacologic and mechanical prophylaxis for prevention of venous thromboembolism (VTE) are being used extensively to prevent VTE after surgery. Many health care professionals, including nurses, believe that pharmacologic prophylaxis is more effective and more important than mechanical prophylaxis. However, some patients cannot use pharmacologic prophylaxis. This integrative review of the literature sought to determine the evidence for best practices related to mechanical prophylaxis to prevent surgical-related venous thromboembolism (VTE) events. Variables compared included the types of mechanical prophylaxis, timing of application, the effects of combining prophylaxis methods, and the use of unilateral prophylaxis for some orthopedic procedures.

A variety of research reports and previous meta-analyses from appropriate sources were reviewed. The criteria and need for mechanical prophylaxis and its optimal initiation varied by institution and profession. Most surgeons followed the SCIP guidelines, whereas experienced perioperative nurses expanded the risk factors to include history of VTE events, level of general immobility, and presence of varicosities. Also examined were issues related to availability of prescribed devices and the timing of their application.

Results of the study indicated that use of mechanical prophylaxis for VTE is increasing, although the timing and duration of application is not consistent. Overall, the best outcomes were obtained when devices, whether they were graduated compression stockings or intermittent pneumatic compression devices, were applied correctly in the preoperative period rather than intraoperatively or postoperatively. No evidence supports the combination of devices to be more effective than either type of device alone. In addition, patients with issues not listed in the SCIP guidelines were also at risk for VTE and could benefit from perioperative mechanical prophylaxis. These include older age, decreased general mobility, irritable bowel syndrome, oral contraceptive use, malignant disease, severe infection, and presence of varicose veins.

Level of Evidence: 1

The study is an analysis of previous research studies on the use of mechanical prophylaxis for perioperative prevention of VTE, examining practices and specific devices. The methods used were appropriate to answer the question posed, and the large numbers of human subjects resulted in credible evidence to support the need for practice consistency.

Commentary: Implications for Practice and Research

The current SCIP criteria for VTE mechanical prophylaxis are beginning points, not end points, for this evolving prevention strategy. Nurses can contribute to the desired outcome of reducing surgical-related VTE events by identifying patients who have other risk factors for VTE that may be less obvious or are not included in the SCIP criteria. By partnering with surgeons to ensure that such patients are prescribed mechanical prophylaxis and that the devices are applied correctly during the preoperative period, the goal of VTE as a "never" event is closer to being achieved.

to use the bed siderails safely for turning and how to protect the surgical wound by splinting when turning. Assure patients that assistance and pain drugs will be given as needed to reduce any anxiety and pain they may have with this activity.

For certain surgical procedures, such as some brain, spinal, and orthopedic procedures, the surgeon may prescribe turning restrictions. Ask the surgeon about other interventions to prevent complications of immobility in patients with turning restrictions. During teaching before surgery, inform the patient of anticipated turning restrictions.

Most patients are allowed and encouraged to get out of bed the day of or the day after surgery. Assist the patient into a chair or with ambulation after the surgery, the next day, or when the surgeon specifies. If a patient must remain in bed, help him or her turn, deep breathe, and perform leg exercises at least every 2 hours to prevent complications from immobility.

Minimizing Anxiety

Planning: Expected Outcomes. Before surgery, the patient is expected to have manageable anxiety as indicated by consistently demonstrating these behaviors:
- Expressing a reduced level of anxiety
- Showing an absence of body language indicators of anxiety (e.g., hand wringing, facial tension, restlessness, dilated pupils, sweating, elevated blood pressure, elevated pulse rate)

Interventions. Anxiety often causes restlessness and sleeplessness. The patient may perceive the surgical experience as a threat to life and function. Assess the patient's level of anxiety, as discussed on p. 222 in the Psychosocial Assessment section. Interventions such as teaching and communicating with the patient before surgery, enabling the patient to use previously successful coping mechanisms, and giving antianxiety drugs help reduce the anxiety. Incorporate available support systems into the plan of care.

Preoperative teaching involves first assessing the patient's knowledge about the surgical experience (see p. 225 in the Providing Information section) and then providing factual information to promote his or her understanding. Allow ample time for questions. Respond to the questions accurately, and refer unanswered questions to the proper professional. During the discussion, continually assess the patient's responses and anxiety level. Be careful not to provide information that might increase anxiety. The informed, educated patient is better able to anticipate events and maintain self-control and is thus less anxious.

Encouraging communication by having the patient state feelings, fears, and concerns can help reduce anxiety. Use an honest and open approach so that the patient can express feelings freely without fear of ridicule or judgment. Keep the patient informed by clarifying information, answering questions, and allaying fears about the surgery.

Promoting rest is helpful because the stress and anxiety of impending surgery often interfere with the patient's ability to sleep and rest the night before surgery. The period before surgery is physically and emotionally stressful. To help the patient relax, determine what he or she usually does to relax and fall asleep. If the patient is able, urge him or her to continue these methods of relaxation. A back rub is relaxing and can be performed by a nurse, unlicensed assistive personnel (UAP), or family member. The surgeon may prescribe a sedative or hypnotic drug to help the patient be well rested for surgery.

Distraction may be used as an intervention for anxiety, especially in the 24 hours immediately before surgery. Listening to music may decrease anxiety, as may watching television, reading, or visiting with friends and family members.

Teaching family members helps reduce anxiety by increasing the likelihood of support and involvement in the patient's care. Assess the readiness and desire of the family to take an active part in the patient's care. A positive sign of family interest is that of members asking questions about the surgical experience. After family readiness is determined, keep family members informed and encourage their involvement in all aspects of education. Emphasize the important role of the family before surgery, but guide discussions and practice sessions so that the patient is the focus of the discussion. Family members can encourage and help the patient practice exercises to be performed after surgery.

Inform the family of the time for surgery, if known, and of any schedule changes. If the patient is an outpatient, provide clear directions to the patient and family regarding any specific night-before procedures, what time and where to report, and what to bring with them. Encourage the family to stay with the patient before surgery for support.

Most families are anxious about the surgery planned for their loved one. To reduce their anxiety, explain the routines expected before, during, and after surgery. Tell the family that after the patient leaves the hospital room or admission area, there is usually a 30- to 60-minute preparation period in the operating area (holding room, treatment area) before the surgery actually begins. After surgery, the patient is taken to the postanesthesia care unit (PACU) usually for 1 to 2 hours before returning to the hospital room or discharge area. The length of stay in the PACU depends on the type of surgery, the type of anesthesia, any complications, and the patient's responses. Tell the family about the best place to wait for the patient or surgeon according to the facility's policy and the surgeon's preference. Many hospitals and surgical centers have surgical waiting areas so that families can wait in comfortable surroundings and be easily located when the procedure is completed. Often families are provided with a beeper to let them know when to report to a specific area to receive updates about the patient's status, meet with the surgeon, or see the patient.

Preoperative Chart Review. Review the patient's chart to ensure that all documentation, preoperative procedures, and orders are completed. Check the surgical informed consent form and, if indicated, any other special consent forms to see that they are signed and dated and that they contain the witnesses' signatures. Confirm that the scheduled procedure, including the identification of left versus right when necessary, is what is listed on the consent form. Even though it might be obvious, inform the patient that the site for surgery will be marked before the procedure begins. If possible, encourage the patient to assist with the marking, as suggested by The Joint Commission's NPSGs. Document allergies according to facility policy. Accurate measuring and recording of height and weight are important for proper dosage of the anesthetic agents. Ensure that the results of all laboratory, radiographic, and diagnostic tests are on the chart. Document any abnormal results, and report them to the surgeon and the anesthesia provider. If the patient is an autologous blood donor or has had directed blood donations made, those special slips must be included in the chart. Record a current set of vital signs (within 1 to 2 hours of the scheduled surgery time), and document any significant physical or psychosocial observations.

Report special needs, concerns, and instructions (including advance directives) to the surgical team, as required by The Joint Commission's NPSGs. For example, advise the surgical team if the patient is a member of Jehovah's Witnesses and does not accept blood products or if the patient is hard of hearing and does not have his or her hearing aid. This information assists the surgical team in providing personalized care while the patient is in the surgical area.

Preoperative Patient Preparation. Facilities usually require the patient to remove most clothing and wear a hospital gown into the OR; however, underpants may be worn in above-the-waist surgery and socks may be worn, except in foot or leg surgery. If prescribed by the surgeon, apply antiembolism stockings or pneumatic compression devices before surgery. In some ambulatory settings, such as for cataract surgery, no or minimal clothes are removed.

Patients are advised to leave all valuables at home. If he or she has valuables, including jewelry, money, or clothes, they are given to a family member or locked in a safe place, according to the facility's policy. If rings cannot be removed, tape them in place. Depending on the type and location of surgery, pierced jewelry may need to be removed. Religious emblems may be pinned or fastened securely to the patient's gown. Some facilities have paper emblems from a religious leader.

The patient wears an identification band that clearly gives the first and last name, hospital number, surgeon, and birth date. An additional bracelet, usually red, identifies any allergies. A bracelet indicating that a blood sample for type and screen has been drawn may be worn, depending on the facility's policy.

If dentures are to be removed, including partial dental plates, place them in a labeled denture cup. Denture removal is a safety measure to prevent aspiration and obstruction of the airway. If a patient has any capped teeth, document this finding on the checklist.

All prosthetic devices, such as artificial eyes and limbs, are removed and given to a family member or safely stored, as are contact lenses, glasses, wigs, and toupees. Check and remove hairpins and clips, which can conduct electrical current used during surgery and cause scalp burns.

Some facilities allow hearing aids in the surgical suite to help communication before and after surgery. If the patient is sent to surgery with a hearing aid, communicate this to the surgical nurse to prevent accidental loss of or damage to the device. Some facilities allow dentures, wigs, and glasses to be worn into the operating suite to prevent embarrassment to the patient. These items are removed when absolutely necessary.

The removal of fingernail polish or artificial nails is controversial. Polish and artificial nails have been thought to affect the accuracy of pulse oximetry readings. Recent studies have indicated that pulse oximetry readings taken on fingers are affected by brown or blue polish but not by red or lighter color polish. In addition, pulse oximetry does not have to be measured on fingers only. Some facilities still require that at least one artificial nail must be removed to monitor oxygen saturation by pulse oximetry.

After the patient is prepared for surgery and the operating suite is ready to receive him or her, ask him or her to empty the bladder. This action prevents incontinence or overdistention and is a starting point for intake and output measurement. A full bladder may hinder access to the surgical site. Answer questions, offer reassurance as needed, and give prescribed drugs.

Preoperative Drugs. Preoperative drugs may be prescribed regardless of the type of planned anesthesia. Various drugs reduce anxiety, promote relaxation, prevent laryngospasm, reduce vagal-induced bradycardia, inhibit oral and gastric secretions, and decrease the amount of anesthetic needed for the induction and maintenance of anesthesia. Drug selection is based on the patient's age, physical and psychological condition, medical history, and height and weight; other drugs the patient takes routinely; test results; and the type and extent of the planned surgical procedure. If more than one response is required, combination therapy may be prescribed.

Drug types for preoperative purposes may include sedatives (e.g., hydroxyzine [Atarax, Vistaril]); hypnotics (e.g., lorazepam [Ativan]); anxiolytics (e.g., midazolam [Versed]); opioid analgesics (e.g., morphine, hydromorphone); and an anticholinergic agent (e.g., atropine). Other specific-purpose drugs also may be added. For example, if rapid emptying of the stomach is needed, metoclopramide (Reglan) may be prescribed. When procedures are long or stress ulcers are likely, an H_2 histamine blocker (e.g., cimetidine [Tagamet]; ranitidine [Zantac]) is used.

Preoperative drugs may be given when the patient is "on call" to the surgical suite. After positively identifying the patient as required by The Joint Commission's NPSGs (using the armband and asking the patient to state his or her name and birth date) and making sure the operative permit is signed, give the correct drugs in the correct doses. Then raise the siderails, place the call light within easy reach of the patient, and remind him or her not to try to get out of bed. Place the bed in a low position. Tell the patient that he or she may become drowsy and have a dry mouth as a result of the drugs.

A more common practice is for the preoperative drugs to be given *after* the patient is transferred to the preoperative area. This practice permits the surgical team and anesthesia personnel to make more accurate assessments and have last-minute discussions with a patient not yet affected by drugs. In addition, after the patient is in the preoperative area, drugs can be given by the IV route. Monitoring equipment such as continuous pulse oximetry and ECG are more readily available in this area. The oral or IM route is used less often because of variable absorption rates. The surgeon may order a prophylactic antibiotic to be given right before or during surgery to reduce the risk for a surgical site INFECTION (SSI), as suggested by The Joint Commission's NPSGs. When needed, the antibiotic is given within 60 minutes before the incision is made, as mandated by the Surgical Care Improvement Project (SCIP) core measures, SCIP Inf-1 (see Table 14-1).

Patient Transfer to the Surgical Suite. In the immediate preoperative period, review and update the patient's chart, reinforce teaching, ensure that the patient is correctly dressed for surgery, and give prescribed preoperative drugs. Use an electronic or hardcopy preoperative checklist for a smooth, efficient transfer to the surgical suite (Fig. 14-6). The patient, along with the signed consent form, the completed preoperative checklist, the chart, and the patient identification card, is transported to the surgical suite.

Most patients in the hospital setting are transferred to the surgical suite on a stretcher with the siderails up. In special circumstances (e.g., patients requiring traction, those having some types of orthopedic surgery, those who should be moved as little as possible), the patient is transferred in the hospital bed. Other factors that influence the decision to transfer in a

PREOPERATIVE CHECKLIST

PATIENT INFORMATION

Date and Time of Arrival to Presurgical Holding Area:

INITIAL APPROPRIATELY

1. Hospital identification band intact and legible including patient name, date of birth, medical record number _____ Yes _____ No

   A. If yes, which arm? _____

   B. If no, make and apply arm band

   C. Is the extremity involved in the surgery? _____ Yes _____ No

   D. If yes, change to another extremity _____ Yes _____ No

	IN PLACE	REMOVED
2. Glasses, contact lenses		
3. Hearing aid(s)		
4. Jewelry, piercings, religious medals, ring taped to finger		
5. Dentures (full, partial)		
6. Other prostheses (list)		
7. Hairpiece, wig, pins/combs		
8. Makeup, nail polish		
9. Clothing		

	YES	NO
10. Antiembolic stockings, compression devices		
11. Patient voided		
12. Advance directives on MR		
13. IV started by:		
14. Permission for surgeon to speak to family		
15. Family has pager #		
16. Informed consent signed, witnessed, on chart		

INITIAL APPROPRIATE COLUMN

	YES	NO
17. Site of site-specific surgery verified by patient and surgeon		
18. History and physical on chart		
19. Pregnancy test date within the past 10 days for females age 11–55 (unless documented hysterectomy)		
20. Type and screen verified with blood bank		
21. Test results (circle those on chart) CBC H&H UA EPI PT/PTT METAPNL ECG CXR		
22. OR notified of latex allergy		
23. ID plate on chart		
24. NPO with appropriate meds		

LIST KNOWN ALLERGIES

PRE-OP MEDS & DOSAGES	TIME

VITAL SIGNS	TIME
BP Pulse	
Resp O2 sat	
Temp Ht Wt	

MISCELLANEOUS	YES/NO
Risk for falls	
Communication barrier	

COMMENTS _____

RN _____ PHONE/PAGER _____ DATE _____ TIME _____

FIG. 14-6 A preoperative checklist.

bed are the patient's age, size, and physical condition. In ambulatory settings, patients either walk or are transferred to the surgical suite on a stretcher or in a wheelchair.

◆ *Evaluation: Outcomes*

Evaluate the care of the preoperative patient based on the identified patient problems. The expected outcomes include that the patient:

- States understanding of the informed consent and preoperative procedures
- Demonstrates postoperative exercises and techniques for prevention of complications
- Has reduced anxiety

Specific indicators for these outcomes are listed for each patient problem in the Planning and Implementation section (see earlier).

NURSING CONCEPTS AND CLINICAL JUDGMENT REVIEW

What might you NOTICE in a patient who is preparing for surgery and has adequate body defenses related to INFECTION?

Vital signs:
- Body temperature within normal range
- No sweating or chills

Physical assessment:
- Skin intact (no rashes, abnormal lesions, open areas, or drainage)
- Skin color normal for ethnicity
- Lymph nodes normal, no enlargement or pain
- Absence of sore throat, pain or burning on urination, productive cough
- Lung sounds clear to auscultation

Psychological assessment:
- Oriented, not confused

Laboratory assessment:
- White blood cell levels within normal limits for age and gender
- All cultures negative for pathogenic organisms
- Urinalysis result shows clear urine, no bacteria, white blood cells, or nitrates present
- Chest x-ray clear

GET READY FOR THE NCLEX® EXAMINATION!

KEY POINTS

Review these Key Points for each NCLEX Examination Client Needs Category.

Safe and Effective Care Environment
- Determine the purpose of surgery for each patient in your care.
- Assess each patient's personal factors for threats to safety.
- Ensure that the patient is wearing proper identification.
- Use at least two appropriate identifiers (e.g., hospital number, the identification band, asking the patient to state his or her name and birthdate) to identify the patient when providing instruction, administering drugs, marking surgical sites, and performing any procedure. *Do not use room number or bed number to identify the patient.* **Safety** QSEN
- Check that the informed consent has been properly signed by the patient and witness and that the presurgical checklist is complete and accurate. **Safety** QSEN
- Ask the patient to explain in his or her own words what surgical procedure is being done and why.
- Check that documentation for any procedure to be performed on one of a paired organ or extremity clearly indicates which organ or extremity is involved. **Safety** QSEN
- If the patient's explanation of the scheduled surgery is not consistent with the documentation, notify the surgeon and request that he or she speak to the patient. **Safety** QSEN

- Ensure that the patient is not asked to sign an operative permit or any other legal document after the preoperative drugs have been given.
- After the patient has received preoperative drugs, keep the siderails up and the bed in the low position.
- Communicate during hand-off to the operating room personnel all care that has been provided and what care may still be needed.

Health Promotion and Maintenance
- Teach patients about dietary restrictions, preoperative preparations, and specific interventions to perform after surgery to prevent complications (incision splinting, deep-breathing exercises, range-of-motion exercises—as described in Charts 14-5 and 14-6). **Patient-Centered Care** QSEN

Psychosocial Integrity
- Assess the extent of the patient's and family members' knowledge about the scheduled surgical procedure to identify learning needs. **Patient-Centered Care** QSEN
- Encourage the patient to express his or her feelings regarding the surgical procedure or its possible outcome.
- Explain and provide written information for all diagnostic procedures, restrictions, and follow-up care to the patient and his or her family.

- Communicate to the surgeon and anesthesia personnel any concerns, fears, or preferences the patient has. **Patient-Centered Care** QSEN
- Apply appropriate interventions to reduce patient anxiety.

Physiological Integrity
- Perform a complete and accurate preoperative assessment.
- If required, ensure that dentures and any other personal items are removed from the patient before he or she is transferred to the surgical suite.

- Apply prescribed antiembolic stockings, sequential compression boots, or other devices to reduce or prevent vascular complications. **Evidence-Based Practice** QSEN
- Communicate to the surgeon and anesthesia personnel any physical or laboratory change that may alter the patient's response to drugs, anesthesia, or surgery.

15 | CHAPTER

Care of Intraoperative Patients

Robin Chard

 http://evolve.elsevier.com/Iggy/

PRIORITY CONCEPTS

- INFECTION
- GAS EXCHANGE
- SENSORY PERCEPTION
- CLOTTING
- THERMOREGULATION

LEARNING OUTCOMES

Safe and Effective Care Environment
1. Differentiate the roles and responsibilities of various intraoperative personnel.
2. Use appropriate patient identifiers when administering drugs, ensuring informed consent, and verifying surgical sites during the intraoperative period.
3. Protect the patient from injury, poor THERMOREGULATION, and INFECTION during the intraoperative period.
4. Communicate care provided and needed at each transition in care during the intraoperative period.

Psychosocial Integrity
5. Reduce the psychological impact for the patient and family regarding the intraoperative experience.

6. Ensure patient concerns and needs are communicated to other members of the health care team during the intraoperative period.

Physiological Integrity
7. Use knowledge of anatomy, physiology, and principles of aging to modify and prioritize patient care during the intraoperative period to prevent skin breakdown and positioning injury.
8. Coordinate appropriate care for the patient with malignant hyperthermia.

The *intraoperative period* begins when the patient enters the surgical suite and ends at the time of transfer to the postanesthesia recovery area, same-day surgery unit, or the intensive care unit. The main concerns of perioperative nurses are safety and patient advocacy by preventing, reducing, controlling, and managing many hazards. In the operating room (OR) the patient is at risk for INFECTION, impaired skin integrity, increased anxiety, poor THERMOREGULATION and altered body temperature, and injury related to positioning and other hazards. The surgical phase is filled with unfamiliar experiences and uncertain outcomes. Nursing care during this period affects the patient's physical needs, spiritual needs, comfort, safety, dignity, and psychological status. Specific procedures and policies may differ among agencies but should all reflect the standards and recommended practices as published by the Association of periOperative Registered Nurses (AORN) (2014a). Perioperative nurses practice within a specific, patient-focused model that incorporates professional practice with attainable, measurable outcomes.

OVERVIEW

Members of the Surgical Team

The surgical team usually consists of the surgeon, one or more surgical assistants, the anesthesia provider, and the OR nursing staff. Perioperative, or OR, nurses include the holding area nurse, circulating nurse, scrub nurse or a non-nurse "scrub person," and specialty nurse. The number of assistants, circulating nurses, and scrub nurses depends on the complexity and length of the surgical procedure. For some minor procedures, only a circulating nurse and scrub person may be needed in addition to the surgeon. More complex procedures may require additional nursing staff to either circulate or scrub.

Surgeon and Surgical Assistant

The *surgeon* is a physician who is responsible for the surgical procedure and any surgical judgments about the patient. The *surgical assistant* might be another surgeon (or physician, such as a resident or intern) or an advanced practice nurse, physician assistant, certified registered nurse first assistant (CRNFA), or surgical technologist. Under the direction of the surgeon and within the legal scope of practice for each state, the assistant may hold retractors, suction the wound (to improve viewing of the operative site), cut tissue, suture, and dress wounds.

Anesthesia Providers

The *anesthesiologist* is a physician who specializes in giving anesthetic agents. A *certified registered nurse anesthetist (CRNA)* is an advanced practice registered nurse with additional education and credentials who delivers anesthetic agents under the supervision of an anesthesiologist, surgeon, dentist, or podiatrist. The anesthesia provider gives anesthetic drugs to induce and maintain anesthesia and delivers other drugs to support the patient during surgery.

The anesthesia provider monitors the patient during surgery by assessing and monitoring:

- The level of anesthesia (i.e., by using a peripheral nerve stimulator or electroencephalogram [EEG] bispectral analysis)
- Cardiopulmonary function (using electrocardiographic [ECG] monitoring, pulse oximetry, end-tidal carbon dioxide monitoring, arterial blood gases [ABGs], and hemodynamic monitoring via arterial lines and/or pulmonary artery catheters)
- Capnography (monitors ventilation for non-intubated patients)
- Vital signs
- Intake and output

Depending on the patient's needs, anesthesia personnel give IV fluids, including blood products.

Perioperative Nursing Staff

Perioperative nursing staff have several roles during surgery, depending on their education, experience, skill, and job responsibilities. Regardless of their role, the OR nurse uses clinical decision-making skills, develops a plan of nursing care, and coordinates care delivery to patients and their family members.

Holding area nurses work in those operating suites that have a presurgical holding area next to the main ORs. The holding area nurse coordinates and manages the care while the patient waits in this area until the OR is ready. Responsibilities include greeting the patient on arrival, reviewing the medical record and preoperative checklist, verifying that the operative consent forms are signed, and documenting the risk assessment (Fig. 15-1). This nurse also assesses the patient's physical and emotional status, gives emotional support, answers questions, and provides additional education as needed.

The holding area is busy, with many staff members performing different procedures before surgery (e.g., starting IV lines, inserting catheters). The nurse promotes comfort, privacy, and confidentiality. In some facilities, family members may wait here with the patient.

Circulating nurses, or "circulators," are registered nurses who coordinate, oversee, and are involved in the patient's nursing care in the OR. This nurse's actions are vital to the smooth flow of events before, during, and after surgery. He or she coordinates all activities within that particular OR. The circulator sets up the OR and ensures that needed supplies, including blood products and diagnostic support, are available. All anticipated equipment is gathered and inspected by the circulator to ensure safety and function before surgery. Depending on the procedure and position required, the circulator makes up the operating bed (OR table) with gel pads (to prevent pressure ulcers), safety straps and armboards, and either heating pads under the sheets or disposable warming blankets placed over the patient as needed to prevent hypothermia.

If there is no holding area nurse, the circulator also assumes the responsibilities of that role. Even when there is a holding area nurse, the circulator also greets the patient and reviews findings with the holding area nurse.

Once the patient is moved into the OR, the circulating nurse, along with the OR team, assists the patient in transferring to the OR table. The nurse positions the patient, protecting bony areas with padding while providing comfort and reassurance. While observing the patient, the circulating nurse also assists the anesthesia provider with the induction of anesthesia by positioning the patient and applying cricoid pressure, when requested. The circulator then may assist with additional positioning, insert a Foley catheter if needed, apply the grounding pad, test equipment, and "prep" (scrub) the surgical site before the patient is draped with sterile drapes.

Throughout the surgery, the circulating nurse:
- Protects the patient's privacy
- Ensures the patient's safety
- Monitors traffic in the room
- Assesses the amount of urine and blood loss
- Reports findings to the surgeon and anesthesia provider
- Ensures that the surgical team maintains sterile technique and a sterile field
- Anticipates the patient's and surgical team's needs, providing supplies and equipment
- Communicates information about the patient's status to family members during long or unique procedures
- Documents care, events, interventions, and findings

Depending on facility policy, the circulating nurse may record drugs, blood, and blood components given. (This also may be a function of the anesthesia provider.)

Before the procedure is over, the circulating nurse completes documentation in the OR and nursing records, including the presence of drains or catheters, the length of the surgery, and a count of all sponges, "sharps" (needles, blades), and instruments. He or she notifies the postanesthesia care unit (PACU) of the patient's estimated time of arrival and any special needs.

Scrub nurses or scrub persons set up the sterile table (Fig. 15-2), drape the patient, and hand sterile supplies, sterile equipment, and instruments to the surgeon and the assistant. Knowledge of the surgical procedure allows the scrub person to anticipate which instruments and types of sutures the surgeon will need, which reduces the duration of anesthesia. Collaboration and coordination of activities between the surgeon and the scrub person help promote the best surgical outcome for the patient. Throughout the procedure, the scrub person (with the circulating nurse) maintains an accurate count of sponges, sharps, and instruments and amounts of irrigation fluid and drugs used.

A specially trained person who is not a nurse may perform the scrub role. Such people are called *operating room technicians (ORTs)* or *surgical technologists.* Often certified surgical technologists (CSTs) are used in the OR.

Specialty nurses may be in charge during some types of specialty surgery (e.g., orthopedic, cardiac, ophthalmologic) and provide specific nursing care during surgery. This nurse assesses, maintains, and recommends equipment, instruments, and supplies used in that specialty.

Identification of Patient, Procedure, and Surgical Side/Sites, and Fire Risk Assessment

Procedure: _____   Date of Procedure _____   Side 1

Preoperative verification process to be completed by assigned personnel in designated areas. Mark appropriate blocks.

PEP	Sending Unit	Prep & Holding/Admission Area	Surgical Site Marking Verification
Posting Card	Patient verbalizes	Patient verbalizes	* Not applicable (N/A) meets exemption criteria (see instructions on side 2)
Patient verbalizes	ID Bracelet (e.g., Name & DOB)	ID Bracelet (e.g., Name & DOB)	* After 2 methods of verification (patient verbalized, consent, H & P, other), the patient (in presence of RN) will write "Yes" with a permanent marker on or as near to surgical site:
Other	OR Schedule	OR Schedule	☐ RIGHT ☐ LEFT
	Surgical Consent	Surgical Consent	☐ N/A
	Site marked with "Yes" ☐ N/A	Site marked with "Yes" ☐ N/A	
	H & P	H & P	Signature _____ Print Name _____ Date / Time _____
	X-ray Report / X-ray	X-ray Report / X-ray	Side/Sites Marked by: _____
	Other studies	Other studies	
Signature:	Signature:	Signature:	**COMMENTS**
Print Name:	Print Name:	Print Name:	
Date/Time:	Date/Time:	Date/Time:	Signature _____ Date/Time _____

ANESTHESIA (Time-out)   CONFIRMATION OF PATIENT IDENTIFICATION, PROCEDURE, & SURGICAL SITE PRIOR TO THE START OF ANESTHESIA BLOCK

The anesthesiologist _____ (Provider Name(s)) and the identification assistant (perianesthesia nurse, operating room RN, another anesthesia provider, another physician or physician assistant) have verbally agreed that _____ (Patient Name) will have the following block performed: _____   Identification Assistant _____

Re-verification completed _____   Re-verification completed _____

SURGICAL TEAM (Time-out)   CONFIRMATION OF PATIENT IDENTIFICATION, PROCEDURE, SURGICAL SITE, AND IMPLANT WITH START OF PROCEDURE AS APPLICABLE,

The surgical team (Surgeon/Resident, Anesthesia Provider, and Circulating RN) has verbally agreed that _____ Patient Name will have the above procedure performed.

Document procedure/site only if the procedure/site is different or left blank at top of form. _____

Circulating RN: _____

Re-verification completed _____   Signature / Print Name _____ Date / Time _____

SURGICAL TEAM   SURGICAL SITE FIRE RISK ASSESSMENT SCORE

Alcohol based prep solution had sufficient time for fumes to dissipate. ☐ YES ☐ NO ☐ N/A   Verified by: _____

(Circle appropriate option)	Y	N	
Surgical site or incision above the xiphoid	1	0	(Circulating RN Signature)
Open oxygen source (Patient receiving supplemental oxygen via any variety of face mask or nasal cannula)	1	0	Print Name: _____
Available ignition source (i.e., electrosurgery unit, laser, fiberoptic light source)	1	0	☐ High Risk Fire Protocol initiated

Scoring 3 = High risk; 2 = Low risk w/potential to convert to high risk; 1 = Low risk   Total Score _____

(Complete this section if Risk Score increases to "3" during procedure)

☐ High Risk Fire Protocol Initiated   Signature/Title: _____   Print Name: _____   Time: _____

FIG. 15-1 Identification of patient, procedure, and surgical side/sites, and fire risk assessment.

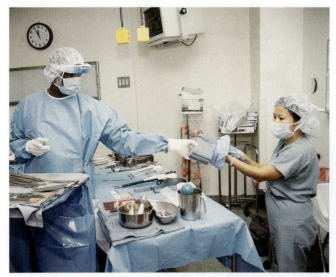

FIG. 15-2 Setting up the sterile table.

FIG. 15-3 **A,** A typical operating room. **B,** A typical anesthesia station with an anesthesia machine.

If the facility uses laser technology, a nurse specially trained in the use, care, and maintenance of the laser is needed (laser specialty nurse or a laser nurse coordinator). (**Laser** is an acronym for **l**ight **a**mplification by the **s**timulated **e**mission of **r**adiation.) A laser creates intense heat, rapidly clots blood vessels or tissue, and turns target tissue (e.g., a tumor) into vapor. All personnel must observe safety measures (e.g., wear eye shields, read door signs) during laser procedures to prevent injury to the patient and staff (AORN, 2014h).

Preparation of the Surgical Suite and Team Safety

The patient is unable to protect himself or herself during surgery; protection is provided by all members of the surgical team. The OR layout helps prevent INFECTION by reducing contaminants through air exchanges in the room, maintaining recommended temperature and humidity levels, and limiting the traffic and activities in the OR. Safety straps are used for the patient, and the OR bed is locked in place. Blankets or warming units are used to prevent hypothermia from poor THERMOREGULATION, and interventions are used to prevent skin breakdown.

The nurse ensures electrical safety through proper placement of grounding pads and use of electrical equipment that meets safety standards. All equipment used during surgery must be functional and in proper working condition as determined by the safety procedure of that facility. Equipment is cleaned and, when required, sterilized before use. The scrub and circulating nurses together ensure a correct count of surgical instruments, sharps, and sponges. Counts are performed before the procedure, during the procedure as items are added or when personnel are relieved from that assignment, at closure of the first layer of the surgical wound, and immediately before complete skin closure (AORN, 2014l).

All OR personnel work to prevent fire and complications from the use of hazardous or toxic substances. Ignition sources, oxidizers, and fuels are present in the OR and increase the risk for fires. Such events are rare but can occur during any procedure. A cool room temperature (between 68° and 73° F [20° and 23° C]) with low humidity (30% to 60%) is optimal. The nurse is aware of emergency measures to take in the event of a fire or spill.

Layout

The surgical suite is located out of the mainstream of the hospital and near the PACU and support services (e.g., blood bank, pathology, and laboratory departments). Traffic flow is patterned to reduce contamination from outside the suite. Within the suite, clean and contaminated areas are separate. The surgical area is divided into three zones—unrestricted, semirestricted, and restricted—to ensure proper movement of patients and personnel.

Most suites contain staff areas as well as areas related to patient care, surgery, and surgical support. Staff areas include locker rooms and staff lounges. Patient care areas include an admission or holding area and operating rooms (ORs). Support areas include ORs, cabinets for sterile supplies, separate utility rooms for clean and soiled equipment, and a clean linen room.

Fig. 15-3 shows a typical OR. The number of tables and equipment in a room is based on the needs of each patient. A

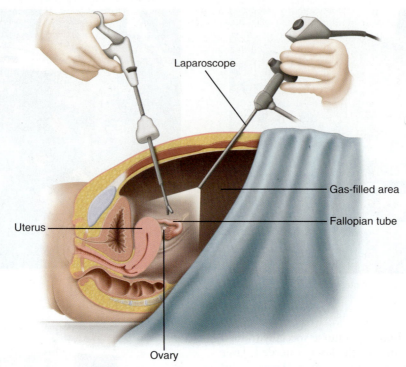

FIG. 15-4 How an operative laparoscope is used.

communication system links the OR with the main desk of the surgical suite and includes an intercom with separate systems for routine and emergency calls.

New OR designs use computers with the surgical equipment, lights, OR bed, and communications. These "hi-tech" rooms are similar to traditional ORs but larger with the addition of computer equipment. Many have voice-activated command systems to operate some equipment instead of manual operation.

Minimally Invasive and Robotic Surgery

Minimally invasive surgery (MIS) is a common practice and now is the preferred technique for many types of surgery, including cholecystectomy, cardiac surgery, splenectomy, and spinal surgery. It is even being used for cancer surgeries, such as the removal of a lung lobe (lobectomy) or even the entire lung (pneumonectomy) and colectomy. Benefits of MIS include reduced surgery time for some surgeries, smaller incisions, reduced blood loss, faster recovery time, and less pain after surgery.

During MIS, one or more small incisions is made in the surgical area and an **endoscope** (a tube that allows viewing and manipulation of internal body areas) is placed through the opening (Fig. 15-4). These instruments may be rigid, semirigid, or flexible and may have self-contained light sources. Endoscopes have different names and shapes for different surgical purposes. For example, laparoscopes are used for abdominal surgery, arthroscopes are used for joint surgery, and ureteroscopes are used for urinary tract surgery.

In addition to being used for examination and obtaining specimens for biopsy, endoscopes can be used for organ removal, reconstruction, blood vessel grafting, and many other procedures. Cutting, suturing, stapling, cautery, and laser surgery can all be performed through or with endoscopes. An important part of MIS for abdominal surgery, pelvic surgery, and surgery in some other body cavity areas is injecting gas or air into the cavity before the surgery to separate organs and improve visualization. This injection is known as **insufflation** and may contribute to complications and patient discomfort. This factor is considered when deciding whether to perform a procedure by traditional surgery or by endoscopy.

Patient preparation for endoscopic surgery is similar to the preparation for the same procedure when performed by open surgical methods. An endoscopic surgical procedure has a chance for becoming an open surgical procedure depending on what patient-related or procedure-related variables are discovered or develop during the surgery.

Robotic technology takes MIS to a new level and is changing how surgery is performed and how the OR is organized. Many gynecologic, urologic, and cardiovascular procedures are being performed by using robotics. The robotic system consists of a console, surgical arm cart, and video cart (Fig. 15-5). The surgeon first inserts the required instruments and positions the articulating arms; he or she then breaks scrub and performs the surgery while sitting at the console. A three-dimensional (3-D) view of the patient's anatomy allows precise control and dexterity. The vision cart holds the monitors, cameras, and recorder equipment. This new technology requires a perioperative robotics nurse specialist who teaches patients and family and trains members of the surgical team.

Mechanical trauma and thermal injury are two types of injury that a patient can incur during MIS and robotic surgery (Ulmer, 2010). Both MIS and robotic surgery are limited by the cost of special equipment, OR settings, and the lengthy training and practice periods for the surgeon to become proficient in even one procedure using these methods.

Health and Hygiene of the Surgical Team

People are a source of contamination in the surgical setting from the bacteria on the skin and the hair and in the airways.

Assistant monitor

Interchangeable instruments with EndoWrist™ technology simultaneously follow surgeon's hand and wrist movements

Surgical cart

Nurse

Anesthesiologist

Assistant

Surgeon uses open-surgery hand movements that are precisely replicated in the operative field by the instruments

Surgeon at operative console

FIG. 15-5 The operating room layout for robotic surgery with the da Vinci Surgery System.

To avoid transmitting these organisms to the patient, policies and procedures for special health standards and dress must be followed. All members of the surgical team and support personnel in the surgical suite must be free of communicable diseases. No one who has an open wound, cold, or any INFECTION should participate in surgery.

Good personal hygiene and frequent handwashing help prevent and control INFECTION. Jewelry carries many organisms and should be minimal. All personnel must wash their hands between touching patients and performing procedures. Hands of surgical personnel may be cultured on a regular basis to assess for potential **nosocomial** (health care–acquired) infections and to identify sources of pathogens. Further interventions or cultures are needed if quality reports indicate a problem. Routine cultures are usually obtained every 3 to 6 months. Surgical attire and the surgical scrub help prevent contaminations.

Surgical Attire

All members of the surgical team and all OR personnel must wear scrub attire while in the surgical suite. Scrub attire, provided by the hospital, is clean (not sterile) and is worn to reduce contamination and risk for INFECTION from areas outside of the surgical setting. Basic surgical attire is a shirt and pants and a cap or hood (Fig. 15-6). Shoe coverings may be worn only to protect the shoes. *Staff change into clean surgical attire in the OR suite locker rooms, not at home* (AORN, 2014o). All members of the surgical team must cover their hair, including any facial hair.

In addition to basic attire, everyone must wear protective attire (mask, eyewear, gloves, and gown). Everyone who enters an OR where a sterile field is present must wear a mask. Surgical team members who are scrubbed and at the bedside during the surgery must also wear a sterile fluid-resistant gown, sterile gloves, and eye protectors or face shields. Team members who are *not* scrubbed (e.g., anesthesia provider, circulator) may wear cover scrub jackets that are snapped or buttoned closed and eyewear, as warranted. For some procedures, the surgical team wears what amounts to surgical "space suits" to prevent wound contamination.

Surgical Scrub

The surgeon, assistants, and the scrub nurse perform a surgical scrub after putting on a mask and before putting on a sterile gown and gloves (Fig. 15-7). *The scrub does not make the skin sterile.* Correctly performed, the scrub reduces the number of organisms from the hands, arms, and nails. Rings, watches, and bracelets are removed before scrubbing. Fingernails are kept short, clean, and healthy. Artificial nails, which have been proven to harbor organisms even after appropriate

FIG. 15-6 Typical attire for all scrubbed personnel. Note complete hair covering, eye shields, mask, sterile gloves over the sleeves of the sterile gown, and shoe coverings. Note that when not in use, the hands are typically folded in front of the body, never below the waist.

❓ NCLEX EXAMINATION CHALLENGE
Safe and Effective Care Environment

While at the scrub sink, the scrub person informs the circulating nurse that she now wears artificial nails because her own nails break frequently posing a risk for a glove puncture. What is the nurse's best response?

A. Ask the scrub person to wear double-gloves to prevent puncture or contamination.

B. Confirm with the scrub person that artificial nails are acceptable and do not affect hand hygiene.

C. Support the scrub person's rationale that broken nails are a serious source of cross-contamination.

D. Remind the scrub person that artificial nails alter skin flora, impede hand hygiene, and are not permitted.

Anesthesia

Anesthesia reduces or temporarily eliminates SENSORY PERCEPTION. Anesthesia delivery is a precise science. It requires the skill of an anesthesiologist, a certified registered nurse anesthetist (CRNA) working under the direction of an anesthesiologist or another physician, or an anesthesiologist assistant (AA—similar to a physician assistant working under the direction of an anesthesiologist).

Anesthesia is an induced state of partial or total loss of SENSORY PERCEPTION, with or without loss of consciousness. The purpose of anesthesia is to block nerve impulse transmission, suppress reflexes, promote muscle relaxation, and, in some cases, achieve a controlled level of unconsciousness. Anesthesia providers use a separate anesthesia record for documentation.

Usually the anesthesia provider selects the type of anesthesia to be used after consulting with the patient and surgeon and after considering specific patient factors. The nurse and patient communicate preferences and fears about anesthesia to the anesthesia provider. Patient health problems are factors in the selection and dose of anesthetic. Selection is also influenced by:

- Type and duration of the procedure
- Area of the body having surgery
- Safety issues to reduce injury, such as airway management
- Whether the procedure is an emergency
- Options for management of pain after surgery
- How long it has been since the patient ate, had any liquids, or had any drugs
- Patient position needed for the surgical procedure
- Whether the patient must be alert enough to follow instructions during surgery
- The patient's previous responses and reactions to anesthesia

The physical status of a patient is ranked according to a classification system developed by the American Society of Anesthesiologists (ASA). The anesthesiologist assesses the patient and assigns him or her to one of six categories based on current health and the presence of diseases and disorders. The categories rank patients in a range from a totally healthy patient (P1 ranking) to a patient who is brain dead (P6 ranking) (Johnson, 2011). This system is used to estimate potential risks during surgery and patient outcomes.

Anesthesia delivery begins with selecting and giving preoperative drugs (see Chapter 14). The nurse must know the actions of the drugs used and their effects during and after surgery.

scrub techniques are used, are not worn (World Health Organization, 2014).

A surgical antimicrobial solution is used for the surgical scrub. Plain or antimicrobial soap is used for washing hands immediately before the surgical scrub. Vigorous rubbing that creates friction is used from the fingertips to the elbow. The scrub continues for 3 to 5 minutes, followed by a rinse. For rinsing, hands and arms are positioned so that water runs off, rather than up or down, the arms (AORN, 2014p). After scrubbing, personnel enter the OR with their hands held higher than the elbows and thoroughly dry their hands and forearms with a sterile towel. This person is then assisted into a sterile gown ("gowning") and puts on sterile gloves ("gloving"). Newer, alcohol-based surgical scrub agents may or may not require the use of water. Operating room personnel wash and dry their hands with soap and water before applying the agent to their hands and forearms, rubbing thoroughly until dry.

Gowns, gloves, and materials used at the operative field must be sterile. These items are changed between procedures and as they become contaminated. The surgical gown is considered sterile only on the front from the chest to the level of the sterile field. The entire sleeves of the gown are considered sterile from 2 inches above the elbow to the cuff. The back of the gown is not considered sterile because it cannot be seen by the wearer. Only when they are properly scrubbed and attired do members of the surgical team handle sterile drapes and equipment.

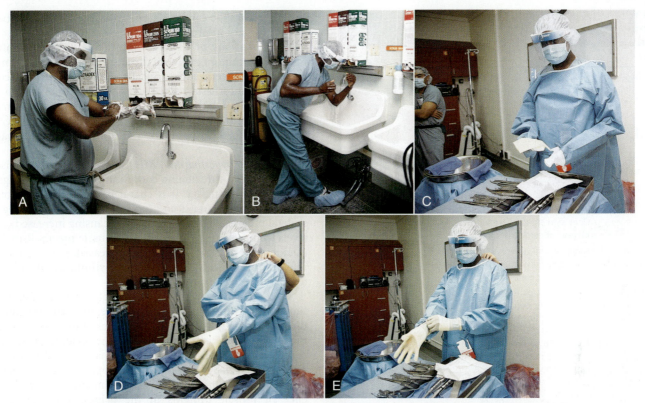

FIG. 15-7 The scrubbing, gowning, and gloving process. **A,** The surgical scrub. **B,** Rinsing. Note the water falling off the hands and arms. Also note the foot-operated handle that controls the water flow. (After scrubbing and rinsing, the scrub nurse dries his hands and arms with a sterile towel inside the operating room and then is assisted into a sterile gown.) **C,** The scrub nurse prepares sterile gloves. Note that the scrub nurse's hands are *inside* the sleeve of the gown and that he is touching the sterile gloves only with the sterile sleeve. **D,** The scrub nurse puts on his first sterile glove while the sterile gown is being tied in the back. Note again that his hand never emerges from under the sterile sleeve. **E,** The scrub nurse puts on his second sterile glove.

Anesthetic agents affect many systems and can worsen other health problems. For example, most anesthetics are metabolized by the liver and excreted by the kidneys. Liver or kidney impairment increases anesthetic effects and the risk for toxicity. In addition, interactions may occur between the anesthetics and other drugs the patient has received.

Anesthesia can be induced in many ways. The most common forms of anesthesia used in North America include general, regional, and local anesthesia (Table 15-1). Less commonly used forms include hypnosis, cryothermia (use of cold), and acupuncture.

General Anesthesia

General anesthesia is a reversible loss of consciousness induced by inhibiting neuronal impulses in several areas of the central nervous system (CNS). This state can be achieved with a single agent or a combination of agents. General anesthesia depresses the CNS, resulting in analgesia (pain relief or pain suppression), amnesia (memory loss of the surgery), and unconsciousness, with loss of muscle tone and reflexes. The patient is unconscious and has no SENSORY PERCEPTION. General anesthesia is used most often in surgery of the head, neck, upper torso, and abdomen.

Stages of General Anesthesia. Induction of general anesthesia involves four stages. Table 15-2 lists the expected patient responses and nursing care for each stage. The speed of emergence (recovery from the anesthesia) depends on the anesthetic

agent, the duration of anesthesia administration, and whether a reversal agent is used. Retching, vomiting, and restlessness may occur during emergence, although not all patients have these responses. Suction equipment must be available to prevent aspiration. During recovery, shivering, rigidity, and slight cyanosis may occur. These responses are caused by a temporary change in the body's THERMOREGULATION. The nurse provides warm blankets, radiant heat, and oxygen to decrease the effects of emergence.

Administration of General Anesthesia. General anesthesia agents are administered by inhalation and IV injection. A combination of types of agents (balanced anesthesia) is used to provide hypnosis, amnesia, analgesia, muscle relaxation, and reduced reflexes with minimal disturbance of physiologic function. This method provides safe and controlled anesthetic delivery, especially for older and high-risk patients. An example of balanced anesthesia is the use of thiopental or propofol for induction, morphine for analgesia, and pancuronium for muscle relaxation. Agent selection is based on the individual patient and the specific surgical procedure.

Other drugs, such as hypnotics, opioid analgesics, and neuromuscular blocking agents, may be used as part of the anesthesia regimen. Hypnotics and opioid analgesics can be used for sedation before surgery, for IV moderate sedation for short procedures, and as an adjunct to general anesthesia during surgery. The neuromuscular blocking agents are used to relax the jaw and vocal cords immediately after induction so that the

TABLE 15-1 Features of Various Types of Anesthesia

TYPE	FEATURES
Inhalation	Most controllable method Induction and reversal accomplished with pulmonary ventilation Must be used in combination with other agents for painful or prolonged procedures Limited muscle relaxant effects Postoperative nausea and shivering common
Intravenous	Rapid and pleasant induction Low incidence of postoperative nausea and vomiting Must be metabolized and excreted from the body for complete reversal Contraindicated in presence of liver or kidney disease Increased cardiac and respiratory depression
Balanced	Minimal disturbance to physiologic function Can be used with older and high-risk patients Drug interactions can occur
Regional or Local	Gag and cough reflexes stay intact Allows participation and cooperation by the patient Less disruption of physical and emotional body functions No way to control agent after administration Increased nervous system stimulation (overdose) Not practical for extensive procedures because of the amount of drug that would be required to maintain anesthesia

endotracheal tube can be placed. These drugs also may be used during surgery to provide continued muscle relaxation.

Complications of General Anesthesia. Complications can range from minor (e.g., sore throat) to death. Improvement in anesthesia delivery and surgical techniques has resulted in a decline in anesthesia-related deaths, even among higher-risk patients. Although the anesthesia provider has the main responsibility for monitoring patient responses during surgery, the circulating nurse also remains alert for changes in the patient's condition.

Malignant hyperthermia (MH), an inherited muscle disorder, is an acute, life-threatening complication of certain drugs used for general anesthesia. It is characterized by many problems, including poor THERMOREGULATION. The reaction begins in skeletal muscle exposed to the drugs, causing increased calcium levels in muscle cells and increased muscle metabolism. Serum calcium and potassium levels are increased, as is the metabolic rate, leading to acidosis, cardiac dysrhythmias, and a high body temperature.

Onset of MH may occur immediately after anesthesia induction, several hours into the procedure, or even after the anesthetic has been terminated. Manifestations are caused by increased muscle calcium level and the greatly increased body metabolism. These include tachycardia, dysrhythmias, muscle rigidity (especially of the jaw and upper chest), hypotension, tachypnea, skin mottling, cyanosis, and myoglobinuria (presence of muscle proteins in the urine). *The most sensitive*

TABLE 15-2 The Four Stages of General Anesthesia and Related Nursing Interventions

DESCRIPTION	NURSING INTERVENTIONS	RATIONALES
Stage 1 (Analgesia and Sedation, Relaxation)		
Begins with induction and ends with loss of consciousness. Patient feels drowsy and dizzy, has a reduced sensation to pain, and is amnesic. Hearing is exaggerated.	Close operating room doors, dim the lights, and control traffic in the operating room. Position patient securely with safety belts. Keep discussions about the patient to a minimum.	Avoiding external stimuli in the environment promotes relaxation. Using safety measures in stage 1 prepares for stage 2. Being sensitive to the patient maintains his or her dignity.
Stage 2 (Excitement, Delirium)		
Begins with loss of consciousness and ends with relaxation, regular breathing, and loss of the eyelid reflex. Patient may have irregular breathing, increased muscle tone, and involuntary movement of the extremities. Laryngospasm or vomiting may occur. Patient is susceptible to external stimuli.	Avoid auditory and physical stimuli. Protect the extremities. Assist the anesthesiologist or CRNA with suctioning as needed. Stay with patient.	Sensory stimuli can contribute to the patient's response. Safety measures help prevent injury. Adequate suctioning of vomitus can prevent aspiration. Staying with the patient is emotionally supportive.
Stage 3 (Operative Anesthesia, Surgical Anesthesia)		
Begins with generalized muscle relaxation and ends with loss of reflexes and depression of vital functions. The jaw is relaxed, and breathing is quiet and regular. The patient cannot hear. Sensations (i.e., to pain) are lost.	Assist the anesthesiologist or CRNA with intubation. Place patient into operative position. Prep (scrub) the patient's skin over the operative site as directed.	Providing assistance helps promote smooth intubation and prevent injury. Performing procedures as soon as possible promotes time management to minimize total anesthesia time for the patient.
Stage 4 (Danger)		
Begins with depression of vital functions and ends with respiratory failure, cardiac arrest, and possible death. Respiratory muscles are paralyzed; apnea occurs. Pupils are fixed and dilated.	Prepare for and assist in treatment of cardiac and/or pulmonary arrest. Document occurrence in the patient's chart.	Teamwork and preparedness help decrease injuries and complications and promote the possibility of a desired outcome for the patient.

CRNA, Certified registered nurse anesthetist.

indication is an unexpected rise in the end-tidal carbon dioxide level with a decrease in oxygen saturation and tachycardia. Extremely elevated temperature, as high as 111.2° F (44° C), is a late sign of MH. Survival depends on early diagnosis and the immediate actions of the entire surgical team. Dantrolene sodium, a skeletal muscle relaxant, is the drug of choice along with other interventions (Mitchell-Brown, 2012).

! NURSING SAFETY PRIORITY (QSEN)
Critical Rescue

Monitor patients for the cluster of elevated end-tidal carbon dioxide level, decreased oxygen saturation, and tachycardia related to malignant hyperthermia. If these changes begin, alert the surgeon and anesthesia provider immediately.

When the patient has a known history or risk for MH, treatment with dantrolene can begin before, during, and after surgery to prevent it. Chart 15-1 lists best practices for care of the patient with MH. The AORN recommends that all operating rooms have a dedicated MH cart containing drugs for management (normal saline, dantrolene, sodium bicarbonate, insulin, 50% dextrose, lidocaine, and calcium chloride), a protocol card listing interventions, and the MH hotline number. Additional nursing support is needed during this true perioperative emergency.

🧬 GENETIC/GENOMIC CONSIDERATIONS
Patient-Centered Care (QSEN)

MH is a genetic disorder with an autosomal dominant pattern of inheritance. The patient with a genetic predisposition for MH is at risk for this complication from halothane, enflurane, isoflurane, desflurane, sevoflurane, and succinylcholine. This rare problem is most common in young adults. Males are affected more often than females (despite the autosomal dominant pattern of inheritance) because of gender differences in muscle mass. The muscle biopsy tested with the caffeine halothane contracture test (CHCT) is still considered the most commonly used MH testing even though this disorder is inherited and only five centers are approved to perform the test (Online Mendelian Inheritance in Man [OMIM], 2013). There is also a genetic test that is performed on blood to assess whether a mutation in the *RYR1* gene is present. Usually, the cost of the genetic test is not covered by insurance. Always ask the patient about any previous problems or difficulties with anesthesia.

Overdose of anesthetic can occur if the patient's metabolism and drug elimination are slower than expected, such as with patients who are older or who have liver or kidney problems. Other drugs (e.g., antihypertensives) also alter metabolism, and interactions can occur between the anesthetic and the patient's regular drugs. Accurate information about the patient's height, weight, and medical history, especially liver and kidney function, is vital in determining the anesthetic type and dosage.

Unrecognized hypoventilation is an anesthesia-induced complication. Failure of adequate GAS EXCHANGE can lead to cardiac arrest, permanent brain damage, and death. Monitoring standards include the use of an end-tidal carbon dioxide monitor to confirm carbon dioxide levels in the patient's expired gas and

CHART 15-1 Best Practice for Patient Safety & Quality Care (QSEN)
Emergency Care of the Patient with Malignant Hyperthermia

- Stop all inhalation anesthetic agents and succinylcholine.
- If an endotracheal tube (ET) is not already in place, intubate immediately.
- Ventilate the patient with 100% oxygen, using the highest possible flow rate.
- Administer dantrolene sodium (Dantrium) IV at a dose of 2 to 3 mg/kg.
- If possible, terminate surgery. If termination is not possible, continue surgery using anesthetic agents that do not trigger malignant hyperthermia (MH).
- Assess arterial blood gases (ABGs) and serum chemistries for metabolic acidosis and hyperkalemia.
- If metabolic acidosis is evident by ABG analysis, administer sodium bicarbonate IV.
- If hyperkalemia is present, administer 10 units of regular insulin in 50 mL of 50% dextrose IV.
- Use active cooling techniques:
  - Administer iced saline (0.9% NaCl) IV at a rate of 15 mL/kg every 15 minutes as needed.
  - Apply a cooling blanket over the torso.
  - Pack bags of ice around the patient's axillae, groin, neck, and head.
  - Lavage the stomach, bladder, rectum, and open body cavities with sterile iced normal saline.
- Insert a nasogastric tube and a rectal tube.
- Monitor core body temperature to assess effectiveness of interventions and to avoid hypothermia.
- Monitor cardiac rhythm by electrocardiography (ECG) to assess for dysrhythmias.
- Insert a Foley catheter to monitor urine output.
- Treat any dysrhythmias that do not resolve on correction of hyperthermia and hyperkalemia with antidysrhythmic agents *other than* calcium channel blockers.
- Administer IV fluids at a rate and volume sufficient to maintain urine output above 2 mL/kg/hr.
- Monitor urine for presence of blood or myoglobin.
- If urine output falls below 2 mL/kg/hr, consider using osmotic or loop diuretics, depending on the patient's cardiac and kidney status.
- Contact the Malignant Hyperthermia Association of the United States (MHAUS) hotline for more information regarding treatment: (800) 644-9737.
- Transfer the patient to the intensive care unit (ICU) when stable.
- Continue to monitor the patient's temperature, ECG, ABGs, electrolytes, creatine kinase, coagulation studies, and serum and urine myoglobin levels until they have remained normal for 24 hours.
- Instruct the patient and family about testing for MH risk.
- Refer the patient and family to the Malignant Hyperthermia Association of the United States at (800) 986-4287 or www.mhaus.org.
- Report the incident to the North American Malignant Hyperthermia Registry at the Malignant Hyperthermia Association of the United States: (800) 644-9737.

Data from Malignant Hyperthermia Association of the United States. (2014). *Emergency therapy for MH acute phase treatment.* Retrieved April 2014, from www.mhaus.org/healthcare-professionals/#.UPGIEGeN58F

a breathing system disconnect monitor to detect any break in the breathing circuit equipment.

Intubation complications can include many problems (e.g., broken teeth and caps, swollen lip, vocal cord trauma). Difficult intubation may be caused by anatomic issues or disease presence (e.g., small oral cavity, tight jaw joint, tumor). Improper neck extension during intubation may cause injury. The surgeon should be in the OR during the intubation process in case a tracheotomy is needed when the endotracheal tube (ET) is placed. Intubation causes tracheal irritation and edema. Often the patient has a sore throat after surgery.

Local or Regional Anesthesia

Local or regional anesthesia briefly disrupts sensory nerve impulse transmission from a specific body area or region, thus reducing SENSORY PERCEPTION in a limited area. Motor function may or may not be affected. The patient remains conscious and can follow instructions. The gag and cough reflexes remain intact, and the risk for aspiration is low. This type of anesthesia may be supplemented with sedatives, opioid analgesics, or hypnotics to reduce anxiety and increase comfort. The OR nurse provides the patient with information, directions, and emotional support before, during, and after the procedure.

Local Anesthesia. **Local anesthesia** is delivered topically (applied to the skin or mucous membranes of the area to be anesthetized) and by local infiltration (injected directly *into* the tissue around an incision, wound, or lesion). Sometimes when the term *local* is used, it means *any* form of anesthesia that is not general or monitored anesthesia.

Regional Anesthesia. **Regional anesthesia** is a type of local anesthesia that blocks multiple peripheral nerves and reduces SENSORY PERCEPTION in a specific body region. It can be used under a variety of conditions and surgeon and patient preferences. It is often used when pain management after surgery is enhanced by regional anesthesia, such as after a total knee replacement. If the patient has eaten and the surgery is an emergency, it may be possible to perform surgery with the patient under regional anesthesia to decrease the risk for aspiration. Regional anesthesia includes field block, nerve block, spinal, and epidural (Table 15-3). Figs. 15-8 and 15-9 show common sites of nerve blocks, spinal anesthesia, and epidural anesthesia.

The nurse's role in the delivery of regional anesthesia consists of:
- Assisting the anesthesia provider
- Observing for breaks in sterile technique
- Providing emotional support for the patient
- Staying with the patient
- Offering information and reassurance
- Positioning the patient comfortably and safely

TABLE 15-3	Types of Regional Anesthesia
ANESTHESIA TYPE	**DEFINITION AND COMMON USE**
Field block	A series of injections *around* the operative field Most commonly used for chest procedures, hernia repair, dental surgery, and some plastic surgeries
Nerve block	Injection of the local anesthetic agent *into or around* one nerve or group of nerves in the involved area Most commonly used for limb surgery or to relieve chronic pain
Spinal anesthesia	Injection of an anesthetic agent into the cerebrospinal fluid in the subarachnoid space (see Fig. 15-9) Most commonly used for lower abdominal, pelvic, hip, and knee surgery
Epidural anesthesia	Injection of an agent into the epidural space (see Fig. 15-9) Most commonly used for anorectal, vaginal, perineal, hip, and lower extremity surgeries

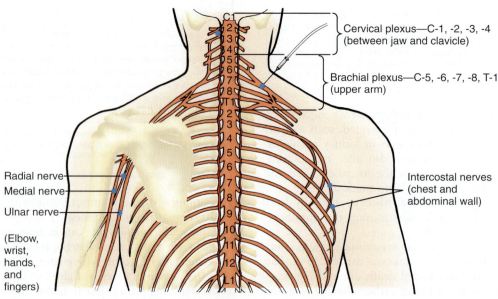

Cervical plexus—C-1, -2, -3, -4 (between jaw and clavicle)

Brachial plexus—C-5, -6, -7, -8, T-1 (upper arm)

Radial nerve
Medial nerve
Ulnar nerve

(Elbow, wrist, hands, and fingers)

Intercostal nerves (chest and abdominal wall)

FIG. 15-8 Nerve block sites.

FIG. 15-9 Administration of spinal and epidural anesthesia. **A,** Spinal or epidural anesthesia is administered by inserting a spinal needle between the second and third or the third and fourth lumbar vertebrae (L2-3 or L3-4). The patient is placed in the flexed lateral (fetal) position *(shown here)* or seated on the edge of the operating bed with the back arched and the chin tucked to the chest. **B,** Spinal anesthesia *(viewed from the side).* A large needle is inserted to the surface of the dura mater, and a second, smaller needle is passed through the first to penetrate the dura mater and arachnoid mater. An anesthetic is injected, sometimes through an indwelling catheter, directly into the cerebrospinal fluid in the subarachnoid space. **C,** Epidural anesthesia *(viewed from the side).* The needle is inserted to the surface of the dura mater, and the anesthetic is injected, usually through an indwelling catheter, into the epidural space.

Complications of Local or Regional Anesthesia. Complications of local or regional anesthesia are related to patient sensitivity to the anesthetic agent (anaphylaxis), incorrect delivery technique, systemic absorption, and overdose. The nurse observes for central nervous system (CNS) stimulation followed by CNS and cardiac depression, which are indications of a systemic toxic reaction. The nurse also assesses for restlessness, excitement, incoherent speech, headache, blurred vision, metallic taste, nausea, tremors, seizures, and increased pulse, respiration, and blood pressure. Interventions include establishing an open airway, giving oxygen, and notifying the surgeon. Usually a fast-acting barbiturate is needed for treatment. If the toxic reaction is untreated, unconsciousness, hypotension, apnea, cardiac arrest, and death may result.

Cardiac arrest may occur as a rare complication of spinal anesthesia. Epinephrine is given to prevent cardiac arrest in patients who develop sudden, unexplained bradycardia.

Local early complications include edema and inflammation. Abscess formation, tissue necrosis, and/or gangrene may occur later. Abscesses result from contamination during injection of the agent. Necrosis and gangrene may occur as a result of prolonged blood vessel constriction in the injected area.

Moderate Sedation

Moderate sedation (conscious sedation) is the IV delivery of sedative, hypnotic, and opioid drugs to reduce SENSORY PERCEPTION but allow the patient to maintain a patent airway. The amnesia action is short, and the patient has a rapid return to ADLs. Etomidate (Amidate), diazepam (Valium, Vivol♣, Novo-Dipam ♣), midazolam (Versed), fentanyl (Sublimaze), alfentanil (Alfenta), propofol (Diprivan), and morphine sulfate are the most commonly used drugs. Moderate sedation is used to reduce the level of consciousness during endoscopy, cardiac catheterization, closed fracture reduction, cardioversion, and other short procedures.

Selection of patients for moderate sedation is based on specific criteria. The physician determines whether the patient is a candidate. In most states, a credentialed registered nurse may deliver moderate sedation under physician supervision and within the state-defined scope of nursing practice. Credentialing includes advanced training in IV drug delivery, airway management, and advanced cardiac life support (ACLS).

The nurse monitors the patient during and after the procedure for response to the procedure and the drugs. The airway, level of consciousness, oxygen saturation, capnography (measure of carbon dioxide level), ECG status, and vital signs are monitored every 15 to 30 minutes until the patient is awake and oriented and vital signs have returned to baseline levels (AORN, 2014i).

Evaluation of consciousness for recovery sedation is performed using a sedation scale. The Ramsay Sedation Scale (RSS) lists specific patient responses or behaviors to a continuum of environmental stimulation demonstrating degree of arousal from sedation (Table 15-4).

The patient receiving IV moderate sedation can be discharged to go home with a responsible adult if capnography indicates GAS EXCHANGE is adequate and arousal from sedation is at an RSS 2 level. If the patient returns to the general medical-surgical nursing unit, the unit nurses continue monitoring. The patient is expected to be sleepy but arousable for several hours after the procedure. Oral intake is not permitted until 30 minutes after the patient has received the sedation or according to the physician's prescription. If the patient was intubated or had oral endoscopy, return of the gag reflex is required before oral intake. When fluids are permitted, the nurse makes sure that the patient is awake and positioned to avoid aspiration.

TABLE 15-4 Ramsay Sedation Scale for Assessing Post-Sedation Consciousness

RAMSAY SCORE	RESPONSE DESCRIPTORS
RSS 1	Patient is anxious and agitated or restless, or both.
RSS 2	Patient is cooperative, oriented, and tranquil (calm, not agitated).
RSS 3	Patient responds quickly, but only to commands.
RSS 4	Patient exhibits brisk response to stimulus.
RSS 5	Patient exhibits a sluggish response to stimulus.
RSS 6	Patient exhibits no response to stimulus. The RSS must be reapplied at intervals until full consciousness is achieved.

Data from Dawson, R., von Fintel, N., & Naim, S. (2010). Sedation assessment using the Ramsay scale. *Emergency Nurse, 18*(3), 18-20.
RSS, Ramsay Sedation Scale.

❖ PATIENT-CENTERED COLLABORATIVE CARE

◆ Assessment

History. On arrival in the surgical suite, the patient is taken to the holding area or directly into the operating suite. The holding area nurse or the circulating nurse greets the patient on arrival. As indicated in The Joint Commission's National Patient Safety Goals (NPSGs), *correct identification of the patient is the responsibility of every member of the health care team.* Check the patient's identification bracelet and ask, "What is your name and birth date?" This practice prevents errors by drowsy or confused patients. For example, if a patient is asked "Are you Mr. Gates?," he may respond inappropriately if he is anxious or sedated. The nurse always validates identification using the medical record and identification bracelet and by asking the patient or family.

> ⚠ **NURSING SAFETY PRIORITY** (QSEN)
> **Critical Rescue**
>
> The Joint Commission's NPSGs require that you verify the patient's identity with two types of identifiers (name, medical record number, telephone number, or other person-specific identifier). Ask the patient to tell you his or her name.

After completing the identification process, the nurse validates that the surgical consent form has been signed and witnessed. The nurse asks "What kind of operation are you having today?" to ascertain that the patient's perception of the procedure, the surgical consent, the surgeon's order, and the operative schedule are the same. *When the procedure involves a specific site, validating the side on which a procedure is to be performed (e.g., for amputation, cataract removal, hernia repair) is the responsibility of each health care professional before and at the time of surgery. The Joint Commission now recommends that the patient and the licensed independent practitioner who is ultimately accountable for the procedure and will be present during the procedure (usually the surgeon performing the surgery) mark the*

surgical site (The Joint Commission [TJC], 2014). Before proceeding, each health care professional thoroughly investigates *any* discrepancy and notifies the surgeon and anesthesia provider. The Joint Commission (TJC) has developed a Universal Protocol for Preventing Wrong Site, Wrong Procedure, Wrong Person Surgery, and the Association of periOperative Registered Nurses has developed recommendations based on this protocol (AORN, 2014r). The nurse asks the patient about any allergies and determines whether autologous blood was donated. A special allergy bracelet on the patient's wrist and the medical record must be verified with what has been communicated.

> ⚠ **NURSING SAFETY PRIORITY** (QSEN)
> **Critical Rescue**
>
> If the patient's description of the surgical site is different from that listed on the informed consent, form a time-out with the patient, yourself, and the surgeon to ascertain and mark the correct site.

The nurse checks the patient's attire to ensure adherence with facility policy. Dentures and dental prostheses, jewelry (including body piercing), eyeglasses, contact lenses, hearing aids, wigs, and other prostheses are removed. Denture removal before anesthesia is controversial because, although the denture plate may come loose and obstruct the airway, the anesthesia provider may request that dentures be left in place to ensure a snug fit of the bag-mask. In some facilities, patients may wear eyeglasses and hearing aids until after anesthesia induction.

Medical Record Review. The circulating nurse and anesthesia provider review the patient's medical record in the holding area or the operating room (OR). This record provides information to identify patient needs during surgery and allows the nurse to assess and plan specific care during and after surgery. It is the main source of information on the type and location of the planned surgery. The nurse checks the medical record to ensure required data are present before surgery is started.

Advance Directives and Do-Not-Resuscitate Orders. Ethical dilemmas may occur during or after surgery. As a patient advocate, the nurse may have to intervene on behalf of the patient's rights and wishes. The nurse must be familiar with the advance directives and do-not-resuscitate (DNR) orders for each patient. It is difficult for some health care providers to not treat the patient in the OR for an emergency situation, and they may ignore an advance directive or living will. Some agencies suspend DNR orders while a patient is undergoing a surgical procedure. The position statement of the Association of periOperative Registered Nurses regarding the care of patients with DNR orders states that automatically suspending a DNR or allow-natural-death order during surgery undermines a patient's right to self-determination (AORN, 2014c).

> ⚠ **NURSING SAFETY PRIORITY** (QSEN)
> **Action Alert**
>
> Advance directives are to be honored in the surgical environment regardless of the situation.

Allergies and Previous Reactions to Anesthesia or Transfusions. The nurse asks about allergies and previous reactions to anesthesia or blood transfusions. Allergies to iodine products or shellfish indicate a risk for a reaction to the agents used to clean the surgical area. Latex allergies are assessed with all patients because anaphylaxis can occur with latex contact during surgery. Latex-free equipment and supplies are used when there is a latex allergy. The nurse documents the allergy in the medical record and notifies the OR team.

The patient's previous experience with anesthesia helps the nurse and anesthesia provider anticipate needs and plan interventions. For example, if a patient is restless or agitated as a reaction to anesthesia, the nurse can have padding for the siderails and protective restraints available. The use of blood products during surgery may be influenced by the patient's history, religious beliefs, preferences, and past transfusion reactions.

Autologous Blood Transfusion. Autologous blood transfusion (reinfusing the patient's own blood) may be used for surgery. Chapters 14 and 40 discuss autologous transfusion in more detail. Chart 15-2 outlines best practices for autologous blood transfusion using blood salvage techniques during surgery.

Laboratory and Diagnostic Test Results. The OR nurse reviews the most recent laboratory findings and test results to inform the surgical team about the patient's health and to alert them for potential problems. These results are usually obtained within 24 to 48 hours before surgery for hospitalized patients and within 4 weeks for ambulatory surgery patients. The nurse reports all abnormal findings or results to the surgeon and anesthesia provider. Laboratory values greater than or less than the normal range are potentially life threatening during surgery (see Chapter 14). For example, if the hemoglobin level is less than 10 g/dL, oxygen transport and GAS EXCHANGE are reduced, affecting the amount and type of anesthesia used.

Medical History and Physical Examination Findings. The nurse performs a final assessment for threats to patient safety, starting with the patient's age and general physical condition. Older patients and those who are thin or overweight are at greater risk for skin injury. Assessing mental status is important because confused patients and those who are unable to either follow instructions or communicate may not be able to tell you when a problem exists. Patients who have impaired SENSORY PERCEPTION of any type are at increased risk for injury. Specific drugs, such as long-term steroid use (which increases capillary fragility and thins the skin), as well as limitations of range or motion, require modification during positioning and threaten patient safety.

The OR nurse checks that the medical history and examination findings, including usual pulse and blood pressure, are recorded. This information provides baseline data to assess the patient's reaction to the surgery and anesthesia. Drugs taken before surgery may affect the patient's reaction to surgery and wound healing. For example, aspirin and other NSAIDs that can increase CLOTTING time and the risk for hemorrhage.

Knowing the patient's medical history and age allows the nurse to plan interventions for the care and safety of high-risk patients (Chart 15-3). The nurse carefully monitors older patients and those with cardiac disease for potential fluid overload.

After completing the medical record review, the nurse may insert an IV catheter and perform a surgical skin preparation. He or she provides emotional support and explains procedures to the patient. If the patient is in the holding area, he or she is moved to the OR after the preoperative routine is completed.

! NURSING SAFETY PRIORITY (QSEN)
Action Alert

Once the patient has been moved into the holding area or the OR, do not leave him or her alone.

? CLINICAL JUDGMENT CHALLENGE
Ethical/Legal; Safety; Teamwork and Collaboration; Quality Improvement (QSEN)

A patient scheduled for a palliative, pain-relieving procedure has a do-not-resuscitate (DNR) order confirmed in the medical record. However, after being premedicated, the patient requests the order be suspended during the procedure and that a family member be contacted.

1. Is the patient permitted to suspend the DNR order in light of the fact that he has already received premedication?
2. What principle of ethical behavior guides your response? (You may need to review the ethical principles in Chapter 1.)
3. How should the OR nurse proceed with the patient request?
4. What steps could be taken to ensure that patient requests and revisions of requests can be handled appropriately in the future?

CHART 15-3 Nursing Focus on the Older Adult
Intraoperative Nursing Interventions

- Allow patients to retain eyeglasses, dentures, and hearing aids until anesthesia has begun.
- Use a small pillow under the patient's head if his or her head and neck are normally bent slightly forward.
- Lift patients into position to prevent shearing forces on fragile skin.
- Position arthritic and artificial joints carefully to prevent postoperative pain and discomfort from strain on those joints.
- Pad bony prominences to prevent pressure sores.
- Provide extra padding for those patients with decreased peripheral circulation.
- Use warming devices to prevent hypothermia.
- Cover the patient's head and feet.
- Warm IV and irrigation fluids as indicated by agency policy and manufacturer's recommendations.
- Follow strict aseptic technique.
- Carefully monitor intake and output, including blood loss.

Data from Clayton, J. (2008). Special needs of older adults undergoing surgery. *AORN Journal, 88*(3), 557-570.

CHART 15-2 Best Practice for Patient Safety & Quality Care (QSEN)
Intraoperative Autologous Blood Salvage and Transfusion

- Be aware of the cell-processing method to be used.
- Make sure that collection containers are labeled for the patient.
- Assist with sterile setup as necessary.
- Assist with processing and reinfusing procedures as needed.
- Document the transfusion process.
- Monitor the patient's vital signs during the transfusion procedure.

FIG. 15-10 Common surgical positions.

◆ **Analysis**

The priority NANDA-I nursing diagnoses and collaborative problems for patients during surgery include:

1. Risk for Perioperative Positioning Injury related to improper positioning (NANDA-I)
2. Risk for Infection related to invasive procedures (NANDA-I)
3. Impaired Gas Exchange related to anesthesia, pain, reduced respiratory effort (NANDA-I)

◆ **Planning and Implementation**

Preventing Injury

Planning: Expected Outcomes. The patient is expected to be free of injury as indicated by:

- Adequate capillary refill and peripheral pulses in all extremities
- SENSORY PERCEPTION and motor function after surgery at the same level as before surgery
- Absence of skin redness or open skin areas
- Absence of bruising

Interventions. Interventions are needed to prevent injury from positioning because of anesthesia and the narrow OR bed. The patient cannot guard against nerve or joint damage and muscle stretch or strain. In addition, pressure ulcers often start to develop during surgery. Thus proper positioning is important. The circulating nurse pads the operating bed with foam and/or silicone gel pads and properly places the grounding pads. He or she coordinates the transfer to the operating bed and helps the patient to a comfortable position. The skin is assessed, especially of older patients, for bruising or injury, and extra padding is placed as indicated.

The patient is usually in a supine position after transfer to the operating bed. Anesthesia may be initiated with the patient supine, and the patient then may be repositioned for surgery (Fig. 15-10).

The circulating nurse coordinates positioning of the patient for surgery and modifies the position according to the patient's safety and special needs. The OR nurse ensures that there is an adequate number of personnel to assist in positioning the patient.

Factors influencing the *timing* of repositioning include:

- The surgical site
- The age and size of the patient
- The anesthetic delivery technique
- Pain on movement (conscious patient)

Factors influencing the actual *position* include:

- The specific procedure being performed
- The surgeon's preference
- The patient's age, size, and weight
- Any pulmonary, skeletal, or muscular limitations, such as arthritis, joint replacements, emphysema, or implanted devices

Chart 15-4 lists best practices to prevent complications related to prolonged immobility during surgery.

The dorsal recumbent (supine), prone, lithotomy, and lateral positions are most often used for surgery. Fig. 15-10 shows many surgical positions and the use of protective padding. When general anesthesia is used, the nurse positions the patient slowly to prevent hypotension from blood vessel dilation. Proper positioning is ensured by assessing for:

- Anatomic alignment
- Interference with circulation and breathing
- Protection of skeletal and neuromuscular structures

CHART 15-4 Best Practice for Patient Safety & Quality Care QSEN

Prevention of Complications Related to Intraoperative Positioning

Prevention of Brachial Plexus Complications (Paralysis, Loss of Sensation in Arm and Shoulder)
- Pad the elbow if tucked at the side.
- Avoid excessive abduction.
- Secure the arm firmly on a padded armboard, positioned at shoulder level, and extended less than 90 degrees.

Prevention of Radial Nerve Complications (Wrist Drop)
- Support the wrist with padding.
- Be careful not to overtighten wrist straps.

Prevention of Medial or Ulnar Nerve Complications (Hand Weakness, Claw Hand)
- Place the safety strap above or below the nerve locations.

Prevention of Peroneal Nerve Complications (Foot Drop)
- Pad knees and ankles.
- Maintain minimal external rotation of the hips.
- Support the lower extremities.
- Be careful not to overtighten leg straps.

Prevention of Tibial Nerve Complications (Loss of Sensation on the Plantar Surface of the Foot)
- Place the safety strap above the ankle.
- Do not place equipment on lower extremities.
- Urge operating room (OR) personnel to avoid leaning on the patient's lower extremities.

Prevention of Joint Complications (Stiffness, Pain, Inflammation, Limited Motion)
- Place a pillow or foam padding under bony prominences.
- Maintain the patient's extremities in good anatomic alignment.
- Slightly flex joints and support with pillows, trochanter rolls, or pads.

Data from Association of periOperative Registered Nurses. (2010). Recommended practices for positioning the patient in the perioperative practice setting. In *Perioperative standards and recommended practices* (pp. 327-350). Denver: Author.

- Optimal exposure of the operative site and IV line
- Adequate access to the patient for the anesthesia provider
- The patient's comfort, safety, and dignity

Care is modified to reduce the potential complications from specific positions. For example, patients in the lithotomy position may develop leg swelling, pain in the legs or back, reduced foot pulses, or reduced SENSORY PERCEPTION from compression of the peroneal nerve. The nurse ensures proper padding and position changes at regular intervals. He or she continually assesses circulation adequacy by checking pulses and capillary refill below pressure points. Throughout surgery, the nurse prevents obstruction of circulation, respiration, or nerve conduction caused by tight straps, poorly placed pads and pillows, or the position of the bed.

Preventing Infection

Planning: Expected Outcomes. The patient is expected to have an uninfected surgical wound or wounds. Indicators include:
- Wound edges are closed and not excessively red or swollen
- Wound is free from purulent drainage
- White blood cell counts remain at expected levels after surgery
- Patient is afebrile

Interventions. Surgical wound INFECTIONS interfere with recovery, delay wound healing, contribute to rising health care costs, and are a source of nosocomial infections. The Centers for Disease Control and Prevention (CDC) defines surgical site infections as occurring 30 days post-surgery (CDC, 2014). Aseptic technique must be strictly practiced by all OR personnel to ensure that the patient is free from infection, as required by The Joint Commission's NPSGs. The Surgical Care Improvement Project (SCIP), as described in Table 14-1 of Chapter 14, has core measures related for the prevention of surgical site infections.

Assess the risk for INFECTION by identifying patients with health problems such as diabetes mellitus, immunodeficiency, obesity, and kidney disease. The nurse performs the prescribed skin preparation, protects against cross-contamination, keeps traffic to a minimum, and administers prescribed antimicrobial prophylaxis. Surgery increases risk for wound complications (e.g., incisional tears, lacerations), infection, and loss of body fluids. Sterile surgical technique and the use of protective drapes, skin closures, and dressings reduce complications and promote wound healing. When a wound is already infected or is at high risk for infection, antibiotics may be used directly in the wound before wound closure.

Skin and tissue closures include sutures, staples, special tape, and tissue adhesive (surgical "glue"). Fig. 15-11 shows commonly used wound closures. They are used to:
- Hold wound edges in place until wound healing is complete
- Occlude blood vessels, preventing poor CLOTTING and hemorrhage
- Prevent wound contamination and INFECTION

Sutures are absorbable or nonabsorbable. *Absorbable sutures* are digested over time by body enzymes. *Nonabsorbable sutures* become encapsulated in the tissue during the healing process and remain in the tissue unless they are removed. Body enzymes do not affect nonabsorbable sutures. Retention (stay) sutures (see Fig. 15-11) may be used in addition to standard sutures for patients at high risk for impaired wound healing (obese patients, patients with diabetes, and those taking steroids).

After the incision is closed, the surgeon may inject a local anesthetic or instill an antibiotic into the wound. A gauze or spray dressing may be applied to protect the incision from contamination. A variety of dressings are used to absorb drainage and support the incision. A pressure dressing may be applied to prevent poor CLOTTING and bleeding. One or more drains (see Chapter 16) may be inserted to remove secretions and fluids around the surgical area. These secretions, if not drained, slow healing and promote bacterial growth, which could result in wound INFECTION.

The nurse coordinates the surgical team in positioning and transferring the patient. When needed, a roller board or a lift sheet is used to move the patient from the operating bed to a stretcher or bed. The circulating nurse and anesthesia provider go with the patient to the PACU and report his or her surgical experience to the PACU nurse (see Chapter 16).

Preventing Hypoventilation

Planning: Expected Outcomes. The patient is expected to be free of damaging events related to impaired GAS EXCHANGE and hypoventilation as indicated by:
- Maintenance of Sao_2, Pao_2, and blood pH within normal limits

Interrupted sutures   Continuous sutures (interlocking stitch)   Staples

Tapes   Retention bridge   Stay (retention) sutures

FIG. 15-11 Common skin closures.

- Vital signs within normal limits
- Return to presurgical level of cognitive function

Interventions. The purpose of interventions is to prevent injury resulting from the anesthesia effect on breathing and GAS EXCHANGE. The nurse, surgeon, and anesthesia provider monitor the patient according to official standards. These standards, adopted by both the American Society of Anesthesiologists and the American Association of Nurse Anesthetists, include continuous monitoring of breathing, circulation, and cardiac rhythms; blood pressure and heart rate recordings every 5 minutes; and the constant presence of an anesthesia provider during the case.

◆ Evaluation: Outcomes

The nurse evaluates the care of the patient during surgery based on the identified priority patient problems. The expected outcomes are that the patient:

- Is safely anesthetized without complications
- Does not experience any injury related to surgical positioning or equipment
- Is free of skin or tissue contamination and INFECTION during surgery
- Is free of skin tears, bruises, redness, or other injury over pressure points and elsewhere
- Maintains normal THERMOREGULATION and body temperature

Specific indicators for these outcomes are listed for each priority patient problem under the Planning and Implementation section (see earlier).

NURSING CONCEPTS AND CLINICAL JUDGMENT REVIEW

What might you NOTICE in a patient during surgery who has adequate body defenses related to INFECTION?

Vital signs:
- Body temperature within normal range
- No sweating or chills

Physical assessment:
- Skin color normal for ethnicity
- Any drainage is not purulent
- Urine is clear

GET READY FOR THE NCLEX® EXAMINATION!

KEY POINTS

Review these Key Points for each NCLEX Examination Client Needs Category.

Safe and Effective Care Environment

- Review preoperative checklist and informed consent forms, including any allergies.
- Highlight any known allergies. **Safety** `QSEN`
- Ensure that all personnel entering the OR are wearing proper OR attire for their role.
- Observe for and inform OR personnel of any break in sterile field or sterile technique. **Safety** `QSEN`
- Use appropriate patient identifiers when administering drugs or marking surgical sites. **Safety** `QSEN`
- Report to the surgeon any discrepancy between what type of surgery the patient says is going to be performed and what the informed consent form indicates. **Safety** `QSEN`
- Apply grounding pads as needed. **Safety** `QSEN`
- Complete any needed skin preparation.
- Perform an accurate "sharps," sponge, and instrument count with the scrub nurse or surgical technologist. **Safety** `QSEN`

Psychosocial Integrity

- Communicate patient preferences or fears about anesthesia to the anesthesia provider. **Patient-Centered Care** `QSEN`
- Preserve the patient's privacy and dignity by keeping body exposure to a minimum.

- Stay with the patient during induction of anesthesia.
- Communicate information about the patient's status to waiting family members.
- Ensure that the patient's wishes, as expressed in the advance directives statement, are honored in the surgical setting. **Patient-Centered Care** `QSEN`

Physiological Integrity

- Apply padding to the OR bed to maintain the patient's skin integrity. **Evidence-Based Practice** `QSEN`
- Position the patient comfortably and safely.
- Maintain the malignant hyperthermia cart.
- Monitor the patient's airway, level of consciousness, oxygen saturation, ECG, and vital signs during and immediately after moderate sedation.
- Assess the patient for tachycardia, increased end-tidal carbon dioxide level, and increased body temperature as indicators of malignant hyperthermia.
- Assess all skin areas and document findings before transferring the patient to the postanesthesia care unit.
- Communicate clearly and accurately information about the patient's surgical experience when handing off the patient to the postanesthesia care nurse. **Teamwork and Collaboration** `QSEN`

16 CHAPTER

Care of Postoperative Patients

Robin Chard

 http://evolve.elsevier.com/Iggy/

PRIORITY CONCEPTS

- GAS EXCHANGE
- PAIN
- CLOTTING
- INFECTION
- TISSUE INTEGRITY

LEARNING OUTCOMES

Safe and Effective Care Environment

1. Protect the patient from injury and INFECTION during the postoperative period.
2. Communicate care provided and needed at each transition in care during the postoperative period.

Health Promotion and Maintenance

3. Evaluate patient risk for complications of wound healing, INFECTION, and development of venous thromboembolism.
4. Continue to provide perioperative education for patients and family members after surgery.

Psychosocial Integrity

5. Reduce the psychological impact for the patient and family regarding the postoperative experience.

Physiological Integrity

6. Perform an ongoing head-to-toe assessment of the postoperative patient.
7. Implement appropriate PAIN relief strategies for the postoperative patient.
8. Apply knowledge of anatomy, physiology, and pathophysiology to monitor the patient for the complications of shock, respiratory depression, and impaired wound healing.
9. Prioritize nursing interventions for the patient during the postoperative period.
10. Collaborate with health care team members to perform emergency procedures for surgical wound dehiscence or wound evisceration.

The **postoperative period** starts with completion of surgery and transfer of the patient to a specialized area for monitoring such as the postanesthesia care unit (PACU) and may continue after discharge from the hospital until all activity restrictions have been lifted. The period of postanesthesia care is divided into three phases that are based on the level of care needed, not the physical place of care. Not every patient will need all three phases.

Phase I care occurs immediately after surgery, most often in a PACU, although care in an ambulatory care unit is becoming common. For those patients who have very complicated procedures or many serious health problems, phase I care may occur in an intensive care unit (ICU). The length of time the patient remains at a phase I level of observation depends on his or her health status, the surgical procedure, anesthesia type, and rate of progression to complete alertness and hemodynamic stability. It can range from less than 1 hour to days. This level features very close monitoring of the airway, vital signs, and indicators of recovery that varies from every 5 to 15 minutes initially. The

time between assessments gradually increases as the patient progresses toward recovery.

Phase II postoperative recovery focuses on preparing the patient for care in an extended care environment, such as a medical-surgical unit, step-down unit, skilled nursing facility, or home. This phase can occur in a PACU, on a medical-surgical unit, or in the same-day surgery (SDS) unit (ambulatory care unit) and may last only 15 to 30 minutes, although 1 to 2 hours is more typical. Patients are discharged from this phase when presurgery level of consciousness has returned, oxygen saturation is at baseline, and vital signs are stable. Some patients achieve this level of recovery in phase I and can be discharged directly to home. Others may require further observation.

The third phase of postoperative recovery, known as the *extended-care environment,* most often occurs on a hospital unit or in the home. For patients who have continuing care needs that cannot be met at home, discharge may be from the hospital unit to an extended-care facility. Although vital signs continue to be monitored in this type of environment, the frequency ranges from several times daily to just once daily.

The actual time spent away from home after surgery varies according to age, physical health, self-care ability, support systems, type and length of surgical procedure, anesthesia, any complications, home environmental conditions, and community resources. The core measures recommended by the Surgical Care Improvement Project (SCIP) that were initiated during the preoperative period to prevent certain surgical complications are continued or re-evaluated during the postoperative period. (See Chapter 14 and Table 14-1 for an explanation of these measures.)

OVERVIEW

The purpose of a **postanesthesia care unit (PACU)** (recovery room) is the ongoing evaluation and stabilization of patients to anticipate, prevent, and manage complications after surgery. The PACU is usually located close to the surgical suite for ease of access and patient transfer. The unit is usually a large and open room to provide direct observation of all patients and easy access to supplies and emergency equipment. The patient area may be divided into individual cubicles. So that each patient can be observed continuously, privacy curtains or screens are partially open and are fully closed only during bedside procedures. Each cubicle has equipment to monitor and care for the patient, such as oxygen, suction equipment, cardiac monitors, pulse oximetry, airway equipment, and emergency drugs.

After the surgery is completed, the circulating nurse and the anesthesia provider accompany the patient to the PACU. For patients in critical condition, transfer may be directly from the operating room (OR) to the ICU. On arrival, the anesthesia provider and the circulating nurse give the PACU nurse a verbal "hand-off" report to communicate the patient's condition and care needs.

A hand-off report that meets The Joint Commission's National Patient Safety Goals requires effective communication between health care professionals. It is at least a two-way verbal interaction between the health care professional giving the report and the nurse receiving it. The language used to give the report is clear and cannot be interpreted in more than one way. The nurse receiving the report focuses on the report and is not distracted by the environment or other responsibilities. Standardizing the information reported helps prevent omission of critical patient-centered information and helps avoid irrelevant details (Association of periOperative Registered Nurses [AORN], 2014). The receiving nurse takes the time to restate (report back) the information to verify what was said and to make certain he or she has the same understanding as the reporting person. The receiving nurse takes the time to ask questions and the reporting professional must respond to the questions until a common understanding is established. Chart 16-1 gives an example of critical information to include in a standard hand-off report.

The PACU nurse is skilled in the care of patients with multiple medical and surgical problems immediately after a surgical procedure. This area requires in-depth knowledge of anatomy and physiology, anesthetic agents, pharmacology, PAIN management, extubation, surgical procedures, and advanced cardiac life support (ACLS). The PACU nurse is skilled in assessment and can make knowledgeable, quick decisions if

---

CHART 16-1 **Best Practice for Patient Safety & Quality Care** QSEN

Postoperative Hand-off Report

- Type and extent of the surgical procedure
- Type of anesthesia and length of time the patient was under anesthesia
- Allergies (especially to latex or drugs)
- Any health problems or pathologic conditions
- Status of vital signs, including temperature and oxygen saturation
- Type and amount of IV fluids and drugs administered
- Estimated blood loss (EBL)
- Any intraoperative complications, such as a traumatic intubation
- Primary language, any sensory impairments, any communication difficulties
- Special requests that were verbalized by the patient preoperatively
- Preoperative and intraoperative respiratory function and dysfunction
- Location and type of incisions, dressings, catheters, tubes, drains, or packing
- Intake and output, including current IV fluid administration and estimated blood loss
- Prosthetic devices
- Joint or limb immobility while in the operating room, especially in the older patient
- Other intraoperative positioning that may be relevant in the postoperative phase
- Intraoperative complications, how managed, patient responses (e.g., laboratory values)

---

emergencies or complications occur. The patient is monitored closely. The anesthesia provider and surgeon are consulted as needed.

❖ PATIENT-CENTERED COLLABORATIVE CARE

◆ Assessment

History. Use the surgical team's report to plan the care for an individual patient. After receiving the report and assessing the patient, review the medical record for information about the patient's history, physical condition, and emotional status. If the patient remains as an inpatient, the surgical and anesthesia information is incorporated into the postoperative plan of care. Chapter 14 identifies factors that increase the risk for the potential complications listed in Table 16-1.

Physical Assessment/Clinical Manifestations. Assess the patient, and record data on a PACU flow chart record (Fig. 16-1). Assessment data include level of consciousness, temperature, pulse, respiration, oxygen saturation, and blood pressure. Examine the surgical area for bleeding. Monitor vital signs as often as your facility's policy states, the patient's condition warrants, and the surgeon prescribes. Once the patient is discharged from the PACU, vital signs are measured as prescribed or as often as the patient's condition indicates.

! **NURSING SAFETY PRIORITY** QSEN

Action Alert

Respiratory assessment is the most critical assessment to perform after surgery for any patient who has undergone general anesthesia or moderate sedation or has received sedative or opioid drugs.

TABLE 16-1 General Potential Complications of Surgery

Respiratory System Complications
- Atelectasis
- Pneumonia
- Pulmonary embolism (PE)
- Laryngeal edema
- Ventilator dependence
- Pulmonary edema

Cardiovascular Complications
- Hypertension
- Hypotension
- Hypovolemic shock
- Dysrhythmias
- Venous thromboembolism (VTE), especially deep vein thrombosis (DVT)
- Heart failure
- Sepsis
- Disseminated intravascular coagulation (DIC)
- Anemia
- Anaphylaxis

Skin Complications
- Pressure ulcers
- Wound infection
- Wound dehiscence
- Wound evisceration
- Skin rashes or contact allergies

Gastrointestinal Complications
- Paralytic ileus
- Gastrointestinal ulcers and bleeding

Neuromuscular Complications
- Hypothermia
- Hyperthermia
- Nerve damage and paralysis
- Joint contractures

Kidney/Urinary Complications
- Urinary tract infection
- Acute urinary retention
- Electrolyte imbalances
- Acute kidney injury (AKI)
- Stone formation

CHART 16-2 Focused Assessment

The Patient on Arrival at the Medical-Surgical Unit After Discharge from the Postanesthesia Care Unit

Airway
- Is it patent?
- Is the neck in proper alignment?

Breathing
- What is the quality and pattern of the breathing?
- What is the respiratory rate and depth?
- Is the patient using accessory muscles to breathe?
- Is the patient receiving oxygen? At what setting? What is the pulse oximetry reading?

Mental Status
- Is the patient awake, able to be aroused, oriented, and aware?
- Does the patient respond to verbal stimuli?

Surgical Incision Site
- How is it dressed?
- Review the amount of drainage on the dressing immediately.
- Is there any bleeding or drainage under the patient?
- Are any drains present?
- Are the drains set properly (e.g., compressed if they should be compressed, not kinked, patient not lying on them)?
- How much drainage is present in the drainage container?

Temperature, Pulse, and Blood Pressure
- Are these values within the patient's baseline range?
- Are these values significantly different from when the patient was in the postanesthesia care unit (PACU)?

Intravenous Fluids
- What type of solution is infusing and with what additives?
- How much solution was remaining on arrival?
- How much solution infused in the transport time from PACU?
- At what rate is the infusion supposed to be set? Is it?

Other Tubes
- Is there a nasogastric or intestinal tube?
- What is the color, consistency, and amount of drainage?
- Is suction applied to the tube if ordered? Is the suction setting correct?
- Is there a Foley catheter?
- Is the Foley draining properly?
- What is the color, clarity, and volume of urine output?

The health care team determines the patient's readiness for discharge from the PACU by the presence of a recovery score rating of 9 to 10 on the recovery scale (see Fig. 16-1). Other criteria for discharge (e.g., stable vital signs; normal body temperature; no overt bleeding; return of gag, cough, and swallow reflexes; the ability to take liquids; and adequate urine output) may be specific to the facility. After you determine that all criteria have been met, the patient is discharged by the anesthesia provider to the hospital unit or to home. If an anesthesia provider has not been involved, which may be the case with local anesthesia or moderate sedation, the surgeon or nurse discharges the patient once the discharge criteria have been met.

Assessment continues from the PACU to the intensive care or medical-surgical nursing unit. If the patient is to be discharged from the PACU to home, assessment and any needed nursing care are continued by home care nurses or by the patient or family members after health teaching. When the patient is transferred to an inpatient unit, complete an initial assessment on arrival (Chart 16-2).

During the postoperative period, all patients remain at risk for pneumonia, shock, cardiac arrest, respiratory arrest, CLOTTING and venous thromboembolism (VTE), and GI bleeding. These serious complications can be prevented or the consequences reduced with collaborative care. Nursing observations and interventions are part of critical rescue management for patient safety and quality care.

Respiratory System. *When the patient is admitted to the PACU, immediately assess for a patent airway and adequate GAS EXCHANGE. Although some patients may be awake and able to speak, talking is not a good indicator of adequate gas exchange. An artificial airway, such as an endotracheal tube*

FORREST GENERAL HOSPITAL
POST ANESTHESIA CARE UNIT RECORD

POST ANESTHESIA RECOVERY SCORE			MINUTES				
		in	30	60	90	out	
Activity							
Able to move 4 extremities voluntarily or on command	= 2						
Able to move 2 extremities voluntarily or on command	= 1						
Able to move 0 extremities voluntarily or on command	= 0						
Respiration							
Able to deep breathe and cough freely	= 2						
Dyspnea or limited breathing	= 1						
Apneic	= 0						
Circulation							
BP ± 20 of Preanesthetic level	= 2						
BP ± 20-50 of Preanesthetic level	= 1						
BP ± 50 of Preanesthetic level	= 0						
Consciousness							
Fully Awake	= 2						
Arousable on calling	= 1						
Not Responding	= 0						
O₂ Saturation							
Able to maintain O₂ Sat > 92% on room air	= 2						
Needs O₂ to maintain O₂ Sat > 90%	= 1						
O₂ Sat < 90% even with O₂	= 0						
TOTAL							

Pre-op B.P. _____
Allergy

Airway: On Adm.
Jawthrust _____
Chin Hold _____
Endotracheal _____
Oral Airway _____
Mask Oxygen _____
Nasal Oxygen _____
Trach _____
T-Tube _____
Nasal Airway _____
Ventilator Settings _____

Addressograph

Time In _____ Time Out _____

Accompanied by _____

Type of anesthesia _____

Surgical Procedure:

PULSE - RESPIRATION - BLOOD PRESSURE

| | 15 | 30 | 45 | 15 | 30 | 45 | 15 | 30 | 45 | 15 | 30 | 45 |
240 / 220 / 200 / 180 / 160 / 140 / 120 / 100 / 80 / 60 / 40 / 20

O2 Sat.
Pain score
PAP

CODES ⊥ A-line / T B.P.   V Manual or / ∧ NBP   Pulse • / Resp. o   Siderails: Yes / No   Restraints:: Yes / No

IV Type _____

Total IV in OR _____ cc
Blood in OR _____ units
Urinary Output in OR _____ cc
Est. Blood Loss _____ cc

Foley Cath. _____
Suprapubic _____
Ureteral _____
Levine _____
DRAINS

RN Signature _____

RN Signature _____

MEDICATIONS AND TREATMENTS

	AMT.	ROUTE	TIME
Demerol			
Morphine			
Phenergan			
Droperidol			
Zofran			
Toradol			

FIG. 16-1 Example of a postanesthesia care unit record.

(ET), a nasal trumpet, or an oral airway, may be in place. If the patient is receiving oxygen, document the type of delivery device and the concentration or liter flow of the oxygen. Continuously monitor pulse oximetry for oxygen saturation (Spo₂) while the patient is in the PACU. The Spo₂ should be above 95% (or at the patient's presurgery baseline).

! **NURSING SAFETY PRIORITY** (QSEN)

Critical Rescue

If the oxygen saturation drops below 95% (or below the patient's pre-surgery baseline), notify the surgeon or anesthesia provider. If it drops by 10 percentage points and you are certain it is an accurate measure, call the Rapid Response Team.

Assess the rate, pattern, and depth of breathing to determine adequacy of GAS EXCHANGE. A respiratory rate of less than 10 breaths per minute may indicate anesthetic- or opioid analgesic–induced respiratory depression. Rapid, shallow respirations may signal shock, cardiac problems, increased metabolic rate, or PAIN.

Listen to the lungs over all lung fields to assess breath sounds. Also check symmetry of breath sounds and chest wall movement. If, for example, the patient has an ET tube, it could move down into the right bronchus and prevent left lung expansion. In this case, lung sounds on the left are absent or decreased and only the right chest wall rises and falls with breathing.

Perform ongoing inspection of the chest wall for accessory muscle use, sternal retraction, and diaphragmatic breathing. These manifestations may indicate an excessive anesthetic effect, airway obstruction, or paralysis, which could result in hypoxia. Listen for snoring and **stridor** (a high-pitched crowing sound). Snoring and stridor occur with airway obstruction resulting from tracheal or laryngeal spasm or edema, mucus in the airway, or blockage of the airway from edema or tongue relaxation. When neuromuscular blocking agents are retained, the patient has muscle weakness, which could impair GAS EXCHANGE. Indicators of muscle weakness include the inability to maintain a head lift, weak hand grasps, and an abdominal breathing pattern.

If the patient returns to an inpatient unit, complete an initial assessment on arrival (see Chart 16-2) and then continue to assess for respiratory depression or hypoxemia. Listen to the lungs to check for effective expansion and for abnormal breath sounds. Check the lungs at least every 4 hours during the first 24 hours after surgery and then every 8 hours, or more often, as indicated. Older patients, smokers, and patients with a history of lung disease are at greater risk for respiratory complications after surgery and need more frequent assessment (Sullivan, 2011). Obese patients are also at high risk for respiratory complications.

Cardiovascular System. *Vital signs* and heart sounds are assessed on admission to the PACU and then at least every 15 minutes until the patient's condition is stable. Automated blood pressure cuffs and cardiac monitoring assist in continuous assessment.

Review vital signs after surgery for trends, and compare them with those taken before surgery. Report blood pressure changes that are 25% higher or lower than values obtained before surgery (or a 15- to 20-point difference, systolic or diastolic) to the anesthesia provider or the surgeon. Decreased blood pressure and pulse pressure and abnormal heart sounds indicate possible cardiac depression, fluid volume deficit, shock, hemorrhage, or the effects of drugs (see Chapters 11 and 37). Bradycardia could indicate an anesthesia effect or hypothermia. Older patients are at risk for hypothermia because of age-related changes in the hypothalamus (the temperature regulation center), low levels of body fat, and coolness of the OR suite (Sullivan, 2011; Touhy & Jett, 2014). An increased pulse rate could indicate hemorrhage, shock, or PAIN.

Cardiac monitoring is maintained until the patient is discharged from the PACU. For patients at risk for dysrhythmias, monitoring may continue either on telemetry units or on general medical-surgical units. In assessing the vital signs of a patient who is not being monitored continuously, compare the rate, rhythm, and quality of the apical pulse with the rate, rhythm, and quality of a peripheral pulse, such as the radial pulse. A **pulse deficit** (a difference between the apical and peripheral pulses) could indicate a dysrhythmia.

Peripheral vascular assessment needs to be performed because anesthesia and positioning during surgery (e.g., the lithotomy position for genitourinary procedures) may impair the peripheral circulation and contribute to CLOTTING and venous thromboembolism (VTE), especially deep vein thrombosis (DVT). Compare distal pulses on both feet for pulse quality, observe the color and temperature of extremities, evaluate sensation and motion, and determine the speed of capillary refill. Palpable pedal pulses indicate adequate circulation and perfusion of the legs.

In adherence with The Joint Commission's Surgical Care Improvement Project (SCIP) core measures for prevention of inappropriate CLOTTING and VTE, continue the prophylactic measures initiated before surgery (Myles, 2012). Although these measures vary in type (e.g., drug therapy with anticoagulants or antiplatelet drugs, sequential compression devices, antiembolic stockings or elastic wraps, early ambulation) depending on the patient's specific risk factors and the type and extent of surgery, any preventive strategies started before surgery are usually needed for at least the first 24 hours after surgery. Reassess the patient's risk for CLOTTING and VTE and the effectiveness of the preventive strategies daily. Assess the feet and legs for redness, pain, warmth, and swelling, which may occur with DVT. Foot and leg assessment may be performed once during a nursing shift or once daily depending on the patient's risk for complications and the facility's or agency's policy. (See Chapters 14 and 36 for more information on prevention of inappropriate CLOTTING and VTE.)

Neurologic System. *Cerebral functioning* and the level of consciousness or awareness must be assessed in *all* patients who have received general anesthesia (Table 16-2) or any type of sedation. Observe for lethargy, restlessness, or irritability, and test coherence and orientation. Determine awareness by observing responses to calling the patient's name, touching the patient, and giving simple commands such as "Open your eyes" and "Take a deep breath." Eye opening in response to a command indicates wakefulness or arousability but not necessarily awareness. Determine the degree of orientation to person, place, and time by asking the conscious patient to answer questions such as "What is your name?" (person), "Where are you?" (place), and "What day is it?" (time).

TABLE 16-2   **Immediate Postoperative Neurologic Assessment: Return to Preoperative Level**

Order of Return to Consciousness After General Anesthesia
1. Muscular irritability
2. Restlessness and delirium
3. Recognition of pain
4. Ability to reason and control behavior

Order of Return of Motor and Sensory Functioning After Local or Regional Anesthesia
1. Sense of touch
2. Sense of pain
3. Sense of warmth
4. Sense of cold
5. Ability to move

CLINICAL JUDGMENT CHALLENGE

Patient-Centered Care QSEN

The patient is a 71-year-old woman who came from the operating room to the postanesthesia recovery unit about an hour ago after a short procedure (dilation and curettage) under general anesthesia for dysfunctional uterine bleeding. She awakens when her name is called, but she does not know where she is or why. In addition, she has pulled off her oxygen cannula and keeps trying to pull out her IV. Her last vital signs, taken 15 minutes ago, were BP, 140/92; pulse, 88; respirations, 18. When you check her vital signs now, they are BP, 128/102; pulse 110; respirations 24. She is saying she is thirsty and wants some water.

1. Are any of the changes in vital signs a cause for concern? If so which ones?
2. Given her surgery, where should you look for bleeding? (Check Chapter 71 for information about this procedure.)
3. Should you apply oxygen? Why or why not?
4. Should you give her sips of water? Why or why not?
5. Should you notify the surgeon or anesthesia provider? Why or why not?

CONSIDERATIONS FOR OLDER ADULTS

Patient-Centered Care QSEN

For an older adult, a rapid return to his or her level of orientation before surgery may not be realistic. Preoperative drugs and anesthetics may delay the older patient's return of orientation.

Reassure family members that most episodes of postoperative confusion or delirium resolve within a day or two (Brooks, 2012).

Compare the patient's baseline neurologic status (obtained before surgery) with the findings after surgery. Patients who had altered cerebral functioning before surgery because of another condition usually continue to have that alteration after surgery. After the patient is alert (and all other criteria have been met), he or she is discharged from the PACU. On the medical-surgical nursing unit, assess the level of consciousness every 4 to 8 hours or as indicated by the patient's condition and the facility's policy.

Motor function and sensory function after general anesthesia are altered and must be assessed. General anesthesia depresses all voluntary motor function. Regional anesthesia alters the motor and sensory function of only part of the body. (See Chapter 15 for more information on anesthesia.)

Motor and sensory function after spinal and epidural anesthesia are profoundly affected and critical to assess. Assess the level of sensation loss remaining by lightly pricking the patient's skin with a needle or pin and having the patient indicate when the sensation feels sharp rather than dull (just pressure). Evaluate motor function by asking the patient to move each extremity. The patient who had epidural or spinal anesthesia remains in the PACU until sensory function (feeling) and voluntary motor movement of the legs have returned (see Table 16-2). Also assess the strength of each limb, and compare the results on both sides. Test for the return of sympathetic nervous system tone by gradually elevating the patient's head and monitoring for hypotension. Begin this evaluation after the patient's sensation has returned to at least the spinal dermatome level of T10.

Specific assessment findings for complications of spinal and epidural anesthesia are listed in Chart 16-3. After the patient is transferred to the nursing unit, continue neurologic assessment as indicated.

CHART 16-3 Best Practice for Patient Safety & Quality Care QSEN

Recognizing Serious Complications of Spinal and Epidural Anesthesia

Respiratory Depression (can occur if the anesthetic agent moves higher in the epidural or subarachnoid space)

- What is the quality and pattern of the breathing?
- What is the respiratory rate and depth?
- Is the patient receiving oxygen? At what setting? What is the pulse oximetry result?
- Notify the anesthesia provider if pulse oximetry drops or if the patient is unable to increase the depth of respiration.

Hypotension (can occur when regional anesthesia causes widespread vasodilation)

- What is the patient's blood pressure?
- Is the blood pressure now lower than in the preoperative or operative period?
- Has the pulse pressure widened?
- Notify the anesthesia provider if systolic blood pressure remains more than 10 mm Hg below the patient's baseline or if other manifestations of shock are present.
- Notify the anesthesia provider if hypotension is accompanied by other manifestations of autonomic nervous system blockade (bradycardia, nausea, vomiting).

Epidural Hematoma

- Assess for delayed or regressing return of sensory and motor function.
- If return is delayed or is taking longer than usual, alert the anesthesia provider.
- Determine whether sensory or motor deficits are improving, remaining the same, or worsening.
- If motor deficits are worsening or decreasing after brief improvement, notify the anesthesia provider immediately.
- Assess for return of deep tendon reflexes of extremities on both sides.
- Compare reflexes from one side of the body with the other.
- If reflexes regress, notify the anesthesia provider immediately.
- Assess pain level in the back.
- If the patient feels pressure or increasing back pain while coughing or straining, notify the anesthesia provider immediately.

Infection (Meningitis)

- Assess for mental status changes.
- Assess for increasing temperature.
- Assess for ability to turn the neck.
- Notify the anesthesia provider immediately for temperature elevations above 101° F (38.3° C), inability to move the neck, acute confusion.

Postdural Puncture Headache

- Assess for report of headache in the occipital region, especially when the patient is permitted to sit upright.

NCLEX EXAMINATION CHALLENGE

Physiological Integrity

Which assessment parameter is most important for the nurse to employ for the client admitted to the postanesthesia care unit (PACU) for recovery after surgery under epidural anesthesia?
A. Determining the client's level of consciousness
B. Checking for pain on dorsi and plantar flexion of the foot
C. Assessing the response to pinprick stimulation from feet to mid-chest level
D. Comparing blood pressure taken in the right arm with blood pressure taken in the left arm

Fluid, Electrolyte, and Acid-Base Balance. Fasting before and during surgery, the loss of fluid during the procedure, and the type and amount of blood or fluid given affect the patient's fluid and electrolyte balance after surgery. Fluid volume deficit or fluid volume overload may occur after surgery. Sodium, potassium, chloride, and calcium imbalances also may result, as may changes in other electrolyte levels. Fluid and electrolyte imbalances occur more often in older or debilitated patients and in those with health problems such as diabetes mellitus, Crohn's disease, or heart failure.

Intake and output measurement is part of the operative record and is reported by the circulating nurse to the PACU nurse. Record any intake or output, including IV fluid intake, vomitus, urine, wound drainage, and nasogastric (NG) tube drainage. You must know the total intake and output from both the OR and the PACU to assess fluid balance accurately and to complete the 24-hour intake and output record.

Hydration status is assessed in the PACU and the medical-surgical unit. To determine hydration status, inspect the color and moisture of mucous membranes; the turgor, texture, and "tenting" of the skin (test over the sternum or forehead of an older patient); the amount of drainage on dressings; and the presence of axillary sweat. Measure and compare total output (e.g., NG tube drainage, urine output, wound drainage) with total intake to identify a possible fluid imbalance. Consider insensible fluid loss, such as sweat, when reviewing total output. Continue to assess intake and output as long as the patient is at risk for fluid imbalances. Some facilities require intake and output to be measured if the patient receives IV fluids or has a catheter, drains, or an NG tube. In addition, patients who have heart disease or kidney disease may need a longer period of intake and output measurement.

IV fluids are closely monitored to promote fluid and electrolyte balance. Isotonic solutions such as lactated Ringer's (LR), 0.9% sodium chloride (normal saline), and 5% dextrose with lactated Ringer's (D_5/LR) are used for IV fluid replacement in the PACU. After the patient returns to the medical-surgical unit, the type and rate of IV infusions are based on need.

Acid-base balance is affected by the patient's respiratory status; metabolic changes during surgery; and losses of acids or bases in drainage. For example, NG tube drainage or vomitus causes a loss of hydrochloric acid and leads to metabolic alkalosis. Examine arterial blood gas (ABG) values and other laboratory values. (See Chapter 12 for more detailed information on acid-base imbalances.)

Kidney/Urinary System. Control of urination may return immediately after surgery or may not return for hours after general or regional anesthesia. The effects of preoperative drugs (especially atropine), anesthetic agents, or manipulation during surgery can cause urine retention. Assess for urine retention by inspection, palpation, and percussion of the lower abdomen for bladder distention or by the use of a bladder scanner (see Chapter 65). Assessment may be difficult to perform after lower abdominal surgery. Urine retention is common early after surgery and requires intervention, such as intermittent (straight) catheterization, to empty the bladder.

When the patient has an indwelling urinary (Foley) catheter, assess the urine for color, clarity, and amount. If the patient is voiding, assess the frequency, amount per void, and any manifestations. Urine output should be close to the total intake for a 24-hour period. Consider sweat, vomitus, or diarrhea stools as sources of output. Report a urine output of less than 30 mL/

hr (240 mL per 8-hour nursing shift) to the surgeon. Decreased urine output may indicate hypovolemia or renal complications. (See Chapter 65 for kidney/urinary assessment.)

Gastrointestinal System. *Postoperative nausea and vomiting (PONV)* are among the most common reactions after surgery. Many patients who receive general anesthesia have some form of GI upset within the first 24 hours after surgery; however, some patients are more at risk than others (Tinsley & Barone, 2013). Patients with a history of motion sickness are more likely to develop nausea and vomiting after surgery. Obese patients may be at risk because many anesthetics are retained by fat cells and remain in the body longer. Abdominal surgery and the use of opioid analgesics reduce intestinal peristalsis after surgery. These problems increase the risk for prolonged nausea and vomiting after surgery. Preventive drug therapy, often started in the preoperative period, is effective in reducing the incidence. Drugs often used are a serotonin antagonist such as ondansetron (Zofran), a sedating H_1 histamine antagonist such as dimenhydrinate (Dramamine), and an anticholinergic agent such as scopolamine.

PONV can stress and irritate abdominal and GI wounds, increase intracranial pressure in patients who had head and neck surgery, elevate intraocular pressure in patients who had eye surgery, and increase the risk for aspiration. Assess the patient continuously for PONV. Often patients have nausea as the head of the bed is raised early after surgery. Help reduce this distressing symptom by having the patient in a side-lying position before raising the head slowly.

Intestinal peristalsis may be delayed because of prolonged anesthesia time, the amount of bowel handling during surgery, and opioid analgesic use. In the PACU and later on the medical-surgical unit, assess for the return of peristalsis. *Patients who are recovering from abdominal surgery often have decreased or no peristalsis for at least 24 hours.* This problem may persist for several days for those who have GI surgery.

Listen for bowel sounds in all four abdominal quadrants and at the umbilicus. If NG suction is being used, turn off the suction before listening to prevent mistaking the sound of the suction for bowel sounds. *The presence of active bowel sounds usually indicates return of peristalsis; however, the absence of bowel sounds does not confirm a lack of peristalsis. The best indicator of intestinal activity is the passage of flatus or stool* (Massey, 2012). Abdominal cramping along with distention denotes trapped, nonmoving gas—not peristalsis.

Decreased peristalsis occurs in patients who have a paralytic ileus. The abdominal wall is distended with no visible intestinal movement. Assess for the manifestations of paralytic ileus (distended abdomen, abdominal discomfort, vomiting, no passage of flatus or stool). In some patients, bowels sounds can be heard even when a true paralytic ileus is present. The passage of flatus or stool is the best indicator of resolution of a paralytic ileus. See the Evidence-Based Practice box.

A nasogastric (NG) tube may be inserted during surgery to decompress and drain the stomach, to promote GI rest, and to allow the lower GI tract to heal. It may also be used to monitor any gastric bleeding and to prevent intestinal obstruction. Usually low suction is applied to promote drainage. Suction is either continuous or intermittent.

Record the color, consistency, and amount of the NG drainage every 8 hours (Table 16-3). In some instances, an occult blood test (Gastroccult) may be performed. Normal NG drainage fluid is greenish yellow. Red or pink drainage fluid

EVIDENCE-BASED PRACTICE (QSEN)

Evidence-Based Practice or Sacred Cow?

Massey, R. (2012). Return of bowel sounds indicating an end of postoperative ileus: Is it time to cease this long-standing nursing tradition? *MEDSURG Nursing, 21*(3), 146-150.

Abdominal surgery, especially surgery involving bowel anastomosis, is known to reduce or stop intestinal peristalsis and result in postoperative ileus (POI) with a duration of 3 to 5 days. POI causes a cluster of patient symptoms, which include abdominal pain, distention, nausea, and vomiting. In addition, POI delays nutrition and lengthens hospital stay. For more than a century, the classic indicator for return of bowel function after POI was the presence of bowel sounds. Recommended assessment is auscultation of the four abdominal quadrants for 5 minutes each, a total time task of 20 minutes. A variety of previous research suggests that assessment of bowel sounds for return of function after POI is an unreliable "tradition" that wastes nursing care time and may, in fact, cause harm.

Problems associated with assessment of bowel sounds as an indicator of bowel function return include the fact that the small intestine usually recovers bowel sounds ahead of the colon but that the sounds do not always correlate to peristaltic movement of retained gas and fluids. This means that positive bowel sounds in some quadrants may result in early enteral feeding of a patient before true peristalsis returns. Also, some patients have no loss of bowel sounds after abdominal surgery but do experience the symptom cluster associated with POI, again making the presence of bowel sounds an unreliable indicator of peristalsis. Moreover, studies indicate that most nurses auscultate the abdomen for only 30 to 60 seconds in each quadrant, not the recommended but unvalidated time of 5 minutes per quadrant. Even this smaller amount of time represents unproductive nursing activity.

The current study examined the return of bowel sounds and other manifestations as indicators for resolution of POI among 66 patients who all had intestinal surgery with anastomosis for cancer. The average return of bowel sounds among these 66 patients was 2.23 days and was not related to the average time to first passage of flatus.

Level of Evidence: 3

This quasi-experimental study with a two-group, post-test only design was randomized and had sufficient subjects to provide result validity. The use of objective measurements added to study strength.

Commentary: Implications for Practice and Research

This study provides evidence for the rational elimination of 20 minutes of nursing time spent in auscultation of bowel sounds several times daily after abdominal surgery. The findings of this study support other studies that recommend using the practice of using passage of flatus or stool as the marker for the end of POI rather than the time-honored but unsupported practice of auscultating bowel sounds for 20 minutes. Actual passage of flatus or stool demonstrates an end of POI and complete return of peristalsis with forward propulsion of intestinal contents for the entire GI tract. Additional positive indicators for evidence of an end to POI include elimination of abdominal distention, nausea, and vomiting and the tolerance of oral intake. Nurses need to understand the physiologic basis for why return of bowel sounds may be an unreliable indicator of an end to POI and may result in inappropriate initiation of dietary intake.

indicates active bleeding, and brown liquid or drainage with a "coffee-ground" appearance indicates old bleeding. Assess that the NG tube is securely taped to the nose, and note any skin irritation.

Assess the patient for complications related to NG tube use, such as fluid and electrolyte imbalances, aspiration, and nares

TABLE 16-3 Calculating Nasogastric Tube Drainage

Formula

$$\text{Drainage in collection device} - \text{Amount of irrigant}$$
$$= \text{True (actual) amount of drainage}$$

Example

A patient's drainage container was marked at 150 mL at 7 AM. At 3 PM, there was 525 mL in the container. During the nursing shift, the nurse instilled 30 mL of saline as an irrigant into the tube four times, as prescribed by the physician.

$$525\,\text{mL} - 150\,\text{mL} = 375\,\text{mL of drainage}$$
$$30\,\text{mL} \times 4 = 120\,\text{mL of irrigant}$$
$$375\,\text{mL} - 120\,\text{mL} = 255\,\text{mL of actual drainage}$$

discomfort. To prevent aspiration, check the tube placement every 4 to 8 hours and before instilling any liquid, including drugs, into the tube. (See Chapter 55 for information on tube placement and care.) Electrolyte imbalances can result from NG drainage and tube irrigation with water instead of saline. Imbalances include fluid volume deficit, hypokalemia and hyponatremia (see Chapter 11), hypochloremia, and metabolic alkalosis (see Chapter 12).

! NURSING SAFETY PRIORITY (QSEN)

Action Alert

After gastric surgery, do not move or irrigate the NG tube unless prescribed by the surgeon.

Constipation may occur after surgery as a result of anesthesia, analgesia (especially opioids), decreased activity, and decreased oral intake. Assess the abdomen by inspection, auscultation, palpation, and percussion and record the elimination pattern to determine whether intervention is needed. *Auscultate before palpation or percussion because these two maneuvers can affect peristalsis.* Increased dietary fiber intake, the use of mild laxatives or bulk-forming agents, or the use of enemas may be needed.

? NCLEX EXAMINATION CHALLENGE

Safe and Effective Care Environment

The assessment findings for the nasogastric tube drainage of a client recently transferred from the PACU include the presence of 140 mL of greenish yellow drainage. What is the nurse's best action?

A. Instruct the client to drink water until the drainage is clear.
B. Reposition the tube to increase the drainage.
C. Call and report this finding to the surgeon.
D. Document the finding as the only action.

Skin Assessment. The clean surgical wound regains TISSUE INTEGRITY (heals) at skin level in about 2 weeks in the absence of trauma, connective tissue disease, malnutrition, or the use of some drugs, such as steroids. Smokers and patients who are older, obese, or have diabetes or whose immunity is reduced have delayed wound healing. Complete tissue integrity (healing) of all layers within the surgical wound may take 6 months to 2 years. The physical health and age of the patient, size and location of the wound, and stress on the wound all affect healing time. Head and facial wounds heal more quickly than abdominal and leg wounds because of the better blood flow to the head and neck.

Normal Wound Healing. During the first few days of normal wound healing, the incised tissue regains blood supply and begins to bind together. Fibrin and a thin layer of epithelial cells seal the incision. After 1 to 4 days, epithelial cells continue growing in the fibrin and strands of collagen begin to fill in the wound gaps. *This process continues for 2 to 3 weeks. At that time, TISSUE INTEGRITY appears regained; however, healing is not complete for up to 2 years, until the scar is strengthened.* (See Chapters 24 and 25 for discussion of wound healing and wound infection.)

When the patient is an inpatient, the surgeon usually removes the original dressing on the first or second day after surgery. Assess the TISSUE INTEGRITY of the incision on a regular basis, at least every 8 hours, for redness, increased warmth, swelling, tenderness or PAIN, and the type and amount of drainage. Some drainage, changing from **sanguineous** (bloody) to serosanguineous to **serous** (serum-like, or yellow), is normal during the first few days. Serosanguineous drainage continuing beyond the fifth day after surgery or increasing in amount instead of decreasing alerts you to the possibility of dehiscence (discussed below), and the surgeon should be notified. Crusting on the incision line is normal, as is a pink color to the line itself, which is caused by inflammation from the surgical procedure. Slight swelling under the sutures or staples is also normal. Redness or swelling of or around the incision line, excessive tenderness or pain on palpation, and purulent or odorous drainage indicate wound INFECTION and must be reported to the surgeon.

Impaired Wound Healing. Impaired wound healing with loss of TISSUE INTEGRITY may be caused by INFECTION, distention, stress at the surgical site, and health problems that cause delayed wound healing (e.g., diabetes). Wound **dehiscence** is a partial or complete separation of the outer wound layers, sometimes described as a "splitting open of the wound." **Evisceration** is the total separation of all wound layers and protrusion of internal organs through the open wound (Fig. 16-2). Both of these problems occur most often between the fifth and tenth days after surgery. Wound separation occurs more often in obese patients and those with diabetes, immune deficiency, or malnutrition or who are using steroids. Dehiscence or evisceration may follow forceful coughing, vomiting, or straining and when not splinting the surgical site during movement. The patient may state, "Something popped" or "I feel as if I just split open."

Dressings and Drains. Assess all dressings, including casts and elastic (Ace) bandages, for bleeding or other drainage on admission to the PACU and then hourly thereafter. When the patient is on the nursing unit, assess the dressing each time vital signs are taken (at least every 8 hours). During dressing inspection, check for drainage and record its amount, color, consistency, and odor. If drainage is present on a dressing or cast, monitor its progression by outlining it with a pencil and indicating the date and time. Check the area underneath the patient also, because drainage or blood may leak from the side of the dressing and not appear on the dressing itself.

Ensure that the dressing does not restrict circulation or sensation. This problem is most likely to occur when dressings are tight or completely encircle an arm or a leg. Chest dressings that are too tight or that encircle the chest can restrict breathing.

The surgeon inserts a drain into or close to the wound if more than a minimal amount of drainage is expected. A Penrose drain (a single-lumen, soft, open, latex tube) is a gravity-type drain under the dressing. Drainage on the dressing is expected with open tube drains but is not expected with closed drainage systems. Assess closed-suction drains, such as Hemovac, Vacu-Drain, and Jackson-Pratt drains, for maintenance of suction. Specialty drains, such as a T-tube, may be placed for specific drainage purposes. For example, a T-tube drains bile after a cholecystectomy. Chronic wounds or wounds that heal by delayed primary intention are drained with a negative pressure wound device. Fig. 16-3 shows commonly used drains.

Assess all drains for patency when the patient is admitted to the PACU and every time vital signs are taken. Monitor the amount, color, and type of drainage while the patient is in the PACU and at least every 8 hours after he or she is transferred to the medical-surgical nursing unit. Large amounts of sanguineous drainage may indicate poor CLOTTING and possible internal bleeding.

Discomfort/Pain Assessment. The patient almost always has PAIN or discomfort after surgery. Pain is a subjective experience and may be more intense than you can appreciate. Pain after surgery is related to the surgical wound, tissue manipulation, drains, positioning during surgery, presence of an endotracheal tube, and the patient's experience with pain (Ward, 2014). In accordance with The Joint Commission's National Patient Safety Goals, assess the patient's discomfort and need for medication by considering the type, extent, and length of the surgical procedure. Assess for physical and emotional signs of acute pain, such as increased pulse and blood pressure, increased respiratory rate, profuse sweating, restlessness, confusion (in the older adult), wincing, moaning, and crying. When possible, ask the patient to rate the pain before and after drugs are given (e.g., on a scale of 0 to 10, with 0 being no pain and 10 being extreme pain). Plan the patient's activities around the timing of analgesia to improve mobility. Observe for a return of baseline physical and emotional behaviors. (See Chapter 3 for further discussion of pain assessment.)

PAIN assessment is started by the PACU nurse. After the patient is transferred from the PACU, the medical-surgical nurse continues to assess the patient's comfort level. Pain usually reaches its peak on the second day after surgery, when the

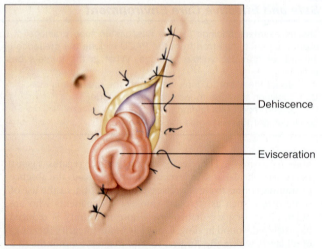

FIG. 16-2 Complications of surgical wound healing.

Dehiscence

Evisceration

FIG. 16-3 Types of surgical drains. Gravity drains, such as the Penrose **(A)** and the T-tube **(B)** drain directly through a tube from the surgical area. In closed wound drainage systems, such as the Jackson-Pratt **(C)** and Hemovac **(D)**, drainage collects in a collecting vessel by means of compression and re-expansion of the system.

patient is more awake and more active and the anesthetic agents and drugs given during surgery have been excreted.

Psychosocial Assessment. Consider the psychological, social, and cultural issues of the patient after surgery as you provide physical care. This assessment may be delayed or difficult to perform in the PACU when the patient is drowsy or confused. Consider the patient's age and medical history, the surgical procedure, and the impact of surgery on recovery, body image, roles, and lifestyle.

Indications of anxiety include restlessness; increased pulse, blood pressure, and respiratory rate; and crying. The patient may be anxious and ask questions about the results or findings of the surgical procedure. Reassure the patient that the surgeon will speak with him or her after he or she is fully awake. If the surgeon has already spoken with the patient, reinforce what was said.

After the patient returns to the medical-surgical unit, continue the psychosocial assessment and also assess family members for psychological discomfort.

Laboratory Assessment. Laboratory tests are performed after surgery to monitor for complications. Tests are based on the surgical procedure, the patient's medical history, and clinical manifestations after surgery. Common tests include analysis of electrolytes and a complete blood count (see Chart 14-3 in Chapter 14). Changes in electrolyte, hematocrit, and hemoglobin levels often occur during the first 24 to 48 hours after surgery because of blood and fluid loss and the body's reaction to the surgical process. Fluid loss with minimal blood loss may cause elevated laboratory values. Such test results appear increased but actually are concentrated normal values.

An indication of INFECTION is an increase in the band cells (immature neutrophils) in the white blood cell differential count, known as a "left-shift" or *bandemia*. The source of infection may be the respiratory system, urinary tract, surgical wound, or IV site. Obtain specimens for culture and sensitivity testing, and monitor the culture reports at 24, 48, and 72 hours. Notify the surgeon of positive culture results. (See Chapters 17 and 23 for information on infection.)

Arterial blood gas (ABG) tests may be needed for patients who have respiratory or cardiac disease, those undergoing mechanical ventilation after surgery, and those who had chest surgery. Review ABG results, and notify the surgeon of any acid-base imbalance or hypoxemia that indicates poor GAS EXCHANGE. (For more discussion on arterial blood gases and acidosis, see Chapter 12.)

Urine and kidney laboratory tests also may be obtained (e.g., urinalysis, urine electrolyte levels, serum creatinine levels). Other laboratory tests depend on the diagnosis, type of surgical procedure, and other health problems. Examples are a serum amylase level for a patient who had pancreatic surgery and a blood glucose level for a patient with diabetes.

◆ Analysis

The priority NANDA-I nursing diagnoses and collaborative problems for patients after surgery include:

1. Potential for hypoxemia related to the effects of anesthesia, pain, opioid analgesics, and immobility
2. Potential for wound infection and delayed healing related to wound location, decreased mobility, drains and drainage, and tubes
3. Acute Pain related to the surgical incision, positioning during surgery, and endotracheal (ET) tube irritation (NANDA-I)

◆ Planning and Implementation

Preventing Hypoxemia

Planning: Expected Outcomes. The patient is expected to attain or maintain optimal lung expansion and breathing patterns after surgery as indicated by:

- Partial pressure of arterial oxygen (Pao_2) within normal range
- Partial pressure of arterial carbon dioxide ($Paco_2$) within normal range
- Oxygen saturation values within normal range

Interventions

Airway Maintenance. After assessing the airway and GAS EXCHANGE, you may need to insert an oral airway if the patient does not already have one. The oral airway pulls the tongue forward and holds it down to prevent obstruction. If the patient had oral surgery or has clenched teeth, a large tongue, or upper airway obstruction, insert a nasal airway (nasal trumpet) to keep the airway open. Keep the manual resuscitation bag and emergency equipment for intubation or tracheostomy nearby. For patients whose only airway is a tracheostomy or laryngectomy stoma, alert other staff members by posting signs in the room and notes on the chart.

Monitoring. Monitor the patient's oxygen saturation (Spo_2) for adequacy of GAS EXCHANGE with pulse oximetry at least every hour or more often, according to the patient's condition. Patients who normally have a low Pao_2, such as those with lung disease or older adults, are at higher risk for hypoxemia. An older adult is often prescribed low-dose oxygen therapy for the first 12 to 24 hours after surgery to reduce confusion from anesthesia and sedation (Sullivan, 2011). A patient who received moderate sedation with a benzodiazepine such as midazolam (Versed) or lorazepam (Ativan, Nu-Loraz ✦) may be overly sedated or have respiratory depression sufficient to need reversal with flumazenil (Romazicon) (Chart 16-4). Hypothermia after surgery causes shivering, which increases oxygen demand and can induce hypoxemia. Many rewarming methods can be

---

CHART 16-4 Best Practice for Patient Safety & Quality Care (QSEN)

Emergency Care of the Patient Experiencing a Benzodiazepine Overdose

- Secure the airway and IV access before starting benzodiazepine antagonist therapy.
- Prepare to administer flumazenil (Romazicon)* in a dose of 0.2 mg to 1 mg IV.
- Repeat drug every 2 to 3 minutes up to 3 mg, as needed, depending on the patient's response.
- Give oxygen if hypoxia is present or if respirations are below 10 breaths per minute.
- Have suction equipment available because flumazenil can trigger vomiting and a drowsy patient is at risk for aspiration.
- Continuously monitor vital signs and level of consciousness for reversal of overdose.
- Do not leave the patient until he or she is fully responsive.
- Continue to monitor the patient's vital signs and level of consciousness every 10 to 15 minutes for the first 2 hours because flumazenil is eliminated from the body more quickly than is the benzodiazepine.
- Determine the need for additional flumazenil therapy 1 to 2 hours after the patient initially becomes fully responsive.
- Observe the patient for tremors or convulsions because flumazenil can lower the seizure threshold in patients who have seizure disorders.
- Assess the IV site every shift because flumazenil can cause thrombophlebitis at the injection site.
- Observe the patient for side effects of flumazenil, including skin rash, hot flushes, dizziness, headache, sweating, dry mouth, and blurred vision. The incidence of these side effects increases with higher total doses of flumazenil.

*There are other benzodiazepine antagonists; however, flumazenil is used most often to manage adult benzodiazepine overdose in the postoperative period.

---

used, although prevention is more important. The highest incidence of hypoxemia after surgery occurs on the second postoperative day.

Positioning. *In the PACU, immediately position the patient in a semi-Fowler's position unless contraindicated. If the patient cannot have the head of the bed raised, either place him or her in a side-lying position or turn the head to the side to prevent aspiration.*

Oxygen Therapy. Hypoxemia is prevented and managed with oxygen therapy. Apply oxygen by face tent, nasal cannula, or mask to eliminate inhaled anesthetic agents, increase oxygen levels, raise the level of consciousness, and reduce confusion. After the patient is fully reactive and stable, raise the head of the bed to promote respiratory function.

For some patients, oxygen therapy may continue through the second day after surgery. When hypoxemia occurs despite preventive care, interventions such as respiratory treatments and mechanical ventilation may be used to manage the cause of the hypoxemia.

Breathing Exercises. After the patient regains the gag and cough reflexes and meets the agency's criteria for extubation (if intubated), remove the airway or ET tube. Usual extubation criteria include the ability to raise and hold the head up and evidence of thoracic breathing. Help the patient splint the incision, cough, and deep breathe to promote GAS EXCHANGE and eliminate anesthetic agents. Chart 14-5 in Chapter 14 reviews breathing exercises and splinting of the surgical area. As soon as the patient is awake enough to follow commands, urge him or her to cough, use the incentive spirometer, and take deep breaths hourly while awake throughout the postoperative period. The patient who is unable to remove mucus or sputum requires oral or nasal suctioning. Perform mouth care after removing secretions.

Movement. Assist the patient out of bed and to ambulate as soon as possible to help remove secretions and promote ventilation. Even when the patient has had extensive surgery, the expectation may be to get out of bed the day of or the first day after surgery. If this is not possible, assist him or her to turn at least every 2 hours (side to side) and ensure that breathing exercises and leg exercises are performed (see Charts 14-5 and 14-6 in Chapter 14). Early ambulation reduces the risk for pulmonary complications, especially after abdominal, pelvic, or spinal surgery. It increases circulation to extremities and reduces the risk for CLOTTING and venous thromboembolism (VTE), especially deep vein thrombosis (DVT). The patient may resist getting up, but you must stress the importance of activity to prevent complications. When indicated, offer pain medication 30 to 45 minutes before he or she gets out of bed.

Preventing Wound Infection and Delayed Healing

Planning: Expected Outcomes. The patient is expected to have incision healing without wound complications as indicated by:

- Wound edges remaining together
- No purulent drainage, induration, or redness in, from, or around the incision

Interventions. Nursing assessment of the surgical area is critical (see the discussion of skin assessment on p. 263). Although most wound complications do not require additional surgical intervention, emergency surgical procedures may be needed.

Nonsurgical Management. Wound care includes reinforcing the dressing, changing the dressing, assessing the wound for healing and infection, and caring for drains, including emptying drainage containers/reservoirs, measuring drainage, and documenting drainage features. Emphasize the importance of early deep-breathing exercises to prevent forceful coughing. Urge the patient to bend the hips when in the supine position to reduce tension on a chest or abdominal wound. Remind him or her to always splint the chest or abdominal incision when coughing. Promote wound healing and protection of the skin, especially for the older patient (Sullivan, 2011). Chart 16-5 lists best practices for skin care of the older patient after surgery.

Dressings. The surgeon usually performs the first dressing change to assess the wound, remove any packing, and advance (pull partially out) or remove drains. Before the first dressing change, reinforce the dressing (add more dressing material to the existing dressing) if it becomes wet from drainage. Document the added material, as well as the color, type, amount, and odor of drainage fluid and time of observation. Assess the surgical site at least every shift, and report any unexpected findings to the surgeon.

After removal of the dressing, the surgeon may leave the suture or staple line open to the air, which allows easy assessment of the wound and early detection of poor wound edge adherence, drainage, swelling, or redness. Some surgeons believe that air-drying promotes healing. A draining wound, however, is always covered with a dressing.

Dressing changes are prescribed by the surgeon; however, the facility or unit may have standards or policies that dictate specific protocols for dressing changes and incision care. An unchanged wet or damp dressing is a source of INFECTION. Change dressings using aseptic technique until the sutures or staples are removed.

FIG. 16-4 Patient with a dressing held in place with Montgomery straps.

Dressings vary with the surgical procedure and the surgeon's preference. Common dressings for large incisions consist of gauze or nonadherent pads covered with a larger absorbent pad held in place by tape, a tubular stretchy net, or Montgomery straps (Fig. 16-4). Some incisions may be covered with a transparent plastic surgical dressing (e.g., OpSite) or a spray in the operating room. This type of dressing stays intact for 3 to 6 days, allows direct observation of the wound, prevents contamination, and eliminates the need for dressing changes.

Wound or suture line care consists of changing gauze dressings at least once during a nursing shift or daily and may include cleaning the area with sterile saline or some other solution. Some suture lines are left open to air without any dressing to cover the incision. The hospital's policy, the unit's standards, and the surgeon's preference determine what solution, if any, is used to clean the wound and how often dressings are changed. For large dressing changes or drain removal, offer the patient a prescribed analgesic before the procedure. Always assess the skin for redness, rash, or blisters in areas where tape has been used. Tape can cause a skin reaction after surgery even among patients who are not known to be tape sensitive.

Skin sutures or staples are usually removed 5 to 10 days after surgery, although this varies up to 30 days depending on the type of surgery and the patient's health. After sutures or staples are removed, the incision may then be secured with Steri-Strips, which stay in place until they fall off on their own. The surgeon or the nurse removes the sutures or staples, depending on the agency's policy. Clean the incision with the prescribed solution before removing sutures or staples. Before removing sutures, examine the condition and healing stage of the wound. First remove every other suture or staple and re-assess the wound for integrity. If wound healing is progressing normally, the rest of the sutures or staples may then be removed. If the wound does not appear to be healing well or if any manifestations of INFECTION are present, notify the surgeon before removing any sutures.

Drains. Drains (see Fig. 16-3) may be placed in the wound or through a separate small incision (known as a "stab" wound) close to the incision during surgery. Drains provide an exit route for air, blood, and bile. Drains also help prevent deep INFECTION and abscess formation during healing.

The Penrose drain is placed into the external aspect of the incision and drains directly onto the dressing and skin around the incision. Change a damp or soiled dressing, and carefully clean under and around the Penrose drain. Then place absorbent pads under and around the exposed drain to prevent skin irritation, wound contamination, and INFECTION. Whether sutured in place or not, the drain can be dislodged or pulled out accidentally during a dressing change. It is also possible for the drain to slip back through the wound into the patient. Usually this complication is prevented when the drain is first placed in the OR. The surgeon pins a sterile safety pin through the drain at an angle perpendicular to the drain and the wound, which prevents the drain from slipping. As the wound heals, the surgeon or nurse shortens (advances) the drain by pulling it out a short distance and trimming off the excess external portion so that only 2 to 3 inches of drain protrudes through the incision. The safety pin must be repositioned each time the drain is advanced. The drain remains in place until drainage stops.

Jackson-Pratt and Hemovac drains are two self-contained drainage systems that drain wounds directly through a tube via gravity and vacuum. These drains are sutured in place with a suture that seals the area when the drain is removed. Use sterile technique to empty the reservoir. Record the amount and color of drainage during every nursing shift or more often if prescribed. After emptying and compressing the reservoir to restore suction, secure the drain to the patient's gown (never to the sheet or mattress) to prevent pulling and stress on the surgical wound.

Drug Therapy. Wound INFECTION is a major complication after surgery. It usually results from contamination during surgery, preoperative infection, debilitation, or immunosuppression. In accordance with the Surgical Care Improvement Project (SCIP) core measures for prevention of surgical site infection, a patient at risk for wound infection may have received antibiotic therapy with drugs that are effective against organisms common to the specific surgical site both before and

during surgery. The need for these antibiotics is re-evaluated at 24 hours after surgery. If manifestations of infection are not present, the antibiotic is discontinued at that time (SCIP Infection-3, see Table 14-1 in Chapter 14). If manifestations of wound infection are present, they are documented to justify continuation of antibiotic therapy.

Wounds that become infected and open are treated with dressing changes and systemic antibiotic therapy. Depending on the surgeon's prescription, irrigate the wound (e.g., with sterile saline, hydrogen peroxide, povidone-iodine, or acetic acid), loosely pack it with solution-soaked gauze (e.g., neomycin, gentamicin, iodoform, povidone-iodine, saline, or acetic acid), and cover the wound with dry, sterile dressings. These wet-to-damp dressing changes, done 1 to 3 times daily, promote healing from within the wound and **débridement** (removal of the infected or dead tissue) as the wound heals. Negative pressure wound care systems such as Wound VAC may be prescribed to help close the wound. Chapter 25 discusses these systems.

Surgical Management. Poorly healing wounds, infected wounds, or complicated wounds may require surgical intervention.

Management of Dehiscence. If dehiscence (wound opening) occurs, apply a sterile nonadherent (e.g., Telfa) or saline dressing to the wound and notify the surgeon. Instruct the patient to bend the knees and to avoid coughing. A wound that becomes infected dehisces by itself, or it may be opened by the surgeon through an incision and drainage (I&D) procedure. In either case, the wound is left open and is treated as described previously.

Management of Evisceration. An **evisceration** *(a wound opening with protrusion of internal organs) is a surgical emergency.* Chart 16-6 lists best practices for emergency care of the patient with surgical wound evisceration. Provide support by explaining what happened and reassuring the patient that the emergency will be handled competently.

! NURSING SAFETY PRIORITY (QSEN)
Critical Rescue

When a surgical wound evisceration occurs, one nurse tends to the patient while another nurse immediately notifies the surgeon.

The surgeon may prescribe a nasogastric (NG) tube to decompress the stomach and relieve internal pressure or to remove the stomach's contents if the patient has been eating and general anesthesia is needed. Prepare the patient for surgery (see Chapter 14) to close the wound. Regional or local anesthesia may be used, depending on the location and type of wound. Nausea and vomiting, which stress the already fragile incision, are reduced when regional or local anesthesia is used. To increase the incision's integrity, stay or retention sutures of wire or nylon are used along with standard sutures or staples (see Fig. 15-11 in Chapter 15).

Prevention. Patients also are at risk for developing pressure ulcers from positioning during surgery, from contact with damp surgical linens, and from unpadded surfaces. Pressure ulcers acquired during the surgical period prolong stays and increase the risk for complications. Early intervention of pressure ulcers can prevent progression and complications.

Examine the patient's skin for areas of redness or open areas. Document and report any abnormalities. Use padding and

Emergency Care of the Patient with Surgical Wound Evisceration

1. Call for help! Instruct the person who responds to notify the surgeon or Rapid Response Team immediately and to bring any needed supplies into the patient's room.
2. Stay with the patient.
3. Cover the wound with a nonadherent dressing premoistened with warmed sterile normal saline. **NOTE:** The supplies needed for this emergency should be in the patient's room, especially if the patient is at high risk for dehiscence or evisceration.
4. If premoistened dressings are not available, moisten sterile gauze or sterile towels in a sterile irrigation tray with sterile saline and then cover the wound.
5. If saline is not immediately available, cover the wound with gauze and then moisten with sterile saline using a sterile irrigation tray as soon as someone brings saline.
6. Do not attempt to reinsert the protruding organ or viscera.
7. While covering the wound, note the patient's response and assess for manifestations of shock.
8. Place the patient in a supine position with the hips and knees bent.
9. Raise the head of the bed 15 to 20 degrees.
10. Take vital signs, and document them. **NOTE:** If the person who answered the call for help is back in the room before this, instruct him or her to take vital signs while you focus on covering the wound and repositioning the patient.
11. Provide support and reassurance to the patient.
12. Continue assessing the patient, including vital signs assessment, every 5 to 10 minutes until the surgeon arrives.
13. Keep dressings continuously moist by adding warmed sterile saline to the dressing as often as necessary. Do not let the dressing become dry.
14. When the surgeon arrives, report your finding and your interventions. Then follow the surgeon's directions.
15. Document the incident, the activity the patient was engaged in at the time of the incident, your actions, and your assessments.

positioning to relieve pressure. Treat any open areas according to facility guidelines and the surgeon's prescription. Ensure that information about the patient's skin condition in the PACU is communicated to the medical-surgical nurse. For patients at high risk, collaborate with a certified Wound, Ostomy, and Continence registered nurse (WOCRN) to plan preventive or interventional skin care.

Managing Pain

Planning: Expected Outcomes. The postoperative patient is expected to attain or maintain optimal comfort levels. Indicators include:
- Reporting that pain is controlled
- Absence of physiologic indicators of acute pain (increased heart rate and blood pressure)
- Absence of facial grimacing, teeth clenching
- Willingness to move and participate in self-care

Interventions. PAIN management after surgery includes drug therapy and other methods of management, such as positioning, massage, relaxation techniques, and diversion. Often the patient has better pain relief from a combination of approaches. Assess the patient's comfort level and the effectiveness of the therapies. See Chapter 3 for discussion of pain assessment and management. The patient who has optimal pain control is better able to cooperate with the therapies and exercises to prevent complications and promote rehabilitation.

Drug Therapy. The use of opioids or other analgesics for pain management may mask or increase the severity of symptoms of an anesthesia reaction. Therefore give these drugs with caution, especially in the PACU when the patient's condition is not stable. When pain drugs are used in the PACU, they are usually given IV in small doses. After receiving any drug for PAIN, the patient remains in the PACU for a defined period (often 45 to 60 minutes). Assess for hypotension, respiratory depression, and other side effects. Within 5 to 10 minutes after an IV injection, assess the effectiveness of the drug (i.e., on a rating scale) in relieving pain.

Opioid analgesics are given during the first 24 to 48 hours after surgery to control acute PAIN. Around-the-clock scheduling or the use of patient-controlled analgesia (PCA) systems is more effective than "on demand" scheduling because more constant blood levels are achieved. Drugs commonly used include morphine (Statex ✦), hydromorphone (Dilaudid), ketorolac (Toradol), codeine, butorphanol (Stadol), and oxycodone with aspirin (Percodan) or oxycodone with acetaminophen (Tylox, Percocet).

! NURSING SAFETY PRIORITY (QSEN)
Drug Alert

The usual dosage for hydromorphone is much smaller (about one-fifth to one-tenth) that of morphine.

Assess the type, location, and intensity of the pain before and after giving medication (see also Discomfort/Pain Assessment, p. 264). Monitor the patient's vital signs for hypotension and hypoventilation after giving opioid drugs. Chart 16-7 lists more information about analgesics used after surgery.

Patient-controlled analgesia (PCA) by IV infusion or internal pump (the catheter is sutured into or near the surgical area) and epidural analgesia are often used for better pain control. In PCA, the patient adjusts the dosage of the analgesic based on the pain level and response to the drug. This method allows more consistent pain relief and more control by the patient. The maximum dose per hour is "locked in" to the pump so that the patient cannot accidentally overdose. Common drugs used in PCA include morphine and hydromorphone.

Epidural analgesia can be given intermittently by the anesthesia provider or by continuous infusion through an epidural catheter left in place after epidural anesthesia. Drugs given by epidural catheter include the opioids *fentanyl (Sublimaze), preservative-free morphine (Duramorph),* and *bupivacaine (Marcaine).*

Take care not to overmedicate or undermedicate, especially with older patients. In assessing for overmedication, monitor vital signs, especially blood pressure and respiratory rate, and level of consciousness. Complications from the use of opioid analgesics include respiratory depression, hypotension, nausea, vomiting, and constipation. An opioid antagonist, such as naloxone (Narcan), may be needed to reverse the acute effects of opioid depression. Because of the short effect of the opioid antagonist, monitor the patient's blood pressure and respirations every 15 to 30 minutes until the full effect of the opioid analgesic has passed. You may need to give more doses of the antagonist during this time because it is eliminated from the body more quickly than is the opioid. (See Chart 16-8 for more information on using opioid antagonists to reverse opioid

CHART 16-7 Common Examples of Drug Therapy
Management of Postoperative Pain

DRUG	USUAL DOSAGE	NURSING INTERVENTIONS	RATIONALES
Morphine sulfate (Epimorph ✤, Statex ✤)	2-15 mg IM or IV incrementally 10-30 mg orally every 4 hr	Monitor respiratory status. Monitor blood pressure. Assess for GI motility and urine output.	Respiratory depression can be severe and require medical intervention. Hypotension, constipation, and urinary retention can occur.
Hydromorphone hydrochloride (Dilaudid)	1-4 mg IV or IM every 3-4 hr 2-4 mg orally every 3-4 hr	Monitor respirations. Monitor blood pressure. Monitor for food intolerance. Monitor fluid and electrolyte balance. Assess GI motility.	Respiratory depression, hypotension, anorexia, nausea, vomiting, and constipation can occur.
Codeine sulfate, codeine phosphate (Paveral ✤)	15-60 mg IM or orally every 4 hr	Monitor respiratory status. Monitor for food intolerance. Monitor fluid and electrolyte balance. Assess GI motility.	Respiratory depression, nausea, and vomiting can occur. Constipation is common; prophylactic interventions may be indicated.
Butorphanol tartrate (Stadol)	1-4 mg IM every 3-4 hr 0.5-2 mg IV	Monitor neurologic status and changes in level of consciousness. Monitor respiratory status.	Butorphanol can cause increased intracranial pressure and respiratory depression.
Oxycodone hydrochloride and aspirin (Percodan, Endodan ✤, Oxycodan ✤)	1-2 tablets (5-10 mg) orally every 3-4 hr	Assess GI tolerance of medication. Assess for GI bleeding. Monitor GI motility. Monitor coagulation studies (PT, aPTT). Monitor respiratory status.	The aspirin component can irritate the stomach and could cause GI bleeding. Bleeding times and other coagulation study results may be increased because of the aspirin component. Respiratory depression and constipation can be caused by the oxycodone component.
Oxycodone hydrochloride and acetaminophen (Tylox, Percocet, Endocet ✤, Oxycocet ✤)	1-2 tablets (5-10 mg) orally every 3-4 hr	Monitor blood pressure and respiratory status. Assess for GI motility.	Respiratory depression, hypotension, and constipation can occur.
Ketorolac tromethamine (Toradol)	15-60 mg IM or IV every 6 hr	Monitor for GI bleeding. Monitor for kidney effects, especially in older adults.	GI bleeding, ulceration, and perforation can occur. Decreased urine output, increased serum creatinine, hematuria, and proteinuria can occur. Ketorolac is cleared more slowly in older adults. Older persons are more sensitive to the kidney effects of NSAIDs.
Ibuprofen (Motrin, Amersol ✤, Novoprofen ✤)	300-800 mg orally every 4-6 hr	Monitor upper GI tolerance of medication. Give with food or milk. Monitor coagulation studies (PT, aPTT). Assess for signs of bleeding or delayed clotting.	Food or milk helps decrease irritation of the stomach. Bleeding times and other coagulation study results may be increased. Monitoring leads to early detection of complications.

aPTT, Activated partial thromboplastin time; *GI,* gastrointestinal; *NSAID,* nonsteroidal anti-inflammatory drug; *PT,* prothrombin time.

overdose.) In addition, the patient has breakthrough PAIN after the opioid antagonist is given, so other interventions to promote comfort are needed.

Assess for undermedication by asking the patient about degree of PAIN relief and observing for other cues of discomfort (e.g., restlessness, increased confusion, "picking" at bedcovers). Offer prescribed drug(s) after checking for hypotension and respiratory depression.

As recovery progresses, reduce the doses and frequency of drugs for PAIN control. Drugs are changed from injectable or PCA to oral as soon as the patient can tolerate oral agents. Non-opioid analgesics, such as acetaminophen (Tylenol, Atasol ✤),

and NSAIDs, such as ibuprofen (Motrin, Novo-Profen ✤) and ketorolac (Toradol), are used alone or with an opioid analgesic. Antianxiety drugs may be given with an opioid analgesic to decrease pain-related anxiety, reduce muscle tension, and control nausea.

⚠ NURSING SAFETY PRIORITY (QSEN)
Drug Alert

Do not confuse Toradol with Tramadol (a drug used for central analgesia).

Emergency Care of the Patient Experiencing an Opioid Overdose

- Prepare to administer naloxone hydrochloride (Narcan)* in a dose of 1 to 2 mg IV.
- Repeat naloxone every 2 to 3 minutes up to 10 mg, as needed, depending on the patient's response.
- Maintain an open airway.
- Give oxygen if hypoxia is present or if respirations are below 10 breaths per minute.
- Have suction equipment available because naloxone can trigger vomiting and a drowsy patient is at risk for aspiration.
- Continuously monitor vital signs and level of consciousness for reversal of overdose.
- Do not leave the patient until he or she is fully responsive.
- Assess the patient for pain because reversal of the opioid overdose also reverses the analgesic effects.
- Continue to monitor the patient's vital signs and level of consciousness every 10 to 15 minutes for the first hour. Naloxone is eliminated from the body more quickly than is the opioid, and it may induce side effects, including blood pressure changes, tachycardia, and dysrhythmias.
- Determine the need for additional antagonist therapy 1 hour after the patient initially becomes fully responsive.

*There are other opioid antagonists; however, naloxone hydrochloride is used most often to manage adult opioid overdose in the postoperative period.

Complementary and Alternative Therapies. Provide other comfort measures that may lower the amount of drugs needed to control PAIN. These measures, such as positioning, massage, relaxation, and diversion, reduce anxiety and allow the patient to relax and rest.

In positioning the patient, consider the position during surgery, the location of the surgical incision and drains, and problems such as arthritis and chronic lung disease. Assist the patient to a position of comfort. Support the extremities with pillows. Turn or help the patient turn at least every 2 hours while he or she is bedridden to prevent complications of immobility.

Action Alert

Unless the surgeon prescribes pillow support, place no pillows under the knees, and do not raise the knee gatch, because this position could restrict circulation and increase the risk for venous thromboembolism.

Based on the surgeon's prescription and your assessment of the patient's tolerance, urge the patient to increase activity progressively to prevent complications. When he or she is first allowed out of bed, assist the patient to the side of the bed and into a chair. Teach him or her to splint the surgical wound for support and comfort during the transfer.

Use gentle massage on stiff joints or a sore back to decrease discomfort. Assist the patient to a side-lying position, and apply lotion with smooth, gentle strokes to increase blood flow to the area and promote relaxation. *Do not massage the calves because of the risk for loosening a clot and causing a life-threatening pulmonary embolus.*

Nonpharmacologic Interventions to Reduce Postoperative Pain and Promote Comfort

- Control or remove noxious stimuli.
- Cushion and elevate painful areas; avoid tension or pressure on those areas.
- Provide adequate rest to increase pain tolerance.
- Encourage the patient's participation in diversional activities.
- Instruct the patient in relaxation techniques; use audio recordings or CDs and breathing exercises.
- Provide opportunities for meditation.
- Help the patient stimulate sensory nerve endings near the painful areas to inhibit ascending pain impulses.
- Use ice to reduce and prevent swelling, as indicated.
- Find a general position of comfort for the patient.
- Help the patient stimulate the area contralateral (opposite) to the painful area.

Relaxation and diversion are also used to control acute episodes of PAIN during dressing changes and injections. (See Chapter 3 for how to instruct and guide the patient through these pain control methods.) Music and noise reduction may help decrease awareness of discomfort. Chart 16-9 lists other interventions that may help reduce pain and promote comfort.

Psychosocial Integrity

The nurse is about to give the prescribed pain medication to a client 30 minutes before a scheduled dressing change. The client states that the drug makes him feel sick and he would rather "tough it out." What is the nurse's best first response?
A. "Tell me more about the sick feeling."
B. "That's fine. You have the right to refuse any drug."
C. "Your surgeon would not have prescribed the drug if it wasn't needed."
D. "Remember that the pain of the dressing change would be worse than feeling sick."

Community-Based Care

Many patients are discharged after a brief hospital stay or directly from the PACU to home. Because of the shortened length of hospital stays, discharge planning, teaching, and referral begin before surgery and continue after surgery.

Home Care Management. If the patient is discharged directly to home, assess information about the home environment for safety, patient accessibility, cleanliness, and availability of caregivers. Use the data obtained on admission before surgery to determine the patient's needs. For example, if the patient is unable or not allowed to climb stairs and lives in a two-story house with only one bathroom, advise the patient to rent a bedside commode. Collaborate with the social worker or discharge planner to identify needs related to care after surgery, including meal preparation, dressing changes, drain management, drug administration, equipment rental, physical therapy, and personal hygiene. A referral to a home care nursing agency may be indicated.

The patient is usually concerned about complications, PAIN, changes in the usual activity level, or payment of the hospital bill. The more extensive the surgical procedure is, the more fearful the patient is of assuming self-care. Support the patient and family members as they make discharge plans. The patient with visible scars after surgery may need more emotional support from and acceptance by his or her family. The patient may be angry about the surgical outcome or about role changes. He or she may be concerned about financial matters and work. The surgical outcome may not have met the patient's expectations, and further interventions may be needed to assist in resolving his or her feelings. Ensure that referrals are made for additional counseling as indicated.

Self-Management Education. The teaching plan for the patient and family after surgery includes:

- Prevention of infection
- Care and assessment of the surgical wound
- Management of drains or catheters
- Nutrition therapy
- Pain management
- Drug therapy
- Progressive increase in activity

If dressing changes and drain or catheter care are needed, instruct the patient and family members on the importance of proper handwashing to prevent infection. Explain and demonstrate wound care to the patient and family, who then perform a return demonstration. During teaching sessions, evaluate learning and promote adherence after discharge. At the same time, teach about the manifestations of complications such as wound INFECTION. Also instruct the patient and family about what to do if complications occur.

A diet high in protein, calories, and vitamin C promotes wound healing. Supplemental vitamin C, iron, zinc, and other vitamins are often prescribed after surgery to aid in wound healing and red blood cell formation. Instruct the patient who needs dietary restrictions about the importance of following the prescribed diet while recovering from surgery. Encourage the older adult or debilitated patient to continue using dietary supplements, if prescribed, between meals until the wound is completely healed and the energy levels are restored.

Teach the patient about drugs for PAIN, especially about the proper dosage and frequency. Instruct the patient to notify the surgeon if pain is not controlled or if the pain suddenly increases. If antibiotics or other drugs are prescribed, stress the importance of completing the entire prescription.

Surgery stresses the body, and time and rest are needed for healing. Teach the patient to increase activity level slowly, rest often, and avoid straining the wound or the surrounding area. The surgeon decides when the patient may climb stairs, return to work, drive, and resume other usual activities, such as sexual intercourse. The amount of weight that the patient can lift safely after surgery is specifically defined by the surgeon (i.e., in pounds or kilograms). Remind patients of the weights of grocery bags, women's handbags, and common items in the home.

Instruct the patient in the use of proper body mechanics. A patient whose work involves a moderate amount of physical labor may return to work about 6 weeks after abdominal surgery. Stress the importance of adherence to prevent complications or disability. A referral for a home care nurse may be needed for follow-up.

> **! NURSING SAFETY PRIORITY** (QSEN)
>
> **Action Alert**
>
> Always ensure that the patient and family receive written discharge instructions to follow at home. Assess the patient's and family's understanding of the instructions by having them explain the instructions in their own words.

Health Care Resources. After returning home, the patient may need supplies or equipment and assistance with dressing changes, ADLs, and meal preparation. Referral to a home care agency is made if needed. Home care may be paid for by third-party insurance payers, including Medicare, if the patient is homebound and requires skilled care such as dressing changes or physical therapy. The home care nurse provides skilled nursing assessments, dressing supplies, education in self-care, and referrals for services as needed. Such referrals include Meals on Wheels, support groups, and homemaker services (e.g., for housekeeping, food shopping).

◆ **Evaluation: Outcomes**

Evaluate the care of the patient after surgery based on the identified priority patient problems. The expected outcomes include that the patient:

- Attains and maintains adequate lung expansion and respiratory function
- Has complete wound healing without complications
- Has acceptable comfort levels after surgery

Specific indicators for these outcomes are listed for each priority patient problem in the Planning and Implementation section (see earlier).

NURSING CONCEPTS AND CLINICAL JUDGMENT REVIEW

What might you NOTICE in a patient after surgery who has a surgical wound INFECTION?

- Elevated body temperature
- Heart rate elevated above the patient's baseline
- Sweating and chills present
- Wound edges are red for 1 cm or more on each side of the wound
- Incision line is swollen, and skin adjacent to the incision is warmer to the touch than is the skin further away from the incision
- Purulent drainage is present
- An odor may emanate from the incision
- An open area or areas may be present within the incision

What should you INTERPRET and how should you RESPOND to a patient who has a wound INFECTION after surgery?

Perform and interpret physical assessment, including:

- Assessing vital signs with temperature at least every 4 hours
- Assessing for increase in pain perception
- Assessing cognition
- Assessing the wound for pain, size, open areas, and drainage

- Assessing the skin immediately surrounding the wound for redness and swelling
- Assessing serial white blood cell counts with differential for changes, including elevations above normal, decreases below normal, and presence of a "left shift"

Respond by:
- Documenting wound features
- Notifying the surgeon or health care provider
- Cleansing the wound (obtaining cultures, if within agency policy)
- Maintaining or starting IV line

- Administering prescribed drug therapy
- Monitoring laboratory test results to determine therapy effectiveness
- Continuing to assess for changes in the patient's condition, especially indications of infection in any other body area.

On what should you REFLECT?
- Identify the patient's personal factors that could have contributed to the wound infection.
- Think about what steps could be taken to identify the problem earlier.

GET READY FOR THE NCLEX® EXAMINATION!

KEY POINTS

Review these Key Points for each NCLEX Examination Client Needs Category.

Safe and Effective Care Environment
- Examine individual patient factors for potential threats to safety, especially risk for surgical site INFECTION, hypoventilation, and venous thromboembolism. **Safety** QSEN
- Use aseptic technique during all dressing changes. **Safety** QSEN
- Use established criteria to determine when a patient is ready to leave the postanesthesia care unit (PACU) for discharge to home or a medical-surgical nursing unit.
- Keep suction equipment, oxygen, and artificial breathing equipment near the patient in the PACU. **Safety** QSEN

Health Promotion and Maintenance
- Reinforce to the patient and family after surgery the specific interventions to use to prevent complications (incision splinting, deep-breathing exercises, range-of-motion exercises—as described in Charts 14-5 and 14-6 in Chapter 14).
- Encourage early ambulation.
- Stress the need for following the activity restrictions prescribed by the surgeon.
- Teach the patient and family about any drugs to be continued after discharge from the facility. **Patient-Centered Care** QSEN

- Instruct the patient and family about the clinical manifestations of complications and when to seek assistance. **Patient-Centered Care** QSEN

Psychosocial Integrity
- Keep family members informed of the patient's progress during the time that he or she is in the postanesthesia recovery area.
- Reassure patients and family members that taking pain medication when needed, even opioids, does not make them drug abusers. **Patient-Centered Care** QSEN

Physiological Integrity
- Begin every assessment of the patient after surgery by checking the airway and breathing effectiveness. **Safety** QSEN
- Assess the incision site each shift (on the medical-surgical nursing unit).
- Offer alternative therapies for relaxation, pain reduction, and distraction, such as massage, music therapy, and guided imagery.
- In the event of wound dehiscence or evisceration, have the patient lie flat (supine) with knees bent to reduce intra-abdominal pressure; apply sterile, nonadherent dressing materials to the wound; and follow the steps outlined in Chart 16-6. **Evidence-Based Practice** QSEN

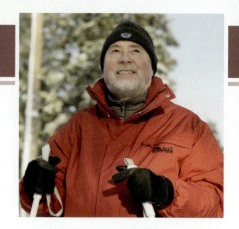

CONCEPT OVERVIEW

Protection

The human need for protection is provided through the actions of the concepts of INFLAMMATION and IMMUNITY (Giddens, 2013). The body works best when the internal environment is kept separate from the external environment. This is especially important for substances and organisms that could harm body cells, tissues, and organs. Normal protection is provided by three types of defenses—similar to how people living in a castle are protected against invaders (Fig. 1).

FIG. 1 Three levels of protection (moat, castle wall, knights and soldiers) for people.

The first defense is the moat surrounding the castle walls. Although the moat seldom kills invaders directly, it at least slows them down and sometimes repels them. The human "moat" is the normal flora on the surface of the skin and mucous membranes, sometimes referred to as types of general or innate IMMUNITY. This normal flora is made up of bacteria and other organisms that belong on the skin, live peacefully with the human host, and help repel more harmful microorganisms. When the normal flora is changed as a result of some types of

drug therapy, procedures, diseases, excessive dryness, and normal aging, this small protection is damaged or lost.

The second defense is the castle wall and the "watchers" and alarm systems embedded within it. When it is tall, thick, and intact and when the watchers and alarms are working, penetration of the castle by invaders is greatly reduced. In humans, this type of protection is provided by intact skin and mucous membranes, which are also part of innate IMMUNITY. These structures are a formidable barrier to invaders and help prevent dangerous changes in the internal environment. However, the castle walls do suffer some damage over time and must be repaired and maintained to provide continuing protection.

The last and strongest defense consists of the knights and soldiers within the castle. These individuals have the skills to capture or kill invaders. Some of these skills are common to all the knights and soldiers, and others are unique to different groups. In humans, the white blood cells (leukocytes) and the substances they produce serve as knights and soldiers, which provide the responses of INFLAMMATION and IMMUNITY. In addition to the work related directly to the invaders, this defense helps repair and maintain the castle walls. It is important to remember that this level of protection relies on the alarms of the castle wall and its physical barrier to recognize invaders and trigger the protective responses of the knights and soldiers.

Protection occurs best when all three defenses are intact and are working at their highest functional levels. These defenses of INFLAMMATION and IMMUNITY begin at birth and are at the maximum function in early to middle adulthood. The defenses decline slowly over time, making an older adult at greater risk for illnesses related to invasion and a decreased ability to repair damage. External factors and health status can reduce the ability of INFLAMMATION and IMMUNITY to provide complete protection. Specific nursing strategies can help reduce risk and protect the person whose defenses are less than perfect.

CHAPTER | **17**

Inflammation and Immunity

M. Linda Workman

 http://evolve.elsevier.com/Iggy/

The immune system involves the concepts of both INFLAMMATION and IMMUNITY to work with other defenses in providing *protection* from harmful microorganisms and cells. As indicated in the Concept Overview defining the issue of *protection* using the concepts of inflammation and immunity, the cells and cell products of inflammation and immunity are represented mostly by the knights and soldiers behind the castle walls. The products made by cells (e.g., cytokines, growth factors, antibodies) are the weapons of the knights and soldiers. Some of these cells serve as watchers and alarm systems within the castle walls (skin and mucous membranes) and help repair these walls when damage occurs.

Although infectious diseases are common, most people are healthy more often than they are ill. INFLAMMATION and IMMUNITY are the major defenses that protect against disease when the body is invaded by organisms. These same defenses also help the body recover after tissue damage. Thus inflammation and immunity are critical to maintaining health and preventing disease. When all the different parts and functions of inflammation and immunity are working well, the person is **immunocompetent** and has maximum protection against infection.

IMMUNITY is reduced by many diseases, injuries, and medical therapies. *Whether immunity is reduced temporarily or perma-* *nently, it always endangers the patient's health.* Chapter 19 discusses inadequate immunity and inflammatory responses. Other problems occur when immunity and inflammation are excessive or occur at inappropriate times. Chapters 18 and 20 discuss issues related to excess or inappropriate inflammatory or immune responses.

OVERVIEW

IMMUNITY is composed of many cell functions that protect against the effects of injury or invasion. People interact with many other large and small living organisms (bacteria, viruses, molds, spores, pollens, protozoa, and cells from other people or animals). As long as organisms do not enter the body, they pose no health threat. Body defenses to prevent organisms from entering include intact skin and mucous membranes, skin surface normal flora, and natural chemicals that inhibit bacterial growth. These defenses are not perfect, and invasion can occur. However, most invasions do not result in disease or illness because of proper immunity.

The purpose of INFLAMMATION and IMMUNITY is to provide *protection* by neutralizing, eliminating, or destroying organisms that invade the body. To protect without harming the body,

FIG. 17-1 Proteins on human cell plasma membranes.

FIG. 17-2 Determination by immune system cell of self versus non-self cells.

immune system cells exert these actions only against non-self proteins and cells. Immune system cells can distinguish between the body's own healthy self cells and non-self proteins and cells.

Self Versus Non-Self

Non-self proteins and cells include infected body cells, cancer cells, cells from other people, and invading organisms. Recognizing self versus non-self, which is necessary to prevent healthy body cells from being destroyed along with the invaders, is called self-tolerance. The immune system cells are the only cells capable of determining self from non-self. Self-tolerance is possible because of the different proteins present on cell membranes.

Each cell is surrounded by a plasma membrane with different proteins protruding through the surface (Fig. 17-1). For example, in liver cells, many different protein types are present on the liver cell membranes. The amino acid sequence of each protein type differs from that of all other protein types. Some of these protein types are found only on human cells, because these protein types are specific markers for human tissues. Also, each person's cells have surface proteins that are specific to that person. These unique proteins would be identical only to the proteins of an identical sibling. These unique proteins, known as human leukocyte antigens (HLAs), are found on the surface of all body cells of that person and serve as a "universal product code" for that person. One person's HLAs are recognized as "foreign," or non-self, by the immune system of another person. Because the cell-surface proteins are non-self to another person's immune system, they are antigens, which are proteins capable of stimulating an immune response.

Human leukocyte antigens are on the surfaces of most body cells—not just leukocytes. They are a normal part of the person and determine the *tissue type* of a person. Other names for these HLAs are *human histocompatibility antigens* and *class I antigens.*

There are many different human major HLAs that are determined by a set of genes called the *major histocompatibility complex (MHC).* However, each human expresses only six of the major HLAs. The specific antigens that any person has (of a large number of possible antigens) are determined by which MHC gene alleles were inherited from his or her parents.

The HLAs are key for recognition and self-tolerance. The immune system cells constantly come into contact with other body cells and with any invader that enters the body. At each encounter, the immune system cells compare the surface protein HLAs to determine whether the encountered cell belongs in the body (Fig. 17-2). If the encountered cell's HLAs perfectly match the HLAs of the immune system cell, the encountered cell is "self" and is not attacked. If the encountered cell's HLAs do not perfectly match the HLAs of the immune system cell, the encountered cell is non-self, or foreign. The immune system cell then takes action to neutralize, destroy, or eliminate this foreign invader.

IMMUNITY changes during a person's life as a result of nutrition status, environmental conditions, drugs, disease, and age. Immunity is most efficient when people are in their 20s and 30s and slowly declines with increasing age (Touhy & Jett, 2014). Older adults have decreased immune function, increasing their risk for many health problems (Chart 17-1).

Organization of the Immune System

The immune system is present throughout the body and is influenced by the nervous system, the endocrine system, and the GI system. Most immune system cells come from the bone marrow. Some cells mature in the bone marrow; others leave the bone marrow and mature in different body sites. When mature, many immune system cells are released into the blood, where they circulate to most body areas and have specific effects.

The bone marrow is the source of all blood cells, including most immune system cells. The bone marrow produces immature, undifferentiated cells called stem cells. Stem cells are pluripotent, meaning that each cell has more than one potential outcome. When the stem cell is first generated in the bone marrow, it is undifferentiated, not yet committed to maturing into a specific blood cell type. This stem cell is flexible (pluripotent) and could become any one of many mature blood cells. Fig. 17-3 shows the possible outcomes for maturation of stem cells. The type of mature cell that the stem cell becomes depends on which pathway it follows.

The maturational pathway of any stem cell depends on body needs and on the presence of specific growth factors that direct the cell to a pathway. For example, erythropoietin is a growth factor for red blood cells (erythrocytes [RBCs]). When immature stem cells are exposed to erythropoietin, they commit to the erythrocyte pathway and eventually become mature RBCs.

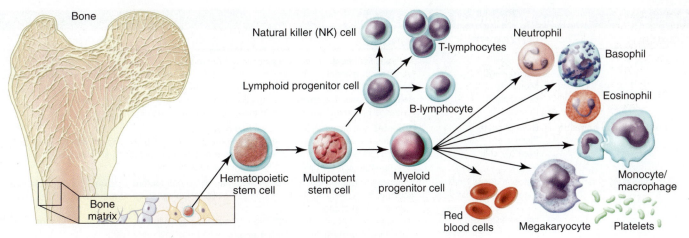

FIG. 17-3 Stem cell differentiation and maturation.

CHART 17-1 Nursing Focus on the Older Adult

Changes in Immune Function Related to Aging

IMMUNE COMPONENT	FUNCTIONAL CHANGE	NURSING IMPLICATIONS
Inflammation	Reduced neutrophil function. Leukocytosis does not occur during acute infection. Older adults may not have a fever during inflammatory or infectious episodes.	Neutrophil counts may be normal, but activity is reduced, increasing the risk for infection. Patients may have an infection but not show expected changes in white blood cell counts. Not only is there potential loss of protection through inflammation, but also minor infections may be overlooked until the patient becomes severely infected or septic.
Antibody-mediated immunity	The total number of colony-forming B-lymphocytes and the ability of these cells to mature into antibody-secreting cells are diminished. There is a decline in natural antibodies, decreased response to antigens, and reduction in the amount of time the antibody response is maintained.	Older adults are less able to make new antibodies in response to the presence of new antigens. Thus they should receive immunizations, such as "flu shots," the pneumococcal vaccination, and the shingles vaccination. Older adults may not have sufficient antibodies present to provide protection when they are re-exposed to microorganisms against which they have already generated antibodies. Thus older patients need to avoid people with viral infections and need to receive "booster" shots for old vaccinations and immunizations, especially tetanus and pertussis (whooping cough).
Cell-mediated immunity	The number of circulating T-lymphocytes decreases.	Skin tests for tuberculosis may be falsely negative. Older patients are more at risk for bacterial and fungal infections, especially on the skin and mucous membranes, in the respiratory tract, and in the genitourinary tract.

White blood cells (**leukocytes [WBCs]**) protect the body from the effects of invasion by organisms. These cells are the immune system cells, the knights and soldiers protecting the castle inhabitants after invaders get through the castle wall. Table 17-1 lists the functions of different immune system cells. The leukocytes provide protection through these defensive actions:

- Recognition of self versus non-self
- Destruction of foreign invaders, cellular debris, and unhealthy or abnormal self cells
- Production of antibodies directed against invaders
- Complement activation
- Production of cytokines that stimulate increased formation of leukocytes in bone marrow and increase specific leukocyte activity

The three processes needed for human protection through IMMUNITY are (1) INFLAMMATION, (2) antibody-mediated immunity (AMI), and (3) cell-mediated immunity (CMI). Each process uses different defensive actions, and each influences or requires assistance from the other two processes (Fig. 17-4). *Therefore full immunity (immunocompetence) requires the function and interaction of all three processes.*

INFLAMMATION

INFLAMMATION, also called *innate-native immunity* or *natural immunity,* provides immediate protection against the effects of tissue injury and invading foreign proteins. Innate-native immunity is any natural protective feature of a person. It can be a barrier to prevent organisms from entering the body or can be an attacking force that eliminates organisms that have already entered the body. This type of IMMUNITY cannot be transferred from one person to another and is not an adaptive response to exposure or invasion by foreign proteins.

TABLE 17-1   Immune Functions of Specific Leukocytes

VARIABLE	LEUKOCYTE	FUNCTION
Inflammation	Neutrophil	Nonspecific ingestion and phagocytosis of microorganisms and foreign protein
	Macrophage	Nonspecific recognition of foreign proteins and microorganisms; ingestion and phagocytosis
	Monocyte	Destruction of bacteria and cellular debris; matures into macrophage
	Eosinophil	Releases vasoactive amines during allergic reactions to limit these reactions
	Basophil	Releases histamine and heparin in areas of tissue damage
Antibody-mediated immunity	B-lymphocyte	Becomes sensitized to foreign cells and proteins
	Plasma cell	Secretes immunoglobulins in response to the presence of a specific antigen
	Memory cell	Remains sensitized to a specific antigen and can secrete increased amounts of immunoglobulins specific to the antigen on re-exposure
Cell-mediated immunity	Helper/inducer T-cell	Enhances immune activity through secretion of various factors, cytokines, and lymphokines
	Cytotoxic/cytolytic T-cell	Selectively attacks and destroys non-self cells, including virally infected cells, grafts, and transplanted organs
	Natural killer cell	Nonselectively attacks non-self cells, especially body cells that have undergone mutation and become malignant; also attacks grafts and transplanted organs

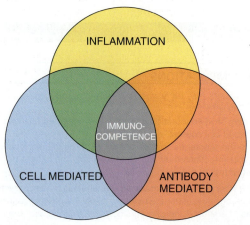

FIG. 17-4 The three divisions of immunity: inflammation, antibody-mediated immunity, and cell-mediated immunity. Optimal function of all three divisions is necessary for complete immunity.

The inflammatory responses are part of innate IMMUNITY. Other parts of innate immunity include skin, mucosa, antimicrobial chemicals on the skin, complement, and natural killer cells.

The ability to respond with inflammation is critical to health and well-being. INFLAMMATION differs from AMI and CMI in two important ways:

- Inflammatory protection is immediate but short-term. It does not provide true immunity on repeated exposure to the same organisms.
- Inflammation is a *nonspecific* body defense to invasion or injury and can be started quickly by almost any event, regardless of where it occurs or what causes it.

So, inflammation triggered by a scald burn to the hand is the same as inflammation triggered by bacteria in the middle ear. How widespread the manifestations of INFLAMMATION are depends on the intensity, severity, and duration of exposure to the initiating event. For example, a splinter in the finger triggers inflammation only at the splinter site, whereas a burn injuring 50% of the skin leads to an inflammatory response involving the entire body.

INFLAMMATION starts tissue actions that cause visible and uncomfortable manifestations that are important in ridding the body of harmful organisms. However, if the inflammatory response is excessive, tissue damage may result. Inflammation also helps start both antibody-mediated and cell-mediated actions to activate full IMMUNITY.

Infection

A confusing issue about INFLAMMATION is that this process occurs in response to tissue injury, as well as to infection by organisms. *Infection is usually accompanied by inflammation; however, inflammation can occur without infection.* Examples of inflammation without infection include joint sprain injuries, myocardial infarction, and blister formation. Examples of inflammation caused by noninfectious invasion include allergic rhinitis, contact dermatitis, and other allergic reactions. Inflammations from infection include otitis media, appendicitis, and viral hepatitis, among many others. *Inflammation does not always mean that an infection is present.*

Cell Types Involved in Inflammation

The leukocytes (white blood cells [WBCs]) involved in INFLAMMATION are neutrophils, macrophages, eosinophils, and basophils. An additional cell type important in inflammation is the tissue mast cell. Neutrophils and macrophages destroy and eliminate foreign invaders. Basophils, eosinophils, and mast cells release chemicals that act on blood vessels to cause tissue-level responses that help neutrophil and macrophage actions.

Neutrophils

Mature neutrophils make up between 55% and 70% of the normal total WBC count. Neutrophils come from the stem cells and complete the maturation process in the bone marrow (Fig. 17-5). They are also called *granulocytes* because of the large number of granules present inside each cell. Other names for neutrophils are based on their appearance and maturity. Mature neutrophils are also called *segmented neutrophils* ("segs") or *polymorphonuclear cells* ("polys," PMNs) because of their segmented nucleus. Less mature neutrophils are called *band neutrophils* ("bands" or "stabs") because of their nuclear shape.

Usually, growth of a stem cell into a mature neutrophil requires 12 to 14 days. This time is shortened by the presence of specific growth factors (cytokines), such as granulocyte-macrophage colony-stimulating factor (GM-CSF) and granulocyte colony-stimulating factor (G-CSF). The purpose and action of cytokines are described on p. 286 in the Cytokines section.

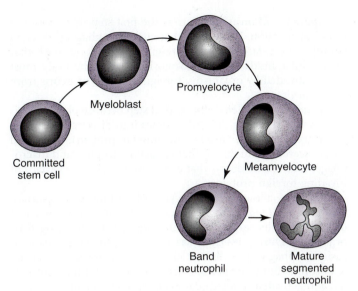

FIG. 17-5 Stem cell maturation into fully functional segmented neutrophils.

TABLE 17-3	Tissue Macrophages
TISSUE	**MACROPHAGE**
Lung	Alveolar macrophage
Connective tissue	Histiocyte
Brain	Microglial cell
Liver	Kupffer cell
Peritoneum	Peritoneal macrophage
Bone	Osteoclast
Joint	Synovial type A cell
Kidney	Mesangial cell

TABLE 17-2   Values of a White Blood Cell Differential for Peripheral Blood Representing a Normal Count

WBC TYPE	%	/MM³
Total WBC	**100**	**10,000**
Segs	62	6200
Bands	5	500
Monos	3	300
Lymphs	28	2800
Eosins	1.5	150
Basos	0.5	50

WBC, White blood cell.

In the healthy person with full IMMUNITY, more than 100 billion fresh, mature neutrophils are released from the bone marrow into the circulation daily. This huge production is needed because the life span of each neutrophil is short—about 12 to 18 hours.

Neutrophil function provides protection after invaders, especially bacteria, enter the body. This powerful army of small cells destroys invaders by phagocytosis and enzymatic digestion, although each cell is small and can take part in only one episode of phagocytosis.

Mature neutrophils are the only stage of this cell capable of phagocytosis. Because this cell type is responsible for continuous, instant, nonspecific protection against organisms, the percentage and actual number of mature circulating neutrophils are used to measure a patient's risk for infection: the higher the numbers, the greater the resistance to infection. This measurement is the **absolute neutrophil count (ANC),** also called the *absolute granulocyte count* or *total granulocyte count.*

The differential of a normal white blood cell count shows the number and percent of the different types of circulating leukocytes (Table 17-2). Usually, most neutrophils released into the blood from the bone marrow are segmented neutrophils; only a small percentage are band neutrophils or other less

mature forms. Some problems, such as sepsis, cause the neutrophils in the blood to change from being mostly segmented neutrophils to being less mature forms. This situation is termed a **left shift** or *bandemia* because the segmented neutrophil (at the far right of the neutrophil pathway in Fig. 17-5) is no longer the most numerous type of circulating neutrophils. Instead, more of the circulating cells are bands—the less mature cell type found farther left on the neutrophil pathway.

A left shift indicates that the patient's bone marrow cannot produce enough mature neutrophils to keep pace with the continuing infection and is releasing immature neutrophils into the blood. These immature cells are of no benefit because they are not capable of phagocytosis.

Macrophages

Macrophages come from the committed myeloid stem cells in the bone marrow and form the mononuclear-phagocyte system. The stem cells first form monocytes, which are released into the blood at this stage. Until they mature, monocytes have limited activity. Most monocytes move from the blood into body tissues, where they mature into macrophages. Some macrophages become "fixed" in position within the tissues, whereas others can move within and between tissues. Macrophages in various tissues have slightly different appearances and names (Table 17-3). The liver, spleen, and intestinal tract contain large numbers of these cells.

Macrophage function protects the body in several ways. These cells are important in immediate inflammatory responses and also stimulate the longer-lasting immune responses of antibody-mediated IMMUNITY (AMI) and cell-mediated IMMUNITY (CMI). Macrophage functions include phagocytosis, repair, antigen presenting/processing, and secretion of cytokines for immune system control.

The inflammatory function of macrophages is phagocytosis. Macrophages can easily distinguish between self and non-self, and their large size makes them very effective at trapping invading cells. They have long life spans and can take part in many phagocytic events.

Basophils

Basophils come from myeloid stem cells and make up only about 1% of the total circulating WBC count. These cells cause the manifestations of INFLAMMATION.

Basophil function acts on blood vessels with basophil chemicals (vasoactive amines), which include heparin, histamine, serotonin, kinins, and leukotrienes. Basophils have sites that bind the base portion of immunoglobulin E (IgE) molecules, which binds to and is activated by allergens. When allergens bind to the IgE on the basophil, the basophil membrane opens and releases the vasoactive amines into the blood, where most of them act on smooth muscle and blood vessel walls. Heparin inhibits blood and protein clotting. Histamine constricts small veins, inhibiting blood flow and decreasing venous return. This effect causes blood to collect in capillaries and arterioles. Kinins dilate arterioles and increase capillary permeability. These actions cause blood plasma to leak into the interstitial space (*vascular leak syndrome*). Thus basophils stimulate both general INFLAMMATION and the inflammation of allergy and hypersensitivity reactions.

Eosinophils

Eosinophils come from the myeloid line and contain many vasoactive chemicals. Only 1% to 2% of the total WBC count normally is composed of eosinophils.

Eosinophil function is very active against infestations of parasitic larvae and also limits inflammatory reactions. The eosinophil granules contain many different substances. Some are enzymes that degrade the vasoactive chemicals released by other leukocytes. This is why the number of circulating eosinophils increases during an allergic response.

Tissue Mast Cells

Tissue mast cells look like and have functions very similar to basophils and eosinophils. Although mast cells do originate in the bone marrow, they come from a different parent cell than leukocytes and do not circulate as mature cells (Abbas et al., 2012). Instead, they differentiate and mature in tissues, especially those near blood vessels, nerves, lung tissue, skin, and mucous membranes. Like basophils, mast cells have binding sites for the base of IgE molecules and are involved in hypersensitivity reactions. Some mast cells also respond to the inflammatory products made and released by T-lymphocytes. The tissue mast cells have important roles in maintaining and prolonging inflammatory and hypersensitivity reactions.

Phagocytosis

A key process of INFLAMMATION is **phagocytosis**, the engulfing and destruction of invaders, which also rids the body of debris after tissue injury. Neutrophils and macrophages are most efficient at phagocytosis. Phagocytosis involves the seven steps shown in Fig. 17-6.

1. Exposure/invasion   2. Attraction   3. Adherence
4. Recognition   5. Cellular ingestion
6. Phagosome formation   7. Degradation

FIG. 17-6 Steps of phagocytosis. *M*, Macrophage.

Exposure and invasion occur as the first step in response to injury or invasion. Leukocytes that engage in phagocytosis and stimulate INFLAMMATION are present in the blood and other extracellular fluids. For phagocytosis to start, the body must first be invaded by organisms, foreign proteins, or debris from damaged tissues.

Attraction is needed as the second step because phagocytosis can occur only when the WBC comes into direct contact with the target (antigen, invader, or foreign protein). Damaged tissues secrete chemotaxins that attract neutrophils and macrophages and release debris that can combine with the surface of invading foreign proteins.

Adherence allows the phagocytic cell to bind to the surface of the target. *Opsonins* are substances that increase contact of the cell with its target by coating the target cell (antigen or organism). During INFLAMMATION, coating the target makes it easier for phagocytic cells to stick to it. Many substances can act as opsonins. Some are particles from dead neutrophils, antibodies, and activated (fixated) complement components.

Complement activation and fixation are part of opsonization and help with adherence. Twenty different inactive complement proteins are present in the blood. When stimulated, each complement protein is activated, joins other activated complement proteins, surrounds an antigen, and "fixes" or sticks to the antigen. Complement fixation occurs quickly as a cascade.

Recognition occurs when the phagocytic cell sticks to the target cell and "recognizes" it as non-self. The phagocytic cells examine the universal product codes (human leukocyte antigens [HLAs]) of whatever they encounter. Recognition of non-self is made easier by opsonins on the target cell surface. Phagocytic cells start phagocytosis only when the target cell is recognized as non-self or debris.

Cellular ingestion is needed because phagocytic destruction occurs inside the cell. The target cell is brought inside the phagocytic cell by phagocytosis (engulfment).

Phagosome formation occurs when the phagocyte's granules break and release enzymes that attack the ingested target.

Degradation is the final step. The enzymes in the phagosome digest the engulfed target.

Sequence of Inflammation

INFLAMMATION (inflammatory responses) occurs in a predictable three-stage sequence. The sequence is the same regardless of the triggering event. Responses at the tissue level cause the **five cardinal manifestations of inflammation**: warmth, redness, swelling, pain, and decreased function. The timing of the stages may overlap.

Stage I is the vascular part of the inflammatory response that first involves changes in blood vessels. Injured tissues and the leukocytes and tissue mast cells in this area secrete histamine, serotonin, and kinins that constrict the small veins and dilate the arterioles in the area of injury. These blood vessel changes cause redness and warmth of the tissues. This increased blood flow increases delivery of nutrients to injured tissues.

Blood flow to the area increases (**hyperemia**), and swelling (**edema**) forms at the site of injury or invasion. Capillary leak also occurs, allowing blood plasma to leak into the tissues. This response causes swelling and pain. Edema at the site of injury or invasion protects the area from further injury by creating a cushion of fluid. The duration of these responses depends on the severity of the initiating event, but usually they subside within 24 to 72 hours.

The macrophage is the major cell involved in stage I of INFLAMMATION. The action is rapid because macrophages are already in place at the site of injury or invasion. This action is limited because the number of macrophages is so small. To enhance the inflammatory response, the tissue macrophages secrete several cytokines. One cytokine is colony-stimulating factor (CSF), which triggers the bone marrow to shorten the time needed to produce white blood cells (WBCs) from 14 days to a matter of hours. Some cytokines cause neutrophils from the bone marrow to move to the site of injury or invasion, which leads to the next stage of inflammation.

Stage II is the cellular exudate part of the response. In this stage, neutrophilia (an increased number of circulating neutrophils) occurs. Exudate in the form of pus occurs, containing dead WBCs, necrotic tissue, and fluids that escape from damaged cells.

The most active cells in stage II are the neutrophils, basophils, and tissue mast cells. Under the influence of cytokines, the neutrophil count can increase hugely within 12 hours after inflammation starts. Neutrophils attack and destroy organisms and remove dead tissue through phagocytosis. Basophils and tissue mast cells continue or sustain the initial responses.

In acute INFLAMMATION, the healthy person produces enough mature neutrophils to keep pace with invasion and prevent the organisms from growing. At the same time, the WBCs and inflamed tissues secrete cytokines, which allow tissue macrophages to increase and trigger bone marrow production of monocytes. This reaction begins slowly, but its effects are long lasting.

During this phase, the arachidonic acid cascade starts to increase the inflammatory response. This action begins by the conversion of fatty acids in plasma membranes into arachidonic acid (AA). The enzyme *cyclooxygenase* (COX) converts AA into many chemicals that are further processed into the substances (mediators) that promote the continued inflammatory response in the tissues. These mediators include histamine, leukotrienes, prostaglandins, serotonin, and kinins. Many anti-inflammatory drugs, including NSAIDs, stop this cascade by preventing cyclooxygenase from converting AA into inflammatory mediators.

When an infection stimulating INFLAMMATION lasts longer than just a few days, the bone marrow begins to release immature neutrophils, reducing the number of circulating mature neutrophils. This reduction of mature neutrophils limits the helpful effects of inflammation and increases the risk for sepsis.

Stage III features tissue repair and replacement. Although this stage is completed last, it begins at the time of injury and is critical to the final function of the inflamed area.

Some of the WBCs involved in INFLAMMATION start the replacement of lost tissues or repair of damaged tissues by inducing the remaining healthy cells to divide. In tissues that cannot divide, WBCs trigger new blood vessel growth and scar tissue formation. Because scar tissue does not act like the tissue it replaces, function is lost wherever scar tissue forms. The degree of function lost depends on how much normal tissue is replaced by scar tissue. For example, when heart muscles are destroyed because of a myocardial infarction (heart attack), scar tissue forms in the area to prevent a hole from forming in the muscle wall as the ischemic cells die. (Remember that heart muscle is non-dividing tissue and the heart cannot replace these muscle cells.) The scar tissue serves only as a patch; it does not contract or act in any way like heart muscle. So, if 20% of the left ventricle is replaced with scar tissue, the effectiveness of left ventricular contraction is reduced by at least 20%.

INFLAMMATION alone cannot provide IMMUNITY. Inflammatory cells must interact with lymphocytes to provide long-lasting immunity. Long-lasting immune actions develop through antibody-mediated immunity (AMI) and cell-mediated immunity (CMI).

? NCLEX EXAMINATION CHALLENGE

Safe and Effective Care Environment

The white blood cell count with differential of a client undergoing preadmission testing before surgery indicates a total count of 10,000 cells per cubic millimeter (mm^3) of blood. Which differential counts or percentages does the nurse report to the physician?
A. Eosinophils 200/mm^3
B. Monocytes 2000/mm^3
C. Segmented neutrophils 5700/mm^3
D. Lymphocytes 2100/mm^3

IMMUNITY

IMMUNITY is an *adaptive* internal protection that results in long-term resistance to the effects of invading microorganisms. This means that the responses are not automatic. The body has to learn to generate specific immune responses when it is infected by or exposed to specific organisms. Lymphocytes develop actions and products that provide the protection of true immunity. These cells develop specific actions in response to specific invasion (Fig. 17-7).

Antibody-Mediated Immunity

Antibody-mediated immunity (AMI), also known as *humoral immunity,* involves antigen-antibody interactions to neutralize, eliminate, or destroy foreign proteins. Antibodies are produced by sensitized B-lymphocytes (B-cells).

B-cells become sensitized to a specific foreign protein (antigen) and produce antibodies directed specifically against that protein. The antibody, rather than the actual B-cell, then causes one of several actions to neutralize, eliminate, or destroy that antigen.

B-cells have the most direct role in AMI. Macrophages and T-lymphocytes (discussed on p. 285 in the Cell-Mediated Immunity section) work with B-cells to start and complete antigen-antibody interactions. *For optimal AMI, the entire immune system must function adequately.*

B-cells start as stem cells in the bone marrow, the primary lymphoid tissue, that commit to the lymphocyte pathway (see Fig. 17-3) and are then restricted in development. The lymphocyte stem cells are released from the bone marrow into the blood. They then migrate into many secondary lymphoid tissues to mature. The secondary lymphoid tissues for B-cell maturation are the spleen, parts of lymph nodes, tonsils, and the mucosa of the intestinal tract.

Antigen-Antibody Interactions

The body learns to make enough of any specific antibody to provide long-lasting immunity against specific organisms or toxins. The seven steps needed to produce a specific antibody directed against a specific antigen whenever the person is

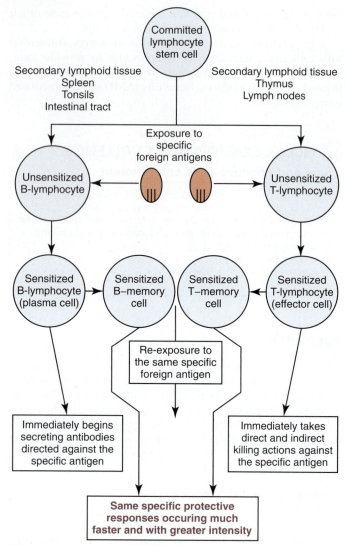

FIG. 17-7 B-lymphocyte and T-lymphocyte differentiation, maturation, and function.

disease is developing, the baby-sitter's white blood cells are taking part in antibody-antigen actions to prevent him or her from having influenza A more than once.

Antigen recognition is the next step to begin making antibodies against an antigen. The unsensitized B-cell must first recognize the antigen as non-self. B-cells need the help of macrophages and helper/inducer T-cells to recognize an antigen.

Recognition is started by the macrophages. After the antigen surface has been altered by opsonization (see discussion of "adherence" on p. 280), the macrophage recognizes the invading antigen as non-self and attaches itself to the antigen. This attachment allows the macrophage to "present" the attached antigen to the helper/inducer T-cell. Then the helper/inducer T-cell and the macrophage together process the antigen to expose the antigen's recognition sites (universal product code). After processing the antigen, the helper/inducer T-cell brings the antigen into contact with the B-cell so that the B-cell can recognize the antigen as non-self.

Sensitization occurs when the B-cell recognizes the antigen as non-self and is now "sensitized" to this antigen. A single unsensitized B-cell can become sensitized only once. *So, each B-cell can be sensitized to only one type of antigen.*

Sensitizing allows this B-cell to respond to any substance that carries the same antigens (codes) as the original antigen. The sensitized B-cell always remains sensitized to that specific antigen. In addition, all cells produced by that sensitized B-cell also are already pre-sensitized to that same specific antigen.

Immediately after it is sensitized, the B-cell divides and forms two types of B-lymphocytes, each one remaining sensitized to that specific antigen (see Fig. 17-7). One new cell becomes a **plasma cell,** which starts immediately to produce antibodies against the sensitizing antigen. The other new cell becomes a memory cell. The **memory cell** is a sensitized B-cell but does not produce antibodies until the next exposure to the same antigen (see discussion of sustained immunity (memory) on p. 284).

Antibody production and release allow the antibodies to search out specific antigens. Antibodies are produced by plasma cells, and each plasma cell can make as many as 300 molecules of antibody per second. Each plasma cell produces antibody specific only to the antigen that originally sensitized the parent B-cell. For example, in the case of the baby-sitter who was invaded by the influenza A virus, the plasma cells from those B-cells sensitized to the influenza A virus can make only anti–influenza A antibodies. The antibody class (e.g., immunoglobulin G [IgG] or immunoglobulin M [IgM]) that the plasma cell produces may vary, but the antibody can be forever directed only against the influenza A virus.

Antibody molecules made by plasma cells are released into the blood and other body fluids as free antibody. Because the antibody is in body fluids (or body "humors") and is separate from the B-cells, this type of IMMUNITY is sometimes called **humoral immunity.** *Circulating antibodies can be transferred from one person to another to provide the receiving person with immediate immunity of short duration.*

Antibody-antigen binding is needed for anti-antigen actions. Antibodies are Y-shaped molecules (Fig. 17-9). The tips of the short arms of the Y recognize the specific antigen and bind to it. Because each antibody molecule has two tips (Fab fragments, or arms), each antibody can bind either to two separate antigens or to two areas of the same antigen.

exposed to that antigen are shown in Fig. 17-8 and described below.

Exposure or invasion is needed because antibody actions occur inside the body or on a few body surfaces. Thus the antigen must first enter the person to generate an antibody, although not all exposures result in antibody production. Invasion by the antigen must occur in such large numbers that some of the antigen evades detection by the body's natural nonspecific defenses or overwhelms the ability of the inflammatory response to get rid of the invader.

For example, a person who has never been exposed to the viral disease *influenza A* now baby-sits for three children who develop influenza symptoms within the next 10 hours. These children, in the pre-symptomatic stage, shed many millions of live influenza A virus particles by droplets from the upper respiratory tract. They expose the baby-sitter by drinking out of the baby-sitter's cup, kissing him or her directly on the lips, and sneezing and coughing directly into his or her face. During the 5 hours spent with the children, the baby-sitter is heavily invaded by the influenza A virus and will become sick with this disease within 2 to 4 days. While the virus is growing and the

1. Invasion of the body by new antigens in sufficient numbers to stimulate an immune response.

2. Interaction of macrophage (M) and helper/inducer T-cell (T$_H$) in the processing and presenting of the antigen to the unsensitized "virgin" B-lymphocyte (B).

3. Sensitization of the virgin B-lymphocyte to the new antigen.

7. On re-exposure to the same antigen, the sensitized lymphocytes and their progeny produce large quantities of the antibody specific to the antigen. In addition, new "virgin" B-lymphocytes become sensitized to the antigen and also begin antibody production.

4. Antibody production by the B-lymphocyte. These antibodies are directed specifically against the initiating antigen. The antibodies are released from the B-lymphocyte and float freely in the blood and some other fluids.

6. Antibody binding causes cellular events and attracts other leukocytes to the complex. The interaction of other leukocytes along with the cellular events results in the neutralization, destruction, or elimination of the antigen.

5. Antibodies bind to the antigen, forming an immune complex.

FIG. 17-8 Sequence of the seven steps required to stimulate antibody-mediated immunity.

Fc receptors

Antigen recognition site

Fc fragment

Leukocyte with Fc receptors

Antibody molecules

Antibodies bound to a leukocyte by an Fc fragment, leaving antigen-binding sites open

FIG. 17-9 Antibody structure and the Fc receptors on leukocytes.

Antigen   Antibody

LARGE antigen-antibody complex

SMALL antigen-antibody complex

FIG. 17-10 Formation of large and small antigen-antibody complexes (immune complexes).

The binding of antibody to antigen may not be lethal to the antigen. Instead, antibody-antigen binding starts other actions that neutralize, eliminate, or destroy the antigen.

Antibody-binding actions are triggered by binding of antibody to antigen. The resulting reactions of agglutination, lysis, complement fixation, precipitation, and inactivation can then neutralize, eliminate, or destroy the bound antigen.

Agglutination is a clumping action that results from the antibody linking antigens together, forming large and small immune complexes (Fig. 17-10). Agglutination slows the

The stem of the Y is the "Fc fragment." This area can bind to Fc receptor sites on white blood cells (WBCs). The WBC then not only has its own means of attacking antigens but also has the added power of having surface antibodies that can stick to antigens (see Fig. 17-9).

movement of the antigen in body fluids. Also, the irregular shape of the antigen-antibody complex (see Fig. 17-10) increases the actions of macrophages and neutrophils.

Lysis is cell membrane destruction, and it occurs now because of antibody binding to membrane-bound antigens of some invaders. The actual binding makes holes in the invader's membrane, weakening the invader, especially bacteria and viruses. This response usually requires that complement be activated and "fixed" to the immune complex.

Complement activation and fixation are actions triggered by the IgG and IgM classes of antibodies that can remove or destroy antigen. (See discussion of adherence on p. 280 for an explanation of how complement assists in immunity.) Binding of either IgG or IgM to an antigen provides a binding site for the first component of complement. Once the first complement molecule is activated, other proteins of the complement system are activated in a cascade.

Precipitation is similar to agglutination but has a larger response. With precipitation, antibody molecules bind so much antigen that large antigen-antibody complexes are formed. These complexes cannot stay in suspension in the blood. Instead, they form a large precipitate, which then can be acted on and removed by neutrophils and macrophages.

Inactivation (neutralization) is the process of making an antigen harmless without destroying it. Usually only a small area of the antigen, the active site, causes the harmful effects. When an antibody binds to an antigen's active site, covering it up, the antigen is made harmless without destroying it.

Sustained immunity (memory) provides us with long-lasting IMMUNITY to a specific antigen. Sustained immunity results from memory B-cells made during the lymphocyte sensitization stage. These memory cells remain sensitized to the specific antigen to which they were originally exposed. On re-exposure to the same antigen, the memory cells rapidly respond by first dividing and forming new sensitized blast cells and plasma cells. The blast cells continue to divide, producing many more sensitized plasma cells. These new sensitized plasma cells rapidly make large amounts of the antibody specific for the sensitizing antigen.

This ability of the memory cells to respond on re-exposure to the same antigen that originally sensitized the B-cell allows a rapid and large immune response *(anamnestic response)* to the antigen. Because so much antibody is made, often the invading organisms are removed completely and the person does not become ill. This process prevents people from becoming ill with chickenpox or any infectious disease more than once, even though they are exposed many times to the causative organism. Without immunologic memory, people would remain susceptible to specific diseases on subsequent exposure to the organisms and no long-term IMMUNITY would be generated (Abbas et al., 2012; McCance et al., 2014).

Antibody Classification

All antibodies are immunoglobulins, also called *gamma globulins.* These names are based on the structure and function of antibodies. A globulin is a protein that is globular rather than straight. Because antibodies are globular proteins, they are "globulins." The term **immunoglobulin** is used for antibodies because they are globular proteins that provide IMMUNITY. Antibodies also are called **gamma globulins** because all free antibodies in the plasma separate out in the gamma fraction of plasma proteins during electrophoresis. The five antibody types

TABLE 17-4	Antibody Classification
ANTIBODY	**FUNCTION**
IgA	"Secretory" antibody that is present in high concentrations in the secretions of mucous membranes and in the intestinal mucosa Very low circulating levels Most responsible for preventing infection in the upper and lower respiratory tracts, the GI tract, and the genitourinary tract
IgD	Present in low blood concentrations in conjunction with IgM
IgE	Variable concentration in blood Associated with antibody-mediated hypersensitivity reactions Binds to mast cells and causes their degranulation when an allergen (antigen) binds to IgE antigen recognition sites
IgG	Composes at least 75% of circulating antibody population Is heavily expressed on second and subsequent exposures to antigens to provide sustained, long-term immunity against invading microorganisms Activates classic complement pathway, and enhances neutrophil and macrophage actions
IgM	First antibody formed by a newly sensitized B-lymphocyte plasma cell Composes about 10% to 15% of circulating antibody population Especially effective at the antibody actions of agglutination and precipitation because of having 10 potential binding sites per molecule Activates complement pathway

are classified by differences in size, location, amount, function, and timing (Table 17-4).

On first exposure to an antigen, the newly sensitized B-cell produces the IgM antibody type against the antigen. IgM is special because it forms itself into a five-member group. Each IgM group, then, has ten antigen binding sites. So, even though antibody production is slow on first exposure, the antibody type produced forms groups that are very efficient at antigen binding. This process ensures that the initial illness, like influenza A, lasts only 5 to 10 days. On re-exposure to the same antigen, the already sensitized B-cell makes large amounts of the IgG type of antibody against that antigen. Although IgG does not form groups of five, the enormous amounts produced make IgG antibodies efficient at clearing the antigen and protecting the person from becoming ill with the disease again.

Acquiring Antibody-Mediated Immunity

Antibody-mediated IMMUNITY (AMI) is a type of **adaptive immunity** in which a person's body learns to make as an adaptive response to invasion by organisms or foreign proteins. Thus antibody-mediated immunity is an *acquired immunity.* Adaptive immunity occurs either naturally or artificially through lymphocyte responses and can be either active or passive.

Active immunity occurs when antigens enter a person's body and it responds by making specific antibodies against the antigen. This type of IMMUNITY is *active* because the body takes an active part in making antibodies. Active immunity occurs under natural or artificial conditions.

Natural active IMMUNITY occurs when an antigen enters the body naturally without human assistance and the body responds by actively making antibodies against that antigen (e.g., influenza A virus). Usually, the invasion that triggers antibody production also causes the disease. However, processes occurring in the body at the same time as infection create immunity to that antigen. Thus the person will not become ill after a second exposure to the same antigen. *Natural active immunity is the most effective and the longest lasting.*

Artificial active IMMUNITY is the protection developed by vaccination or immunization. This type of immunity is used to prevent serious and potentially deadly illnesses (e.g., tetanus, diphtheria, polio). Small amounts of specific antigens are placed as a vaccination into a person. The person's immune system responds by actively making antibodies against the antigen. Because antigens used for this procedure have been specially processed to make them less likely to grow in the body (**attenuated**), this exposure usually does not cause the disease. Artificial active immunity lasts many years, although repeated but smaller doses of the original antigen are required as a "booster" to retain the protection.

Passive IMMUNITY occurs when the antibodies against an antigen are transferred to a person's body after first being made in the body of another person or animal. Because these antibodies are foreign to the receiving person, they are recognized as non-self and eliminated quickly. For this reason, passive immunity provides only immediate, short-term protection against a specific antigen. It is used when a person is exposed to a serious disease for which he or she has little or no actively acquired immunity. Instead, the injected antibodies are expected to inactivate the antigen. Artificial passive immunity may be used to prevent disease or death for patients exposed to rabies, tetanus, and poisonous snake bites.

Natural passive IMMUNITY occurs when antibodies are passed from the mother to the fetus via the placenta or to the infant through colostrum and breast milk.

AMI works with INFLAMMATION to protect against infection. However, AMI can provide the most effective long-lasting IMMUNITY only when its actions are combined with those of cell-mediated immunity.

Cell-Mediated Immunity

Cell-mediated IMMUNITY (CMI), or cellular immunity, involves many white blood cell (WBC) actions and interactions. CMI is another type of adaptive or acquired true immunity that is provided by lymphocyte stem cells that mature in the secondary lymphoid tissues of the thymus and pericortical areas of lymph nodes (see Fig. 17-7). Certain CMI responses influence and regulate the activities of antibody-mediated immunity (AMI) and INFLAMMATION by producing and releasing cytokines. For total or full immunity, CMI must function optimally.

Cell Types Involved in Cell-Mediated Immunity

The WBCs with the most important roles in CMI include several specific T-lymphocytes (T-cells) along with a special population of cells known as *natural killer (NK) cells*. T-cells have a variety of subsets, each of which has a specific function.

Different T-cell subsets can be identified by the presence of "marker proteins" (antigens) on the cell membrane's surface. More than 200 different T-cell proteins have been identified on the cell membrane, and some of these are commonly used clinically to identify specific cells (Abbas et al., 2012). Most T-cells have more than one antigen on their cell membrane. For example, all mature T-cells contain T1, T3, T10, and T11 proteins.

The names used to identify specific T-cell subsets include the specific membrane antigen and the overall actions of the cells in a subset. The three T-lymphocyte subsets that are critically important for the development and continuation of CMI are helper/inducer T-cells, suppressor T-cells, and cytotoxic/cytolytic T-cells. An additional cell, the natural killer cell, although not a true T-cell, also contributes to CMI.

Helper/inducer T-cells have the T4 protein on their membranes. These cells are usually called *T4+ cells* or T_H *cells*. The most correct name for helper/inducer T-cells is *CD4+* (cluster of differentiation 4).

Helper/inducer T-cells easily recognize self cells versus non-self cells. When they recognize non-self (antigen), helper/inducer T-cells secrete cytokines that can enhance the activity of other WBCs and increase overall immune function. These cytokines increase bone marrow production of stem cells and speed up their maturation. Thus helper/inducer T-cells act as organizers in "calling to arms" various squads of WBCs involved in inflammatory, antibody, and cellular protective actions.

Suppressor T-cells have the T8-lymphocyte antigen on membrane surfaces. These cells are commonly called *T8+ cells, CD8+ cells,* or T_S-*cells*. Suppressor T-cells help regulate CMI.

Suppressor T-cells prevent **hypersensitivity** (immune overreactions) on exposure to non-self cells or proteins. This function is important in preventing the formation of antibodies directed against normal, healthy self cells, which is the basis for many autoimmune diseases. The suppressor T-cells secrete cytokines that have an overall *inhibitory* action on most cells of the immune system.

Suppressor T-cells have the opposite action of helper/inducer T-cells. For optimal function of CMI, then, a balance between helper/inducer T-cell activity and suppressor T-cell activity must be maintained. This balance occurs when the helper/inducer T-cells outnumber the suppressor T-cells by a ratio of 2:1. When this ratio increases, indicating that helper/inducer T-cells vastly outnumber the suppressor cells, overreactions can occur, some of which are tissue damaging as well as unpleasant. When the helper/suppressor ratio decreases, indicating fewer-than-normal helper/inducer T-cells, IMMUNITY is suppressed and the person's risk for infections increases.

Cytotoxic/cytolytic T-cells are also called T_C-*cells*. Because they have the T8 protein present on their surfaces, they are a subset of suppressor cells. Cytotoxic/cytolytic T-cells destroy cells that contain a processed antigen's human leukocyte antigens (HLAs). This activity is most effective against self cells infected by parasites, such as viruses or protozoa.

Parasite-infected self cells have both self HLA proteins (universal product code) and the parasite's antigens on the cell surface. This allows the person's immune system cells to recognize the infected self cell as abnormal, and the cytotoxic/cytolytic T-cell can bind to it, punch a hole, and deliver a "lethal hit" of enzymes to the infected cell, causing it to lyse and die.

Natural killer (NK) cells are also known as *CD16+ cells* and are very important in providing CMI. The actual site of NK cell differentiation and maturation is unknown, and it is not a true T-cell subset (Abbas et al., 2012).

NK cells have direct cytotoxic effects on some non-self cells without first being sensitized. They conduct "seek and destroy" missions in the body to eliminate non-self cells.

NK cells are most effective in destroying unhealthy or abnormal self cells. The non-self cells most often harmed by NK cells are cancer cells and virally infected body cells.

Cytokines

Cell-mediated IMMUNITY (CMI) regulates the immune system by the production and activity of cytokines. Cytokines are small protein hormones produced by the many WBCs (and some other tissues). Cytokines made by the macrophages, neutrophils, eosinophils, and monocytes are called monokines. Those produced by T-cells are called lymphokines. In addition, we now know that many other body cell types can produce and respond to cytokines.

Cytokines work like hormones: one cell produces a cytokine, which in turn exerts its effects on other cells of the immune system and on other body cells. The cells responding to the cytokine may be located close to or remote from the cytokine-secreting cell. Thus cytokines act like "messengers" that tell specific cells how and when to respond. The cells that change their activity when a cytokine is present are "responder" cells. For a responder cell to respond to the presence of a cytokine, the responder cell must have a specific receptor to which the cytokine can bind. Once the cytokine binds to its receptor, the responder cell changes its activity.

Cytokines control many inflammatory and immune responses and are controlled by interactions with other systems, especially the nervous system. Cytokines include the interleukins (ILs), interferons (IFNs), colony-stimulating factors, tumor necrosis factors (TNFs), and transforming growth factors (TGFs). The interleukins are the largest group of cytokines, with interleukin-33 (IL-33) being the most recently defined. There are many cytokines, and cytokine classification is undergoing changes. Some are considered "proinflammatory" and increase the actions of natural immunity (INFLAMMATION). These currently include TNF-α, IL-1, IL-10, IL-12, and interferons (α [alpha], β [beta], and γ [gamma]). Other cytokines have a major influence on AMI and CMI activities. These include IL-2, IL-4, IL-5, IL-10, TGF-β, and IFN-γ. Although there are many cytokines, not all their functions are known or clinically useful at this time; however, this is an area of continuing research and discovery. Table 17-5 lists the cytokines that have current clinical importance. Chapters discussing specific diseases (e.g., lymphoma, rheumatoid arthritis) caused by or treated with certain cytokines have more information about the role of specific cytokines in the disease and its treatment.

Protection Provided by Cell-Mediated Immunity

Cell-mediated IMMUNITY (CMI) helps protect the body through the ability to differentiate self from non-self. The non-self cells most easily recognized by CMI are cancer cells and those self cells infected by organisms that live within host cells, especially viruses. CMI watches for and rids the body of self cells that might potentially harm the body. *CMI is important in preventing the development of cancer and metastasis after exposure to carcinogens.*

Transplant Rejection

Natural killer (NK) cells and cytotoxic/cytolytic T-cells also destroy cells from other people or animals. Although this action is normal and is usually helpful, it is also responsible for rejection of tissue grafts and transplanted organs (also termed *grafts*). Because the solid organ transplanted into the recipient

TABLE 17-5	**Activity of Selected Cytokines**
CYTOKINE	**ACTIONS**
Pro-inflammatory Cytokines	
Interleukin-1 (IL-1)	Induces fever
	Stimulates production of prostaglandins
	Increases growth of CD4+ T-cells
Interleukin-2 (IL-2)	Increases growth and differentiation of T-lymphocytes
	Enhances natural killer cell activity against cancer cells
Interleukin-6 (IL-6)	Stimulates liver to produce fibrinogen and protein C
	Increases rate of bone marrow production of stem cells
	Increases numbers of sensitized B-lymphocytes
Tumor Necrosis Factor (TNF)	Induces fever
	Major cytokine involved in rheumatoid arthritis damage
	Major cytokine involved in the acute inflammatory response to infectious bacteria and starts many of the systemic complications of severe infection or sepsis
	Participates in graft rejection
	Induces cell death
	Stimulates delayed hypersensitivity reactions and allergy
Growth Factors	
Granulocyte Colony-Stimulating Factor (G-CSF)	Increases numbers and maturity of neutrophils
Granulocyte-Macrophage Colony-Stimulating Factor (GM-CSF)	Increases growth and maturation of myeloid stem cells
Erythropoietin	Increases growth and differentiation of erythrocytes
Thrombopoietin	Increases growth and differentiation of platelets

is seldom a perfectly identical match of human leukocyte antigens (unless the organ is obtained from an identical sibling) between the donated organ and the recipient host, the patient's immune system cells recognize a newly transplanted organ as non-self. Without intervention, the recipient's immune system starts inflammatory and immunologic actions to destroy or eliminate these non-self cells. This activity causes rejection of the transplanted organ. Rejection of transplanted solid organs and other grafts is a result of a complex series of responses that change over time and involve different components of the immune system. Rejection can be hyperacute, acute, or chronic.

Hyperacute Rejection

Hyperacute rejection begins immediately on transplantation and is an antibody-mediated response. Antigen-antibody complexes form in the blood vessels of the transplanted organ. The recipient's (host's) blood has pre-existing antibodies to one or more of the antigens (including blood group antigens) present in the donated organ. The antigen-antibody complexes adhere to the lining of blood vessels and activate complement. The activated complement in the blood vessel linings triggers the blood clotting cascade, causing small clots to form throughout the new organ. Widespread clotting occludes blood vessels and leads to ischemic necrosis, INFLAMMATION with phagocytosis of the necrotic blood vessels, and release of lytic enzymes into the new organ. These enzymes cause massive cellular destruction within the transplanted organ and graft loss.

Hyperacute rejection occurs mostly in transplanted kidneys but is less common now as a result of greater efforts in HLA matching. The patients at greatest risk for hyperacute rejection are those who have received donated organs of an ABO blood type different from their own, have received multiple blood transfusions at any time in life before transplantation, have a history of multiple pregnancies, or have received a previous transplant.

The manifestations of hyperacute rejection are apparent within minutes of attachment of the donated organ to the recipient's blood supply. The process cannot be stopped once it has started, and the rejected organ is removed as soon as hyperacute rejection is diagnosed.

Acute Rejection

Acute rejection first occurs within 1 week to 3 months after transplantation and may occur sporadically after that. Two mechanisms are responsible. The first mechanism is antibody mediated and results in vasculitis within the transplanted organ. This reaction differs from hyperacute rejection in that blood vessel necrosis (not occlusion) leads to organ destruction.

The second mechanism is cellular. The recipient's cytotoxic/cytolytic T-cells and NK cells enter the transplanted organ through the blood, penetrate the organ cells, start an inflammatory response, and cause lysis of the organ cells.

Diagnosis of acute rejection is made by laboratory tests that show impaired function of the donated organ and by biopsy of the donated organ. Manifestations of acute rejection vary with each patient and with the specific organ transplanted. For example, when acute rejection occurs in a transplanted kidney, the patient usually has some tenderness in the kidney area and may have other general manifestations of INFLAMMATION.

An episode of acute rejection after solid organ transplantation does not automatically mean that the patient will lose the new organ. Drug management of the recipient's immune responses at this time may limit the damage to the organ and allow the graft to be maintained.

Chronic Rejection

The origin of *chronic rejection* is similar to chronic INFLAMMATION and scarring. The smooth muscles of blood vessels overgrow and occlude the vessels. The donated organ tissues are replaced with fibrotic, scarlike tissue. Because this fibrotic tissue is not organ tissue, the transplanted organ's function is reduced in proportion to the amount of normal tissue that is replaced by fibrotic tissue. This type of reaction is long-standing and occurs continuously as a response to chronic ischemia caused by blood vessel injury. The results of chronic rejection are unique to different transplanted organs. For example, in transplanted lungs, chronic rejection thickens small airways. In transplanted livers, chronic rejection destroys bile ducts. In transplanted hearts, this process is called *accelerated graft atherosclerosis (AGA)* and is the major cause of death in patients who have survived 1 or more years after heart transplantation.

Although good control over the recipient's immune function can delay this type of rejection, the process probably occurs to some degree with all transplanted solid organs obtained from donors who are not identical siblings of the recipients. Because the fibrotic changes are permanent, there is no cure for chronic graft rejection. When the fibrosis increases to the extent that the transplanted organ can no longer function, the only recourse is retransplantation.

Management of Transplant Rejection

Rejection of transplanted solid organs involves all three components of IMMUNITY, although cell-mediated immune (CMI) responses contribute the most to the rejection process. Approved drugs used to manage transplant rejection are listed in Chart 17-2.

Maintenance therapy is the continuous immunosuppression used after a solid organ transplant. The drugs used for routine therapy after solid organ transplantation are combinations of a calcineurin inhibitor, a corticosteroid, and an antiproliferative agent (Alexander & Susla, 2013). Which drugs are used depends on the transplant type and other patient-specific conditions. These are all oral agents and must be taken for the life of the transplanted organ. All are immunosuppressive to some degree, and the dosage is adjusted to the immune response of each patient. Treatment with these agents increases the risk for bacterial and fungal infections and for cancer development.

Rescue therapy is used to treat acute rejection episodes. The drug categories for this purpose are the monoclonal and polyclonal antibodies (see Chart 17-2). The drugs used for maintenance are often also used during rejection episodes at much higher dosages than for maintenance.

CHART 17-2	Common Examples of Drug Therapy		
Transplant Rejection			

DRUG/CLASS	ROUTE OF ADMINISTRATION		SIDE EFFECTS
Corticosteroids			
Broadly inhibit cytokine production in most leukocytes, resulting in generalized immunosuppression			
Prednisone (Deltasone)	Oral		Hypertension
			Hyperlipidemia
			Osteoporosis
			Weight gain
			Cushingoid appearance
			Opportunistic infection
			Glaucoma
			GI ulcer formation
			Hyperglycemia
Prednisolone (Millipred, Orapred, Veripred)	Oral		Same as for prednisone

Continued

CHART 17-2   Common Examples of Drug Therapy—cont'd

Transplant Rejection

DRUG/CLASS	ROUTE OF ADMINISTRATION	SIDE EFFECTS
Calcineurin Inhibitors		
The inhibition of calcineurin stops the production and secretion of IL-2, which then prevents the activation of lymphocytes involved in transplant rejection.		
Cyclosporine (Sandimmune, Neoral, Gengraf)	Oral	Nephrotoxic Hypertension Tremor Coronary artery disease Hirsutism Gingival hyperplasia Opportunistic infections Malignancies Hyperuricemia Hepatoxicity
Tacrolimus (Prograf)	Oral	Nephrotoxic Hypertension Hyperkalemia Hypomagnesemia Hyperglycemia Opportunistic infections Malignancies
Antiproliferatives		
The main action of all antiproliferatives is to inhibit something essential to DNA synthesis, which prevents cell division in activated lymphocytes. Some have additional immune suppressive actions.		
Azathioprine (Imuran)	Oral	Bone marrow suppression Thrombocytopenia Anemia Pancreatitis Hepatotoxicity Malignancies
Mycophenolate (CellCept, Myfortic)	Oral	Leucopenia Thrombocytopenia Nausea Opportunistic infection Malignancies
Sirolimus (Rapamune)	Oral	Leucopenia Thrombocytopenia Hypercholesterolemia Hypertriglyceridemia
Everolimus (Afinitor, Zortress)	Oral	Acne GI upsets Hepatoxicity Cushingoid appearance Gingival hyperplasia Hyperglycemia Hyperlipidemia Hypertension Leucopenia
Monoclonal Antibodies		
Specifically target the activation sites of T-lymphocytes, increasing their elimination from circulation		
Muromonab-CD3 (Orthoclone OKT3)	IV	Systemic inflammatory responses Aseptic meningitis Opportunistic infections Malignancies Hypersensitivity reactions
Basiliximab (Simulect)	IV	GI disturbances
Daclizumab (Zenapax)	IV	GI disturbances
Polyclonal Antibodies		
Antibodies derived from other animals (horses or rabbits) that bind to and eliminate most T-lymphocytes, thus stopping a transplant rejection episode.		
Antithymocyte globulin–equine (Atgam)	IV	Leukopenia Serum sickness Thrombocytopenia Pruritus Fever Arthralgias Opportunistic infections Malignancies
Antithymocyte globulin–rabbit (RATG, Thymoglobulin)	IV	Same as for antithymocyte globulin–equine

⚲ CLINICAL JUDGMENT CHALLENGE

Patient-Centered Care; Safety **QSEN**

A patient comes to the emergency room after stepping on a rusty nail while fixing a fence on his horse farm. He tells you that his last tetanus toxoid booster vaccination was about 12 years ago. The health care provider prescribes an injection of HyperTET, which contains concentrated pre-formed antibodies to the tetanus bacterium. The patient is instructed to return to his health care provider in 10 days to receive a tetanus "booster" vaccination.

1. What type of immunity is provided by the booster vaccination the patient received 12 years ago? Explain your choice.
2. Why does this patient need HyperTET now, and what type of immunity does it provide?
3. Why does the patient have to wait 10 days to receive the next tetanus booster?

NURSING CONCEPTS AND CLINICAL JUDGMENT REVIEW

What might you NOTICE in a patient with adequate protection as a result of appropriate responses for INFLAMMATION and IMMUNITY?

Vital signs:
- Body temperature within normal range

Physical assessment:
- Skin intact (no rashes, abnormal lesions)
- Skin color normal (no redness)

- No edema or excessively warm body areas
- All body areas fully functional with no pain
- No indicators of infection or illness

Laboratory assessment:
- White blood cell count and differential within the normal range
- No positive cultures of skin, blood, urine, sputum
- No evidence of allergic reactions

GET READY FOR THE NCLEX® EXAMINATION!

■ KEY POINTS

Review these Key Points for each NCLEX Examination Client Needs Category.

Physiological Integrity
- INFLAMMATION and IMMUNITY are provided through the actions and products of white blood cells (WBCs), also called *leukocytes.*
- Different types of WBCs provide different types of immune or inflammatory protection.
- The differential of the WBC count can be used to determine the patient's risk for infection, the presence or absence of infection, the presence or absence of an allergic reaction, and whether an infection is bacterial or viral.
- WBCs are the only body cells able to recognize non-self cells and to attack them.
- Self-tolerance is the special ability of WBCs to recognize healthy self cells and not attempt to attack or destroy them.
- Human leukocyte antigens (HLAs) are a person's tissue type and are inherited from parents.
- Immunocompetence requires that all three parts of INFLAMMATION and IMMUNITY have optimal functioning.
- INFLAMMATION is a general, nonspecific protective response also known as *innate immunity.*
- The five cardinal manifestations of INFLAMMATION are redness, warmth, swelling, pain, and loss of function.
- INFLAMMATION and infection are not the same thing. Infection almost always is accompanied by inflammation, but inflammation often occurs without infection.

- The tissue responses to INFLAMMATION are helpful if confined to the area of invasion or infection and do not extend beyond the acute phase.
- Chronic INFLAMMATION can damage tissues and reduce function.
- The cells and actions of cell-mediated IMMUNITY control and coordinate the entire inflammatory and immune responses.
- Inflammatory protection cannot be transferred from one person to another.
- Immune function declines with age, making the older adult at increased risk for infection and cancer development.
- Antibody-mediated IMMUNITY (also known as *humoral immunity*) can be transferred from one person or animal to another.
- Antibodies transferred from one person into another person have a short-term effect.
- Natural, active IMMUNITY is the most beneficial and long-lasting type of immunity.
- Vaccinations cause artificial active IMMUNITY and require "boosting" for best long-term effects.
- A person's normal membrane proteins would be antigens in another person.
- Transplant rejection is a normal response of the immune system that can damage or destroy the transplanted organ.
- Patients who receive transplanted organs (unless from an identical sibling) need to take immunosuppressive drugs daily to prevent transplant rejection.
- Patients who take immunosuppressive drugs have an increased risk for infection and cancer development.

18 | CHAPTER

Care of Patients with Arthritis and Other Connective Tissue Diseases

Donna D. Ignatavicius

ⓔ http://evolve.elsevier.com/Iggy/

PRIORITY CONCEPTS

- PAIN
- MOBILITY
- INFECTION

- IMMUNITY
- INFLAMMATION

LEARNING OUTCOMES

Safe and Effective Care Environment

1. Identify interdisciplinary team members who collaborate to ensure quality care for patients with connective tissue diseases (CTDs).
2. Prioritize collaborative evidence-based interventions for patients with osteoarthritis (OA) and rheumatoid arthritis (RA).

Health Promotion and Maintenance

3. Identify community resources to help patients achieve or maintain independence in ADLs.
4. Describe risk factors for the development of arthritis and other CTDs.
5. Teach patients how to protect and exercise their joints to prevent injury.
6. Teach patients evidence-based strategies for how to prevent osteoarthritis.
7. Teach patients how to prevent Lyme disease and detect it early if it occurs.

Psychosocial Integrity

8. Assess the patient's and family's response to arthritis or other CTD, their support systems, and available resources.
9. Assess the patient's and family's sources of stress and coping mechanisms when living with arthritis or other CTD.

Physiological Integrity

10. Compare and contrast the pathophysiology and clinical manifestations of OA and RA, including those caused by joint INFLAMMATION and degenerative changes.
11. Interpret laboratory findings for patients with RA and other CTDs that affect IMMUNITY.
12. Assess presence and extent of PAIN and suffering in patients with arthritis.
13. Apply knowledge of pathophysiology to monitor for and prevent complications of total hip and knee arthroplasty.
14. Teach patients and their families about the postoperative care required after a total joint arthroplasty.
15. Provide information for patients and families about the use and side effects of drug therapy for arthritis or other CTD.
16. Identify the nursing implications associated with drug therapy for patients with rheumatoid arthritis and other CTDs.
17. Document and plan patient care in the electronic health care record for the patient with arthritis.
18. Differentiate between discoid lupus erythematosus and systemic lupus erythematosus.
19. Prioritize nursing interventions for patients who have systemic sclerosis.
20. Describe the patient-centered collaborative care of gout based on knowledge of pathophysiology.
21. Explain the differences between polymyositis, systemic necrotizing vasculitis, polymyalgia rheumatica, ankylosing spondylitis, Reiter's syndrome, and Sjögren's syndrome.
22. Describe current treatment strategies for patients with fibromyalgia syndrome and psoriatic arthritis.

Connective tissue disease (CTD) is the major focus of *rheumatology,* the study of rheumatic disease. A **rheumatic disease** is any disease or condition involving the musculoskeletal system. In this text, CTDs are discussed separately from other musculoskeletal conditions because most CTDs are classified as autoimmune disorders. In autoimmune disease, antibodies attack healthy normal cells and tissues. For reasons that are unclear, the immune system does not recognize body cells as self and therefore triggers an immune response. The usual *protective* nature of the immune system does not function properly in patients with autoimmune CTDs.

Most common CTDs are characterized by chronic PAIN and progressive joint deterioration, which results in decreased function and impaired MOBILITY. Some of these disorders have additional localized clinical manifestations, whereas others are systemic. The economic and social costs of these diseases are staggering and will increase steadily as "baby boomers" continue to age. Patient care usually requires an interdisciplinary approach, including medicine, surgery, nursing, rehabilitation therapy, pharmacy, and/or case management.

Arthritis means INFLAMMATION of one or more joints. In clinical practice, however, arthritis is categorized as either non-inflammatory or inflammatory. Noninflammatory, localized arthritis such as osteoarthritis (OA) is not systemic; OA is not an autoimmune disease. Systemic autoimmune diseases such as rheumatoid arthritis (RA) and systemic lupus erythematosus (SLE) are inflammatory disorders.

OSTEOARTHRITIS

❖ PATHOPHYSIOLOGY

Osteoarthritis is the most common arthritis and a major cause of disability among adults in the United States and the world. It is sometimes called *osteoarthrosis* or *degenerative joint disease (DJD)*.

Osteoarthritis is the progressive deterioration and loss of cartilage and bone in one or more joints. Articular cartilage, also known as *hyaline cartilage,* contains water and a matrix of:

- Proteoglycans (glycoproteins containing chondroitin, keratin sulfate, and other substances)
- Collagen (elastic substance)
- Chondrocytes (cartilage-forming cells)

As people age or experience joint injury, proteoglycans and water decrease in the joint. The production of synovial fluid, which provides joint lubrication and nutrition, also declines because of the decreased synthesis of hyaluronic acid and less body fluid in the older adult (Antonelli & Starz, 2012).

In patients of any age with OA, enzymes, such as stromelysin, break down the articular matrix. In early disease, the cartilage changes from its normal bluish white, translucent color to an opaque and yellowish brown appearance. As cartilage and the bone beneath the cartilage begin to erode, the joint space narrows and osteophytes (bone spurs) form (Fig. 18-1). As the disease progresses, fissures, calcifications, and ulcerations develop and the cartilage thins. Inflammatory cytokines

(enzymes) such as interleukin-1 (IL-1) enhance this deterioration. The body's normal repair process cannot overcome the rapid process of degeneration (McCance et al., 2014). Secondary joint INFLAMMATION can occur when joint involvement is severe.

Eventually the cartilage disintegrates and pieces of bone and cartilage "float" in the diseased joint causing crepitus, a grating sound caused by the loosened bone and cartilage. The resulting joint pain and stiffness can lead to decreased mobility and muscle atrophy. Muscle tissue helps support joints, particularly those that bear weight (e.g., hips, knees).

Etiology and Genetic Risk

The cause of OA is a combination of many factors. For patients with *primary* OA, the disease is caused by aging and genetic factors. Weight-bearing joints (hips and knees), the vertebral column, and the hands are most commonly affected, probably because they are used most often or bear the mechanical stress of body weight and many years of use.

Secondary OA occurs less often than primary disease and results from joint injury and obesity (Antonelli & Starz, 2012). Injury to the joints from excessive use, trauma, or other joint disease (e.g., rheumatoid arthritis) predisposes a person to OA. Heavy manual occupations (e.g., carpet laying, construction, farming) cause high-intensity or repetitive stress to the joints. The risk for hip and knee OA is increased in professional athletes, especially football players, runners, and gymnasts. Fractures or other joint tissue injuries can lead to OA years after the trauma. Certain metabolic diseases (e.g., diabetes mellitus, Paget's disease of the bone) and blood disorders (e.g., hemophilia, sickle cell disease) can also cause joint degeneration.

Obesity is a common contributing factor to osteoarthritis. Weight-bearing joints, such as hips and knees, are most often affected in obese people.

Incidence and Prevalence

The prevalence of OA varies among different populations but is a universal problem. Most people older than 60 years have joint changes that can be seen on x-ray examination, although not all of those people actually develop the disease. According to Arthritis Foundation (2013b) estimates, 27 million people in the United States have symptomatic osteoarthritis.

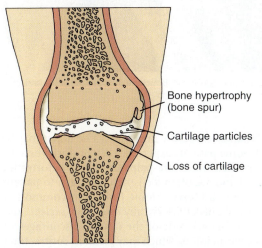

Bone hypertrophy (bone spur)

Cartilage particles

Loss of cartilage

FIG. 18-1 Joint changes in degenerative joint disease.

GENDER HEALTH CONSIDERATIONS

Patient-Centered Care QSEN

More men than women younger than 55 years have AO, but after 55, women have it more often than men (Antonelli & Starz, 2012). Although the cause for this difference is not known, contributing factors may include increased obesity in women after having children, broader hips in women than men, and more athletic injuries in young men as compared with young women (Arthritis Foundation, 2013b).

Lesbian women and bisexuals are more likely to be overweight or obese when compared with other populations. Although the reason for this difference is not known, it is possible that lesbian women and bisexual people use food as a coping strategy because many have fears and concerns about "coming out" about their sexual orientation, especially to health care professionals and family members (Pettinato, 2012). Be sure to assess all patients in the hospital or community-based setting, particularly those who are older and obese, for clinical manifestations of osteoarthritis.

Health Promotion and Maintenance

The Arthritis Foundation's Osteoarthritis Intervention Working Group produced an evidence-based document that proposed the Public Health Agenda needed to prevent and manage osteoarthritis.

❖ PATIENT-CENTERED COLLABORATIVE CARE

◆ Assessment

History. Patients with OA usually seek medical attention in ambulatory care settings for their joint pain. However, you will also care for those who have OA as a secondary diagnosis in acute and chronic care facilities. Ask the patient about the course of the disease. Collect information specifically related to OA, such as the nature and location of joint PAIN and how much pain and suffering he or she is experiencing. *Remember that older patients may underreport pain, resulting in inadequate management.* Use a 0-to-10 scale or other assessment tool to assess PAIN intensity. Chapter 3 discusses pain assessment in detail.

Other questions to ask include:

- If joint stiffness has occurred, where and for how long?
- When and where has any joint swelling occurred?
- What do you do to control the PAIN or stiffness?
- Do you have any loss of MOBILITY or difficulty in performing ADLs?

Because this disease occurs more often in older women, age and gender are important factors for the nursing history. Ask patients about their occupation, nature of work, history of injury (including falls), weight history, and current or previous involvement in sports. A history of obesity is significant, even for those currently within the ideal range for body weight. Document any family history of arthritis. Determine whether the patient has a current or previous medical condition that may cause joint symptoms.

Physical Assessment/Clinical Manifestations. In the early stage of the disease, the clinical manifestations of OA may appear similar to those of rheumatoid arthritis (RA). The distinction between OA and RA becomes more evident as the disease progresses. Table 18-1 compares the major characteristics of both diseases and their common drug therapy.

The typical patient with OA is a middle-aged or older woman who reports *chronic joint pain and stiffness.* Early in the course of the disease, the PAIN diminishes after rest and worsens after activity. Later the pain occurs with slight motion or even when at rest. Because cartilage has no nerve supply, the pain is caused by joint and soft-tissue involvement and by spasms of the surrounding muscles. During the joint examination, the patient may have tenderness on palpation or when putting the joint through range of motion. Crepitus may be felt or heard as the joint goes through range of motion. One or more joints may be affected. The patient may also report joint stiffness that usually lasts less than 30 minutes after a period of inactivity.

On inspection, the joint is often enlarged because of bony hypertrophy. The joint feels hard on palpation. The presence of INFLAMMATION in patients with OA indicates a secondary synovitis. About half of patients with hand involvement have Heberden's nodes (bony nodules at the distal interphalangeal [DIP] joints) and Bouchard's nodes (bony nodules at the proximal interphalangeal [PIP] joints) (Fig. 18-2). Although OA is *not* a bilateral, symmetric disease, these large bony nodes appear

CHARACTERISTIC	RHEUMATOID ARTHRITIS	OSTEOARTHRITIS
Typical onset (age)	35-45 yr	Older than 60 yr
Gender affected	Female (3:1)	Female (2:1)
Risk factors or cause	Autoimmune (genetic basis) Emotional stress (triggers exacerbation) Environmental factors	Aging Genetic factor (possible) Obesity Trauma Occupation
Disease process	Inflammatory	Degenerative
Disease pattern	Bilateral, symmetric, multiple joints Usually affects upper extremities first Distal interphalangeal joints of hands spared Systemic	May be unilateral, single joint Affects weight-bearing joints and hands, spine Metacarpophalangeal joints spared Nonsystemic
Laboratory findings	Elevated rheumatoid factor, antinuclear antibody, ESR	Normal or slightly elevated ESR
Common drug therapy	NSAIDs (short-term use) Methotrexate Leflunomide (Arava) Corticosteroids Biological response modifiers Other immunosuppressive agents	NSAIDs (short-term use) Acetaminophen Other analgesics

TABLE 18-1   **Differential Features of Rheumatoid Arthritis and Osteoarthritis**

ESR, Erythrocyte sedimentation rate; *NSAIDs,* nonsteroidal anti-inflammatory drugs.

FIG. 18-2 Heberden's and Bouchard's nodes are enlarged bony nodules affecting the joints of the hand.

on both hands, especially in women. The nodes may be painful and red. Some patients experience discomfort when developing nodes or when nodes are palpated. These deformities tend to be familial and are often a cosmetic concern to patients.

Joint effusions (excess joint fluid) are common when the knees are inflamed. Observe any *atrophy of skeletal muscle* from disuse. The vicious cycle of the disease discourages the movement of painful joints, which may result in contractures, muscle atrophy, and further PAIN. *Loss of function* or MOBILITY may result, depending on which joints are involved. Hip or knee pain may cause the patient to limp and restrict walking distance.

Osteoarthritis (OA) can affect the spine, especially the lumbar region at the L3-4 level or the cervical region at C4-6 (neck). Compression of spinal nerve roots may occur as a result of vertebral facet bone spurs. The patient typically reports radiating PAIN, stiffness, and muscle spasms in one or both extremities.

Severe pain and deformity interfere with ambulation and self-care. In addition to performing a musculoskeletal assessment, collaborate with the physical and occupational therapists to conduct a functional assessment. Assess the patient's MOBILITY and ability to perform ADLs. Chapter 6 describes functional assessment.

Psychosocial Assessment. OA is a chronic condition that may cause permanent changes in lifestyle. An inability to care for oneself in advanced disease can result in role changes and other losses. Constant PAIN interferes with quality of life. Chronic pain can also affect sexuality. Patients may not have the energy for sexual intercourse or may find positioning uncomfortable.

Patients with continuous PAIN from arthritis may develop depression or anxiety. The patient may also have a role change in the family, workplace, or both. To identify changes that have been or need to be made, ask his or her roles before the disease developed. Identify coping strategies to help live with the disease. Ask the patient about his or her expectations regarding treatment for OA.

In addition to role changes, joint deformities and bony nodules often alter body image and self-esteem. Observe the patient's response to body changes. Does he or she ignore them or seem overly occupied with them? Ask patients directly how they perceive their body image. Document your assessment findings in the interdisciplinary electronic health record per agency policy.

Laboratory Assessment. The health care provider uses the history and physical examination to make the diagnosis of OA. The results of routine laboratory tests are usually normal but can be helpful in screening for associated conditions. The erythrocyte sedimentation rate (ESR) and high-sensitivity C-reactive protein (hsCRP) may be slightly elevated when secondary synovitis (synovial INFLAMMATION) occurs. The ESR also tends to rise with age, infection, and other inflammatory disorders.

Imaging Assessment. Routine x-rays are useful in determining structural joint changes. Specialized views are obtained when the disease cannot be visualized on standard x-ray film but is suspected. Magnetic resonance imaging (MRI) and computed tomography (CT) may be used to determine vertebral or knee involvement.

◆ **Analysis**

The priority NANDA-I nursing diagnoses and collaborative problems for patients with osteoarthritis (OA) include:
1. Chronic Pain related to cartilage deterioration (NANDA-I)
2. Impaired Mobility related to joint pain and muscle atrophy (NANDA-I)

◆ **Planning and Implementation**

In 2010, the Osteoarthritis Research Society International (OARSI) committee updated its evidence-based expert consensus guidelines for patients with knee, hand, and hip OA (Zhang et al., 2010). These interdisciplinary best practice guidelines were also supported by the Arthritis Foundation and have major implications for nursing care.

Managing Chronic Pain

Planning: Expected Outcomes. The patient with OA is expected to have PAIN control that is acceptable to the patient (e.g., at a 3 on a pain intensity scale of 0 to 10).

Interventions. No drug therapy can influence the course of OA. Optimal management of patients with OA requires a multimodal approach (combination of therapies) to manage PAIN. If these measures are ineffective, surgery may be performed to reduce pain (Zhang et al., 2010). Perform a pain assessment before and after implementing interventions.

Nonsurgical Management. Management of chronic joint PAIN can be challenging for both the patient and the health care professional. Drug therapy and a variety of nonpharmacologic therapies are used to manage the patient with OA. Chapter 3 elaborates on interventions for chronic non-cancer pain.

Drug Therapy. The purpose of drug therapy is to reduce PAIN caused by cartilage destruction, muscle spasm, and/or secondary joint INFLAMMATION. The American Pain Society, American Geriatrics Society, and OARSI committee recommend regular *acetaminophen* (Tylenol, Atasol♦) as the primary drug of choice because OA is not a primary anti-inflammatory disorder (Davies, 2011).

> ! **NURSING SAFETY PRIORITY** (QSEN)
> **Drug Alert**
>
> Patients are at risk for liver damage if they take more than 3000 mg daily of acetaminophen, have alcoholism, or have liver disease. *Older adults are particularly at risk because of normal changes of aging, such as slowed excretion of drug metabolites.* Remind patients to read the labels of over-the-counter (OTC) or prescription drugs that could contain acetaminophen before taking them. Teach them that their liver enzyme levels will be monitored while taking this drug.

Topical drug applications may help with temporary relief of PAIN. Prescription lidocaine 5% patches (Lidoderm) have been approved by the Federal Drug Administration (FDA) for postherpetic neuralgia (nerve pain) but may also relieve joint PAIN (especially the knee) for some patients. Teach the patient to apply the patch on clean, intact skin for 12 hours each day. Up to three patches may be applied to painful joints at one time. Remind him or her that Lidoderm can cause skin irritation. Teach the patient that the lidocaine patch is contraindicated in those patients taking class I antidysrhythmics. Topical salicylates, such as OTC Aspercreme patch, gel, or cream, are also useful for some patients as a temporary pain reliever, especially for knee pain. Buspirone HCl (Buspar) topical cream may also relieve local joint pain for some patients.

If acetaminophen or topical agents do not relieve PAIN, the analgesic drug class of choice is *nonsteroidal anti-inflammatory drugs (NSAIDs)* if the patient can tolerate them. These traditional drugs supported by OARSI guidelines include oral COX-2 nonselective and selective NSAIDs and topical NSAIDs.

Before beginning oral NSAID therapy, baseline laboratory information is obtained, including a complete blood count (CBC) and kidney and liver function tests. Celecoxib (Celebrex), a COX-2 inhibitor, is usually the first choice unless the patient has hypertension, kidney disease, or cardiovascular disease.

Topical NSAIDs are considered to be safe and effective non-systemic drugs for pain relief. For example, the diclofenac-epolamine patch and diclofenac solution are used for patients with signs and symptoms associated with knee OA.

When topical or systemic drugs are not effective and for temporary relief of PAIN in a single joint, the health care provider may inject an individual joint with cortisone, a commonly used steroid. Patients may have the same joint injected up to 4 times a year, or once every 3 months. Frequently injected joints include the knee, base of the thumb, shoulder, and trochanteric bursa, which people often call the *hip*.

Other agents, such as hyaluronate (Hyalgan) and hylan G-F 20 (Synvisc), are specific injections for knee and hip PAIN associated with OA. These synthetic joint fluid implants replace or supplement the body's natural hyaluronic acid, which is broken down by inflammation and aging.

Other oral drugs that can be given to patients with OA include muscle relaxants and opioids. Muscle relaxants, such as cyclobenzaprine hydrochloride (Flexeril), are sometimes given for painful muscle spasms, especially those occurring in the back from OA of the vertebral column. *These drugs should be used with caution in older adults because they can cause acute confusion. Remind any patient not to drive or operate dangerous machinery when taking muscle relaxants.* Weak opioid drugs such as tramadol (Ultram or Ultram ER) may also be given for patients with OA. Chapter 3 discusses drug therapy for pain relief in more detail.

Nonpharmacologic Interventions. In addition to analgesics, many nonpharmacologic measures can be used for patients with OA, such as rest balanced with exercise, joint positioning, heat or cold applications, weight control, and a variety of complementary and alternative therapies.

Teach the patient to *position joints in their functional position.* For example, when in a supine position (recumbent), he or she should use a small pillow under the head or neck but avoid the use of other pillows. The use of large pillows under the knees or head may result in flexion contractures. If needed, the legs may be elevated 8 to 12 inches (20 to 30 cm) to reduce back discomfort. Remind him or her to use proper posture when standing and sitting to reduce undue strain on the vertebral column. Teach the patient to wear supportive shoes; foot insoles may help relieve pressure on painful metatarsal joints. Collaborate with the physical therapist (PT) to plan a program for muscle-strengthening exercises to better support the joints.

Most patients apply *heat* or *cold* for temporary relief of PAIN, but not all patients find these modalities effective. Heat may help decrease the muscle tension around the tender joint and thereby decrease pain. Suggest hot showers and baths, hot packs or compresses, and moist heating pads. *Regardless of treatment, teach him or her to check that the heat source is not too heavy or so hot that it causes burns.* A temperature just above body temperature is adequate to promote comfort.

If needed, collaborate with the PT to provide special heat treatments, such as paraffin dips, diathermy (using electrical current), and ultrasonography (using sound waves). A 15- to 20-minute application usually is sufficient to temporarily reduce PAIN, spasm, and stiffness. Cold packs or gels that feel hot and cold at the same time may also be used.

Cold therapy has limited use for most patients in controlling PAIN. Cold works by numbing nerve endings and decreasing secondary joint inflammation, if present.

There is no one food that causes or cures arthritis. Instead, a well-balanced diet is recommended. Gradual *weight loss* for obese patients may lessen the stress on weight-bearing joints, decrease pain, and perhaps slow joint degeneration. If needed, collaborate with the registered dietitian to provide more in-depth teaching and meal planning or make referrals to community resources.

Complementary and Alternative Therapies. Some patients with OA have reported that a variety of complementary and alternative medicine (CAM) therapies are useful. However, the evidence supporting their effectiveness is often inconsistent and inconclusive (see the Evidence-Based Practice box).

Topical *capsaicin* products are safe over-the-counter (OTC) drugs. They work by blocking or modifying substance P and other neurotransmitters for PAIN. Tell the patient using capsaicin to expect a burning sensation for a short time after applying it. Recommend the use of plastic gloves for application. To prevent burning of eyes or other body areas, wash hands immediately after applying the substance.

Dietary supplements may complement traditional drug therapies. Glucosamine and chondroitin are widely used and are the most effective nonprescription supplements taken to decrease PAIN and improve functional ability. However, the evidence to support their use is inconsistent (Fouladbakhsh, 2012).

EVIDENCE-BASED PRACTICE QSEN

Which Complementary and Alternative Methods Best Relieve Osteoarthritis Symptoms?

Fouladbakhsh, J. (2012). Complementary and alternative modalities to relieve osteoarthritis symptoms. *Orthopaedic Nursing, 31*(2), 115-121.

The author conducted a systematic review of current literature to determine the effectiveness and safety of commonly used complementary and alternative medicine (CAM) therapies in patients with osteoarthritis (OA), including mind-body therapies, supplements, and body-based treatments.

Research findings related to mind-body therapies revealed limited evidence for the use of yoga and a moderate level of evidence supporting the use of tai chi for patients with OA. According to the literature review, the only energy therapy that is moderately effective for OA is acupuncture for pain relief. Evidence for the use of glucosamine and chondroitin sulfate supplement is inconsistent. No evidence exists to support the use of most other supplements except for pycnogenol (pine bark extract). Research shows that massage therapy, a body-based treatment, for patients with OA is moderately effective for the relief of back pain.

Level of Evidence: 1

The author conducted a systematic literature review (previous 10 years) to draw conclusions about the effectiveness of selected CAM therapies for patients who have OA.

Commentary: Implications for Practice and Research

Further study is needed to examine the effectiveness of commonly used CAM therapies by patients with OA. Consistency in studies is needed to provide clearer answers and explore the complexity of these therapies. Nurses caring for patients with OA need to provide information about the evidence or lack of evidence for CAM therapies. Before patients take supplements such as glucosamine, remind them to check with their health care provider about their safety.

CHART 18-1 Patient and Family Education: Preparing for Self-Management

Considerations for Taking Glucosamine Supplements

- Tell your health care provider if you decide to take glucosamine.
- Do not take glucosamine if you have hypertension.
- Do not take glucosamine if you are pregnant or breast-feeding.
- Monitor for bleeding if you take chondroitin with glucosamine or chondroitin alone if you are on anticoagulant therapy.
- If diabetic, monitor your blood glucose levels carefully because taking glucosamine for a prolonged time can increase them.
- Be aware that glucosamine can cause adverse effects such as a rash; GI disturbances, especially diarrhea; drowsiness; and headache.
- Be sure to take the recommended dosage based on your weight.
- Read drug labels to ensure that you do not take too much glucosamine for your weight; some drug names may not indicate they contain glucosamine (e.g., Bioflex, Arth-X Plus, Nutri-Joint).

These natural products are found in and around bone cartilage for repair and maintenance. **Glucosamine** may decrease inflammation, and **chondroitin** may play a role in strengthening cartilage. These supplements are used topically or taken in oral form. Chart 18-1 summarizes what you should teach your patients about glucosamine, with or without chondroitin.

CLINICAL JUDGMENT CHALLENGE

Patient-Centered Care; Evidence-Based Practice QSEN

A 66-year-old woman visits a new health care provider for a physical examination. She tells you that she works in a school cafeteria and has to stand most of the day. When you take an admission history, she tells you that she has pain and stiffness in her knees, feet, hands, and cervical spine. She takes ibuprofen when needed with some pain relief but has frequent indigestion for which she takes OTC Zantac. The patient is 5'4" tall and weighs 183 pounds today.

During her physical assessment, you note that the patient has multiple Heberden's and Bouchard's nodes on both hands and a swollen right knee. She has a joint effusion in her right third PIP, and she is right-handed. The health care provider diagnoses her joint involvement as osteoarthritis (OA).

1. What additional physical assessment do you need to perform to determine the patient's level of functioning?
2. What risk factors contribute to her diagnosis of OA?
3. What OTC, nonpharmacologic, or CAM therapies for joint pain and stiffness might you recommend? What evidence supports those recommendations?
4. How might this patient's OA affect her ability to continue working in her current job?
5. What health teaching is needed for this patient to help manage her OA?

Surgical Management. Surgery may be indicated when conservative measures or drug therapy no longer provides PAIN control, when MOBILITY becomes so restricted that the patient cannot participate in activities he or she enjoys, and when he or she cannot maintain the desired quality of life. The most common surgical procedure performed for *older adults* with OA is **total joint arthroplasty (TJA)** (surgical creation of a joint), also known as **total joint replacement (TJR)**. Almost any synovial joint of the body can be replaced with a prosthetic system that consists of at least two parts—one for each joint surface. TJAs are expected to increase exponentially as baby boomers age over the next 20 years.

Total joint arthroplasty is a procedure used most often to manage the PAIN of OA and to improve MOBILITY, although other conditions causing cartilage destruction may require the surgery. These disorders include RA, congenital anomalies, trauma, and osteonecrosis. **Osteonecrosis** is bony necrosis secondary to lack of blood flow, usually from trauma or chronic steroid therapy. Hip and knee joints are most commonly replaced, but finger and wrist joint, elbow, shoulder, toe joint, and ankle replacements have been improved in the past 15 years.

The *contraindications* for TJA are active infection anywhere in the body, advanced osteoporosis, and rapidly progressive inflammation. An infection elsewhere in the body or from the joint being replaced can result in an infected TJA and subsequent prosthetic failure. Therefore if a patient has a urinary tract infection, for example, the physician treats the infection before surgery. Advanced osteoporosis can cause bone shattering during insertion of the prosthetic device. Severe medical problems, such as uncontrolled diabetes or hypertension, put the patient at risk for major postoperative complications and possible death.

Total Hip Arthroplasty. The number of total hip arthroplasty (THA) procedures (also known as *total hip replacement [THR]*) has steadily increased over the past 35 years. The first time a patient receives any total joint arthroplasty, it is referred to as primary arthroplasty. If the implant loosens, revision arthroplasty may be performed. Availability of improved joint implant materials and better custom design features allow longer life of a replaced hip. Although patients of any age can undergo THR, the procedure is performed most often in those older than 60 years. *The special needs and normal physiologic changes of older adults often complicate the perioperative period and may result in additional postoperative complications.*

Preoperative Care. As with any surgery, preoperative care begins with assessing the patient's level of understanding about the surgery and his or her ability to participate in the postoperative plan of care. The surgeon explains the procedure and postoperative expectations (including possible complications) during the office visit, but this patient education may have occurred weeks or months before the scheduled surgery. Some patients may not know what questions to ask or may forget the important information that was taught. Information may be provided in a notebook or DVD format that the patient can take home to review and share with family. This is particularly useful to patients with poor reading skills or poor memory. Written materials or other media provided in the patient's language appropriate for the patient's educational level are essential.

In some hospitals or orthopedic office practices, the physical therapist (PT) may have the patient practice transfers, positioning, and ambulation. An occupational therapist (OT) may partner with the PT to assist in exercises or learning to ambulate with an assistive device, such as crutches or a walker. The OT may also help obtain assistive/adaptive equipment that will be needed after surgery. The cost of some items, such as an elevated toilet seat, is covered by Medicare and other insurers because they are essential to prevent hip dislocation. Other helpful equipment, such as grab bars and shower chairs, may not be paid for by third-party payers and can be purchased at local pharmacies or medical supply stores, based on the patient's specific needs.

All patients are also told to visit a dentist and have any necessary dental procedures done before surgery. After surgery, he or she must take extreme care not to acquire an infection that could migrate to the surgical area and cause prosthetic failure. *Remind the patient to tell any future health care provider that he or she has had any total joint arthroplasty.*

In addition to usual preoperative laboratory tests, the surgeon may ask the patient with RA to have a cervical spine x-ray if he or she is having general anesthesia. Those with RA often have cervical spine disease that can lead to subluxation during intubation. Hip x-rays, CT scan, and/or MRI may be done to assess the operative joint and surrounding soft tissues.

Because venous thromboembolism (VTE) is a serious postoperative complication, especially for hip surgery, assess the patient's risk factors for clotting problems, including history of previous clotting, obesity, smoking, and advanced age. *Teach patients that drugs that increase the risks for clotting and bleeding, such as NSAIDs, vitamins C and E, and hormone replacement therapy (HRT) or oral contraceptive drugs, must be discontinued about a week before surgery.*

Patients are also assessed for the need for possible blood transfusion after surgery. For patients who are at risk for postoperative anemia, one or more blood transfusions may be needed. Autologous (patient's own) or banked blood can be used. If desired, the patient may donate blood several weeks before surgery to be used after surgery. This pre-deposit autologous blood donation is a safe and cost-effective blood replacement alternative for those who are undergoing elective surgeries. It also decreases the risk for blood transfusion reactions.

For some patients, the surgeon may prescribe several weeks of epoetin alfa (Epogen, Procrit, Eprex ✦) with or without iron to prevent anemia that can occur after hip or knee replacement. Epoetin alfa is recombinant human erythropoietin, a substance that is essential for developing red blood cells. This drug is particularly useful for older adults, who frequently have mild anemia before surgery.

Remind patients that they will likely be asked to take a shower with special antiseptic soap the night before surgery to decrease bacteria that could cause infection after surgery. Tell them to wear clean nightwear after their shower and sleep on clean linen. Review which drugs are safe to take or necessary the morning of the operation, such as antihypertensives, and which ones should be avoided. Medication should be taken with a very small amount of water to prevent vomiting and aspiration during surgery. See Chapter 14 for additional preoperative care for any type of surgery.

Operative Procedures. Similar to other orthopedic surgeries, the patient receives an IV antibiotic, usually a cephalosporin such as cefazolin (Ancef), within an hour before the initial surgical incision to help prevent INFECTION.

The anesthesiologist or nurse anesthetist places the patient under general or neuraxial (epidural/spinal) anesthesia for lower extremity surgery. Neuraxial induction reduces blood loss and the incidence of deep vein thrombosis. Intraoperative blood loss with hypotensive neuraxial anesthesia is usually less than that with general anesthesia, thereby decreasing the need for postoperative blood transfusions. Patients receiving general anesthesia may have a regional nerve block, which lasts up to 24 hours after surgery.

Some patients are candidates for *minimally invasive surgery* (MIS) using a smaller incision with special instruments to reduce muscle cutting. This newer technique cannot be used for patients who are obese or those with osteoporosis. It is done only for primary THAs, not for revision surgeries. Like those of any MIS, the benefits of minimally invasive THA are decreased soft tissue damage and postoperative PAIN. Patients often have a shorter hospital stay and quicker recovery. They are generally satisfied with the cosmetic appearance of the incision because there is less scarring. Postoperative complications are not as common in patients having minimally invasive ("mini") hip replacements when compared with those having the traditional technique.

Regardless of procedure type, two components are used in the THA—the acetabular component and the femoral component (Fig. 18-3). A non-cemented prosthesis is most often used. Bone surfaces are smoothed as they are prepared to receive the artificial components. The non-cemented components are press-fitted into the prepared bone. The acetabular cup may be placed using computer or robotic assistance. If the prosthesis is cemented, polymethyl methacrylate (an acrylic fixating substance) is used. A closed wound drainage system may be placed in the wound before the surgeon closes the incision.

Considerations of a non-cemented prosthesis include protection of weight-bearing status to allow bone to grow into the prosthesis and decreased problems with loosening of the prosthesis. With a cemented prosthesis, cement can fracture or deteriorate over time, leading to loosening of the prosthesis, which causes pain and can lead to the need for a revision arthroplasty.

FIG. 18-3 A, Two major components of total hip arthroplasty. **B,** X-ray showing the components in place.

In revision arthroplasty, the old prosthesis is removed and new components are replaced. Bone graft may be placed if bone loss is significant. Outcomes from revision arthroplasty may not be as positive as with primary arthroplasty.

Postoperative Care. In addition to providing the routine postoperative care discussed in Chapter 16, assess for and help prevent possible postoperative complications. Table 18-2 summarizes these complications, including nursing measures for prevention, assessment, and intervention. Chart 18-2 highlights special concerns for the care of older adults in the postoperative period. Collaborate with your patient and his or her family to become safety partners to keep the patient free from harm, including complications, such as:

- Hip dislocation
- Venous thromboembolism (VTE)
- Infection
- Anemia
- Neurovascular compromise

Preventing Hip Dislocation. A major complication of THA is sub-luxation (partial dislocation) or total dislocation.

> **! NURSING SAFETY PRIORITY** (QSEN)
>
> **Action Alert**
>
> Teach patients to maintain correct positioning at all times. When the patient returns from the postanesthesia care unit (PACU), place him or her in a supine position with the head slightly elevated. Place a regular or abduction pillow between the patient's legs to prevent adduction beyond the midline of the body according to agency policy or surgeon preference.

In some hospitals, abduction devices with straps are placed on patients who are restless or cannot follow instructions, especially older adults with delirium or dementia. One or two regular bed pillows are used in most cases to remind patients to keep their legs abducted. For devices with straps, be sure to loosen the straps every 2 hours and check the patient's skin for irritation or breakdown.

TABLE 18-2 Nursing Interventions to Prevent Complications of Lower Extremity Total Joint Arthroplasty

COMPLICATION	PREVENTION/INTERVENTION
Dislocation	Position correctly. For hip, keep leg slightly abducted. For hip, prevent hip flexion beyond 90 degrees. Assess for acute PAIN, rotation, and extremity shortening. Report immediately to physician.
Infection	Use aseptic technique for wound care and emptying of drains. Wash hands thoroughly when caring for patient. Culture drainage fluid, if change. Monitor temperature. Report excessive inflammation or drainage to physician.
Venous thromboembolism	Have patient wear elastic stockings and/or sequential compression device per agency policy. Teach leg exercises to patient. Encourage fluid intake. Observe for signs of thrombosis (redness, swelling, or pain). Observe patient for changes in mental status. Administer anticoagulant as prescribed. Do not massage legs. Do not flex knees for a prolonged period of time.
Hypotension, bleeding, or infection	Take vital signs at least every 4 hours. Observe patient for bleeding. Report excessively low blood pressure or bleeding to physician.

> **CHART 18-2** **Nursing Focus on the Older Adult**
>
> **Postoperative Care of the Older Adult with a Total Hip Arthroplasty**
>
> - Use an abduction pillow or splint to prevent adduction after surgery if the patient is very restless or has an altered mental state.
> - Keep the patient's heels off the bed to prevent pressure ulcers.
> - Do not rely on fever as a sign of infection; older patients often have infection without fever. Decreasing mental status typically occurs when the patient has an infection.
> - When assisting the patient out of bed, move him or her slowly to prevent orthostatic (postural) hypotension.
> - Encourage the patient to deep breathe and cough and to use the incentive spirometer every 2 hours to prevent atelectasis and pneumonia.
> - As soon as permitted, get the patient out of bed to prevent complications of immobility.
> - Anticipate the patient's need for pain medication, especially if he or she cannot verbalize the need for pain control.
> - Expect a temporary change in mental state immediately after surgery as a result of the anesthetic and unfamiliar sensory stimuli. Reorient the patient frequently.

Place and support the affected leg in neutral rotation. *Keep the patient's heels off the bed to prevent skin breakdown, particularly older adults.* The procedure for postoperative turning is controversial and specified by agency policy or surgeon preference. In most cases, you are safe to turn the patient if the pillow

FIG. 18-4 Correct (**A, B**) and incorrect (**C**) hip flexion after a total hip replacement.

is in place. Some surgeons allow only turning directly onto one side or the other, depending on the surgical approach.

Teach the patient and family about other precautions to prevent dislocation as outlined in Chart 18-3. In addition to preventing adduction, remind them that the patient should avoid flexing the hips more than 90 degrees at all times. Use diagrams or demonstrate correct positioning to help reinforce this information before the patient gets out of bed (Fig. 18-4).

! NURSING SAFETY PRIORITY (QSEN)

Critical Rescue

> Observe for possible signs of hip dislocation, which include severe hip PAIN, shortening of the affected leg, and leg rotation. If any of these clinical manifestations occur, keep the patient in bed and notify the surgeon immediately!

If the hip is dislocated, the surgeon manipulates and relocates the affected hip after the patient receives moderate sedation. The hip is then immobilized by an abduction splint or other device until healing occurs—usually in about 6 weeks.

Preventing Venous Thromboembolism. The most potentially life-threatening complication after THA is venous thromboembolism (VTE), which includes deep venous thrombosis (DVT) and pulmonary embolism (PE). *Older patients are especially at increased risk for VTE because of age and decreased circulation before surgery. Obese patients and those with a history of VTE are also at high risk for thrombi.* Apply sequential compression devices (SCDs) and/or antiembolism stockings according to agency policy.

Anticoagulants, such as warfarin (Coumadin, Warfilone ✦), subcutaneous low-molecular-weight heparin (LMWH), or factor Xa inhibitors, help prevent VTE. Patients are usually on anticoagulants for 3 to 6 weeks after surgery, depending on the patient's response and risk factors. The use of subcutaneous LMWHs has markedly increased for patients with total hip and

CHART 18-3 Patient and Family Education: Preparing for Self-Management

Care of Patients with Total Hip Arthroplasty After Hospital Discharge

Hip Precautions
- Do not sit or stand for prolonged periods.
- Do not cross your legs beyond the midline of your body.
- Do not bend your hips more than 90 degrees.
- Do not twist your body when standing.
- Use an ambulatory aid, such as a walker, when walking.
- Use assistive/adaptive devices for dressing, such as for putting on shoes and socks.
- Do not put more weight on your affected leg than allowed.
- Resume sexual intercourse as usual on the advice of your surgeon.

Pain Management
- Report increased hip pain to the surgeon immediately.
- Take oral analgesics as prescribed and only as needed.
- Do not overexert yourself; take frequent rests.

Incisional Care
- Inspect your hip incision every day for redness, heat, or drainage; if any of these are present, call your physician immediately.
- Cleanse your hip incision with a mild soap and water every day; be sure to dry it thoroughly.

Other Care
- Continue walking and performing the leg exercises as you learned in the hospital.
- Do not cross your legs to help prevent blood clots.
- Report pain, redness, or swelling in your legs to your physician immediately.
- Call 911 for acute chest pain or shortness of breath.
- If you are taking an anticoagulant, follow the precautions learned in the hospital to prevent bleeding; avoid using a straight razor, avoid injuries, and report bleeding or excessive bruising to your surgeon immediately.
- Perform postoperative exercises as instructed, including straight leg raises, gluteal sets, ankle pumps, and "ham" sets.

knee replacements. Examples include enoxaparin (Lovenox), dalteparin (Fragmin), and tinzaparin (Innohep).

As an alternative to LMWHs, subcutaneous fondaparinux (Arixtra), a factor Xa inhibiting agent, may be prescribed for some patients undergoing hip and knee arthroplasty. A newer Xa inhibitor, rivaroxaban (Xarelto), is given orally once a day. You do not need to monitor the international normalized ratio (INR), prothrombin time (PT), or activated partial thromboplastin time (aPTT) for patients receiving these drugs because they do not affect coagulation values. Like other anticoagulants, however, patients are at risk for bleeding. A complete discussion of nursing care associated with patients taking anticoagulants and VTE is found in Chapter 36. The Joint Commission's *VTE Core Measures* are also discussed in that chapter.

Early ambulation and exercise help prevent VTE. Teach the patient about leg exercises, which should begin in the immediate postoperative period and continue through the rehabilitation period. These exercises include plantar flexion and dorsiflexion (heel pumping), circumduction (circles) of the feet, gluteal and quadriceps muscle setting, and straight-leg raises (SLRs). Teach the patient to perform gluteal exercises by pushing the heels into the bed and achieve **quadriceps-setting exercises** ("quad sets") by straightening the legs and pushing the back of the knees into the bed. In addition to preventing clots, these exercises improve muscle tone, which helps restore the function of the extremity.

Preventing Infection. INFECTION can occur during hospitalization or months or years later after a hip replacement. Most infections are caused by contamination during surgery and are considered "deep" infections.

Monitor the surgical incision and vital signs carefully—every 4 hours for the first 24 hours and every 8 to 12 hours thereafter. Observe for signs of INFECTION, such as an elevated temperature and excessive or foul-smelling drainage from the incision. *An older patient may not have a fever with infection but, instead, may experience an altered mental state.* If you suspect this problem, obtain a sample of any drainage for culture and sensitivity to determine the offending organisms and the antibiotics that may be needed for treatment.

Assessing for Bleeding and Managing Anemia. Observe the surgical hip dressing for bleeding or other type of drainage at least every 4 hours or when vital signs are taken. Empty and measure the bloody fluid in the surgical drain(s) every shift. The total amount of drainage is usually less than 50 mL/8 hr. Patients who have the minimally invasive procedure may not have a drain. The surgeon usually removes the drains and operative dressing 24 to 48 hours after surgery. *Take special care when removing tape from the skin to prevent tape burns and skin tears as the surgical dressing is changed, especially for older adults.*

The surgeon also requests periodic hemoglobin and hematocrit (H&H) tests to assess for anemia. Although some patients receive several units of blood during surgery, the H&H levels may continue to fall; in this case, additional blood is given 1 to 2 days after surgery. Blood pressure may be lower than usual because of blood loss during surgery.

Assessing for Neurovascular Compromise. As with other musculoskeletal surgery, monitor neurovascular assessments frequently for a possible compromise in circulation to the affected distal extremity.

In addition to implementing interventions to prevent potential postoperative complications and monitoring for early signs of complications, the interdisciplinary team plans care to

---

! **NURSING SAFETY PRIORITY** (QSEN)
Action Alert

Check and document color, temperature, distal pulses, capillary refill, movement, and sensation. Remember to compare the operative leg with the nonoperative leg. These assessments are performed at the same time the vital signs are checked. Report any changes in neurovascular assessment to the surgeon, and carefully monitor for changes. Early detection of changes in neurovascular status can prevent permanent tissue damage.

---

manage PAIN, improve MOBILITY and activity, and promote self-management.

Managing Pain. Although hip arthroplasty is performed to relieve joint PAIN, patients experience pain related to the surgical procedure. Many state that their pain is different and less severe than before surgery. Immediate pain control is typically achieved by extended-release epidural morphine (EREM) or patient-controlled analgesia (PCA) with morphine or another opioid. An NSAID should be taken with the opioid to decrease INFLAMMATION. Chapter 3 contains information on the nursing care associated with these acute pain modalities. *Keep in mind that the patient may also receive additional analgesic drugs for chronic arthritic pain in other joints.*

Regardless of the PAIN management method used, most patients do not require parenteral analgesics after the first day. Oral opioids, such as oxycodone plus acetaminophen (Percocet, Tylox), are then commonly prescribed until the pain can be controlled by NSAIDs such as ketorolac (Toradol, Acular) or ibuprofen (Motrin, Apo-Ibuprofen ✦).

Nonpharmacologic methods for acute and chronic PAIN control can also be used to decrease the amount of drug therapy used (see Chapter 3). A study by Thomas and Sethares (2010) found that guided imagery can be helpful in controlling pain in patients with total joint arthroplasty.

Promoting Mobility and Activity. Depending on the time of day that the surgery is performed, the patient with a THA gets out of bed with assistance the night of surgery to prevent problems related to impaired MOBILITY (e.g., atelectasis, pneumonia), especially in older adults.

! **NURSING SAFETY PRIORITY** (QSEN)
Action Alert

Be sure to assist the patient the first time he or she gets out of bed to prevent falls and observe for dizziness. When getting the patient out of bed, stand on the same side of the bed as the affected leg. After the patient sits on the side of the bed, remind him or her to stand on the unaffected leg and pivot to the chair with guidance. *To avoid injury, do not lift the patient!*

Remind the patient to avoid flexing the hips beyond 90 degrees as discussed earlier (see Fig. 18-4). Raised toilet seats and reclining chairs help prevent hyperflexion of the replaced hip joint. Be sure to teach the patient to also *avoid* twisting the body or crossing his or her legs to prevent hip dislocation.

The surgeon, type of prosthesis, and surgical procedure determine the amount of weight bearing that can be applied to the affected leg. A patient with a cemented implant is usually allowed immediate partial weight bearing (PWB) and progresses to full weight bearing (FWB). Typically, only "toe-touch" or minimal weight bearing is permitted for patients with uncemented prostheses. When x-ray evidence of bony ingrowth can be seen, the patient can progress to PWB and then to FWB.

In collaboration with the physical therapist (PT), teach the patient how to follow weight-bearing restrictions. Most patients use a walker (may be a rolling walker), but younger adults may use crutches. They are usually advanced to a single cane or crutch if they can walk without a severe limp 4 to 6 weeks after surgery. When the limp disappears, they no longer need an ambulatory/assistive device and may be permitted to sit in chairs of normal height, use regular toilets, and drive a car.

❓ NCLEX EXAMINATION CHALLENGE

Physiological Integrity

A client had a right total hip arthroplasty 2 days ago. Which precautions will the nurse teach the client to prevent surgical complications? **Select all that apply.**
A. "Stand on your right leg and pivot to the chair."
B. "Do not bend your hips more than 90 degrees."
C. "Cross your legs to be most comfortable."
D. "Avoid twisting your body when moving."
E. "Use a long-handled shoe horn to put on your shoes."

Promoting Self-Management. The hospital's occupational therapy department may supply assistive/adaptive devices to help with ADLs, especially for those having traditional surgery. Particularly important are devices designed for reaching to prevent patients from bending or stooping and flexing the hips more than 90 degrees. Extended handles on shoehorns and dressing sticks may be very useful to achieve ADL independence. Third-party payers may or may not pay for these devices, depending on the patient's status.

For those who have *traditional surgery,* the length of stay in the acute care hospital is typically 2 to 3 days, but older adults or those experiencing postoperative complications may stay longer. Those who have the *minimally invasive THA* are discharged on the second postoperative day or the day of surgery (23-hour stay). Those patients are discharged to home on crutches to practice their own rehabilitative exercises. Most of them are able to return to work in 2 weeks. For that reason, some hospitals have started Rapid Recovery Hip Replacement programs for patients who are candidates for MIS.

Discharge for patients having *traditional surgery* may be to the home, a rehabilitation unit, a transitional care unit, or a skilled unit or long-term care facility for continued rehabilitation before discharge to home. The interdisciplinary team provides written instructions for posthospital care and reviews them with patients and their family members (see Chart 18-3). Be sure to provide a copy of these instructions for the patient.

In some acute care settings, postoperative classes are provided to the caregivers of patients who have joint replacements to improve the quality of the postoperative experience (Mazaleski, 2011). These classes are provided by the interdisciplinary team and include pain management, new medications, activity level, discharge instructions, and home preparation (see the Quality Improvement box).

Acute rehabilitation usually takes 1 to 2 weeks or longer, depending on the patient's age and tolerance and the type of prosthesis used. However, it often takes 6 weeks or longer for complete recovery. Some patients who are discharged to their

QUALITY IMPROVEMENT (QSEN)

Improving Postoperative Total Joint Replacement Education for Caregivers

Mazaleski, A. (2011). Postoperative total joint replacement class for support persons: Enhancing patient and family centered care using a quality improvement model. *Orthopaedic Nursing, 30*(6), 361-364.

Postoperative education is essential to ensure positive patient outcomes and increase patient satisfaction. The orthopedic clinical nurse specialist for an active orthopedic unit suggested a postoperative class on the unit for caregivers of patients who had total joint replacements. The ultimate goal of the education was to promote patient- and family-centered care.

The Plan, Do, Study, Act (PDSA) quality improvement (QI) model was used to guide the planning and implementation of the project. A review of patient and family satisfaction scores revealed poor understanding of drug therapy and its side effects. The class included information on new medications, pain management, activity level, and home preparation. A post-class survey was given to class attendees and used to improve future classes. For example, specific discharge instruction sheets were developed for oxycodone and Warfarin. Since the classes were started, patient and family satisfaction scores increased and over 90% of the class attendees strongly agreed that the information was helpful.

Readmission rates will be monitored for patients whose caregivers attended the class. In addition, questions and concerns related to office staff during follow-up visits will be tracked.

Commentary: Implications for Practice and Research

Research indicates that discharge teaching after surgery improves quality of care and improves patient and family satisfaction. This QI project planned and implemented a class for caregivers of patients who had total joint replacements to educate them on postoperative care at home. The attendees for each class were surveyed to determine their satisfaction with the class. The staff made changes to subsequent classes based on those findings.

Other outcome data are needed to evaluate the effectiveness of the classes. The authors plan to collect these data, including hospital readmission rate and postoperative complications.

home are able to attend physical therapy sessions in an office or ambulatory care setting. Others have no means or cannot use community resources and need physical therapy in the home, depending on their health insurance coverage. *Collaborate with the case manager to determine which option is best for your patient.*

Total Knee Arthroplasty. Although many adults require total knee arthroplasty (TKA, also known as *total knee replacement [TKR]),* those who have a knee replaced are often younger than those who have a hip replaced. Continued improvements in total knee implants have increased the expected life of a TKA to 20 years or more, depending on the age and activity level of the patient. An increasing number of patients who have TKAs are overweight or obese. Obesity increases wear and tear on weight-bearing joints, which can lead to revision surgeries. Unilateral (one joint) or bilateral joint replacements done at the same time may be performed, depending on the patient.

Preoperative Care. TKA, like hip replacement, is performed when joint PAIN cannot be managed by conservative measures. When limited MOBILITY severely prevents patients from participating in work or activities they enjoy, this procedure can restore a high quality of life. The preoperative care and teaching for patients undergoing a TKA are similar to that for total hip replacement. However, precautions for positioning are not the same. Differences in patient and family teaching depend on the procedure used by the orthopedic surgeon.

Like the minimally invasive surgery (MIS) for the hip, the knee can also be replaced using MIS. Candidates for mini–knee replacement cannot have severe bone loss, obesity, or previous knee surgery. They should be in good general health. Patients having MIS usually have less blood loss during surgery, less pain, more joint range of motion (less stiffness from scarring), and a faster recovery, leading to a shorter hospital stay. Rapid Recovery Knee Replacement programs for patients having minimally invasive TKA are becoming popular in a number of hospitals.

All patients are given verbal and either written or video preoperative instructions, which include the activity protocol to follow after surgery. The PT and OT provide information about transfers, ambulation, postoperative exercises, and ADL assistance. Patients may practice walking with walkers or crutches to prepare them for ambulation after TKA. Teach patients about the possible need for assistive-adaptive devices to assist with ADLs, including an elevated toilet seat, safety handrails, and dressing devices like a long-handled shoehorn. Some third-party payers cover these devices, depending on the patient's condition and age; however, other insurers may not pay for them. Teach the patient and family how and where this equipment can be obtained to have it available after surgery.

Some surgeons prescribe a continuous passive motion (CPM) machine after knee surgery to increase joint MOBILITY. Others have found that the range of motion for the surgical knee is not improved by using this device. If the patient will have a CPM machine after surgery, be sure to explain what it is and how it is used.

Routine diagnostic testing is requested, as well as any additional tests, such as cervical spine x-rays for patients with rheumatoid arthritis (RA) to determine if the patient can be intubated for anesthesia. Cervical spine involvement occurs in about half of all patients with RA. Changes in the cricoarytenoid joint of the larynx can also make intubation difficult (Nelson, 2011). Knee x-rays, CT scan, and/or MRI may be done to assess the joint and surrounding soft tissues. Rheumatoid arthritis is discussed later in this chapter.

Teach patients that they will need to shower with a special antiseptic soap the night before surgery to decrease bacteria on the skin that could cause INFECTION after surgery. Remind them to wear clean nightwear and sleep on clean linen. Ask them to check with their surgeon about what medications they can take the morning of surgery, including antihypertensives and corticosteroids (taken by many patients with RA). Take these drugs with a small amount of water to prevent vomiting and aspiration during surgery. See Chapter 14 for additional preoperative care for any type of surgery.

Operative Procedures. As with the hip, the knee can be replaced with the patient under general or neuraxial (epidural or spinal) anesthesia. An antibiotic, usually an IV cephalosporin, is given shortly before surgical opening to help prevent INFECTION. In the *traditional surgery,* the surgeon makes a central longitudinal incision about 8 inches (20 cm) long. Osteotomies of the femoral and tibial condyles and of the posterior patella are performed, and the surfaces are prepared for the prosthesis. The femoral component is often non-cemented (using a press-fit) with the tibial component being cemented. The surgeon typically inserts a surgical drain and applies a pressure dressing to decrease edema and bleeding.

Minimally invasive TKA may be performed using a shorter incision and special instruments to spare muscle and other soft tissue. Computer-guided or robotic equipment may be used to ensure accurate positioning of the knee implants. This procedure is referred to as a *computer-assisted TKA.*

Complementary and Alternative Therapies. A newer intervention to reduce the severe PAIN that occurs after knee arthroplasty is the intraoperative insertion of Adlea, a refined capsaicin product, directly into the surgical joint. Most patients who were given Adlea during knee surgery have less acute postoperative pain when compared with others who did not receive the treatment.

Postoperative Care. Postoperative nursing care of the patient with a TKA is similar to that for the patient with a total hip arthroplasty; however, maintaining hip abduction is not necessary. The surgeon may prescribe a CPM machine, which can be applied in the postanesthesia care unit (PACU) or soon after the patient is admitted to the postoperative unit (Fig. 18-5). The CPM machine keeps the prosthetic knee in motion and may prevent the formation of scar tissue, which could decrease knee mobility and increase postoperative pain. In the immediate postoperative period, the surgeon may also prescribe ice packs or an ice machine to decrease swelling at the surgical site. Swelling and bruising are more common with this type of surgery than with hip surgery.

The surgeon, PT, or technician presets the CPM machine for the appropriate range of motion and cycles per minute. A typical initial setting is 20 to 30 degrees of flexion and full extension (0 degrees) at two cycles per minute, but this setting varies according to surgeon preference. The machine is generally used on an intermittent schedule of a designated number of hours several times a day, with the range of motion increased gradually. Observe and document the patient's response to the device, and follow the surgeon's protocol for settings. Chart 18-4 outlines your responsibility when caring for a patient using the CPM machine.

In general, pain control measures for patients with TKA are similar to those with total hip arthroplasty. Many patients report high ratings on the PAIN intensity scale and require IV opioid medications longer than patients with THA, particularly if they have had bilateral surgery. *Be sure to manage your patient's pain to provide comfort, increase his or her participation in physical therapy, and improve joint mobility.*

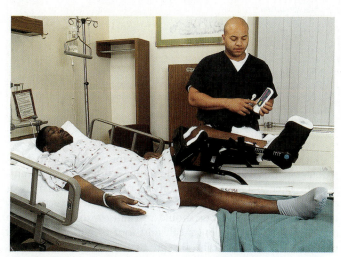

FIG. 18-5 A continuous passive motion (CPM) machine in use.

One of the most recent advances in postoperative PAIN management for lower extremity total joint arthroplasty is *peripheral nerve blockade (PNB)*. In this procedure, the anesthesiologist injects the femoral or sciatic nerve with local anesthetic; the patient may receive a continuous infusion of the anesthetic by portable pump. This method not only decreases pain but also allows patients to participate in rehabilitation earlier than when using opioid analgesia alone. Patients having continuous femoral nerve blockade (CFNB) after TKA require less opioids and antiemetics when compared with patients receiving no CFNB and those who had a single-shot femoral nerve blockade (FNB).

When caring for a patient receiving a CPNB, perform neurovascular assessments every 2 to 4 hours or according to hospital protocol. The patient should be able to plantarflex and dorsiflex the affected foot but not feel PAIN in the lower leg. Check for movement, sensation, warmth, color, pulses, and capillary refill.

! NURSING SAFETY PRIORITY (QSEN)

Critical Rescue

Monitor the patient for signs and symptoms that could indicate that the local anesthetic is getting into the patient's system, such as:

- Metallic taste
- Tinnitus
- Nervousness
- Slurred speech
- Bradycardia
- Hypotension
- Decreased respirations
- Seizures

Report any of these new signs and symptoms to the surgeon or anesthesiologist immediately, and carefully continue monitoring the patient for changes.

Because dislocation is a rare problem for a patient with TKA, special positioning to prevent adduction is not required. Maintain the knee in a neutral position and not rotated internally or externally. If a CPM machine is not used, the surgeon may recommend that the knee should rest flat on the bed or with one pillow under the lower calf and foot to encourage slight extension of the knee joint. Be sure that the surgical knee does not hyperextend.

Some complications that affect patients with total hip arthroplasty may also affect those having TKA, such as venous thromboembolism, infection, anemia, and neurovascular compromise. Assessments and interventions associated with these complications are described in the Postoperative Care section of the discussion of Total Hip Arthroplasty on pp. 297-300.

The desired outcome for discharge from the acute hospital unit is that the patient can walk independently with crutches, walker, or cane and has adequate flexion in the operative knee for ambulation. Patients who had minimally invasive TKA are discharged to home in 1 to 2 days with instructions for postoperative exercises, weight bearing, and activity progression. Many of these instructions (except for preventing hip dislocation) are similar to those provided for teaching patients after a total hip arthroplasty (see Chart 18-3).

Patients are able to partially weight bear unless the prosthesis is not cemented. During the home rehabilitation phase, the use of a stationary bicycle or CPM machine may help gain flexion. These patients can return to work and other usual activities in 2 to 3 weeks, depending on their age and other health status factors.

Acute rehabilitation for *traditional* TKA usually takes about 1 to 2 weeks longer, depending on the age and tolerance of the patient. These patients may be discharged to their home or to an acute rehabilitation unit, transitional care unit, skilled unit, or long-term care facility for therapy. They may also be instructed to use a continuous passive motion (CPM) machine at home. If able, they may attend physical therapy sessions in an office or ambulatory care setting. If not, home care services can provide physical therapy and nursing care in their home, depending on the insurance available. *Collaborate with the case manager to determine which option is best for your patient.* Total recovery from traditional TKA takes 6 weeks or longer, especially for those older than 75 years.

? NCLEX EXAMINATION CHALLENGE

Safe and Effective Care Environment

A nursing technician is assigned to care for a client who has a CPM machine in place after a total knee arthroplasty. Which statement by the "tech" indicates a need for further teaching and supervision by the nurse?
A. "I will turn off the machine if the client has any pain."
B. "I will turn off the machine when the client eats."
C. "I will store the machine on a chair when not used."
D. "I will check to make sure the client's leg is correctly placed."

Other Joint Arthroplasties. After the hip and knee, the shoulder and hand are the most common joints replaced for severe OA, RA, or trauma. Elbow, wrist, ankle, and foot replacements are not performed as often as other types of arthroplasties. The shoulder and other upper extremity joints do not bear weight and therefore tend to have less degeneration and subsequent PAIN. Preoperative teaching for patients having any of these surgeries depends on the surgeon's technique and postoperative protocols. For example, the continuous passive motion (CPM) machine may be prescribed postoperatively in the hospital and in the posthospital setting (home or other facility). These devices are available for almost any joint surgery in the body. Some surgeons find that the CPM machine is not helpful in promoting joint mobility and may be uncomfortable for patients.

Total shoulder arthroplasty (TSA) has gained popularity as newer prostheses and technology have been developed. This procedure usually decreases arthritic PAIN and increases the patient's ability to perform ADLs. Because the shoulder joint is complex and has many **articulations** (joint surfaces), **subluxation** (partial dislocation) or complete dislocation is a major potential complication. Usually the glenohumeral joint, created by the glenoid cavity of the shoulder blade (scapula) and the head of the humerus, is replaced because it moves the most and is therefore most affected by arthritis. A **hemiarthroplasty** (replacement of part of the joint), typically the humeral component, may be performed as an alternative to TSA.

The surgeon makes an incision to replace the joint while the patient is under general anesthesia. The implant may be cemented or press-fitted without cement. Some surgeons perform *minimally invasive TSA,* which decreases postoperative complications like infection and nerve damage. A sling is applied to immobilize the joint until therapy begins.

In addition to dislocation, postoperative complications are similar to those for other total joint replacements and include infection and neurovascular compromise. Active and passive exercises are needed to begin shoulder movement. *As for any other total joint arthroplasty, perform frequent neurovascular assessments, at least every 4 to 8 hours.* The hospital stay for TSA is shorter than for a total hip or knee replacement. Rehabilitation with an occupational therapist generally takes several months.

Total elbow arthroplasty (TEA) is performed most often for patients with rheumatoid arthritis (RA), but it is done for anyone whose severe arthritis limits MOBILITY and causes uncontrolled PAIN. TEA may be successful in increasing range of motion, but infection and loosening may occur because of extensive tissue cutting during surgery. Active and passive exercises are used postoperatively. In general, elbow motion is allowed as tolerated. Occupational therapy may not be necessary, but the need depends on the individual patient. Lifting is usually restricted on a long-term basis after TEA. Generalized swelling usually resolves in 3 to 6 months.

Any joint of the hand or foot can be replaced *(phalangeal joint, metacarpal or metatarsal arthroplasties),* often for patients with RA. Hand prostheses are implanted without the use of cement because they stay in place and do not bear weight.

For the hand, a bulky dressing is used temporarily after surgery and is then replaced with a dynamic splint. Edema is controlled by having the patient elevate the arm as much as possible. The rehabilitation program for phalangeal joint arthroplasties may last for many weeks until normal function and strength return. These procedures are typically performed in specialized hand centers. Joint replacements in the toe usually require less rehabilitation.

Any bone of the *wrist* can also be replaced, including the heads of the radius and ulna. The postoperative pressure dressing is removed in 1 to 2 days, and a splint is applied. The patient usually regains full function within 6 to 12 weeks, but lifting may be restricted for a longer period. Special hand therapists work with these patients for the extensive rehabilitation that is required for phalangeal and wrist replacements.

Because the ankles support about 25% of the body's weight and are complex joints, developing an implant that is both small enough and strong enough has been difficult. Although total ankle arthroplasties (TAAs) have been problematic for more than three decades, newer non-cemented prosthetic systems have renewed interest in ankle replacements. Surgeons who specialize in foot and ankle surgeries are available in some parts of the country.

Postoperative complications include infection, delayed wound healing, nerve injuries, and loosening. Therefore TAA is not as successful as total hip or knee replacements. Noncemented prostheses seem to be preferred over cemented ones to prevent loosening. The patient is allowed to begin weight bearing at about 6 weeks, and rehabilitation continues for about 3 months.

Improving Mobility

Planning: Expected Outcomes. The patient with osteoarthritis (OA) is expected to maintain or improve a level of MOBILITY and activity that allows him or her to function independently with or without an assistive ambulatory device.

Interventions. Management of the patient with OA is an interdisciplinary effort. If needed, collaborate with the physical therapist (PT) and occupational therapist (OT) to meet the outcome of independent function and MOBILITY. Major interventions include therapeutic exercise and the promotion of ADLs and ambulation by teaching about health and the use of assistive devices.

Certain recreational activities may also be therapeutic, such as swimming to enhance chest and arm muscles. Aerobic exercises (e.g., walking, biking, swimming, aerobic dance) are also recommended. Kim et al. (2012) reported the effectiveness of an aquarobic (water exercise) program for patients with osteoarthritis in increasing MOBILITY and reducing PAIN. Exercises may be prescribed by rehabilitation therapists for the patient with OA, but you will need to reinforce their techniques and principles. The ideal time for exercise is immediately after the application of heat. To prevent further joint damage, teach patients to carefully follow the instructions for exercise outlined in Chart 18-5.

Collaborate with the PT to evaluate the patient's need for ambulatory aids such as canes, walkers, or platform crutches. Although some patients do not like to use these aids or may forget how to use them, they can help prevent further joint deterioration and PAIN. Collaborate with the OT, if needed, to provide suggestions and devices for assistance for ADLs.

CHART 18-5 Patient and Family Education: Preparing for Self-Management

Exercises for Patients with Osteoarthritis or Rheumatoid Arthritis

- Follow the exercise instructions that have been prescribed specifically for you. There are no universal exercises; your exercises have been specifically tailored to your needs.
- Do your exercises on both "good" and "bad" days. Consistency is important.
- Respect pain. Reduce the number of repetitions when the inflammation is severe and you have more pain.
- Use active rather than active-assist or passive exercise whenever possible.
- Do not substitute your normal activities or household tasks for the prescribed exercises.
- Avoid resistive exercises when your joints are severely inflamed.

Community-Based Care

The patient with OA is not usually hospitalized for the disease itself but is admitted for surgical management. Expect that any patient older than 60 years will have some degree of arthritis and possibly chronic pain that needs to be managed.

Home Care Management. If weight-bearing joints are severely involved, the patient may have difficulty going up or down stairs. Making arrangements to live on one floor with accessibility to all rooms is often the best solution. A home care nurse or case manager may collaborate with a rehabilitation therapist to assess the need for structural alterations to the home to accommodate ambulatory aids and enable the patient to perform ADLs. For example, a kitchen counter may need to be lowered or a seat and handrails may need to be installed in the shower. If the patient has undergone a total hip replacement, an elevated toilet seat is necessary for several weeks postoperatively to prevent excessive hip flexion. Patients who have TKAs may also find elevated toilet seats easier to use.

Self-Management Education. Self-management education (SME) is an effective psychosocially focused nonpharmacologic intervention (Shin & Kolanowski, 2010). Learning how to protect joints is the most important part of patient and family education. Preventing further damage to joints slows the progression of OA and minimizes PAIN. Explain the general principles of joint protection, and give practical examples (Chart 18-6).

As with other diseases in which drugs and nutritional therapy are used, teach the patient and family the drug therapy protocol, desired effects and potential side effects, and toxic effects. Emphasize the importance of reducing weight and eating a well-balanced diet to promote tissue healing.

Many patients with arthritis look for a cure after becoming frustrated and desperate about the course of the disease and treatment. Better control of arthritis is possible, but cure is not yet available. Unfortunately, tabloids, books, media, and the Internet often report "curative" remedies. People spend billions of dollars each year on quackery, including liniments, special diets, and copper bracelets. More hazardous substances, such as snake venom and industrial cleaners, are also advertised as remedies. Refer the patient to the Arthritis Foundation for up-to-date information about these "cures." The practice of wearing a copper bracelet will not cure arthritis, but it will not cause harm. If the patient is using a potentially harmful substance or method, however, reinforce the need to avoid the unproven remedy and explain why it should not be used. Respect the patient's preferences, values, and beliefs for using benign remedies that do not cause harm.

With most types of arthritis and connective tissue disease (CTD), patients must live with a chronic, unpredictable, and painful disorder. Their roles, self-esteem, and body image may be affected by these diseases. Body image is often not as devastating in OA as in the inflammatory arthritic diseases, such as RA. The psychosocial component associated with having arthritis is discussed in more detail later in this chapter in the Rheumatoid Arthritis section.

Health Care Resources. The patient who has undergone surgery may need help from community resources. After an arthroplasty, he or she may need assistance with MOBILITY. The patient may be discharged to home or an inpatient unit. Collaborate with the case manager and surgeon to determine the best placement. If the patient is discharged to home, home care nurses may be approved for third-party payment for several visits, depending on the presence of any existing systemic diseases. A home care aide may visit the home to help with hygiene-related needs, and a physical therapist may work with ambulatory and mobility skills. For older patients, a family member, significant other, or other caregiver should be in the home for at least the first few weeks when the patient needs the most assistance. Emphasize the need for patient safety, especially interventions to prevent falls as described in Chapter 2.

Provide written instructions about the required care, regardless of whether the patient goes home or to another inpatient facility. As required by The Joint Commission's National Patient Safety Goals (NPSGs) and other health care accrediting organizations, hand-off communication with the new care provider is essential for seamless continuity of care.

The Arthritis Foundation (www.arthritis.org) is an important community resource for all patients with arthritis and other CTDs. This organization provides information to lay people and health care professionals and refers patients and their families to other resources as needed. Local support groups can help them cope with these diseases.

◆ Evaluation: Outcomes

Evaluate the care of the patient with OA on the basis of the identified priority problems. The expected outcomes are that he or she:

- Achieves PAIN control to a pain intensity level of 3 to 4 on a scale of 0 to 10 or at a level that is acceptable to the patient
- Moves and functions in his or her own environment independently with or without assistive devices

RHEUMATOID ARTHRITIS

❖ PATHOPHYSIOLOGY

Rheumatoid arthritis (RA) is a chronic, progressive, systemic inflammatory autoimmune disease process that affects primarily the synovial joints. **Systemic** means this disease affects the body system, affecting many joints and other tissues. RA affects over 1.3 million people, and Euro-Americans have the disease

---

CHART 18-6 **Patient and Family Education: Preparing for Self-Management**

Evidence-Based Instructions for Joint Protection

- Use large joints instead of small ones; for example, place your purse strap over your shoulder instead of grasping the purse with your hand.
- Do not turn a doorknob clockwise. Turn it counterclockwise to avoid twisting your arm and promoting ulnar deviation.
- Use two hands instead of one to hold objects.
- Sit in a chair that has a high, straight back.
- When getting out of bed, do not push off with your fingers; use the entire palm of both hands.
- Do not bend at your waist; instead, bend your knees while keeping your back straight.
- Use long-handled devices, such as a hairbrush with an extended handle.
- Use assistive/adaptive devices, such as Velcro closures and built-up utensil handles, to protect your joints.
- Do not use pillows in bed except a small one under your head.
- Avoid twisting or wringing your hands.

more often than other groups (Arthritis Foundation, 2013c). The cause for this trend is not known.

In RA, transformed autoantibodies (rheumatoid factors [RFs]) are formed that attack healthy tissue, especially synovium, causing inflammation. The disease then begins to involve the articular cartilage, joint capsule, and surrounding ligaments and tendons. IMMUNITY and INFLAMMATION factors cause cartilage damage in patients with RA (McCance et al., 2014):

- CD4 T–helper cells and other immune cells in synovial fluid promote cytokine release, especially interleukin-1 (IL-1) and tumor necrosis factor–alpha (TNFA), which attack cartilage.
- Neutrophils and other inflammatory cells in the joint are activated and break down the cartilage.
- Immune complexes deposit in synovium, and osteoclasts are activated.
- B- and T-lymphocytes of the immune system are stimulated and increase the inflammatory response. (Also see Chapter 17 for a complete discussion of the inflammatory response.)

The synovium then thickens and becomes hyperemic, fluid accumulates in the joint space, and a pannus forms. The **pannus** is vascular granulation tissue composed of inflammatory cells; it erodes articular cartilage and eventually destroys bone. As a result, in late disease, fibrous adhesions, bony ankylosis, and calcifications occur; bone loses density, and secondary osteoporosis occurs.

Permanent joint changes may be avoided if RA is diagnosed early. Early and aggressive treatment to suppress synovitis may lead to a remission. RA is a disease characterized by natural remissions and exacerbations. Interdisciplinary health care team management helps control the disease to decrease the intensity and number of exacerbations. Preventing flares helps prevent joint erosion and permanent joint damage.

Because rheumatoid arthritis is a systemic disease, areas of the body besides the synovial joints can be affected. Inflammatory responses similar to those occurring in synovial tissue may occur in any organ or body system in which connective tissue is prevalent. If blood vessel involvement (**vasculitis**) occurs, the organ supplied by that vessel can be affected, leading to eventual failure of the organ or system in late disease.

The etiology of RA remains unclear, but research suggests a *combination of environmental and genetic factors.* Some researchers also suspect that female reproductive hormones influence the development of RA because it affects women more often than men—usually young to middle-aged women. Others suspect that infectious organisms may play a role, particularly the Epstein-Barr virus (McCance et al., 2014). Physical and emotional stresses have been linked to exacerbations of the disorder and may be contributing factors or "triggers" to its development.

GENETIC/GENOMIC CONSIDERATIONS

Patient-Centered Care QSEN

Research has shown that there is a strong association between RA and several human leukocyte antigen (HLA)-DR alleles. The cause of this association is not clear, but most HLA diseases are autoimmune (Nussbaum et al., 2007). *DR* alleles, especially *DR4* and *DRB1,* are the primary genetic factors contributing to the development of RA. *DR4* is associated with more severe forms of the disease. Other contributing factors are being researched.

CHART 18-7   Key Features

The Patient with Rheumatoid Arthritis

Early Manifestations
Joint
- Inflammation

Systemic
- Low-grade fever
- Fatigue
- Weakness
- Anorexia
- Paresthesias

Late Manifestations
Joint
- Deformities (e.g., swan neck or ulnar deviation)
- Moderate to severe pain and morning stiffness

Systemic
- Osteoporosis
- Severe fatigue
- Anemia
- Weight loss
- Subcutaneous nodules
- Peripheral neuropathy
- Vasculitis
- Pericarditis
- Fibrotic lung disease
- Sjögren's syndrome
- Kidney disease
- Felty's syndrome

❖ PATIENT-CENTERED COLLABORATIVE CARE

◆ Assessment

The onset of rheumatoid arthritis (RA) may be acute and severe or slow and progressive; patients may have vague symptoms that last for several months before diagnosis. The onset of the disease is more common in the winter months than in the warmer months. The manifestations of RA can be categorized as early or late disease and as articular (joint) or extra-articular (Chart 18-7).

Physical Assessment/Clinical Manifestations

Early Disease Manifestations. The patient with RA typically reports joint signs and symptoms of joint INFLAMMATION, generalized weakness, and fatigue. Anorexia and a weight loss of about 2 to 3 pounds (1 kg) usually occur early in the disease process. Persistent low-grade fever may accompany these manifestations. In patients with early disease, the upper-extremity joints are involved initially—often the proximal interphalangeal (PIP) and metacarpophalangeal (MCP) joints of the hands. These joints may be slightly reddened, warm, stiff, swollen, and tender or painful, particularly on palpation (caused by synovitis). The typical pattern of joint involvement in RA is bilateral and symmetric (e.g., both wrists). The number of joints involved usually increases as the disease progresses. In early disease, the patient may report migrating symptoms known as **migratory arthritis**.

The presence of only *one* hot, swollen, painful joint (out of proportion to the other joints) may mean the joint is infected. *Refer the patient to the health care provider (generally the rheumatologist) immediately if this is the case.* Single hot, swollen joints are considered infected until proven otherwise and require immediate long-term antibiotic treatment.

Late Disease Manifestations. As the disease worsens, the joints become progressively inflamed and very painful. The patient usually has frequent morning stiffness (also called the **gel phenomenon**), which lasts for 45 minutes to several hours after awakening. On palpation, the joints feel soft and look puffy because of synovitis and **effusions** (joint swelling with fluid, especially the knees). The fingers often appear spindle-like. Note any muscle atrophy (which can result from disuse secondary to joint pain) and a decreased range of motion in the affected joints.

Most or all synovial joints are eventually affected. The temporomandibular joint (TMJ) may be involved in severe disease, but such involvement is uncommon. When the TMJ is affected, the patient may have PAIN when chewing or opening the mouth.

When the spinal column is involved, the cervical joints are most likely to be affected. During clinical examination, gently palpate the posterior cervical spine and identify it as cervical pain, tenderness, or loss of motion.

> ## ! NURSING SAFETY PRIORITY (QSEN)
> ### *Critical Rescue*
>
> Cervical disease may result in subluxation, especially of the first and second vertebrae. This complication may be life threatening because branches of the phrenic nerve that supply the diaphragm are restricted and respiratory function may be compromised. The patient is also in danger of becoming quadriparetic (weak in all extremities) or quadriplegic (paralyzed in all extremities). If a person with RA reports cervical PAIN (may radiate down one arm) or loss of range of motion in the cervical spine, notify the health care provider immediately.

Joint Involvement. *Joint deformity* occurs as a late, articular manifestation, and secondary osteoporosis can cause bone fractures. Observe common deformities, especially in the hands and feet (Fig. 18-6). Extensive wrist involvement can result in carpal tunnel syndrome (see Chapter 51 for assessment and management of carpal tunnel syndrome).

Gently palpate the tissues around the joints to elicit PAIN or tenderness associated with other rheumatoid complications, unless the patient is having severe joint pain. For example, Baker's cysts (enlarged popliteal bursae behind the knee) may occur and cause tissue compression and pain. Tendon rupture is also possible, particularly rupture of the Achilles tendon.

Systemic Complications and Associated Syndromes. Numerous extra-articular clinical manifestations are associated with advanced disease. Assess the patient to ascertain systemic involvement. In addition to increased joint swelling and tenderness, *moderate to severe weight loss, fever, and extreme fatigue* are common in late disease exacerbations, often called "flare-ups." Some patients have the characteristic round, movable, nontender subcutaneous nodules, which usually appear on the ulnar surface of the arm, on the fingers, or along the Achilles tendon. These nodules can disappear and reappear at any time and are associated with severe, destructive disease. Rheumatoid nodules usually are not a problem themselves; however, they occasionally open and become infected and may interfere with ADLs. Accidentally bumping the nodules may cause discomfort. Occasionally, nodules occur in the lungs.

Inflammation of the blood vessels results in *vasculitis*, particularly of small to medium-size vessels. When arterial involvement occurs, major organs can become ischemic and malfunction. Assess for ischemic skin lesions that appear in groups as small, brownish spots, most commonly around the nail bed (periungual lesions). Monitor the number of lesions, note their location each day, and report vascular changes to the health care provider. Increased lesions indicate increased vasculitis, and a decreased number indicates decreased vasculitis. Also carefully assess any larger lesions that appear on the lower extremities. These lesions can lead to ulcerations, which heal slowly as a result of decreased circulation. Peripheral neuropathy associated with decreased circulation can cause footdrop and paresthesias (burning and tingling sensations), usually in older adults.

Respiratory complications may manifest as *pleurisy, pneumonitis, diffuse interstitial fibrosis, and pulmonary hypertension.* Cardiac complications include *pericarditis and myocarditis.* These health problems are discussed elsewhere in this text. Assess for eye involvement, which typically manifests as *iritis and scleritis.* If either of these complications is present, the sclera of one or both eyes is reddened and the pupils have an irregular shape. Visual disturbances may occur.

Several syndromes are seen in patients with advanced RA. The most common is Sjögren's syndrome, which includes a triad of:
- Dry eyes (keratoconjunctivitis sicca [KCS], or the sicca syndrome)
- Dry mouth (xerostomia)
- Dry vagina (in some cases)

Note the patient's report of dry mouth or dry eyes. Some patients state that their eyes feel "gritty," as if sand is in their eyes. Inspect the mouth for dry, sticky membranes and the eyes for redness and lack of tearing.

Less commonly observed is Felty's syndrome, which is characterized by RA, hepatosplenomegaly (enlarged liver and spleen), and leukopenia. Caplan's syndrome is characterized by the presence of rheumatoid nodules in the lungs.

Psychosocial Assessment. Rheumatoid arthritis (RA) and other inflammatory types of arthritis are chronic diseases that can be crippling if not well controlled. Fear of becoming disabled and dependent, uncertainty about the disease process, altered body image, devaluation of self, frustration, and depression are common psychosocial problems. Physical limitations and PAIN caused by disease may limit MOBILITY and ADLs. These limitations can result in role changes in the family and society. For example, the person may not be able to cook for the family or be an active sexual partner. In addition, extreme fatigue often causes patients to desire an early bedtime and may result in a reluctance to socialize.

Body changes caused by joint changes and steroid therapy (if used) may also cause poor self-esteem and body image. Because many societies value people with physically fit, attractive bodies, the patient with RA may be embarrassed to be seen in public places. The patient may grieve or experience degrees of depression. He or she may have feelings of helplessness

FIG. 18-6 Common joint deformities seen in rheumatoid arthritis.

caused by a loss of control over a disease that can "consume" the body. Fortunately, newer drugs have improved the treatment of RA and provide the patient with hope and better disease control. Only a small percentage of patients with RA become wheelchair dependent.

Living with a chronic disease and its PAIN is difficult for the patient and family. Chronic suffering and pain affect quality of life. Assess the patient's emotional and mental status in relation to the disease and its problems. Evaluate his or her support systems and resources. Patients who are knowledgeable about their disease and treatment options feel emotionally stronger to cope with their disease and better able to discuss treatment options with their health care provider.

Laboratory Assessment. Laboratory tests help support a diagnosis of RA, but no single test or group of tests can confirm it. Chart 18-8 summarizes the most common laboratory tests that the health care provider may use for diagnosing connective tissue diseases.

The test for *rheumatoid factor (RF)* measures the presence of unusual antibodies of the immunoglobulins G (IgG) and M (IgM) types that develop in a number of connective tissue diseases. Many patients with RA have a positive titer (greater than 1:80), but not all positive results indicate the disease, *especially in older adults* (Pagana & Pagana, 2014).

The *antinuclear antibody (ANA)* test measures the titer of a group of antibodies that destroy the nuclei of cells and cause tissue death in patients with autoimmune disease. The fluorescent method is sometimes referred to as *FANA*. If this test result is positive (a value higher than 1:40), various subtypes of this antibody are identified and measured.

When RA patients also have Sjögren's syndrome (SS) or if the syndrome occurs as a separate disease, several unusual anti–SS antibody types may be present. In particular, *anti–SS-A (Ro)* and *anti–SS-B (La)* antibodies are present in about 60% to 70%

of those with Sjögren's syndrome or those with secondary Sjögren's and RA (Pagana & Pagana, 2014).

Serum *complement proteins*, especially C3 and C4, are usually decreased in autoimmune diseases, including RA and lupus. An elevated *erythrocyte sedimentation rate (ESR)*, or "sed rate," can confirm INFLAMMATION or INFECTION anywhere in the body. An elevated ESR helps support a diagnosis of an unspecified inflammatory disease. The test is most useful to monitor the course of a disease, especially for inflammatory autoimmune diseases. In general, the more severe the disease gets, the higher the ESR rises; as the disease improves or goes into remission, the ESR level decreases.

The *high-sensitivity C-reactive protein*, or *hsCRP*, is another useful test to measure INFLAMMATION and may be done with or instead of the ESR. As the name implies, it is more sensitive to inflammatory changes than the ESR. It is also very useful for detecting infection anywhere in the body.

The presence of most chronic diseases usually causes mild to moderate anemia, which contributes to the patient's fatigue. Therefore monitor the patient's complete blood count (CBC) for a low hemoglobin, hematocrit, and red blood cell (RBC) count. An increase in white blood cell (WBC) count is consistent with an inflammatory response. A decrease in the WBC count may indicate Felty's syndrome, a complication associated with late RA. Thrombocytosis (increased platelets) can also occur in patients with late RA. Additional laboratory tests may be performed depending on the body systems and organs that may be affected by the disease. For example, if heart involvement is suspected, the health care provider may request cardiac enzymes.

Other Diagnostic Assessment. A standard x-ray is used to visualize the joint changes and deformities typical of RA. A CT scan may help determine the presence and degree of cervical spine involvement.

CHART 18-8 Laboratory Profile

Connective Tissue Disease

TEST	NORMAL RANGE FOR ADULTS	SIGNIFICANCE OF ABNORMAL FINDINGS
Rheumatoid factor	Negative	Positive or increase indicative of possible RA or other CTD; may also be elevated in leukemia, liver disease, and kidney disease
ANA (total)	Negative (if positive, types of ANA identified [e.g., anti-ENA, anti-Smith, anti-ss-A (Ro)] to indicate what part of cells are involved)	Elevations common in SLE, SSc, RA, and other inflammatory CTDs (5% of healthy adults have positive ANA results)
Serum complement	*Total:* 30-75 units/mL (*C3:* 75-175 mg/dL; *C4:* 22-45 mg/dL)	Decreased values indicative of active autoimmune disease, such as SLE, and other problems like anemia, infection, and malnutrition
Erythrocyte sedimentation rate (ESR)	*Male:* up to 15 mm/hr *Female:* up to 20 mm/hr	Increased in inflammatory diseases, like RA, SLE, PMR, temporal arteritis; also elevated in patients with bacterial infections or severe anemias
SPEP	*Total:* 6.4-8.3 g/dL	
Albumin	3.5-5.0 g/dL	Decreased level occurs with chronic inflammation or infection; also decreased in malnutrition and advanced cirrhosis
Globulin	2.3-3.4 g/dL	
Alpha$_1$ globulin	0.1-0.3 g/dL	Increased level possible in RA
Alpha$_2$ globulin	0.6-1.0 g/dL	
Beta globulin	0.7-1.1 g/dL	
Gamma globulin	0.8-1.6 g/dL	Increased levels indicative of CTD (inflammatory type)
HLA testing (*HLA-B27*)	None	Presence of *HLA-B27* indicative of Reiter's syndrome or ankylosing spondylitis

ANA, Antinuclear antibody; *CTD,* connective tissue disease; *ENA,* extractable nuclear antigens; *HLA,* human leukocyte antigen; *PMR,* polymyalgia rheumatica; *RA,* rheumatoid arthritis; *SLE,* systemic lupus erythematosus; *SPEP,* serum protein electrophoresis; *SSc,* systemic sclerosis.

An *arthrocentesis* is an invasive procedure that may be used for patients with joint swelling caused by excess synovial fluid (effusion). It may be performed at the bedside or in a health care provider's office or clinic. After administering a local anesthetic, the provider inserts a large-gauge needle into the joint (usually the knee) to aspirate a sample of synovial fluid to relieve pressure. The fluid is analyzed for inflammatory cells and immune complexes, including RF. Fluid from patients with RA typically reveals increased WBCs, cloudiness, and volume.

Teach the patient to use ice and rest the affected joint for 24 hours after arthrocentesis. Often the health care provider will recommend acetaminophen as needed for PAIN. If increased pain or swelling occurs, teach the patient or family to notify the health care provider immediately.

! NURSING SAFETY PRIORITY (QSEN)
Action Alert

After an arthrocentesis, monitor the insertion site for bleeding or leakage of synovial fluid. Notify the health care provider if either of these problems occurs.

A bone scan or joint scan can also assess the extent of joint involvement. MRI may be performed to assess spinal column disease or other joint involvement.

Because RA can affect multiple body systems, tests to diagnose specific systemic manifestations are performed as necessary. For example, electromyography helps confirm peripheral neuropathy. Pulmonary function tests help determine the presence of lung involvement.

? NCLEX EXAMINATION CHALLENGE
Physiological Integrity

Which assessment findings will the nurse expect for the client with early-stage rheumatoid arthritis? **Select all that apply.**
A. Heberden's nodes
B. Elevated erythrocyte sedimentation rate (ESR)
C. Positive antinuclear antibody (ANA) titer
D. Severe weight loss
E. Joint inflammation
F. Red, swollen joints

◆ Interventions

As in other types of arthritis, the interdisciplinary health care team manages PAIN by using a combination of pharmacologic and nonpharmacologic measures. A synovectomy to remove inflamed synovium may be needed for joints like the knee or elbow. Total joint arthroplasty (TJA) may be indicated when other measures fail to relieve PAIN. TJA is discussed in the Osteoarthritis section of this chapter.

Managing Inflammation and Pain. The expected outcome is that the disease goes into remission and its progression slows to decrease PAIN, prevent joint destruction, and increase MOBILITY. Drug therapy and nonpharmacologic interventions are used to help meet this outcome.

Drug Therapy. Some drugs prescribed for RA have antiinflammatory and/or analgesic actions. Other drugs are immunosuppressive and disease modifying, which may cause remission of the illness and prevent erosive joint changes.

Biological response modifiers make up the newest class of disease-modifying drugs that help reduce signals for the immune system to cause INFLAMMATION (Chart 18-9). Patients with inflammatory diseases other than RA are also using various biological response modifying drugs successfully. Although RA is a chronic disease and no cure is yet available, drugs now used can better control the disease and prevent further deterioration.

The health care provider, often a rheumatologist, makes decisions about appropriate drug therapy for patients with rheumatoid disease based on the severity of the disease. Initially, most patients are managed with **disease-modifying antirheumatic drugs (DMARDs)**. As the name implies, these drugs are given to slow the progression of the disease.

First-Line Disease-Modifying Antirheumatic Drugs. Methotrexate (MTX) (Rheumatrex), an immunosuppressive medication, in a low, once-a-week dose (generally 25 mg or less per week orally) is the mainstay of therapy for RA because it is effective and relatively inexpensive. It is a slow-acting drug, taking 4 to 6 weeks to begin to control joint INFLAMMATION. Observe for desired therapeutic drug effects, such as a decrease in joint PAIN and swelling.

Monitor patients for potential adverse effects, such as decreasing WBCs and platelets (as a result of bone marrow suppression) or elevations in liver enzymes or serum creatinine.

! NURSING SAFETY PRIORITY (QSEN)
Drug Alert

Patients taking MTX are at risk for INFECTION. Teach them to avoid crowds and people who are ill. Remind patients to avoid alcoholic beverages while taking MTX to prevent liver toxicity. Teach them to observe and report other side and toxic effects, which include mouth sores and acute dyspnea from pneumonitis. Rarely, lymph node tumor (lymphoma) has been associated in those who have RA and are taking MTX. Folic acid, one of the B vitamins, is often given to those who are taking MTX to help decrease some of the drug's side effects.

Pregnancy is not recommended while taking methotrexate because birth defects are possible. *Strict birth control is recommended for childbearing women who are in need of MTX to control their RA.* If pregnancy is ever desired, instruct the patient to consult the rheumatologist as well as an obstetric/gynecologic (OB/GYN) health care provider. Generally, the health care provider will discontinue the drug at least 3 months before planned pregnancy. MTX may be restarted after birth if the patient does not breast-feed (Lilley et al., 2014).

Leflunomide (Arava) may be prescribed for some patients. It is a slow-acting immune-modulating medication that helps diminish inflammatory symptoms of joint swelling and stiffness and improves MOBILITY. The drug is generally prescribed as a loading dose of 100 mg orally daily for 3 days followed by 20 mg orally daily thereafter. Inform the patient that Arava takes 4 to 6 weeks and sometimes up to 3 months before maximum benefit is realized.

Arava is a potent medication that is generally tolerated, but side effects of hair loss, diarrhea, decreased WBCs and platelets, or increased liver enzymes have been reported. *Teach patients to report these changes, and monitor laboratory results carefully. Remind them to avoid alcohol. Inform them that Arava can cause birth defects, and therefore recommend strict birth control to*

CHART 18-9 Common Examples of Drug Therapy

Biological Response Modifiers Used for Rheumatoid Arthritis and Other Connective Tissue Diseases*

DRUG AND USUAL DOSAGE	PURPOSE OF DRUG	NURSING INTERVENTIONS	RATIONALES
For *all* biological response modifiers (BRMs) (also called *biologics*)	Neutralize biologic activity of tumor necrosis factor–alpha (TNFA), interleukins (IL), T-lymphocytes, or tyrosine kinase (TK) to decrease immune response and inflammation	Do not give BRMs if patient has a serious infection, TB, or MS. Teach patients taking BRMs to avoid getting live vaccines. Teach patient to avoid crowds and people with infections.	Drugs may exacerbate infections, MS, or lupus. Serious infections, especially respiratory infections, can lead to hospitalization or cause death.
Etanercept (Enbrel): Usually 25 mg subcutaneously twice weekly	TNFA inhibitor	Teach patient to report site reaction. Teach patient how to self-administer drug.	Site reactions can be painful. Patients need to self-administer the drug at home or have another person learn how to give the injections.
Infliximab (Remicade): 3 mg/kg of body weight as IV infusion, followed by the same dose at Weeks 2 and 6. If patient responds, maintenance infusions are given at the same dose every 8 weeks.	TNFA inhibitor	Refrigerate all BRMs except Remicade. Teach patient to report chest pain or difficulty breathing during infusion; monitor blood pressure and infusion site.	Refrigeration prevents drug decomposition. Severe allergic reaction is potentially life threatening; infusion reactions usually subside.
Adalimumab (Humira): 40 mg subcutaneously every 2 weeks	TNFA inhibitor	Teach patient to report site reaction.	Site reactions may occur to indicate local allergic response.
Anakinra (Kineret): Typically 100 mg subcutaneously daily	IL-1 receptor antagonist	Teach patient to monitor site for reaction (occurs more commonly when compared with other BRMs). Monitor WBC count. Teach patient to report respiratory symptoms, such as cough and fever. Teach patient that malignancies can result from taking this drug.	Site reactions may occur. Drug can cause a severe decrease in WBC count and make patient very susceptible to infection. Drug can cause serious respiratory infections and various types of cancers.
Abatacept (Orencia): Based on body weight from 500 to 1000 mg IV each week for 2 wks, and then may be given at longer intervals for maintenance	Selective T-lymphocyte co-stimulator modulator (T-cell inhibitor)	Report cough, dizziness, and sore throat; do not receive live vaccines while taking the drug. Monitor for dyspnea, wheezing, flushing, itching.	Serious respiratory infections can occur. This drug can cause a mild to moderate allergic reaction.
Rituximab (Rituxan): Two 1000-mg IV doses given 2 weeks apart initially, followed by the same dosing every 4-6 months depending on the patient's response	Monoclonal antibody	Observe for infusion reaction as above.	Drug can cause a local allergic response.
Golimumab (Simponi): 50 mg subcutaneously once a month	TNFA inhibitor	Teach patient to report signs and symptoms of infection, including fever and malaise; teach patient to avoid live vaccines while taking drug. Teach patient about adverse drug effects including hypertension, GI distress, and infection from opportunistic pathogens; report signs and symptoms of these problems to the health care provider.	Drug has a black box warning about serious infections from opportunistic pathogens that can lead to hospitalizations or death. These adverse drug effects can lead to serious illness.
Tocilizumab (Actemra): Dose varies based on weight; given IV initially at 4 mg/kg and then increased to 8 mg/kg of body weight; drug may also be self-administered as a subcutaneous prefilled injection; dosing intervals depend on the patient's response and route of administration	IL-6 inhibitor	Teach patient the importance of having frequent WBC, platelet, and liver enzyme testing.	Drug can cause decreased WBCs and platelets, and liver dysfunction.

MS, Multiple sclerosis; *TB*, tuberculosis; *TNF*, tumor necrosis factor; *WBC*, white blood cell.

*This is not a comprehensive list; this chart lists only the common biological response modifiers (BRMs) used for rheumatoid arthritis and other connective tissue diseases.

women of childbearing age. Tell patients to contact the health care provider immediately if pregnancy occurs while taking the drug. Cholestyramine (Questran) is available to help block the drug's action.

Another DMARD sometimes used for RA is hydroxychloroquine (Plaquenil). This drug slows the progression of mild rheumatoid disease before it worsens (see Chart 18-9). It is an antimalarial drug that helps decrease joint and muscle PAIN. Patients generally tolerate Plaquenil quite well. In a few cases, mild stomach discomfort, light-headedness, or headache has been reported.

⚠ NURSING SAFETY PRIORITY (QSEN)

Drug Alert

The most serious adverse effect of Plaquenil is retinal damage. Teach patients to report blurred vision or headache. Remind them to have an eye examination before taking the drug and every 6 months to detect changes in the cornea, lens, or retina. If this rare complication occurs, the health care provider discontinues the drug (Lilley et al., 2014).

Nonsteroidal Anti-inflammatory Drugs. NSAIDs are sometimes used for RA to relieve PAIN and INFLAMMATION. The choice of which one to prescribe depends on the patient's needs and tolerance, as well as the scientific evidence supporting the drug therapy. To decrease GI problems, the NSAID may be given with an H2-blocking agent, such as ranitidine (Zantac) or misoprostol (Cytotec). If there is no clinical change after 6 to 8 weeks, the health care provider may discontinue the current NSAID and try another one or change to a different drug class.

It was once thought that celecoxib (Celebrex), a COX-2 inhibiting NSAID, should be given rather than the older NSAIDs like ibuprofen. However, all COX-2 inhibiting drugs have recently been associated with cardiovascular disease, such as myocardial infarction, and some have been taken off the market. The risk for GI bleeding is also high in patients taking Celebrex, and the drug cannot be given to those who have had recent open heart surgery.

Biological Response Modifiers. As a group, **biological response modifiers (BRMs),** sometimes called **biologics,** are one of the newest classes of DMARDs. Most BRMs neutralize the biologic activity of tumor necrosis factor–alpha (TNFA) by inhibiting its binding with TNF receptors. Any one of the BRMs may be tried. If one drug is not effective, the health care provider prescribes another drug in the same class. All these drugs are extremely expensive at this time, and insurance companies may not completely pay for their use. Some patients receive one of these drugs in addition to the drugs in this Drug Therapy section.

Teach patients receiving any one of the BRMs that they are at a high risk for developing INFECTION. Instruct them to stay away from people with infections and to avoid large crowds if possible. Remind patients with multiple sclerosis (MS), tuberculosis (TB), or a positive TB test that they should not receive TNF inhibitors because they make patients susceptible to flare-ups of these diseases. Determine whether the patient has had a recent negative purified protein derivative (PPD) test for TB. If not, a PPD skin test is typically administered and the selected BRM is not started until a negative test result is confirmed. Collaborate with the health care provider to ensure that this process is complete.

Etanercept (Enbrel) is given subcutaneously as 25 mg twice weekly for most patients. Immunosuppression with medications such as methotrexate is generally tried before using Enbrel or other biological response modifiers. Methotrexate is often given in combination with biologic therapies because the combination may be more effective than either drug alone (Cranwell-Bruce, 2011). Most patients tolerate Enbrel or Enbrel and methotrexate together; however, laboratory monitoring is important. Combination therapy requires CBC, serum creatinine, and a liver panel to be drawn regularly, generally every 4 to 8 weeks. In general, clinical outcomes with Enbrel have been excellent.

Teach the patient or family member how to self-administer Enbrel injections. Injection site reaction and systemic INFECTION (especially respiratory) are possible adverse effects. Ice and hydrocortisone 1% cream can be used if a red, itchy rash at the injection site develops. Teach the patient to notify the health care provider if infection or a delay in wound healing occurs.

Infliximab (Remicade), first approved to treat Crohn's disease, is given in a single IV infusion over several hours. The initial dose generally used for RA is 3 mg/kg of body weight. The drug dosage is repeated at weeks 2 and 6. After these first three infusions, a maintenance dose of 3 mg/kg of body weight is given every 8 weeks, depending on the response of the patient. For patients who do not respond to the first three infusions, the drug dosage may be increased up to 10 mg/kg of body weight given at 4-week intervals. The risk of side effects and adverse effects increases at higher doses. Patients typically take methotrexate before starting Remicade and continue on combination therapy.

⚠ NURSING SAFETY PRIORITY (QSEN)

Drug Alert

Teach the patient to report and observe for symptoms of Remicade infusion reaction: chest discomfort, tachycardia, shortness of breath, or light-headedness. If any of these symptoms are reported, decrease the IV rate or discontinue it!

The symptoms of infusion reaction generally subside, but the health care provider must be notified in case medical assistance is needed. Dose, rate, and interval changes may be needed. Acetaminophen and Benadryl are medications often given before the start of Remicade and are often used at the time of reported infusion reaction. Those who experience serious adverse effects, such as hypertension or anaphylaxis, require permanent discontinuation of the drug.

Adalimumab (Humira) is the first fully human TNFA inhibitor and is given by subcutaneous injection. Symptoms of inflammatory arthritis tend to decrease with the use of Humira, including less joint swelling, less stiffness, and better MOBILITY. Injection site reactions and adverse effects similar to the other TNFA inhibitors have been reported. Careful monitoring, especially with combination therapy of Humira and methotrexate or other drug that affects the body's IMMUNITY, is important and similar to combination therapy with other BRMs.

Anakinra (Kineret) is another biological response modifier. Instead of affecting tumor necrosis factor–alpha (TNFA), however, it works to inhibit a different protein signal of the immune system called *interleukin-1 (IL-1).* IL-1 is also a pro-inflammatory protein that signals the immune system to increase INFLAMMATION (Cranwell-Bruce, 2011). It is thought that IL-1 is a weaker protein than TNF, but having an alternative drug that targets a different receptor site is helpful when a patient cannot take other biologics. Those who have multiple sclerosis or tuberculosis cannot take TNF inhibitors, but Kineret can be used with this population.

Injection site reactions occur more often with Kineret compared with other BRMs. Ice and hydrocortisone 1% cream are recommended. Remind patients to rotate injection sites. Kineret is administered with a simple jet for self-administration. The patient has the option to use the simple jet or administer the subcutaneous injection traditionally.

Abatacept (Orencia) and *rituximab (Rituxan, MabThera)* require IV infusions every 2 weeks to start and then may be more spread out, depending on the drug. Like the results of the other BRMs, patients usually report feeling a benefit from these drugs in 2 weeks, but it may take months for the maximum benefit to be seen. *Golimumab (Simponi)* is the first biologic that is administered only once each month for both RA and psoriatic arthritis. Teach patients that this drug has a black box warning for serious INFECTIONS that may lead to hospitalization or death from opportunistic pathogens (Cranwell-Bruce, 2011).

Tocilizumab (Actemra) is given when the patient cannot tolerate other drugs. Tocilizumab is different from other biologics because it is the first humanized interleukin-6 (IL-6) receptor-inhibiting monoclonal antibody that is available for patients with RA. It can be used alone or in combination with other DMARDs. Teach patients about adverse drug effects, including hypertension, GI distress, infection, and an increase in low-density lipoproteins (LDLs) and liver enzymes. Like for other biologics, teach the patient about the high risk of infection (e.g., tuberculosis) when taking Actemra.

One of the newest biologics is *tofacitinib (Xeljanz),* which has been approved for moderate to severe RA as monotherapy or in combination with methotrexate. This drug is a tyrosine kinase inhibitor (TKI). Tyrosine kinases usually facilitate cytokine-mediated (e.g., interleukin) signals that promote the inflammatory process. Teach patients that tofacitinib carries a black box warning alerting patients about its potential for serious opportunistic INFECTIONS, tuberculosis, lymphoma, and other cancers.

Other Drugs. A few drugs may be given as adjuncts to or instead of the previously described drugs. It is not unusual for a patient to be taking several disease-modifying drugs, such as methotrexate, a BRM, and an adjunct medication. Each drug works differently to relieve symptoms and slow the progression of the disease.

Glucocorticoids (steroids)—usually prednisone (Deltasone)—are given for their fast-acting anti-inflammatory and immunosuppressive effects. Prednisone may be given in high dose for short duration (pulse therapy) or as a low chronic dose. Moderate-dose short-term tapering bridge therapy may be used when inflammation is symptomatic and other RA medications are insufficient or have not yet had an effect.

Chronic steroid therapy can result in numerous complications, such as:
- Diabetes mellitus
- INFECTION
- Fluid and electrolyte imbalances
- Hypertension
- Osteoporosis
- Glaucoma

Some drug effects are dose related, whereas others are not. Observe the patient for complications associated with chronic steroid therapy, and report them to the health care provider. For example, if blood pressure becomes elevated or significant laboratory values change, notify the health care provider.

Instruct patients taking chronic steroids to take calcium 1200 to 1500 mg daily plus vitamin D 400 mg daily to help prevent osteoporosis. Bisphosphonate drugs may also be prescribed. Bone density measurements (DEXA [dual-energy x-ray absorptiometry] scans) are done every 2 to 3 years to monitor for bone loss.

Patients with RA may experience one or a few joints that have more PAIN and INFLAMMATION than the others. Cortisone injections in single joints may be used to relieve local pain and inflammation. Have the patient ice and rest the joint for 24 hours after the procedure. Oral analgesics also are sometimes needed during that time.

Other immunosuppressive agents that may be used as a last resort are *azathioprine (Imuran)* and *cyclophosphamide (Cytoxan).* Cyclophosphamide is sometimes given specifically to control RA vasculitis. Such immunosuppressive drugs may cause bone marrow suppression and occasionally leukemia or lymphoma. White blood cell counts are expected to decrease 7 to 14 days after the administration of IV cyclophosphamide; therefore monitor laboratory results closely to ensure safe limits. Hemorrhagic cystitis is a concern more with oral cyclophosphamide. Instruct the patient to drink water and void frequently (about every 2 hours while awake), which dilutes the urine and empties the bladder, thus decreasing opportunity for bladder irritation from residual drug. Hair thinning or loss can be seen with immunosuppressive medications. Cyclophosphamide may also cause sterility; strict birth control is recommended.

Nonpharmacologic Interventions. Adequate rest, proper positioning, and ice and heat applications are important in pain management. If acute INFLAMMATION is present, ice packs may be applied to "hot" joints for PAIN relief until the inflammation lessens. The ice pack should not be too heavy. At home, the patient can use a small bag of frozen peas or corn as an ice pack.

Heated paraffin (wax) dips may help increase comfort of arthritic hands. Finger and hand exercises are often done more easily after paraffin treatment. To relieve morning stiffness or the pain of late-stage disease, recommend a hot shower rather than a sponge bath or a tub bath. It is often difficult for the patient with RA to get into and out of a bathtub, although special hydraulic lifts and tub chairs are available to allow the patient to bathe. Safety (grab) bars and nonskid tread in the tub or shower floor are important safety features to discuss with all patients. Some older adults prefer using shower chairs and a walk-in shower that does not have a ledge that could cause falls.

Hot packs applied directly to involved joints may be beneficial. Most physical therapy departments have machines that keep hot packs ready anytime they are needed. Teach patients to use the microwave or stovetop heating instructions to warm heat packs at home. Remind them to follow the instructions given with each heating device used.

Plasmapheresis (sometimes called *plasma exchange*) is an in-hospital procedure prescribed by a health care provider in which the patient's plasma is treated to remove the antibodies causing the disease. Although not commonly done, this procedure may be combined with steroid pulse therapy for patients with severe, life-threatening disease.

Complementary and Alternative Therapies. Some patients may have pain relief from hypnosis, acupuncture, imagery, music therapy, or other technique. Stress management is also popular as a PAIN relief intervention. Chapter 3 discusses these therapies in more detail.

Adequate nutrition is an important part of the management of RA. Obesity should be avoided or treated if present. The inflammatory state may place a greater burden on the metabolism of some essential nutrients. This catabolic state may be related to increased cytokine production, specifically tumor necrosis factor.

According to the National Center for Complementary and Alternative Medicine, some supplements have been found to help decrease INFLAMMATION and include:

- Cold water fish or fish oil capsules containing omega-3 fatty acids at 2.5 to 5 g daily (should not be taken if the patient is taking anticoagulant therapy)
- Gamma-linolenic acid (GLA), an omega-6 fatty acid found in the oils of certain plant seeds, such as primrose and black currant

According to the Arthritis Foundation, no one food causes or cures RA; however, healthy nutrition in general is important. Refer the patient to the Arthritis Foundation's pamphlet regarding diet and arthritis. Refer him or her to the dietitian for vitamin- and nutrition-specific questions or recommendations. Teach patients to take any herbal or nutrition supplement under the supervision of a qualified health care provider to prevent adverse events and drug-food or drug-drug interactions.

Other complementary and alternative medicine (CAM) therapies are safe and have been scientifically proven to be effective to help control RA PAIN for most people. Examples include mind-body therapies, such as relaxation techniques, imagery, and spiritual practices. For information about these techniques, see Chapter 3.

Promoting Self-Management. Although the physical appearance of a patient with severe RA may create the image that ADL independence is not possible, a number of alternative and creative methods can be used to perform these activities. *Do not perform these activities for the patient unless asked. Those with RA do not want to be dependent.* For example, hand deformities often prevent a patient from opening packages of food, such as a box of crackers; however, he or she may prefer to use the teeth to open the crackers rather than depend on someone else.

In the hospital or long-term care facility, a patient may not eat because of the barriers of heavy plate covers, milk cartons, small packages of condiments, and heavy containers. Styrofoam or paper cups may bend and collapse as he or she attempts to hold them. A china or heavy plastic cup with handles may be easier to manipulate. Collaborate with the dietitian to assist with access to food and total independence in eating.

When fine motor activities (e.g., squeezing a tube of toothpaste) become impossible, larger joints or body surfaces can substitute for smaller ones. For example, teach how to use the palm of the hand to press the paste onto the brush. Devices such as long-handled brushes can help patients brush their hair; dressing sticks can assist with putting on pants. These examples illustrate the need to assess the problem area, suggest alternative methods, and refer the patient to an occupational or physical therapist for special assistive and adaptive devices if necessary.

Managing Fatigue. Nursing interventions depend in part on identifying the factors contributing to fatigue. For example, increases in PAIN, sleep disturbances, and weakness are posi-

tively associated with increased fatigue. Anemia may also be a contributing factor and may be treated with iron (if an iron deficiency anemia is present), folic acid, or vitamin supplements prescribed by the health care provider. Chronic normochromic or chronic hypochromic anemia often occurs in most chronic systemic diseases. Assess for drug-related blood loss, such as that caused by NSAIDs, by checking the stool for gross or occult blood. *Older white women are the most likely to experience GI bleeding as a result of taking these medications. The reason for this trend is not known.*

When fatigue results from muscle atrophy, the health care provider prescribes an aggressive physical therapy program to strengthen muscles and prevent further atrophy. Patients experience increased fatigue when pain prevents them from getting adequate rest and sleep. Measures to facilitate sleep include promoting a quiet environment, giving warm beverages, and administering hypnotics or relaxants as prescribed, if necessary.

In addition to identifying and managing specific reasons for fatigue, determine the patient's usual daily activities and teach principles of energy conservation, including:

- Pacing activities
- Allowing rest periods
- Setting priorities
- Obtaining assistance when needed

Chart 18-10 lists specific suggestions for conserving energy and thus increasing activity tolerance and MOBILITY.

Enhancing Body Image. Body image may be affected by both the disease process and drug therapy. Steroids can cause a moonfaced appearance, acne, striae, "buffalo humps," and weight gain. Determine the patient's perception of these changes and the impact of the reactions of family and significant others. The most important intervention is communicating acceptance of the patient. When a trusting relationship is established, encourage him or her to express personal feelings.

As a reaction to body image disturbance and the presence of a chronic, painful disease, some patients display behaviors indicative of loss. They may use coping strategies that range from denial or fear to anger or depression. In an attempt to regain control over the effects of the disease process, they may appear to be "manipulative and demanding" and sometimes may be referred to as having an "arthritis personality." *This personality, which represents a negative label, is a myth; using these terms should be avoided.* Patients are trying to cope with the effects of their illness and should be treated with patience and understanding. Continually assess and accept these behaviors, but remain realistic in discussing goals to improve self-esteem. Emphasize their strengths, and help them identify previously successful coping strategies.

CHART 18-10 **Patient and Family Education: Preparing for Self-Management**

Energy Conservation for the Patient with Arthritis

- Balance activity with rest. Take one or two naps each day.
- Pace yourself; do not plan too much for one day.
- Set priorities. Determine which activities are most important, and do them first.
- Delegate responsibilities and tasks to your family and friends.
- Plan ahead to prevent last-minute rushing and stress.
- Learn your own activity tolerance, and do not exceed it.

Community-Based Care

Patients with rheumatoid arthritis (RA) are usually managed at home but, in a few cases, may be institutionalized in a long-term care facility if they become restricted to bed or a wheelchair. Some patients may be transferred to a rehabilitation facility for several weeks to aid in developing strategies, techniques, and skills for independent living at home.

Home Care Management. The amount of home care preparation depends on the severity of the disease. Structural changes may be necessary if there are deficits in ADLs or MOBILITY. Doors must be wide enough to accommodate a wheelchair or walker if one is used. Ramps are needed to prevent the patient in a wheelchair from becoming homebound. If the person cannot use stairs, he or she must have access to facilities for all ADLs on one floor. Handrails should be available in the bathroom and halls.

To promote continued homemaking functions, countertops and appliances may require structural changes. The patient may also require handrails and elevated chairs and toilet seats, which facilitate transfers (Fig. 18-7). *These devices are especially important for older adults with arthritis.*

Self-Management Education. Self-management education (SME) is a vital role for nurses in collaborative management of arthritis. Many people have signs and symptoms of joint INFLAMMATION but do not seek medical attention. Teach them to seek professional health care to reduce PAIN and disability.

Teach patients to discuss any questions with their health care provider before trying any over-the-counter or home remedies. Some remedies may be harmful. Check with the Arthritis Foundation for the latest information on arthritis myths and quackery (www.arthritis.org).

Provide information to the patient and family about drug therapy, as well as joint protection, energy conservation, rest, and exercise. This SME is summarized in Charts 18-5, 18-6, and 18-10.

Assess the patient's coping strategies. The patient with RA often reports being on an "emotional roller coaster" from coping with a chronic illness every day. Control over one's life is an important human need. The patient with an unpredictable chronic disease may lose this control, and this lowers self-esteem. Health care providers must allow the patient to make decisions about care. Families and significant others must also include him or her in decision making. Although the patient's behavior may be perceived as demanding or manipulative, his or her self-esteem cannot be improved without this important aspect of interpersonal relationships.

Increased dependency also affects a sense of control and self-esteem. Some people ignore their health needs and portray a tough image for others by insisting that they need no assistance. Emphasize to the patient and family that asking for help may be the best decision at times to prevent further joint damage and disease progression.

RA may also affect work and social roles. The patient may have physical difficulty doing tasks that require lifting, climbing, grasp, or gross or fine motor activities. The severity of RA disease may cause difficulty with total number of hours worked. Some people with RA can do their jobs well without problem; others may have varying degrees of difficulty. Those who can no longer do their job at work may need to discuss with their employer having a lighter workload, but some may need to file for disability with their company and Social Security office.

Health Care Resources. The need for health care resources for the patient with RA is similar to that for the patient with osteoarthritis. A home care nurse or aide, physical therapist, or occupational therapist may be needed during severe exacerbations or as the disease progresses. In collaboration with the case manager, identify these resources and make sure they are available as needed. The Arthritis Foundation is an excellent source of information and support.

Arthritis support groups and self-help courses provide the education and the support that patients, families, and friends need. Refer the patient to a psychological counselor or religious or spiritual leader for emotional support and guidance during times of crisis or as needed. Identify and recommend other support systems within the family and community when necessary.

❓ CLINICAL JUDGMENT CHALLENGE

Teamwork and Collaboration; Safety QSEN

An 81-year-old woman with RA has been controlled with methotrexate for 18 years. Recently she experienced increased joint pain and swelling in her right knee that have affected her mobility and activity level. She walks with a cane in the community but uses a walker at home. Earlier in the week, she almost fell while walking to her car after she left the bank. The rheumatologist plans to add etanercept (Enbrel) to her drug regimen.

1. With what members of the health care team might you collaborate as part of her plan of care?
2. What safety measures are needed before she begins taking Enbrel?
3. What self-management education will she need before starting Enbrel?
4. What home and community assessment might be needed to ensure her safety?

LUPUS ERYTHEMATOSUS

❖ PATHOPHYSIOLOGY

The two main classifications of lupus are discoid lupus erythematosus (DLE) and systemic lupus erythematosus (SLE). A small percentage of patients with lupus have the DLE type, which affects only the skin.

Unlike DLE, systemic lupus erythematosus is a chronic, progressive, inflammatory connective tissue disorder that can

FIG. 18-7 Handrails and an elevated toilet seat make transfers easier for the patient.

cause major body organs and systems to fail. It is characterized by spontaneous remissions and exacerbations ("flare-ups"), and the onset may be acute or insidious (slow). The condition is potentially fatal, but most patients with SLE live many years after diagnosis and lead productive lives. Improvements in determining the cause, diagnosis, and treatment of lupus account for the prolonged survival.

Lupus is thought to be an autoimmune process. Antinuclear antibodies (ANAs) primarily affect the DNA, ribonucleic acid (RNA), and other components within the cell nuclei. As a result, immune complexes form in the serum and organ tissues, which cause INFLAMMATION, damage, and destruction (McCance et al., 2014). These complexes invade organs directly or cause vasculitis (vessel inflammation), which deprives the organs of arterial blood and oxygen.

Autoimmune complexes in SLE tend to be most attracted to the glomeruli of the kidneys. Therefore many of these patients have some degree of kidney involvement, called *lupus nephritis*—the leading cause of death from the disease. Other causes of death are cardiac and central nervous system involvement.

🌐 CULTURAL CONSIDERATIONS

Patient-Centered Care QSEN

Lupus affects women 10 times more often than men; women of color are affected far more often than Euro-Americans. The reason for this difference is unknown (McCance et al., 2014). The disease also occurs among American Indians, Asian Americans, and Hispanics (Lupus Foundation of America, 2014).

The onset of the disease occurs most often during the child-bearing years (ages 20 to 40 years), but it has been reported in young children and older adults. A genetic predisposition is based on the trend to develop the disease in some twins and the occurrence of autoimmune disease in some families of patients who have lupus. However, it is not the only basis of the disease. Like RA, lupus is probably caused by a complex *combination of genetic and environmental factors.*

A transient lupus-like syndrome can occur in some patients taking select medications, especially procainamide (Pronestyl) and hydralazine (McCance et al., 2014). When these drugs are discontinued, the syndrome usually resolves. Neither of these drugs is commonly used.

❖ PATIENT-CENTERED COLLABORATIVE CARE

◆ Assessment

It is impossible to describe a typical textbook picture of a patient with lupus because of the extreme range of symptoms. There is no classic presentation of this disease. When lupus is in remission, the patient may appear healthy and have few or no activity limitations. When the disease flares, some patients may be so ill that admission to a critical care unit is needed. Chart 18-11 highlights the clinical manifestations that can occur with systemic lupus.

Physical Assessment/Clinical Manifestations

Skin Involvement. *The major skin manifestation of DLE and SLE is a dry, scaly, raised rash on the face* ("butterfly" rash) (Fig. 18-8). This rash may also appear on other sun-exposed areas. The rash is initially nonscarring and may increase in a lupus flare and disappear when the disease is in remission.

CHART 18-11 Key Features
Systemic Lupus Erythematosus (SLE) and Systemic Sclerosis (SSc)

SYSTEMIC LUPUS ERYTHEMATOSUS	SYSTEMIC SCLEROSIS
Skin Manifestations	
Inflamed, red rash	Inflamed
Discoid lesions	Fibrotic
	Sclerotic
	Edematous
Renal Manifestations	
Nephritis	Kidney failure
Cardiovascular Manifestations	
Pericarditis	Myocardial fibrosis
Raynaud's phenomenon	Raynaud's phenomenon
Pulmonary Manifestations	
Pleural effusions	Interstitial fibrosis
	Pulmonary hypertension
Neurologic Manifestations	
CNS lupus	Not common
Gastrointestinal Manifestations	
Abdominal pain	Esophagitis
	Ulcers
Musculoskeletal Manifestations	
Joint inflammation	Joint inflammation
Myositis	Myositis
Other Manifestations	
Fever	Fever
Fatigue	Fatigue
Anorexia	Anorexia
Vasculitis	Vasculitis

CNS, Central nervous system.

FIG. 18-8 The characteristic "butterfly" rash of systemic lupus erythematosus.

Individual round **discoid** (coinlike) **lesions** are the scarring lesions of discoid lupus. The lesions are especially evident when the patient is exposed to sunlight or ultraviolet light. Alopecia is also common in lupus. Observe and document all skin changes, and monitor them daily while the patient is in an acute care setting or during an ambulatory care or home visit. Mouth ulcers are not uncommon.

Other Manifestations. In addition to skin changes, *polyarthritis* occurs in most patients with SLE. The early joint changes are similar to those seen in rheumatoid arthritis (RA), but severe deformities are not common even in late disease. Small joints and the knees are most commonly inflamed. **Osteonecrosis** (bone necrosis from lack of oxygen) is often seen in those who have been treated for at least 5 years with steroids like prednisone. Chronic steroid therapy may cause the constriction of small blood vessels supplying the joint, which causes the tissue to die. The hip is most commonly affected, and reports of PAIN and decreased MOBILITY result. As a result, a total hip arthroplasty may be done.

Observe for *muscle atrophy,* which can result from disuse, from skeletal muscle invasion by the immune complexes (**myositis**), or from chronic steroid therapy. Myalgia (muscle pain) may also occur. Inspect and palpate the major muscles, especially those in the extremities.

Because SLE is an inflammatory condition, *fever* and *fatigue* are common findings. *Fever is the classic sign of a flare, or exacerbation.* Various degrees of generalized weakness, fatigue, anorexia, and weight loss may occur. These signs may be the only evidence of disease, which makes diagnosis by the health care provider difficult. Therefore some patients have a diagnosis of "probable SLE."

Any or all body systems may be affected by SLE. Because lupus nephritis is the leading cause of death, carefully assess for signs of renal involvement (e.g., changes in urine output, proteinuria, hematuria, fluid retention).

Pleural effusions or *pneumonia* is found in almost half of all cases of SLE, but this complication is usually not life threatening. Pulmonary restrictive or obstructive changes may not result in overt clinical signs; however, progressive involvement can lead to dyspnea and arterial blood gas abnormalities. Perform a complete respiratory assessment to determine any abnormalities in respiratory pattern or breath sounds.

Pericarditis is the most common cardiovascular manifestation and causes tachycardia, chest pain, and myocardial ischemia. Monitor the vital signs at least every 4 hours while the patient is in the hospital, and report chest pain immediately to the physician. *Anemia, leukopenia, and thrombocytopenia* are also common in patients with SLE.

Raynaud's phenomenon occurs in a small portion of lupus patients. On exposure to cold or extreme stress, the patient reports the characteristic red, white, and blue color changes and severe pain in the digits; these changes are caused by arteriolar vasospasm. Ask patients whether color changes occur when their hands or feet are exposed to cold or when they are extremely stressed.

Neurologic manifestations are varied. Central nervous system effects include psychoses, paresis, seizures, migraine headaches, and cranial nerve palsies. Peripheral neuropathies are also common. Perform a neurologic assessment as described in Chapter 41.

Monitor *abdominal* PAIN, which usually results from **serositis** (peritoneal involvement). Mesenteric arteritis, pancreatitis

from arteritis of the pancreatic artery, and colonic ulcers also can cause abdominal pain with lupus. Jaundice is rare. Many patients have lymph enlargement, and a few have splenomegaly (enlarged spleen). Palpate the lymph nodes, and document findings. Vasculitis affecting any major or small vessels can lead to organ failure.

Psychosocial Assessment. The psychosocial results of lupus can be devastating. With either DLE or SLE, the rash can be disfiguring and embarrassing. Young adult women who never had a blemish are confronted with a rash that cannot be completely covered with makeup. If chronic steroid therapy is used, side effects such as acne, striae, fat pads, and weight gain intensify the problem of an already altered body image.

Chronic fatigue and generalized weakness may prevent the patient from being as active as in the past. He or she may avoid social gatherings and may withdraw from family activities. The unpredictability and chronicity of SLE can cause fear and anxiety. Fear may increase if the patient knows another person with the disease, particularly if the other person has more advanced severe disease. Unfortunately, the myth that lupus is fatal is still common. Inform the patient and family that control of lupus is generally possible with regular medical monitoring, medications, and healthy practices, such as limiting sun exposure to prevent exacerbation of the disease.

Assess the patient's and family's feelings about the illness to identify areas requiring intervention. Determine their usual coping mechanisms and support systems before developing a plan of care. See p. 293 in the Psychosocial Assessment section of the Rheumatoid Arthritis section for additional information.

Laboratory Assessment. Because discoid lupus erythematosus (DLE) is not a systemic condition, the only significant test is a *skin biopsy.* The physician gently scrapes skin cells from the rash for microscopic evaluation. The characteristic lupus cell and a number of inflammatory cells confirm the diagnosis.

Some of the immunologic-based laboratory tests used to diagnose SLE are the same as those performed for rheumatoid arthritis (RA): rheumatoid factor, antinuclear antibody, erythrocyte sedimentation rate, serum protein electrophoresis, serum complement (especially C3 and C4), and immunoglobulins (see Chart 18-8). A false-positive Venereal Disease Research Laboratory (VDRL) syphilis test is common with lupus (Pagana & Pagana, 2014).

More specific immunologic tests, such as anti–SS-a (Ro), anti–SS-b (La), anti-Smith (anti-Sm), anti-DNA, and extractable nuclear antigens (ENAs), are also performed (Pagana & Pagana, 2014). High titers of some of these antibodies are associated with lupus.

A CBC commonly shows **pancytopenia** (a decrease of all cell types), probably caused by direct attack of the blood cells or bone marrow by immune complexes. Serum electrolyte levels, kidney function, cardiac and liver enzymes, and clotting factors are also routinely assessed to determine other body system functioning.

◆ Interventions

The health care provider often prescribes potent drugs that are used topically and systemically. In addition, precautions are taken to prevent further skin impairment and exacerbations. Many of the skin lesions do not disappear, even with treatment, but they usually fade when the disease is in remission.

Managing Lupus with Drug Therapy. With DLE, the patient's major concern is the rash or discoid lesions. Patients with SLE are also concerned about skin changes. Topical cortisone preparations help reduce inflammation and promote fading of the skin lesions. Acetaminophen (Tylenol) or NSAIDs may be used to treat joint and muscle PAIN and INFLAMMATION.

In addition, the health care provider may prescribe the anti-malarial agent *hydroxychloroquine* (Plaquenil) for some patients. Plaquenil decreases the absorption of ultraviolet light by the skin and therefore decreases the risk for skin lesions. *Teach patients to have frequent eye examinations (before starting the drug and every 6 months thereafter) if they are receiving Plaquenil.*

The health care provider often prescribes chronic steroid therapy to treat the systemic disease process. For renal or central nervous system lupus, he or she may also prescribe immunosuppressive agents, such as methotrexate (Rheumatrex) or azathioprine (Imuran). Although clinical manifestations improve during remission, maintenance doses of these drugs are usually continued to prevent further exacerbations of the disease. These drugs make patients susceptible to INFECTION.

⚠ NURSING SAFETY PRIORITY (QSEN)

Drug Alert

When patients are taking steroids and/or immunosuppressants, stress the importance of avoiding large crowds and people who are ill. Teach patients to report any early sign of INFECTION to their health care provider. Observe for side effects and toxic effects of these drugs, and report their occurrence immediately. Remind patients to take their medication early in the morning before breakfast because that is the time when the body's natural corticosteroid level is the lowest.

For severe renal involvement, immunosuppressants may be given in combination with steroids. For patients who do not respond to this regimen, a high-dose IV bolus of glucocorticoids, cyclophosphamide, and plasmapheresis may be tried for 3 consecutive days. Kidney transplantation has been successful for some patients.

The first drug approved for SLE in 60 years is *belimumab* (Benlysta). In SLE, abnormal B-cells contribute to autoantibodies. Belimumab is an IV human monoclonal antibody (mAb) that prevents B-lymphocyte stimulator protein from binding to B-cell receptor sites, thus decreasing B-cell survival. It is given with other drugs to treat SLE. Like for other biologics, teach patients that the drug increases their risk for serious INFECTIONS. Teach patients not to receive live vaccines for 30 days before treatment.

Protecting the Skin. Teach patients to protect their skin to prevent an exacerbation of the disease.

⚠ NURSING SAFETY PRIORITY (QSEN)

Action Alert

Instruct patients to avoid prolonged exposure to sunlight and other forms of ultraviolet lighting, including certain types of fluorescent light. Remind them to wear long sleeves and a large-brimmed hat when outdoors. Patients should use sun-blocking agents with a sun protection factor (SPF) of 30 or higher on exposed skin surfaces.

In addition, teach patients to clean the skin with mild soap (e.g., Ivory) and to avoid harsh, perfumed substances. The skin should be rinsed and dried well and lotion applied. Excess powder and other drying substances should be avoided. Cosmetics must be carefully selected and should include moisturizers and sun protectors. If desired, refer the patient to a medical cosmetologist who specializes in applying makeup for skin lesions of all types.

Patients' hair should receive special attention because alopecia (hair loss) is common. Recommend the use of mild protein shampoos and the avoidance of harsh treatments (e.g., permanents or highlights) until the hair regrows during remission.

Community-Based Care

Community-based care for the patient with lupus is similar to that for RA. In general, the patient is home but may need repeated hospitalizations during exacerbations of disease. He or she usually does not need rehabilitation unless having surgery, because severe joint deformity and prolonged immobility are not common in lupus.

Two major differences exist between SLE and RA in terms of education of the patient and family or significant others. First, instruct patients with SLE how to protect the skin (Chart 18-12). Second, teach them to monitor body temperature. Fever is the major sign of an exacerbation, during which they can become seriously ill. Teach the importance of reporting any other unusual or new clinical manifestations to the health care provider immediately.

Many patients become frustrated that family members, significant others, and lay people do not have a thorough understanding of lupus. When lupus is in complete remission, patients appear to be healthy; however, an exacerbation can lead to a critical care admission. This unpredictability disrupts the patient's life and can cause fear and anxiety. Help him or her identify coping strategies and support systems that can help with functioning in the community.

Teach the possible effects of the disease on lifestyle, including fatigue. Women of childbearing age need to know that pregnancy can be a stressor and can cause an exacerbation of the disease, either during pregnancy or after delivery. The pregnant woman also has an increased risk for miscarriage, stillbirth, or premature birth. Pregnancy is not recommended for those with cardiac, renal, or central nervous system involvement. Sexual counseling regarding contraception options may be necessary.

The Arthritis Foundation is a general resource for all patients with connective tissue disease. The Lupus Foundation

---

CHART 18-12 Patient and Family Education: Preparing for Self-Management

Evidence-Based Practice for Skin Protection in Patients with Lupus Erythematosus

- Cleanse your skin with a mild soap, such as Ivory.
- Dry your skin thoroughly by patting rather than rubbing.
- Apply lotion liberally to dry skin areas.
- Avoid powder and other drying agents, such as rubbing alcohol.
- Use cosmetics that contain moisturizers.
- Avoid direct sunlight and any other type of ultraviolet lighting, including tanning beds.
- Wear a large-brimmed hat, long sleeves, and long pants when in the sun.
- Use a sun-blocking agent with a sun protection factor (SPF) of at least 30.
- Inspect your skin daily for open areas and rashes.

(www.lupus.org) is a resource specific for patients with lupus. It is a national organization and has chapters in every state to provide information and assistance for patients with lupus and their families. Local support groups and services are offered free of charge.

SYSTEMIC SCLEROSIS

❖ PATHOPHYSIOLOGY

Systemic sclerosis (SSc), also called *scleroderma,* is an uncommon chronic, inflammatory, autoimmune connective tissue disease. Formerly called *progressive systemic disease,* or *PSS,* this illness is not always progressive. **Scleroderma** means hardening of the skin, which is only one clinical manifestation of the problem. Some patients, often children, have only skin involvement, or localized scleroderma (also called *linear scleroderma*). However, adults usually have skin and other body system involvement. SSc is less common than systemic lupus erythematosus (SLE) but is associated with a higher mortality rate. See Chart 18-11 for a comparison of the clinical manifestations of these two diseases. The manifestations for both diseases vary widely from person to person.

The early inflammatory process of SSc is so similar to that of lupus that patients may first be diagnosed as having probable SLE until the disease progresses or until antibody testing supports the diagnosis. The inflamed tissue in patients with SSc becomes fibrotic and then **sclerotic** (hard). Renal involvement is the leading cause of death. Respiratory involvement and hypertension are also common. Patients with SSc do not respond well to the steroids and immunosuppressants used for lupus, and therefore the mortality rate is higher.

The classification for systemic sclerosis is:
- **Diffuse cutaneous SSc**—skin thickening on the trunk, face, and proximal and distal extremities (over most of the body)
- **Limited cutaneous SSc**—thickened skin limited to sites distal to the face, neck, and distal extremities

Patients with the *limited* form of the disease often have the **CREST syndrome:**
- **C**alcinosis (calcium deposits)
- **R**aynaud's phenomenon (first symptom that occurs)
- **E**sophageal dysmotility
- **S**clerodactyly (scleroderma of the digits)
- **T**elangiectasia (spider-like hemangiomas)

The first symptom that usually occurs in patients with the *diffuse* form of the disease is hand and forearm edema, which may exist with bilateral carpal tunnel syndrome. Gastroesopha-

geal reflux disease (GERD) is commonly present in patients with either type of the disease.

Little is known about the cause of SSc, but autoimmunity is suspected. The occurrence of more than one case per family is uncommon, but other connective tissue diseases may be noted in the family history. At this time, specific genetic causes have not been confirmed.

Systemic sclerosis has been described in people of all races and in all geographic areas and affects over 300,000 people. Women are affected more often than men. The onset of the disease is usually between 25 and 55 years of age, with most women getting it in their 40s (Scleroderma Foundation, 2013).

❖ PATIENT-CENTERED COLLABORATIVE CARE

◆ Assessment

Physical Assessment/Clinical Manifestations. **Arthralgia** (joint PAIN) and stiffness are common manifestations that you can assess during the musculoskeletal examination. The acute joint INFLAMMATION that occurs with rheumatoid arthritis (RA) is not common, and deformities are rare.

Findings on inspection of the skin depend on the stage of the scleroderma. Typically, a painless, symmetric, pitting edema of the hands and fingers is present, especially in patients with the diffuse form of the disease. The edema may progress to include the entire upper and lower extremities and face. In this phase, the fingers are described as *sausage-like.* The skin is taut, shiny, and free of wrinkles. If diffuse scleroderma occurs, swelling is replaced by tightening, hardening, and thickening of skin tissue; this phase is sometimes called the *indurative phase* (Fig. 18-9). The skin loses its elasticity, and range of motion is markedly decreased; ulcerations may occur. Joint contractures may develop, and the patient may be unable to perform ADLs independently.

Major organ damage is likely to develop with diffuse scleroderma, specifically affecting the renal and cardiopulmonary systems. The initial GERD symptoms progress into other problems, especially affecting the esophagus. The esophagus loses its motility, resulting in *dysphagia (difficulty swallowing).* Assess for the ability of the patient to swallow before allowing him or her to drink or eat food. A small, sliding hiatal hernia may be present, and swallowing may be difficult. Reflux of the gastric contents can cause esophagitis and subsequent ulceration, particularly in the lower two thirds of the esophagus. Intestinal changes are similar to those of the esophagus. Peristalsis is diminished, which causes clinical manifestations similar to a partial bowel obstruction. Malabsorption is a common complication, causing malodorous *diarrheal stools.*

In addition to assessing problems of the digestive tract, observe for *cardiovascular manifestations. Raynaud's phenomenon* occurs in various degrees in most patients with SSc. On exposure to cold or emotional stress, the small arterioles in the digits of both hands and feet rapidly constrict, which causes decreased blood flow. In severe cases, the patient experiences digit necrosis, excruciating pain, and **autoamputation of the distal digits** (the tips of the digits fall off spontaneously). In many patients, vasculitic lesions, often around the nail beds **(periungual lesions),** are evident. *Myocardial fibrosis,* another common problem, is evidenced by electrocardiographic (ECG) changes, cardiac dysrhythmias, and chest pain.

Lung involvement in the patient with SSc may go undetected until late in the disease or sometimes until autopsy. *Fibrosis of*

FIG. 18-9 Late-stage skin changes seen in patients with systemic sclerosis.

the alveoli and interstitial tissues is present in almost all cases of the disease, but clinical manifestations may not be present. Patients with scleroderma and *pulmonary arterial hypertension* have a more serious prognosis. *Renal involvement* is an important aspect of the overall disease process and often causes malignant hypertension and death. Assess for signs of impending organ failure, such as changes in urine output and increased blood pressure.

Laboratory Assessment. The laboratory findings for SSc are similar to those for SLE. Clinical findings and the patient's response to drug therapy help the health care provider differentiate between the two diseases. Additional tests depend on which organs seem to be affected. Upper and lower GI series are commonly performed because of the frequency of GI clinical manifestations.

◆ Interventions

The medical management of SSc aims to force the disease into remission and thus slow disease progression. The health care provider uses drug therapy primarily for this purpose, but it is often unsuccessful. Systemic steroids and immunosuppressants are used in large doses and often in combination. Another desired outcome of disease management is to identify early organ involvement and treat it before it becomes severe and irreversible. For example, a patient who has lung involvement receives aggressive respiratory therapy and other treatments as the condition requires.

Recently, bosentan (Tracleer), the first of a new class of drugs called *endothelin receptor antagonists,* demonstrated improved walk tests for patients with class III or class IV pulmonary arterial hypertension. Various doses improved patients' breathing during exercise, but the potential for liver injury at the highest dose caused recommended doses to be lowered. Teach the patient the desired and potential adverse effects, including liver toxicity and birth defects. Remind him or her of the importance of follow-up testing for liver enzyme levels.

New oral tyrosine kinase inhibitors (TKIs), including nilotinib (Tasigna) and imatinib mesylate (Gleevec), are being tested for use for patients with systemic sclerosis. These drugs work to decrease INFLAMMATION and slow the progression of the disease. They are currently approved in the United States for use in certain types of cancer.

Local skin protective measures can help maintain skin integrity. Teach the patient to use mild soap and lotions and gentle

---

CHART 18-13　Best Practice for Patient Safety & Quality Care　QSEN

The Patient with Systemic Sclerosis and Esophagitis

- Keep the patient's head elevated at least 60 degrees during meals and for at least 1 hour after each meal.
- Provide small, frequent meals rather than three large meals each day.
- Give the patient small amounts of food for each bite, and explain the importance of chewing each bite carefully before swallowing.
- Provide semisoft foods, such as mashed potatoes and pudding or custard; liquids are most likely to cause choking.
- Collaborate with the dietitian about the patient's diet.
- Teach the patient to avoid foods that increase gastric secretion, such as caffeine, pepper, and other spices.
- Give antacids or histamine antagonists as needed.

---

cleaning techniques. Inspect the skin for further changes or open lesions. Skin ulcers are treated according to their type and location.

In addition to drug therapy to control the overall disease process, specific measures can provide comfort. The patient with SSc not only experiences chronic joint PAIN but also has severe, acute pain during episodes of Raynaud's phenomenon. Remind unlicensed nursing personnel to use a bed cradle and foot board to keep bed covers away from the skin in severe cases. Adjust the room temperature to prevent chilling, which can precipitate digit vasospasm. The patient who can tolerate touching of the affected areas can wear gloves and socks to increase warmth. Because cigarette smoking and extreme emotional stress can also cause symptoms to recur, teach the patient to avoid or minimize these factors as much as possible.

If the patient has esophageal involvement, collaborate with the speech and language pathologist to schedule a swallowing study. The patient may need small, frequent meals rather than the traditional three meals daily. He or she should minimize the intake of foods and liquids that stimulate gastric secretion (e.g., spicy foods, caffeine, alcohol). Teach the patient to keep his or her head elevated for 1 to 2 hours after meals. He or she may need to be in this position continuously. Histamine antagonists and antacids help reduce and neutralize gastric acid. To help prevent choking, collaborate with the dietitian for dietary changes (Chart 18-13).

Nursing care for the patient with joint PAIN and decreased MOBILITY is very similar to that for rheumatoid arthritis (see the Interventions section of the Rheumatoid Arthritis section on p. 293). NSAIDs are given for INFLAMMATION and pain. Joint protection and energy conservation are also important for these patients.

Community-Based Care

Community-based care for the person with SSc is similar to that for lupus. The patient is treated at home but may need frequent hospitalizations if major organ involvement occurs during exacerbations. The Arthritis Foundation (www.arthritis.org) and Scleroderma Foundation (www.scleroderma.org) are excellent resources for more information about the disease and how to manage it.

GOUT

❖ PATHOPHYSIOLOGY

Gout, or gouty arthritis, is a systemic disease in which urate crystals deposit in the joints and other body tissues, causing inflammation. It is the most common inflammatory arthritis in older adults, affecting an estimated 6.1 million people (Arthritis Foundation, 2013a). The cause and treatment of gout have been firmly established. The classic case of well-advanced disease is seldom seen today unless the patient does not adhere to the therapeutic regimen. The two major types of gout are primary and secondary.

Primary gout is the most common type and results from one of several inborn errors of purine metabolism. An end product of purine metabolism is uric acid, which is usually excreted by the kidneys. In primary gout, the production of uric acid exceeds the excretion capability of the kidneys. Sodium urate is deposited in synovium and other tissues, resulting in inflammation. For some patients, primary gout is inherited as an X-linked trait; males are affected through female carriers. A number of patients have a family history of gout. Primary gout affects middle-aged and older men and postmenopausal women. The peak time of onset in men is between 40 and 50 years of age (McCance et al., 2014).

Secondary gout involves **hyperuricemia** (excessive uric acid in the blood) caused by another disease or factor. Secondary gout affects people of all ages. Renal insufficiency, diuretic therapy, "crash" diets, and certain chemotherapeutic agents decrease the normal excretion of uric acid and other waste products. Disorders such as multiple myeloma and certain carcinomas result in increased production of uric acid because of a greater turnover of cellular nucleic acids. Treatment involves management of the underlying disorder.

Hyperuricemia and gout are often seen in older patients with cardiovascular health problems, obese people, and postmenopausal women. The incidence of gout is increasing as the baby boomer generation reaches 65 years of age.

The three clinical stages of the primary disease process are asymptomatic hyperuricemia, acute gouty arthritis, and chronic or tophaceous gout (McCance et al., 2014). The patient is usually unaware of the *asymptomatic hyperuricemic stage* unless he or she has had a serum uric acid level determination. The serum level is elevated, but no obvious signs of the disease are present. No treatment is needed in this stage.

The first "attack" of gouty arthritis begins the *acute stage*. The patient experiences excruciating PAIN and INFLAMMATION

in one or more small joints, usually the metatarsophalangeal joint of the great toe, called **podagra.** The erythrocyte sedimentation rate (ESR) is usually increased as a result of the inflammatory process. Months or years may pass before additional attacks occur. The patient is asymptomatic, and no abnormalities are found during examination of the joints.

After repeated episodes of acute gout, deposits of urate crystals develop under the skin and within the major organs, particularly in the renal system. The patient is then classified as having *chronic tophaceous gout.* In chronic gout, urate kidney stone formation is more common than renal insufficiency. Chronic gout can begin anywhere between 3 and 40 years after the initial gout symptoms occur (McCance et al., 2014).

❖ PATIENT-CENTERED COLLABORATIVE CARE

◆ Assessment

Note the patient's age, gender, and family history of gout. A complete history is needed to determine whether gout has been caused by another problem. Some women overuse diuretics, which can lead to secondary gout.

Overt manifestations are present in the acute and chronic phases of gout. You will likely encounter a patient with acute gout, but chronic gout is not as common in the United States today. *Joint INFLAMMATION is the most common finding of acute gout. The joint is usually so painful that the patient seeks medical care immediately.* Inspect the inflamed area. It is usually too painful and swollen to be touched or moved.

The health care provider requests a serum uric acid level to check for hyperuricemia. Because the level can be altered by food intake, several measurements may be obtained. A consistent level of more than 6.5 mg/dL is generally considered abnormal, depending on the laboratory test used. Urinary uric acid levels are also measured; an overproduction of uric acid is confirmed by an excretion of more than 750 mg/24 hr (Pagana & Pagana, 2014).

The health care provider may request kidney function tests, such as blood urea nitrogen (BUN) and serum creatinine levels, to monitor possible kidney involvement. A definitive diagnostic test for the disease is synovial fluid aspiration (arthrocentesis) to detect the needle-like crystals in the affected joint that are characteristic of the disorder.

With *chronic* gout, inspect the skin for **tophi,** or deposits of sodium urate crystals (Fig. 18-10). Although tophi are rarely

FIG. 18-10 Typical appearance of tophi, which may occur in chronic gout, on an index finger.

seen today, they may appear on the outer ear, arms, and fingers near the joints. The tophi are hard on palpation and are irregular in shape. When the skin over the tophi is irritated, it may break open and a yellow, gritty substance is discharged. Infection may result.

Other manifestations of chronic gout include signs of renal calculi (stones) or renal dysfunction, such as severe PAIN or changes in urinary output. In some cases, urate kidney stones occur before the arthritis is present.

◆ Interventions

Gout is one of the easiest diseases for the health care provider to diagnose and treat in its early phases. If the patient receives treatment and adheres to drug therapy, he or she should experience no further symptoms and no change in body image or lifestyle. The patient with gout is treated on an ambulatory basis, but hospitalized patients may have a secondary diagnosis of the disease.

Drug Therapy. Drug therapy is the key to managing patients with gout. In acute gouty "attacks," the inflammation subsides spontaneously within 3 to 5 days; however, most patients cannot tolerate the pain for that long. The drugs used for acute gout are different from those used for chronic gout. The health care provider typically prescribes a combination of colchicine (Colcrys) and an NSAID, such as indomethacin (Indocin, Novomethacin ♣) or ibuprofen (Motrin, Amersol ♣) for acute gout. IV colchicine works within 12 hours. The patient takes oral medications until the INFLAMMATION subsides, usually for 4 to 7 days.

For patients with repeated acute episodes or with chronic gout, the health care provider prescribes drugs on a continuous, maintenance basis to promote uric acid excretion or to reduce its production. Allopurinol (Zyloprim, Purinol ♣) or febuxostat (Uloric) is the drug of choice. Febuxostat may cause a greater risk to cardiovascular health than allopurinol (Lilley et al., 2014). As xanthine oxidase inhibitors, these drugs prevent the conversion of xanthine to uric acid. Teach patients to take them after meals and drink a glass of water with each dose to prevent GI distress. Drinking at least 8 glasses of water each day helps prevent renal dysfunction. Remind patients that periodic follow-up laboratory tests, including liver enzymes, kidney function studies, and complete blood count, are important because xanthine oxidase inhibitors cause liver dysfunction and bone marrow suppression.

Probenecid can also be effective as a uricosuric drug in gout because it promotes the excretion of excess uric acid. Combination drugs that contain probenecid and colchicine (e.g., Col-BENEMID) are also available. The health care provider and nurse monitor serum uric acid levels to determine the effectiveness of these medications. Aspirin should be avoided because it inactivates the effects of the drug.

For patients with severe gout who do not respond to other drugs (refractory gout), pegloticase (Krystexxa) can be prescribed as an IV dose every 2 weeks. This drug is an enzyme that works directly on uric acid and converts it to allantoin, which can be excreted by the kidneys. Monitor patients carefully for allergic reactions, including anaphylaxis, during and immediately after drug administration because pegloticase is a protein that is foreign to the body.

Nutrition Therapy and Lifestyle Recommendations. The American College of Rheumatology best practice guidelines recommend a strict low-purine diet and suggest that patients avoid foods such as organ meats, shellfish, and oily fish with bones (e.g., sardines). Some health care providers and dietitians believe that limiting protein foods, especially red and organ meats, is sufficient. It is well known, however, that excessive alcohol intake and fad "starvation" diets can cause a gouty attack. *Teach patients to determine which foods precipitate acute attacks and try to avoid them.*

In addition to food and beverage restrictions, patients with gout should avoid all forms of aspirin and diuretics because they may precipitate an attack. Likewise, excessive physical or emotional stress can exacerbate the disease. Surgery or acute illness, like a myocardial infarction, can also trigger an attack. Stress-management techniques may be helpful for the patient with gout.

Teach the patient to drink plenty of fluids to prevent the formation of urinary stones. Increasing fluid intake helps dilute urine and prevent sediment formation. Uric acid is more soluble in urine with a high pH and therefore is less likely to form urinary stones in that environment. The patient's urinary pH can be increased with an intake of alkaline ash foods, such as citrus fruits and juices, milk, and certain other dairy products. The value of adhering to a strict diet rich in these foods is questionable, however. If the patient is overweight, recommend community resources for losing weight, including increasing exercise.

⍰ NCLEX EXAMINATION CHALLENGE
Physiological Integrity

The nurse is preparing to give medications to a group of clients. Which drug is not appropriate to treat the disease with which it is matched?
A. Rheumatoid arthritis—methotrexate (MTX)
B. Osteoarthritis—acetaminophen (Tylenol)
C. Acute gout—allopurinol (Zyloprim)
D. Systemic lupus erythematosus—prednisone (Deltasone)

INFECTIOUS ARTHRITIS

Any infectious agent can invade the joint space and cause PAIN, INFLAMMATION, and tissue destruction. Certain pathogens, such as *Staphylococcus aureus,* destroy tissue rapidly; others, especially viruses, do not cause irreversible damage. The cornerstone of management is local or systemic antibiotic therapy for 6 to 8 weeks.

LYME DISEASE

Lyme disease is a reportable systemic infectious disease caused by the spirochete *Borrelia burgdorferi* and results from the bite of an infected deer tick, also known as the *black-legged tick.* It is the most common vector-borne disease in the United States and Europe. Most cases of the disease in the United States are seen in New England; the mid-Atlantic states, including Maryland and Virginia; the upper Midwest, including Wisconsin and Minnesota; and northern California, especially during the summer months.

In the early and *localized stage I,* the patient appears with *flu-like symptoms,* erythema migrans (round or oval, flat or slightly raised rash), and PAIN *and stiffness in the muscles and joints.* Most patients in the United States tend to have only one

Prevention and Early Detection of Lyme Disease

- Avoid heavily wooded areas or areas with thick underbrush, especially in the spring and summer months.
- Walk in the center of the trail.
- Avoid dark clothing. Lighter-colored clothing makes spotting ticks easier.
- Use an insect repellent (DEET) on your skin and clothes when in an area where ticks are likely to be found.
- Wear long-sleeved tops and long pants; tuck your shirt into your pants and your pants into your socks or boots.
- Wear closed shoes or boots and a hat or cap.
- Bathe immediately after being in an infested area, and inspect your body for ticks (about the size of a pinhead); pay special attention to your arms, legs, and scalp.
- Check your pets for ticks.
- Gently remove with tweezers or fingers covered with tissue or gloves any tick that you find (do not squeeze). Dispose of the tick by flushing it down the toilet (burning a tick could spread infection).
- After removal, clean the tick area with an antiseptic such as rubbing alcohol.
- Wait 4 to 6 weeks after being bitten by a tick before being tested for Lyme disease (testing before this time is not reliable).
- Report symptoms, such as a rash or influenza-like illness, to your physician immediately.

lesion, sometimes referred to as a *"bull's-eye lesion."* Symptoms begin within 3 to 30 days of the tick bite, but most present in 7 to 14 days. Antibiotic therapy, such as doxycycline or amoxicillin, is prescribed during this uncomplicated stage for 14 to 21 days. Erythromycin can be used for patients who are allergic to penicillin. Without treatment, these symptoms may disappear in about 4 to 5 weeks.

If not treated or if treatment is not successful, the patient may progress to the more serious complications of Lyme disease. *Stage II (early disseminated stage)* occurs 2 to 12 weeks after the tick bite. The patient may develop *carditis* with *dysrhythmias, dyspnea, dizziness, or palpitations,* as well as central nervous system disorders such as *meningitis, facial paralysis* (often misdiagnosed as Bell's palsy), and *peripheral neuritis.* For severe disease, IV antibiotics (e.g., ceftriaxone or cefotaxime) are given for at least 30 days.

If Lyme disease is not diagnosed and treated in the earlier stages, later chronic complications (e.g., *arthritis, chronic fatigue, memory/thinking problems*) can result. This *late stage III (chronic persistent stage)* occurs months to years after the tick bite. *For some patients, the first and only sign of Lyme disease is arthritis.* In some cases, the disease may not respond to antibiotics in any stage and the patient develops permanent damage to joints and the nervous system. *Prevention is the best strategy for Lyme disease.* Teach patients to follow the measures outlined in Chart 18-14 to prevent Lyme and other tick-borne diseases. Tell them about community resources such as the Lyme Disease Foundation (www.lyme.org) for more information.

PSORIATIC ARTHRITIS

Psoriatic arthritis (PsA) affects some people who have psoriasis—a skin condition characterized by a scaly, itchy rash, usually on the elbows, knees, and scalp. Fingernail and toenail lifting and pitting may also occur (see Chapter 25 for discussion

of this disease). The joint PAIN associated with psoriasis is often associated with stiffness, especially in the morning. Neck and back pain are particularly common, but various forms of the disease can cause small joint arthritis or involvement of the sacroiliac joints of the spine.

PsA occurs most often in people between 30 and 50 years of age in men and women of all races. Nail symptoms are common in patients who have the associated arthritis. Causes may include genetic and environmental factors, infectious agents, and immune system dysfunction.

Most patients do not experience destructive and deforming arthritis affecting more than three joints, but for those who do, the experience has a major impact on their quality of life. Treatment is focused on managing joint PAIN and INFLAMMATION, controlling skin lesions, and slowing the progression of the disease. Health teaching for skin care is similar to that for lupus. Management of joint inflammation is similar to that for rheumatoid arthritis as described earlier in this chapter. Methotrexate (Rheumatrex), sulfasalazine (Azulfidine), and biological response modifiers (also called *biologics*), such as etanercept (Enbrel) and golimumab (Simponi), are being used with success.

Teach the patient or family member how to self-administer Enbrel injections. Injection site reactions and infections (especially respiratory) are possible adverse effects. Ice and hydrocortisone 1% cream can be used if a red, itchy rash at the injection site develops.

Golimumab (Simponi) is the first biologic that is administered only once each month for psoriatic arthritis. Teach patients that this drug has a black box warning for serious infections that may lead to hospitalization or death from opportunistic pathogens (Cranwell-Bruce, 2011).

Several newer types of biologics have also been approved for psoriatic arthritis. Ustekinumab (Stelara) targets the cytokines *interleukin (IL)-12* and *IL-23* to decrease INFLAMMATION. Alefacept (Amevive) is an IV immunosuppressive drug (T-cell blocker) that is reserved for moderate to severe disease. Teach patients taking these drugs about their risk for INFECTION. Remind them to avoid crowds and anyone with an INFECTION.

Acitretin (Soriatane) is an oral retinoid given for patients with severe disease. Teach patients to take the drug once a day with a meal and follow up with laboratory testing for liver enzymes.

The National Psoriasis Foundation (www.psoriasis.org) is an excellent community resource for patients and their families. Further discussion regarding management of psoriasis can be found in Chapter 25.

FIBROMYALGIA SYNDROME

Fibromyalgia syndrome (FMS), also referred to as simply *fibromyalgia,* is a chronic PAIN syndrome, not an inflammatory disease. However, arthritis and other comorbidities are commonly present in patients diagnosed with FMS. Pain, stiffness, and tenderness are located at specific sites in the back of the neck, upper chest, trunk, low back, and extremities. These tender points are also known as trigger points and can typically be palpated to elicit pain in a predictable, reproducible pattern. The pain is typically described as burning and gnawing. Increased muscle tenderness may be caused by the inability to tolerate pain, possibly related to dysfunction in the brain, especially the thalamus and hypothalamus (McCance et al., 2014).

The PAIN and tenderness tend to come and go but typically worsen in response to stress, increased activity, and weather conditions. The patient reports mild to severe fatigue, and sleep disturbances are common. Some people report numbness or tingling in their extremities, and others are sensitive to noxious odors, loud noises, and bright lights. Headaches and jaw pain are also common. Secondary FMS can accompany any connective tissue disease (CTD), particularly lupus and rheumatoid disease, and may not necessarily be related to sleep patterns.

Other symptoms include:

- Gastrointestinal (GI), including abdominal PAIN, diarrhea and constipation, and heartburn
- Genitourinary, including dysuria, urinary frequency, urgency, and pelvic pain
- Cardiovascular, including dyspnea, chest pain, and dysrhythmias
- Visual, including blurred vision and dry eyes
- Neurologic, including forgetfulness and concentration problems

Many with these symptoms become frustrated because they are not properly diagnosed and are in constant pain and discomfort.

Some patients are diagnosed as having chronic fatigue syndrome (CFS). CFS, migraine headache, irritable bowel syndrome (IBS), and myofascial PAIN are often present in those with FMS. As a result, patients can become depressed and anxious.

Most patients are women between 30 and 50 years of age. It is unlikely that the disease is caused by one factor. Possible precipitating factors include CFS, Lyme disease, trauma, and flu-like illness (McCance et al., 2014). FMS may also be aggravated by deep-sleep deprivation. Teach patients to limit caffeine, alcohol, or other unnecessary substances that could interfere with deep sleep. Establish a regular sleep pattern.

Pregabalin (Lyrica) and duloxetine HCl (Cymbalta), which are antidepressant drugs, are approved for fibromyalgia nerve PAIN. These drugs work to increase the release of serotonin and norepinephrine, neurotransmitters in the brain (Lilley et al., 2014). Teach the patient that these drugs can cause drowsiness and sleepiness and that alcohol should be avoided while taking them.

Tricyclic antidepressive agents, such as amitriptyline (Elavil, Apo-Amitriptyline ✤) or nortriptyline (Pamelor), may promote sleep and reduce pain or muscle spasm. These drugs should be used with caution in older adults because they can cause confusion and orthostatic hypotension. Trazodone (Desyrel) may be preferred for this population because of its minimal side effects. Tramadol (Ultram) is also effective for managing fibromyalgia. This drug has tricyclic effects and opioid properties to help relieve PAIN (see Chapter 3).

Physical therapy along with NSAIDs and possibly muscle relaxants may also be prescribed to help decrease fibromyalgia PAIN. Instruct the patient to exercise regularly. Home exercise should include stretching, strengthening, and low-impact aerobic exercise. Walking, swimming, rowing, biking, and water exercise are good examples of low-impact exercise. Complementary and alternative therapies, such as tai chi, acupuncture, hypnosis, and stress management, may help some patients with symptom relief. Refer patients to the land, water, and walking exercise pamphlets produced by the Arthritis Foundation (www.arthritis.org). Inform them about the National Fibromyalgia Association for additional information and patient and family support (www.fmaware.org).

CHRONIC FATIGUE SYNDROME

Chronic fatigue syndrome (CFS), also known as *chronic fatigue and immune dysfunction syndrome (CFIDS),* is a chronic illness in which patients have severe fatigue for 6 months or longer, usually following flu-like symptoms. In addition, four or more of these criteria must be met for a diagnosis of CFS:

- Sore throat
- Substantial impairment in short-term memory or concentration
- Tender lymph nodes
- Muscle PAIN
- Multiple joint PAIN with redness or swelling
- Headaches of a new type, pattern, or severity (not familiar to the patient)
- Unrefreshing sleep
- Postexertional malaise lasting more than 24 hours

Chronic fatigue syndrome is most common in women and is not limited to any socioeconomic group or age. There is no laboratory test to confirm the diagnosis, and therefore many people with the disease probably have not been diagnosed. The cause is unknown, although immune, endocrine, neurologic, and environmental factors are being studied.

Management of the patient is challenging in that there is no cure for CFS. Treatment is supportive and focuses on alleviation or reduction of symptoms. For example, NSAIDs may help with body aches and PAIN. Low-dose antidepressants, such as pregabalin (Lyrica), may also be effective in promoting sleep and preventing or treating depression. Teach the patient to follow healthy practices, such as adequate sleep, proper nutrition, regular exercise (but not excessive to increase fatigue), stress management, and energy conservation. Complementary and alternative therapies, such as acupuncture, tai chi, massage, and herbal supplements, may be helpful for some patients.

Refer the patient to the National Chronic Fatigue Syndrome and Fibromyalgia Association for information and support groups.

OTHER CONNECTIVE TISSUE DISEASES

Many other connective tissues diseases (CTDs) may be seen, but they are not as common as those health problems previously described. Table 18-3 describes some of these CTDs, their key assessments, and primary collaborative interventions.

OTHER DISEASE-ASSOCIATED ARTHRITIS

A number of other diseases can cause secondary arthritis. Tuberculosis, Crohn's disease, ulcerative colitis, hemophilia, and sickle cell anemia are typical examples. To manage joint involvement, the primary disease is treated. For example, when a patient with Crohn's disease is in remission, joint manifestations also subside. Conditions in which joint involvement can occur are presented in Table 18-4.

MIXED CONNECTIVE TISSUE DISEASE

A diagnosis of mixed CTD is made when a patient presents with clinical manifestations that are not typical of any one CTD.

TABLE 18-3 Other Connective Tissue Diseases That Affect Joints

DISEASE	DESCRIPTION/ PATHOPHYSIOLOGY	ASSESSMENT/CLINICAL MANIFESTATIONS	COLLABORATIVE INTERVENTIONS
Polymyositis/ dermatomyositis	Autoimmune, inflammatory disease that causes symmetric muscle atrophy; when skin rash is also present, disease is called *dermatomyositis (DM)*; women between 30 and 60 years affected most often.	Severe muscle weakness Dysphagia (difficulty swallowing) Periorbital edema and lilac eyelid rash (DM) Malignant neoplasms in older patients	Comfort measures Swallowing precautions Nutritional support PT/OT support Immunosuppressant agents and/ or chronic steroid therapy (Teach about risk for infection.) Health teaching about progression of disease, comfort measures, and dietary needs
Systemic necrotizing vasculitis	A group of autoimmune diseases that result in arteritis (inflammation of arterial walls) causing ischemia in the tissues or organs that are supplied by the arteries.	Peripheral arterial disease causing severe pain and necrosis of toes or fingers Signs and symptoms of organ dysfunction or failure, such as kidney or heart failure; also can cause stroke-like symptoms	Chronic steroid therapy and other immunosuppressants Vasodilators, depending on type of vasculitis Management of organ dysfunction or failure
Polymyalgia rheumatica (PMR) and temporal arteritis (TA)	Autoimmune, genetic-based disease affecting middle-aged and older women most often that causes proximal muscle weakness (shoulder and pelvic girdles) (PMR). TA (also known as *giant cell arteritis*) may occur as a separate disease or with PMR.	Shoulder, neck, pelvic, and hip weakness, stiffness, joint aches, low-grade fever, fatigue, and weight loss caused by inflammation (PMR) Headache and visual disturbances (TA)	Responds well to high-dose steroid therapy to cause remission of disease Symptom management Short-term PT/OT as needed Health teaching about medication and pain modalities, such as heat application for joints
Ankylosing spondylitis	Autoimmune, inflammatory disease affecting the spine that is thought to be genetic (strongly associated with specific variations in the *HLA-27* allele on chromosome 6). Can occur in both men and women, but white men younger than 40 years most commonly affected.	Chronic back pain Compromised respiratory function due to rigid chest wall Visual disturbances caused by iritis (inflammation of the iris) Joint pain and aching Malaise Weight loss	Chronic pain management modalities NSAIDs DMARDs, such as methotrexate and biologic response modifiers Symptom management
Reiter's syndrome	Complex syndrome associated with the *HLA-27* allele causing a triad of arthritis, conjunctivitis, and urethritis (inflammation of the urethra). Triggered by exposure to infection, especially sexually transmitted disease or intestinal infection.	Joint pain Eye infection causing redness, pain, and drainage Pain or burning on urination and changes in urinary pattern	Antibiotic therapy to manage infection Pain management NSAIDs Other symptom management
Marfan syndrome	Autosomal dominant disorder resulting from mutations in the *fibrillin I* gene (FBNI). Fibrillin important in limiting the stretch of elastic connective tissues and allowing them to return to their original resting shape. Disease shortens life expectancy, often with death in the 30s.	Excessive height Elongated hands and feet Joint discomfort or pain Scoliosis Visual problems, such as decreased visual acuity or glaucoma Cardiovascular problems, such as mitral valve prolapse and aortic aneurysm, leading to heart failure or death	Symptom management Frequent echocardiography monitoring and physical examinations to detect heart problems Genetic counseling

DMARDs, Disease-modifying antirheumatic drugs; *OT,* occupational therapy; *PT,* physical therapy.

TABLE 18-4 Common Disorders Associated with Arthritis

- Crohn's disease
- Ulcerative colitis
- Tuberculosis
- Hemophilia
- Whipple's disease
- Intestinal bypass surgery
- Hyperparathyroidism
- Hyperthyroidism
- Diabetes mellitus
- Sickle cell anemia crisis
- Psoriasis
- Infection

About 10% of patients with CTDs are classified as having mixed disease. Some of these are overlap syndromes, in which two or more diseases occur at the same time. Common examples are (1) systemic lupus erythematosus (SLE) plus systemic sclerosis (SSc) and (2) rheumatoid arthritis (RA) plus SLE. Management depends on the clinical manifestations, but often the patient is treated as having SLE.

NURSING CONCEPTS AND CLINICAL JUDGMENT REVIEW

What might you NOTICE if the patient has impaired IMMUNITY as a result of arthritis or other connective tissue disease (CTD)?
- Joint inflammation (redness, swelling, pain)
- Impaired joint mobility and stiffness
- Joint deformity
- Difficulty ambulating
- Fever
- Rash
- Report of weight loss and fatigue
- Other manifestations that indicate organ involvement, such as dysrhythmias (heart) and decreased urinary output (kidneys)

What should you INTERPRET and how should you RESPOND to a patient with impaired IMMUNITY as a result of arthritis or other CTD?

Perform and interpret focused physical assessment findings, including:
- Joint assessment, including range of motion
- ADL ability
- Pain intensity and quality
- Body weight
- Ability to cope with disease
- Vital signs
- Other assessments related to specific organ involvement (e.g., cardiac assessment)

Respond:
- Provide pain control interventions, including drug therapy and nonpharmacologic measures (e.g., heat and cold application).

- Collaborate with members of the health care team to improve mobility and ambulation, if needed.
- Teach about drug therapy, including the expected and adverse effects.
- Teach about nonpharmacologic measures to control pain, including ice and heat, and CAM therapies, such as glucosamine.
- Report manifestations of organ involvement to the health care provider for possible immediate intervention (e.g., drug therapy for severe dysrhythmias).
- Monitor laboratory test results to determine progress of treatment.
- Continue to assess for changes in the patient's condition, including new or additional manifestations of organ involvement.
- Encourage patients and their families to discuss their feelings about chronic illness and possible body image changes.
- Help identify coping strategies, and provide information about community and professional resources and support groups.

On what should you REFLECT?
- Monitor the patient's response to pain control interventions.
- Evaluate the patient's and family's knowledge of the disease and its management.
- Evaluate the patient's and family's stress levels and coping strategies.
- Think about what else you might do to promote mobility.
- Decide whether you need to provide alternative interventions or additional health teaching.

GET READY FOR THE NCLEX® EXAMINATION!

KEY POINTS

Review these Key Points for each NCLEX Examination Client Needs Category.

Safe and Effective Care Environment
- Collaborate with the health care team to manage chronic PAIN and increase MOBILITY for patients with arthritis and other CTDs. **Teamwork and Collaboration** QSEN
- Prioritize care for patients with systemic lupus erythematosus (SLE) and systemic sclerosis (SSc) by monitoring for life-threatening complications, such as kidney failure.

Health Promotion and Maintenance
- Provide information about community resources for patients, especially professional organizations such as the Arthritis Foundation and Lupus Foundation.
- Teach patients to prevent joint trauma and reduce weight as needed to help prevent osteoarthritis. **Evidence-Based Practice** QSEN

- Recall that a combination of environmental, genetic, and immune risk factors can cause arthritis and other connective tissue diseases.
- Reinforce the importance of good health practices, such as adequate sleep, proper nutrition, regular exercise, and stress-management techniques for patients with arthritis and other CTDs.
- Teach patients with arthritis what exercises to do (Chart 18-5), joint protection techniques (Chart 18-6), and energy conservation guidelines (Chart 18-10). **Evidence-Based Practice** QSEN
- Teach patients with SLE to avoid sunlight; exacerbations of the disease may be triggered.
- Remind patients with gout to avoid factors that trigger an attack, such as aspirin, organ meats, and alcohol. **Evidence-Based Practice** QSEN
- Teach people ways to prevent or detect early Lyme disease as listed in Chart 18-14.

Psychosocial Integrity

- Recognize that patients with rheumatoid arthritis (RA) may have body image disturbance as a result of potentially deforming joint involvement and nodules.
- Encourage patients with arthritis and connective tissue diseases to discuss their chronic illness and identify coping strategies that have previously been successful. **Patient-Centered Care** QSEN
- Be aware that chronic, painful diseases affect the patient's quality of life and role performance.
- Recognize that patients with fibromyalgia syndrome (FMS) and chronic fatigue syndrome (CFS) are often frustrated because they have not been diagnosed or have been misdiagnosed.
- Teach patients with FMS and CFS that antidepressant drugs can promote sleep and decrease PAIN, as well as prevent or treat the depression that is common with these illnesses.

Physiological Integrity

- Be aware that most of the connective tissue diseases and arthritic disorders have a genetic basis as part of their etiology; most are also classified as autoimmune diseases and have remissions and exacerbations.
- Differentiate OA as primarily a degenerative joint problem that can affect one or more joints, and RA as a systemic disease that presents as a bilateral symmetric joint INFLAMMATION.
- Realize that older patients have OA more than younger patients; younger patients have RA more than older adults; other differences between the two diseases are summarized in Table 18-1.
- Teach patients who have osteoarthritis (OA) or are prone to the disease to lose weight (if obese), avoid trauma, and limit strenuous weight-bearing activities.
- Instruct patients with arthritic pain to use multiple modalities for pain relief, including ice/heat, rest, positioning, complementary and alternative therapies, and medications as prescribed.
- Teach patients to monitor and report side and adverse effects of drugs used to treat OA and other connective tissue diseases.
- Assess patients with rheumatoid arthritis for early or late clinical manifestations as listed in Chart 18-7.

- Teach patients who are taking hydroxychloroquine (Plaquenil) to have frequent (every 6 months) eye examinations to monitor for retinal changes. **Safety** QSEN
- Remind patients to avoid crowds and other possible sources of INFECTION when they are taking immunosuppressant drugs. **Safety** QSEN
- Implement interventions for patients having total joint arthroplasty (TJA) to prevent venous thromboembolitic complications (e.g., anticoagulants, exercises, sequential compression devices); observe the patient for bleeding when he or she is taking anticoagulants.
- Be careful when positioning a patient after a total hip arthroplasty (THA) to prevent dislocation; do not hyperflex the hips or adduct the legs (see Chart 18-3). **Safety** QSEN
- Be aware that disease-modifying antirheumatic drugs (DMARDs) and biological response modifiers (BRMs) slow the progression of connective tissue diseases, especially RA and SLE.
- Remind patients taking methotrexate (Rheumatrex) to avoid people with INFECTIONS; check the patient's PPD test or history of tuberculosis before starting the drug. **Safety** QSEN
- Teach patients receiving BRMs and other disease-modifying agents to avoid crowds and people with INFECTIONS; opportunistic pathogens may cause serious infections or death (see Chart 18-9).
- Monitor and interpret laboratory test results for patients with autoimmune connective tissue diseases as highlighted in Chart 18-8.
- Differentiate clinical manifestations and prognosis for patients with systemic lupus erythematosus (SLE) versus systemic sclerosis (SSc) as listed in Chart 18-11.
- Prioritize care by assessing for swallowing ability in patients who have SSc; collaborate with the dietitian for food modifications if needed. **Teamwork and Collaboration** QSEN
- Monitor for acute joint INFLAMMATION in patients with a history of gout; the great toe and other small joints are most typically affected.
- Keep in mind that patients with psoriatic arthritis have skin and joint involvement that require collaborative management (also see Chapter 25 for discussion of psoriasis).
- Assess for visual symptoms (indicating possible giant cell arteritis) in patients with polymyalgia rheumatica; report changes immediately to the health care provider.
- Be aware that arthritis often accompanies other diseases, such as Crohn's disease and hemophilia.

19 CHAPTER

Care of Patients with HIV Disease and Other Immune Deficiencies

James Sampson and M. Linda Workman

ⓔ http://evolve.elsevier.com/Iggy/

PRIORITY CONCEPTS

- Immunity
- Infection
- Nutrition
- Tissue Integrity
- Pain

LEARNING OUTCOMES

Safe and Effective Care Environment

1. Use appropriate techniques to reduce the risk for INFECTION in an immunosuppressed patient.
2. Prevent human immune deficiency virus (HIV) transmission to yourself and others.

Health Promotion and Maintenance

3. Assess all patients for high-risk behaviors related to HIV INFECTION.

Psychosocial Integrity

4. Reduce the psychological impact of HIV disease or other immune deficiencies for the patient and family.

5. Work with other members of the health care team to ensure that the values, preferences, and expressed needs of patients with HIV disease or other immune deficiencies are respected.

Physiological Integrity

6. Use clinical manifestations and laboratory data to assess for immune deficiencies and their complications.
7. Integrate the contributions of others who play a role in helping the patient/family experiencing HIV disease achieve health goals.
8. Prioritize nursing care for the patient with AIDS.

IMMUNITY is complex and functions to help the body stay healthy by preventing the growth of infectious organisms and abnormal cells, such as cancer cells. Infectious organisms and cancer cells are considered "non-self," as described in Chapter 17. The immune system monitors all cells and substances, maintaining those that are considered "self" (belonging to the body) and attacking and destroying "non-self" (foreign) substances. INFECTION from different organisms is a major threat, and exposure occurs daily. The efficiency of the immune system prevents disease despite this exposure. As discussed in Chapter 17, an important function of the immune system is detecting body cells that undergo changes to cancer cells. When detected early enough, the immune system destroys these precancerous cells before a tumor forms.

When the immune system fails to recognize infectious agents, severe local and systemic INFECTIONS are not suppressed or controlled. Immune system failure can be the result of a primary (congenital) immune deficiency in which one or more parts of the system are not functioning properly from birth. It can also be secondary (acquired after birth) as the result of viral infection, contact with a toxin, or medical therapy that can cause a normal immune system to function less efficiently. Then

the immune system can no longer recognize foreign invaders (non-self). The consequences can range from mild, localized health problems to total IMMUNITY failure, leaving the body open to attack from any foreign pathogen.

ACQUIRED (SECONDARY) IMMUNE DEFICIENCIES

HIV INFECTION AND AIDS

❖ PATHOPHYSIOLOGY

Human immune deficiency virus (HIV) INFECTION and disease can progress to acquired immune deficiency syndrome (AIDS), which is the most common immune deficiency disease and is now a serious worldwide epidemic (World Health Organization [WHO], 2013).

Etiology and Genetic Risk

The cause of HIV INFECTION is a virus—the human immune deficiency virus. HIV is a parasite looking for a way into a cell, to take over the cell, and to force the cell into making more copies of the virus (viral particles). These new viral particles then look for additional cells to infect, repeating the cycle as long as there are new host cells to infect.

The HIV Infectious Process. Viral particle features include an outer envelope with special "docking proteins," known as *gp41* and *gp120,* that assist in finding a host (Fig. 19-1). Inside, the virus has genetic material along with the enzymes *reverse transcriptase (RT)* and *integrase.* The HIV must get inside a host cell. It does this by first entering the host's bloodstream and then "hijacking" certain cells, especially the *CD4+ T-cell,* also known as the *CD4+ cell, helper/inducer T-cell,* or *T4-cell* (see Chapter 17). This cell directs immune system defenses and regulates the activity of all immune system cells. When HIV enters a CD4+ T-cell, it can then create more virus particles.

Virus-host interactions are needed after INFECTION for disease development. When a person is infected with HIV, the virus randomly "bumps" into many cells. The docking proteins on the outside of the virus must find special receptors on a host cell for the virus to bind and then enter the cell. The CD4+ T-cell has surface receptors known as *CD4, CCR5,* and *CXCR4* (Fig. 19-2). Proteins on the HIV particle surface, known as *gp120* and *gp41,* recognize these receptors on the CD4+ T-cell. For the virus to enter this cell, *both* the *gp120* and the *gp41* must bind to the receptors. The *gp120* first binds to the primary CD4 receptor, which changes its shape and allows the *gp120* to bind to either the *CCR5* co-receptor or the *CXCR4* co-receptor. Once co-receptor binding occurs, *gp41* inserts a fusion peptide into the T-cell membrane, boring a hole to allow insertion of viral genetic material and enzymes into the host cell. This attachment allows the virus to then enter the CD4+ T-cell (see Fig. 19-2). *Viral binding to the CD4 receptor and to either of the co-receptors is needed to enter the cell.* (The drug class known as *entry inhibitors* works here to prevent the interaction needed for entry of HIV into the CD4+ T-cell.)

After entering a host cell, HIV must get its genetic material into the host cell's DNA. HIV is a **retrovirus,** which is able to insert its single-stranded ribonucleic acid (ss-RNA) genetic material into the host's DNA. The genetic material of the human cell is double-stranded DNA (ds-DNA). To infect and take over a human cell, the genetic material must be the same. The HIV enzyme *reverse transcriptase (RT)* converts HIV's ss-RNA into ds-DNA, which makes the viral genetic material the same as human DNA. (The drug classes known as *nucleoside reverse transcriptase inhibitors [NRTIs]* and *non-nucleoside reverse transcriptase inhibitors [NNRTIs]* work here to prevent viral replication [Fig. 19-3] by reducing how well reverse transcriptase can convert HIV genetic material into human genetic material.) HIV then uses its enzyme *integrase* to get its DNA into the nucleus of the host's CD4+ T-cell and insert it into the host's ds-DNA. This action completes the infection of the CD4+ T-cell. (The drug class known as *integrase inhibitors* works here to prevent viral DNA from integrating into the host's DNA.)

HIV particles are made within the infected CD4+ T-cell, using all the metabolic machinery of the host. The new virus particle is made in the form of one long protein strand. The strand is clipped by the enzyme *HIV protease* into smaller functional pieces. These pieces are formed into a new finished viral particle. (The drug class known as *protease inhibitors* works here to inhibit HIV protease.) Once the new virus particle is finished, it fuses with the infected cell's membrane and then buds off in search of another CD4+ T-cell to infect (see Fig. 19-3).

Effects of HIV infection are related to the new genetic instructions that now direct CD4+ T-cells to change their role in immune system defenses. The new role is to be an "HIV factory," making up to 10 billion new viral particles daily. In addition, the immune system is made weaker by removing some CD4+ T-cells from circulation. In early HIV infection before HIV disease is evident, the immune system can still attack and destroy most of the newly created virus particles. With time, however, the number of HIV particles overwhelms the immune system. Gradually, CD4+ T-cell counts fall, viral numbers *(viral load)* rise, and without treatment, the patient eventually dies of opportunistic INFECTION or cancer.

Everyone who has AIDS has HIV infection; however, not everyone who has HIV infection has AIDS. The distinction is the number of CD4+ T-cells and whether any opportunistic infections have occurred. A healthy adult usually has at least 800 to 1000 CD4+ T-cells per cubic millimeter (mm^3) of blood. This number is reduced in the person with HIV disease.

Some people develop an acute INFECTION within 4 weeks of first being infected. Manifestations of this acute HIV infection can be fever, night sweats, chills, headache, and muscle aches, which are similar to those of any viral infection—not just HIV. A sore throat and rash also may accompany this acute HIV infection. With time, these symptoms cease and the person feels well again, although a "war is going on" between HIV and the immune system.

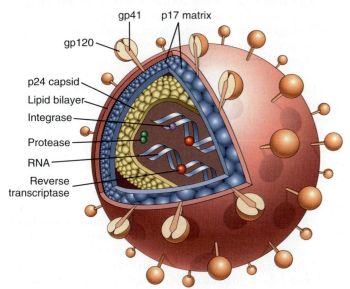

FIG. 19-1 The human immune deficiency virus (HIV).

gp41   p17 matrix
gp120
p24 capsid
Lipid bilayer
Integrase
Protease
RNA
Reverse transcriptase

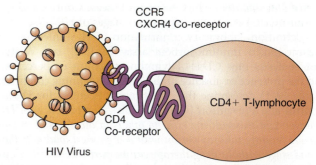

FIG. 19-2 The HIV "docking" proteins and the successful interaction of these proteins with the CD4+ T-lymphocyte receptors.

CCR5
CXCR4 Co-receptor
CD4+ T-lymphocyte
CD4 Co-receptor
HIV Virus

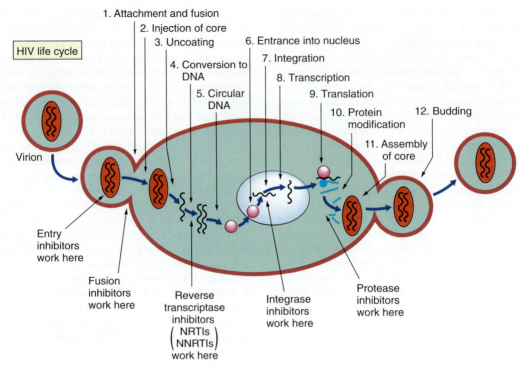

FIG. 19-3 The life cycle of the HIV and sites of action for anti-HIV therapy.

As time passes, more CD4+ T-cells are infected and taken out of service. The count decreases, and those that remain function poorly. Poor CD4+ T-cell function leads to these immune system abnormalities:

- Lymphocytopenia (decreased numbers of lymphocytes)
- Increased production of incomplete and nonfunctional antibodies
- Abnormally functioning macrophages

As the CD4+ T-cell level drops, the patient is at risk for bacterial, fungal, and viral INFECTIONS, as well as opportunistic cancers. **Opportunistic infections** are those caused by organisms that are present as part of the body's normal environment and are kept in check by normal immune function. They occur because of the profound immunosuppression in the person with AIDS.

A diagnosis of AIDS requires that the person be HIV positive and have either a CD4+ T-cell count of less than 200 cells/mm³ or less than 14% (even if the total CD4+ count is above 200 cells/mm³) or an opportunistic infection. Once AIDS is diagnosed, even if the patient's T-cell count goes higher than 200 cells/mm³ or if the percentage rises above 14%, or the infection is successfully treated, the AIDS diagnosis remains and the patient does not revert to being just HIV positive.

HIV Classification. The Centers for Disease Control and Prevention (CDC) currently defines four stages of HIV disease. In this definition, laboratory confirmation of HIV infection (by enzyme-linked immunosorbent assay [ELISA] and Western blot analysis) plus CD4+ T-lymphocyte count or percentage and the presence or absence of the 27 AIDS-defining conditions (Table 19-1) determine the classification (Centers for Disease Control and Prevention [CDC], 2013b). *The person with HIV infection can transmit the virus to others at all stages of disease, but the recently infected person with a high viral load and those at end stage without drug therapy can be particularly infectious.*

Stage 1 CDC Case Definition describes a patient with a CD4+ T-cell count of greater than 500 cells/mm³ or a percentage

of 29% or greater. A person at this stage has no AIDS-defining illnesses.

Stage 2 CDC Case Definition describes a patient with a CD4+ T-cell count between 200 and 499 cells/mm³ or a percentage between 14% and 28%. A person at this stage has no AIDS-defining illnesses.

Stage 3 CDC Case Definition describes any patient with a CD4+ T-cell count of less than 200 cells/mm³ or a percentage of less than 14%. A person who has higher CD4+ T-cell counts or percentages but who also has an AIDS-defining illness meets the Stage 3 CDC Case Definition.

Stage 4 CDC Case Definition is used to describe any patient with a confirmed HIV infection but no information regarding CD4+ T-cell counts, CD4+ T-cell percentages, and AIDS-defining illnesses is available.

HIV Progression. The time from the beginning of HIV INFECTION to development of AIDS ranges from months to years. The range depends on how HIV was acquired, personal factors, and interventions. For people who have been transfused with HIV-contaminated blood, for example, AIDS often develops quickly. For those who become HIV positive as a result of a single sexual encounter, the period is much longer before progression to AIDS. Other personal factors that influence progression to AIDS include frequency of re-exposure to HIV, presence of other sexually transmitted diseases (STDs), nutrition status, and stress.

Incidence and Prevalence

Since the beginning of the epidemic in the United States, more than 636,000 people have died of AIDS. Currently, about 50,000 people are diagnosed yearly and more than 1,148,200 people in the United States are living with HIV/AIDS (CDC, 2013b). Worldwide, about 40 to 60 million people are currently infected with HIV, at least 30 million deaths from AIDs have occurred, and 33 million people are living with AIDS (WHO, 2013).

TABLE 19-1 Centers for Disease Control and Prevention Classification of Aids-Defining Conditions in Adults

- Bacterial infections, multiple or recurrent
- Candidiasis of bronchi, trachea, or lungs
- Candidiasis of esophagus
- Cervical cancer, invasive
- Coccidioidomycosis, disseminated or extrapulmonary
- Cryptococcosis, extrapulmonary
- Cryptosporidiosis, chronic intestinal (>1-month's duration)
- Cytomegalovirus disease (other than liver, spleen, or nodes)
- Cytomegalovirus retinitis (with loss of vision)
- Encephalopathy, HIV-related
- Herpes simplex: chronic ulcers (>1-month's duration) or bronchitis, pneumonitis, or esophagitis
- Histoplasmosis, disseminated or extrapulmonary
- Isosporiasis, chronic intestinal (>1-month's duration)
- Kaposi's sarcoma
- Lymphoid interstitial pneumonia or pulmonary lymphoid hyperplasia complex
- Lymphoma, Burkitt's (or equivalent term)
- Lymphoma, immunoblastic (or equivalent term)
- Lymphoma, primary, of brain
- *Mycobacterium avium* complex or *Mycobacterium kansasii,* disseminated or extrapulmonary
- *Mycobacterium tuberculosis* of any site, pulmonary, disseminated, or extrapulmonary
- *Mycobacterium,* other species or unidentified species, disseminated or extrapulmonary
- *Pneumocystis jiroveci* pneumonia
- Pneumonia, recurrent (two instances within 12 months)
- Progressive multifocal leukoencephalopathy
- *Salmonella* septicemia, recurrent
- Toxoplasmosis of brain
- Wasting syndrome attributed to HIV

From Schneider, E., Whitmore, S., Glynn, K.M., Dominguez, K., Mitsch, A., McKenna, M.T.; Centers for Disease Control and Prevention. (2008). Revised surveillance case definitions for HIV infection among adults, adolescents, and children aged <18 months and for HIV infection and AIDS among children aged 18 months to <13 years—United States, 2008. *Morbidity and Mortality Weekly Report: Recommendations and Reports, 57*(RR-10), 9. Retrieved December 2013 from www.cdc.gov/mmwr/preview/mmwrhtml/rr5710a2.htm

GENETIC/GENOMIC CONSIDERATIONS

Patient-Centered Care [QSEN]

About 1% of people with HIV infection are long-term nonprogressors (LTNPs). These people have been infected with HIV for at least 10 years and have remained asymptomatic, with CD4+ T-cell counts within the normal range and a viral load that is either undetectable or very low.

A genetic difference for this population is that their *CCR5/CXCR4* co-receptors on the CD4+ T-cells are abnormal and nonfunctional as a result of gene mutations for these co-receptors. The mutation creates defective co-receptors that do not bind to the HIV docking proteins. Cells with this defective co-receptor successfully resist the entrance of HIV. People who have only one mutated co-receptor gene allele have fewer normal co-receptors and can be infected with HIV, although disease progression is relatively slow.

Most AIDS cases in North America occur among men who have sex with men (MSM) (59%-69%) or people of either gender who have used injection drugs (16%) (CDC, 2013b). *The changing demographics of the infection indicate that the perception that HIV/AIDS is only a problem for homosexual white men is false (Kirton, 2011).*

CULTURAL CONSIDERATIONS

Patient-Centered Care [QSEN]

Most new HIV infections reported in the United States occur in racial and ethnic minority groups, particularly among African Americans and Hispanics (CDC, 2013b). These two groups show an increasing trend in HIV infection and disease compared with a leveling off among white people.

GENDER HEALTH CONSIDERATIONS

Patient-Centered Care [QSEN]

About 25% of newly diagnosed cases are women. In less affluent countries, 50% of cases occur in women (WHO, 2013). The largest risk factor is sexual exposure. Strategies specifically targeted to reducing sexual exposures of HIV to women may help prevent an increase in HIV infection in that group. Women with HIV disease have a poorer outcome with shorter mean survival time than that of men. This outcome may be the result of late diagnosis and social or economic factors that reduce access to medical care.

Gynecologic problems, especially persistent or recurrent vaginal candidiasis, may be the first signs of HIV disease in women. Other problems include pelvic inflammatory disease, genital herpes, other sexually transmitted diseases (STDs), and cervical dysplasia or cancer.

The effect of HIV on pregnancy outcomes includes higher incidence of premature delivery, low-birth-weight infants, and transmission of the disease to the infant. Appropriate antiretroviral drug therapy during pregnancy reduces the risk for transmitting the infection to the infant. (See the discussion on p. 332 in the Perinatal Transmission section.)

CONSIDERATIONS FOR OLDER ADULTS

Patient-Centered Care [QSEN]

Infection with HIV can occur at any age. Assess the older patient for risk behaviors, including a sexual and drug use history (Foster et al., 2012). (See the Evidence-Based Practice box for specific risky behaviors often practiced by older adults.) Age-related decline in immunity increases the likelihood that the older adult will develop the infection after an HIV exposure.

Health Promotion and Maintenance

AIDS is a disease with a mortality rate of at least 60% for adults. Although a very few people who have been given high doses of antiretroviral drugs immediately upon diagnosis have subsequently shown no detectable virus, there are too few cases to indicate whether such therapy can result in an enduring cure. Thus, at this time, there is no available cure for AIDS and a major focus for health care worldwide is prevention of HIV INFECTION.

HIV has been found in blood, semen, vaginal secretions, breast milk, amniotic fluid, urine, feces, saliva, tears, cerebrospinal fluid, lymph nodes, cervical cells, corneal tissue, and brain tissue of infected patients. The fluids with the highest concentrations of HIV are semen and blood. HIV is transmitted most often in these three ways:

- Sexual: genital, anal, or oral sexual contact with exposure of mucous membranes to infected semen or vaginal secretions
- Parenteral: sharing of needles or equipment contaminated with infected blood or receiving contaminated blood products

EVIDENCE-BASED PRACTICE (QSEN)

How Are Older Adults at Risk for HIV Infection?

Foster, V., Clark, P., Holstad, M., & Burgess, E. (2012). Factors associated with risky sexual behaviors in older adults. *Journal of the Association of Nurses in AIDS Care, 23*(6), 487-499.

The incidence of human immune deficiency virus (HIV) infection is significant among adults over 50 years of age in North America and contributes to earlier mortality and morbidity in this age-group. Many programs for HIV risk reduction focus on younger adults, teenagers, and racial/ethic minorities. However, the older adult age-group continues to develop HIV infection. This correlational study sought to (1) determine whether higher levels of HIV knowledge and higher levels of motivation to practice safer sex were associated with lower levels of risky sexual behaviors and (2) identify what factors were associated with continued practice of risky sexual behaviors among adults ages 50 years and older.

A convenience sample of 106 sexually active, community-dwelling, single men and women ranging in age from 50 to 74 years were recruited into the study. (Some participants planned to be sexually active, whereas others were sexually active during the study period.)

Level of Evidence: 4

The study method was prospective, cross-sectional, and correlational. Statistical evaluation methods were appropriate for the design.

Commentary: Implications for Practice and Research

The study is important for many reasons. First, it established the incidence of sexual behaviors in a relatively large group of older adult participants. It also highlighted the fact that many health care professionals, as well as older adult patients, are reluctant to discuss sexual behaviors and risk for HIV infection in the defined age-group. In addition, the knowledge of correct condom use, a well-established deterrent to HIV transmission, is lacking among many older adults.

The study defined important areas for future nursing research. Among these are the need for nurses and other health care professionals to understand that aging does not limit the risks for HIV transmission and the absolute need for consistently addressing sexuality in older adults. Strategies to increase correct condom use among sexually active older adults (who may only see the use as a no-longer-needed form of birth control) need to be developed and tested.

• Perinatal: from the placenta, from contact with maternal blood and body fluids during birth, or from breast milk from an infected mother to child

Teach everyone about the transmission routes and ways to reduce their exposure (discussed next). Also stress that HIV is not transmitted by casual contact in the home, school, or workplace. Sharing household utensils, towels and linens, and toilet facilities does not transmit HIV. In addition, HIV is not spread by mosquitoes or other insects.

! NURSING SAFETY PRIORITY (QSEN)

Action Alert

Teach all people, regardless of age, gender, ethnicity, or sexual orientation, that they are susceptible to HIV infection.

Sexual Transmission

Safer sex methods of *A, abstinence; B, be faithful;* and *C, condom use* can reduce HIV transmission. *Abstinence and mutually monogamous sex with a noninfected partner are the only absolutely safe methods of preventing HIV INFECTION from sexual contact.* Many forms of sexual expression can spread HIV infection if one partner is infected. *The risk for becoming infected from a partner who is HIV positive is always present,* although some sexual practices are more risky than others. Because the virus concentrates in blood and seminal fluid and is also present in vaginal secretions, risk differs by gender, sexual act, and the viral load of the infected partner.

Gender affects HIV transmission, like all other sexually transmitted diseases (STDs), and it is more easily transmitted from infected male to uninfected female than vice versa. This is because HIV is most easily transmitted when infected body fluids come into contact with mucous membranes or nonintact skin. The vagina has more surface area of mucous membrane than does the penis. Teach women the importance of always either using a vaginal or dental dam or female condom or having their male partners use a condom.

Sexual acts or practices that permit infected seminal fluid to come into contact with mucous membranes or nonintact skin are the most risky for sexual transmission of HIV. The practice with the highest risk is anal intercourse with the penis and seminal fluid of an infected person coming into contact with the mucous membranes of the uninfected partner's rectum. *Anal intercourse in which the semen depositor (inserting or active partner) is infected is a very risky sexual practice regardless of whether the semen receiver (receiving partner) is male or female.* Anal intercourse not only allows seminal fluid to make contact with the mucous membranes of the rectum but also tears the mucous membranes, making INFECTION more likely. Teach patients who engage in anal intercourse that the semen depositor needs to wear a condom during this act.

Viral load, or the amount of virus present in blood and other body fluids, affects transmission. The higher the blood level of HIV (**viremia**), the greater the risk for sexual and perinatal transmission. Current highly active antiretroviral therapy (HAART) has caused the viral load of some infected patients to drop below detectable levels. *Although there is less virus in seminal or vaginal fluids of people receiving HAART, the risk for transmission still exists.*

Safer sex practices are those that reduce the risk for nonintact skin or mucous membranes coming in contact with infected body fluids and blood. Teach everyone the importance of consistently using these safer sex practices:
• A latex or polyurethane condom for genital and anal intercourse
• A condom or latex barrier (dental dam) over the genitals or anus during oral-genital or oral-anal sexual contact
• Latex gloves for finger or hand contact with the vagina or rectum

New research for prevention of sexual transmission has resulted in the use of drug therapy for *pre-exposure prophylaxis* (Aschenbrenner, 2012). The use of the combination drug *Truvada* (emtricitabine and tenofovir) by HIV-1–negative sexual partners of known HIV-1–positive people appears to reduce HIV transmission.

For those who believe they have been exposed to HIV as a result of sexual relations or other types of non-occupational

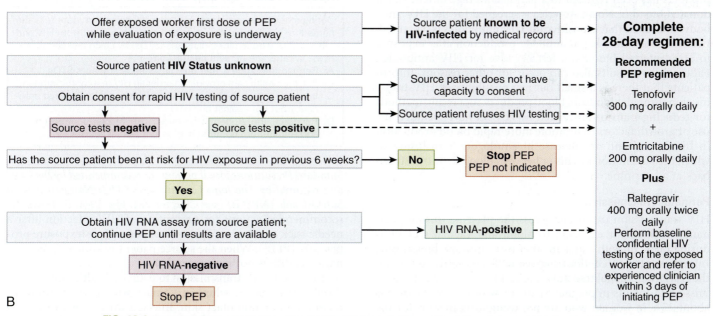

FIG. 19-4 New York State Health Department HIV guidelines. **A,** Recommendations for non-occupational postexposure prophylaxis for HIV infection. **B,** Recommendations for occupational postexposure prophylaxis for HIV infection.

exposure, the CDC has guidelines for *postexposure prophylaxis.* The length and type of prophylaxis therapy depend on the nature of the exposure (Fig. 19-4, *A*).

Parenteral Transmission

Preventive practices to reduce transmission among injection drug users (IDUs) include the use of proper cleaning of "works" (needles, syringes, other drug paraphernalia). Instruct IDUs to clean a used needle and syringe by first filling and flushing them with clear water. Next, the syringe should be filled with ordinary household bleach. The bleach-filled syringe should be shaken for 30 to 60 seconds. Advise IDUs to carry a small container with this solution whenever sharing needles. Some communities have a needle exchange program in which needles and

Drug Alert

Pre-exposure prophylaxis does not replace the standard safer sex practices recommended to prevent HIV transmission. Also, if this type of drug therapy is used in patients who become infected with HIV-1, the risk for developing drug resistance greatly increases. Therefore remind people prescribed Truvada to use the safer sex practices previously described and to adhere to an every-3-month HIV testing schedule along with monitoring for side effects of this drug.

? NCLEX EXAMINATION CHALLENGE

Physiological Integrity

Which couple has the highest risk for sexual transmission of HIV without the use of a condom or dental dam?
A. Uninfected male performing vaginal intercourse with an infected female
B. Infected male performing vaginal intercourse with an uninfected female
C. Uninfected male performing anal intercourse with an infected male
D. Infected male performing oral sex on an uninfected male

CHART 19-1   Best Practice for Patient Safety & Quality Care (QSEN)

Recommendations for Preventing HIV Transmission by Health Care Workers

- Workers should adhere to Standard Precautions.
- Workers with exudative lesions or weeping dermatitis should not perform direct patient care or handle patient care equipment and devices used in invasive procedures.
- Workers must follow guidelines for disinfection and sterilization of reusable equipment used in invasive procedures.
- Workers infected with HIV are not restricted from practice of non–exposure-prone procedures, as long as they comply with Standard Precautions and sterilization and disinfection recommendations.
- Workers should identify exposure-prone procedures by institutions where they are performed.
- Workers who perform exposure-prone procedures should know their HIV antibody status.
- Workers who are infected with HIV should seek advice from an expert review panel before performing exposure-prone procedures to determine under what circumstances they may continue to practice these procedures. These circumstances would include notification of prospective patients of HIV positivity.

Adapted from Centers for Disease Control and Prevention. (1991). Recommendations for preventing transmission of human immunodeficiency virus and hepatitis B virus to patients during exposure-prone invasive procedures. *Morbidity and Mortality Weekly Report: Recommendations and Reports, 40*(RR-8), 1-9.

? NCLEX EXAMINATION CHALLENGE

Health Promotion and Maintenance

During a health assessment, a 22-year-old college student tells the nurse that she is sexually active and protects herself from HIV and other sexually transmitted diseases (STDs) by using oral contraceptives. What is the nurse's best action?
A. Remind the student that only abstinence prevents STDs.
B. Ask the health care provider to order an HIV test for this student.
C. Inform the student that oral contraceptives protect against pregnancy but not against any STD.
D. Reinforce the student's preferred use of oral contraceptives, and refrain from commenting on her sexual activity.

syringes are used only once and are then exchanged for clean ones.

The risk for AIDS transmission through blood and blood products has been reduced to a national average of 0.02%. All donated blood in North America is screened for the HIV antibody, and blood that is positive for HIV antibodies is discarded. Because of the time lag in antibody production after exposure to HIV, infected blood can test negative for HIV antibodies. False-negative results also can occur for other reasons. Inform patients that there is a small but real possibility of HIV transmission through blood and blood products. As a result, methods for reducing transfusion-related INFECTION have included the use of growth factors to promote more rapid blood production in the patient and an increase in autologous transfusion in which the patient donates his or her own blood to be transfused back at a later time.

Perinatal Transmission

HIV transmission can occur across the placenta during pregnancy, with infant exposure to blood and vaginal secretions during birth, or with exposure after birth through breast milk. Inform women of childbearing age with HIV infection about the risks for perinatal transmission. The risk for perinatal transmission to infants in pregnant patients with HIV INFECTION is about 25% in woman who are not using drug therapy for the disease compared with about 8% for women who are using drug therapy for HIV. Therefore encourage HIV-positive women who are pregnant to continue the therapy or, if they are not on antiviral therapy, to start the therapy as soon as possible.

Transmission and Health Care Workers

Needle stick or "sharps" injuries are the main means of occupation-related HIV infection for health care workers. In addition, health care workers can be infected through exposure of nonintact skin and mucous membranes to blood and body fluids. *The best prevention for health care providers is the consistent use of*

Standard Precautions for all patients as recommended by the CDC and required by The Joint Commission's (TJC) National Patient Safety Goals (NPSGs) (see Chapter 23). Fig. 19-4, *B* shows the recommended actions for prevention of HIV infection after a needle stick or other occupational exposure (postexposure prophylaxis [PEP]). When the source patient is known to be HIV negative, PEP is not recommended.

To prevent HIV transmission to patients, health care workers should wear gloves when in contact with patients' mucous membranes or nonintact skin. Infected workers with weeping dermatitis or open lesions should not perform direct care. The CDC guidelines for preventing HIV transmission by health care workers during exposure-prone invasive procedures are listed in Chart 19-1. These include any procedure in which there is a risk for broken skin injury to the health care worker and the worker's blood is likely to make contact with the patient's body cavity, subcutaneous tissues, or mucous membranes.

Testing

Testing for HIV antibodies or other features of the virus is complex, requiring interpretation, counseling, and confidentiality. Testing plays a role in prevention because tests are a way

---

CHART 19-2 Patient and Family Education: Preparing for Self-Management

CDC Recommendations for HIV Testing

You should be tested for HIV if you fall within one or more of these groups:

- People with sexually transmitted disease
- Injection drug users
- People who consider themselves at risk
- Women of childbearing age with identifiable risks, including:
  - Used injection drugs
  - Engaged in prostitution
  - Had sexual partners who were infected or at risk
  - Had sexual contact with men from countries with high HIV prevalence
- People who received a transfusion between 1978 and 1985
- People planning to get married
- People undergoing medical evaluation or treatment for manifestations that may be HIV related
- People admitted to hospitals
- People in correctional institutions such as jails and prisons
- Prostitutes and their customers

Adapted from Centers for Disease Control and Prevention. (1987). Public Health Service guidelines for counseling and antibody testing to prevent HIV infection and AIDS. *Morbidity and Mortality Weekly Report, 36*(31), 509-515. *CDC,* Centers for Disease Control and Prevention.

---

of diagnosing HIV INFECTION before immune changes or disease manifestations develop. A primary health care focus for testing is to teach those who test positive to modify their behaviors to prevent transmission to others. *Therefore all sexually active people should know their HIV status.* Chart 19-2 lists additional conditions for which HIV antibody testing is advised.

Pretest and post-test counseling must be performed by personnel trained in HIV issues. These counselors may be nurses, physicians, social workers, health educators, or even lay educators who have specialized training. Counseling helps the patient make an informed decision about testing and provides an opportunity to teach risk-reduction behaviors. Post-test counseling is needed to interpret the results, discuss risk reduction, and provide psychological support and health promotion information for the patient with a positive test result. People who test positive should also be counseled on how to inform sexual partners and those with whom they have shared needles. Testing methods, their accuracy, and indications are presented on p. 336 in the Laboratory Assessment section.

❖ PATIENT-CENTERED COLLABORATIVE CARE

◆ Assessment

The person who has HIV disease is monitored on a regular basis for changes in immune function or health status that indicate disease progression and the need for intervention. The frequency of monitoring varies from every 2 to 6 months based on disease progression and responses to treatment. This continuing assessment of the patient with HIV disease is crucial, because he or she may have problems related to disease in many organ systems and to ensure that the drug continues to work optimally. Assess subtle changes so that INFECTIONS and other problems can be found early and treated.

History. Ask about age, gender, occupation, and where the person lives. Thoroughly assess the current illness, including when it started, the severity of symptoms, associated problems, and any interventions to date. Ask the patient about when the

HIV INFECTION was diagnosed and what manifestations led to that diagnosis. Ask him or her to give a chronologic history of infections and problems since the diagnosis. Assess the patient's health history, including whether he or she received a blood transfusion between 1978 and 1985 in the United States (before routine blood testing for HIV contamination). Because blood testing for HIV contamination is not consistently performed in all parts of the world, ask the immigrant patient about his or her history of transfusion therapy before coming to the United States.

Ask the patient about sexual practices, sexually transmitted diseases (STDs), and major infectious diseases, including tuberculosis and hepatitis. If the patient has hemophilia, ask about treatment with clotting factors. Determine whether the patient has engaged in past or present injection drug use, including needle sharing. Assess the patient's level of knowledge regarding the diagnosis, symptom management, diagnostic tests, treatments, community resources, and modes of HIV transmission. Also assess his or her understanding and use of safer sex practices. If knowledge deficits are found, provide the appropriate patient teaching.

Physical Assessment/Clinical Manifestations. HIV disease and AIDS are a progression continuum. The patient with HIV disease may either have few manifestations and problems or may have problems that are acute rather than chronically present. As the disease progresses, however, more severe health problems occur and the patient may not realize that the disease is progressing. Assess for clusters of symptoms that may indicate disease progression (Chart 19-3).

Opportunistic Infections. The patient with HIV/AIDS often develops pathogenic INFECTIONS and opportunistic infections. *Pathogenic infections* are caused by virulent organisms and occur even among people with normal IMMUNITY. *Opportunistic infections* are those caused by organisms that are present as part of the body's normal environment and are kept in check by normal immune function. Only when immunity is depressed are such organisms capable of causing infection.

Opportunistic INFECTIONS occur because of the profound immunosuppression of the person with HIV disease. They may result from primary infection or reactivation of a latent infection. Opportunistic infections account for many of the clinical manifestations observed in HIV infection and can be protozoan, fungal, bacterial, or viral. More than one infection may be present at the same time. The presence of opportunistic infections may represent disease progression or a temporary further reduction of immune status. *In either case, these infections can result in death if appropriate treatment is not started quickly.* Priority nursing actions when caring for a patient who is HIV positive are continually assessing for and documenting the presence of an opportunistic infection and monitoring the patient's response to therapy. Report to the health care provider those manifestations that may indicate an infection.

Opportunistic infections do not pose a threat to the immunocompetent health care worker caring for a patient with HIV disease or AIDS. When the patient with HIV disease or AIDS has a pathogenic infection, however, health care personnel must use precautions appropriate to the specific disease to prevent disease spread. For example, when the person with HIV/AIDS also has tuberculosis at a transmissible stage, Airborne Precautions are needed in addition to Standard Precautions. See Chapter 23 for a more complete discussion on Transmission-Based Precautions for specific infectious diseases.

CHART 19-3 Key Features

AIDS

Immunologic Manifestations
- Low white blood cell counts:
  - CD4+/CD8+ ratio <2
  - CD4+ count <200/mm³
- Hypergammaglobulinemia
- Opportunistic infections
- Lymphadenopathy
- Fatigue

Integumentary Manifestations
- Dry skin
- Poor wound healing
- Skin lesions
- Night sweats

Respiratory Manifestations
- Cough
- Shortness of breath

Gastrointestinal Manifestations
- Diarrhea
- Weight loss
- Nausea and vomiting

Central Nervous System Manifestations
- Confusion
- Dementia
- Headache
- Fever
- Visual changes
- Memory loss
- Personality changes
- Pain
- Seizures

Opportunistic Infections
- Protozoal infections:
  - Toxoplasmosis
  - Cryptosporidiosis
  - Isosporiasis
  - Microsporidiosis
  - Strongyloidiasis
  - Giardiasis
- Fungal infections:
  - Candidiasis
  - *Pneumocystis jiroveci* pneumonia
  - Cryptococcosis
  - Histoplasmosis
  - Coccidioidomycosis
- Bacterial infections:
  - *Mycobacterium avium* complex infection
  - Tuberculosis
  - Nocardiosis
- Viral infections:
  - Cytomegalovirus infection
  - Herpes simplex virus infection
  - Varicella-zoster virus infection

Malignancies
- Kaposi's sarcoma
- Non-Hodgkin's lymphoma
- Hodgkin's lymphoma
- Invasive cervical carcinoma

FIG. 19-5 Oral candidiasis (thrush).

Candida fungus) occurs because the immune system can no longer control fungal growth. *Candida* stomatitis or esophagitis occurs often in AIDS. Patients may report food tasting "funny," mouth pain, difficulty in swallowing, and pain behind the sternum. On examination of the mouth and throat, you may see cottage cheese–like, yellowish white plaques and inflammation (Fig. 19-5). Esophagitis is diagnosed by endoscopic examination with biopsy and culture. Women with HIV disease or AIDS may have persistent vaginal candidiasis with severe pruritus (itching), perineal irritation, and a thick, white vaginal discharge.

Cryptococcosis, caused by *Cryptococcus neoformans*, is a debilitating meningitis and can be a widely spread infection in AIDS. Ask about fever, headache, blurred vision, nausea and vomiting, neck stiffness, confusion, and other mental status changes. Patients may have seizures and other neurologic problems, or they may have mild malaise, fever, and headaches.

Histoplasmosis, caused by *Histoplasma capsulatum*, begins as a respiratory INFECTION and progresses to widespread infection in the person with AIDS. Assess for dyspnea, fever, cough, and weight loss. Check for enlargement of lymph nodes, the spleen, or the liver.

Bacterial infections are acquired from other people or sources and as overgrowth of skin flora. *Mycobacterium avium* complex (MAC) is the most common bacterial INFECTION associated with AIDS. This problem is caused by *M. intracellulare* or *M. avium*, which infects the respiratory or GI tract. MAC is a systemic infection. Assess for fever, debility, weight loss, malaise, and sometimes swollen lymph glands or organ disease.

Tuberculosis (TB), caused by *Mycobacterium tuberculosis*, occurs in 2% to 10% of persons with AIDS (CDC, 2009). More than 50% of all patients with AIDS and TB have extrapulmonary disease sites, including the central nervous system, bones, liver, spleen, skin, and intestinal tract. Ask about cough, dyspnea, chest pain, fever, chills, night sweats, weight loss, and anorexia. Manifestations of extrapulmonary infection vary with the site. *The person with TB and a CD4+ T-cell count below 200/mm³ may not have a positive TB skin test (purified protein derivative [PPD]) because of an inability to mount an immune response to the antigen, a condition known as anergy.* Blood analysis by the fully automated nucleic acid amplification test (NAAT) for tuberculosis with results available in less than 2 hours is the most

Protozoal and fungal infections are common among patients with AIDS. *Pneumocystis jiroveci* pneumonia (PCP) is the most common opportunistic INFECTION in persons infected with HIV. This organism is now considered a fungus. Assess for dyspnea on exertion, tachypnea, a persistent dry cough, and a persistent low-grade fever. The patient may report fatigue and weight loss. Auscultate breath sounds for crackles.

Toxoplasmosis encephalitis, caused by *Toxoplasma gondii*, is acquired through contact with contaminated cat feces or by ingesting infected undercooked meat. Assess the patient for subtle changes in mental status, neurologic deficits, headaches, and fever. Additional changes may include difficulties with speech, gait, and vision; seizures; lethargy; and confusion. Perform a comprehensive mental status examination and monitor the patient to detect subtle changes.

Cryptosporidiosis is an intestinal INFECTION caused by *Cryptosporidium* organisms. In AIDS, this illness ranges from a mild diarrhea to a severe wasting with electrolyte imbalance. Diarrhea may result in fluid loss of up to 15 to 20 L/day. Ask the patient about the presence of diarrhea and whether he or she has had an unplanned weight loss of 5 pounds or more.

Fungal INFECTION occurs by overgrowth of normal body flora. *Candida albicans* is part of the intestinal tract's natural flora. In the person with AIDS, candidiasis (overgrowth of the sensitive and rapid test for the presence of *M. tuberculosis.* It is very useful in the acute care setting to determine whether a symptomatic patient actually has TB. Other diagnostic tests include a chest x-ray, acid-fast sputum smear, and sputum culture.

> ### ❗ NURSING SAFETY PRIORITY (QSEN)
> **Action Alert**
>
> Until parameters other than a skin test come back negative for TB in a patient with AIDS who also has TB manifestations, maintain Airborne Precautions along with Standard Precautions.

The tuberculosis bacillus is spread by airborne routes. When particles from the patient's respiratory tract are aerosolized, anyone near him or her is at risk for inhaling the particles and the bacillus. Therefore the nurse or respiratory therapist who gives cough-inducing aerosol treatments, such as pentamidine isethionate, to patients with AIDS should be screened with a PPD skin test or QuantiFERON blood test every 6 months to determine whether he or she has been infected with TB.

Pneumonia from bacterial INFECTION recurs often among patients with AIDS, and two or more episodes of any type of bacterial pneumonia in a 12-month period are an AIDS case definition. Assess for chest pain, productive cough, fever, and dyspnea.

Viral infection from a virus other than HIV is common among people with HIV disease that has progressed to AIDS. Cytomegalovirus (CMV) can infect many sites in persons with AIDS, including the eye (CMV retinitis), respiratory and GI tracts, and the central nervous system. CMV INFECTION can also cause many nonspecific problems such as fever, malaise, weight loss, fatigue, and swollen lymph nodes. CMV retinitis impairs vision, ranging from slight impairment to total blindness. CMV can also cause diarrhea, abdominal bloating and discomfort, and weight loss. Ask the patient whether he or she has any of these manifestations. In addition, CMV can cause encephalitis, pneumonitis, adrenalitis, hepatitis, and disseminated infection.

Herpes simplex virus (HSV) INFECTION in people with HIV disease or AIDS occurs in the perirectal, oral, and genital areas. The manifestations are more widespread and of longer duration among patients with HIV/AIDS than among those who are immunocompetent. Numbness or tingling at the site of infection occurs up to 24 hours before blisters form. Lesions are painful, with chronic open areas after blisters rupture. Assess for fever, pain, bleeding, and enlarged lymph nodes in the affected area. Also assess for headache, myalgia, and malaise.

Varicella-zoster virus (VZV) infection (*shingles*) is not a new INFECTION for people with AIDS. This virus causes chickenpox and then remains present in the nerve ganglia. When people who have had chickenpox previously are immunocompromised, VZV leaves the nerve ganglia and enters other tissue areas, causing shingles. Ask whether the patient has pain and burning along sensory nerve tracts (see Chapter 41 for the dermatomes of sensory nerve locations), headache, and low-grade fever. Examine the skin for fluid-filled blisters with or without crusts.

Malignancies. Weakened IMMUNITY increases the risk for some cancers. These include Kaposi's sarcoma, lymphomas,

FIG. 19-6 Kaposi's sarcoma lesions.

invasive cervical cancer, lung cancer, GI cancer, and anal cancer (Kirton, 2011).

Kaposi's sarcoma (KS) is the most common AIDS-related malignancy. The risk for KS appears to be related to co-infection with human herpes virus-8.

KS develops as small, purplish brown, raised lesions that are usually not painful or itchy. The skin and mucous membrane lesions can occur anywhere on the body (Fig. 19-6). In some patients, lesions develop in the lymph nodes, mouth and throat, intestinal tract, or lungs. KS is diagnosed by biopsy and histologic examination of the lesion. Assess KS lesions for number, size, location, and whether they are intact, and monitor their progression.

Malignant lymphomas occurring with AIDS are Hodgkin's lymphoma, non-Hodgkin's B-cell lymphomas (such as Burkitt's lymphoma), immunoblastic lymphoma, and primary brain lymphoma. Manifestations include swollen lymph nodes, weight loss, fever, and night sweats.

Human papilloma virus (HPV) INFECTION results in multiple types of malignancies and manifestations, but the most common in HIV infection are cervical and anal cancers. Cervical Papanicolaou (Pap) testing every 6 months is the standard of care for HIV-positive patients. In MSM patients, performing an anal Pap test, using the same medium as for a cervical Pap test, is now becoming standard of care and is being extended to both male and female patients for the early detection and treatment of cervical and anal cancers.

Endocrine Complications. Patients with HIV disease may have disease-related and treatment-related endocrine problems, such as gonadal dysfunction, body shape changes, adrenal insufficiency, diabetes mellitus, and elevated triglycerides and cholesterol (which increase the risk for cardiovascular problems).

Many HIV-positive men have low testosterone levels, and HIV-positive women often have irregular menstrual cycles. With this gonadal dysfunction comes a decrease in body muscle mass for both genders, with a decrease in weight, and a change in libido, accompanied by a decrease in energy and an increase in fatigue.

Body shape changes from fat redistribution or fat disposition (known as *lipodystrophy*) are common in patients receiving antiretroviral therapies, especially protease inhibitors and nucleoside reverse transcriptase inhibitors. Manifestations include "buffalo humps" or cervical (neck) fat development and large abdominal fat accumulations. Other body areas, such as the face, arms, and legs, have a wasted appearance and show prominent vein patterns or sunken facial cheeks from loss of subcutaneous fat, known as *lipoatrophy.*

Adrenal dysfunction can result from the glands being infected by opportunistic infections, resulting in adrenal insufficiency. This problem manifests as fatigue, weight loss, nausea, vomiting, low blood pressure, and electrolyte disturbances and can be life threatening.

Patients taking protease inhibitors have a higher-than-expected incidence of type 1 diabetes and hyperlipidemia. These problems are seen even among patients who have no other risks for these problems or the associated heart disease.

Other Clinical Manifestations. All body systems are affected in AIDS. *AIDS dementia complex (ADC),* also called *HIV-associated dementia complex,* refers to the manifestations of central nervous system involvement. ADC occurs in about 70% of people with AIDS and is a result of infection of cells within the central nervous system by HIV. ADC causes cognitive, motor, and behavioral impairments. Manifestations range from barely noticeable to severe dementia. (See Chapter 42 for more discussion on dementia.)

Some neurologic problems may be a result of HIV INFEC-TION or drug side effects, including peripheral neuropathies and myopathies. Assess for manifestations of peripheral neuropathies, which include paresthesias and burning sensations, reduced sensory perception, pain, and gait changes. Myopathies are accompanied by leg weakness, ataxia, and muscle pain.

AIDS wasting syndrome is not due to any single factor. It may be a result of altered metabolism from cancer or INFECTION. Diarrhea, malabsorption, anorexia, and oral and esophageal lesions can all contribute to persistent weight loss, and the patient may appear quite emaciated.

Skin changes include dry, itchy, irritated skin and many types of rashes. Folliculitis, eczema, or psoriasis may occur. Ask the patient about skin sensation changes, and examine any rash or irritation. When the platelet count is low, petechiae or bleeding gums may be present.

Kidney problems, including HIV-associated nephropathy (HIVAN) are common. These problems range from discrete glomerular injury to acute and chronic kidney diseases. Compared with the general population, patients with HIV have a sixteenfold higher risk for requiring a renal replacement intervention.

Psychosocial Assessment. Psychosocial data collection for a patient with AIDS is very important. Ask about the patient's social support system, including family, significant others, and friends. To protect confidentiality, learn who in this support system is aware of the diagnosis so that it is not inadvertently mentioned. Health care professionals must respect the patient's choices as much as possible without compromising care. Offer resources to help with disclosure to sexual partners or significant others.

The patient may be closest to a lover or a friend who is not legally recognized as next of kin. Obtain the name and telephone number of that person, and learn whether a health care proxy or durable power-of-attorney document has been signed.

Ask about the patient's ADLs and any changes that may have occurred since the diagnosis. Assess his or her employment status and occupation, immigration status, social activities and hobbies, living arrangements, and financial resources, including health insurance. Ask whether he or she uses drugs,

including tobacco, alcohol, supplements, opioids, benzodiaze-pines, cocaine, crystal methamphetamine, or injection drugs.

To plan care and monitor changes, assess the patient's anxiety level, mood, cognitive ability, and energy level. Ask about any experiences with discrimination and how they were handled. After assessing the patient's level of self-esteem and changes in body image, work with him or her to identify strengths and coping strategies. Gather information about any suicidal ideation, depression, or other psychological problems. Also ask about the use of support groups or other community resources.

The patient with HIV disease has less energy as the disease progresses, and there are many causes. Pace interviews, assessments, and interventions to match his or her energy level. When the patient is greatly fatigued, postpone or eliminate nonurgent tests or care activities.

Laboratory Assessment

Lymphocyte Counts. Lymphocyte counts are performed as part of a complete blood count (CBC) with differential (see Chapter 17). The normal white blood cell (WBC) count is between 5000 and 10,000 cells/mm^3, with a differential of about 30% to 40% lymphocytes (an absolute number of 1500 to 4500). Patients with AIDS are often leukopenic, with a WBC count of less than 3500 cells/mm^3, and lymphopenic (<1500 lymphocytes/mm^3).

CD4+ T-cell and CD8+ T-cell counts and percentages are part of an immune profile. People with HIV disease and AIDS usually have a lower-than-normal number of CD4+ T-cells, whereas the number of CD8+ T-cells remains normal. The normal ratio of CD4+ to CD8+ T-cells is 2:1. In HIV disease and AIDS, because of the low number of CD4+ T-cells, this ratio is low. Low CD4+ T-cell counts and a low ratio are associated with more disease manifestations.

Antibody Tests. Antibody tests are used to measure the patient's response to the virus (the antigen) rather than to measure parts of the virus. When the body is infected with HIV, the body makes an antibody to the virus, usually within 3 weeks to 3 months after the INFECTION first occurs. In some people, antibodies are not made until 36 months after initial infection.

HIV antibodies can be measured by enzyme-linked immu-nosorbent assay (ELISA) and Western blot analysis. False-negative results (incorrectly indicating the absence of HIV infection) have been reported early in the infection, in people with cancer, and in people receiving long-term immunosup-pressive therapy.

ELISA is an inexpensive and accurate test. The patient's serum is mixed with HIV grown in culture. If the patient has antibodies to HIV, they bind to the HIV antigens and can be detected (a positive test). However, this test can be negative even when the person has HIV INFECTION if the test is performed before antibodies are made in sufficient amounts. The time between when a person is first infected with the virus and when viral replication is occurring but the immune system has not yet started making antibodies is called the "window period." *So, if the patient has unprotected sex with an HIV-positive person one night and comes in for testing a week later, the ELISA will be negative even though the patient may have active HIV. Thus testing during the window does not provide useful information.*

False-positive test results (incorrectly indicating HIV infec-tion) occur in about 0.1% (1 of 1000) of those tested with ELISA. False-positive results sometimes occur in pregnant women and women who have had children, injection drug users, people who have had malaria, patients with lymphomas, and other conditions. Therefore anyone who has a positive ELISA needs to have additional testing to confirm or rule out INFECTION.

Western blot is used to confirm the diagnosis when the results of an ELISA are positive. This test is more sophisticated and expensive than the ELISA. The Western blot detects serum antibodies to four specific major HIV antigens. A positive Western blot result is based on the presence of antibodies to at least two of the major HIV antigens.

The result is inconclusive if two of the major antibodies are not detected but other antibodies to HIV are. The person should then be retested. *If a person has a positive test result for HIV antibodies, it does not mean that he or she has HIV disease or AIDS—only that he or she has been infected with the virus.*

Both the ELISA and Western blot are blood-based tests. This requires special equipment and trained personnel to test for HIV infection. Some HIV testing is simpler, using techniques that are not blood-based so that testing can be done anywhere, even at home. One test involves oral testing for HIV antibody. This test uses a device that is placed against the gum and cheek for 2 minutes. Fluid (called *transmucosal exudate*, not saliva) is drawn into an absorbable pad, which, in an HIV-positive person, contains HIV-specific antibodies. The pad is placed in a solution; a positive result shows a change similar to a positive result in a urine pregnancy test. Total testing time is about 20 minutes. This test has the same accuracy as blood testing and can provide results quickly. If results are positive for HIV, a blood test is needed to confirm the result.

Home test kits require that a drop of blood be placed on a test card with a special code number. The card is mailed to a laboratory where the blood is tested for HIV antibodies. A special telephone number is called and the code entered. Test results are then given.

A newly approved HIV home test kit is the OraQuick In-Home HIV Test. This test uses oral transmucosal exudate and results are ready in 20 to 40 minutes. The manufacturer recommends that the test be performed at least 3 months after a risk event has occurred. A positive result indicates the need for additional testing. The manufacturer provides a 24-hour telephone support service for correct use of the product and general counseling.

Viral Load Testing. Viral load testing (also called *viral burden testing*) measures the presence of HIV viral genetic material (RNA) or other viral proteins in the patient's blood rather than the body's response to the virus. These tests are quantitative and indicate the level of viral burden or viral load, which is useful to monitor disease progression and treatment effectiveness.

Quantitative RNA assays quantify viral load. These assays are the reverse transcriptase-polymerase chain reaction (RT-PCR), the branched DNA (bDNA) method, and the nucleic acid sequence–based assay (NASBA). All three assays use gene amplification to determine the amount of HIV RNA present in a patient's serum, and all have a specificity of 100%. Even if only a few infected cells are present in a serum sample, tiny amounts of the HIV RNA are amplified to allow detection and diagnosis of people who have no indication of INFECTION. These tests are used to monitor therapy effectiveness and the need to change drug regimens.

Other Laboratory Assessment. Other laboratory tests monitor the patient's overall health and detect or diagnose any infections or other problems related to HIV disease. These tests include blood chemistries, a CBC with differential and platelets, toxoplasmosis antibody titer, liver function tests, a serologic test for syphilis (STS), antigens and antibodies to hepatitis viruses A, B, and C, lipid profile, QuantiFERON TB testing or PPD, and cervical and anal Pap testing. Other tests to evaluate the immune profile may include bone marrow aspiration with biopsy and cultures. Other tests may be performed to monitor toxicities from antiretroviral drugs.

GENETIC/GENOMIC CONSIDERATIONS
Patient-Centered Care QSEN

The HIV genotype test is used to determine whether any mutations exist in the strain of HIV that has infected the patient. This test is useful before starting antiretroviral therapy to learn whether the patient is infected with a resistant strain of HIV. The test helps the clinician choose which antiretroviral drugs are most likely to be effective against viral replication. It is also useful in patients who demonstrate initial success in antiretroviral therapy and then have rapid disease progression. The human leukocyte antigen (HLA) *B5701* allele test is a genetic test to determine how a person will respond to a drug. Patients with a variant of this gene allele have a hypersensitivity reaction to abacavir (Ziagen) that ranges from mild fever, rash, nausea, and vomiting to fatal anaphylaxis. Abacavir should not be used without first testing for *B5701*, and if positive, abacavir is never used either as an individual drug or in combined drug preparations.

Other Diagnostic Assessment. Other diagnostic tests are performed on the basis of the patient's manifestations. These may include testing stool for ova and parasites; biopsies of the skin, lymph nodes, lungs, liver, GI tract, or brain; a chest x-ray; gallium scans; bronchoscopy, endoscopy, or colonoscopy; liver and spleen scans; CT scans; pulmonary function tests; and arterial blood gas (ABG) analysis.

◆ Analysis

The priority NANDA-I nursing diagnoses and collaborative problems for patients with AIDS include:
1. Risk for Infection related to immune deficiency (NANDA-I)
2. Inadequate oxygenation related to anemia, respiratory infection (*P. jiroveci* pneumonia [PCP], cytomegalovirus [CMV] pneumonitis), pulmonary Kaposi's sarcoma (KS), or anemia
3. Chronic Pain related to neuropathy, myelopathy, cancer, or infection (NANDA-I)
4. Imbalanced Nutrition: Less Than Body Requirements related to high metabolic need, nausea and vomiting, diarrhea, difficulty chewing or swallowing, or anorexia (NANDA-I)
5. Diarrhea related to infection, food intolerance, or drugs (NANDA-I)
6. Impaired Skin Integrity related to KS, infection, altered nutritional state, incontinence, immobility, hyperthermia, or cancer (NANDA-I)
7. Confusion (Acute and Chronic) related to AIDS dementia complex (ADC), central nervous system infection, or cancer (NANDA-I)
8. Reduced self-esteem related to changes in body image, role, or independence

◆ Planning and Implementation

Preventing Infection. The patient with AIDS is susceptible to opportunistic other INFECTIONS because of immune

CHART 19-4 Patient and Family Education: Preparing for Self-Management

Prevention of Infection

During the times when your white blood cell counts are low:

- Avoid crowds and other large gatherings of people who might be ill.
- Do not share personal toilet articles, such as toothbrushes, toothpaste, washcloths, or deodorant sticks, with others.
- If possible, bathe daily, using an antimicrobial soap. If total bathing is not possible, wash the armpits, groin, genitals, and anal area twice a day with an antimicrobial soap.
- Clean your toothbrush at least weekly by either running it through the dishwasher or rinsing it in liquid laundry bleach (and then rinsing out the bleach with hot running water).
- Wash your hands thoroughly with an antimicrobial soap before you eat or drink, after touching a pet, after shaking hands with anyone, as soon as you come home from any outing, and after using the toilet.
- Avoid eating salads; raw fruits and vegetables; undercooked meat, fish, and eggs; and pepper and paprika.
- Wash dishes between use with hot, sudsy water, or use a dishwasher.
- Do not drink water, milk, juice, or other cold liquids that have been standing for longer than an hour.
- Do not reuse cups and glasses without washing.
- Do not change pet litter boxes. If unavoidable, use gloves and wash hands immediately.
- Avoid turtles and reptiles as pets.
- Do not feed pets raw or undercooked meat.
- Take your temperature at least once a day and whenever you do not feel well.
- Report any of these manifestations of infection to your physician immediately:
  - Temperature greater than 100° F (37.8° C)
  - Persistent cough (with or without sputum)
  - Pus or foul-smelling drainage from any open skin area or normal body opening
  - Presence of a boil or abscess
  - Urine that is cloudy or foul smelling or that causes burning on urination
- Take all prescribed drugs.
- Do not dig in the garden or work with houseplants.
- Wear a condom (if you are a man) when having sex. If you are a woman having sex with a male partner, ensure that he wears a condom or use a female vaginal polyurethane condom.
- Avoid travel to areas of the world with poor sanitation or less-than-adequate health care facilities.

CHART 19-5 Best Practice for Patient Safety & Quality Care QSEN

Care of the Hospitalized Immunosuppressed Patient

- Place the patient in a private room whenever possible.
- Use good handwashing technique or use alcohol-based hand rubs before touching the patient or any of his or her belongings.
- Ensure that the patient's room and bathroom are cleaned at least once each day.
- Do not use supplies from common areas for neutropenic patients. For example, keep a dedicated box of disposable gloves in his or her room and do not share this box with any other patient. Provide single-use food products, individually wrapped gauze, and other individually wrapped items.
- Limit the number of health care personnel entering the patient's room.
- Monitor vital signs, including temperature, every 4 hours.
- Inspect the patient's mouth at least every 8 hours.
- Inspect the patient's skin and mucous membranes (especially the anal area) for the presence of fissures and abscesses at least every 8 hours.
- Inspect open areas, such as IV sites, every 4 hours for manifestations of infection.
- Change gauze-containing wound dressings daily.
- Obtain specimens of all suspicious areas for culture (as specified by the agency), and promptly notify the physician.
- Assist the patient in performing coughing and deep-breathing exercises.
- Encourage activity at a level appropriate for the patient's current health status.
- Keep frequently used equipment in the room for use with this patient only (e.g., blood pressure cuff, stethoscope, thermometer).
- Limit visitors to healthy adults.
- Use strict aseptic technique for all invasive procedures.
- Avoid the use of indwelling urinary catheters.
- Keep fresh flowers and potted plants out of the patient's room.
- Teach the patient to eat a low-bacteria diet (e.g., avoiding raw fruits and vegetables; undercooked meat, eggs, and fish; pepper and paprika as seasonings sprinkled on food right before eating).

deficiency. Initial management focuses on supporting the patient's IMMUNITY by controlling the HIV infection with antiretroviral therapy. When the patient's immunity declines, management includes both prophylaxis and treatment of opportunistic infections.

Planning: Expected Outcomes. The patient is expected to remain free of opportunistic diseases and other INFECTION. Indicators include:

- Absence of chills, fever, or temperature instability
- Absence of purulent drainage or sputum
- Absence of diarrhea
- Absence of chest x-ray infiltration
- Maintenance of white blood cell (WBC) count within the patient's normal range

Interventions. The person who has HIV infection and is immunosuppressed is at greater risk for any type of INFECTION. Teach him or her to avoid exposure to infection (Chart 19-4). Chart 19-5 outlines best practices for prevention of infection in a hospitalized patient with decreased immune function.

Drug Therapy. All currently licensed antiretroviral drugs have excellent activity against HIV; however, *it is important to remember that antiretroviral therapy only inhibits viral replication and does not kill the virus.* Treatment with only one antiretroviral agent (i.e., *monotherapy*) promotes drug resistance and does not improve the patient's life span. Instead, multiple drugs are used together in combinations from different classes of antiretroviral agents. This approach is termed *highly active antiretroviral therapy (HAART)* and has reduced viral load, improved CD4+ T-cell counts, and slowed disease progression. As a general rule, patients are told they must take the drugs correctly 90% of the time, making sure that out of 10 doses, 9 are taken on time and correctly. This is a tall order when considering that this drug therapy is for the rest of one's life.

An important issue with HAART is the development of drug-resistant mutations in the HIV organism. When resistance develops, viral replication is no longer suppressed by the drugs. Testing is now possible to determine whether a strain of HIV has developed resistance to specific drugs (see the Genetic/Genomic Considerations box on p. 337). Several factors contribute to the development of drug resistance to HAART, with the most important being missed doses of drugs. When doses are missed, the blood drug concentrations become lower than what are needed for inhibition of viral replication (often called the *minimum inhibitory concentration*). When this concentration is too low, the HIV can replicate and produce new viral particles that are resistant to the drugs being used.

An important understanding about HIV resistance to one or more drugs is that once a patient has HIV with resistant mutations, the resistant virus is stored in the body indefinitely, a process known as *archiving*. The drugs to which the virus is resistant are no longer used for that patient. Even years later, if the drug to which the HIV demonstrated resistance is tried again, the viruses with the resistant mutation come out of archival storage to defeat the drug.

> ⚠ **NURSING SAFETY PRIORITY** (QSEN)
> **Drug Alert**
>
> Ensure that HAART drugs are not missed, delayed, or administered in lower-than-prescribed doses in the inpatient setting. Teach patients the importance of taking their drugs exactly as prescribed to maintain the effectiveness of HAART drugs. Even a few missed doses per month can promote drug resistance (remember the 90% rule).

The main actions of each drug category and representative drugs in each category are presented in Chart 19-6. These categories are nucleoside reverse transcriptase inhibitors (NRTIs), non-nucleoside reverse transcriptase inhibitors (NNRTIs), protease inhibitors (PIs), integrase inhibitors, fusion inhibitors, and entry inhibitors. Drawbacks to HAART include the expense of the drugs, food and timing requirements, and the number of daily drugs. Newer combination drug formulations have reduced the number of tablets and capsules that need to be taken daily; however, the daily regimen is lifelong and burdensome.

Most antiretroviral drugs have significant side effects and many possible drug interactions. Be sure to consult a drug reference book for usual dosages, side effects, and nursing interventions.

An interesting complication of effective HAART in some patients whose CD4+ T-cell counts rise and immune responses return to normal is the development of immune reconstitution inflammatory syndrome (IRIS) (Carr & Traufler, 2011). As the drugs begin to suppress HIV replication and the T-cells slowly

CHART 19-6   Common Examples of Drug Therapy

HIV Infection

DRUG CATEGORY	MECHANISM OF ACTION	REPRESENTATIVE DRUGS
Nucleoside Reverse Transcriptase Inhibitors (NRTIs)	Drugs have a similar structure to the four nucleoside bases of DNA, making them "counterfeit" bases. Fools the HIV enzyme *reverse transcriptase* into using these counterfeit bases so that viral DNA synthesis and replication are suppressed.	Abacavir (Ziagen) Didanosine (Videx EC) Emtricitabine (Emtriva) Lamivudine (Epivir) Stavudine (Zerit) Tenofovir (Viread) Zidovudine (Retrovir)
Non-Nucleoside Reverse Transcriptase Inhibitors (NNRTIs)	Drugs bind directly to the HIV-1 enzyme *reverse transcriptase*, preventing viral cell DNA replication, RNA replication, and protein synthesis. This action suppresses viral replication of the HIV-1 virus but does not affect HIV-2 viral replication.	Delavirdine (Rescriptor) Efavirenz (Sustiva) Etravirine (INTELENCE) Nevirapine (Viramune, Viramune XR) Rilpivirine (EDURANT)
Protease Inhibitors (PIs)	Drugs competitively block the HIV protease enzyme, preventing viral replication and release of viral particles. The HIV initially produces all of its proteins in one long strand, which must be broken down into separate smaller proteins by HIV protease to be active. Thus, when inhibited, viral proteins are not functional and viral particles cannot leave the cell to infect other cells.	Atazanavir (Reyataz) Darunavir (Prezista) Fosamprenavir (Lexiva) Indinavir (Crixivan) Lopinavir/ritonavir (Kaletra) Nelfinavir (Viracept) Saquinavir (Invirase) Tipranavir (Aptivus)
Integrase Inhibitors	Drugs inhibit the HIV enzyme *integrase*, which the virus uses to insert the viral DNA into the host cell's human DNA. Without this action, viral proteins are not made and viral replication is inhibited.	Dolutegravir (TIVICAY) Elvitegravir (EVG) Raltegravir (Isentress)
Fusion Inhibitors	Drugs block the fusion of HIV with a host cell by blocking the ability of *gp41* to fuse with the host cell's CD4 receptor. Without fusion, infection of new cells does not occur.	Enfuvirtide (Fuzeon)
Entry Inhibitors/CCR5 Antagonists	Drug works to prevent infection by blocking the *CCR5* receptor on CD4+ T-cells. (The virus's *gp120* must bind to the CD4 receptor and its *gp41* must bind to the *CCR5* receptor or to the *CXCR4* receptor for entry into host cells. This class of drug prevents cellular infection with HIV.	Maraviroc (Selzentry)
Combination Products	Each ingredient has the same mechanism of action as the parent drug class.	Atripla (emtricitabine, tenofovir, & efavirenz) Combivir (lamivudine & zidovudine) Complera (emtricitabine, rilpivirine, & tenofovir) Epzicom (lamivudine & abacavir) Stribild (elvitegravir, cobicistat, emtricitabine, & tenofovir) Truvada (emtricitabine & tenofovir) Trizivir (lamivudine, zidovudine, & abacavir)

begin to rebound, the T4-cells "recognize" several opportunistic INFECTIONS (e.g., tuberculosis, cryptococcosis, *Mycobacterium avium* complex, pneumocystis pneumonia, cytomegalovirus, hepatitis, and others) that were present before but not recognized because of severe immunosuppression. With the T-cells now in sufficient numbers and active, they begin to sound the alarm about the presence of these opportunistic infections. The T4-cells generate an inflammatory reaction, high fever, chills and, depending on which opportunistic infection the immune system is reacting against, worsening disease. For example, IRIS is common with those co-infected with HIV and TB. TB manifestations initially become much worse after starting HAART. Because some of these manifestations are similar to those of drug therapy side effects and other problems, IRIS may go undiagnosed and untreated, increasing the risk for death. When IRIS is recognized, short-term therapy with corticosteroids can reduce the inflammatory responses.

❓ CLINICAL JUDGMENT CHALLENGE

Safety; Evidence-Based Practice; Patient-Centered Care QSEN

J.L. and C.R. are two men in a 2-year monogamous relationship, who were recently married in Washington state. J.L. has been HIV-positive for 4 years. C.R. is HIV-negative and in good health. J.L. is currently an inpatient for an elective cholecystectomy this afternoon. His HIV infection is well controlled on a three-drug cocktail, which he is tolerating well. During the assessment, you ask J.L. how they keep C.R. HIV-negative. A sheepish grin follows. J.L. is generally the insertive (active) partner and C.R. and J.L. have mutually agreed to not use condoms for either oral or rectal sex, as that affects the quality of their sexual pleasure. They continue to make sure that J.L.'s viral load is kept undetectable and he always "pulls out" prior to ejaculation.
1. How safe are their sexual practices for C.R. if he chooses to remain HIV-negative?
2. What should you tell them about condom use?
3. Is C.R. an appropriate candidate for pre-exposure prophylaxis (Pr-EP)?
4. After checking out the information about Pr-EP, what can you tell them about the pros and cons of this therapy?

Immune Enhancement. Research is being conducted to evaluate treatments that may enhance or replenish the immune system of patients with AIDS. Some of these methods include bone marrow transplantation, lymphocyte transfusion, and infusions of lymphokines, white blood cell colony-stimulating factors, and red blood cell growth factors.

Complementary and Alternative Therapies. Complementary therapies are often used by people with HIV/AIDS. Such therapies include vitamins, shark cartilage, and botanical products available at health food stores. The usefulness of these products has yet to be established through well-controlled clinical trials. In addition, some botanicals alter the effects of prescription drugs. Ask the patient which botanicals or homeopathic agents he or she is using, and check with the pharmacist to determine known drug interactions with HAART therapy.

Enhancing Oxygenation

Planning: Expected Outcomes. The patient is expected to maintain adequate gas exchange with oxygenation and perfusion and to have minimal dyspnea. Indicators include:
• Rate and depth of respiration within the normal range
• Pulse oximetry within the normal range

❓ NCLEX EXAMINATION CHALLENGE
Safe and Effective Care Environment

What is the most important question the nurse asks the client prescribed to begin highly active antiretroviral therapy?
A. Do you have any symptoms now of active infection?
B. Is there any possibility that you are pregnant?
C. Are you currently sexually active?
D. What other medications do you take?

• Absence of cyanosis or pallor and abnormal breath sounds

Interventions. The nurse or respiratory therapist uses drug therapy, respiratory support and maintenance, comfort, and rest to enhance oxygenation.

Drug therapy is a mainstay for gas exchange problems resulting from INFECTION. Drug therapy is started after an infectious cause for respiratory difficulty is identified. A common respiratory infection among people with HIV disease is *P. jiroveci* pneumonia (PCP). The treatment of choice for PCP is trimethoprim with sulfamethoxazole (Apo-Sulfatrim ✦, Bactrim, Cotrim, Septra). Many patients have adverse reactions to this drug, including nausea, vomiting, hyponatremia, rashes, fever, leukopenia, thrombocytopenia, and hepatitis.

Pentamidine isethionate (Pentacarinat ✦, Pentam), usually given IV or IM, is also used to treat PCP. Aerosolized pentamidine isethionate is used as prophylaxis for patients with CD4+ T-cell counts below 200 (or 14%), as well as for those who have already had PCP.

Other drug therapies include bronchodilators to improve airflow, as well as dapsone (Avlosulfon) and atovaquone (Mepron), which can be used as alternative therapies to trimethoprim-sulfamethoxazole for existing PCP or as prophylaxis. For moderate to severe PCP, steroids may be used to reduce the inflammation.

Respiratory support and maintenance help maintain respiratory function and avoid complications. Assess the respiratory rate, rhythm, and depth, breath sounds, and vital signs and monitor for cyanosis at least every 8 hours. Apply oxygen and humidify the room as prescribed. Also monitor mechanical ventilation, perform suctioning and chest physical therapy as needed, and evaluate blood gas results.

Comfort can help improve gas exchange. Assess the patient's comfort. The patient with difficulty breathing is often more comfortable with the head of the bed elevated. Pace activities to reduce shortness of breath and fatigue.

Rest and activity changes are needed when gas exchange is impaired. Most patients with HIV/AIDS have fatigue, especially when respiratory problems also are present. Some treatments worsen fatigue. Consult with the patient to pace activities to conserve energy. Guide the patient in active and passive range-of-motion (ROM) exercises. Schedule non–time-critical activities, such as bathing, so that he or she is not fatigued at mealtime.

Managing Pain. The patient with severe HIV disease or AIDS often has PAIN from many causes. Pain can result from enlarged organs stretching the viscera or compressing nerves. Tumor invasion of bone and other tissues can cause pain, as can compression of nerves from swollen lymph nodes. Many patients with AIDS have peripheral neuropathy–induced pain from the disease or drug therapies (Anastasi et al., 2013). Many have generalized joint and muscle pain.

Planning: Expected Outcomes. The patient is expected to achieve an acceptable level of comfort and PAIN reduction. Indicators include:

- Reporting that pain is controlled to a level that is acceptable to him or her
- Absence of indicators of acute pain (increased heart rate and blood pressure)
- Absence of facial grimacing, teeth clenching
- Willingness to move and participate in self-care

Interventions. Drug therapy and other approaches are used together to manage PAIN in the patient with HIV/AIDS, depending on the cause of the pain.

Comfort measures include the use of pressure-relieving mattress pads, warm baths or other forms of hydrotherapy, massage, and applying heat or cold to painful areas to reduce PAIN levels, with or without drug therapy. Take care when moving or assisting the patient. Use lift sheets to avoid pulling or grasping the patient with joint pain. The patient may be thin and have poor circulation, contributing to pain and discomfort. Help him or her change positions often.

Drug therapy with different drug classes is used to manage different types of PAIN. For arthralgia and myalgia, NSAIDs may reduce inflammation and increase comfort. Pregabalin (Lyrica) may provide some relief from muscle and joint pain. Neuropathic pain may respond to tricyclic antidepressants such as amitriptyline (Elavil) or to anticonvulsant drugs such as gabapentin (Neurontin), phenytoin (Dilantin), or carbamazepine (Tegretol), although these drugs often interact with antiretroviral drugs. These drugs may take days to weeks before a full effect is seen. During this time, opioids may be needed to control pain.

When opioids are used, assess the patient for PAIN intensity and quality. Mild to moderate pain is treated with weaker opioids such as hydrocodone, tramadol, or codeine. More intense pain is treated with stronger opioids such as oxycodone, morphine, hydromorphone (Dilaudid), or fentanyl transdermal (Duragesic). Combinations of weak and strong opioids along with non-opioid drugs may be used to provide the best sustained pain relief and allow the patient to participate in activities to the extent that he or she wishes.

Complementary and alternative therapies are used by many patients with PAIN from HIV/AIDS. These include acupuncture, massage, guided imagery, distraction, progressive relaxation, body-talk, and biofeedback and can be used with traditional and pharmacologic measures to improve comfort.

Enhancing Nutrition. Many patients with AIDS have difficulty maintaining their weight and NUTRITION status. This problem may be caused by fatigue, anorexia, nausea and vomiting, difficult or painful swallowing, diarrhea, intestinal malabsorption, or wasting syndrome.

Planning: Expected Outcomes. The patient is expected to maintain optimal weight through adequate NUTRITION and hydration. Indicators include:

- Selecting foods high in calories and protein
- Maintaining current weight or gaining weight
- Drinking at least 2 to 3 L of fluids per day
- Maintaining normal blood levels of ferritin, albumin, prealbumin, and hemoglobin

Interventions. Because there are many factors for poor NUTRITION in AIDS, diagnostic procedures are needed to determine the cause. Once the cause is determined, appropriate therapy is initiated. For example, in candidal esophagitis, nutrition is affected by swallowing difficulties.

Drug therapy can include ketoconazole (Nizoral) or fluconazole (Diflucan) orally, or IV amphotericin B (Fungizone). Administer the drug as prescribed, and monitor for side effects such as nausea and vomiting, which also affect NUTRITION. Provide mouth care and ice chips, and keep unpleasant odors out of the patient's environment. Antiemetics are used as needed.

Nutrition therapy includes monitoring weight, intake and output, and calorie count. Assess food preferences and dietary cultural or religious practices. Teach the patient about the need for a high-calorie and high-protein diet. Encourage him or her to avoid dietary fat, because fat intolerance often occurs as a result of the disease and as a side effect of some antiretroviral drugs. Collaborate with the registered dietitian to provide an appropriate diet, including small, frequent meals (better tolerated than large meals). Supplemental vitamins and fluids are indicated in some cases. For the patient who cannot achieve adequate NUTRITION through food, tube feedings or total parenteral nutrition may be needed.

Mouth care can improve appetite. When this nursing action is delegated to unlicensed assistive personnel (UAP), instruct them to offer the patient rinses of sodium bicarbonate with sterile water or normal saline several times a day. Explain to UAP why the patient should use a soft toothbrush and the need to drink plenty of fluids. For oral pain, general analgesics or oral anesthetic gels and solutions may be needed. Avoid the use of alcohol-based mouthwashes.

Complementary and alternative therapies to promote healing of mouth sores can help improve food intake. Some patients have found relief from oral thrush with the use of lemon juice and lemongrass infusions.

Minimizing Diarrhea. Patients with AIDS often suffer from diarrhea. Sometimes an infectious cause (e.g., *Giardia, Cryptosporidium,* or amoeba) can be determined and treated, or the cause is determined but no effective therapy is available. Many patients are lactose intolerant, and HIV disease worsens the condition. Diarrhea may occur as a side effect of drug therapy. In some cases, no cause can be identified.

Planning: Expected Outcomes. The patient is expected to have decreased diarrhea; to maintain fluid, electrolyte, and NUTRITION status; and to reduce incontinence. Indicators include:

- Has a stool amount and character that are appropriate for the diet
- Recognizes urge to defecate
- Maintains control of stool passage

Interventions. For most patients with AIDS and diarrhea, symptom management is all that is available. Antidiarrheals, such as diphenoxylate hydrochloride (Diarsed ✦, Lomotil) or loperamide (Imodium), given on a regular schedule, provide some relief. Consult with the dietitian, and teach about appropriate foods. Recommended dietary changes include less roughage; less fatty, spicy, and sweet food; and no alcohol or caffeine. Some patients obtain relief when they eliminate dairy products or eat smaller amounts of food more often and drink plenty of fluids, especially between meals.

Assess the perineal skin every 8 to 12 hours for a change in skin TISSUE INTEGRITY. Provide the patient with a bedside commode or a bedpan if needed because some patients cannot reach the bathroom in time. Teach UAP performing this care to provide the patient with privacy, support, and understanding. Explain the need to keep the patient's perineal area clean and dry. Instruct UAP to report any skin changes in the perineal area, including persistent redness, rashes, blisters, or open areas. Collaborate with a wound care specialist for more interventions to manage anal excoriation and discomfort.

💡 NCLEX EXAMINATION CHALLENGE

Health Promotion and Maintenance

> Which dietary change does the nurse suggest for the client who has diarrhea associated with HIV disease?
> A. "Avoid fatty foods."
> B. "Increase your intake of fiber."
> C. "Take an antacid 30 minutes before each meal."
> D. "Restrict your intake of fluids to 1 liter per day."

Restoring Skin Integrity. Impaired TISSUE INTEGRITY in AIDS may be related to Kaposi's sarcoma (KS) of the skin, mucous membranes, and internal organs. Lesions may be localized or widespread. Large lesions can cause pain, restrict movement, and impede circulation, causing open, weeping, painful lesions. Another cause of impaired tissue integrity may be skin INFECTION with herpes simplex virus (HSV) or varicella zoster virus (VZV) (shingles).

Planning: Expected Outcomes. The patient is expected to have healing of any existing lesions and avoid increased skin breakdown or secondary INFECTION. Indicators include:

- Absence of new lesions or open skin areas
- Existing lesions become smaller in diameter
- Absence of pus, induration, or redness in, from, or around skin lesions

Interventions. Often, KS responds well to effective antiretroviral drug therapy. With time and HAART, many lesions disappear and do not reappear as long as the patient remains on HAART. For lesions that do not respond to HAART, KS can be treated with local radiation, intralesional or systemic chemotherapy, cryotherapy, or topical retinoids. Systemic therapy with chemotherapy or interferon is used in patients with rapidly progressive disease or with major involvement of the intestinal tract, lungs, or other organs.

Treatment of painful KS lesions includes analgesics and comfort measures. Keep open, weeping KS lesions clean and dressed to prevent infection. Many patients with KS are concerned about their appearance and the risk for being identified as HIV positive. Makeup (if lesions are closed), long-sleeved shirts, and hats may help maintain a normal appearance.

For the patient with a herpes simplex virus (HSV) outbreak, provide good skin care directly or delegate this care to UAP. Stress the importance of keeping the area clean and dry. Teach UAP to clean abscesses at least once per shift with normal saline and allow them to air-dry. This infection is painful and requires analgesics, assistance with position, and other comfort measures. Modified Burow's solution (Domeboro) soaks promote healing for some patients. HSV infection is treated with acyclovir (Zovirax) or valacyclovir (Valtrex).

Minimizing Confusion. Neurologic changes and confusion are major areas of concern for patients with HIV disease or AIDS. These changes may be due to psychological stressors accompanying the disease or to organic disorders caused by opportunistic INFECTIONS, cancer, or HIV encephalitis.

Planning: Expected Outcomes. The patient is expected to show improved mental status. Indicators include that the patient demonstrates these behaviors:

- Identifies self and significant others
- Identifies correct month and year
- Recalls immediate, recent, and remote information accurately

Interventions. Patients with AIDS suffer from enormous loss and psychological stress, which complicates the assessment of changes in behavior or affect. Assess baseline neurologic and mental status by using neurologic assessment tools (see Chapter 41) to compare any changes. Evaluate the patient for subtle changes in memory, ability to concentrate, affect, and behavior. It is important to determine whether the cause of the neurologic changes is treatable.

Reorient the confused patient to person, time, and place as needed. Coordinate with all members of the health care team to ensure that reorientation methods are performed by everyone who interacts with the patient. Remind the patient of your identity and explain what is to be done at any given time. Give simple directions; use short, uncomplicated sentences; explain activities in simple language; and involve him or her in daily planning. Ask significant others to bring in familiar items from home. When possible, arrange all items in the patient's environment in the same location as at home. Calendars, clocks, radios, and putting the bed close to a window may help keep the patient oriented.

Drug therapy is used for different conditions that can cause confusion in the person with AIDS. Psychotropic drugs are used to manage ongoing behavioral problems or emotional disorders. Antidepressants and anxiolytics may be prescribed.

Safety measures are crucial to the well-being of the confused patient. He or she may not be aware of activities or surroundings and may need help with bathing, dressing, eating, ambulating, and other ADLs. Make the environment, whether a hospital room or long-term care facility, safe and comfortable.

Some patients with AIDS have seizures. Institute seizure precautions, including keeping siderails in the up position and having oxygen and suctioning equipment available. Anticonvulsants may be added to the drug therapy.

Assess the patient with neurologic manifestations for increased intracranial pressure (ICP). If not recognized and managed early, ICP can lead to permanent brain damage and death. Increased ICP in patients with HIV disease is most commonly managed with corticosteroids.

⚠ NURSING SAFETY PRIORITY (QSEN)

Critical Rescue

> Document and report immediately any changes in level of consciousness (one of the earliest signs of increased ICP), vital signs, pupil size or reactivity, or limb strength to the health care provider for appropriate intervention.

Support the family and friends of the patient who has neurologic impairment. There is great trauma in seeing a loved one unable to care for himself or herself or showing childlike behavior. Answer questions honestly and sensitively. Teach UAP, the family, and significant others how to reorient the patient. Encourage them to continue to provide the patient with news of family happenings or current events. Coordinate with the social worker to identify community resources for the patient and family.

Supporting Self-Esteem. The patient with AIDS may have changes in self-esteem resulting from dramatic changes in appearance. Many patients also have significant changes in their relationships and in day-to-day activities, including a job. All changes can reduce self-esteem.

Planning: Expected Outcomes. The patient is expected to identify his or her positive aspects and accept himself or herself. Indicators include that he or she often or consistently demonstrates these behaviors:

- Maintains eye contact
- Accepts compliments from others
- Expresses feelings of self-worth

Interventions. Provide a climate of acceptance for patients with AIDS by promoting a trusting relationship. Help them express feelings, and identify positive aspects of themselves. Allow for privacy, but do not avoid or isolate the patient. Encourage self-care, independence, control, and decision making by helping him or her set short-term, attainable goals and offering praise when goals are achieved.

Guided imagery is used by many patients to increase their sense of control and enhance self-esteem. Imagery can focus on helping them cope with distressing side effects or painful procedures. Some patients picture battle scenes in which HIV is killed by immune system cells.

Community-Based Care

HIV disease is manageable and chronic (Starr & Bradley-Springer, 2014). The usual course of illness is one of intermittent acute INFECTIONS and periods of relative wellness over years. This period is often followed by chronic, progressive debilitation. Because of the cyclic nature of HIV disease and AIDS, the patient often spends long periods at home between hospital admissions. In some instances, especially as the illness becomes more severe, he or she may need referral to a long-term care facility, home care agency, or hospice. In collaboration with the social worker, dietitian, and others, work with patients to plan what will be needed and how they will manage at home with self-care and ADLs.

Home Care Management. Before the patient is discharged to home, assess his or her status, ability to perform self-care activities, and plans to maintain communication with primary care providers. Home care can range from help with ADLs for those with weakness, debility, or limited function to around-the-clock nursing care, drugs, and nutrition support for severely or terminally ill patients. Assess available resources, including family members and significant others willing and able to be caregivers. Help the family make arrangements for outside caregivers or respite care, if needed. Patients may need referrals or help in planning housing, finances, insurance, legal services, and spiritual counseling. Coordinate with the case manager to ensure these issues are addressed.

Usually a home care nurse makes an initial visit to the patient with AIDS for assessment purposes, and care is followed up by home care aides. If the patient becomes more debilitated, a nurse re-assesses his or her status. Chart 19-7 lists focused assessment areas for the patient with AIDS at home.

Self-Management Education. Teaching the patient, family, and friends is a high priority when preparing for discharge. Instruct about modes of transmission and preventive behaviors (e.g., guidelines for safer sex; not sharing toothbrushes, razors,

---

CHART 19-7 Focused Assessment

The Person with AIDS

Assess cardiovascular and respiratory status:
- Vital signs
- Presence of acute chest pain or dyspnea
- Presence of cough
- Presence of fever
- Activity tolerance

Assess nutritional status:
- Food intake
- Weight loss or gain
- General condition of skin
- Financial resources

Assess neurologic status:
- Cognitive changes
- Motor changes
- Sensory disturbances

Assess gastrointestinal status:
- Mouth and oropharynx
- Presence of dysphagia
- Presence of abdominal pain
- Presence of nausea, vomiting, diarrhea, constipation

Assess psychological status:
- Presence of anxiety
- Presence of depression

Assess activity and rest:
- Activities of daily living (ADLs)
- Mobility and ambulation
- Fatigue
- Sleep pattern
- Presence of pain

Assess home environment:
- Safety hazards
- Structural barriers affecting functional ability

Assess patient's and caregiver's adherence and understanding of illness and treatment, including:
- Manifestations to report to nurse
- Medication schedule and side or toxic effects

Assess patient's and caregiver's coping skills.

---

and other potentially blood-contaminated articles). Caregivers also need instruction about best practices for Infection Control Precautions to prevent transmission while caring for the patient in the home (Chart 19-8), nursing techniques to use in the home, and coping or support strategies.

Teach the patient, family, and friends how to protect the patient from INFECTION, how to identify the presence of infections, and what to do if these appear. Teach about the use of self-care strategies, such as good hygiene, balanced rest and exercise, skin care, mouth care, and safe administration and potential side effects of all prescribed drugs. During diet teaching, stress good NUTRITION; the need to avoid raw or rare fish, fowl, or meat; thorough washing of fruits and vegetables; and proper food refrigeration.

Teach the patient to avoid large crowds, especially in enclosed areas, not to travel to countries with poor sanitation, and to avoid cleaning pet litter boxes. Chart 19-4 lists more strategies to teach the patient and family how to avoid INFECTION.

Psychosocial Preparation. Patients with AIDS often fear social stigma and rejection. Be aware that this fear is realistic, and help identify ways to avoid problems, as well as identify coping strategies for difficult situations. Support family members and friends in efforts to help the patient and provide protection from discrimination.

Encourage patients to continue as many usual activities as possible. Except when too ill or too weak, they can continue to work and participate in most social activities. Support them in their selection of friends and relatives with whom to discuss the diagnosis. Stress that sexual partners and care providers should be informed; beyond that, it is up to the patient. Some patients have depression or anxiety about the future. Almost all feel the burden of having a fatal disease widely considered unacceptable and feel compelled to maintain some secrecy about the illness. Referrals to community resources, mental health/behavioral health professionals, and support groups can help the patient verbalize fears and frustrations and cope with the illness.

Infection Control for Home Care of the Person with AIDS

Direct Care
- Follow Standard Precautions and good handwashing techniques.
- Do not share razors or toothbrushes.

Housekeeping
- Wipe up feces, vomitus, sputum, urine, or blood or other body fluids and the area with soap and water. Dispose of solid wastes and solutions used for cleaning by flushing them down the toilet. Disinfect the area by wiping with a 1:10 solution of household bleach (1 part bleach to 10 parts water). Wear gloves during cleaning.
- Soak rags, mops, and sponges used for cleaning in a 1:10 bleach solution for 5 minutes to disinfect them.
- Wash dishes and eating utensils in hot water and dishwashing soap or detergent.
- Clean bathroom surfaces with regular household cleaners, and then disinfect them with a 1:10 solution of household bleach.

Laundry
- Rinse clothes, towels, and bedclothes if they become soiled with feces, vomitus, sputum, urine, or blood. Then dispose of the soiled water by flushing it down the toilet. Launder these clothes with hot water and detergent with 1 cup of bleach added per load of laundry.
- Keep soiled clothes in a plastic bag.

Waste Disposal
- Dispose of needles and other "sharps" in a labeled puncture-proof container such as a coffee can with a lid or empty liquid bleach bottle, using Standard Precautions, to avoid needle stick injuries. Decontaminate full containers by adding a 1:10 bleach solution. Then seal the container with tape and place it in a paper bag. Dispose of the container in the regular trash.
- Remove solid waste from contaminated trash (e.g., paper towels or tissues, dressings, disposable incontinence pads, disposable gloves); then flush the solid waste down the toilet. Place the contaminated trash items in tied plastic bags, and dispose of them in the regular trash.

Health Care Resources. In many cities, community groups and volunteers assist people with AIDS. The types and number of services vary by agency and city, but many include HIV testing and counseling, clinic services, buddy systems, support groups, respite care, education and outreach, referral services, and housing. Patients may need referrals to other local resources, such as home care agencies, companies that provide home IV therapy, community mental health/behavioral health agencies, Meals on Wheels, transportation services, and others. In addition, educational materials and support groups are available through Internet access.

◆ *Evaluation: Outcomes*

The overall outcomes for care of patients with AIDS are to maintain the highest possible level of function for as long as possible, reduce INFECTIONS, and maintain quality of life and dignity during the course of progressive illness. Evaluate the care of the patient with AIDS on the basis of the identified priority problems. Expected outcomes include that he or she should:
- Adhere to the prescribed drug therapy regimen at least 90% of the time
- Practice safer sex techniques all of the time

- Remain free from opportunistic INFECTIONS
- Have adequate respiratory function
- Achieve an acceptable level of physical comfort
- Attain adequate weight and NUTRITION and fluid status
- Maintain TISSUE INTEGRITY
- Remain oriented
- Maintain self-esteem
- Maintain a support system and involvement with others

Specific indicators for these outcomes are listed for each patient problem in the Planning and Implementation section (see earlier).

💡 CLINICAL JUDGMENT CHALLENGE
Ethical/Legal

Mark S. is a 24-year-old man who was diagnosed with HIV 3 years ago. He has been followed in the HIV clinic and has not been adherent to his medication regimen. In addition, he has struggled off and on with substance abuse. He currently lives with his mother and came to the emergency department today with severe pneumocystis pneumonia. He required intubation and admission to the ICU. On his first day in the unit, his mother asked about his condition. She was told that he had a severe pneumonia, but that it was likely he would recover. The staff ask the nurse manager whether Mark's mother has a right to know his HIV status since he lives with her and might be at risk for exposure to the virus.
1. What is the nurse manager's responsibility in this situation?
2. Is Mark's mother likely to be at risk for exposure to HIV? Why or why not?
3. Should the staff inform Mark's mother about his HIV status? Why or why not?
4. If his mother is informed about Mark's HIV status, what, if any, ethical issues/principles would be violated?

THERAPY-INDUCED IMMUNE DEFICIENCIES

Some acquired secondary immune deficiencies may be related to other conditions that cause the loss of immunoglobulins or destruction of lymphocytes. The most common cause of secondary immune deficiency is the use of drugs and other treatment modalities for various diseases. Sometimes immunosuppression is a desired effect, as in organ transplantation or for the treatment of autoimmune disorders. Often immunosuppression is an undesirable, complicating side effect of therapy that is used for another intent, such as cancer chemotherapy, and may even require changing the therapeutic regimen. Various therapies cause different types and degrees of immunosuppression. The challenge is to have maximum therapeutic effect without leaving the patient overly susceptible to serious complications.

Drug-Induced Immune Deficiencies

Several drug classes have major immunosuppressive effects. Some induce general immunosuppression; others are more specific and target one part of the immune system more than another.

Cytotoxic drugs are mostly those used in the treatment of cancer and autoimmune disorders. These drugs interfere with all rapidly dividing cells, especially the white blood cells (WBCs), which are responsible for providing IMMUNITY and protection against INFECTION. The result is a decrease in the number of these important cells, especially the neutrophils, greatly increasing the patient's risk for infection. Cytotoxic drugs also interfere with the ability of lymphocytes to produce and release products such as lymphokines and antibodies, causing general immunosuppression.

Corticosteroids are hormones that have both anti-inflammatory and immunosuppressive effects that are used to treat many autoimmune diseases, neoplasms, and endocrine disorders. They inhibit inflammation by blocking the movement of many WBCs. These drugs disrupt the synthesis of arachidonic acid, the main precursor for a variety of inflammatory chemicals.

Corticosteroids reduce the number of circulating T-cells and result in suppressed cell-mediated immunity. They also interfere with immunoglobulin G (IgG) production and reduce antibody-antigen binding. These drugs have many effects that alter disease activity, as well as numerous side effects, including:

- Central nervous system changes, such as euphoria, insomnia, or psychosis
- Cardiovascular changes, such as edema and hypertension
- GI effects, such as gastric irritation, ulcers, and increased appetite (with weight gain)
- Other changes (e.g., hyperglycemia, muscle weakness, delayed wound healing, bone density loss, body fat redistribution, adrenal suppression)

Cyclosporine (Sandimmune, Neoral) is a drug that selectively suppresses the CD4+ T-cells by blocking their growth and development. It is used to prevent organ transplant rejection and graft-versus-host disease and occasionally is used for autoimmune disorders.

Disease-modifying immunosuppressive drugs represent a large group of newer agents that specifically slow the damage caused by a variety of autoimmune diseases. Examples include alefacept (Amevive), etanercept (Enbrel), infliximab (Remicade), and many others. Regardless of their specific action in reducing cell damage, they always decrease the general immune responses to some degree and increase the risk for INFECTION, both newly acquired infections and dormant pre-existing infections. The health problems for which these drugs are most commonly prescribed are rheumatoid arthritis and psoriasis. Specific disease-modifying drugs are discussed in the chapters presenting the health problems for which they are prescribed.

Radiation-Induced Immune Deficiencies

Although chemotherapy suppresses IMMUNITY and inflammation more than radiotherapy does, radiation also is toxic to white blood cells (WBCs), especially lymphocytes and neutrophils. Some radiation exposures can induce profound general immunosuppression. Whether immune deficiency occurs after radiation therapy depends on the location and dose of radiation. Exposure to the ilium and femur in adults can cause generalized immunosuppression because these bone areas are the primary blood cell–producing sites.

Management of the patient with treatment-induced immune deficiency aims to improve immune function and prevent INFECTION. The most severe immunosuppression occurs while he or she is receiving the immunosuppressive drugs or during radiation treatment. The severity and duration of the immunosuppression are related to the dosage of specific drugs. Although this impairment is usually temporary, with good recovery of IMMUNITY and inflammation within weeks or months of

therapy completion, the potential for severe infections makes this problem a major treatment concern. Common infections occurring during this period include those of fungal origin, especially yeast, residual viral breakthrough, and a variety of bacteria.

Coordinate with other health care professionals to provide safe care to patients at risk for INFECTION. Chart 19-5 lists specific actions to prevent infection among patients with any type of immunosuppression. Good handwashing by all health care personnel before contact with the patient is essential for infection prevention. Aseptic technique must be used with any invasive procedure as required by The Joint Commission's National Patient Safety Goals (NPSGs).

In some instances, drug-induced immunosuppression can be reduced or avoided by giving hematopoietic growth factors to stimulate bone marrow production of immune system cells. Although not appropriate for all types of disorders, this treatment can reduce the patient's risk for INFECTION during drug therapy. See Chapters 22 and 40 for discussion about this therapy.

Many patients remain at home during periods of immunosuppression. Teach the patient and family best practices to reduce the patient's risk for INFECTION (see Chart 19-4).

For patients receiving long-term therapy with immunosuppressive drugs, drug dosages are altered according to their responses. The lowest dose that achieves the desired effect is given.

CONGENITAL (PRIMARY) IMMUNE DEFICIENCIES

Congenital, or primary, immune deficiencies are rare disorders in which the person is born with a defect in the development or function of one or more immune components. Thus IMMUNITY does not adequately protect him or her from INFECTION or cancer.

Some congenital immune deficiencies are inherited as an X-linked trait (e.g., Bruton's agammaglobulinemia or Wiskott-Aldrich syndrome), and some are recessive (e.g., ataxia-telangiectasia). For many congenital immune deficiencies there is no identified genetic defect.

Congenital immune deficiencies are classified according to the type of immune function that is impaired: antibody-mediated, cell-mediated, or combined. Because cell-mediated and combined immune deficiencies are so severe and rare that the affected person is usually managed in a pediatric setting, only antibody-mediated problems (seen in adults) are discussed in this chapter.

SELECTIVE IMMUNOGLOBULIN A DEFICIENCY

Selective immunoglobulin A (IgA) deficiency is the most common congenital immune deficiency seen in adults, occurring in 1 per 600 to 800 people (McCance et al., 2014). The patient may be asymptomatic or have chronic recurrent INFECTIONS of the upper respiratory tract, skin, urinary tract, vaginal tract, and GI tract. Selective IgA deficiency does not reduce life span. Because IgA is the major antibody in secretions, bacterial infections are seen mostly in the respiratory, GI, and urogenital tracts.

Treatment for IgA deficiency is limited to vigorous treatment of INFECTIONS. Unlike other immunoglobulin deficiencies, IgA deficiency is not managed with exogenous immunoglobulin for two reasons. First, exogenous immunoglobulin contains little IgA and would not help boost IgA levels. Second, because patients with IgA deficiency make normal amounts of all other antibodies, they are at high risk for severe allergic reactions to exogenous immunoglobulin.

> ### ! NURSING SAFETY PRIORITY (QSEN)
> *Drug Alert*
>
> Never administer intravenous immunoglobulin (IVIG) to a patient who has selective immunoglobulin A deficiency.

BRUTON'S AGAMMAGLOBULINEMIA

A classic congenital antibody-mediated immune deficiency is Bruton's disease or Bruton's agammaglobulinemia. Boys born with this disease start to have recurrent INFECTIONS at about 6 months of age, after maternal antibodies, transferred through the placenta, have been lost. These infections include otitis, sinusitis, pneumonia, furunculosis, meningitis, and septicemia. Laboratory assessment shows an absence of circulating immunoglobulin (antibodies).

The prognosis for many patients with Bruton's disease is good if antibody replacement with immune serum globulin is started early. The globulin is regularly given to these patients, usually about 100 to 400 mg/kg IV every 3 to 4 weeks. The dosage and schedule are individualized. Antibiotics are used for specific infections. Long-term prophylactic antibiotic therapy may be used.

COMMON VARIABLE IMMUNE DEFICIENCY

The patient with common variable immune deficiency, or hypogammaglobulinemia, has recurrent bacterial INFECTIONS similar to those seen with Bruton's disease. The patient has low levels of circulating antibodies (immunoglobulins) of all classes.

Hypogammaglobulinemia differs from Bruton's disease in that it usually first appears later (in adolescence or young adulthood), it occurs almost equally in men and women, and the infections are less severe. Common problems include giardiasis (intestinal infection with *Giardia lamblia*), pneumonia, sinusitis, gastric cancer, bronchiectasis, and gallstones.

Treatment is similar to that for Bruton's disease. Regular infusions of immune serum globulin and regular or intermittent use of antibiotics protect the affected person against infection.

NURSING CONCEPTS AND CLINICAL JUDGMENT REVIEW

What might you NOTICE if the patient has impaired protection and increased INFECTION risk as a result of HIV disease and AIDS?
- Chronic or recurrent infections
- History or presence of opportunistic infections
- Decreasing CD4+ T-cell count
- Decreasing CD4+ T-cell to CD8+ T-cell ratio
- Diarrhea
- Report of weight loss and fatigue
- Swollen lymph nodes
- Poor wound healing
- Skin lesions
- Headache
- Fever
- Memory loss

What should you INTERPRET and how should you RESPOND to a patient who has impaired protection and increased INFECTION risk as a result of HIV disease and AIDS?

Perform and interpret focused physical assessment findings including:
- Assess cardiovascular and respiratory status:
  Vital signs
  Presence of acute chest pain or dyspnea
  Presence of cough
  Presence of fever
  Activity tolerance
- Assess nutrition status:
  Food intake
  Weight loss or gain
  General condition of skin

- Assess neurologic status:
  Cognitive changes
  Sensory disturbances
- Assess gastrointestinal status:
  Mouth and oropharynx
  Presence of dysphagia
  Presence of nausea, vomiting, diarrhea
- Assess psychological status:
  Presence of anxiety
  Presence of depression
- Assess activity and rest:
  Activities of daily living (ADLs)
  Fatigue
  Sleep pattern
  Presence of pain

Respond:
- Collaborate with members of the health care team to protect the patient from infection.
- Monitor laboratory test results to determine therapy effectiveness, progression of disease, indications of opportunistic infection.
- Teach the patient and significant other about highly active antiretroviral therapy (HAART) including dosages, schedule, side effects, and the need to take all drugs exactly as prescribed.
- Teach the patient and significant other how to avoid infection in the home environment.
- Teach the patient how to avoid transmission of the HIV.
- Continue to assess for changes in the patient's condition, especially indications of infection in any body area.

On what should you REFLECT?

- Consider your personal views on sexuality, lifestyle choices, what constitutes family membership, gender identification, and fear of HIV transmission.
- Evaluate the patient's, family's, and significant other's knowledge of the disease and its management.
- Evaluate the patient's, family's, and significant other's stress levels, use of coping strategies, and knowledge of community resources.

- Assess the knowledge and proficiency of unlicensed assistive personnel (UAP) in carrying out infection control measures.
- Evaluate the degree of compassion and interaction that UAP display toward patients with HIV infection and AIDS.

GET READY FOR THE NCLEX® EXAMINATION!

KEY POINTS

Review these Key Points for each NCLEX Examination Client Needs Category.

Safe and Effective Care Environment

- Use Standard Precautions for all patients regardless of age, gender, race or ethnicity, sexual orientation, education level, and profession. **Safety** QSEN
- Follow the best practices outlined in Chart 19-5 to protect the hospitalized immunosuppressed patient from INFECTION. **Evidence-Based Practice** QSEN
- Use good handwashing techniques before providing any care to a patient who is immune deficient.
- Ensure the confidentiality of the patient's HIV status. **Patient-Centered Care** QSEN
- Teach unlicensed assistive personnel (UAP) to use Standard Precautions. **Teamwork and Collaboration** QSEN
- Teach unlicensed assistive personnel (UAP) the differences in care required for a patient with a pathogenic infection versus a patient with an opportunistic INFECTION. **Teamwork and Collaboration** QSEN

Health Promotion and Maintenance

- Identify patients at high risk for INFECTION because of work environment or leisure activities.
- Urge all patients who are HIV positive to use condoms and other precautions during sexual intimacy even if the partner is also HIV positive.
- Teach patients with protein-calorie malnutrition what foods to include in the diet to promote better NUTRITION.
- Teach the patient and family to protect against INFECTION by following the recommendations in Chart 19-4.
- Teach the patient and family about the manifestations of INFECTION and when to seek medical advice.
- Urge patients to adhere to their antiviral drug regimen.

Psychosocial Integrity

- Treat all patients, regardless of diagnosis, with dignity.
- Do not assume that any visitor or family member knows the patient's diagnosis.
- Urge all patients who are HIV positive to inform their sexual partners of their HIV status.

- Respect the patient's right to inform or not to inform family members about his or her HIV status. **Patient-Centered Care** QSEN
- Use a nonjudgmental approach when discussing sexual practices, sexual behaviors, and recreational drug use.
- Pace your interview to match the learning needs and energy level of each patient.
- Encourage the patient to express his or her feelings about a change in health status or the diagnosis of an "incurable" disease.
- Refer patients newly diagnosed with HIV INFECTION to local resources and support groups.
- Teach family members reorientation techniques to use when the patient is confused.
- Explain all diagnostic procedures, restrictions, and follow-up care to the patient scheduled for tests.
- Allow patients who have a change in physical appearance to mourn this change.

Physiological Integrity

- Use prescribed oxygen therapy, drug therapy, and respiratory support to improve gas exchange and oxygenation for the patient with respiratory problems related to reduced IMMUNITY.
- Use pharmacologic and nonpharmacologic therapies to reduce pain for the patient with HIV disease and AIDS. **Patient-Centered Care** QSEN
- Pace nonurgent health care activities to reduce the risk for fatigue for patients with AIDS.
- Assess the immune-deficient patient every shift for manifestations of INFECTION. Document the assessment findings, and report any manifestation of infection immediately to the health care provider. **Safety** QSEN
- Assess the TISSUE INTEGRITY of the perianal region of a patient with AIDS-related diarrhea after every bowel movement.
- Collaborate with the health care provider, registered dietitian, respiratory therapist, pharmacist, social worker, and case manager to individualize patient care for the person with HIV disease and AIDS in any care setting. **Teamwork and Collaboration** QSEN

Care of Patients with Immune Function Excess: Hypersensitivity (Allergy) and Autoimmunity

M. Linda Workman

 http://www.elsevier.com/Iggy/

PRIORITY CONCEPTS

- INFLAMMATION
- IMMUNITY

LEARNING OUTCOMES

Safe and Effective Care Environment

1. Protect the patient who has hypersensitivities from injury related to INFLAMMATION.
2. Coordinate with other members of the health care team to ensure a safe environment for the patient with a latex allergy.

Health Promotion and Maintenance

3. Teach patients with allergies how to protect themselves against harm from a hypersensitivity reaction.

Psychosocial Integrity

4. Reduce the psychological impact for patients and families of patients who have IMMUNITY or INFLAMMATION excess.

Physiological Integrity

5. Assess all patients for the potential to have a severe hypersensitivity reaction.
6. Prioritize care for the patient experiencing anaphylaxis.

Usually, INFLAMMATION and IMMUNITY are protective and helpful responses. However, when inflammation or immunity is prolonged or excessive or occurs at an inappropriate time, normal tissues are damaged. These responses are "overreactions" to invaders and foreign antigens and are known as *hypersensitivity* or *allergic responses*. When these responses fail to recognize and protect self cells, normal body tissues are attacked and harmed. This type of reaction is known as an *autoimmune response*. Hypersensitivity and autoimmune responses can severely damage cells, tissues, and organs (Abbas et al., 2012).

HYPERSENSITIVITIES/ALLERGIES

Hypersensitivity or **allergy** is excessive INFLAMMATION occurring in response to the presence of an **antigen** (foreign protein or allergen) to which the patient usually has been previously exposed. It can cause problems that range from uncomfortable (e.g., itchy, watery eyes or sneezing) to life threatening (e.g., allergic asthma, anaphylaxis, bronchoconstriction, or circulatory collapse). The terms *hypersensitivity* and *allergy* are used interchangeably. Hypersensitivity reactions are classified into four basic types, determined by differences in timing, pathophysiology, and manifestations (Table 20-1). Each type may occur alone or along with one or more other types (McCance et al., 2014).

TYPE I: RAPID HYPERSENSITIVITY REACTIONS

Type I, or rapid hypersensitivity, also called *atopic allergy*, is the most common type of hypersensitivity from excess IMMUNITY. This type results from the increased production of the immunoglobulin E (IgE) antibody class. Acute INFLAMMATION occurs when IgE responds to an antigen, such as pollen, and causes the release of histamine and other vasoactive amines from basophils, eosinophils, and mast cells. Examples of type I reactions include anaphylaxis and allergic asthma (discussed in Chapter 30); atopic allergies such as hay fever and allergic rhinitis; and allergies to substances such as latex, bee venom, peanuts, iodine, shellfish, drugs, and thousands of other environmental allergens. Allergens can be contacted in these ways:

- Inhaled (plant pollens, fungal spores, animal dander, house dust, grass, ragweed)
- Ingested (foods, food additives, drugs)
- Injected (bee venom, drugs, biologic substances such as contrast dyes)
- Contacted (latex, pollens, foods, environmental proteins)

Some reactions occur just in the areas exposed to the antigen, such as the mucous membranes of the nose and eyes, causing symptoms of rhinorrhea, sneezing, and itchy, red, watery eyes. Other reactions may involve all blood vessels and bronchiolar smooth muscle causing widespread blood vessel dilation,

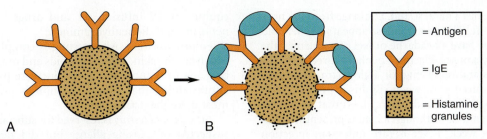

FIG. 20-1 Degranulation and histamine release. **A,** Mast cell with IgE. **B,** Mast cell degranulation and histamine release when allergen binds to IgE.

TABLE 20-1	Mechanisms and Examples of Types of Hypersensitivities
MECHANISM	**CLINICAL EXAMPLES**
Type I: Immediate	
Reaction of IgE antibody on mast cells with antigen, which results in release of mediators, especially histamine	Hay fever Allergic asthma Anaphylaxis
Type II: Cytotoxic	
Reaction of IgG with host cell membrane or antigen adsorbed by host cell membrane	Autoimmune hemolytic anemia Goodpasture's syndrome Myasthenia gravis
Type III: Immune Complex–Mediated	
Formation of immune complex of antigen and antibody, which deposits in walls of blood vessels and results in complement release and inflammation	Serum sickness Vasculitis Systemic lupus erythematosus Rheumatoid arthritis
Type IV: Delayed	
Reaction of sensitized T-cells with antigen and release of lymphokines, which activates macrophages and induces inflammation	Poison ivy Graft rejection Positive TB skin tests Sarcoidosis

IgE, Immunoglobulin E; *IgG,* immunoglobulin G; *TB,* tuberculosis.

decreased cardiac output, and bronchoconstriction. This condition is known as anaphylaxis, which is a medical emergency and must be treated immediately (see the Anaphylaxis section on p. 351).

ALLERGIC RHINITIS
❖ *PATHOPHYSIOLOGY*

Allergic rhinitis, or *hay fever,* is triggered by IMMUNITY and INFLAMMATION reactions to airborne allergens, especially plant pollens, molds, dust, animal dander, wool, food, and air pollutants. Some acute episodes are "seasonal," recurring at the same time each year and lasting only a few weeks. Chronic rhinitis, or perennial rhinitis, occurs intermittently (with no predictable seasonal pattern) or continuously when a person is exposed to certain allergens. In "nonallergic rhinitis," the same manifestations are present although no allergic cause is identified and the immune system does not appear to be involved.

On first exposure to an allergen (an antigen that causes allergic sensitization), the person responds by making antigen-specific IgE. This IgE binds to the surface of basophils and mast cells (see Fig. 17-9 on p. 283 in Chapter 17). These cells have many granules containing vasoactive amines (including histamine) that are released when stimulated. Once the antigen-specific IgE is formed, the person is sensitized to that allergen.

In a type I allergic reaction, the already sensitized person is re-exposed to the allergen. The resulting response has a primary phase and a secondary phase. In the primary phase, the allergen binds to two adjacent IgE molecules on the surface of a basophil or mast cell, which breaks the cell membrane. The membrane opens and releases the vasoactive amines into tissue fluids (Fig. 20-1).

The most common vasoactive amine is *histamine,* a short-acting biochemical. Histamine causes capillary leak, nasal and conjunctival mucus secretion, and itching (pruritus), often occurring with erythema (redness). These manifestations of INFLAMMATION last for about 10 minutes after histamine is first released. When the allergen is continuously present, mast cells continuously release histamine and other proteins, prolonging the response.

The secondary phase results from the release of other cellular proteins. These other proteins draw more white blood cells to the area and stimulate a more general inflammatory reaction through actions of leukotriene and prostaglandins (other mediators of INFLAMMATION; see Chapter 17). This reaction occurs in addition to the allergic reaction stimulated in the primary phase. The resulting inflammation increases the clinical manifestations and continues the response.

The production of high IgE levels in response to antigen exposure is genetically based on the inheritance of many genes. Although allergic tendencies are inherited, specific allergies are *not* inherited. For example, a mother who has an allergy to penicillin but not to peanuts may have a child with an allergy to peanuts but not to penicillin. Atopic allergies affect about 10% of the population in North America (McCance et al., 2014).

❖ *PATIENT-CENTERED COLLABORATIVE CARE*
◆ *Assessment*

History. An accurate and detailed history helps identify possible allergic rhinitis (Holmes & Scullion, 2012). Ask the patient to describe the onset and duration of problems in relation to possible allergen exposure. Ask about work, school, and home environments and about possible exposures through hobbies, leisure time, or sports activities. Because a tendency toward type I allergic responses can be inherited, ask about the presence of allergies among parents and siblings.

Physical Assessment/Clinical Manifestations. The patient with allergic rhinitis has rhinorrhea (a "runny" nose), a "stuffy" nose, and itchy, watery eyes. He or she may breathe through the mouth, and the voice has a nasal sound. Drainage from the nose is usually clear or white. The nasal mucosa appears swollen and pink. The patient may have a headache or feel pressure over the frontal and maxillary sinuses. Placing a penlight directly on the skin over the sinuses and observing for a glow (transillumination) often shows reduced glow when rhinitis is present. With postnasal drip, the patient has a dry, scratchy throat and pharyngitis. He or she often feels as though a cold is present that has lasted longer than a week. Fever is rare unless an infection occurs with the rhinitis.

Laboratory Assessment. A white blood cell (WBC) count and differential indicate the presence of excess IMMUNITY with an allergic response by an increase in eosinophils. A patient with severe seasonal allergic rhinitis may have an eosinophil count as high as 12% (normal being 1% to 2%). Some patients have an increased total WBC count, but the percentage of neutrophils remains normal (55% to 70%). If an acute infection occurs with allergic rhinitis, both the total WBC count and the neutrophils increase.

Other laboratory tests indicating an allergic reaction include serum immunoglobulin E (IgE) levels measured by enzyme-linked immunosorbent assay (ELISA) and the radioallergosorbent test (RAST) (Pagana & Pagana, 2014). A normal level of IgE for adults is about 39 IU/ mL (or less than 100 IU/mL). This level increases greatly with allergies. The usual IgE test does not indicate the specific allergen—only the tendency to have allergic responses. The radioimmunosorbent test (RIST) shows the blood level of IgE directed against a specific antigen and can determine specific allergies. The expense of this study limits its use in allergy testing.

Allergy Testing. Skin testing can show which specific allergens are the cause of a type I reaction. Skin testing is performed as scratch testing or intradermal testing. Patch testing is often reserved for contact dermatitis.

A scratch or prick test can show an *immediate* hypersensitivity reaction to an allergen and is used in routine allergy testing for type I reactions. Allergens introduced through a scratch or prick cause a localized reaction (wheal) when the test result is positive. Results are usually determined after 15 to 20 minutes.

Patient Preparation. Systemic glucocorticoids and antihistamines are discontinued 2 weeks before the test to avoid suppressing the test response. Nasal sprays to reduce mucous membrane swelling are permitted, except for sprays that contain an antihistamine.

Procedure. The best site for scratch testing is the inside of the forearm or on the back. Other sites are used if a rash or skin problem is present on the arms or back. Gently clean the skin with soap and water, and remove surface oils with alcohol.

Small drops of sera containing different known allergens are placed on the skin. The skin is scratched or pricked through the drop with a skin testing needle. Control drops are also applied to determine how a person reacts to substances that do not normally stimulate a reaction (negative control) and to substances that normally should stimulate an excess IMMUNITY reaction (positive control). The allergen-tested areas are examined for the presence and size of reactions. These areas are then compared with the control areas. Areas with erythema and wheal formation are positive for that antigen. Degree of sensitivity is estimated by the size of the response.

Although serious reactions in response to scratch testing are rare, ensure that emergency equipment is available during testing. This includes manual resuscitation bag, oxygen, suction equipment, IV infusion set, and drugs for anaphylaxis (epinephrine and diphenhydramine).

Follow-up Care. After testing is completed, wash the solution from the skin. Topical steroids and oral antihistamines may be given to reduce itching and increase patient comfort. If an antihistamine that causes sedation is given, another person must drive the patient home.

Intradermal testing is reserved for substances that are strongly suspected of causing allergy but did not test positive with scratch testing. Intradermal testing increases the risk for an adverse reaction, including anaphylaxis. Ensure that emergency equipment is in the room with the patient. Small amounts of testing sera (0.1 mL) are injected intradermally on the upper arm, and the area is observed for erythema and wheal formation. The degree of allergy is estimated by the size of the response. Preparation and follow-up care are the same as for scratch testing.

Oral food challenges are used for patients who have allergic rhinitis when the allergen is eaten rather than inhaled. This type of testing is used to identify specific allergens if skin testing is not conclusive and if keeping a food diary has failed to determine the offending food items. The test requires the patient to eliminate suspected foods for 7 to 14 days before testing. After this time, the patient is directed to eat a specific suspected food for at least 1 day and to monitor for manifestations of allergy. When many food allergies are present, the patient may have to eat only one food type per day of testing. *Oral food challenges are not performed using foods that have previously caused a serious or anaphylactic reaction in the patient being tested.*

◆ Interventions

Interventions for allergy management include avoidance therapy, drug therapy, complementary therapies, and desensitization therapy. Many patients use a combination of these therapies for management of allergic rhinitis and other manifestations of type I allergy.

Avoidance Therapy. Avoidance therapy can be successful when specific allergens have been identified. Teach the patient to avoid direct or close contact with these agents. Some allergens, such as foods or drugs, may be easy to avoid. Other allergens, such as pollen, mold, or dust mites, may require environmental changes.

Teach patients that airborne allergens can be reduced by air-conditioning and air-cleaning units. Removing cloth drapes, upholstered furniture, and carpeting also reduces airborne allergens. Covering mattresses and pillows with plastic or an ultra-mesh cover reduces exposure to dust mites and mold, as does laundering bed linens weekly in hot water and detergent.

Pet-induced allergies pose special challenges. Simple interventions, such as keeping pets out of the bedroom and thorough cleaning of the room to remove animal hair and dander, may reduce symptoms. Frequent bathing of the pet or keeping the pet outdoors can decrease allergen exposure. Depending on the severity of the allergy and how well other methods provide relief, pets with fur, feathers, or dander may need to be removed from the household.

Drug Therapy. Drug therapy for symptom relief can be effective in reducing the allergic response and making the patient more comfortable. This therapy involves the use of steroidal and nonsteroidal agents (to reduce inflammation), vasoconstrictors, antihistamines, mast cell stabilizers, and drugs that inhibit the release or action of leukotrienes.

Decongestants are available as systemic oral drugs or nasal sprays. These drugs do not clear the allergen or prevent the release of mediators such as histamine. They work by causing vasoconstriction in the inflamed tissue, thereby reducing the edema. Decongestants often contain ephedrine, phenylephrine, or pseudoephedrine. Secretions are reduced when vasoconstricting drugs are combined with an anticholinergic drug, such as scopolamine or atropine. Many decongestants are available by prescription and as over-the-counter cold and allergy drugs. Side effects include dry mouth, increased blood pressure, and sleep difficulties.

! NURSING SAFETY PRIORITY (QSEN)
Drug Alert

Because effects are systemic, teach patients with high blood pressure, glaucoma, or urinary retention to consult with a health care professional before taking any decongestant.

Antihistamines block histamine from binding to the receptor. This action prevents vasodilation and capillary leak. Many antihistamines also decrease secretions. Some antihistamines, such as diphenhydramine (Benadryl, Allerdryl ✦) and chlorpheniramine (Allergy, Aller-Chlor, Chlor-Trimeton), often induce sedation. Others, such as desloratadine (Clarinex), cetirizine (Zyrtec), and fexofenadine (Allegra), are less sedating.

Corticosteroids decrease INFLAMMATION and excess IMMUNITY in many ways, one of which is by preventing the synthesis of mediators. Corticosteroid nasal sprays (topical intranasal steroids) can prevent the symptoms of rhinitis. Systemic corticosteroids can produce severe side effects and are used only on a short-term basis for serious problems associated with type I reactions, rarely for rhinitis.

Mast cell stabilizing drugs include nasal sprays, such as cromolyn sodium (Nasalcrom), that prevent mast cell membranes from opening when an allergen binds to IgE. Thus these drugs prevent the symptoms of allergic rhinitis but are not useful during an acute episode.

Leukotriene antagonists may be used to manage and prevent allergic rhinitis. Zileuton (Zyflo) prevents leukotriene synthesis. (See Chapter 17 for a discussion of the role of leukotriene in INFLAMMATION and allergy.) Zafirlukast (Accolate) blocks the leukotriene receptor.

Complementary and Alternative Therapies. Complementary and alternative therapies have helped some patients with rhinitis obtain relief, especially through the use of aromatherapy. Possible mechanisms of action include competition and desensitization. Some patients with pollen allergies report decreased problems after eating unprocessed honey.

Desensitization Therapy. Desensitization therapy, commonly called "allergy shots," may be needed when allergens are identified and cannot be avoided easily. It involves subcutaneous injections of very dilute solutions of the identified allergen or allergens. A 0.05-mL dose of this solution is injected subcutaneously. Usually an increasing dose is given weekly until the patient is receiving a 0.5-mL dose. The patient is then started on the lowest dose of the next higher concentration of allergen solution. The process is repeated with increasing concentrations of allergen solutions until the patient is receiving the maximum dose of the greatest concentration (usually 1:100), depending on his or her response. The recommended full course of treatment is about 5 years.

Desensitization appears to reduce allergic responses by competition. In theory, the very small amounts of allergen first injected are too low to bind to the IgE already present but are enough to induce immunoglobulin G (IgG) production against that allergen. IgG is not attached to either mast cells or basal cells, and allergens that bind to IgG do not trigger allergic responses. IgG then clears the allergen from the body (see Chapter 17). By gradually increasing the allergen injection, large amounts of IgG are produced against the allergen. When the patient is then exposed to the allergen in the environment, the IgG binds to it and clears it from the body before IgE can bind to it and trigger an allergic reaction. Because so much more IgG can be produced compared with IgE, IgG is successful in the competition to bind the allergen (Abbas et al., 2012).

ANAPHYLAXIS

❖ PATHOPHYSIOLOGY

Anaphylaxis, the most life-threatening example of a type I hypersensitivity reaction, occurs rapidly and systemically. It affects many organs within seconds to minutes after allergen exposure. Anaphylaxis is not common, episodes can vary in severity, and *it can be fatal. The major factor in fatal outcomes for anaphylaxis is a delay in the administration of epinephrine* (Simons et al., 2011). Many substances can trigger anaphylaxis in a susceptible person (Table 20-2). Drugs and dyes are more

TABLE 20-2 Common Agents That Cause Anaphylaxis

Drugs/Foreign Proteins
- Antibiotics (penicillin, cephalosporins, tetracycline, sulfonamides [especially Bactrim and Septra]), streptomycin, vancomycin, chloramphenicol, amphotericin B, others)
- Adrenocorticotropic hormone, insulin, vasopressin, protamine*
- Allergen extracts, muscle relaxants, hydrocortisone, vaccines, local anesthetics (lidocaine, procaine)*
- Angiotensin-converting enzyme (ACE) inhibitors
- Angiotensin receptor blockers (ARBs)
- Chemotherapy agents (antineoplastic drugs)
- Monoclonal antibodies
- Whole blood, cryoprecipitate, immune serum globulin*
- Radiocontrast media*
- Opiates

Foods
- Peanuts
- Shellfish
- Eggs
- Legumes, nuts
- Grains
- Berries
- Preservatives
- Bananas

Other Agents
- Pollens
- Molds
- Latex
- Other

Insects/Animals
- Hymenoptera: bees, wasps, hornets
- Fire ants
- Snake venom

*Anaphylaxis caused by these substances is probably a result of direct mast cell degranulation rather than an immunoglobulin E (IgE)-mediated hypersensitivity event.

FIG. 20-2 EpiPen and EpiPen Jr. self-injectors for epinephrine.

CHART 20-1 Patient and Family Education: Preparing for Self-Management

Care and Use of Automatic Epinephrine Injectors

- Practice assembly of injection device with a non–drug-containing training device provided through the injection device manufacturer.
- Keep the device with you at all times.
- When needed, inject the drug into the top of your thigh, slightly to the outside, holding the device so that the needle enters straight down.
- You can inject the drug right through your pants; just avoid seams and pockets where the fabric is thicker.
- Use the device when *any* symptom of anaphylaxis is present and call 911. It is better to use the drug when it is not needed than to not use it when it is needed!!!
- Whenever you need to use the device, get to the nearest hospital for monitoring for at least the next 4 to 6 hours.
- Have at least two drug-filled devices on hand in case more than one dose is needed.
- Protect the device from light and avoid temperature extremes.
- Carry the device in the case provided by the manufacturer.
- Keep safety cap in place until you are ready to use the device.
- Check the device for:
  - Expiration date—If the date is close to expiring or has expired, obtain a replacement device.*
  - Drug clarity—If the drug is discolored, obtain a replacement device.
  - Security of cap—If the cap is loose or comes off accidently, obtain a replacement device.

*Some manufacturers have an automatic notification service to let you know your device is about to expire.

---

common causes of anaphylaxis in acute care settings; food and insect stings/bites are common causes in community settings.

Health Promotion and Maintenance

Anaphylaxis has a rapid onset and a potentially fatal outcome (even with appropriate medical intervention); thus prevention and early intervention are critical. *Teach the patient with a history of allergic reactions to avoid allergens whenever possible, to wear a medical alert bracelet, and to alert health care personnel about specific allergies.* Some patients must carry an emergency anaphylaxis kit (e.g., a kit with injectable epinephrine, sometimes called a "bee sting kit") or an epinephrine injector, such as the EpiPen or Twinject automatic injector. The EpiPen device is a spring-loaded injector that delivers 0.3 mg of epinephrine per 2-mL dose directly into the subcutaneous tissue or intramuscularly (Fig. 20-2). Teach patients prescribed the device how to care for and use it (Chart 20-1).

The medical records of patients with a history of anaphylaxis should prominently display the list of specific allergens. Ask the patient about drug allergies before giving any drug or agent. If he or she has a known allergy, be sure to document in the medical

FIG. 20-3 Angioedema of the face, lips, and mouth.

record the allergen and the typical response produced and communicate the allergy and its response to other members of the health care team. *Skin tests should be performed before giving any substance that has a high incidence of causing anaphylactic reactions, such as iodine-containing dyes.* Be aware of common cross-reacting agents. For example, a patient who is allergic to penicillin is also likely to react to cephalosporins because both have a similar chemical structure. People who have an allergy to bananas, avocados, and some nuts are more likely to have a latex allergy, although this is not universal.

Take precautionary measures if a drug or agent must be used despite a history of allergic reactions. Start an IV, and place intubation equipment and a tracheostomy set at the bedside. The patient is often premedicated with diphenhydramine (Benadryl, Allerdryl ✤) or a corticosteroid. The allergy-causing substance is given first intradermally, then subcutaneously, and then intramuscularly in increasing doses at 20- to 30-minute intervals so the initial dose by the next route does not exceed the final dose by the previous route.

❖ PATIENT-CENTERED COLLABORATIVE CARE

◆ Assessment

A major problem with anaphylaxis management is that initial manifestations may be subtle, such as sudden severe abdominal cramping and diarrhea. A set of three criteria, listed in Chart 20-2, is used for diagnosis of anaphylaxis. A patient is considered to have anaphylaxis whenever any *one* of these three criteria is met.

A patient having an anaphylactic reaction first has feelings of uneasiness, apprehension, weakness, and impending doom. Often he or she is anxious and frightened. These feelings are followed, often quickly, by generalized itching and urticaria (hives). Erythema and sometimes angioedema (diffuse swelling) of the eyes, lips, or tongue occur next (Fig. 20-3). Intensely itchy skin wheals or hives may appear and sometimes merge to form large, red blotches.

Histamine and other mediators cause INFLAMMATION, bronchoconstriction, mucosal edema, and excess mucus production.

CHART 20-2 Key Features

Anaphylaxis

Clinical Criteria 1

Onset within minutes to hours of skin or mucous membrane problems involving swollen lips, tongue, soft palate, uvula; widespread hives; pruritus; or flushing along with any *one* of these new onset symptoms:

- Respiratory distress or ineffectiveness:
  - Dyspnea
  - Bronchospasms
  - Wheezes
  - Stridor
  - Hypoxia
  - Cyanosis
  - Peak expiratory rate flow lower than the patient's usual
- Hypotension or any indication of reduced perfusion resulting in organ dysfunction:
  - Loss of consciousness
  - Incontinence
  - Hypotonia
  - Absent deep tendon reflexes

Clinical Criteria 2

Onset within minutes to hours of *two* or more of these symptoms after a patient has been exposed to a potential allergen:

- Skin or mucous membrane problems involving swollen lips, tongue, soft palate, uvula; widespread hives; pruritus; or flushing
- Respiratory distress or ineffectiveness as evidenced by any dyspnea, bronchospasms, wheezes, stridor, hypoxia, cyanosis, or peak expiratory rate flow lower than the patient's usual
- Hypotension or any indication of reduced perfusion resulting in organ dysfunction, such as loss of consciousness, incontinence, hypotonia, or absent deep tendon reflexes
- Persistent GI problems such as nausea or vomiting, cramping, abdominal pain

Clinical Criteria 3

Onset within minutes to hours of hypotension with systolic blood pressure lower than 90 mm Hg or 30% lower than the patient's baseline systolic pressure.

Adapted from Simons, E., Ardusso, L., Bilo, M.B., El-Gamal, Y., Ledford, D., Ring, J., et al. (2011). World Allergy Organization guidelines for the assessment and management of anaphylaxis. *WAO Journal, 4*(2), 13-37.

CHART 20-3 Best Practice for Patient Safety & Quality Care (QSEN)

Emergency Care of the Patient with Anaphylaxis

- Immediately assess the respiratory status, airway, and oxygen saturation of patients who show any symptom of an allergic reaction.
- Call the Rapid Response Team.
- Ensure that intubation and tracheotomy equipment is ready.
- Apply oxygen using a high-flow, non-rebreather mask at 90% to 100%.
- Immediately discontinue the IV drug or infusing solution of a patient having an anaphylactic reaction to that drug or solution. **Do not** discontinue the IV, but change the IV tubing and hang normal saline.
- If the patient does not have an IV, start one immediately and run normal saline.
- Be prepared to administer epinephrine IV (preferred) or IM.
  - Epinephrine 1:1000 concentration, 0.3 to 0.5 mL IV push or IM
  - Repeat drug administration as needed every 5 to 15 minutes until the patient responds
- Keep the head of the bed elevated about 10 degrees if hypotension is present; if blood pressure is normal, elevate the head of the bed to 45 degrees or higher to improve ventilation.
- Raise the feet and legs.
- Stay with the patient.
- Reassure the patient that the appropriate interventions are being instituted.

! NURSING SAFETY PRIORITY (QSEN)

Critical Rescue

Immediately call the Rapid Response Team if you suspect anaphylaxis, because most anaphylactic deaths are related to treatment delay. If the patient is not treated immediately, he or she may lose consciousness. Dysrhythmias, shock, and cardiopulmonary arrest may occur within minutes as intravascular volume is lost and the heart becomes hypoxic.

---

quickly impairs airflow and leads to hypoxemic arrest. Immediately establish or stabilize the airway. If an IV drug is suspected to be causing the anaphylaxis, stop the drug immediately but do not remove the venous access because restarting an IV may be very difficult when the patient becomes severely hypotensive. Change the IV tubing and hang normal saline. Additional emergency interventions for patients with anaphylaxis are listed in Chart 20-3.

The patient with anaphylaxis is usually anxious or frightened and often expresses a sense of impending doom. Stay with the patient and reassure him or her that the appropriate interventions are being instituted.

Epinephrine (1:1000) 0.3 to 0.5 mL is the first-line drug for anaphylaxis. It is given IM or IV when manifestations appear (see Chart 20-3). This drug constricts blood vessels, improves cardiac contraction, and dilates the bronchioles. The same dose may be repeated every 5 to 15 minutes if needed (Vacca & McMahon-Bowen, 2013). Other drugs used to treat anaphylaxis are listed in Chart 20-4.

! NURSING SAFETY PRIORITY (QSEN)

Critical Rescue

Administer epinephrine as quickly as possible. Most deaths from anaphylaxis are related to delay in epinephrine administration.

Respiratory symptoms include congestion, rhinorrhea, dyspnea, and increasing respiratory distress with audible wheezing.

On auscultation, crackles, wheezing, and reduced breath sounds are heard. Patients may have laryngeal edema as a "lump in the throat," hoarseness, and stridor (a crowing sound). Distress increases as the tongue and larynx swell and more mucus is produced. Stridor increases as the airway begins to close. Increasing bronchoconstriction can lead to reduced chest movement and impaired airflow. Respiratory failure may follow from laryngeal edema, suffocation, or lower airway constriction causing hypoxemia (poor blood oxygenation).

The patient is usually hypotensive and has a rapid, weak, irregular pulse from extensive capillary leak and vasodilation. He or she is faint and diaphoretic with increasing anxiety and confusion.

◆ Interventions

Assess respiratory function first. Emergency respiratory management is critical during an anaphylactic reaction, because the severity of the reaction increases with time. The upper airways and lower airways are affected by bronchoconstriction that

CHART 20-4   Common Examples of Drug Therapy
Anaphylaxis

DRUG	MECHANISM	SIDE EFFECTS
Sympathomimetics (First-Line Drugs)		
Epinephrine (Adrenalin)	Rapidly stimulates alpha- and beta-adrenergic receptors of autonomic nervous system (alpha: vasoconstriction; beta: bronchodilation).	Pallor, tachycardia and palpitations, nervousness, muscle twitching, sweating, anxiety, insomnia, hypertension, headache, hyperglycemia.
Isoproterenol (Isuprel)	Stimulates beta-adrenergic receptors, relaxing bronchial smooth muscles and dilating vessels.	Same as for epinephrine.
Ephedrine sulfate (Vatronol)	Similar to isoproterenol but with longer duration of action.	Same as for epinephrine.
Antihistamines (Second-Line Drugs)		
Diphenhydramine HCl (Allerdryl , Benadryl)	Competes with histamine for H₁ receptors on effector cells, thus blocking effects of histamine on bronchioles, gastrointestinal tract, and blood vessels.	Drowsiness, confusion, insomnia, headache, vertigo, photosensitivity, diplopia, nausea, vomiting, dry mouth.
Corticosteroids (Second-Line Drugs)		
Hydrocortisone sodium succinate (Solu-Cortef) (IV/IM) Dexamethasone (Decadron) (IV/IM) Methylprednisolone sodium succinate (Solu-Medrol) (IV/IM) Prednisone (orally)	Anti-inflammatory—inhibits production of many inflammatory mediators; inhibits mast cell degranulation.	Fluid and sodium retention, hypertension, cushingoid state, gastric distress, adrenal suppression, psychosis, osteoporosis, susceptibility to infection.
Vasopressors (Support Drugs)		
Norepinephrine (Levophed)	Raises blood pressure and cardiac output in severely decompensated states.	Headache, tachycardia, fibrillation, decreased urine output, hypertension, metabolic acidosis.
Dopamine (Intropin)	Raises blood pressure and cardiac output in severely decompensated states.	Dysrhythmias, tachycardia, hypertension, dyspnea, nausea and vomiting, azotemia, headache.

Antihistamines such as diphenhydramine (Benadryl, Allerdryl) 25 to 100 mg are second-line drugs and are given IV or IM for angioedema and urticaria. If needed, an endotracheal tube may be inserted or an emergency tracheostomy may be performed.

If the patient can breathe independently, give oxygen to reduce hypoxemia. Start oxygen therapy via a high-flow non-rebreather facemask at 90% to 100% before arterial blood gas results are obtained. Monitor pulse oximetry to determine oxygenation adequacy. Arterial blood gases may be drawn to determine therapy effectiveness. Use suction to remove excess mucus and other secretions, if indicated. Continually assess the respiratory rate and depth, and assess breath sounds continually for bronchospasm, wheezing, crackles, and stridor. Elevate the bed to 45 degrees unless severe hypotension is present.

For bronchospasms, the patient may be given an inhaled beta-adrenergic agonist such as metaproterenol (Alupent) or albuterol (Proventil) via high-flow nebulizer every 2 to 4 hours. Corticosteroids are added to emergency interventions, but they are not effective immediately. Oral steroids are continued (at lower doses) after the anaphylaxis is under control to prevent the late recurrence of manifestations.

Continually assess for changes in any body system or for adverse effects of drug therapy. For severe anaphylaxis, the patient is admitted to a critical care unit for cardiac, pulmonary arterial, and capillary wedge pressure monitoring. Observe the patient for fluid overload from the rapid drug and IV fluid infusions, and report changes to the health care provider immediately. The patient is discharged from the hospital when respiratory and cardiovascular systems have returned to baseline.

🔘 NCLEX EXAMINATION CHALLENGE
Safe and Effective Care Environment

The client having an intravenous injection of radiocontrast material (dye) for an angiogram starts to have skin wheals at the injection site and difficulty breathing. What is the nurse's best first action?
A. Administer oxygen by mask or nasal cannula.
B. Stop the infusion of the contrast material.
C. Prepare an injection of epinephrine.
D. Notify the Rapid Response Team.

LATEX ALLERGY

Latex allergy is a type I hypersensitivity reaction in which the specific allergen is a processed natural latex rubber protein. When the allergen enters the body through inhalation or direct contact with blood vessels (e.g., as might occur during surgery), interaction with IgE occurs, leading to a type I reaction and INFLAMMATION. For some people, latex allergen contact is limited to the skin or mucous membranes, causing contact dermatitis, a type IV hypersensitivity reaction (see p. 355). Others may have a "mixed" allergic response to latex, with symptoms of both type I and type IV hypersensitivities.

The incidence of latex hypersensitivity in the general population is increasing. People at greatest risk are those with a high exposure to natural latex products, such as patients with spina bifida, people who routinely use latex condoms, and health care workers who use latex gloves, especially gloves that are powdered (Wade, 2012).

Ask all patients about their use of and known reactions to natural latex products. Document all food allergies because some have cross-reactivity for latex allergy. In addition, consider your own exposure and risk for reactions to natural latex products.

Avoiding products that contain natural latex proteins can prevent reactions and initial sensitivity. Most surgical gloves, tubing, and vial closures are now being made from synthetic substances that do not contain latex proteins. Interventions for the patient who has a type I or a type IV reaction to latex are the same as for reactions caused by other allergens.

> ? **NCLEX EXAMINATION CHALLENGE**
>
> **Safe and Effective Care Environment**
>
> With which client is it most important for the nurse to use latex-free gloves?
> A. 38-year-old woman taking oral contraceptives
> B. 68-year-old man with total hip replacement
> C. 38-year-old man allergic to shellfish and nuts
> D. 28-year-old woman with spina bifida

TYPE II: CYTOTOXIC REACTIONS

In a type II (cytotoxic) reaction, the body makes autoantibodies directed against self cells that have some form of foreign protein attached to them. The autoantibody binds to the self cell and forms an immune complex (see Fig. 17-10 on p. 283 in Chapter 17). The self cell is then destroyed along with the attached protein. Clinical examples of type II reactions include immune hemolytic anemias, immune thrombocytopenic purpura, hemolytic transfusion reactions (when a patient receives the wrong blood type during a transfusion), Goodpasture's syndrome, and drug-induced hemolytic anemia.

Management of type II reactions begins with discontinuing the offending drug or blood product. Plasmapheresis (filtration of the plasma to remove specific substances) to remove autoantibodies may be beneficial. Otherwise, treatment is symptomatic. Complications such as hemolytic crisis and kidney failure can be life threatening.

TYPE III: IMMUNE COMPLEX REACTIONS

In a type III reaction, excess antigens cause immune complexes to form in the blood (Fig. 20-4). These circulating complexes usually lodge in small blood vessel walls of the kidneys, skin, and joints. The complexes trigger INFLAMMATION, and tissue or vessel damage results.

Many immune complex disorders (mostly connective tissue disorders) are caused by type III reactions. For example, the manifestations of rheumatoid arthritis are caused by immune complexes that lodge in joint spaces followed by tissue destruction, scarring, and fibrotic changes. Systemic lupus erythematosus (SLE) has immune complexes lodged in the vessels

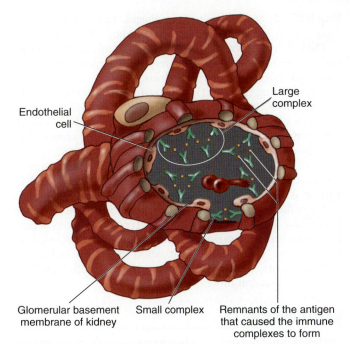

FIG. 20-4 An immune complex in a type III hypersensitivity reaction.

(vasculitis), the glomeruli (glomerulonephritis), the joints (arthralgia, arthritis), and other organs and tissues. (See Chapter 18 for a discussion of SLE.)

Serum sickness is a group of manifestations that occurs after receiving serum or certain drugs. Immune complexes are deposited in blood vessel walls of the skin, joints, and kidneys. Common causes of serum sickness are penicillin, other antibiotics, and some animal serum–based drugs. Other agents known to cause serum sickness include antilymphocyte globulin and antithymocyte globulin, used to treat organ transplant rejection.

The patient with serum sickness has fever, arthralgia (achy joints), rash, malaise, lymphadenopathy (enlarged lymph nodes), and possibly polyarthritis and nephritis about 7 to 12 days after receiving the causative agent. Teach him or her about the possibility of serum sickness and what manifestations to look for whenever you give a foreign serum. Also keep emergency equipment and drugs close at hand in case he or she has an anaphylactic reaction.

Serum sickness is usually self-limiting, and manifestations subside after several days. Management is symptomatic; antihistamines are given for itching and aspirin for arthralgias. Prednisone is given if manifestations are severe.

TYPE IV: DELAYED HYPERSENSITIVITY REACTIONS

In a type IV reaction, the reactive cell is the T-lymphocyte (T-cell). Antibodies and complement are not involved. Sensitized T-cells (from a previous exposure) respond to an antigen by releasing chemical mediators and triggering macrophages to destroy the antigen. A type IV response typically occurs hours to days after exposure. It consists of edema, induration, ischemia, and tissue damage at the site.

An example of a small type IV reaction is a positive purified protein derivative (PPD) test for tuberculosis (TB). In a patient previously exposed to TB, an intradermal injection of this agent causes sensitized T-cells to clump at the injection site, release lymphokines, and activate macrophages. Induration and erythema at the injection site appear after about 24 to 72 hours.

Other examples of type IV reactions include contact dermatitis, poison ivy skin rashes, local response to insect stings, tissue transplant rejections, and sarcoidosis.

Patch testing for type IV hypersensitivity involves applying test chemicals that contain the allergen(s) to which the patient has been exposed. The patches remain in place for 48 hours. After removal, the skin areas in contact with the chemical are examined for localized redness, swelling, and blisters.

Removal of the offending antigen is the major focus of management. The reaction is self-limiting in 5 to 7 days, and the patient is treated symptomatically. Monitor the reaction site and sites distal to the reaction for circulation adequacy. Diphenhydramine (Benadryl) is not useful for type IV reactions because histamine is not the main mediator. Because IgE does not cause this type of reaction, desensitization does not reduce the response. Corticosteroids can reduce the discomfort and help resolve the reaction more quickly.

AUTOIMMUNITY

Autoimmunity is a process whereby a person develops an inappropriate IMMUNITY. In this response, antibodies or lymphocytes are directed against healthy normal cells and tissues. (Antibodies directed against self tissues or cells are known as autoantibodies.) For unknown reasons, the immune system fails to recognize certain body cells or tissues as self and thus triggers immune reactions. The responses, both antibody- and cell-mediated responses, are directed against normal body cells (McCance et al., 2014).

Examples of diseases that have an autoimmune cause include systemic lupus erythematosus (SLE), polyarteritis nodosa, scleroderma, rheumatoid arthritis, autoimmune hemolytic anemia, rheumatic fever, and Hashimoto's thyroiditis (Table 20-3). Other diseases, such as type 1 diabetes mellitus, may have multiple causes, one of which is autoimmune.

Management of autoimmunities depends on the organ or organs affected. *There is no cure.* Anti-inflammatory drugs and immunosuppressive drugs are commonly used along with symptomatic treatment to suppress the excess IMMUNITY.

GENDER HEALTH CONSIDERATIONS
Patient-Centered Care QSEN

Virtually all autoimmune disorders, especially rheumatic disorders, occur much more commonly among women than men (McCance et al., 2014). The risk for autoimmune disease among women compared with men ranges from 5:1 to 20:1.

SJÖGREN'S SYNDROME

❖ PATHOPHYSIOLOGY

Sjögren's syndrome (SS) is a group of problems that often appear with other autoimmune disorders. Problems include dry eyes, dry mucous membranes of the nose and mouth (xerostomia), and vaginal dryness. These problems are caused by autoimmune destruction (excess IMMUNITY) of the lacrimal, salivary, and vaginal mucus-producing glands. Often, the patient with SS also has rheumatoid arthritis or fibromyalgia.

TABLE 20-3 Known or Probable Autoimmune Disorders

DISORDER	AUTOANTIGEN
Systemic or Non–Organ Specific	
Systemic lupus erythematosus	DNA, DNA proteins
Rheumatoid arthritis	IgG, possibly cartilage
Progressive systemic sclerosis	DNA proteins
Mixed connective tissue disorder	DNA proteins
Scleroderma	Endothelial cells; epithelial cells
Organ Specific	
Autoimmune hemolytic anemia	Erythrocytes
Autoimmune thrombocytopenic purpura	Platelets
Crohn's disease	Crypt epithelial cells
Diabetes mellitus, type I	Islet cells, insulin, insulin receptor
Dermatomyositis	Unknown
Glomerulonephritis	Glomerular basement membranes
Goodpasture's syndrome	Glomerular basement membranes, pulmonary basement membranes
Graves' disease	Thyroid-stimulating hormone receptor
Hashimoto's thyroiditis	Thyroid cell surface
Idiopathic Addison's disease	Adrenal cell
Myasthenia gravis	Acetylcholine receptor, acetylcholine
Pernicious anemia	Intrinsic factor, parietal cell, B_{12} complexes
Psoriasis	Stratum corneum
Reiter's syndrome	Possibly collagen, conjunctival cells
Sjögren's syndrome	Salivary gland cells, vaginal mucous cells, lacrimal gland cells
Uveitis	Uveal tract cells (eye)
Vasculitis	Unknown, possibly collagen or endothelial cells

IgG, Immunoglobulin G.

Most patients with SS are women 35 to 45 years old. SS occurs more frequently among patients with certain tissue types, specifically HLA-DRW52, HLA-DR3, and HLA-B8. Although an exact triggering agent has not been identified, viral infection is strongly suspected, especially human immunodeficiency virus type 1 (HIV-1), human T-cell lymphotrophic virus type 1 (HTLV-1), and Epstein-Barr virus (EBV).

Insufficient tears cause INFLAMMATION and ulceration of the cornea. Insufficient saliva decreases digestion of carbohydrates, promotes tooth decay, and increases the risk for oral and nasal infections. Vaginal dryness increases the risk for infection and causes painful sexual intercourse.

❖ PATIENT-CENTERED COLLABORATIVE CARE

The patient with Sjögren's syndrome (SS) usually has blurred vision, burning and itching of the eyes, and thick mattering in the conjunctiva. Difficulty swallowing food is common, as are changes in taste. Ask about nosebleeds (epistaxis) and frequent upper respiratory infections (Catanzaro & Dinkel, 2014).

Examination reveals enlarged lymph nodes. If rheumatoid arthritis (RA) accompanies SS, the patient has swollen, painful joints and limited joint mobility (see Chapter 18 for a discussion of RA). Laboratory assessment may show increased amounts of general antinuclear antibodies, anti–SS-A or anti–SS-B antibodies, and elevated levels of IgM rheumatoid factor.

There is no cure for SS. The intensity and the progression of the disorder can be slowed by suppressing IMMUNITY and INFLAMMATION. Drugs used to modulate the immune system in patients with SS include low-dose chemotherapy with methotrexate (Rheumatrex) or cyclophosphamide (Cytoxan). Both drugs have serious long-term side effects, especially on liver and bone marrow function. Other immunosuppressive drugs used to manage SS are corticosteroids, cyclosporine (Gengraf, Neoral, Sandimmune), and hydroxychloroquine (Plaquenil). The monoclonal antibody *rituximab* (Rituxan) has been beneficial for patients with severe inflammatory manifestations of SS (Poetzsch, 2012).

A variety of artificial tears and artificial saliva can help reduce the dry eye and dry mouth manifestations. Teach patients to use humidifiers in the home to increase environmental moisture. Use of water-soluble vaginal lubricants and moisturizers can increase patient comfort and reduce vaginitis. Some patients relieve dry mouth with drugs that increase salivation, such as systemic pilocarpine (Salagen). A drug that increase tears production is cyclosporine (Restasis) eyedrops.

Another intervention for dry eyes is to block the tear outflow channel with small plugs or close it surgically. Then, tears produced remain in contact with the eye longer.

💡 CLINICAL JUDGMENT CHALLENGE

Patient-Centered Care; Evidence-Based Practice QSEN

The patient is a 49-year-old secretary who has just been diagnosed with Sjögren's syndrome (SS) when her health care provider investigated possible causes for her sudden increase in dental caries (15 in 1 year). Upon hearing about the possible dry eyes and vaginal dryness that often accompany SS, she tells you that she has noticed the dry eyes and thought it was just "old age" catching up with her. She also says that she has noticed some vaginal dryness but is not concerned about it because she is not sexually active. She then tells you that she feels bad about this diagnosis because it means that she probably has a poor immune system and is at a greater risk for infections and cancer.

1. Is she correct about her assessment of her immune function? Why or why not?
2. What should you tell her about the vaginal dryness even though she is not concerned?
3. In addition to follow-up by her primary health care provider for the SS, what other health promotion activities would be important for her?

GOODPASTURE'S SYNDROME

❖ *PATHOPHYSIOLOGY*

Goodpasture's syndrome is an autoimmune disorder in which autoantibodies attack the glomerular basement membrane and neutrophils. The two organs with the most damage are the lungs and the kidneys. A person with the disorder may have lung and/or kidney problems. Lung damage is manifested as pulmonary hemorrhage. Kidney damage shows as glomerulonephritis that may rapidly progress to complete kidney failure (see Chapters 67 and 68). Goodpasture's syndrome is most common in adolescent males or young men (McCance et al., 2014).

❖ *PATIENT-CENTERED COLLABORATIVE CARE*

Goodpasture's syndrome often is not diagnosed until serious lung or kidney problems are present. Manifestations include shortness of breath, hemoptysis (bloody sputum), decreased urine output, weight gain, generalized edema, hypertension, and tachycardia. Chest x-rays show areas of consolidation. The most common cause of death is uremia as a result of kidney failure.

Spontaneous resolution of Goodpasture's syndrome has occurred but is rare. Interventions focus on reducing damage from excess IMMUNITY and performing some type of renal replacement therapy.

Drug therapy is the mainstay of treatment for Goodpasture's syndrome. High-dose corticosteroids are most often used. Other drug therapy to suppress the autoimmune response is the same as that for Sjögren's syndrome (SS).

Additional therapy to reduce the excessive IMMUNITY involves plasmapheresis (filtration of the plasma to remove some proteins) to remove the autoantibodies. If the lungs and kidneys do not have permanent damage, patients undergoing plasmapheresis have shown clinical improvement. Some patients using plasmapheresis need infusions of intravenous immunoglobulin (IVIG) to maintain antibody protection against infection.

Depending on the level of kidney function remaining, the patient may need ongoing renal replacement therapy. Peritoneal dialysis or hemodialysis may be used, depending on the patient's health status, ability to self-manage the therapy, and lifestyle (see Chapter 68).

Kidney transplantation is an option for some patients with Goodpasture's syndrome. After transplantation, kidney function is normal and a few patients have been completely disease-free. In others, the kidney problems are improved but the lung destruction continues. Some of the drugs used to prevent kidney rejection also suppress the autoimmune response.

NURSING CONCEPTS AND CLINICAL JUDGMENT REVIEW

What might you NOTICE if the patient is experiencing excess IMMUNITY and loss of protective response in the form of a severe allergic reaction?

- Possible skin rash, blisters, wheals, especially on the skin at the IV site
- Swelling of the face, lips, tongue (angioedema)
- Difficulty breathing, hoarseness, stridor, wheezing
- Cyanosis
- Increasing anxiety

What should you INTERPRET and how should you RESPOND to a patient experiencing excess IMMUNITY and loss of protection as a result of a severe allergic reaction?

Perform and interpret physical assessment, including:
- Taking vital signs, especially respiratory rate and depth and blood pressure
- Auscultating all lung fields
- Monitoring oxygen saturation by pulse oximetry
- Assessing cognition
- Assessing for the use of accessory muscles
- Assessing for the presence of thick or excessive secretions
- Assessing the patient's ability to cough and clear the airway

Respond by:
- Removing or discontinuing the offending agent
- Ensuring a patent airway
- Notifying the Rapid Response Team
- Applying oxygen, and assessing the patient's responses to this intervention

- Maintaining IV access, changing IV tubing, hanging normal saline
- Keeping the patient's head elevated between 10 and 45 degrees
- Preparing to administer IV diphenhydramine and epinephrine
- Staying with the patient

On what should you REFLECT?
- Observe patient for evidence of drug therapy and oxygen therapy effectiveness (adequate tissue perfusion and oxygenation [see Chapter 27]).
- Think about what may have precipitated this episode and what steps could be taken to either prevent a similar episode or identify it earlier.
- Think about what additional resources could improve the nursing response to this situation.

GET READY FOR THE NCLEX® EXAMINATION!

KEY POINTS

Review these Key Points for each NCLEX Examination Client Needs Category.

Safe and Effective Care Environment
- Ensure that only latex-free products are used for a patient who has a known latex allergy. **Safety** QSEN
- Verify that all allergies are documented in a prominent place in the patient's medical record.
- Keep emergency equipment and drugs (epinephrine, Benadryl, cortisol) in or near the room of a patient with known severe allergies or a history of anaphylaxis. **Safety** QSEN

Health Promotion and Maintenance
- Urge all patients with severe allergies or those who have a history of anaphylaxis to wear a medical alert bracelet.
- Teach the patient and family about the manifestations of allergic reactions and when to seek medical help. **Patient-Centered Care** QSEN
- Teach the patient who has a known drug allergy about which other drugs are likely to stimulate the same reactions. **Patient-Centered Care** QSEN
- Teach the patient who carries an automatic epinephrine injector how to care for, assemble, and use the device. Obtain a return demonstration. **Patient-Centered Care** QSEN

Psychosocial Integrity
- Explain all diagnostic procedures, restrictions, and follow-up care to the patient scheduled for tests related to hypersensitivities.
- Stay with the patient in anaphylaxis.
- Reassure patients who are in anaphylaxis that the appropriate interventions are being instituted.

Physiological Integrity
- Identify patients at risk for hypersensitivity reactions, especially anaphylaxis. **Safety** QSEN
- Communicate a patient's allergies to all members of the health care team.
- Immediately assess the respiratory status and airway of patients who show any manifestations of an allergic reaction. **Evidence-Based Practice** QSEN
- Immediately discontinue the IV drug or solution of a patient having an anaphylactic reaction to that drug or solution. **Do not** discontinue the IV, but change the IV tubing and hang normal saline. **Evidence-Based Practice** QSEN
- Hold the dose of any prescribed drug when a patient develops angioedema. **Safety** QSEN
- Give oxygen to any patient in anaphylaxis.

CHAPTER 21

Cancer Development

M. Linda Workman

 http://evolve.elsevier.com/Iggy/

PRIORITY CONCEPTS

- CELLULAR REGULATION

LEARNING OUTCOMES

Health Promotion and Maintenance

1. Help people identify behaviors that reduce the risk for cancer development and cancer death.
2. Teach the recommended screening practices and schedules for specific cancer types.

Physiological Integrity

3. Explain why causes of specific cancers can be hard to establish.
4. Use knowledge of basic biology to understand how normal cells can lose CELLULAR REGULATION and become malignant.
5. Distinguish the features of normal cells from those of benign tumors and cancer cells.

6. Discuss the roles of oncogenes and suppressor genes in cancer development.
7. Compare the cancer development processes of initiation and promotion.
8. Interpret cancer grading, ploidy, and staging reports.
9. Explain how cancer metastasis occurs and the expected sites of distant metastasis for common cancers.
10. Discuss the role of immunity in protection against cancer.
11. Assess the individual patient's need for genetic testing for cancer predisposition based on family history.

Abnormal cell growth includes moles or skin tags, which are **benign** (harmless) and do not require intervention, as well as **malignant cell growth** (cancer). Cancer is serious and without intervention leads to death. It is a common health problem in the United States and Canada. Over 1.8 million people are newly diagnosed with cancer each year (American Cancer Society [ACS], 2014; Canadian Cancer Society, 2014). Some types of cancer can be prevented; others have better cure rates if diagnosed early. As a nurse, you can have a vital impact in educating the public about cancer prevention and early detection methods.

Although cancer is common today, it is not a new disorder. Some types of cancer are more common today, especially among more affluent societies, than in centuries past. Two reasons for this increase are the longer life expectancy of people in more affluent countries and increased exposure to substances that cause cancer.

Cancer will occur in about 1 of every 3 people currently living in North America (ACS, 2014; Canadian Cancer Society, 2014), although cancer risk differs for each person. More than 13 million Americans with a history of cancer are alive today (ACS, 2014).

PATHOPHYSIOLOGY

During infancy and childhood, growth of cells and tissues is normal, and many body cells continue to "grow" by **mitosis** (cell division) long after maturation is complete. Such cells are located in tissues in which constant damage or wear is likely and continued cell growth is needed to replace dead tissues. Cells of the skin, hair, mucous membranes, bone marrow, and linings of organs such as the lungs, stomach, intestines, bladder, and uterus, among others have the ability to divide throughout a person's life span. The growth is well controlled through CELLULAR REGULATION, ensuring that the right number of cells is always present in any tissue or organ.

Some tissues and organs stop growing by cell division after development is complete. For example, heart muscle cells no longer divide after fetal life; the number of heart muscle cells is fixed at birth. The size of the heart increases as the person grows because each cell gets larger, but the number of heart muscle cells does not increase. Growth that causes tissue to increase in size by enlarging each cell is **hypertrophy**. Growth that causes tissue to increase in size by increasing the number of cells is **hyperplasia** (Fig. 21-1).

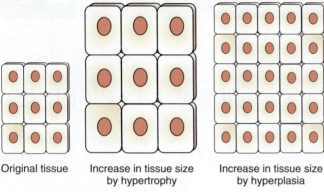

FIG. 21-1 Tissue growth by hypertrophy and hyperplasia.

Original tissue   Increase in tissue size   Increase in tissue size
                   by hypertrophy   by hyperplasia

Neuron   Skin fibroblast   Mature red
                                         blood cell

FIG. 21-2 Distinctive morphology of some normal cells.

Any new or continued cell growth not needed for normal development or replacement of dead and damaged tissues is called neoplasia. This cell growth is always abnormal even if it causes no harm. Whether the new cells are benign or cancerous, neoplastic cells develop from normal cells *(parent cells)*. Thus cancer cells were once normal cells but underwent genetic mutations to no longer look, grow, or function normally. The strict processes controlling normal growth and function, CEL-LULAR REGULATION, have been lost (Beery & Workman, 2012). To understand how cancer cells grow, it is helpful to first understand the regulation and function of normal cells.

Biology of Normal Cells

Many different normal cells work together to make the whole person function at an optimal level. For optimal function, each cell must perform in a predictable manner.

Specific morphology is the feature in which each normal cell type has a distinct and recognizable appearance, size, and shape, as shown in Fig. 21-2.

A smaller nuclear-to-cytoplasmic ratio means that the nucleus of a normal cell does not take up much space inside the cell. As shown in Fig. 21-2, the size of the normal cell nucleus is relatively small compared with the size of the rest of the cell, including the cytoplasm.

Differentiated function means that every normal cell has at least one function it performs to contribute to whole-body function. For example, skin cells make keratin, liver cells make bile, cardiac muscle cells contract, and red blood cells make hemoglobin.

Tight adherence occurs because normal cells make proteins that protrude from the membranes, allowing cells to bind closely and tightly together. One such protein is fibronectin, which keeps most normal tissues bound tightly to each other. Exceptions are blood cells. Red blood cells and white blood cells produce no fibronectin and do not usually adhere together.

Nonmigratory means that normal cells do not wander throughout the body (except for blood cells). This occurs in normal cells because they are tightly bound together, which prevents cell wandering from one tissue into the next.

Orderly and well-regulated growth or CELLULAR REGULATION is a very important feature of normal cells. They divide (undergo mitosis) for only two reasons: (1) to develop normal tissue or (2) to replace lost or damaged normal tissue. Even when they are capable of mitosis, normal cells divide only when body conditions are just right. Cell division (mitosis), occurring in a well-recognized pattern, is described

by the cell cycle. Fig. 21-3 shows the phases of the cell cycle. Living cells not actively reproducing are in a reproductive resting state termed G_0. During the G_0 period, cells actively carry out their functions but do not divide. Normal cells spend most of their lives in the G_0 state rather than in a reproductive state.

Mitosis makes one cell divide into two new cells that are identical to each other and to the cell that began mitosis. The steps of entering and completing the cell cycle are tightly controlled. This CELLULAR REGULATION occurs through proteins produced by "suppressor genes."

Whether a cell enters and completes the cell cycle to form two new cells depends on the presence and absence of specific CELLULAR REGULATION proteins. Proteins that promote cells to enter and complete cell division are produced by oncogenes and are known as *cyclins*. When cyclins are activated, they allow a cell to leave G_0 and enter the cycle. These activated cyclins then drive the cell to progress through the different phases of the cell cycle and divide. Proteins produced by suppressor genes control the amount of cyclins present and ensure that cell division occurs only when it is needed. *Thus CELLULAR REGULATION of division is a balance between the proteins that promote cell division (cyclins) and the proteins that limit cell division (suppressor gene products).*

Fig. 21-4 shows the activities of the phases of the cell cycle (described below):

- **G_1.** In this phase, the cell is getting ready for division by taking on extra nutrients, making more energy, and growing extra membrane. The amount of cytoplasm also increases.
- **S.** Because making one cell into two cells requires twice as much of everything, including DNA, the cell must double its DNA content through DNA synthesis. This process occurs in S phase.
- **G_2.** In this phase, the cell makes important proteins that will be used in actual cell division and in normal physiologic function after cell division is complete.
- **M.** The single cell splits apart into two cells (actual mitosis) during M phase.

Contact inhibition is CELLULAR REGULATION that stops further rounds of cell division when the dividing cell is completely surrounded and touched (contacted) by other cells. Of the normal cells that can divide, each cell divides only when some of its surface is not in direct contact with another cell. Once a normal cell is in direct contact on all surface areas with other cells, it no longer undergoes mitosis. Thus normal cell division is contact inhibited.

Apoptosis is programmed cell death. Not only do normal cells have to divide only when needed and perform their specific differentiated functions, to ensure optimum body function, some cells also have to die at the appropriate time. Thus normal cells have a finite life span. With each cell division, the telomeric DNA at the ends of the cell's chromosomes shortens (see Chapter 4). When this DNA is gone, the cell responds to CEL-LULAR REGULATION signals for apoptosis. This ensures that each organ has an adequate number of cells at their functional peak.

Normal chromosomes (known as **euploidy**) is a feature of most normal human cells. These cells have 23 pairs of chromosomes, the correct number for humans.

Biology of Abnormal Cells

Body cells are exposed to a variety of conditions that can alter how the cells grow or function. When either cell growth or cell function is changed, the cells are considered abnormal. Table 21-1 compares features of normal, benign tumor, and cancer (malignant) cells.

Features of Benign Tumor Cells

Benign tumor cells are normal cells growing in the wrong place or at the wrong time as a result of a small problem with CEL-LULAR REGULATION. Examples include moles, uterine fibroid tumors, skin tags, endometriosis, and nasal polyps. Benign tumor cells have these characteristics:

- *Specific morphology* occurs with benign tumors. They look like the tissues they come from, retaining the specific morphology of parent cells.
- *A smaller nuclear-to-cytoplasmic ratio* is a feature of benign tumors just like completely normal cells.
- *Specific differentiated functions* continue to be performed by benign tumors. For example, in endometriosis, a type of benign tumor, the normal lining of the uterus (endometrium) grows in an abnormal place (e.g., on an ovary or in the chest cavity). This displaced endometrium acts just like

normal endometrium by changing each month under the influence of estrogen. When the hormone level drops and the normal endometrium sheds from the uterus, the displaced endometrium, wherever it is, also sheds.
- *Tight adherence* of benign tumor cells to each other occurs because they continue to make fibronectin.
- *No migration* or wandering of benign tissues occurs because they remain tightly bound and do not invade other body tissues.
- *Orderly growth* with normal growth patterns occurs in benign tumor cells even though their growth is not needed. The fact that growth continues beyond an appropriate time or occurs in the wrong place indicates some problem with CELLULAR REGULATION, but the rate of growth is normal. The benign tumor grows by hyperplastic expansion. *It does not invade.*
- *Normal chromosomes* are usually found in benign tumor cells, with a few exceptions. Most of these cells have 23 pairs of chromosomes, the correct number for humans.

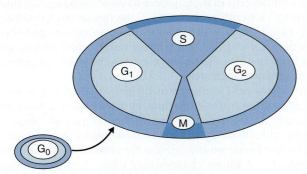

FIG. 21-3 The cell cycle.

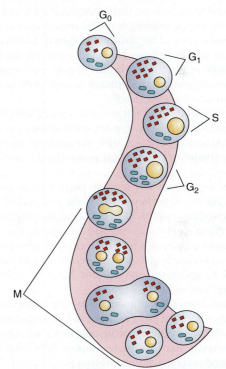

FIG. 21-4 Cellular events during mitotic cell division.

TABLE 21-1	**Characteristics of Normal and Abnormal Cells**		
CHARACTERISTIC	**NORMAL CELL**	**BENIGN TUMOR CELL**	**MALIGNANT CELL**
Cell division	None or slow	Continuous or inappropriate	Rapid or continuous
Appearance	Specific morphologic features	Specific morphologic features	Anaplastic
Nuclear-to-cytoplasmic ratio	Smaller	Smaller	Larger
Differentiated functions	Many	Many	Some or none
Adherence	Tight	Tight	Loose
Migratory	No	No	Yes
Growth	Well regulated	Expansion	Invasion
Chromosomes	Diploid (euploid)	Diploid (euploid)	Aneuploid*
Mitotic index	Low	Low	High*

*Depends on the degree of malignant transformation.

Features of Cancer Cells

Cancer (**malignant**) cells are abnormal, serve no useful function, and are harmful to normal body tissues. Cancers commonly have these features:

- *Anaplasia* is the cancer cells' loss of the specific appearance of their parent cells. As a cancer cell becomes more malignant, it becomes smaller and rounded. Thus many different types of cancer cells look alike under the microscope.
- *A larger nuclear-cytoplasmic ratio* occurs because the cancer cell nucleus is larger than that of a normal cell and the cancer cell is smaller than a normal cell. The nucleus occupies much of the space within the cancer cell, creating a larger nuclear-to-cytoplasmic ratio.
- *Specific functions are lost* partially or completely in cancer cells. *Cancer cells serve no useful purpose.*
- *Loose adherence* is typical for cancer cells because they do not make fibronectin. As a result, cancer cells easily break off from the main tumor.
- *Migration* occurs because cancer cells do not bind tightly together and have many enzymes on their cell surfaces. These features allow the cells to slip through blood vessel walls and between tissues, spreading from the main tumor site to many other body sites. The ability to spread (**metastasize**) is unique to cancer cells and a major cause of death. Cancer cells invade other tissues, both close by and more remote from the original tumor. Invasion and persistent growth make untreated cancer deadly.
- *Contact inhibition does not occur* in cancer cells because of lost CELLULAR REGULATION, even when all sides of these cells are in continuous contact with the surfaces of other cells. This persistence of cell division makes the disease difficult to control.
- *Rapid or continuous cell division* occurs in many types of cancer cells because they re-enter the cell cycle for mitosis almost continuously because CELLULAR REGULATION is lost. These cells also do not respond to signals for apoptosis. Most cancer cells have a lot of the enzyme *telomerase,* which maintains telomeric DNA. As a result, cancer cells do not respond to apoptotic signals and have an unlimited life span (are "immortal").
- *Abnormal chromosomes* (**aneuploidy**) are common in cancer cells as they become more malignant. Chromosomes are lost, gained, or broken; thus cancer cells can have more than 23 pairs or fewer than 23 pairs. Cancer cells also may have broken and rearranged chromosomes.

CANCER DEVELOPMENT

Carcinogenesis/Oncogenesis

Carcinogenesis and **oncogenesis** are other names for cancer development. The process of changing a normal cell into a cancer cell is called **malignant transformation**, occurring through loss of CELLULAR REGULATION leading to the steps of initiation, promotion, progression, and metastasis (Beery & Workman, 2012).

Initiation is the first step in carcinogenesis. Normal cells can become cancer cells if they lose CELLULAR REGULATION by having their genes promoting cell division, **oncogenes**, turn on excessively (overexpressed). Initiation is a change in gene expression caused by anything that can penetrate a cell, get into the nucleus, and mutate the DNA, leading to loss of cellular regulation. Such changes can activate oncogenes that should

have only limited expression and can damage suppressor genes, which normally limit oncogene activity. Thus initiation leads to excessive cell division through DNA damage that results in loss of cellular regulation by either loss of suppressor gene function or enhancement of oncogene function.

Initiation is an irreversible event that can lead to cancer development. After initiation, a cell can become a cancer cell if the CELLULAR REGULATION loss that occurred during initiation continues. *If growth conditions are right, widespread metastatic disease can develop from just one cancer cell.*

Substances that change the activity of a cell's genes so that the cell becomes a cancer cell are **carcinogens**. Carcinogens may be chemicals, physical agents, or viruses. More than 100 agents, substances, mixtures, and exposures are known or reasonably anticipated to cause cancer in humans, and about another 200 are suspected to be carcinogens. The National Toxicology Program's website (http://ntp.niehs.nih.gov/) lists these substances (U.S. Department of Health and Human Services [USDHHS], 2011). Chapters presenting the care of patients with specific cancers discuss specific known carcinogens within the Etiology sections.

Promotion is the enhanced growth of an initiated cell by substances known as **promoters**. Once a normal cell has been initiated by a carcinogen and is a cancer cell, it can become a tumor if its growth is enhanced. Many normal hormones and body proteins, like insulin and estrogen, can act as promoters and make cells divide more frequently. The time between a cell's initiation and the development of an overt tumor is called the **latency period**, which can range from months to years. Exposure to promoters can shorten the latency period.

Progression is the continued change of a cancer, making it more malignant over time. After cancer cells have grown to the point that a detectable tumor is formed (a 1-cm tumor has at least 1 billion cells in it), other events must occur for this tumor to become a health problem. First, the tumor must develop its own blood supply. The tumor makes vascular endothelial growth factor (VEGF) that triggers nearby capillaries to grow new branches into the tumor, ensuring the tumor's continued nourishment and growth.

As tumor cells continue to divide, some of the new cells change features from the original, initiated cancer cell and form different groups. Some of the differences provide these cell groups with advantages *(selection advantages)* that allow them to live and divide no matter how the conditions around them change. These tumor changes may allow it to become more malignant. Over time, the tumor cells have fewer and fewer normal cell features.

The original tumor is called the **primary tumor**. It is usually identified by the tissue from which it arose *(parent tissue),* such as in breast cancer or lung cancer. When primary tumors are located in vital organs, such as the brain or lungs, they can grow and either lethally damage the vital organ or interfere with that organ's ability to perform its vital function. At other times, the primary tumor is located in soft tissue that can expand without damage as the tumor grows. One such site is the breast. The breast is not a vital organ, and even with a large tumor, the primary tumor alone would not cause the patient's death. When the tumor spreads from the original site into vital areas, life functions can be disrupted and death may follow.

Metastasis occurs when cancer cells move from the primary location by breaking off from the original group and establishing remote colonies. These additional tumors are called

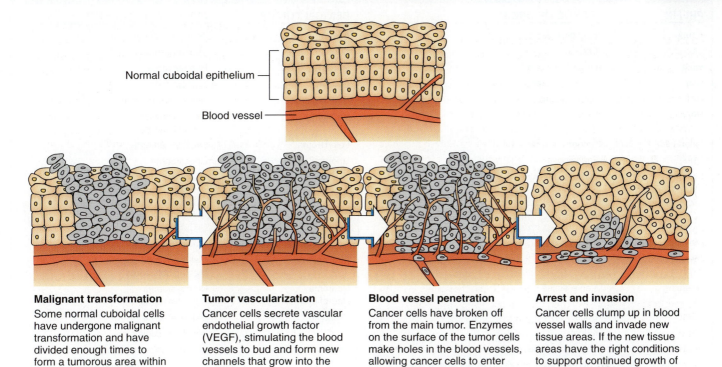

Normal cuboidal epithelium

Blood vessel

Malignant transformation
Some normal cuboidal cells have undergone malignant transformation and have divided enough times to form a tumorous area within the cuboidal epithelium.

Tumor vascularization
Cancer cells secrete vascular endothelial growth factor (VEGF), stimulating the blood vessels to bud and form new channels that grow into the tumor.

Blood vessel penetration
Cancer cells have broken off from the main tumor. Enzymes on the surface of the tumor cells make holes in the blood vessels, allowing cancer cells to enter blood vessels and travel around the body.

Arrest and invasion
Cancer cells clump up in blood vessel walls and invade new tissue areas. If the new tissue areas have the right conditions to support continued growth of cancer cells, new tumors (metastatic tumors) will form at this site.

FIG. 21-5 The steps of metastasis.

metastatic or secondary tumors. *Even though the tumor is now in another organ, it is still a cancer from the original altered tissue. For example, when breast cancer spreads to the lung and the bone, it is still breast cancer in the lung and bone—not lung cancer and not bone cancer.* Metastasis occurs through many steps, as shown in Fig. 21-5.

Tumors first extend into surrounding tissues by secreting enzymes that open up areas of surrounding tissue. Pressure, created as the tumor increases in size, forces tumor cells to invade new territory.

Spread to distant organs and tissues requires cancer cells to penetrate blood vessels. Bloodborne metastasis (tumor cell release into the blood) is the most common cause of cancer spread. Enzymes secreted by tumor cells also make large pores in the patient's blood vessels, allowing tumor cells to enter the blood and circulate. Because tumor cells are loosely held together, clumps of cells break off of the primary tumor into blood vessels for transport.

Tumor cells circulate through the blood and enter tissues at remote sites. Clumps of cancer cells can become trapped in capillaries. These clumps damage the capillary wall and allow cancer cells to leave the capillary and enter the surrounding tissue.

When conditions in the remote site can support tumor cell growth, the cells stop circulating (arrest) and invade the surrounding tissues, creating secondary tumors. Table 21-2 lists the common sites of metastasis for specific tumor types.

Another way cancers metastasize is by *lymphatic spread*. Lymphatic spread is related to the number, structure, and location of lymph nodes and vessels. Primary sites that are rich in lymphatics have more early metastatic spread than areas with few lymphatics.

TABLE 21-2	Common Sites of Metastasis for Different Cancer Types	
Breast Cancer		**Prostate Cancer**
Bone*		Bone (especially spine and legs)*
Lung*		Pelvic nodes
Liver		
Brain		**Melanoma**
		GI tract
Lung Cancer		Lymph nodes
Brain*		Lung
Bone		Brain
Liver		
Lymph nodes		**Primary Brain Cancer**
Pancreas		Central nervous system
Colorectal Cancer		
Liver*		
Lymph nodes		
Adjacent structures		

*Most common site of metastasis for the specific malignant neoplasm.

Cancer Classification

Cancers are classified by the type of tissue from which they arise (e.g., glandular, connective) (McCance et al., 2014), as described in Table 21-3. Other ways to classify cancer include biologic behavior, anatomic site, and degree of differentiation.

About 100 different types of cancer arise from various tissues or organs. Fig. 21-6 compares cancer distribution by site and gender. Cancers are either solid or hematologic. Solid tumors develop from specific tissues (e.g., breast cancer and lung cancer). Hematologic cancers arise from blood cell–forming tissues (e.g., leukemias and lymphomas).

TABLE 21-3 Classification of Tumors By Tissue of Origin

PREFIX	TISSUE OF ORIGIN	BENIGN TUMOR	MALIGNANT TUMOR*
Adeno	Epithelial glands	Adenoma	Adenocarcinoma
Chondro	Cartilage	Chondroma	Chondrosarcoma
Fibro	Fibrous connective	Fibroma	Fibrosarcoma
Glio	Glial cells (brain)	Glioma	Glioblastoma
Hemangio	Blood vessel	Hemangioma	Hemangiosarcoma
Hepato	Liver	Hepatoma	Hepatocarcinoma Hepatoblastoma
Leiomyo	Smooth muscle	Leiomyoma	Leiomyosarcoma
Lipo	Fat/adipose	Lipoma	Liposarcoma
Lympho	Lymphoid tissues		Malignant lymphomas Hodgkin's lymphoma Non-Hodgkin's lymphoma Burkitt's lymphoma Cutaneous T-cell
Melano	Pigment-producing skin		Melanoma
Meningioma	Meninges	Meningioma	Malignant meningioma Meningioblastoma
Neuro	Nerve tissue	Neuroma Neurofibroma	Neurosarcoma Neuroblastoma
Osteo	Bone	Osteoma	Osteosarcoma
Renal	Kidney		Renal cell carcinoma
Rhabdo	Skeletal muscle	Rhabdomyoma	Rhabdomyosarcoma
Squamous	Epithelial layer of skin, mucous membranes, and organ linings	Papilloma	Squamous cell carcinoma of skin, bladder, lungs, cervix

*Carcinomas are tumors of glandular tissue; sarcomas are tumors of connective tissue; blastomas are tumors of less differentiated, embryonal tissues.

Leading Sites of New Cancer Cases and Deaths for the United States and Canada – 2014 Estimates*

Estimated New Cases*		Estimated Deaths	
Male	**Female**	**Male**	**Female**
Prostate 256,600 (27%)	Breast 257,070 (29%)	Lung and bronchus 97,730 (28%)	Lung and bronchus 82,030 (26%)
Lung and bronchus 129,400 (14%)	Lung and bronchus 120,910 (13%)	Prostate 33,480 (10%)	Breast 45,000 (15%)
Colon and rectum 85,335 (8%)	Colon and rectum 75,800 (8%)	Colon and rectum 31,370 (8%)	Colon and rectum 28,240 (9%)
Urinary bladder 62,390 (7%)	Uterine corpus 58,630 (6%)	Pancreas 22,370 (7%)	Pancreas 21,620 (7%)
Melanoma of the skin 47,390 (5%)	Thyroid 52,390 (6%)	Liver and intrahepatic bile duct 16,690 (5%)	Ovary 16,020 (5%)
Kidney and renal pelvis 42,940 (5%)	Non-Hodgkin's lymphoma 36,130 (4%)	Leukemia 15,590 (5%)	Non-Hodgkin's lymphoma 9,720 (3%)
Non-Hodgkin's lymphoma 42,670 (4%)	Melanoma of the skin 35,210 (4%)	Esophagus 14,000 (4%)	Leukemia 11,150 (4%)
Oral cavity and pharynx 33,120 (4%)	Kidney and renal pelvis 27,080 (3%)	Urinary bladder 12,720 (4%)	Uterine corpus 9,510 (3%)
Leukemia 34,500 (4%)	Leukemia 24,880 (3%)	Non-Hodgkin's lymphoma 11,910 (3%)	Liver and intrahepatic bile duct 7,380 (3%)
Liver and intrahepatic bile duct 26,200 (3%)	Pancreas 25,190 (3%)	Kidney and renal pelvis 10,000 (3%)	Brain and other nervous system 7,030 (3%)
All sites 952,920 (100%)	All sites 903,920 (100%)	All sites 350,010 (100%)	All sites 312,310 (100%)

*Excludes basal and squamous cell skin cancers and in situ carcinoma except urinary bladder.
Note: Percentages may not total 100% due to rounding.

FIG. 21-6 Cancer incidence and death by site and gender. (Data from American Cancer Society, 2014 and Canadian Cancer Statistics, 2014.)

TABLE 21-4 Grading of Malignant Tumors

GRADE	CELLULAR CHARACTERISTICS
G_x	Grade cannot be determined.
G_1	Tumor cells are well differentiated and closely resemble the normal cells from which they arose. This grade is considered a low grade of malignant change. These tumors are malignant but are relatively slow growing.
G_2	Tumor cells are moderately differentiated; they still retain some of the characteristics of normal cells but also have more malignant characteristics than do G_1 tumor cells.
G_3	Tumor cells are poorly differentiated, but the tissue of origin can usually be established. The cells have few normal cell characteristics.
G_4	Tumor cells are poorly differentiated and retain no normal cell characteristics. Determination of the tissue of origin is difficult and perhaps impossible.

TABLE 21-5 Staging of Cancer—TNM Classification

Primary Tumor (T)	
T_x	Primary tumor cannot be assessed
T_0	No evidence of primary tumor
T_{is}	Carcinoma in situ
T_1, T_2, T_3, T_4	Increasing size and/or local extent of the primary tumor
Regional Lymph Nodes (N)	
N_x	Regional lymph nodes cannot be assessed
N_0	No regional lymph node metastasis
N_1, N_2, N_3	Increasing involvement of regional lymph nodes
Distant Metastasis (M)	
M_x	Presence of distant metastasis cannot be assessed
M_0	No distant metastasis
M_1	Distant metastasis

Cancer Grading, Ploidy, and Staging

Systems of grading and staging have been developed to help standardize cancer diagnosis, prognosis, and treatment. **Grading** of a tumor classifies cellular aspects of the cancer. **Ploidy** classifies tumor chromosomes as normal or abnormal. **Staging** classifies clinical aspects of the cancer.

Grading is needed because some cancer cells are "more malignant" than others, varying in their aggressiveness and sensitivity to treatment. Some cancer cells barely resemble the tissue from which they arose, are aggressive, and spread rapidly. These cells are a "high-grade" cancer. On the basis of cell appearance and activity, grading compares the cancer cell with the normal parent tissue from which it arose. It is a means of evaluating the patient with cancer for prognosis and appropriate therapy. Grading also allows health care professionals to evaluate the results of management.

Different clinical groups have established different grading systems for different types of cancer cells, but overall, they resemble the standard system listed in Table 21-4. This system rates cancer cells with the lowest rating given to those cells that closely resemble normal cells and the highest rating given to cancer cells that barely resemble normal cells. Grading systems for different cancers are presented in the clinical chapters in which care is discussed.

Ploidy is the description of cancer cells by chromosome number and appearance. Normal human cells have 46 chromosomes (23 pairs), the normal diploid number (**euploidy**). When malignant transformation occurs, changes in the genes and chromosomes also occur. Some cancer cells gain or lose whole chromosomes and may have structural abnormalities of the remaining chromosomes, a condition called **aneuploidy**. The degree of aneuploidy usually increases with the degree of malignancy. Some specific chromosome changes are associated with specific cancers, and their presence is used for diagnosis and prognosis. One example is the "Philadelphia" chromosome abnormality often present in chronic myelogenous leukemia cells (see Chapter 40).

Staging determines the exact location of the cancer and its degree of metastasis at diagnosis. Cancer stage influences selection of therapy. Staging is done by clinical staging, surgical staging, and pathologic staging. *Clinical staging* assesses the patient's clinical manifestations and evaluates them for tumor size and possible spread. *Surgical staging* assesses the tumor size, number, sites, and spread by inspection at surgery. *Pathologic staging* is the most definitive type, determining the tumor size, number, sites, and spread by pathologic examination of tissues obtained at surgery.

The **tumor, node, metastasis (TNM)** system is used to describe the anatomic extent of cancers. The TNM staging systems have specific prognostic value for each solid tumor type. Table 21-5 shows a basic TNM staging system. TNM staging is not useful for leukemia or lymphomas (see Chapter 40). Additional specific staging systems include Dukes' staging of colon and rectal cancer and Clark's levels method of staging skin cancer.

Tumor growth is assessed in terms of **doubling time** (the amount of time it takes for a tumor to double in size) and **mitotic index** (the percentage of actively dividing cells within a tumor). The smallest detectable tumor is about 1 cm in diameter and contains 1 billion cells. To reach this size, it must undergo at least 30 doublings. A tumor with a mitotic index of less than 10% is a slow-growing tumor; a tumor with an index of 85% is fast growing. Tumors have a wide range of growth rates.

? NCLEX EXAMINATION CHALLENGE
Physiological Integrity

Which pathologic description of a client's tumor does the nurse interpret as being the "most malignant" or "high grade" cancer?
A. Poorly differentiated; mitotic index = 20%, euploid
B. Moderately differentiated; mitotic index = 50%, euploid
C. Undifferentiated; mitotic index = 50%, aneuploid
D. Highly differentiated; mitotic index = 10%, aneuploid

Cancer Etiology and Genetic Risk

Carcinogenesis takes years and depends on several tumor and patient factors (Santos et al., 2013). Three interacting factors influence cancer development: exposure to carcinogens, genetic predisposition, and immune function. These factors account for variation in cancer development from one person to another, even when each person is exposed to the same hazards.

Oncogene activation is the main mechanism of carcinogenesis regardless of the specific cause. These oncogenes are turned on (expressed) under controlled conditions for CELLU-LAR REGULATION when cells divide for normal growth and replacement of dead or damaged tissues. At other times they are turned off, controlled, or suppressed by products of "suppressor genes."

When a normal cell is exposed to any carcinogen (initiator), the normal cell's DNA can be damaged and mutated. The mutations damage suppressor genes, preventing them from producing proteins that control CELLULAR REGULATION for the expression of oncogenes. As a result, the oncogenes are overexpressed and can cause the cells to change from normal cells to cancer cells. When oncogenes are overexpressed in a cell, excessive amounts of cyclins are produced and upset the balance between cell growth enhancement and cell growth limitation. The effect of these excessive cyclins is greater than the effect of the suppressor gene products, thus losing cellular regulation and allowing uncontrolled cell division.

Oncogenes are not abnormal genes but are part of every cell's normal makeup. Oncogenes become a problem only if they are overexpressed as a result of exposure to carcinogenic agents or events with loss of CELLULAR REGULATION. Both external and personal factors can activate oncogenes.

External Factors Causing Cancer

External factors, including environmental exposure, are responsible for about 80% of cancer in North America (ACS, 2014). Environmental carcinogens are chemical, physical, or viral agents that cause cancer (USDHHS, 2011).

Chemical carcinogenesis can occur from exposures to many known chemicals, drugs, and other products used in everyday life. Chemicals vary in how carcinogenic they are. For example, tobacco and alcohol appear to be only mildly carcinogenic. For these substances, chronic, long-term exposure to large amounts is required before CELLULAR REGULATION is lost and a cancer develops. However, these two substances can act as *co-carcinogens,* meaning that when they are taken together, they enhance each other's carcinogenic activity.

Not all cells are susceptible to carcinogenesis to the same degree. Normal cells that have the ability to divide are at greater risk for cancer development than are normal cells that are not capable of cell division. For example, cancers commonly arise in bone marrow, skin, lining of the GI tract, ductal cells of the breast, and lining of the lungs. All of these cells normally undergo cell division. Cancers of nerve tissue, cardiac muscle, and skeletal muscle are rare. These cells do not normally undergo cell division.

About 30% of cancers diagnosed in North America are related to tobacco use (ACS, 2014; Canadian Cancer Society, 2014). Tobacco is the single most preventable source of carcinogenesis. It contains many different carcinogens and co-carcinogens. Long-term tobacco use first initiates and then promotes cancer. The risk for cancer development from tobacco use depends on a person's immune function, genetic susceptibility, and amount and types of tobacco exposure.

Tissues with the greatest risk for tobacco-induced cancer are those that have direct contact with tobacco or tobacco smoke. Cigarette smoking and tobacco use also promote the development of other cancers. Table 21-6 lists the specific cancers that are associated with tobacco use.

Physical carcinogenesis from physical agents or events also causes cancer by DNA damage. Two physical agents that are known to cause cancer are radiation and chronic irritation.

TABLE 21-6 **Cancer Types Associated with Tobacco Use**	
• Lung	• Uterine cervix
• Oral cavity	• Kidney
• Pharynx	• Bladder
• Larynx	• Liver
• Esophagus	• Stomach
• Pancreas	• Myeloid leukemia

Data from American Cancer Society. (2014). *Cancer facts and figures—2014.* Report No. 00-300M–No. 500814. Atlanta: Author.

TABLE 21-7 **Cancers Associated with a Known Viral Origin**	
VIRUS	**MALIGNANCIES**
Epstein-Barr virus	Burkitt's lymphoma, B-cell lymphoma, nasopharyngeal carcinoma
Hepatitis B virus	Primary liver carcinoma
Hepatitis C virus	Primary liver carcinoma, possibly B-cell lymphomas
Human papilloma virus	Cervical carcinoma, vulvar carcinoma, penile carcinoma, and other anogenital carcinomas
Human lymphotrophic virus type I	Adult T-cell leukemia
Human lymphotrophic virus type II	Hairy cell leukemia

From U.S. Department of Health and Human Services, Public Health Service, National Toxicology Program. (2011). *Report on carcinogens* (12th ed.). Retrieved January 2014, from http://ntp.niehs.nih.gov/go.roc12.

Even small doses of radiation affect cells to some degree. Some effects are temporary and are self-repaired. Other effects cannot be repaired and may induce cancer in the damaged cell. The two types of radiation that cause cancer are ionizing and ultraviolet (UV). Some ionizing radiation is found naturally in such elements as radon, uranium, and radium found in rocks and soil. Other sources of ionizing radiation include x-rays for diagnosis and treatment of disease, as well as cosmic radiation. UV radiation is a type of solar radiation, coming from the sun. Other sources of UV radiation include tanning beds and germicidal lights. UV rays do not penetrate deeply, and the most common cancer type caused by UV exposure is skin cancer.

Both ionizing and UV radiation mutate genes. Although radiation exposure induces cancers more often among cells that can divide, it can cause cancer also among nondividing cells.

Chronic irritation and tissue trauma are suspected to cause cancer. The incidence of skin cancer is higher in the scars of people with burn scars or other types of severe skin injury. Chronically irritated tissues undergo frequent cell division and thus are at an increased risk for DNA mutation.

Viral carcinogenesis occurs when viruses infect body cells and break DNA strands. Viruses then insert their own genetic material into the human DNA. Breaking the DNA, along with viral gene insertion, mutates the cell's DNA and can either activate an oncogene or damage suppressor genes. Viruses that cause cancer are **oncoviruses**. Table 21-7 lists cancers of known viral origin.

Dietary factors related to cancer development are poorly understood although dietary practices are suspected to alter cancer risk. Suspected dietary factors include low fiber intake and a high intake of red meat or animal fat. Preservatives,

CHART 21-1 Patient and Family Education: Preparing for Self-Management

Dietary Habits to Reduce Cancer Risk

- Avoid excessive intake of animal fat.
- Avoid nitrites (prepared lunch meats, sausage, bacon).
- Minimize your intake of red meat.
- Keep your alcohol consumption to no more than one or two drinks per day.
- Eat more bran.
- Eat more cruciferous vegetables, such as broccoli, cauliflower, Brussels sprouts, and cabbage.
- Eat foods high in vitamin A (e.g., apricots, carrots, leafy green and yellow vegetables) and vitamin C (e.g., fresh fruits and vegetables, especially citrus fruits).

preparation methods, and additives (dyes, flavorings, sweeteners) may have cancer-promoting effects. Chart 21-1 lists dietary habits that may reduce cancer risk.

Personal Factors and Cancer Development

Personal factors, including immune function, age, and genetic risk, also affect whether a person is likely to develop cancer.

Immune function protects the body from foreign invaders and non-self cells (see Chapter 17). Non-self cells include cells that are no longer normal, such as cancer cells. Cell-mediated immunity, especially natural killer (NK) cells and helper T-cells, provides immune surveillance.

Cancer incidence increases among immunosuppressed people. Adults older than 60 years have immune systems with reduced function and a higher incidence of cancer compared with that of the general population. Organ transplant recipients taking immunosuppressive drugs to prevent organ rejection also have a higher incidence of cancer. In patients with acquired immune deficiency syndrome (AIDS), cancer incidence may be as high as 70%.

Advancing age is the single most important risk factor for cancer (ACS, 2013b). As a person ages, immune protection decreases and external exposures to carcinogens accumulate. Teach older adults to be aware of and report manifestations such as the seven warning signs of cancer (Table 21-8) to health care providers. Health care providers should investigate all manifestations suggestive of disease. Cancer assessment considerations for the older adult are listed in Chart 21-2.

GENETIC/GENOMIC CONSIDERATIONS

Patient-Centered Care QSEN

Genetic risk for cancer occurs only in a small percent of the population; however, people who have a genetic predisposition are at very high risk for cancer development (Beery & Workman, 2012). Mutations in suppressor genes or oncogenes can be inherited when they occur in germline cells (sperm and ova) and are then passed on to one's children, in whom all cells contain the inherited mutations. Thus for some people, tight CELLULAR REGULATION is compromised by a mutation in a suppressor gene, which reduces or halts its function and allows oncogene overexpression. In other people, the suppressor genes are normal and the oncogene is mutated and does not respond to suppressor gene signals, thus reducing cellular regulation and increasing the risk for cancer development. Table 21-9 lists conditions associated with an increased genetic risk for cancer development. Be sure to include questions about these conditions when performing a family history.

TABLE 21-8 The Seven Warning Signs of Cancer

C	**C**hanges in bowel or bladder habits
A	**A** sore that does not heal
U	**U**nusual bleeding or discharge
T	**T**hickening or lump in the breast or elsewhere
I	**I**ndigestion or difficulty swallowing
O	**O**bvious change in a wart or mole
N	**N**agging cough or hoarseness

CHART 21-2 Nursing Focus on the Older Adult

Cancer Assessment

CANCER TYPE	ASSESSMENT CONSIDERATION
Colorectal cancer	Ask the patient whether bowel habits have changed over the past year (e.g., in consistency, frequency, color). Is there any obvious blood in the stool? Test at least one stool specimen for occult blood during the patient's hospitalization. Encourage the patient to have a baseline colonoscopy. Encourage the patient to reduce dietary intake of animal fats, red meat, and smoked meats. Encourage the patient to increase dietary intake of bran, vegetables, and fruit.
Bladder cancer	Ask the patient about the presence of: Pain on urination Blood in the urine Cloudy urine Increased frequency or urgency
Prostate cancer	Ask the patient about: Hesitancy Change in the size of the urine stream Pain in the back or legs History of urinary tract infections
Skin cancer	Examine skin areas for moles or warts. Ask the patient about changes in moles (e.g., color, edges, sensation).
Leukemia	Observe the skin for color, petechiae, or ecchymosis. Ask the patient about: Fatigue Bruising Bleeding tendency History of infections and illnesses Night sweats Unexplained fevers
Lung cancer	Observe the skin and mucous membranes for color. How many words can the patient say between breaths? Ask the patient about: Cough Hoarseness Smoking history Exposure to inhalation irritants Exposure to asbestos Shortness of breath Activity tolerance Frothy or bloody sputum Pain in the arms or chest Difficulty swallowing

TABLE 21-9   Conditions Associated with a Genetic Predisposition for Cancer

CONDITION	SPECIFIC CANCER TYPE
Inherited cancers*	Breast cancer
	Prostate cancer
	Ovarian cancer
Familial clustering	Breast cancer
	Melanoma
Bloom syndrome	Leukemia
Familial polyposis	Colorectal cancer
Chromosomal aberrations	
Down syndrome (47 chromosomes)	Leukemia
Klinefelter syndrome (47,XXY)	Breast cancer
Turner's syndrome (45,XO)	Leukemia
	Gonadal carcinoma
	Meningioma
	Colorectal cancer

*Not all breast, prostate, or ovarian cancers are inherited.

Genetic testing for cancer predisposition is available to confirm or rule out a person's genetic risk for some specific cancer types. These tests are performed on blood and are expensive, and the cost often is not covered by insurance. Genetic testing should not be performed unless a family history clearly indicates the possibility of increased genetic risk and the patient wants to have the test results. *These tests do not diagnose the presence of cancer; they only provide risk information.*

A variety of issues and potential problems exist with genetic testing for cancer risk. Correct interpretation of the results is critical. Ideally, a genetic counselor is involved in giving the patient information before, as well as after, testing is performed. *When a patient tests positive for a known cancer-causing gene mutation, his or her risk for cancer development is greatly increased; however, the cancer still may never develop.*

Other issues regarding genetic testing include who will have access to the information and whether to share the test results with family members. Genetic testing has implications for the entire family, not just the patient being tested. For more information on genetic testing, see Chapter 4.

CULTURAL CONSIDERATIONS
Patient-Centered Care QSEN

The incidence of cancer varies among races. American Cancer Society (ACS) data (2012; 2013) show that African Americans have a higher incidence of cancer than white people do and the death rate is higher for African Americans. Since 1960, the overall incidence among African Americans has increased 27% whereas for white people it has increased only 12%. Cancer sites and cancer-related mortality vary along racial lines as well. One explanation for this difference is that more African Americans have less access to health care. Thus they are more often diagnosed with later-stage cancer that is more difficult to cure or control. However, this disparity in health care access does not explain all differences.

When risks for cancer development are assessed, behavior and socioeconomic factors are assessed along with ethnicity and genetic predisposition. The American Cancer Society (2013) reports that cancer incidence and survival are often related to socioeconomic factors. These factors include the availability of health care services or the belief that seeking early health care has a positive effect on the outcome of cancer diagnosis.

CANCER PREVENTION

Cancer prevention activities focus on primary prevention and secondary prevention. **Primary prevention** is the use of strategies to prevent the actual occurrence of cancer. This type of cancer prevention is most effective when there is a known cause for a cancer type. **Secondary prevention** is the use of screening strategies to detect cancer early, at a time when cure or control is more likely.

Primary Prevention

Avoidance of known or potential carcinogens is an effective prevention strategy when a cause of cancer is known and avoidance is easily accomplished. For example, teach people to use skin protection during sun exposure to avoid skin cancer. Much lung cancer can be avoided by not using tobacco and by eliminating environmental asbestos exposure. Teach everyone about the dangers of cigarette smoking and other forms of tobacco use (see the *Health Promotion and Maintenance* feature in Chapter 27). Teach people who are exposed to carcinogens in the workplace to use personal protective equipment that reduces direct contact with this substance. As more cancer causes are identified, avoidance may become even more effective.

Modifying associated factors appears to have a positive influence in reducing cancer risk. Absolute causes are not known for many cancers, but some conditions appear to increase risk. Examples are the increased incidence of cancer among people who consume alcohol; the association of a diet high in fat and low in fiber with colon cancer, breast cancer, and ovarian cancer; and a greater incidence of cervical cancer among women who have multiple sexual partners. Modifying behavior to reduce the associated factor may decrease the risk for cancer development. Therefore teach all people to limit their intake of alcohol to no more than one ounce per day and to include more fruits, vegetables, and whole grains in their diets. Instruct women about the importance of limiting the number of sexual partners and to use safer sex practices to avoid exposure to viruses that can increase the risk for cervical cancer (see Table 21-7 for a listing of cancer-causing viruses).

Removal of "at risk" tissues reduces cancer risk for a person who has a known high risk for developing a specific type of cancer. Examples include removing moles to prevent conversion to skin cancer, removing colon polyps to prevent colon cancer, and removing breasts to prevent breast cancer. Not all "at risk" tissues can be removed (e.g., those that are part of essential organs).

Chemoprevention is a strategy that uses drugs, chemicals, natural nutrients, or other substances to disrupt one or more steps important to cancer development. These agents may be able to reverse existing gene damage or halt the progression of the transformation process. Currently, hundreds of agents are under investigation for chemoprevention. At this time, only a few agents have been found effective and are commonly prescribed. These include the use of aspirin and celecoxib (Celebrex) to reduce the risk for colon cancer, the use of vitamin D and tamoxifen to reduce the risk for breast cancer, and the use of lycopene to reduce the risk for prostate cancer (ACS, 2014).

Vaccination is a new method of primary cancer prevention. Although vaccines against colon cancer and others are being explored, currently the only vaccine approved for cancer prevention prevents infection from several forms of the human papilloma virus (HPV). These vaccines are Gardasil and Cervarix. As more viruses are identified as being cancer causing, it is hoped that vaccines will be developed to prevent those viral infections.

Secondary Prevention

Regular screening for cancer does not reduce cancer incidence but can greatly reduce some types of cancer deaths. Teach all adults the benefits of participating in specific routine screening techniques annually as part of health maintenance. General screening recommendations are listed in chapters discussing cancers by organ system. The age and type of participation in specific screening tests are different for people who have an identified increased risk for a specific cancer type. In addition, there is some controversy about when the age and frequency for screening has the greatest benefit. Examples of recommended screenings include (ACS, 2014):

- Yearly mammography for women older than 40 years
- Yearly clinical breast examination for women older than 40 years; every 3 years for women ages 20 to 39 years
- Colonoscopy at age 50 years and then every 10 years
- Yearly fecal occult blood for adults of all ages
- Digital rectal examination (DRE) for men older than 50 years

Because cancer development clearly involves gene changes (either inherited gene mutations or acquired damage-induced gene mutations), people can be screened for some gene mutations that increase the risk for cancer. A few examples of these known gene mutations are mutations in the *BRCA1* gene, which increases the risk for both breast and ovarian cancer; mutations

in the *BRCA2* gene, which increases the risk for breast cancer; and mutations in the *APC*, *MLH1*, and *MSH2* genes, which increase the risk for colon cancer.

When taking a patient history and the person appears to have a strong family history of either breast cancer or colon cancer, create a three-generation pedigree to more fully explore the possibility of genetic risk. If a pattern of risk emerges, inform the person about the possible benefits of genetic screening and advise him or her to talk with an oncologist or genetics professional for more information. Screening can help a person at increased genetic risk for cancer to alter lifestyle factors, participate in early detection methods, or even have at-risk tissue removed. Genetic screening has some personal risks as well as potential benefits (see Chapter 4).

❓ NCLEX EXAMINATION CHALLENGE
Health Promotion and Maintenance

A 65-year-old client tells the nurse she does not have mammograms because there is no history of breast cancer in her family. What is the nurse's best response?
A. "You are correct. Breast cancer is an inherited type of malignancy and your family history indicates a low risk for you."
B. "Performing breast self-examination monthly at home is sufficient screening for someone with your family history."
C. "Because your breasts are no longer as dense as they were when you were younger, your risk for breast cancer is now decreased."
D. "Breast cancer can be found more frequently in families; however, the risk for general, nonfamilial breast cancer increases with age."

GET READY FOR THE NCLEX® EXAMINATION!

KEY POINTS

Review these Key Points for each NCLEX Examination Client Needs Category.

Health Promotion and Maintenance
- Teach all people to avoid tanning beds and to use sunscreen and to wear protective clothing during sun exposure. **Patient-Centered Care** QSEN
- Encourage patients to participate in the recommended cancer-screening activities for their age-group and cancer risk category. **Patient-Centered Care** QSEN
- Inform all patients who smoke that smoking increases the risk for development of many cancer types.
- Assist anyone interested in smoking cessation to find an appropriate smoking cessation program (see Chapter 27). **Patient-Centered Care** QSEN
- Assess the patient's knowledge about causes of cancer and his or her screening/prevention practices. **Patient-Centered Care** QSEN
- Assist patients who fear a cancer diagnosis to understand that finding cancer at an early stage increases the chances for cure.

- Ask all patients about their exposures to environmental agents that are known or suspected to impair CELLULAR REGULATION and increase the risk for cancer.
- Obtain a detailed family history (at least three generations), and use this information to create a pedigree to assess the patient's risk for familial or inherited cancer. **Patient-Centered Care** QSEN
- Teach anyone, especially older adults, the "seven warning signs of cancer" (see Table 21-8).

Physiological Integrity
- Be aware of these facts regarding cancer risk and cancer development:
  - Cancer cells originate from normal body cells.
  - Transformation of a normal cell into a cancer cell involves mutation of the genes (DNA) of the normal cell and results in the loss of CELLULAR REGULATION.
  - Oncogenes that are overexpressed can cause a cell to develop into a tumor.
  - Only one cell has to undergo malignant transformation for cancer to begin.

- Benign tumors grow by expansion, whereas malignant tumors grow by invasion.
- Most tumors arise from cells that are capable of cell division.
- A key feature of cancer cells is the loss of CELLULAR REGULATION and apoptosis. These cells have an "infinite" life span.
- Primary prevention of cancer involves avoiding exposure to known causes of cancer.

- Secondary prevention of cancer involves screening for early detection.
- Tobacco use is a causative factor in 30% of all cancers.
- Tumors that metastasize from the primary site into another organ are still designated as tumors of the originating tissue.

Care of Patients with Cancer

June Eilers

PRIORITY CONCEPTS

- INFECTION
- PAIN
- CLOTTING

LEARNING OUTCOMES

Safe and Effective Care Environment

1. Modify the environment to protect patients who have neutropenia, thrombocytopenia, or peripheral neuropathy from INFECTION and injury.
2. Protect yourself and others from cytotoxic agents and radiation.

Health Promotion and Maintenance

3. Teach patients and family members how to avoid injury and INFECTION when blood counts are low.
4. Teach patients and family members how to manage side effects of cancer treatment.

Psychosocial Integrity

5. Reduce the psychological impact of cancer treatment for the patient and family.
6. Work with other members of the health care team to ensure that patient values, preferences, and expressed needs related to cancer and its treatment are respected.

Physiological Integrity

7. Interpret laboratory data and clinical manifestations to determine the presence of cancer treatment side effects and oncologic emergencies.
8. Ensure that the patient with cancer has his or her PAIN effectively managed.
9. Prioritize nursing interventions for the patient with neutropenia or thrombocytopenia.
10. Prioritize nursing care for the patient receiving radiation therapy.
11. Prioritize nursing care for the patient receiving hormonal manipulation therapy.
12. Prioritize nursing care for the patient receiving biological response modifiers and growth factors as supportive therapy in the treatment of cancer.
13. Prioritize nursing care for the patient receiving targeted therapy for cancer.
14. Prioritize care for patients who experience an oncologic emergency.

Cancer is a serious common problem in all parts of the world. Most people fear cancer and associate a cancer diagnosis with PAIN, suffering, and death. In affluent countries, more than 68% of people diagnosed with cancer are cured and thousands of others live 5 years or longer (American Cancer Society, 2014; Canadian Cancer Society, 2014). *Regardless of treatment type, cancer always affects a person's physical and psychological functioning and stresses the family.*

Providing care to patients experiencing cancer and their families is complex and challenging. This chapter describes the general interventions for cancer and the problems associated with cancer treatment. For treatments and patient problems that occur with specific cancer types, consult the chapters in which the cancer is described. Table 22-1 lists common cancer types and the specific locations within this text where the interventions are presented.

GENERAL DISEASE-RELATED CONSEQUENCES OF CANCER

Cancer can develop in any organ or tissue and destroys normal tissue, which decreases function of that tissue or organ. Even when cancers occur in nonvital tissues or organs, they can cause death by metastasizing (spreading) into vital organs and disrupting critical physiologic processes (see Chapter 21). Advanced cancers often cause:

- Reduced immunity and blood-producing functions
- Altered GI structure and function

TABLE 22-1 Text Location of Specific Cancer Content	
CANCER TYPE	**CHAPTER**
Bladder (urothelial)	66
Brain	45
Breast	70
Cervical	71
Colorectal	56
Esophageal	54
Head and Neck	29
Leukemia	40
Lung	30
Lymphoma	40
Ovarian	71
Prostate	72
Renal cell carcinoma	67
Skin	25
Stomach (gastric)	55

- Motor and sensory deficits
- Decreased respiratory function

REDUCED IMMUNITY AND BLOOD-PRODUCING FUNCTIONS

Impaired immune and blood-producing functions occur most often in patients with leukemia and lymphoma but can also occur with any cancer that invades the bone marrow. Tumor cells enter the bone marrow and reduce the production of healthy white blood cells (WBCs), which are needed for normal immune function. Thus patients who have cancer, especially leukemia, are at an increased risk for INFECTION (McCance et al., 2014).

When cancer invades the bone marrow, it also causes anemia by decreasing the number of red blood cells (RBCs) and causes thrombocytopenia by decreasing the number of platelets. These changes may be caused by the cancer itself or by cancer treatment, especially chemotherapy. The patient feels weak and fatigued and is at risk for impaired CLOTTING with bleeding. In addition, patients with anemia may be short of breath, especially if they also have respiratory involvement related to cancer.

ALTERED GI STRUCTURE AND FUNCTION

Abdominal tumors may obstruct or compress structures anywhere in the GI tract, reducing the ability to absorb nutrients and eliminate wastes. Tumors often also increase metabolic rate and the need for nutrients at a time when the patient has less energy for meal preparation or eating.

Tumors that invade the liver profoundly damage this organ, which has many important metabolic functions. This damage leads to malnutrition and death.

Many patients with cancer have anorexia that often interferes with their ability to meet energy needs. Cachexia (extreme body wasting and malnutrition) develops from an imbalance between food intake and energy use (increased catabolism). This problem may occur even when nutritional intake appears adequate.

Changes in taste resulting from the cancer or the treatment can reduce appetite and cause food aversions. Some patients experience early satiety or a sense of fullness and inability to eat even though they have eaten only a small volume of food.

Nutrition support for the patient with cancer, especially one undergoing cancer therapy, is complex. A diet high in protein and carbohydrates is often prescribed to help him or her maintain weight and to provide the nutrients needed for energy and cellular repair. Patients and families often believe cancer can be cured more easily if weight is gained or maintained. Currently no one nutrition plan meets the needs of all patients with cancer. Challenges related to food intake often become an emotional problem for family members who struggle with watching nutrition changes in their loved ones.

MOTOR AND SENSORY DEFICITS

Motor and sensory deficits occur when cancers invade bone or the brain or compress nerves. In patients with bone metastasis, the primary cancer started in another organ (e.g., lung, prostate, breast). Bones become thinner with an increased risk for *pathologic fractures* that can occur with minimal trauma. Bone metastasis causes PAIN, fractures, spinal cord compression, and hypercalcemia, each of which reduces mobility.

Patients have sensory changes if the spinal cord is damaged or if nerves are compressed. Sensory, motor, and cognitive functions are impaired when cancer spreads to the brain. Any tumor, cancer or benign, growing in the brain can destroy healthy brain tissue and cause death.

Cancer treatments also contribute to sensory and motor deficits. Certain chemotherapy agents cause peripheral neuropathy that leads to altered sensation, PAIN, and modified gait. "Chemo brain" is an alteration of cognitive function experienced by some patients.

The patient with cancer may also have PAIN, especially chronic pain. Pain does not always accompany cancer, but it can be a major problem for those with terminal cancer. Chapter 3 provides an in-depth discussion of the causes and management of cancer pain. The concept map in Chapter 3 (p. 27) presents nursing care issues related to chronic cancer pain.

REDUCED GAS EXCHANGE

Cancer can disrupt oxygenation in several ways and often results in death. Tumors in the airways cause airway obstruction. If lung tissue is involved, lung capacity is decreased, leading to hypoxemia. Tumors can also press on blood and lymph vessels in the chest, which results in pulmonary edema and dyspnea. Tumors can thicken the alveolar membrane and damage pulmonary blood vessels, reducing gas exchange. With any lung tumor (primary or metastatic), patients are at risk for hypoxia, poor gas exchange, and poor tissue oxygenation.

CANCER MANAGEMENT

The purpose of cancer management is to prolong survival time and improve quality of life. Without cancer therapy, many patients with cancer would die within months of diagnosis. Cancer therapy includes surgery, radiation, chemotherapy, immunotherapy (biological response modifiers), molecularly targeted therapy, photodynamic therapy, and hormonal therapy. These therapies may be used separately or in combination to kill cancer cells. The types of therapy used depend on the specific type of cancer, whether the cancer has spread, and the health of the patient. Treatment regimens *(protocols)* have been established for most types of cancer.

SURGERY

Surgery is the earliest known treatment for cancer and continues to be a cornerstone of therapy. Most cancers are diagnosed with the assistance of surgery, and it is used as part of therapy in many cancers. For cancer, surgery involves the removal of diseased or suspicious tissue. If cancer is confined to the removed tissue, surgery alone can result in a "cure" for that cancer. Even when surgery cannot result in a cancer cure, it is often a useful part of diagnosis, treatment, follow-up, and rehabilitation. Current types of cancer surgery are used for prophylaxis, diagnosis, cure, control, palliation, assessing therapy effectiveness, and reconstruction.

Prophylactic surgery removes "at-risk" tissue to prevent cancer development. It is performed when a patient has either an existing premalignant condition or a strong predisposition for development of a specific cancer. For example, removing a benign polyp from the colon before it can develop into colon cancer is a prophylactic action.

Diagnostic surgery (biopsy) is the removal of all or part of a suspected lesion for examination and testing. It provides evidence for the presence of cancer. Other forms of therapy are seldom initiated without this confirmation of cancer. The extent of a biopsy varies from a fine needle aspiration to an open incision exploratory surgery.

Curative surgery removes all cancer tissue. Surgery alone can result in a cure rate of about 30% when all visible and microscopic tumor is removed or destroyed. This number could increase with screening and early detection efforts.

Cancer control, or *cytoreductive surgery,* removes part of but not the entire tumor. It is also known as "debulking" surgery and decreases the number of cancer cells, which increases the chances that other therapies can be successful.

Palliative surgery focuses on improving the quality of life during the survival time, not on cure. Examples include removal of tumor tissue that is causing PAIN, obstruction, or difficulty swallowing.

Second-look surgery is a repeat examination after treatment to assess the disease status in patients who have been treated and have no symptoms of remaining tumor. The results of this surgery are used to determine whether a specific therapy should be continued or discontinued.

Reconstructive or *rehabilitative surgery* increases function, enhances appearance, or both. Examples include breast reconstruction after mastectomy, replacement of the esophagus, bowel reconstruction, revision of scars, and cosmetic reconstruction in head and neck cancer.

Side Effects of Surgical Therapy

Unlike surgery performed for many other reasons, cancer surgery often involves the loss of a body part or its function. Sometimes whole organs are removed, such as the kidney, lung, breast, testis, leg, or tongue. *Any organ loss reduces function.* Some cancer surgery results in scarring or disfigurement. Patients are anxious about surviving the cancer and want to be "rid" of it. However, they also may be grieving a change in appearance or lifestyle.

❖ *PATIENT-CENTERED COLLABORATIVE CARE*

The care needs of the patient having surgery for cancer are similar to those related to surgery for other reasons (see Chapters 14, 15, and 16). For cancer surgery, additional priority care needs are psychosocial support and assisting the patient to achieve maximum function.

Often cancer surgery occurs within days of the diagnosis, before the patient and family have time to adjust. Be aware that the stress of the diagnosis can significantly impact the patient's and family's ability to understand any teaching provided at this time. Assess the patient's and family's ability to cope with the uncertainty of cancer and its treatment and with the changes in body image and role. For example, surgery involving the genitals, urinary tract, colon, or rectum may permanently damage these organs, resulting in changes in the patient's means of sexual expression or control of elimination. Procedures to create a urinary or fecal diversion may damage nerves, causing erectile dysfunction in men and painful intercourse in women.

Coordinate with the health care team to support the patient. Encourage the patient and family to express their concerns. Help the patient accept changes in appearance or function by encouraging him or her to look at the surgical site, touch it, and participate in dressing changes. Provide information about support groups such as those sponsored by the American Cancer Society (www.cancer.org) or Canadian Cancer Society (www.cancer.ca). Some cancer organizations have support groups for patients and separate support groups for patients' spouses and children. Discuss having a person who has coped with the same issues come for a visit. Such visits can help show the patient that many aspects of life can be the same after cancer treatment. For patients who have persistent depression as a result of the cancer diagnosis or appearance changes, a referral to a mental health counselor and drug therapy may be indicated.

Physical rehabilitation is often indicated after surgery. Reduced function may be an outcome for some types of cancer surgery. For example, a modified radical mastectomy for breast cancer can lead to muscle weakness and reduced arm function on that side. Performing specific exercises after surgery can reduce functional loss. Head and neck cancer surgery often requires therapy to improve swallowing and speech. Therapy can be painful and challenging. The patient needs encouragement to perform the expected activities. Teach patients about the importance of performing the exercises to regain as much function as possible and prevent complications. Coordinate with the physical therapist, occupational therapist, and family members to plan strategies individualized to each patient to regain or maintain optimal function.

The role of surgery in cancer care continues to change. Laparoscopic and other minimally invasive approaches with smaller incisions and robotic access to internal body cavities have reduced some risks (Yu et al., 2013) (see Chapters 14 and 15). Regardless of the surgical approach, nurses have a critical role in the patient's recovery after surgery. This includes reinforcing the importance of early mobility, PAIN management, and prevention of INFECTION.

The use of surgery in combination with other therapies has increased. Such combinations may include intraoperative radiation therapy, the placement of a radioactive source, or the administration of chemotherapy into a body cavity. Other uses include surgical placement of internal catheters into a specific vessel and placement of electronic pumps for chemotherapy or pain drugs.

RADIATION THERAPY

Radiation therapy (radiotherapy) involves the use of radionuclides, ionizing radiation beams, or discrete gamma ray sources to treat cancer. The purpose of radiation therapy for cancer is to destroy cancer cells, have minimal damaging effects on the surrounding normal cells, and maintain a safe environment. Radiation may be used to cure, control, or palliate the disease.

The effects of radiation are seen only on tissues within the radiation path; thus this type of therapy usually is a *local* treatment. For example, radiation to the chest for lung cancer causes skin changes and hair loss only on the chest area actually being irradiated. The person does *not* lose his or her scalp hair. When total body irradiation (TBI) is used, all body areas are affected. Some effects are apparent within days or weeks, whereas other effects on deeper tissues may not be apparent for months to years after radiation therapy is completed.

Most radiation therapy for cancer is ionizing radiation. When cells are exposed to it, particles within the cell's nucleus are rearranged, resulting in a tremendous release of intracellular energy. Ionizing radiation is given off by many elements, including radium, and radioactive isotopes of specific elements.

As a radioactive element breaks down (decays), radiation energy is released as high energy particles (alpha particles and beta particles) and high energy photons (gamma rays). **X-rays** are radiation that is generated by machine. All types of radiation are identical in their effects on cells.

The energy produced by radioactive elements (gamma rays, alpha particles, beta particles) varies in its ability to penetrate tissues and damage cells (Fig. 22-1). *Gamma rays* are used most commonly for radiation therapy because of their ability to deeply penetrate tissues. *Beta particles* are weaker and must be placed within or very close to the cancer cells for cancer therapy (see discussion of brachytherapy on p. 375). *Alpha particles* are not used as cancer therapy.

The amount of radiation delivered to a tissue is the **exposure**; the amount of radiation absorbed by the tissue is the **radiation dose**. The dose is always less than the exposure because some energy is lost on the way to the tissue. The three factors determining the absorbed dose are the *intensity* of exposure, the *duration* of exposure, and the *closeness* (distance) of the radiation source to the cells. Absorbed radiation doses are described in units called **gray (gy)**. One gy is equal to one joule of energy absorbed by one kg of a material. The total dose of radiation used depends on tumor size and location and on the radiation sensitivity of the tumor and nearby tissues. Some normal tissues are more sensitive than others to radiation. For example, breast tissue tolerates much higher doses of radiation than the liver does. A total dose of 50 to 60 gy might be prescribed for a breast cancer. However, only 12 gy might be prescribed for a liver tumor because a higher dose would destroy healthy liver cells as well as the tumor.

Radiation therapy usually is given as a series of divided doses because of the varying responses of all cancer cells within one tumor. Most often, small doses of radiation are given on a daily basis for a set time period to allow greater destruction of cancer cells while reducing the damage to normal tissues.

The intensity of the radiation decreases with the distance from the radiation emitting source. This factor is known as the *inverse square law*. For example, the radiation dose received at

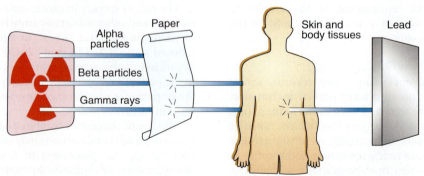

FIG. 22-1 Penetrating capacity of different types of radiation.

a distance of 2 meters from the radiation source is only one fourth of the dose received at a distance of 1 meter from the radiation source; the dose of radiation received at 3 meters is only one ninth of the dose received at 1 meter.

Cells damaged by radiation either die outright or become unable to divide. Radiation damage occurs anytime a cell is exposed to radiation, not just when it is dividing. However, the damage is greater to dividing cells than to non-dividing cells when exposed to radiation. Cancer radiation therapy does not immediately kill all cells within a tumor because these cells absorb the radiation dose slightly differently and their overall response to the radiation is slightly different. A few cells die immediately, and more die within the next few days. Some cells are unable to divide as a result of a single treatment. Still other cells repair the radiation-induced damage and recover.

Radiation may be used as a stand-alone treatment or may be combined with other cancer therapies. Combining therapies requires careful planning of sequencing, timing, and dose of each therapy to maximize tumor kill and limit damage to normal cells. Often, combining radiation with chemotherapy involves first giving agents that radiosensitize and actually enhance the radiation damage and result in a greater cell kill than either therapy used alone.

Radiation Delivery Methods and Devices

Radiation delivery types for cancer therapy are teletherapy and brachytherapy. The type used depends on the patient's general health and on the shape, size, and location of the tumor. The ideal radiation dose is one that kills the cancer cells with an acceptable level of damage to normal tissues (damage to normal tissues cannot be avoided).

Teletherapy is radiation delivered from a source outside of the patient. *Because the source is external, the patient is not radioactive and is not hazardous to others.* Newer teletherapy delivery methods improve the accuracy of the dose delivered. Intensity modulated radiation therapy (IMRT) breaks the single beam into thousands of smaller beams that better focus on the tumor. Stereotactic body radiotherapy (SBRT) uses three-dimensional tumor imaging to identify the exact tumor location, which allows precise delivery of higher radiation doses and spares more of the surrounding tissue. Usually, the total dosage is delivered in one to five separate treatment sessions.

Regardless of the delivery method, the exact tumor location is first determined for therapy accuracy. Once the pattern of radiation delivery is decided, the patient must always be in exactly the same position for all treatments. Ensure that the patient can get into and maintain this position. Position-fixing devices and markings, either on the patient's body or on the devices, ensure the proper position each day of treatment. The markings may be small permanent "tattoos," ink outlines on the skin, or a marked mask laid over the skin. Position-fixing devices include customized external body molds, foam-based body molds, and fiberglass splints.

Brachytherapy means "short" (close) therapy. The radiation source comes into direct, continuous contact with the tumor for a specific time period. This method provides a high dose of radiation in the tumor and a very limited dose in surrounding normal tissues.

Brachytherapy uses radioactive isotopes either in solid form or within body fluids. Isotopes can be delivered to the tumor in several ways. *With all types of brachytherapy, the radiation source is within the patient. Therefore the patient emits radiation for a period of time and is a potential hazard to others.* When the isotopes used are unsealed and suspended in a fluid, they are given by the oral or IV routes or instilled within body cavities. An example of brachytherapy with soluble isotopes is the ingestion or injection of the radionuclide *iodine-131* (^{131}I) (an iodine base with a half-life of 8.05 days) to treat some thyroid cancers. The iodine concentrates in the thyroid gland and destroys the thyroid cancer cells. *When isotopes are unsealed, they enter body fluids and eventually are eliminated in waste products. These wastes are radioactive and should not be directly touched by anyone. They must be handled according to guidelines established by the institution. After the isotope is completely eliminated from the body, neither the patient nor the body wastes are radioactive.*

Solid or sealed radiation sources are implanted within or near the tumor. These sources can be temporary or permanent. Most implants emit continuous, low-energy radiation to tumors. Some devices (e.g., seeds or needles) can be placed into the tumor and stay in place by themselves. Seeds are so small and the half-life of the isotope so short that this device is permanently left in place (often for prostate cancer) and, over time, completely loses its radioactivity. Other devices are removed and reused in other patients. Some sources must be held in place during therapy using special applicators. While the solid implants are in place, the patient emits radiation but excreta are not radioactive. Thus, at this time, the patient poses a hazard to others but the excreta do not.

Traditional implants deliver "low-dose rates" (LDRs) of radiation continuously, and patients are hospitalized for several days. "High-dose rate" (HDR) implant radiation is another delivery type. The patient comes into the radiation therapy department several times a week, and a stronger radiation implant is placed for only an hour or so each time. The patient is radioactive only when the implant is in place (Rupert, 2011). Chart 22-1 lists the best practices for the safety of the personnel providing care to the patient with a sealed radiation implant.

A newer approach of targeted therapy for liver cancers involves interventional radiology to place a catheter in the femoral artery and then position it into the liver. Yttrium-90 radioactive beads are injected into the blood vessels supplying liver tumors. These beads lodge in the tumor vessels and deliver a calculated dose of beta particles directly into the tumor(s). This dose travels only 1 to 2 centimeters, and the beads decay to near zero after about 96 hours. This method can deliver an effective therapy dose to the liver without damaging the healthy liver tissue.

Side Effects of Radiation Therapy

Side effects of radiation therapy include both acute and long-term site-specific changes (Table 22-2). These effects are limited to the tissues exposed to the radiation. Therefore the side effects vary according to the site (Ruppert, 2011). Skin changes and hair loss are local but are often permanent depending on the total absorbed dose.

Altered taste sensations and fatigue are two common systemic side effects noted by patients during radiation, regardless of the radiation site. Taste changes are thought to be caused by metabolites released from dead cells. Many patients develop an aversion to the taste of red meats. Fatigue may be related to the increased energy demands needed to repair damaged cells. Regardless of the cause, radiation-induced fatigue can be debilitating and may last for months (Poirier, 2011). Some degree of bone marrow suppression occurs regardless of the treatment

CHART 22-1　Best Practice for Patient Safety & Quality Care (QSEN)

Care of the Patient with Sealed Implants of Radioactive Sources

- Assign the patient to a private room with a private bath.
- Place a "Caution: Radioactive Material" sign on the door of the patient's room.
- If portable lead shields are used, place them between the patient and the door.
- Keep the door to the patient's room closed as much as possible.
- Wear a dosimeter film badge at all times while caring for patients with radioactive implants. The badge offers no protection but measures a person's exposure to radiation. Each person caring for the patient should have a separate dosimeter to calculate his or her specific radiation exposure.
- Wear a lead apron while providing care. Always keep the front of the apron facing the source of radiation (do not turn your back toward the patient).
- If you are attempting to conceive, do not perform direct patient care regardless of whether you are male or female.
- Pregnant nurses should not care for these patients; do not allow pregnant women or children younger than 16 years to visit.
- Limit each visitor to one-half hour per day. Be sure visitors stay at least 6 feet from the source.
- Never touch the radioactive source with bare hands. In the rare instance that it is dislodged, use a long-handled forceps to retrieve it. Deposit the radioactive source in the lead container kept in the patient's room.
- Save all dressings and bed linens in the patient's room until after the radioactive source is removed. After the source is removed, dispose of dressings and linens in the usual manner. Other equipment can be removed from the room at any time without special precautions and does not pose a hazard to other people.

TABLE 22-2　Acute and Late Site-Specific Effects of Radiation Therapy

ACUTE EFFECTS	LATE EFFECTS
Brain	**Subcutaneous and Soft Tissue**
Alopecia and radiodermatitis of the scalp	Radiation-induced fibrosis
Ear and external auditory canal irritation	**Central Nervous System**
Cerebral edema	Brain necrosis
Nausea and vomiting	Leukoencephalopathy
Somnolence syndrome	Cognitive and emotional dysfunction
	Pituitary and hypothalamic dysfunction
Head and Neck	Spinal cord myelopathies
Oral mucositis	
Taste changes	**Head and Neck**
Oral candidiasis	Xerostomia and dental caries
Oral herpes	Trismus
Acute xerostomia	Osteoradionecrosis
Dental caries	Hypothyroidism
Esophagitis and pharyngitis	
	Lung
Breast and Chest Wall	Pulmonary fibrosis
Skin reactions	
Esophagitis	**Heart**
	Pericarditis
Chest and Lung	Cardiomyopathy
Esophagitis and pharyngitis	Coronary artery disease
Taste changes	
Pneumonia	**Breast/Chest Wall**
	Atrophy, fibrosis of breast tissue
Abdomen and Pelvis	Lymphedema
Anorexia	
Nausea and vomiting	**Abdomen and Pelvis**
Diarrhea and proctitis	Small and large bowel injury
Cystitis	
Vaginal dryness/vaginitis	
Eye	
Conjunctival edema and tearing	

site. The intensity of the suppression is related to the dose, site, and size of the area irradiated.

Radiation damage to normal tissues during therapy can start inflammatory responses that lead to tissue fibrosis and scarring. These effects may appear years after radiation treatment. For example, women who receive HDR therapy for uterine cancer may develop radiation-induced colon changes (which also was irradiated) years later, resulting in constipation and even obstruction. Because any form of radiation can damage and mutate normal cell DNA, radiation therapy increases the risk for development of second malignancies. This risk is lower when delivery methods involve less exposure to normal tissues.

Not all patients experience the same degree of side effects to normal tissues even when receiving the same dose of radiation therapy. Genetic differences appear to influence how sensitive a person's normal tissues are to radiation damage (Proud, 2014).

❖ PATIENT-CENTERED COLLABORATIVE CARE

Most patients and family members are anxious about radiation and look to the nurse to explain the purpose and side effects of radiation therapy. Accurate information about radiation therapy helps patients cope with the treatment (Ruppert, 2011).

Skin in the radiation path becomes dry and may break down. Teaching patients about skin care needs during radiation therapy is a priority intervention. Instruct the patient to not remove temporary ink markings when cleaning the skin until radiation therapy is completed. There are no universal evidence-based interventions for skin care during radiation therapy. It is important to teach patients to avoid skin irritation from

clothing and to follow the radiation-oncology department's policy regarding the use and timing of skin care products. Use of skin care products designed to manage or protect the skin from radiation damage does reduce the degree of skin problems that develop during a full course of radiation therapy (Bergstrom, 2011). Chart 22-2 is an example of an established skin care protocol during external radiation therapy.

❗ NURSING SAFETY PRIORITY (QSEN)

Action Alert

Skin in the radiation path is more sensitive to sunburn and sun damage. Advise against direct skin exposure to the sun during treatment and for at least 1 year after completing radiation therapy.

The normal tissues most sensitive to external radiation are bone marrow cells, skin, mucous membranes, hair follicles, and germ cells (ova and sperm). When possible, these tissues are shielded from radiation during therapy. At times, they cannot be protected from exposure. Some changes caused by radiation are permanent. The long-term problems vary with the location and dose of radiation received (see Table 22-2). For example,

CHART 22-2 Patient and Family Education: Preparing for Self-Management

Skin Protection During Radiation Therapy

- Wash the irradiated area gently each day with either water or a mild soap and water as prescribed by your radiation therapy team.
- Use your hand rather than a washcloth when cleansing the therapy site to be gentler.
- Rinse soap thoroughly from your skin.
- If ink or dye markings are present to identify exactly where the beam of radiation is to be focused, take care not to remove them.
- Dry the irradiated area with patting motions rather than rubbing motions; use a clean, soft towel or cloth.
- Use only powders, ointments, lotions, or creams on your skin at the radiation site that are prescribed by the radiation oncology department.
- Wear soft clothing over the skin at the radiation site.
- Avoid wearing belts, buckles, straps, or any type of clothing that binds or rubs the skin at the radiation site.
- Avoid exposure of the irradiated area to the sun:
  - Protect this area by wearing clothing over it.
  - Try to go outdoors in the early morning or evening to avoid the more intense sun rays.
  - When outdoors, stay under awnings, umbrellas, and other forms of shade during the times when the sun's rays are most intense (10 AM to 7 PM).
- Avoid heat exposure.

radiation to the throat and upper chest can cause difficulty in swallowing and can lead to reduced nutrition. A registered dietitian is part of the radiation oncology team. Head and neck radiation may damage the salivary glands and cause dry mouth (**xerostomia**), which affects quality of life and increases the patient's lifelong risk for tooth decay. Thus teach patients that regular dental visits are essential. Bone exposed to radiation therapy is less dense and breaks more easily (the cause of pathologic fractures). Fatigue remains a common problem during and for some time after radiation therapy. Exercise and sleep interventions may be somewhat beneficial for fatigue. Teach about the symptoms that might be expected from the specific location and dose of radiation (see Table 22-1 for the location of this information for different cancer types).

NCLEX EXAMINATION CHALLENGE

Psychosocial Integrity

The client receiving brachytherapy with implanted radioactive "seeds" for prostate cancer asks the nurse when these seeds will be removed. What is the nurse's best response?
A. "The half-life of radiation in these seeds is so short that it is not necessary to remove them."
B. "They will be removed only if their presence is painful or leads to an enlarged prostate gland."
C. "When we know for certain that all cancerous cells have been killed, the seeds will be removed."
D. "The seeds are small enough to be absorbed by your body and excreted in the urine or stool."

CYTOTOXIC SYSTEMIC AGENT THERAPY

When cancer has spread beyond a localized area that can be removed with surgery or safely treated with radiation therapy, systemic therapy is indicated for optimal results. Systemic therapy has many effects on normal tissues as well as on cancerous tissue.

 GENETIC/GENOMIC CONSIDERATIONS

Patient-Centered Care QSEN

A newer approach to selection of cancer treatment agents to be used is checking the patient's genetic profile to determine the likelihood of experiencing dangerous side effects. This process, known as *pharmacogenomics*, allows a more individualized approach to chemotherapy selection and side effect management. In addition, checking the genetic profile of the tumor can determine its sensitivity to various chemotherapy and targeted therapy agents (Boucher et al., 2014; Santos et al., 2013). This increasingly common practice individualizes cancer therapy and improves therapy outcomes. Expected future outcomes include an economic advantage for cancer care as decisions for treatment can be based on likelihood of effectiveness for an individual rather than on a tumor type or stage of disease. Remind patients that assessing genetic sensitivity can result in a selection of therapy that differs from that of other people with the same cancer type.

Systemic therapy with the use of antineoplastic agents is cytotoxic therapy in that the agents induce cell damaging/cell killing (cytotoxic) actions on cells, including cancer cells. Selection of agents to use as cytotoxic treatment of cancer is based on cellular kinetic concepts that include cell cycle, growth factors, and tumor burden. Most of the cytotoxic agents are not cancer cell specific and thus potentially affect all cells in the body. This effect is especially seen on rapidly dividing cells such as those in the bone marrow. The time when bone marrow activity and white blood cell counts are at their lowest levels after cytotoxic therapy is the **nadir**. It occurs at different times for different drugs. To reduce immunosuppression, combination cytotoxic therapy avoids using drugs with nadirs that occur at or near the same time.

CHEMOTHERAPY

Chemotherapy, the treatment of cancer with chemical agents, is used to cure and to increase survival time. It has some selectivity for killing cancer cells over normal cells. This killing effect on cancer cells is related to the ability of chemotherapy to damage DNA and interfere with cell division. Tumors with rapid growth are often more sensitive to chemotherapy.

As described in Chapter 21, cancer cells can separate from the original tumor, spread to new areas, and establish new cancers at distant sites (**metastasize**). Patients with metastatic cancer will die unless treatment eliminates the metastatic cancer cells along with the original cancer cells. Chemotherapy is useful in treating cancer because its effects are systemic, providing the opportunity to kill metastatic cancer cells that may have escaped local treatment. Chemotherapy used along with surgery or radiation is termed **adjuvant** therapy.

Drugs used for chemotherapy usually are given systemically and exert their cell-damaging (**cytotoxic**) effects against healthy cells as well as cancer cells. The normal cells most affected by chemotherapy are those that divide rapidly, including skin, hair, intestinal tissues, spermatocytes, and blood-forming cells. These drugs are classified by the specific types of action they exert in the cancer cell (Table 22-3).

Chemotherapy Drug Categories

Alkylating agents cross-link DNA, making the DNA strands bind tightly together. This action prevents proper DNA and ribonucleic acid (RNA) synthesis, which inhibits cell division.

TABLE 22-3 Categories of Chemotherapeutic Drugs

Antimetabolites

Azacitidine (Vidaza)
Capecitabine (Xeloda)
Cladribine (Leustatin)
Clofarabine (Clolar)
Cytarabine (Cytosar, ara-C)
Decitabine (Dacogen)
Floxuridine (FUDR)
5-Fluorouracil (Adrucil, Efudex, Fluoroplex)
Fludarabine (Fludara, FLAMP)
Gemcitabine (Gemzar)
6-Mercaptopurine (Purinethol)
Methotrexate (MTX, Mexate)
Nelarabine (Arranon)
Pemetrexed (Alimta)
Pentostatin (Nipent)
6-Thioguanine (Tabloid)

Antitumor Antibiotics

Bleomycin (Blenoxane)
Dactinomycin (Cosmegen)
Daunorubicin (Cerubidine, Daunomycin)
Doxorubicin (Adriamycin, Rubex)
Doxorubicin liposomal (Doxil)
Epirubicin (Ellence)
Idarubicin (Idamycin)
Mitomycin C (Mutamycin)
Mitoxantrone (Novantrone)
Valrubicin (Valstar)

Antimitotics

Cabazitaxel (Jevtana)
Docetaxel (Taxotere)
Etoposide (VP-16, VePesid)
Eribulin mesylate (Halaven)
Paclitaxel (Taxol)
Teniposide (Vumon)
Vinblastine (Velban, Velbe, Velsar)
Vincristine (Oncovin)
Vinorelbine (Navelbine)

Alkylating Agents

Altretamine (Hexalen)
Bendamustine (Treanda)
Busulfan (Busulfex)
Carboplatin (Paraplatin)
Carmustine (BiCNU, Gliadel)
Chlorambucil (Leukeran)
Cisplatin (Platinol)
Cyclophosphamide (Cytoxan, Procytox)
Dacarbazine (DTIC)
Estramustine (Emcyt, Estracyte)
Ifosfamide (Ifex)
Lomustine (CCNU, CeeNU)
Mechlorethamine (Mustargen)
Melphalan (Alkeran) (available in oral or IV form)
Oxaliplatin (Eloxatin)
Streptozocin (Zanosar)
Temozolomide (Temodar)
Thiotepa (Thioplex)

Topoisomerase Inhibitors

Irinotecan (Camptosar)
Topotecan (Hycamtin)

Miscellaneous Agents

Arsenic trioxide (Trisenox)
Asparaginase (Elspar)
Hydroxyurea (Droxia, Hydrea)
Ixabepilone (Ixempra)
Pegaspargase (Oncaspar)
Procarbazine (Matulane, Natulan ✦)
Vorinostat (Zolinza)

Data from the U.S. Food and Drug Administration website at www.fda.gov/cder/index.html; and MD Consult at www.mdconsult.com/php/82925233-2/homepage.

Antimetabolites are similar to normal metabolites needed for vital cell processes. Most cell reactions require metabolites in order to begin or continue the reaction. Antimetabolites closely resemble normal metabolites and are "counterfeit" metabolites that fool cancer cells into using the antimetabolites in cellular reactions. Because antimetabolites cannot function as proper metabolites, their presence impairs cell division.

Antimitotic agents interfere with the formation and actions of microtubules so cells cannot complete mitosis during cell division. As a result, the cancer cell either does not divide at all or divides only once.

Antitumor antibiotics damage the cell's DNA and interrupt DNA or RNA synthesis. Exactly how the interruptions occur varies with each agent.

Topoisomerase inhibitors disrupt an enzyme (topoisomerase) essential for DNA synthesis and cell division. When drugs disrupt the enzyme, proper DNA maintenance is prevented, leading to DNA breakage and cell death.

Miscellaneous chemotherapy drugs are those with mechanisms of action that are either unknown or do not fit those of other drug categories.

Combination Chemotherapy

Successful cancer chemotherapy often involves giving more than one specific anticancer drug in a timed manner (*combination chemotherapy*). Using more than one drug can be more effective in killing cancer cells than using just one drug. However, the side effects and damage caused to normal tissues also increase with combination chemotherapy.

Treatment Issues

Drugs selected for use with a given patient are based on the sensitivity of cancer cells to the drug and the stage or extent of disease. Dosages for most chemotherapy drugs are calculated according to the patient's size. Often, calculations are based on milligrams per square meter of total body surface area (TBSA), which considers the patient's height as well as weight.

Chemotherapy drugs are given on a regular basis and are timed to maximize cancer cell kill and minimize damage to normal cells. The intent is to allow normal cells time to recover from any injury but not allow adequate time for the cancer cells to recover. The schedule may vary slightly to accommodate a patient's response to therapy, but chemotherapy is usually scheduled every 3 to 4 weeks for a specified number of times. Maintaining the intended dosage and timing schedule to ensure the patient receives what was planned is a critical factor in the successful response to chemotherapy. Newer protocols of giving higher doses of chemotherapy more often, called **dose-dense chemotherapy**, may be used for aggressive cancer treatment, especially for breast cancer. This dose-dense therapy also results in more intense side effects.

Patient and family education are critical in helping patients maintain an optimal dosing schedule for best outcomes, reducing side effects, and preventing therapy complications. Many patient problems are managed in the home. Therefore comprehensive and consistent patient education efforts by knowledgeable nurses are key to patient safety (see the Quality Improvement box).

Many chemotherapy drugs are given IV, although other routes may be used. For specific cancer types, the chemotherapy may be infused or instilled into a body cavity. The *intrathecal* route delivers drugs into the spinal canal, and the *intraventricular* route delivers drugs directly into the ventricles of the brain. *Intraperitoneal* instillations place the drugs within the abdominal cavity, most often for ovarian cancer. Drugs for bladder cancer can be instilled directly into the bladder (*intravesicular route*). In some instances, drugs may be applied as a *topical* preparation for skin lesions. *Intra-arterial* infusions may be used to deliver a higher dose locally. For examples, with liver tumors, an interventional radiologist places a catheter into the artery supplying the liver tumor. The concentrated chemotherapy drug, delivered in sponge-like beads, is infused, and the beads become trapped in the small arteries feeding the tumor. The techniques and care needs for different routes are described with the specific cancer type most commonly associated with the specific administration route.

The IV route is the most common for chemotherapy. The standard of care designated by the Oncology Nursing Society (ONS) and supported by the American Society of Clinical Oncologists (ASCO) for safe administration of IV

QUALITY IMPROVEMENT (QSEN)

Use of Checklists Can Help Ensure Important Information is Included in Patient Education

Dalby, C., Nesbitt, M., Frechette, C., Kennerley, K., Lacoursiere, L., & Buswell, L. (2013). Standardization of initial chemotherapy teaching to improve care. *Clinical Journal of Oncology Nursing, 17*(5), 472-475.

Chemotherapy for cancer treatment uses toxic drugs with many side effects and complications, and regimens often last for many months. Patients and families require much education and support to manage side effects and reduce the ongoing risks to patient safety. The oncology nurses at a large, well-known comprehensive cancer center that has multiple satellite ambulatory care sites noted that patients continued to have concerns for how to manage problems at home and when to seek professional help even after completing an initial chemotherapy teaching session. Closer examination of teaching techniques revealed that different satellites employed different resources and that individual oncology nurses used different approaches to patient teaching. To comply with the recently updated standards put forth by the American Society of Clinical Oncology and the Oncology Nursing Society to strengthen patient education, the nurses formed an improvement team consisting of nurse representatives from each treatment satellite, an oncology clinical nurse specialist, and a quality improvement expert. This team first agreed on what categories of patient education were critical and then reached consensus for developing category-specific appropriate checklists for teaching content to cover in each category.

Checklists were developed for content in the categories of (1) patient-specific information, (2) treatment regimen, (3) how and what to communicate (to health care providers), and (4) patient resources. Inclusion of content was determined by vote from experienced oncology nurses. In addition, a treatment-specific calendar for patient/family use was developed, as was a patient education assessment survey. The checklists and other resources were used at the initial chemotherapy visit. The survey was implemented at the third chemotherapy visit to determine checklist effectiveness, reassess patient educational needs, and reinforce key content from earlier teaching sessions.

Survey results at 4 months indicated a high degree of patient satisfaction (97%) with initial chemotherapy teaching. Patients indicated that they were confident in what to expect during chemotherapy and when to contact their providers. The nurses at the satellites involved in this project believed that the checklists helped them provide more consistent and comprehensive education.

Commentary: Implications for Practice and Research

Accurate patient and family education are critical in helping patients maintain an optimal dosing schedule for best outcomes, reducing side effects, and preventing serious therapy complications. This project demonstrated the checklists could help standardize the information and resources presented to patients at initial chemotherapy to ensure adequate patient preparation. Having input from experienced nurses at multiple sites helped ensure no critical information was omitted from teaching plans and helped obtain "buy-in" from all nurses working in these areas. This plan is now being expanded to all satellite clinics of the cancer center.

chemotherapy is that administration of these drugs requires special education and handling (Neuss et al., 2013; Polovich & Martin, 2011). Special education for competency does not mean that only an advanced practice nurse can perform this function; however, it does mean that the person should be a registered nurse who has completed an approved chemotherapy course. Responsibility for monitoring the patient during chemotherapy administration, however, rests with all nurses providing patient care.

FIG. 22-2 Appearance of tissue damage and loss after chemotherapy extravasation.

A serious complication of IV infusion is **extravasation**, which occurs when drug leaks into the surrounding tissues (also called *infiltration*). When the drugs given are **vesicants** (chemicals that damage tissue on direct contact), the results of extravasation can include PAIN, INFECTION, and tissue loss (Fig. 22-2). Surgery is sometimes needed for severe tissue damage.

The most important nursing intervention for extravasation is prevention (Gonzales, 2013; Schulmeister, 2014). Small extravasations resolve without extensive treatment if less than 0.5 mL of the drug has leaked into the tissues. If a larger amount has leaked, extensive tissue damage occurs and surgery may be needed. Careful monitoring of the access site is critical during chemotherapy administration to prevent leakage of larger volumes. Institutions should have established evidenced-based policies and procedures that are drug specific to guide extravasation management. With some drugs, cold compresses to the area are prescribed; for other agents, warm compresses are used. Antidotes may be injected into the site of extravasation. Coordinate with the oncologist and pharmacist to determine the specific antidote needed for the extravasated drug. Increasingly, when vesicants are part of therapy, the use of an implanted port or central line to decrease the risk for extravasation is recommended. Even with these devices, the nurse must observe closely for any indication of leakage and initiate management guidelines immediately.

Most chemotherapy drugs, even oral drugs, are absorbed through the skin and mucous membranes. As a result, the health care workers who prepare or give these drugs (especially nurses and pharmacists) are at risk for absorbing them. Anyone preparing, giving, or disposing of chemotherapy drugs or handling excreta from patients within 48 hours of receiving IV chemotherapy must use extreme caution and wear personal protective equipment (PPE). Such equipment includes eye protection, masks, double gloves or "chemo" gloves, and gown. The Occupational Safety and Health Administration (OSHA)

TABLE 22-4   Current Oral Chemotherapeutic Drugs

AGENT	DRUG CATEGORY	CANCER TYPE
Altretamine (Hexalen)	Alkylating agent	Ovarian cancer
Capecitabine (Xeloda)	Antimetabolite	Breast cancer Colorectal cancer
Chlorambucil (Leukeran)	Alkylating agent	Chronic lymphocytic leukemia; Hodgkin's lymphoma Non-Hodgkin's lymphoma
Dasatinib (Sprycel)	Tyrosine kinase inhibitor	Chronic myelogenous leukemia; acute myelogenous leukemia that is Philadelphia chromosome positive
Erlotinib (Tarceva)	Epidermal growth factor receptor inhibitor	Non–small cell lung cancer Pancreatic cancer
Everolimus (Afinitor)	Angiogenesis inhibitor	Advanced renal cell carcinoma
Gefitinib (Iressa)	Epidermal growth factor receptor inhibitor	Non–small cell lung cancer
Hydroxyurea (Droxia, Hydrea)	Miscellaneous agent	Chronic myelogenous leukemia Head and neck cancer Melanoma Ovarian cancer Sickle cell disease
Imatinib (Gleevec)	Tyrosine kinase inhibitor	Chronic myelogenous leukemia that is Philadelphia chromosome positive Gastrointestinal stromal tumors Myelodysplastic syndrome
Lapatinib (Tykerb)	Tyrosine kinase inhibitor	Breast cancer
Lenalidomide (Revlimid)	Angiogenesis inhibitor	Multiple myeloma; myelodysplastic syndrome
Lomustine (CCNU, CeeNU)	Alkylating agent	Hodgkin's lymphoma Malignant glioma
Melphalan (Alkeran)	Alkylating agent	Multiple myeloma Ovarian cancer
Mercaptopurine (Purinethol)	Antimetabolite	Acute lymphocytic leukemia
Nilotinib (Tasigna)	Tyrosine kinase inhibitor	Chronic myelogenous leukemia that is Philadelphia chromosome positive
Pazopanib (Votrient)	Multikinase inhibitor	Advanced renal cell carcinoma
Procarbazine (Matulane, Natulan ✦)	Miscellaneous agent	Hodgkin's lymphoma
Sorafenib (Nexavar)	Multikinase inhibitor	Advanced renal cell carcinoma; hepatocellular carcinoma
Sunitinib (Sutent)	Multikinase inhibitor	Advanced renal cell carcinoma; gastrointestinal stromal tumor
Temozolomide (Temodar)	Alkylating agent	Brain tumors (primary)
Thioguanine (Tabloid)	Antimetabolite	Acute myelogenous leukemia
Topotecan (Hycamtin)	Topoisomerase inhibitor	Small cell lung cancer
Vorinostat (Zolinza)	Histone inhibitor	Cutaneous T-cell lymphoma

and the Oncology Nursing Society (ONS) have established these practice guidelines and protective standards (Walton et al., 2012).

About two dozen anticancer drugs are available currently as oral agents (Table 22-4). This number is expected to double within the next 10 years. Only a few are actually oral formulations of classic cytotoxic chemotherapy agents; more are classified as specific types of targeted therapy agents (discussed later). Oral drugs are more convenient for the patient, and they can be taken at home. However, there are many problems with oral anticancer drugs. One of the biggest problems is the perception by patients and non-oncology nurses that these drugs are less toxic than those given intravenously (Davey, 2013; Neuss et al., 2013), which is **not** true. *Oral anticancer drugs are just as toxic to the person taking the drug and the person handling the drug as are standard chemotherapy drugs.* The responsibility for administration of these drugs often shifts from the oncology clinic to the home or to non-oncology acute care settings, and issues of protection, correct administration, adherence, and recognition

and management of side effects are major concerns. Patients need education and support to self-manage this therapy, including the accidental ingestion by another person. Not all patients are willing or able to accept the responsibility of self-management, and this must be considered during patient selection for oral chemotherapy.

Because these oral agents can be absorbed through skin and mucous membranes and exert toxic effects, the person who handles and administers them needs to use PPE in the same way as during IV chemotherapy administration. This becomes a more critical issue when non-oncology nurses are administering the drugs. The ONS practice guidelines stress nurse education for competence to administer these drugs. All nurses administering these drugs must know the indications for drug use, dosage ranges, side effects and adverse effects, schedules, and specific precautions (Yagasaki & Komatsu, 2013). In addition, these oral agents must not be crushed, split, broken, or chewed. These drugs are biohazardous and must be discarded in accordance with agency policy.

Adherence to defined oral chemotherapy schedules and dosages is more of a problem than with IV administration (Davey, 2013). Studies have shown that even highly motivated patients with cancer consider that skipping doses or reducing doses of oral drugs has only a minor impact. As with teaching other aspects of self-care, nurses have to be certain that patients and caregivers understand the implications of the decisions they make. Disrupting the schedule or reducing dosages has a negative impact on therapy outcomes and leads to drug resistance among cancer cells, disease progression, and reduced survival.

Side Effects of Chemotherapy

Temporary and permanent damage can occur to normal tissues from chemotherapy because it is systemic and exerts its effects on all cells. Problems include hemorrhagic cystitis, cardiac muscle damage, and loss of bone density. For some cancer drugs, agents that protect specific healthy cells (cytoprotectants or chemoprotectants) are given ahead of or with chemotherapy drugs to decrease the impact of these drugs on normal tissues. For example, amifostine (Ethyol) reduces DNA damage and is used to prevent kidney damage in patients receiving cisplatin; to reduce neutropenia; and to reduce radiation-induced xerostomia for patients receiving radiation therapy for head and neck cancer. Mesna (Mesnex) binds toxic metabolites to decrease bladder toxicity from ifosfamide and high-dose cyclophosphamide use.

Serious short-term side effects occur with cytotoxic chemotherapy. The side effects on the hematopoietic (blood-producing) system can be life threatening and are the most common reason for changing the dosage or the treatment plan. The suppressive effects on the bone marrow blood-forming cells cause anemia (decreased numbers of red blood cells and hemoglobin), neutropenia (decreased numbers of white blood cells leading to immunosuppression), and thrombocytopenia (decreased numbers of platelets). Common distressing side effects include nausea and vomiting, alopecia (hair loss), mucositis (open sores on mucous membranes), many skin changes, anxiety, sleep disturbance, altered bowel elimination, and changes in cognitive function. The emotional impact of these side effects is referred to as *cancer therapy symptom distress,* which can vary from patient to patient.

Drug therapy is used to reduce symptom distress from some of these side effects. For other problems, such as alopecia, no evidence-based prevention strategies exist but the patient can be helped to reduce his or her distress from its presence. Nonpharmacologic nursing interventions for many types of symptom distress experienced include distraction, massage, guided imagery, and other forms of complementary therapy (Serra et al., 2012).

Psychosocial issues can occur during chemotherapy. For many chemotherapy regimens, drugs are given over a period ranging from 2 hours to as long as 8 hours. During this time, the patient may be confined to a treatment area and constantly reminded of the disease and its treatment. Distraction methods such as virtual reality, guided imagery, reading, watching television, and talking with visitors may help reduce the sense of unpleasantness.

❖ *PATIENT-CENTERED COLLABORATIVE CARE*

The priority care issues during chemotherapy are protecting the patient from the life-threatening side effects and managing the associated distressing symptoms. For some patients, the symptoms are so unpleasant that they want to stop treatment.

Bone Marrow Suppression

In addition to killing cancer cells, chemotherapy also destroys circulating blood cells and reduces replacement of these cells by suppressing bone marrow function, also known as *myelosuppression.* The numbers of all circulating leukocytes, erythrocytes, and platelets are decreased. Reduced leukocyte numbers, especially neutropenia, greatly increase the risk for INFECTION. Decreased erythrocytes and platelets cause hypoxia, fatigue, and impaired CLOTTING leading to an increased tendency to bleed.

INFECTION risk results from neutropenia, placing the patient at extreme risk for sepsis. This critical problem is the major dose-limiting side effect of cancer chemotherapy and can lead to death during treatment. Many chemotherapy drugs cause myelosuppression to some degree and decrease the patient's protective responses to infection. The severity of the risk is related to drug dosage. Impairment is temporary, and protection recovers within weeks after therapy completion. However, the seriousness of potential infections makes this problem a major treatment concern (Held-Warmkessel, 2011). The most common infections are fungal, bacterial, and viral breakthrough. Most infections during neutropenia result from overgrowth of the patient's own normal flora and entrance of these organisms into the bloodstream.

INFECTION risk can be managed with the use of biological response modifiers (BRMs) and growth factors to stimulate bone marrow production of immune system cells. Although not appropriate for all types of cancer, this supportive treatment can reduce the risk for infection during chemotherapy. This treatment is discussed in the Immunotherapy section on p. 387. Actual infections are treated with anti-infective drugs, such as antibiotic, antifungal, and antiviral drugs. Just like for any other infection, anti-infective therapy is specific for the organism(s) causing the infection.

CONSIDERATIONS FOR OLDER ADULTS
Patient-Centered Care QSEN

Older adults are at even greater risk for chemotherapy-induced neutropenia because of age-related changes in bone marrow function. Using growth factors, such as filgrastim (Neupogen) and pegfilgrastim (Neulasta), before neutropenia occurs rather than later can reduce the severity of neutropenia and the risk for infectious complications. Be extra vigilant in assessing older adults for early manifestations of infection.

! NURSING SAFETY PRIORITY QSEN
Action Alert

The priority nursing interventions for the patient with neutropenia are protecting him or her from INFECTION within the health care system and teaching the patient and family how to reduce infection risk in the home. Total patient assessment, including skin and mucous membrane inspection, lung sounds, mouth assessment, and inspection of venous access device insertion sites, must be performed every 8 hours by a registered nurse for hospitalized patients.

Explain to the patient the importance of reporting any change in skin and mucous membranes or other health status. Instruct him or her to report any pimple, sore, rash, or open skin area. Also teach him or her to report a cough, burning on urination, PAIN around the venous access site, or new drainage from any body area. Good handwashing before contact with the patient is essential for INFECTION prevention. Use aseptic technique with any invasive procedure. Chart 22-3 lists the best practices to prevent infection in patients with neutropenia.

When delegating any nursing care activity to unlicensed assistive personnel (UAP), teach them the importance of protecting the neutropenic patient from INFECTION. Stress the ways that cross-contamination can occur and how to avoid this source of infection. Also ensure that UAP understand that even when the neutropenic patient is very tired and does not feel well, certain aspects of personal hygiene cannot be deferred. *Teach the importance of mouth care and washing of the axillary and perianal regions at least every 12 hours.*

Monitoring for manifestations of INFECTION is critical for the hospitalized patient with neutropenia. The reduced numbers of neutrophils can limit the presence of common infection manifestations. Often the patient with neutropenia does not develop a high fever or have purulent drainage even when a severe infection is present. Hospital units specializing in care of neutropenic patients often have standard protocols that nurses initiate as soon as infection is suspected, *before* a physician examines the patient, because treatment delay can result in sepsis and death. These protocols specify what types of cultures to obtain (e.g., blood, urine, sputum, central line, wound), what

diagnostic tests to obtain (e.g., chest x-ray), and what antibiotics to start immediately.

> ## ! NURSING SAFETY PRIORITY (QSEN)
> ### Critical Rescue
>
> Consider any temperature elevation in a patient with neutropenia an indication of INFECTION. Report it to the health care provider immediately, and implement standard infection protocols.

Many patients remain at home during periods of neutropenia and are at continuing risk for INFECTION. The focus remains on keeping the patient's own normal flora under control and preventing transmission of organisms from other people to him or her. *The patient with neutropenia but no other manifestations of communicable disease is NOT an infection hazard to other people; however, other people can be an infection hazard to the patient.* Teach patients and families self-care actions to reduce the risk for infection (Chart 22-4), especially handwashing.

Anemia and *thrombocytopenia* also result from the bone marrow suppression caused by some chemotherapy drugs.

CHART 22-3 Best Practice for Patient Safety & Quality Care (QSEN)

Care of the Patient with Myelosuppression and Neutropenia

- Place the patient in a private room whenever possible.
- Use good handwashing technique or use alcohol-based hand rubs before touching the patient or any of the patient's belongings.
- Ensure that the patient's room and bathroom are cleaned at least once each day.
- Do not use supplies from common areas for patients with myelosuppression and neutropenia. For example, keep a dedicated box of disposable gloves in his or her room and do not share this box with any other patient. Provide single-use food products, individually wrapped gauze, and other individually wrapped items.
- Limit the number of health care personnel entering the patient's room.
- Monitor vital signs every 4 hours, including temperature.
- Inspect the patient's mouth at least every 8 hours.
- Inspect the patient's skin and mucous membranes (especially the anal area) for the presence of fissures and abscesses at least every 8 hours.
- Inspect open areas, such as IV sites, every 4 hours for manifestations of infection.
- Change wound dressings daily.
- Obtain specimens of all suspicious areas for culture (as specified by the agency), and promptly notify the physician.
- Assist the patient in coughing and deep-breathing exercises.
- Encourage activity at a level appropriate for the patient's current health status.
- Change IV tubing daily or according to unit protocol.
- Keep frequently used equipment in the room for use with this patient only (e.g., blood pressure cuff, stethoscope, thermometer).
- Limit visitors to healthy adults.
- Use strict aseptic technique for all invasive procedures.
- Monitor the white blood cell count daily.
- Avoid the use of indwelling urinary catheters.
- Follow agency policy for restriction of fresh flowers and potted plants in the patient's room.

CHART 22-4 Patient and Family Education: Preparing for Self-Management

Prevention of Infection

During the times your white blood cell counts are low:

- Avoid crowds and other large gatherings of people who might be ill.
- Do not share personal toilet articles, such as toothbrushes, toothpaste, washcloths, or deodorant sticks, with others.
- If possible, bathe daily, using an antimicrobial soap. If total bathing is not possible, wash the armpits, groin, genitals, and anal area twice a day with an antimicrobial soap.
- Clean your toothbrush at least weekly by either running it through the dishwasher or rinsing it in liquid laundry bleach (and then rinsing the bleach out with hot running water).
- Wash your hands thoroughly with an antimicrobial soap before you eat and drink, after touching a pet, after shaking hands with anyone, as soon as you come home from any outing, and after using the toilet.
- Follow the cancer center's instructions for eating fresh salads; raw fruits and vegetables; meat, fish and eggs; and pepper and paprika.
- Wash dishes between use with hot, sudsy water, or use a dishwasher.
- Do not drink water, milk, juice, or other cold liquids that have been standing at room temperature for longer than an hour.
- Do not reuse cups and glasses without washing.
- Do not change pet litter boxes.
- Take your temperature at least once a day and whenever you do not feel well.
- Report any of these indications of infection to your physician immediately:
  - Temperature greater than 100° F (37.8° C)
  - Persistent cough (with or without sputum)
  - Pus or foul-smelling drainage from any open skin area or normal body opening
  - Presence of a boil or abscess
  - Urine that is cloudy or foul smelling or that causes burning on urination
- Take all prescribed drugs.
- Wear clean disposable gloves underneath gardening gloves when working in the garden or with houseplants.
- Wear a condom (if you are a man) when having sex. If you are a woman having sex with a male partner, ensure that he wears a condom.

Anemia causes patients to feel fatigued from a lack of adequate red blood cells to transport oxygen, and some tissues are hypoxic. Thrombocytopenia increases the risk for excessive bleeding from impaired CLOTTING. When the platelet count is less than 50,000/mm³, small trauma can lead to prolonged bleeding. With a count lower than 20,000 platelets/mm³, spontaneous and uncontrollable bleeding may occur. Both anemia and thrombocytopenia may require transfusion therapy.

The use of growth factors to stimulate production of red blood cells and platelets to improve CLOTTING is common. Erythropoiesis-stimulating agents (ESAs) such as darbepoetin alfa (Aranesp) and epoetin alfa (Epogen and Procrit) can prevent or improve anemia associated with chemotherapy and can reduce the need for transfusions. These drugs increase the production of many blood cell types, not just erythrocytes, increasing the patient's risk for hypertension, blood clots, strokes, and heart attacks, especially among older adults. Also, certain types of cancer cells grow faster in the presence of these ESAs, such as head and neck cancer cells, leukemias, and some lymphomas, and their use may be restricted. Dosing is based on each patient's hemoglobin levels to ensure that just enough red blood cells are produced to avoid the need for transfusion but not necessarily to bring hemoglobin or hematocrit levels up to normal.

An example of growth factor therapy for thrombocytopenia is the use of oprelvekin (Neumega). This drug increases the production of platelets. The drug may cause fluid retention and increase the risk for heart failure and pulmonary edema. Other side effects include conjunctival bleeding, hypotension, and tachycardia. Check whether patients have a working scale, and teach them to weigh themselves daily and keep a record. Remind them to immediately report sudden weight gain or dyspnea to the health care provider.

The priority for nursing care for the patient with thrombocytopenia is to provide a safe environment. Chart 22-5 lists the best practices for Bleeding Precautions for impaired CLOTTING. Teach UAP the importance of using Bleeding Precautions and the need to report any evidence of bleeding immediately. Caregivers at home also need to know these practices.

Teach patients with thrombocytopenia and their families to avoid injury and excessive bleeding when discharge occurs before the platelet count has returned to normal. Chart 22-6 reviews precautions to teach patients to prevent bleeding and what to do if bleeding occurs.

💡 NCLEX EXAMINATION CHALLENGE

Physiological Integrity

The client receiving high-dose chemotherapy who has neutropenia asks the nurse whether he and his wife can have sexual intercourse while he is receiving chemotherapy. What is the nurse's best response?
A. "No, this activity will increase the side effects of the chemotherapy."
B. "No, the danger of impregnating your wife is too great."
C. "Yes, as long as you feel like it and use a condom."
D. "Yes, if you do not have an infection."

Chemotherapy-Induced Nausea and Vomiting

Chemotherapy-induced nausea and vomiting (CINV) arises from a variety of GI and neural mechanisms. It may manifest

---

CHART 22-5 Best Practice for Patient Safety & Quality Care (QSEN)

Prevention of Injury for the Patient with Thrombocytopenia

- Handle the patient gently.
- Use and teach unlicensed assistive personnel (UAP) to use a lift sheet when moving and positioning the patient in bed.
- Avoid IM injections and venipunctures.
- When injections or venipunctures are necessary, use the smallest-gauge needle for the task.
- Apply firm pressure to the needle stick site for 10 minutes or until the site no longer oozes blood.
- Apply ice to areas of trauma.
- Test all urine and stool for the presence of occult blood.
- Observe IV sites every 4 hours for bleeding.
- Instruct patients to notify nursing personnel immediately if any trauma occurs and if bleeding or bruising is noticed.
- Avoid trauma to rectal tissues:
  - Do not administer enemas.
  - If suppositories are prescribed, lubricate liberally and administer with caution.
- Instruct the patient and UAP that the patient should use an electric shaver rather than a razor.
- When providing mouth care or supervising others in providing mouth care:
  - Use a soft-bristled toothbrush or tooth sponges.
  - Do not use water pressure gum cleaners.
  - Make certain that dentures and other dental devices fit and do not irritate.
- Instruct the patient not to blow the nose or insert objects into the nose.
- Instruct UAP and the patient that the patient should wear shoes with firm soles whenever ambulating.
- Practice fall prevention strategies according to the agency's policies.
- Keep pathways and walkways clear and uncluttered.

---

as *anticipatory* (before receiving the chemotherapy, often triggered by thoughts, sights, and sounds related to the anticipated chemotherapy), *acute* (within the first 24 hours after chemotherapy), *delayed* (occurring after the first 24 hours), *breakthrough* (occurring intermittently during therapy for CINV), or a combination of these. Many cancer drugs are **emetogenic** (vomiting inducing) to some degree, depending on the dose. Although evidence-based advances in prevention and control of CINV are helpful, it remains a common and distressing issue (Cherwin, 2012). Nausea often persists even when vomiting is controlled.

Acute CINV is more common than other types. It may persist for 1 to 2 days after chemotherapy is given. A few drugs, such as dacarbazine (DTIC), may trigger CINV almost as soon as the drug is started. Other drugs, such as cisplatin (Platinol), induce delayed nausea and vomiting that can continue as long as 5 to 7 days after receiving it. Patients who have CINV during one round of chemotherapy may begin to have the same manifestations before the next round as a result of sheer anticipation. Once considered the single most distressing side effect of chemotherapy, CINV often can be well controlled with appropriate evidence-based antiemetic therapy, especially with serotonin (5-HT3) antagonist drugs and the use of standardized protocols for its prevention and management.

Drug Therapy. Many antiemetics are available to relieve nausea and vomiting. These drugs vary in the side effects they

Preventing Injury or Bleeding

During the time your platelet count is low:

- Use an electric shaver.
- Use a soft-bristled toothbrush.
- Do not have dental work performed without consulting your cancer health care provider.
- Do not take aspirin or any aspirin-containing products. Read the label to be sure that the product does not contain aspirin or salicylates.
- Do not participate in contact sports or any activity likely to result in your being bumped, scratched, or scraped.
- If you are bumped, apply ice to the site for at least 1 hour.
- Avoid hard foods that would scrape the inside of your mouth.
- Eat only warm, cool, or cold foods to avoid burning your mouth. Be especially cautious with cheese topping on pizza.
- Check your skin and mouth daily for bruises, swelling, or areas with small reddish purple marks that may indicate bleeding.
- Notify your cancer health care provider if you:
  - Are injured and persistent bleeding results
  - Have excessive menstrual bleeding
  - See blood in your vomit, urine, or bowel movement
- Avoid trauma with intercourse.
- Avoid anal intercourse.
- Take a stool softener to prevent straining during a bowel movement.
- Do not use enemas or rectal suppositories.
- Avoid bending over at the waist, which increases pressure in the brain.
- Do not wear clothing or shoes that are tight or that rub.
- Avoid blowing your nose or placing objects in your nose. If you must blow your nose, do so gently without blocking either nasal passage.
- Avoid playing musical instruments that raise the pressure inside your head, such as brass wind instruments and woodwinds or reed instruments.

produce and how well they control CINV. One or more antiemetics are usually given before, during, and after chemotherapy. Drugs commonly used short-term to control CINV are listed in Chart 22-7. *Patient response to antiemetic therapy is variable, and the drug combinations are individualized for best effect (Barak et al., 2013).*

! NURSING SAFETY PRIORITY QSEN

Drug Alert

Do not confuse the antiemetic drug *Anzemet* (dolasetron) with the diabetes drug *Avandamet* (a combination of metformin and rosiglitazone). The drugs have similar sounding names but totally different actions.

Regardless of which drugs are being used to prevent or reduce CINV, they are most effective when used in an evidence-based approach for prevention and management on a scheduled basis (Davidson et al., 2012). Drug therapy for CINV works best when given before the nausea and vomiting are out of control. *The nursing priority is to coordinate with the patient and health care provider to ensure adequate control of CINV. Ensure that antiemetics are given before chemotherapy and are repeated based on the response and duration of CINV.* When patients are

receiving dose-dense chemotherapy, the intensity of CINV also increases and more aggressive antiemetic therapy is needed. Teach patients to continue the therapy, even when CINV appears controlled. *When the patient stops taking the drug(s), teach him or her to start retaking the drug at the first sign of nausea to prevent it from becoming uncontrollable.*

CONSIDERATIONS FOR OLDER ADULTS

Patient-Centered Care QSEN

The older adult can become dehydrated more quickly than a younger adult if CINV is not controlled. Teach older adults to be proactive with taking their prescribed antiemetics and to contact their health care provider if the CINV either does not resolve within 12 hours or becomes worse.

Mucositis

Mucositis (sores in mucous membranes) often develops in the entire GI tract, especially in the mouth (**stomatitis** refers to reactions that involve the other tissues and structures in the oral cavity). Mucositis is believed to be a complex, multiphase process at the cellular level started in response to cytotoxic chemotherapy. Mouth sores cause PAIN and interfere with eating and quality of life. Chart 22-8 lists the patient education for self-management of mucositis.

Frequent mouth assessment and oral hygiene are key in managing mucositis. Stress the importance of good and frequent oral hygiene, including teeth cleaning and mouth rinsing. Because most patients with mucositis also have bone marrow suppression and are at risk for impaired CLOTTING with bleeding, they must take care to avoid traumatizing the oral mucosa. Instruct them to use a soft-bristled toothbrush or disposable mouth sponges. Recommendations include *gentle* flossing once daily. Encourage them to rinse the mouth with plain water or saline at frequent intervals during the day and night when awake. Frequency is guided by the intensity of the mucositis. Initially, the rinses start after meals and at bedtime, then every 2 hours, and then progressing to hourly if needed for comfort. Teach patients to avoid mouthwashes that contain alcohol or other drying agents that may further irritate the mucosa.

Oral hygiene equipment must be kept clean. Remind patients not to share toothbrushes. Toothbrushes can be cleaned weekly by using a home dishwasher or by rinsing them with a solution of liquid bleach or hydrogen peroxide and then rinsing with hot water.

Many compounds are available for PAIN relief from mucositis as "swish and spit" mixtures that contain a local anesthetic combined with anti-inflammatory agents, although their use is not evidence-based. Remind the patient that these mixtures are not to be swallowed. For multiple mouth lesions, most patients require systemic pain medications.

Alopecia

Alopecia, hair loss, may occur as whole-body hair loss or may be as mild as only a thinning of the scalp hair. When body hair loss includes pubic hair, patients may struggle with their sexual identity and may not discuss this problem. Reassure patients that hair loss is temporary. Regrowth usually begins about 1 month after completion of chemotherapy; however, the new hair may differ from the original hair in color, texture, and

CHART 22-7 Common Examples of Drug Therapy

Chemotherapy-Induced Nausea and Vomiting

DRUG/USUAL DOSAGE	PHYSIOLOGIC PURPOSE	NURSING INTERVENTIONS	RATIONALE
Serotonin Antagonists Ondansetron (Zofran) 8 mg IV or orally every 8 hr Granisetron (Kytril) 1 mg IV or orally every 12 hr Granisetron transdermal (Sancuso) 1 patch per day starting 24 to 48 hrs before chemotherapy administration and continuing for up to 7 days after chemotherapy administration Dolasetron (Anzemet) 100 mg IV or orally 30 minutes before chemotherapy administration Palonosetron (Aloxi) 0.25 mg IV as a single dose 30 minutes before chemotherapy administration	Prevent CINV by blocking the 5-HT3 receptors in the brain (chemotrigger zone) and in the intestines. This action prevents serotonin from binding to the receptors and activating the nausea and vomiting centers.	Teach patient to change positions slowly to avoid falls. Assess the patient for headache.	These drugs may induce bradycardia, hypotension, and vertigo. Headache is a common side effect of drugs from this class.
Neurokinin Receptor Antagonists Aprepitant (Emend) *3-day oral regimen:* Day 1, 125 mg 1 hour before chemotherapy administration Days 2 and 3, 80 mg in the morning (no chemotherapy these days) *IV regimen:* Day 1, 115 mg 30 minutes before chemotherapy, followed by oral regimen on Days 2 and 3	Reduce CINV by blocking the substance P neurokinin receptor. When used together with a serotonin antagonist and a corticosteroid, both acute and delayed nausea and vomiting are controlled.	Teach patients who are also taking warfarin (Coumadin) to have their INRs checked before and after the 3 days of this therapy. Teach women who are using oral contraceptives to use an additional form of birth control while on this drug.	This drug interferes with the effectiveness of warfarin. The drug reduces the effectiveness of oral contraceptives, increasing the risk for an unplanned pregnancy.
Corticosteroids Dexamethasone (Decadron) 5-10 mg IV or orally daily	Reduce CINV by decreasing swelling in the brain's chemotrigger zone.	Teach patients to reduce salt intake to about 4 g daily.	Drug causes fluid retention and hypertension.
Prokinetic Agents Metoclopramide (Reglan) 20-40 mg IM or IV twice or three times daily	Reduce CINV by blocking dopamine receptors in the brain's chemotrigger zone.	Teach the patient to avoid driving or operating heavy machinery.	Increased drowsiness is common.
Benzodiazepines Lorazepam (Ativan) 1-3 mg orally or IV twice or three times daily	Reduce CINV by enhancing cholinergic effects and by decreasing the person's awareness.	Teach the patient and family that the patient should avoid driving, operating heavy machinery, making legal decisions, and going up and down staircases unassisted.	The drug induces amnesia and profound drowsiness.

CINV, Chemotherapy-induced nausea and vomiting; *INR,* international normalized ratio.

---

thickness. No known evidence-based treatment safely prevents alopecia. *The priority nursing actions are to teach patients how to avoid scalp injury and to assist them in coping with this body image change.*

The hairless scalp is at risk for injury. Teach the patient to avoid direct sunlight on the scalp by wearing a hat or other head covering. Sunscreen use is essential to prevent sunburn because many drugs increase sun sensitivity, regardless of skin darkness. This skin can be damaged by helmets, headphones, headsets, wigs, and other items that rub the head. Teach the patient to wear some head covering underneath these items. Head coverings also are needed during cold weather and in cool environments to reduce body heat loss and prevent hypothermia.

Assist patients in selecting a type of head covering that suits their income and lifestyle. One recommendation is to coordinate wig purchases with the patient's hairdresser or barber. Having very short hair or a shaved head now is common and socially acceptable for men, and many men choose not to wear a wig during chemotherapy. Cutting the hair very short before chemotherapy begins allows a better wig fit.

Suggest that patients purchase a wig before therapy begins and have their hairdresser shape it to mimic their usual hairstyle to reduce appearance changes. High-quality wigs are expensive but can look very much like the patient's own hair. Many local units of the American Cancer Society (ACS) offer the loan of wigs that other patients have donated to be lent to others with cancer. Patients also can disguise hair loss with caps, scarves, and turbans. The ACS also provides instruction (Look Good-Feel Better) regarding makeup and the use of scarves, for example, to improve appearance and how patients feel about themselves. Patients in control of their appearance may improve their quality of life during therapy (Borsellino & Young, 2011).

Changes in Cognitive Function

Some patients receiving chemotherapy have reported changes in cognitive function—most commonly reduced ability to concentrate, memory loss, and difficulty learning new information during treatment and for months to years after treatment. Although most types of chemotherapy drugs do not cross the blood-brain barrier and were thought not to affect any part of

CHART 22-8 **Patient and Family Education: Preparing for Self-Management**

Mouth Care for Patients with Mucositis

- Examine your mouth (including the roof, under the tongue, and between the teeth and cheek) every 4 hours for fissures, blisters, sores, or drainage.
- If sores or drainage is present, contact your health care provider to determine whether these areas need to be cultured.
- Brush the teeth and tongue with a soft-bristled brush or sponges every 8 hours and after meals.
- Avoid the use of mouthwashes that contain alcohol or glycerin.
- "Swish and spit" room-temperature tap water, normal saline, or salt and soda water on a regular basis (at least 4 times a day) and as needed according to changes in the oral cavity.
- Drink 2 or more liters of water per day if another health problem does not require limiting fluid intake.
- Take antimicrobial drugs as prescribed.
- Use topical analgesic drugs as prescribed.
- Take pain medications on schedule as needed.
- Apply a water-based moisturizer to your lips after each episode of mouth care and as needed.
- Use prescribed "artificial saliva" or mouth moisturizers as needed.
- Avoid using tobacco or drinking alcoholic beverages.
- Avoid spicy, salty, acidic, dry, rough, or hard food.
- Cool liquids to prevent burns or irritation.
- If you wear dentures, use them only during meals. When not in place, soak dentures in an antimicrobial solution. Rinse thoroughly before placing them in your mouth.

CHART 22-9 **Patient and Family Education: Preparing for Self-Management**

Chemotherapy-Induced Peripheral Neuropathy

- Protect feet and other body areas where sensation is reduced (e.g., do not walk around in bare feet or stocking feet; always wear shoes with a protective sole).
- Be sure shoes are long enough and wide enough to prevent creating sores or blisters.
- Buy shoes in the afternoon or evening to accommodate any size change needed for foot swelling.
- Provide a long break-in period for new shoes; do not wear new shoes for longer than 2 hours at a time.
- Avoid pointed-toe shoes and shoes with heels higher than 2 inches.
- Inspect your feet daily (with a mirror) for open areas or redness.
- Avoid extremes of temperature; wear warm clothing in the winter, especially over hands, feet, and ears.
- Test water temperature with a thermometer when washing dishes or bathing. Use warm water rather than hot water (less than 105°F or 40.6°C).
- Use potholders when cooking.
- Use gloves when washing dishes or gardening.
- Do not eat foods that are "steaming hot"; allow them to cool before placing them in your mouth.
- Eat foods that are high in fiber (e.g., fruit, whole grain cereals, vegetables).
- Drink 2 to 3 liters of fluid (nonalcoholic) daily unless your health care provider has told you to restrict fluid intake.
- Use the actions for "Falls Prevention" supplied by the cancer center during all activities.
- Get up slowly from a lying or sitting position. If you feel dizzy, sit back down until the dizziness fades before standing; then stand in place for a few seconds before walking or using the stairs.
- To prevent tripping or falling, look at your feet and the floor or ground where you are walking to assess how the ground, floor, or step changes.
- Avoid using area rugs, especially those that slide easily.
- Keep floors free of clutter that could lead to a fall.
- Use handrails when going up or down steps.

brain function, the drugs can induce inflammation and general biochemical changes that could reduce cognitive function, at least temporarily (Kanaskie, 2012; Myers, 2012).

This problem, termed "chemo brain," is reported most often in women undergoing chemotherapy for breast cancer, although it is not limited either to women or to breast cancer treatment. The fact that it is reported more in this population reflects that breast cancer is very common, it is often treated with high-dose chemotherapy, and most patients with breast cancer survive a long time after therapy.

Comparisons of brain structure and cognitive function before, during, and after high-dose chemotherapy show some anatomic changes in brain white matter and gray matter. These changes are not usually present at 3 years after completion of therapy. It is not known why all patients receiving high-dose chemotherapy do not develop the problem; however, genetic differences may be partly responsible. Not only is the exact cause of this side effect unclear, so are the personal risk factors.

The priority for nursing care is to support the patient who reports this side effect. Listen to the patient's concerns, and tell him or her that other patients have also reported such problems. Providing absolute reassurance is difficult, but the results of early studies indicate that recovery is likely with time. A common sense approach includes that patients should be warned against participating in other behaviors that could alter cognitive functioning, such as excessive alcohol intake, recreational drug use, and activities that increase the risk for head injury. Research about reducing the effects of chemo brain is ongoing.

Chemotherapy-Induced Peripheral Neuropathy

Chemotherapy-induced peripheral neuropathy (CIPN) is the loss of sensory or motor function of peripheral nerves associated with exposure to certain anticancer drugs (Binner et al.,

2011; Tofthagen et al., 2011). Some patients undergoing chemotherapy with nerve-damaging drugs (e.g., antimitotics and platinum-based drugs) have rapid onset of severe CIPN. The degree of CIPN is related to the dosage of the nerve-damaging drugs; higher doses lead to greater neuropathy. The results of CIPN on function are widespread, with the most common problems including loss of sensation in the hands and feet, orthostatic hypotension, erectile dysfunction, neuropathic PAIN, loss of taste discrimination, and severe constipation. CIPN is a long-term consequence and may be permanent in some people. No known interventions prevent CIPN.

The priority for nursing care of patients experiencing CIPN is teaching them to prevent injury. Loss of sensation increases the patient's risk for injury because he or she may not be aware of excessive heat, cold, or pressure. The risk for injury to the feet is very high. Falls are more likely because the patient cannot feel changes in terrain and because of orthostatic hypotension. Chart 22-9 lists teaching priorities for the patient with CIPN.

Some issues, such as erectile dysfunction, may be helped with devices or drug therapy (see Chapter 72 for options for erectile dysfunction). Other issues are not correctable and affect many aspects of quality of life. The loss of hand sensation may make some activities that require very fine motor skills difficult or impossible. Assess the patient's ability to cope with these changes. Coordinate with an occupational therapist to help the patient adjust for sensory deficits in performing activities. Patients who have an altered gait are at increased risk for falls and injury.

IMMUNOTHERAPY: BIOLOGICAL RESPONSE MODIFIERS

Biological response modifiers (BRMs) modify the patient's biologic responses to tumor cells. BRMs can influence cancer cells in a variety of ways. Some have direct antitumor activity, helping the body recognize cancer cells as foreign so that the immune system destroys them. BRMs also can improve immune function and enhance the body's ability to repair or replace cells damaged by cancer treatment.

As discussed in Chapter 17, cytokines released from immune system cells are not usually cytotoxic alone but influence how immune system cells function. The cytokines include the interferons, interleukins, tumor necrosis factors, and colony-stimulating factors. Some cytokines enhance immune function, which plays an important role in cancer prevention (see Chapters 17 and 21). Cytokines and other BRMs work by stimulating the immune system to recognize cancer cells and take actions to eliminate or destroy them. Some BRMs stimulate faster recovery of bone marrow function after treatment-induced suppression. Additional BRMs include the monoclonal antibodies and vaccines.

BRMs as Cancer Therapy

Two common types of BRMs used as cancer therapy are the interleukins and interferons. Some agents can stimulate specific immune system cells to attack and destroy cancer cells; other agents block cancer cell access to an essential function or nutrient.

Interleukins (ILs) are a large group of substances the body makes to help regulate inflammation and immunity. Some are now synthesized as anticancer drugs. In particular, ILs have been useful for renal cell carcinoma and melanoma. ILs help different immune system cells recognize and destroy abnormal body cells. In particular, IL-1, IL-2, and IL-6 appear to "charge up" the immune system and enhance attacks on cancer cells by macrophages, natural killer (NK) cells, and tumor-infiltrating lymphocytes (Abbas et al., 2012).

Interferons (IFNs) are cell-produced proteins that have been effective to some degree in the treatment of melanoma, hairy cell leukemia, renal cell carcinoma, ovarian cancer, and cutaneous T-cell lymphoma. They assist in cancer therapy by:
- Slowing tumor cell division
- Stimulating the growth and activation of NK cells
- Inducing cancer cells to resume a more normal appearance and function
- Inhibiting the expression of oncogenes

TABLE 22-5 Common Biological Response Modifiers Used As Supportive Cancer Therapy

AGENT	CELL TYPE AFFECTED	INDICATIONS
Sargramostim (Leukine, Prokine)	All granulocytes Neutrophils Eosinophils Monocytes Macrophages	Chemotherapy-induced leukopenia
Filgrastim (Neupogen) Pegfilgrastim (Neulasta)	Neutrophils	Chemotherapy-induced neutropenia
Epoetin alfa (Epogen, Procrit) Darbepoetin alfa (Aranesp)	Erythrocytes	Chemotherapy-induced anemia Chemotherapy-induced fatigue Anemia induced by renal failure
Oprelvekin (Neumega)	Platelets	Chemotherapy-induced thrombocytopenia
Sipuleucel-T (Provenge) (product is a vaccine)	T-cells; antigen-processing cells (macrophages)	Hormone-refractory prostate cancer

One drug classified as a BRM that has a different action is thalidomide (Thalomid), which reduces the level of tumor-secreted vascular endothelial growth factor (VEGF). VEGF is needed to maintain blood supply to the tumor. When VEGF is reduced, the tumor is poorly nourished and cancer cells die. This drug is approved for treatment of multiple myeloma.

BRMs as Supportive Therapy

BRMs used for supportive therapy during cancer treatment are the colony-stimulating factors or "growth factors" (Table 22-5). These factors induce more rapid recovery of the bone marrow after suppression by chemotherapy. This effect has two benefits. First, when bone marrow suppression is shortened or less severe, patients are less at risk for life-threatening INFECTIONS, anemia, and impaired CLOTTING with bleeding. Second, because the growth factors allow more rapid bone marrow recovery, patients can receive their chemotherapy as scheduled and may even be able to tolerate higher doses, potentially increasing the chance for cure.

Side Effects of BRM Therapy

Patients receiving interleukins have generalized and often severe inflammatory reactions. Fluid shifts and capillary leak syndrome (CLS) are widespread with edema formation. Tissue swelling affects the function of all organs and can be life threatening. Patients receiving high-dose BRM therapy should receive care in an intensive care or monitoring unit. These effects occur during the period of acute drug infusion and resolve after therapy completion.

Many BRMs and growth factors induce manifestations of inflammation during and just after receiving the drug, including fever, chills, rigors, and flu-like symptoms (general malaise). Problems are worse when higher doses are given, but they seem to become less severe over time. The nursing priorities for patients receiving BRMs include assessing for complications of systemic inflammation and making patients as comfortable as possible. Fever is treated with acetaminophen. Patients with severe rigors are managed with meperidine (Demerol). Patients may also experience nausea, vomiting, diarrhea, and anorexia. Antiemetics are helpful in the management of nausea and vomiting.

Neurologic manifestations associated with BRM use can be significant. These include confusion, fatigue, somnolence, irritation or agitation, hallucinations, vivid dreams, anxiety, and sleep disturbances. Some patients have psychosocial issues of fear, tearfulness, depression, and mood swings. Early identification of these manifestations is an important nursing care activity.

Interferon therapy causes peripheral neuropathy. It is not known whether the neuropathy is temporary or permanent. (See the Chemotherapy-Induced Peripheral Neuropathy section on p. 386.)

Skin dryness, itching, and peeling occur with many types of BRM therapy. The skin problems are more severe with higher doses and when more than one type of BRM is used at the same time. Reactions are temporary but cause much discomfort and distress. Advise patients to apply moisturizers (unscented) to the skin and to use mild soap to clean the skin. Involved areas should be protected from the sun with clothing or the use of sunscreen agents. Teach patients to avoid swimming and to not use topical steroid creams on affected areas.

Monoclonal Antibodies

Monoclonal antibody therapy combines actions from immunotherapy and targeted therapy to help treat specific cancers. The body normally responds to foreign substances with the production of antibodies. These proteins are then able to target the antigen when present in the body, attacking and destroying the foreign antigen (nonself cells). In cancer therapy, human, mouse, and rabbit hybrid cells can produce antibodies against given targets known to be present in or on certain types of cancer cells.

Monoclonal antibodies bind to their target antigens, which are often specific cell surface membrane proteins. Binding prevents the protein from performing its functions. Some cancer cells express cell membrane surface proteins that are unique to cancer cells and have a role in cancer cell division. So, by binding these proteins, monoclonal antibodies prevent cell division. Some monoclonal antibodies actually make tumor cells more sensitive to chemotherapy and increase the effectiveness of immune system attacks on the cancer cells. The most well known monoclonal antibody for targeted therapy is rituximab (Rituxan). It binds to the protein *CD20*, which is often overexpressed on the surface of non-Hodgkin's lymphoma cell membranes. This protein activates an early step of the cell cycle division process. Binding *CD20* with rituximab prevents it from stimulating cell division in the non-Hodgkin's lymphoma cells.

Allergic reactions can be an issue in patients receiving monoclonal antibodies because of the incorporation of non-human proteins. Most of these antibodies initially were developed in mice and express some mouse proteins. Now many of these antibodies have been "humanized," reducing the risk for allergic reactions. Nursing assessment is key for early recognition of a potentially life-threatening allergic reaction.

The monoclonal antibodies to the epidermal growth factor receptor (EGFR) bind to those specific receptors on normal and cancerous cells. Thus side effects also occur in the skin, mucous membranes, and lining of the GI tract.

MOLECULARLY TARGETED THERAPY

Molecularly targeted therapies are technically biologic agents. However, their unique actions and roles in cancer therapy warrant separate discussion. These agents use molecular flaws in some cancer cells to specifically target cancer cells and have less of an impact on normal cells. Generally, molecularly targeted therapies block the growth and spread of cancer by interfering with the specific signals or molecules involved in the growth and progression of cancer cells (Beatty et al., 2011). These agents are providing patients with cancer a new sense of hope against a challenging disease.

As discussed in Chapter 21, normal cells have tightly controlled regulation over when and to what extent a cell divides; cancer cells have escaped this tight control. External events can indicate to a cell that cell division is needed. However, these external events must be communicated to the cell's nucleus to activate the genes that promote cell division (oncogenes) and turn off the genes that normally suppress cell division (suppressor genes). The key to communicating the need for cell division is the presence and activation of signal transduction pathways. Fig. 22-3 shows a segment of a cell with one signal transduction pathway. When this pathway is activated at the cell surface by binding growth factors to their receptors, having certain drugs interact with the cell's plasma membrane, binding of certain adhesion molecules (CAMs), changing movement of calcium and sodium across the membrane, or other cell-to-cell interactions, the first result is an increase in the cell's production of a family of enzymes known as *tyrosine kinases (TKs)*. With increased TKs present, the pro–cell division signal activates many substances, known as *transcription factors,* within the pathway. When the pro–cell division transcription factors reach the cell's nucleus, oncogenes are activated, suppressor genes are inactivated, and a variety of proteins are produced to make cell division occur.

When cell division is not needed, external signals, such as growth factor inhibitors and the surrounding of a cell's plasma membrane with other cells, send signals that inhibit activation of TKs and the signal transduction pathway. As a result, fewer transcription factors are produced, suppressor genes are expressed, and oncogenes are suppressed. The proteins needed for cell division are not produced, and cell division does not occur.

Overall, cancer cells have more active signal transduction pathways and transcription factors that ultimately lead to excessive division of the cancer cells. Targeted therapies take advantage of differences in one or more parts of the signal transduction pathway to block it. Often these parts are overexpressed in cancer cells. Agents used as targeted therapies can disrupt the pathway and slow or stop cell division. They may work by blocking a growth factor receptor, by preventing the activation of tyrosine kinases, by limiting the production of transcription factors, and by other mechanisms that are not yet fully understood. Regardless of how a targeted therapy works, it will work only with those cancer cells that have the actual target. The result is that the signal for turning on cell division genes (oncogenes) does not get through to the cell's nucleus (Fig. 22-4) (Byar & Workman, 2012; Santos et al., 2013).

Drugs for targeted therapy have been approved as treatment for certain cancers. These drugs are classified based on the mechanism of action, and some have more than one action (Table 22-6). Because of the varying mechanisms of action and

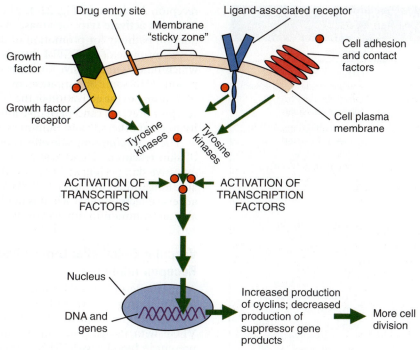

FIG. 22-3 Pro–cell division signal transduction pathway.

FIG. 22-4 Sites of action for targeted therapies that inhibit a signal transduction pathway and greatly reduce cell division.

the relative newness of these therapies, the priority nursing action is careful assessment for adverse reactions to therapy.

It is important to remember that these drugs will not work unless the cancer cell overexpresses the actual target substance. Thus not all patients with the same cancer type would benefit from

the use of targeted therapy. Each person's cancer cells are evaluated to determine whether the cells have enough of a target to be affected by targeted therapy.

The targeted therapy agents are classified based on their action. The first application of these agents was against estrogen

TABLE 22-6 Common Targeted Therapy Agents

CLASSIFICATION	AGENT
Tyrosine kinase inhibitors	Dasatinib (Sprycel)
	Imatinib mesylate (Gleevec)
	Lapatinib (Tykerb)
	Nilotinib (Tasigna)
Epidermal growth factor receptor inhibitors (EGFRIs)	Cetuximab (Erbitux)
	Erlotinib (Tarceva)
	Gefitinib (Iressa)
	Panitumumab (Vectibix)
	Trastuzumab (Herceptin)
Vascular endothelial growth factor receptor inhibitors (VEGFRIs)	Bevacizumab (Avastin)
Multikinase inhibitors	Sorafenib (Nexavar)
	Sunitinib (Sutent)
	Pazopanib (Votrient)
Proteasome inhibitors	Bortezomib (Velcade)
Angiogenesis inhibitors	Everolimus (Afinitor)
	Lenalidomide (Revlimid)
	Temsirolimus (Torisel)
Monoclonal antibodies	Alemtuzumab (Campath)
	Ibritumomab (Zevalin)
	Rituximab (Rituxan)
	^{131}I tositumomab (Bexxar)

in breast cancer (discussed in the Hormonal Manipulation section on p. 391). There now are a group of selective estrogen receptor modulators (SERMs). Aromatase inhibitors (AIs) have been developed to interfere with estrogen's ability to promote the growth of estrogen receptor positive breast cancers. Discussion in this section will focus on the tyrosine kinase inhibitors (TKIs), epidermal growth factor/receptor inhibitors (EGFRIs), vascular endothelial growth factor/receptor inhibitors (VEGFRIs), multikinase inhibitors (MKIs), proteasome inhibitors, and angiogenesis inhibitors.

Tyrosine Kinase Inhibitors

Drugs with the main action of inhibiting activation of tyrosine kinases (TKs) are **tyrosine kinase inhibitors (TKIs)**. There are many different TKs. Some are unique to the cell type; others may be present only in cancer cells that express a specific gene mutation. As a result, the different TKI drugs are effective in disrupting the growth of some cancer cell types and not others. An example of a TKI is imatinib mesylate (Gleevec). This drug binds to the energy site of the enzyme *tyrosine kinase* and prevents its activation. The drug is most useful in cancers that overexpress the *ABL1* oncogene, such as Philadelphia chromosome–positive chronic myeloid leukemia and metastatic gastrointestinal stromal tumors (GISTs).

Side effects common to most TKIs include fluid retention, electrolyte imbalances, and bone marrow suppression. This suppression can be severe enough to cause neutropenia, anemia, and thrombocytopenia. The problems associated with bone marrow suppression are increased when the patient also receives traditional chemotherapy with drugs that suppress bone marrow.

Epidermal Growth Factor/Receptor Inhibitors

The epidermal growth factor/receptor inhibitors (EGFRIs) block epidermal growth factor from binding to its cell surface

receptor. As shown in Fig. 22-4, when this receptor is blocked, it cannot activate tyrosine kinase. As a result, the signal transduction pathway for promotion of cell division is inhibited.

An example of an EGFRI drug is trastuzumab (Herceptin), which binds the excessive amounts of a certain type of EGFR produced by some breast cancer, ovarian, and colon cancer cells in response to the activation of the *HER2/neu* gene. Binding this receptor prevents cancer cell division and increases the sensitivity to chemotherapy and immune system actions.

The most common side effects of EGFRIs include a variety of skin reactions. These may be as mild as a rash or result in excessive skin peeling and fissures. Trastuzumab has been available longer than the other EGFRIs and has been found to have adverse effects on the heart. It is not known if the cardiac effects also are common to other EGFRIs.

Vascular Endothelial Growth Factor/ Receptor Inhibitors

An example of a vascular endothelial growth factor/receptor inhibitor drug is bevacizumab (Avastin). It binds to vascular endothelial growth factor (VEGF) and prevents the binding of VEGF with its receptors on the surfaces of endothelial cells present in blood vessels. This inhibits formation of new blood vessels within a tumor. As a result, tumor cells are poorly nourished and metastasis is inhibited. This drug is used with standard chemotherapy for many cancers that overexpress the receptor.

The most common side effects are hypertension and impaired wound healing. Bone marrow suppression with neutropenia and thrombocytopenia also occur, especially when the drug is used in combination with chemotherapy drugs that cause bone marrow suppression.

Multikinase Inhibitors

The multikinase inhibitors (MKIs) are drugs that inhibit the activity of specific kinases in cancer cells and in tumor blood vessels. An example of an MKI is sunitinib (Sutent). These drugs are most effective in preventing the activation of tyrosine kinases that have a specific gene mutation found most often in some renal cell carcinomas, GI stromal tumors, and pancreatic, colon, and non–small cell lung cancer cells.

A common side effect of this class of drugs is hypertension. Others include nausea and vomiting, diarrhea, constipation, mucositis, and mild neutropenia and thrombocytopenia.

Proteasome Inhibitors

Proteasome inhibitors work by preventing the formation of a large complex of proteins (a proteasome) in cells. The proteasome helps regulate the expression of genes that promote cell division and prevent cell death. Proteasome inhibitors limit the amount of proteasome present, making the cell less likely to divide and more likely to respond to signals for cell death. An example of a proteasome inhibitor is bortezomib (Velcade). Proteasomes are present in normal and cancer cells, but cancer cells are much more sensitive to the effects of proteasome inhibition than are normal cells.

The most common side effects of bortezomib are nausea, vomiting, anorexia, abdominal PAIN, bowel changes, and decreased taste sensation. Peripheral neuropathy is also common. Other side effects include headache, rash, pruritus, back and bone pain, and muscle aches.

Angiogenesis Inhibitors

Angiogenesis inhibitors target a specific protein kinase known as the *mammalian target of rapamycin (mTOR)*. An example of an angiogenesis inhibitor is temsirolimus (Torisel). When the drug binds to an intracellular protein, a protein-drug complex forms that inhibits the activity of mTOR. When mTOR is inhibited, the concentrations of vascular endothelial growth factor (VEGF) are greatly reduced and many pro–cell division signal transduction pathways are disrupted. This drug is especially useful in suppressing the growth of renal cell carcinomas.

Hypersensitivity reactions to these drugs are common and so is hyperglycemia. Bone marrow suppression is moderate to severe with anemia, neutropenia, and thrombocytopenia. Other general side effects include headache, nausea and vomiting, back PAIN, muscle and joint PAIN, mucositis, diarrhea, and skin problems.

PHOTODYNAMIC THERAPY

Photodynamic therapy (PDT) is the selective destruction of cancer cells through a chemical reaction triggered by types of laser light. It can be used to destroy some cancers, reduce the size of tumors and then allow more complete tumor removal by surgery, and shrink tumors in airways or the esophagus to relieve obstruction. PDT is used most often for non-melanoma skin cancers, ocular tumors, GI tumors, and lung cancers located in the upper airways.

An agent that sensitizes cells to light is injected IV along with a dye. The intent is to sensitize cancer cells to destruction by specific wavelengths of laser light administered later. These agents enter all cells but leave normal cells more rapidly than cancer cells. Usually, within 48 to 72 hours, most of the drug has collected in high concentrations in cancer cells. At this time, a laser light is focused on the tumor. The light activates a chemical reaction in those cells retaining the sensitizing drug that induces irreversible cell damage. Some cells die and slough immediately; others continue to slough for several days. Some lesions require only one exposure to the laser, and others must be re-exposed several days after the first treatment (Agostinis et al., 2011).

❖ *PATIENT-CENTERED COLLABORATIVE CARE*

Use of first-generation photosensitizers in PDT was limited by an intense general sensitivity to light for up to 12 weeks. This light sensitivity required strict protection from all light sources for weeks. Newer photosensitizers and laser technologies have less general sensitivity, allowing greater use of this therapy with less need for intense protection.

HORMONAL MANIPULATION

Hormonal manipulation involves changing usual hormone responses. Hormones are natural chemicals secreted by endocrine glands and picked up by capillaries where they circulate to all body areas. Hormones exert their effects only on their specific target tissues. Some hormones make hormone-sensitive tumors grow more rapidly. Thus decreasing the amount of these hormones available to hormone-sensitive tumors can slow the cancer growth rate.

Hormonal manipulation includes steroids, steroid analogues, and enzyme inhibitors (aromatase inhibitors, gonadotropin-releasing hormone analogues, antiandrogens, and antiestrogens). Many of these agents are used to block

TABLE 22-7	Common Agents Used for Hormonal Manipulation of Cancer	
TYPE OF AGENT	**EXAMPLE**
Hormone Agonists	
Androgen	Fluoxymesterone (Halotestin)
	Testolactone (Teslac)
Estrogen	Chlorotrianisene (Tace)
	Conjugated equine estrogen (Premarin)
	Diethylstilbestrol (DES, Stilphostrol)
	Ethinyl estradiol (Estinyl)
Progestin	Medroxyprogesterone (Amen, Provera)
	Megestrol (Megace)
Luteinizing hormone–releasing hormone (LHRH)	Leuprolide (Eligard, Lupron, Viadur)
	Goserelin (Zoladex)
Hormone Antagonists	
Antiandrogens	Bicalutamide (Casodex)
	Flutamide (Eulexin)
Antiestrogens	Fulvestrant (Faslodex)
	Tamoxifen (Nolvadex)
	Toremifene (Fareston)
Hormone Inhibitors	
	Aminoglutethimide (Cytadren, Elipten)
	Anastrozole (Arimidex)
	Exemestane (Aromasin)
	Letrozole (Femara)

receptors and thus prevent the cancer cells from receiving normal hormonal growth stimulation.

Hormonal manipulation can help control some types of cancer for many years but does not cure the disease. If a tumor depends on hormone A for growth and a large quantity of hormone B (similar to A) is given to the patient, hormone B will interfere with the tumor's uptake of hormone A or will limit the amount produced. As a result, tumor growth is slowed and survival time increases. Table 22-7 lists drugs used in hormonal manipulation for cancer therapy.

Some drugs are *hormone antagonists* that compete with natural hormones at the receptors. When hormone antagonists are given, they bind to the specific hormone receptor on or in the tumor cell and prevent the needed hormone from binding to the receptor. If a tumor needs a certain hormone to grow and the hormone can enter or activate the cell only through a receptor, hormone antagonists can slow tumor growth.

The hormone inhibitors also are used for hormonal therapy. These drugs inhibit the normal organ production of some specific hormones. For example, the aromatase inhibitor *anastrozole* (Arimidex) prevents the production of estrogen in the adrenal gland and reduces the blood level of estrogen, which results in slower growth of some breast cancers.

Side effects of hormonal manipulation are different from those of other types of chemotherapy. Androgens and the antiestrogen receptor drugs cause masculinizing effects in women. Chest and facial hair may develop, menstrual periods stop, and breast tissue shrinks. Patients may have some fluid retention. For men and women receiving androgens, acne may develop, hypercalcemia is common, and liver dysfunction may occur with prolonged therapy. Women receiving estrogens or progestins have irregular menses, fluid retention, and breast tenderness. All patients who take estrogen or progestins are at increased risk for venous thromboembolism.

Feminine manifestations appear in men who take estrogens, progestins, or antiandrogen receptor drugs. Facial hair thins, facial skin is smoother, body fat is redistributed, and breast development (**gynecomastia**) can occur. Bone loss is common, which increases the risk for osteoporosis and pathologic bone fractures (Limburg et al., 2014). Testicular and penile atrophy also occur to some degree. Teach patients and families about expected side effects. Encourage them to express their feelings about body changes. Refer them for counseling if needed.

ONCOLOGIC EMERGENCIES

Cancer is a chronic disease. However, a number of acute complications from the cancer and its treatment can occur. There is some controversy regarding which complications are considered oncologic emergencies (Denshar et al., 2011). This chapter includes sepsis and disseminated intravascular coagulation, syndrome of inappropriate antidiuretic hormone, spinal cord compression, hypercalcemia, superior vena cava syndrome, and tumor lysis syndrome as emergencies. Early diagnosis and immediate intervention of these emergency conditions are essential to avoid life-threatening situations. The role of the nurse is to implement interventions to prevent and detect these complications early for immediate treatment.

SEPSIS AND DISSEMINATED INTRAVASCULAR COAGULATION

Sepsis, or *septicemia,* is a condition in which organisms enter the bloodstream (bloodstream infection [BSI]) and can result in septic shock, a life-threatening condition. Patients with cancer are at risk for INFECTION and sepsis because their white blood cell counts are often low and immune function is impaired. Chapter 37 describes the pathophysiology of sepsis and septic shock.

Disseminated intravascular coagulation (DIC) is a problem with the blood-CLOTTING process. DIC is triggered by many severe illnesses, including cancer. In patients with cancer, DIC often is caused by gram-negative sepsis, although viral and other bacterial INFECTIONS can trigger it. A patient's normal flora can enter the bloodstream through any site of skin breakdown and cause a severe infection, especially when neutropenia is present. Additional causes of sepsis include liver disease, intravascular hemolysis, prosthetic devices, or metabolic acidosis.

Extensive, abnormal CLOTTING occurs throughout the small blood vessels of patients with DIC. This widespread clotting depletes the existing clotting factors and platelets. As this happens, extensive bleeding occurs. Bleeding from many sites is the most common problem and ranges from minimal to fatal hemorrhage. Clots block blood vessels and decrease blood flow to major body organs and result in PAIN, strokelike manifestations, dyspnea, tachycardia, reduced kidney function, and bowel necrosis.

DIC is a life-threatening problem with a high mortality rate even when proper therapies are instituted. *Thus the best management of sepsis and DIC is prevention. Identify patients at greatest risk for sepsis and DIC. Practice strict adherence to aseptic technique during invasive procedures and during contact with nonintact skin and mucous membranes. Teach patients and* families the early manifestations of INFECTION and when to seek assistance.

When sepsis is present and DIC is likely, management focuses on reducing the INFECTION and halting the DIC process. IV antibiotic therapy is initiated. During the early phase of DIC, anticoagulants (especially heparin) are given to limit CLOTTING and prevent the rapid consumption of circulating clotting factors. When DIC has progressed and hemorrhage is the primary problem, clotting factors are given. See Chapter 37 for a more detailed discussion of the management of DIC.

SYNDROME OF INAPPROPRIATE ANTIDIURETIC HORMONE

In healthy people, antidiuretic hormone (ADH) is secreted by the posterior pituitary gland only when more fluid (water) is needed in the body, such as when plasma volume is decreased. Certain conditions induce ADH secretion when not needed by the body, which leads to syndrome of inappropriate antidiuretic hormone (SIADH).

Cancer is a common cause of SIADH, especially small cell lung cancer. SIADH also may occur with other cancers, including head and neck, melanoma, gastrointestinal, prostate, and hematologic malignancies, especially when tumors are present in the brain. Some tumors make and secrete ADH, whereas others stimulate the posterior pituitary to secrete ADH. Drugs often used in patients with cancer also can cause SIADH (e.g., morphine sulfate, cyclophosphamide).

In SIADH, water is reabsorbed in excess by the kidney and put into systemic circulation. The retained water dilutes blood sodium levels. Mild manifestations include weakness, muscle cramps, loss of appetite, and fatigue. Serum sodium levels range from 115 to 120 mEq/L or lower (normal range is 135 to 145 mEq/L). With greater fluid retention, weight gain, nervous system changes, personality changes, confusion, and extreme muscle weakness occur. As the sodium level drops toward 110 mEq/L, seizures, coma, and death may follow depending on how rapidly the sodium value is lowered.

SIADH is managed by treating the condition and the cause. Nursing priorities focus on patient safety, restoring normal fluid balance, and providing supportive care. Management includes fluid restriction, increased sodium intake, and drug therapy. One drug, demeclocycline (Declomycin), works in opposition to ADH. Immediate cancer therapy with radiation or chemotherapy may cause enough tumor regression that ADH production returns to normal. Effective treatment of the cancer triggering the syndrome is the only cure for SIADH.

Patient safety includes preventing fluid overload from becoming worse, leading to pulmonary edema and heart failure. The older adult and those with coexisting cardiac problems,

> **! NURSING SAFETY PRIORITY** (QSEN)
> **Action Alert**
>
> Monitor for increasing fluid overload (bounding pulse, increasing neck vein distention (jugular venous distention [JVD]), presence of crackles in lungs, increasing peripheral edema, reduced urine output) at least every 2 hours. *Pulmonary edema can occur very quickly and can lead to death.* Notify the health care provider of any change that indicates the fluid overload from SIADH either is not responding to therapy or is becoming worse.

kidney problems, lung problems, or liver problems are at greater risk for complications with SIADH. See Chapter 62 for a detailed discussion of SIADH management.

SPINAL CORD COMPRESSION

Spinal cord compression (SCC) and damage occur either when a tumor directly enters the spinal cord or the spinal column or when the vertebrae collapse from tumor degradation of the bone. It is a common cause of neurologic complications of cancer. Tumors may begin in the spinal cord but more often spread from the lung, prostate, breast, and colon. SCC may cause back PAIN or other problems before nerve deficits occur. Neurologic problems are specific to the level of spinal compression and can lead to paralysis, which is usually permanent if the compression is not alleviated promptly. Loss of neurologic function has a tremendous negative impact on quality of life for the patient and family.

Early recognition and treatment of spinal cord compression are key to a positive outcome. Assess for neurologic changes, including back PAIN, muscle weakness or a sensation of heaviness in the arms or legs, numbness or tingling in the hands or feet, inability to distinguish hot and cold, and an unsteady gait. Depending on how low the compression occurs, constipation, incontinence, and difficulty starting or stopping urination also may be present. Consider the possibility of SCC with new onset of any of these problems. Teach patients and families the manifestations of early SCC, and instruct them to seek help as soon as problems occur.

Treatment is often palliative with high-dose corticosteroids given first to reduce swelling around the spinal cord and relieve manifestations. High-dose radiation may be used to reduce the size of the tumor in the area and relieve compression. Surgery may be performed to remove the tumor and rearrange the bony tissue so less pressure is placed on the spinal cord. External back or neck braces may be used to reduce the weight borne by the spinal column and to reduce pressure on the spinal cord or spinal nerves.

HYPERCALCEMIA

Hypercalcemia (increased serum calcium level) occurs in up to a third of patients with cancer. At high levels it is regarded an emergency and can lead to death. Breast, lung, and renal cell carcinomas; multiple myeloma; and adult T-cell leukemia and lymphoma are the most common causes among cancer patients. These cancers can secrete parathyroid hormone, causing bone to release calcium. In addition, systemic secretion of vitamin D analogues by the tumor can also cause elevated calcium levels in the bloodstream. Decreased mobility and dehydration worsen hypercalcemia.

Early manifestations of hypercalcemia are nonspecific and lead to delayed recognition, thus worsening the impact of the problem. Common manifestations include skeletal PAIN, kidney stones, abdominal discomfort, and altered cognition. Additional manifestations include fatigue, loss of appetite, nausea, vomiting, constipation, and increased urine output. More serious problems include severe muscle weakness, loss of deep tendon reflexes, paralytic ileus, dehydration, and electrocardiographic (ECG) changes. Severity of manifestations depends on how high the calcium level is and how quickly it rose (see Chapter 11).

Cancer-induced hypercalcemia often develops slowly for many patients, which allows the body time to adapt to this electrolyte change. As a result, manifestations of hypercalcemia may not be evident until the serum calcium level is greatly elevated. Serum ionized calcium levels are the most reliable laboratory test for this complication.

Oral hydration may be enough to reduce calcium levels and relieve manifestations. Normal saline is used when IV hydration is needed. Loop diuretics can promote calcium loss in urine. Many drugs such as bisphosphonates, which block bone resorption of calcium, calcitonin, and oral glucocorticoids, can temporarily lower serum calcium levels. Treatment of the cancer is needed for long-term calcium control. When cancer-induced hypercalcemia is life threatening or occurs with kidney disease, dialysis can temporarily reduce serum calcium levels.

SUPERIOR VENA CAVA SYNDROME

The superior vena cava (SVC), which returns all blood from the cranial, neck, and upper extremity vasculature to the heart, has thin walls, and compression or obstruction by tumor growth or by clots in the vessel leads to congestion of the blood (Fig. 22-5). This is known as *superior vena cava (SVC) syndrome* and can occur quickly or develop gradually over time. With gradual development, increased collateral circulation to handle the blood flow can occur. SVC compression causes PAIN and is life threatening. It occurs most often in patients with lymphomas (especially with tumors in the mediastinum), thymoma, lung cancer, and breast cancer.

The manifestations result from the blockage of venous return from the head, neck, and upper trunk. Early manifestations occur when the patient arises after a night's sleep and include edema of the face, especially around the eyes, and tightness of the shirt or blouse collar. As the compression worsens, the patient develops engorged blood vessels and erythema of the upper body (Fig. 22-6), edema in the arms and hands, dyspnea, and epistaxis. Late manifestations include hemorrhage, cyanosis, mental status changes, decreased cardiac output, and hypotension. Radiographic imaging is essential for diagnosis and treatment planning. Death results if compression is not relieved.

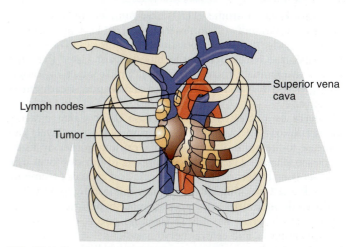

FIG. 22-5 Compression of the superior vena cava by lymph nodes and tumors in superior vena cava syndrome.

FIG. 22-6 Appearance of the face, neck, upper arms, and chest in a patient with superior vena cava syndrome.

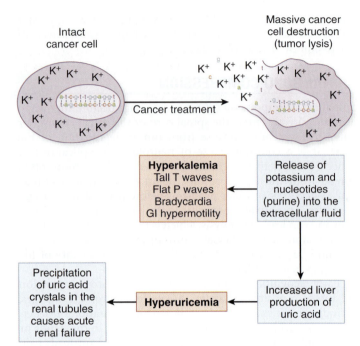

FIG. 22-7 Pathology of tumor lysis syndrome. *K,* Potassium.

SVC syndrome is often a late-stage manifestation; the tumor is usually widespread. High-dose radiation therapy to the upper chest area may be used to provide temporary relief. Chemotherapy may be the only option for long-term control of the cancer causing the compression. Surgery is rarely performed for this condition. A metal stent can be placed in the vena cava in an interventional radiology department to relieve swelling. Follow-up angioplasty can keep this stent open for a longer period.

NCLEX EXAMINATION CHALLENGE

Safe and Effective Care Environment

Which change in health status indicates to the nurse that the client's superior vena cava syndrome is worsening?
A. The client's systolic blood pressure is rising, and the diastolic pressure is decreasing.
B. The client's severe nausea and vomiting no longer respond to antiemetics.
C. The client has experienced four nosebleeds in the past 2 days.
D. Pedal edema is now present.

TUMOR LYSIS SYNDROME

In tumor lysis syndrome (TLS), large numbers of tumor cells are destroyed rapidly (Maloney & Denno, 2011). Their intracellular contents, including potassium and purines (DNA components), are released into the bloodstream faster than the body can eliminate them (Fig. 22-7). Unlike other oncologic emergencies, TLS is a positive sign that cancer treatment is effective.

Severe or untreated TLS can cause tissue damage, acute kidney injury (AKI), and death. Serum potassium levels can increase to the point of hyperkalemia, causing cardiac dysfunction (see Chapter 11). The large amounts of purines form uric acid, causing hyperuricemia. These uric acid crystals precipitate in the kidney, blocking kidney tubules and leading to AKI. The sudden development of hyperkalemia, hyperuricemia, and hyperphosphatemia has life-threatening effects on the heart muscle, kidneys, and central nervous system.

TLS is usually seen in patients receiving radiation or chemotherapy for cancers that are very sensitive to these therapies, including leukemia, lymphoma, small cell lung cancer, germ cell tumors, inflammatory breast cancer, melanoma, and multiple myeloma. Early manifestations include lethargy, nausea, vomiting, anorexia, diarrhea, cloudy urine, flank PAIN, muscle weakness, and cramps.

Hydration prevents and manages TLS by diluting the serum potassium level and increasing the kidney flow rates. These actions prevent the precipitation of uric acid crystals, increase the excretion of potassium, and flush any kidney precipitate.

With tumors known to be very sensitive to cancer therapy, instruct patients to drink at least 3000 mL (5000 mL is more desirable) of fluid the day before, the day of, and for 3 days after treatment. Some fluids should be alkaline (sodium bicarbonate) to help prevent uric acid precipitation. Stress the importance of keeping fluid intake consistent throughout the 24-hour day, and help patients draw up a schedule of fluid intake.

Because some patients have nausea and vomiting after cancer therapy and may not feel like drinking fluids, stress the importance of following the antiemetic regimen. Instruct patients to contact the cancer care provider immediately if nausea prevents adequate fluid intake so parenteral fluids can be started.

Prophylaxis is essential for high-risk patients receiving treatment that is expected to reduce tumor burden quickly. Management becomes more aggressive for patients who become hyperkalemic or hyperuricemic. In addition to fluids, diuretics (especially osmotic types) are given to increase urine flow through the kidney. These agents are used cautiously to avoid dehydration. Drugs that promote purine excretion, such as allopurinol (Aloprim, Zyloprim), rasburicase (Elitek), or febuxostat (Uloric), are given (Mackiewicz, 2012). To reduce serum potassium levels for mild to moderate hyperkalemia, sodium polystyrene sulfonate can be given orally or as a retention enema. For more severe hyperkalemia, IV infusions containing glucose and insulin may be given. Patients who have severe hyperkalemia and hyperuricemia may need dialysis.

NURSING CONCEPTS AND CLINICAL JUDGMENT REVIEW

What might you NOTICE if the patient has impaired protection and increased INFECTION risk as a result of cancer therapy?
- Recurring infections
- Presence of opportunistic infections
- Diarrhea
- Skin lesions
- Headache
- Fever

What should you INTERPRET and how should you RESPOND to a patient who has impaired protection and increased INFECTION risk as a result cancer therapy?

Perform and interpret focused physical assessment findings including:
- Assess cardiovascular and respiratory status:
  - Vital signs
  - Presence of acute chest pain or dyspnea
  - Presence of cough
  - Presence of fever above 100°F (37.8°C)
  - Activity tolerance
- Assess urinary status:
  - Color and clarity of urine
  - Pain or burning on urination
- Assess gastrointestinal status:
  - Mouth, oropharynx, and perineal area for manifestations of infection

- Presence of dysphagia
- Presence of nausea, vomiting, diarrhea

Respond by:
- Collaborating with members of the health care team to protect the patient from infection
- Monitoring laboratory test results to determine indications of infection
- Teaching the patient and family about reporting changes indicating infection immediately
- Teaching the patient and family how to avoid infection in the home environment
- Continuing to assess for changes in the patient's condition, especially indications of infection in any body area

On what should you REFLECT?
- Evaluate the patient's and family's knowledge of neutropenia and its management.
- Evaluate the patient's and family's stress levels, use of coping strategies, and knowledge about community resources.
- Assess the knowledge and proficiency of unlicensed assistive personnel (UAP) in carrying out infection control measures.

GET READY FOR THE NCLEX® EXAMINATION!

KEY POINTS

Review these Key Points for each NCLEX Examination Client Needs Category.

Safe and Effective Care Environment
- Use aseptic technique during care for open skin areas or any invasive procedure to prevent INFECTION. **Safety** QSEN
- Perform good handwashing before providing any care to patients with neutropenia.
- Use Bleeding Precautions for any patient with thrombocytopenia and impaired CLOTTING (see Chart 22-5). **Safety** QSEN
- Use appropriate personal protective equipment (gowns, gloves, masks, eye protection) when mixing or administering IV or oral chemotherapeutic drugs and when handling the excreta of a patient receiving chemotherapy and for 48 hours afterward. **Safety** QSEN
- Position shields properly when patients in inpatient settings are receiving brachytherapy. **Safety** QSEN

Health Promotion and Maintenance
- Teach patients receiving radiation therapy how to care for the skin in the radiation path (see Chart 22-2). **Patient-Centered Care** QSEN
- Teach the patient and family about the manifestations of INFECTION and when to seek medical advice. **Patient-Centered Care** QSEN

- Teach patients at risk for bleeding from impaired CLOTTING the precautions to avoid injury (see Chart 22-6). **Patient-Centered Care** QSEN
- Instruct patients to use prescribed antiemetic drugs on a schedule for maximum relief of nausea and vomiting. **Patient-Centered Care** QSEN

Psychosocial Integrity
- Allow the patient and family the opportunity to express concerns regarding the diagnosis of cancer or the treatment regimen. **Patient-Centered Care** QSEN
- Encourage the patient to verbalize feelings about changes in appearance resulting from cancer therapy. **Patient-Centered Care** QSEN
- Explain all procedures, restrictions, drugs, and follow-up care to the patient and family.
- Encourage patients to use strategies to improve their appearance when alopecia occurs. **Patient-Centered Care** QSEN
- Refer patients and family members to local cancer resources and support groups.
- Ensure that patient preferences are honored whenever possible. **Patient-Centered Care** QSEN

Physiological Integrity
- Perform a total assessment each time the patient with cancer is seen to determine the level of cancer treatment side effects

and whether an oncologic emergency exists. **Patient-Centered Care** QSEN

- Assess the patient's PAIN level on a regular basis. **Patient-Centered Care** QSEN
- Use pharmacologic and nonpharmacologic therapies to reduce PAIN for the patient with cancer. **Patient-Centered Care** QSEN
- Work with other members of the health care team to ensure the implementation of a personalized PAIN management regimen. **Teamwork and Collaboration** QSEN
- Assess the venous access device at least every 30 to 60 minutes during chemotherapy administration. **Safety** QSEN
- Assess the patient receiving chemotherapy for INFECTION at least every 8 hours. **Safety** QSEN
- Inspect the oral mucosa of patients with neutropenia at least every 8 hours. **Evidence-Based Practice** QSEN
- Report any temperature over 100°F (37.8°C) in a patient with neutropenia. **Evidence-Based Practice** QSEN

- Assess the patient with thrombocytopenia and impaired CLOTTING for bleeding. **Safety** QSEN
- Instruct the patient and family caring for skin in the path of radiation therapy.
- Assess the patient receiving hormonal therapy for evidence of blood clot formation. **Safety** QSEN
- Closely monitor patients receiving any type of targeted therapy for manifestations of severe side effects or adverse drug reactions. **Safety** QSEN
- Teach patients and families the manifestations of oncologic emergencies and when to notify the health care provider. **Patient-Centered Care** QSEN
- Assist patients and families experiencing cancer to find appropriate community resources for support, supplies, care, and other assistance.

CHAPTER 23

Care of Patients with Infection

Donna D. Ignatavicius

 http://evolve.elsevier.com/Iggy/

PRIORITY CONCEPTS

- INFECTION
- IMMUNITY

LEARNING OUTCOMES

Safe and Effective Care Environment

1. Describe INFECTION control methods, such as hand hygiene and Transmission-Based Precautions.
2. Apply current principles of INFECTION prevention and control.

Health Promotion and Maintenance

3. Specify health teaching for patients, families, and staff about INFECTION control measures.

Psychosocial Integrity

4. Plan ways to help patients cope with Transmission-Based Precautions.

Physiological Integrity

5. Identify patients most at risk for INFECTION, including older adults.
6. Provide information to patient and family about drug therapy for infections.
7. Identify common clinical manifestations of infections and infectious diseases.
8. Interpret laboratory test findings related to infections and infectious diseases.
9. Evaluate nursing interventions for management of the patient with an INFECTION.
10. Explain why multidrug-resistant organisms are increasing.
11. Identify basic clinical management for common emerging diseases.

The human body has many *protective* systems that promote homeostasis. Physiologic mechanisms are the structural and functional defenses that protect people from stressors such as infection. When these mechanisms fail to work properly or are overcome with microbes, INFECTION can result.

INFECTIONS and infectious diseases have been the major cause of millions of deaths worldwide for centuries. Threats of bioterrorism have been added to the concerns about multidrug-resistant and emerging infections. Global travel and migration have increased exposure to a wider variety of infectious agents than in the past.

Advancing technology and invasive procedures also introduce microorganisms into the body, often resulting in INFECTION. In other environments these microorganisms are harmless. This chapter provides an overview of infection and general principles for prevention and management. Specific infections and their management are described elsewhere in this text.

OVERVIEW OF THE INFECTIOUS PROCESS

A **pathogen** is any microorganism (also called an *agent*) capable of producing disease. Infections can be **communicable** (transmitted from person to person [e.g., influenza]) or not communicable (e.g., peritonitis). Microorganisms with differing levels of **pathogenicity** (ability to cause disease) surround everyone. **Virulence** is a term for pathogenicity. However, virulence is related more to the frequency with which a pathogen causes disease (degree of communicability) and its ability to invade and damage a host. It can also indicate the severity of the disease.

Many microorganisms live in or on the human host without causing disease. Some microbes are beneficial. Each body location harbors its own characteristic bacteria, or **normal flora**. Normal flora often functions to compete with and prevent INFECTION from unfamiliar agents attempting to invade a body site. In some instances, microorganisms that are often pathogenic may be present in the tissues of the host and yet not cause symptomatic disease because of normal flora; this process is called *colonization*.

In the United States, the Centers for Disease Control and Prevention (CDC) collects information about the occurrence and nature of infections and infectious diseases. It then recommends guidelines to health care agencies for infection control and prevention. Certain diseases, such as tuberculosis, must be reported to health departments and the CDC. The infection control practitioner (ICP) for each health care agency is responsible for tracking infections (**surveillance**) and ensuring compliance with federal and local requirements and accreditation standards.

Transmission of Infectious Agents

Transmission of INFECTION requires three factors:
- Reservoir (or source) of infectious agents
- Susceptible host with a portal of entry
- Mode of transmission

Reservoirs (sources of infectious agents) are numerous. Animate reservoirs include people, animals, and insects. Inanimate reservoirs include soil, water, other environmental sources, and medical equipment (e.g., IV solutions, urine collection devices). Stethoscopes used for auscultation by many health care providers carry *Staphylococcus aureus* from the skin of one patient to another. These devices should be cleaned with an antibacterial solution between patients (Alspach, 2014). The host's body can be a reservoir; pathogens colonize skin and body substances (e.g., feces, sputum, saliva, wound drainage). A person with an active INFECTION or an asymptomatic **carrier** (one who harbors an infectious agent without active disease) is a reservoir. Examples of *community* reservoirs include sewage, stagnant or contaminated water, and improperly handled foods.

Bacteria like *Neisseria meningitidis* can exist in the respiratory tract while causing no illness. If the bacteria invade the bloodstream or cerebrospinal fluid, they become extremely pathogenic. Another example is *Enterococcus,* which lives as normal flora in the GI system, where it is nonpathogenic and assists in the digestive process. If it enters the bloodstream, *Enterococcus* can cause disease.

Continued multiplication of a pathogen is sometimes accompanied by toxin production. **Toxins** are protein molecules released by bacteria to affect host cells at a distant site. *Exotoxins* are produced and released by certain bacteria into the surrounding environment. Botulism, tetanus, diphtheria, and *Escherichia coli* 0157:H7–related systemic diseases are attributed to exotoxins. *Endotoxins* are produced in the cell walls of certain bacteria and released only with cell lysis. For example, typhoid and meningococcal diseases are caused by endotoxins.

Host factors influence the development of INFECTION (Table 23-1). Host defenses provide the body with an efficient system for *protection* against pathogens. Breakdown of these defense mechanisms may increase the **susceptibility** (risk) of the host for infection.

The patient's *immune status* plays a large role in determining risk for infection. Congenital abnormalities, as well as acquired health problems (e.g., renal failure, steroid dependence, cancer, acquired immune deficiency syndrome [AIDS]), can result in numerous immunologic deficiencies. Depression of IMMUNITY may make the host more susceptible to infection or impair the ability to combat organisms that have gained entry.

Immunity is resistance to INFECTION; it is usually associated with the presence of antibodies or cells that act on specific microorganisms. **Passive immunity** is of short duration (days or months) and either natural by transplacental transfer from the mother or artificial by injection of antibodies (e.g., immunoglobulin). **Active immunity** lasts for years and is natural by infection or artificial by stimulation of the body's immune defenses (e.g., vaccination). Chapter 17 discusses the immune system and IMMUNITY in detail.

Environmental factors can also influence patients' immune status and thus their susceptibility to or ability to fight

TABLE 23-1	Host Factors That Influence the Development of Infection	
HOST FACTOR	**INCREASED RISK FOR INFECTION**
Natural immunity	Congenital or acquired immune deficiencies
Normal flora	Alteration of normal flora by antibiotic therapy
Age	Infants and older adults
Hormonal factors	Diabetes mellitus, corticosteroid therapy, and adrenal insufficiency
Phagocytosis	Defective phagocytic function, circulatory disturbances, and neutropenia
Skin/mucous membranes/ normal excretory secretions	Break in skin or mucous membrane integrity; interference with flow of urine, tears, or saliva; interference with cough reflex or ciliary action; changes in gastric secretions
Nutrition	Malnutrition or dehydration
Environmental factors	Tobacco and alcohol consumption and inhalation of toxic chemicals
Medical interventions	Invasive therapy such as endoscopy, urinary catheters, IVs; chemotherapy, radiation therapy, and steroid therapy (suppress immune system); surgery

CHART 23-1 Nursing Focus on the Older Adult

Factors That May Increase Risk for Infection in the Older Patient

FACTOR	AGING-ASSOCIATED CHANGES OR CONDITIONS
• Immune system	• Decreased antibody production, lymphocytes, and fever response
• Integumentary system	• Thinning skin, decreased subcutaneous tissue, decreased vascularity, slower wound healing
• Respiratory system	• Decreased cough and gag reflexes
• Gastrointestinal system	• Decreased gastric acid and intestinal motility
• Chronic illness	• Diabetes mellitus, chronic obstructive pulmonary disease, neurologic impairments
• Functional/cognitive impairments	• Immobility, incontinence, dementia
• Invasive devices	• Urinary catheters, feeding tubes, IV devices, tracheostomy tubes
• Institutionalization	• Increased person-to-person contact and transmission

INFECTION. Examples include alcohol consumption, nicotine use, inhalation of bone marrow–suppressing toxic chemicals, and certain vitamin deficiencies. Malnutrition, especially protein-calorie malnutrition, places patients at increased risk for infection. Diseases such as diabetes mellitus also predispose a patient to infection. Older adults have decreased immunity, as well as other physiologic changes that make them very susceptible to infection (Chart 23-1).

Medical and surgical interventions may impair normal immune response. Steroid therapy, chemotherapy, and anti-rejection drugs increase the risk for INFECTION. Medical devices (e.g., intravascular or urinary catheters, endotracheal tubes, synthetic implants) may also interfere with normal host defense mechanisms. Surgery, trauma, radiation therapy, and burns result in nonintact skin. *The body's skin is one of the best barriers or defenses against infection.* When this barrier is broken, infection often results. Microorganisms may enter the body in a variety of ways, including the respiratory tract, GI tract, genitourinary tract, skin and mucous membranes, and bloodstream.

Routes of Transmission

Pathogens may enter the body through the *respiratory tract.* Microbes in droplets are sprayed into the air when people with infected oral or nasal tissues talk, cough, or sneeze. A susceptible host then inhales droplets, and pathogens localize in the lungs or are distributed via the lymphatic system or bloodstream to other areas of the body. Microorganisms that enter the body by the respiratory tract and produce distant infection include influenza virus, *Mycobacterium tuberculosis,* and *Streptococcus pneumoniae.*

Other pathogens enter the body through the *GI tract.* Some stay there and produce disease (e.g., *Shigella* causing self-limited disease). Others invade the GI tract to produce local and distant infection (e.g., *Salmonella enteritidis*). Some produce limited GI symptoms, causing systemic infection (e.g., *Salmonella typhi*) or profound involvement of other organs (e.g., hepatitis A virus). Millions of foodborne illness cases occur each year in the United States. This type of illness results in many hospitalizations and deaths.

Microorganisms also enter through the *genitourinary tract.* *Urinary tract infection (UTI) is one of the most common health care–associated infections (HAIs).* More than half of patients in adult intensive care units (ICUs) have urinary catheters in place. Indwelling urinary catheters are a primary cause of *catheter-associated urinary tract infections (CAUTIs),* especially in older adults. CAUTIs can increase hospital costs by prolonging the patient's length of stay and complicating the patient's recovery. In many settings, nurse-driven protocols have helped decrease the use of urinary catheters and associated infections (see the Quality Improvement box).

Although intact skin is the best barrier to prevent most infections, some pathogens such as *Treponema pallidum* can enter the body through intact *skin* or *mucous membranes.* Most enter through breaks in these normally effective surface barriers. Sometimes a medical procedure creates a break in cutaneous or mucocutaneous barriers, as in catheter-acquired **bacteremia** (bacteria in the bloodstream) and surgical-site infections (SSIs). *Fragile skin of older patients and of those receiving prolonged steroid therapy increases infection risk.*

Microorganisms can gain direct access to the *bloodstream,* especially when invasive devices or tubes are used. The incidence of bloodstream infections (BSIs) continues to increase in hospitals throughout the United States. Central venous catheters (CVCs) are a primary cause of these infections (see Chapter 13 for more discussion of CVC-related BSIs). In the community setting, biting insects can inject organisms into the bloodstream, causing infection (e.g., Lyme disease, West Nile viral encephalitis).

QUALITY IMPROVEMENT (QSEN)

Reducing Catheter-Associated Urinary Tract Infections

Mori, C. (2014). A-voiding catastrophe: Implementing a nurse-driven protocol. *MEDSURG Nursing, 23*(1), 15-21, 28.

In spite of the move to decrease the use of indwelling urinary catheters (e.g., Foley catheters), catheter-associated urinary tract infections (CAUTIs) remain a major cause of sepsis and increased hospital costs. The Centers for Medicare and Medicaid Services (CMS) recently began to link health care reimbursement to quality improvement efforts to prevent CAUTIs.

An interdisciplinary team led by a clinical nurse specialist in a Midwestern community hospital implemented a protocol that decreased the use of urinary catheters and ensured best practices for patients for whom the catheters were indicated. Using a screening checklist, each patient was assessed to determine the need for a Foley catheter. If certain criteria were not met, the catheter was removed by a nurse using a specific protocol during and after removal. For patients who had to have a Foley catheter, the nurse provided care to minimize the chance for urinary infection, including checking that the:

- Catheter was secure
- Tamper-evident seal was intact
- Catheter tubing was not twisted or had a dependent loop
- Catheter bag was positioned lower than the bladder level
- Drainage bag did not touch the floor or was overfilled.

Commentary: Implications for Practice and Research

Research demonstrates that decreasing the use of indwelling urinary catheters is the most important intervention to prevent hospital-acquired CAUTIs. This project used this research and showed how an interdisciplinary team led by a CNS in a community hospital could improve the quality of care by decreasing urinary tract infections. In addition, nurses provided evidence-based care for patients who needed urinary catheters to ensure adequate urinary flow.

A limitation of the project was that incremental changes or strategies to maintain the positive changes were not discussed. More quality improvement activities at a unit or health care agency are needed to use current research, sustain a change in nursing practice, and achieve positive patient outcomes.

Methods of Transmission

For INFECTION to be transmitted from an infected source to a susceptible host, a transport mechanism is required. Microorganisms are transmitted by several routes:

- Contact transmission (indirect and direct)
- Droplet transmission
- Airborne transmission

Contact transmission is the usual mode of transmission of most infections. Many INFECTIONS are spread by direct or indirect contact. With *direct contact,* the source and host have physical contact. Microorganisms are transferred directly from skin to skin or from mucous membrane to mucous membrane. Often called *person-to-person transmission,* direct contact is best illustrated by the spread of the "common cold."

Indirect contact transmission involves the transfer of microorganisms from a source to a host by passive transfer from a contaminated object. Contaminated articles or hands may be sources of infection. For example, patient-care devices like glucometers and electronic thermometers may transmit pathogens if they are contaminated with blood or body fluids. Uniforms, laboratory coats, and isolation gowns used as part of personal protective equipment (PPE) may be contaminated as well.

Indirect transmission may involve contact with infected secretions or *droplets*. Droplets are produced when a person talks or sneezes; the droplets travel short distances. Susceptible hosts may acquire infection by contact with droplets deposited on the nasal, oral, or conjunctival membranes. Therefore the CDC recommends that staff stay at least 3 feet (1 m) away from a patient with droplet infection. An example of droplet-spread INFECTION is influenza.

Airborne transmission occurs when small airborne particles containing pathogens leave the infected source and enter a susceptible host. These pathogens can be suspended in the air for a prolonged time. The particles carrying pathogens are usually contained in droplet nuclei or dust; they are usually propelled from the respiratory tract by coughing or sneezing. A susceptible person then inhales the particles directly into the respiratory tract. For example, tuberculosis is spread via airborne transmission.

Preventing the spread of microbes that are transmitted by the airborne route requires the use of special air handling and ventilation systems in an airborne infection isolation room (AIIR). *M. tuberculosis* and the varicella-zoster virus (chicken-pox) are examples of airborne agents that require one of these systems. In addition to the AIIR, respiratory protection using a certified **powered air purifying respirator (PAPR)** is recommended for health care personnel entering the patient's room. This device has a high efficiency particulate air (HEPA) filter and battery to promote positive-pressure airflow and is more effective than N95 respirators.

Other sources of infectious agents include the environment, such as contaminated food, water, or vectors. Vectors are insects that carry pathogens between two or more hosts, such as the deer tick that causes Lyme disease.

The *portal of exit* completes the chain of INFECTION. Exit of the microbe from the host often occurs through the portal of entry. An organism, such as *M. tuberculosis*, enters the respiratory tract and then exits the same tract as the infected host coughs. Some organisms can exit from the infected host by several routes. For example, varicella-zoster virus can spread through direct contact with infective fluid in vesicles and by airborne transmission.

Physiologic Defenses for Infection

Strong and intact host defenses can prevent microbes from entering the body or can destroy a pathogen that has entered. Impaired host defenses may be unable to defend against microbial invasion, allowing entry of organisms that can destroy cells and cause INFECTION. Common defense mechanisms include:

- Body tissues
- Phagocytosis
- Inflammation
- Immune systems

Intact skin forms the first and most important physical barrier to the entry of microorganisms. In addition to providing a mechanical barrier, the skin's slightly acidic pH (resulting from break-down of lipids into fatty acids), together with normal skin flora, creates an unfriendly environment for many bacteria.

Mucous membranes' mucociliary action provides some mechanical protection against pathogenic invasion. More important, however, mucous membranes are bathed in secretions that inactivate many microorganisms. Lysozymes, which dissolve the cell walls of some bacteria, are present in large quantities in many body secretions, particularly in tears and nasal mucus.

Other body systems provide natural barriers to INFECTION. For instance, the healthy respiratory tract clears most of all inhaled material by upper airway filtration, humidification, mucociliary transport, and coughing. Peristaltic action mechanically empties the GI tract of pathogenic organisms. Stomach acid, intestinal secretions, pancreatic enzymes, and bile, together with the competition from normal bowel flora, provide an environment that protects the GI tract from invasion by harmful organisms. In the genitourinary tract, the flushing action of urine eliminates pathogenic organisms. The low pH of urine also maintains a sterile environment, although some microorganisms, such as *E. coli*, can thrive in an acid medium.

Phagocytosis occurs when a foreign substance evades the first-line mechanical barriers and enters the body. Various leukocyte types function differently in the immune reaction, but neutrophils bear primary responsibility for phagocytosis. This process of engulfing, ingesting, killing, and disposing of an invading organism is an essential mechanism in host defense. Phagocytic dysfunction dramatically increases a patient's risk for INFECTION.

Inflammation is another important nonspecific defense mechanism for preventing the spread of INFECTION. It occurs when tissue becomes damaged. Damaged cells release enzymes, and polymorphonuclear (PMN) leukocytes (neutrophils) are attracted to the infected site from the bloodstream. One important substance, histamine, increases the permeability of the capillaries in inflamed tissues, thus allowing fluid, proteins, and white blood cells to enter an inflamed area. Other enzymes activate fibrinogen, which causes leaked fluid to clot and prevents its flow away from the damaged site into unaffected tissue, essentially "walling off" the inflamed tissue. The process of phagocytosis disposes of the invading microorganism and often dead tissue. If inflammation is caused by infection, the end products of inflammation form pus, which is then absorbed or exits the body through a break in the skin. Chapter 17 discusses the process of inflammation in more detail.

Specific defense responses to specific microorganisms are provided by the antibody- and cell-mediated immune systems. The **antibody-mediated immune system** produces antibodies directed against certain pathogens. These antibodies inactivate or destroy invading microorganisms as well as protect against future infection from that microorganism. Resistance to other microorganisms is mediated by the action of specifically sensitized T-lymphocytes and is called **cell-mediated immunity**. The components of the immune system work both independently and together to protect against infection. Chapter 17 describes the function of the immune system in detail.

HEALTH PROMOTION AND MAINTENANCE

Infections occur most often in high-risk patients, such as older adults and those who have inadequate immune systems (immunocompromised). Implement interventions to prevent infection and detect signs and symptoms as early as possible. Chart 23-2 summarizes nursing interventions for INFECTION prevention and control.

Infection Control in Health Care Settings

INFECTION acquired in the inpatient health care setting (not present or incubating at admission) is termed a **health**

CHART 23-2 Best Practices for Patient Safety & Quality Care (QSEN)

Nursing Interventions for the Patient at Risk for Infection

- Assess patients for risk for infections.
- Monitor for signs and symptoms of infection.
- Monitor laboratory tests results, such as cultures and white blood cell (WBC) count and differential.
- Screen all visitors for infections or infectious disease.
- Inspect skin and mucous membranes for redness, heat, pain, swelling, and drainage.
- Promote sufficient nutritional intake, especially protein for healing.
- Encourage fluid intake to treat fever.
- Teach the patient and family the signs and symptoms of infections and when to report them to the health care provider.
- Teach the patient and family how to avoid infections in health care agencies and the community.

CHART 23-3 Best Practice for Patient Safety & Quality Care (QSEN)

Hand Hygiene

- When hands are visibly soiled or contaminated with proteinaceous material or are visibly soiled with blood or other body fluids, wash hands with soap and water.
- If hands are not visibly soiled, use an alcohol-based hand rub (ABHR) for decontaminating hands or wash hands with soap and water.
- Use either ABHR or wash with soap and water (decontaminate hands) before having direct contact with patients.
- Decontaminate hands before donning sterile gloves to perform a procedure, such as inserting an invasive device (e.g., indwelling urinary catheter).
- Decontaminate hands after contact with a patient's intact skin (e.g., taking a pulse) or with body fluids or excretions/secretions.
- Decontaminate hands after removing gloves.
- Decontaminate hands after contact with inanimate objects (including medical equipment) in the immediate vicinity of the patient.

---

care–associated infection (HAI). When occurring in a hospital setting, they are sometimes referred to as *hospital-acquired infections,* but the former term is more accurate. HAIs can be *endogenous* (from a patient's flora) or *exogenous* (from outside the patient, often from the hands of health care workers, tubes, or implants). HAIs, including surgical site infections (SSIs), cause increased health care costs and many deaths (see discussion in Chapter 16). These infections tend to occur most often because health care workers do not follow basic infection control principles.

Infection control within a health care facility is designed to reduce the risk for HAIs and thus reduce morbidity and mortality, as recommended in The Joint Commission's National Patient Safety Goals (NPSGs). This expected outcome is consistent with the desire for health care facilities to create a *culture of safety* within their environments (see Chapter 1). INFECTION control and prevention is an interdisciplinary effort and includes:

- Facility- and department-specific infection control policies and procedures
- Surveillance and analysis
- Patient and staff education
- Community and interdisciplinary collaboration
- Product evaluation with an emphasis on quality and cost savings
- Bioengineering for designing health care facilities that help control the spread of infections

The INFECTION control program of a hospital is coordinated and implemented by a health care professional certified in infection control (CIC) who has clinical and administrative experience. The Centers for Disease Control and Prevention (CDC) recommends one person with CIC credentials for every 100 occupied acute care beds. Long-term care facilities may not have a practitioner who specializes in infection control. However, every facility must designate a health care professional to be responsible for coordinating and implementing an infection prevention and control program.

Long-term care facilities are unique in that they have a large group of older adults who are together in one setting for weeks to years. Nursing homes, in particular, are required to provide a homelike environment in which residents can move and interact freely. Therefore INFECTION control in these settings can be challenging. As a result, many infectious outbreaks may occur,

such as pneumonia, *Clostridium difficile,* and multidrug-resistant organisms (discussed in the Multidrug-Resistant Organism Infections and Colonizations section on p. 405).

Ambulatory and home health care are the fastest growing segments of the health care system. INFECTION remains a common cause of death for dialysis patients. Little information is available about acquired infections in home health settings because data are not systematically collected, surveillance programs are not established, and best practices for infection prevention and control do not yet exist.

Methods of Infection Control and Prevention

All health care workers who come in contact with patients or care areas are involved in some aspect of the infection control program of the agency. According to the CDC, infections can be prevented or controlled in several ways:

- Hand hygiene
- Disinfection/sterilization
- Standard Precautions
- Transmission-Based Precautions
- Staff and patient placement and cohorting

Hand Hygiene

Health care workers' hands are the primary way in which infection is transmitted from patient to patient or staff to patient. Hand hygiene refers to both handwashing and alcohol-based hand rubs (ABHRs) ("hand sanitizers").

In 2002, the U.S. CDC released a document entitled "CDC Hand Hygiene Recommendations." These recommendations are summarized in Chart 23-3. *Handwashing is still an important part of hand hygiene, but it is recognized that in some health care settings, sinks may not be readily available.* Despite years of education, health care workers do not wash their hands or perform hand hygiene on a consistent basis (Upshaw-Owens & Bailey, 2012). The Quality Improvement box describes one hospital unit's project to improve the percentage of health care workers who perform hand hygiene.

Effective handwashing includes wetting, soaping, lathering, applying friction under running water for at least 15 seconds, rinsing, and adequate drying. Friction is essential to remove skin oils and to disperse transient bacteria and soil from hand surfaces. Performing adequate handwashing takes time that health care workers (HCWs) may not feel they have. Handwashing can

Foulk, K.C., Tocydlowski, P., Snow, T.M., McCloud, K., Cuevas, M., Bishop, D., et al. (2012). Infusing fun into quality and safety initiatives. *Nursing2012, 42*(11), 14-16.

QUALITY IMPROVEMENT (QSEN)

Improving Nursing Staff Compliance with Proper Hand Hygiene

Proper hand hygiene is essential for patient safety to prevent the spread of infection. Nurses on a medical-surgical unit in a large mid-Atlantic hospital recognized that their unit's compliance with using proper hand hygiene was only 71%, lower than the rate for the rest of the hospital. As a result, the unit had a total of 12 *Clostridium difficile* infections over a one-year period. The quality and safety (QI) council of the unit set a goal of achieving 90% compliance with proper hand hygiene and implemented a project to change practice over the next year.

Interventions used to increase compliance included reminders in monthly staff meetings and newsletters, e-mails, and bulletin board postings. A hand hygiene game and music video (entitled "Get Your Clean On") were developed and used by the nursing staff. Each shift's charge nurse gave red laminated hands to any staff member who was not performing proper hand hygiene. The member who collected the most "hot hands" at the end of the shift was considered the most noncompliant. As a result of these interventions, the data for the following year revealed a 98% compliance with proper hand hygiene and a total of only 6 *C. difficile* infections. These data suggest that increased compliance with hand hygiene resulted in a decrease in hospital-acquired infections.

Commentary: Implications for Practice and Research

Research demonstrates that proper hand hygiene is the most important intervention to prevent hospital-acquired infections. This project utilized this research and showed how one group of nurses on a hospital unit could improve the quality of care by decreasing unit infections. The staff took a unit view to develop a variety of approaches to change behaviors. They reported that the project was fun as well as informative.

A limitation of the project was that incremental changes or strategies to maintain the positive changes were not discussed. More quality improvement activities at a unit or health care agency are needed to utilize current research, sustain a change in nursing practice, and achieve positive patient outcomes.

also cause dry skin, and therefore hand moisturizers are essential to maintain good hand health and hygiene.

Alcohol-based hand rubs (ABHRs) allow care providers to spend less time seeking out sinks and more time delivering care. However, these hand rubs have their limitations.

! NURSING SAFETY PRIORITY (QSEN)

Action Alert

If your hands are visibly dirty or soiled or feel sticky or if you have just toileted, *wash your hands instead of using ABHRs.* Keep in mind that ABHRs are also ineffective against spore-forming organisms such as *Clostridium difficile,* a common cause of health care–associated diarrhea, especially in older adults. Do not use an ABHR before inserting eye drops, ointments, or contact lenses because alcohol can irritate the patient's eyes, causing burning and redness. The Joint Commission's National Patient Safety Goals require that health care agencies monitor handwashing practices and the use of ABHRs to make sure that HCWs are performing hand hygiene on a regular basis.

The CDC recommends using antiseptic solutions such as chlorhexidine for handwashing in caring for patients who are at high risk for infection (e.g., those who are immunocompromised).

The classic CDC guidelines (Centers for Disease Control and Prevention [CDC], 2002) also address the issue of artificial fingernails, which have been linked to a number of outbreaks due to poor fingernail health and hygiene. The guidelines recommend that artificial fingernails and extenders not be worn while caring for patients at high risk for infections, such as those in ICUs or operating suites. Most health care agencies have banned artificial nails for all health care workers providing direct patient care and require that natural nails be short. Some agencies also ban the use of nail polish.

Sterilization and Disinfection

Sterilization and disinfection have helped invasive procedures become much more common and safe. **Sterilization** means destroying all living organisms and bacterial spores. Many invasive procedures, such as inserting vascular access devices (VADs) and urinary catheters, require sterile technique. Sterile technique in the operating suite is discussed in detail in Chapter 15.

All items that invade human tissue where bacteria are not commonly found should be sterilized. **Disinfection** does not kill spores and only ensures a reduction in the level of disease-causing organisms. High-level disinfection is adequate when an item is going inside the body where the patient has resident bacteria or normal flora (e.g., GI and respiratory tracts). As with sterilization, no high-level disinfection can occur without first cleaning the item. This can be especially difficult with items that have narrow lumens in which organic debris can become trapped and is not easily visible. For example, endoscopes have been especially challenging to clean and have been linked to a number of infectious outbreaks.

Standard Precautions

The 2007 guidelines from the CDC focus on transmission mechanisms and the precautions needed to prevent the spread of infection. Included in these guidelines are Standard Precautions and Transmission-Based Precautions, including Airborne, Droplet, and Contact Precautions (Tables 23-2 and 23-3).

Standard Precautions are based on the belief that all body excretions, secretions, and moist membranes and tissues, excluding perspiration, are potentially infectious. As barriers to potential or actual infections, **personal protective equipment (PPE)** is used. PPE refers to gloves, isolation gowns, face protection (masks, goggles, face shields), and powered air purifying respirators (PAPRs) or N95 respirators (Fig. 23-1).

! NURSING SAFETY PRIORITY (QSEN)

Action Alert

Remember that gloves are an essential part of INFECTION control and should always be worn as part of Standard Precautions. Either handwashing or use of alcohol-based hand rubs should be done before donning and after removing gloves. The combination of hand hygiene and wearing gloves is the most effective strategy for preventing infection transmission!

Health care settings in the United States and Canada have switched from latex to non-latex gloves. The U.S. National Institute for Occupational Safety and Health (NIOSH) issued a public warning about potential allergic reactions to those exposed to latex in gloves and other medical products. Reactions include rashes, nasal or eye symptoms, asthma, and (rarely) shock. People with **latex allergy** usually have an allergy to foods such as bananas, kiwis, and avocados. Health care

TABLE 23-2 Recommendations for Application of Standard Precautions for the Care of All Patients in All Health Care Settings

COMPONENT	RECOMMENDATIONS
Hand hygiene	Perform hand hygiene after touching blood, body fluids, secretions, excretions, contaminated items; immediately after removing gloves; between patient contacts
Personal protective equipment (PPE)	Use appropriate PPE, including:
• Gloves	For touching blood, body fluids, secretions, excretions, contaminated items; for touching mucous membranes and nonintact skin
• Gown	During procedures and patient-care activities when contact of clothing/exposed skin with blood/body fluids, secretions, and excretions is anticipated
• Mask, eye protection (goggles), face shield*	During procedures and patient-care activities likely to generate splashes or sprays of blood, body fluids, secretions, especially suctioning, endotracheal intubation
Soiled patient-care equipment	Handle in a manner that prevents transfer of microorganisms to others and to the environment; wear gloves if visibly contaminated; perform hand hygiene
Environmental control	Develop procedures for routine care, cleaning, and disinfection of environmental surfaces, especially frequently touched surfaces in patient-care areas
Textiles and laundry	Handle in a manner that prevents transfer of microorganisms to others and to the environment
Needles and other sharps	Do not recap, bend, break, or hand-manipulate used needles; use safety features such as needleless systems when available; place used sharps in puncture-resistant container
Patient resuscitation	Use mouthpiece, resuscitation bag, other ventilation devices to prevent contact with mouth and oral secretions
Patient placement	Prioritize for single-patient room if patient is at increased risk for transmission, is likely to contaminate the environment, does not maintain appropriate hygiene, or is at increased risk for acquiring infection or developing adverse outcome following infection
Respiratory hygiene/cough etiquette (source containment of infectious respiratory secretions in symptomatic patients, beginning at initial point of encounter [e.g., triage and reception areas in emergency departments and physician offices])	Instruct symptomatic persons to cover mouth/nose when sneezing/coughing; use tissues and dispose in no-touch receptacle; observe hand hygiene after soiling of hands with respiratory secretions; wear surgical mask if tolerated or maintain spatial separation, >3 feet if possible

*During aerosol-generating procedures on patients with suspected or proven infections transmitted by respiratory aerosols, wear a powered air purifying respirator (PAPR) (most effective) or N95 mask in addition to gloves, gown, and face/eye protection.

workers (HCWs) have not been as strict with wearing gloves as they should because of poor fit or skin dryness, irritation, and dermatitis. One possible solution to dry skin is the use of aloe vera–coated gloves or moisturizers such as Eucerin or AmLactin products.

The respiratory hygiene/cough etiquette (RH/CE) requirement is directed at patients and visitors with signs of respiratory illness, such as sinus or chest congestion, cough, or rhinorrhea ("runny nose"). The elements for RH/CE include:

- Patient, staff, and visitor education
- Posted signs
- Hand hygiene
- Covering the nose and mouth with a tissue and prompt tissue disposal or using surgical masks (or sneezing/coughing into a shirt sleeve rather than the hand)
- Separation from the person with respiratory INFECTION by more than 3 feet (1 m)

Transmission-Based Precautions

Transmission-Based Precautions may also be referred to as *Isolation Precautions.* But, the word *isolation* implies that the patient is physically separated from everyone, which is not always the case.

Airborne Precautions are used for patients known or suspected to have INFECTIONS transmitted by the airborne transmission route. These infections are caused by organisms that can be suspended in air for prolonged periods. Negative airflow rooms are required to prevent airborne spread of microbes.

Enclosed booths with high-efficiency particulate air (HEPA) filtration or ultraviolet light may be used for sputum induction procedures. Tuberculosis, measles (rubeola), and chickenpox (varicella) are examples of airborne diseases.

Droplet Precautions are used for patients known or suspected to have INFECTIONS transmitted by the droplet transmission route. Such infections are caused by organisms in droplets that may travel 3 feet but are not suspended for long periods. Examples of infectious conditions requiring Droplet Precautions include influenza, mumps, pertussis, and meningitis caused by either *N. meningitidis* or *Haemophilus influenzae* type B.

Contact Precautions are used for patients known or suspected to have INFECTIONS transmitted by direct contact or contact with items in the environment. Patients with significant multidrug-resistant organism (MDRO) infection or colonization, such as methicillin-resistant *Staphylococcus aureus* (MRSA) or vancomycin-resistant *Enterococcus* (VRE), are placed on Contact Precautions. Other infections requiring Contact Precautions include pediculosis (lice), scabies, respiratory syncytial virus (RSV), and *C. difficile.*

Staff and Patient Placement and Cohorting

Adequate staffing of nurses is an essential method for preventing INFECTION. In addition to a ratio of one infection control practitioner to 100 occupied acute care beds, nurse staffing is critical. When possible, bedside nurse staffing should consist of full-time nurses assigned regularly to the unit to ensure consistent practices (Upshaw-Owens & Bailey, 2012).

TABLE 23-3 Transmission-Based Infection Control Precautions

PRECAUTIONS (IN ADDITION TO STANDARD PRECAUTIONS)	EXAMPLES OF DISEASES IN CATEGORY
Airborne Precautions	
1. Private room required with monitored negative airflow (with appropriate number of air exchanges and air discharge to outside or through HEPA filter); keep door(s) closed	Diseases that are known or suspected to be transmitted by air: Measles (rubeola) *Mycobacterium tuberculosis,* including multidrug-resistant TB (MDRTB) Varicella (chickenpox)†; disseminated zoster (shingles)†
2. Special respiratory protection: • Wear PAPR for known or suspected TB • Susceptible persons not to enter room of patient with known or suspected measles or varicella unless immune caregivers are not available • Susceptible persons who must enter room must wear PAPR or N95 HEPA filter*	
3. Transport: patient to leave room only for essential clinical reasons, wearing surgical mask	
Droplet Precautions	
1. Private room preferred: if not available, may cohort with patient with same active infection with same microorganisms if no other infection present; maintain distance of at least 3 feet from other patients if private room not available	Diseases that are known or suspected to be transmitted by droplets: Diphtheria (pharyngeal) Streptococcal pharyngitis Pneumonia Influenza Rubella Invasive disease (meningitis, pneumonia, sepsis) caused by *Haemophilus influenzae* type B or *Neisseria meningitidis* Mumps Pertussis
2. Mask: required when working within 3 feet of patient	
3. Transport: as above	
Contact Precautions	
1. Private room preferred: if not available, may cohort with patient with same active infection with same microorganisms if no other infection present	Diseases that are known or suspected to be transmitted by direct contact: *Clostridium difficile* Colonization or infection caused by multidrug-resistant organisms (e.g., MRSA, VRE) Pediculosis Respiratory syncytial virus Scabies
2. Wear gloves when entering room	
3. Wash hands with antimicrobial soap before leaving patient's room	
4. Wear gown to prevent contact with patient or contaminated items or if patient has uncontrolled body fluids; remove gown before leaving room	
5. Transport: patient to leave room only for essential clinical reasons; during transport, use needed precautions to prevent disease transmission	
6. Dedicated equipment for this patient only (or disinfect after use before taking from room)	

HEPA, High-efficiency particulate air; *MRSA,* methicillin-resistant *Staphylococcus aureus; PAPR,* powered air purifying respirator; *TB,* tuberculosis; *VRE,* vancomycin-resistant *Enterococcus.*
*Before use: training and fit testing required for personnel.
†Add Contact Precautions for draining lesions.

FIG. 23-1 A, Nurse in personal protective equipment (PPE) caring for a patient in a private room. **B,** Powered air purifying respirator (PAPR).

Patient placement has been used as a way to reduce the spread of INFECTION. The CDC does not mandate that all patients with infections have a private room. It does recommend that private rooms always be used for patients on Airborne Precautions and those in a protective environment (PE). A PE is architecturally designed and structured to prevent INFECTION from occurring in patients who are at extremely high risk, such as those having stem cell therapy. The CDC also prefers private rooms for patients who are on Contact and Droplet Precautions. If private rooms are not available, keep these patients at least 3 feet apart. Many hospitals are becoming totally private-room facilities. Large health care systems have biomedical engineers to assist in designing the best environment to reduce the spread of infection, including ventilation systems and physical layout.

Cohorting is another method of patient placement. Cohorting is the practice of grouping patients who are colonized or infected with the same pathogen. This method has been used the most with patients who have an outbreak of a multidrug-resistant organism like methicillin-resistant *Staphylococcus aureus* (MRSA). It is particularly effective in long-term care settings.

INFECTION control principles for *patient transport* include limiting movement to other areas of the facility, using appropriate barriers like covering infected wounds, and notifying other departments or agencies who are receiving the patient about the necessary precautions. Accurate hand-off communication between agencies is also very important to prevent the spread of infection, according to The Joint Commission's NPSGs.

⍰ NCLEX EXAMINATION CHALLENGE

Safe and Effective Care Environment

Which statement by a nursing student indicates a need for further teaching by the nurse regarding infection control for a client who has an open, draining wound?
A. "I will wear an isolation gown when providing direct care."
B. "I will wear gloves when changing the client's dressing."
C. "I will wear a mask each time I enter the client's room."
D. "I will use a hand sanitizer when I can't wash my hands."

MULTIDRUG-RESISTANT ORGANISM INFECTIONS AND COLONIZATIONS

Antibiotics have been available for many years. Unfortunately, these drugs were commonly prescribed for conditions that did not need them or were given at higher doses and for longer periods of time than were necessary. As a result, a number of microorganisms have become resistant to certain antibiotics; that is, drugs that were once useful no longer control these infectious agents (multidrug-resistant organisms [MDROs]). For this reason, a culture of safety related to INFECTION control has been mandated by the CDC, the Institute for Healthcare Improvement (IHI), and The Joint Commission: Standard Precautions must be strictly followed today in all health care settings to prevent more of these difficult and deadly infections.

One of the newest discoveries to explain the increase in health care–acquired infections (HCAIs), especially the rise in drug-resistant infections, is the formation of biofilms. A biofilm, also called *glycocalyx*, is a complex group of microorganisms that functions within a "slimy" gel coating on medical devices such as urinary catheters, orthopedic implants, and enteral feeding tubes; on parts of the body like the teeth (plaque) and tonsils; and in chronic wounds. These reservoirs become sources of INFECTION for which antibiotics and disinfection are not effective. Antibiotic therapy may increase the growth of microbes within biofilms.

Biofilms are extremely difficult to treat, and mechanical disruption strategies are the mainstay of management and research (Ramage et al., 2010). Studies on biofilms that cause the most common HCAIs, such as catheter-associated urinary tract infections (CAUTIs) and wound infections, continue to be conducted. Many specific biofilms have been identified, and methods to remove or disrupt them are being researched.

Patients with *indwelling urinary catheters* are at high risk for pyelonephritis (kidney infection) and septicemia. Current evidence shows that urease-producing bacteria, especially *Proteus mirabilis,* cause crystalline biofilms that create a crust that can block the catheter (Stickler & Feneley, 2010). Therefore indwelling urinary catheters are used only when absolutely necessary. Antimicrobial catheters, either silver-alloy or antimicrobial-coated, are recommended for short-term urinary catheter use to decrease encrustation (Parker et al., 2009). Little evidence is available to demonstrate methods to reduce CAUTIs in long-term indwelling catheters except for frequent catheter changes. In postoperative patients, Palese et al. (2010) found that the regular use of ultrasound bladder scanners reduces urinary tract infections by preventing the inappropriate use of urinary catheters. Nurses can use this information to provide the most current assessment interventions for reducing CAUTIs. Chapter 66 describes evidence-based interventions to prevent urinary tract infections.

Traditional débridement alone is not successful to prevent or manage *chronic wound* infections, often caused by *S. aureus.* A systematic review by Lo et al. (2008) found that silver-releasing dressings were very effective. Biofilms can be disrupted by using dry gauze to mechanically disrupt them after débridement. Antibacterial enzymes may also be used.

The most common MDROs are methicillin-resistant *Staphylococcus aureus,* vancomycin-resistant *Enterococcus,* and carbapenem-resistant *Enterococcus.* Other infections, such as vancomycin-intermediate *S. aureus* (VISA) and vancomycin-resistant *S. aureus* (VRSA), may also occur, which may be effectively treated with antibiotics such as linezolid (Zyvox) and quinupristin-dalfopristin (Synercid).

Methicillin-Resistant *Staphylococcus aureus* (MRSA)

Staphylococcus aureus (S. aureus) is a common bacterium found *on* the skin and perineum and in the nose of many people. It is usually not infectious when in these areas because the number of bacteria is controlled by good hygiene measures. However, when skin or mucous membranes are not intact, minor INFECTIONS, like boils or conjunctivitis, may occur. If the organism enters into deep wounds, surgical incisions, the lungs, or bloodstream, more serious infections occur that require strong antibiotics like methicillin.

Within the past 40 years, more and more *S. aureus* infections have not responded to methicillin or other penicillin-based drugs. Known as *MRSA,* these infections are one of the fastest growing and most common in health care today. In its *5 Million Lives Campaign,* the IHI included reducing MRSA infections as one of its six new goals (see Chapter 1). This type of INFECTION is called *health care–associated MRSA,* or *HA-MRSA.* Patients who have HA-MRSA have increased hospital stays at a very high cost. To add to this problem, about 25% of patients may be colonized with the organism. Health care staff members may also colonize. Patients who develop HA-MRSA pneumonia, abscesses, or bacteremia (bloodstream infection [BSI]) can quickly progress to sepsis and death.

MRSA is spread by direct contact and invades hospitalized patients through indwelling urinary catheters, vascular access devices, and endotracheal tubes. It is susceptible to only a few antibiotics, such as vancomycin (Lyphocin, Vancocin) and linezolid (Zyvox). A newer IV antibiotic, ceftaroline fosamil (Teflaro), is the first cephalosporin approved to treat MRSA.

Current evidence shows that bathing hospitalized patients with pre-moistened cloths or warm water containing chlorhexidine gluconate (CHG) solution can significantly reduce MRSA infection by 23% to 32% (Kassakian, et al., 2011; Powers, et al., 2012). In 2013, the American Association of Critical Care published a recommendation that nurses use CHG to bathe patients in critical care settings as a way to reduce MRSA and other multi-drug–resistant organisms.

⚠ NURSING SAFETY PRIORITY (QSEN)

Action Alert

Patients most at risk for HA-MRSA are older adults and those who have suppressed IMMUNITY, have a long history of antibiotic therapy, or have invasive tubes or lines. ICU patients are especially at risk. Check with your agency policy regarding specific MRSA preventive measures. Examples include bathing patients with chlorhexidine wipes and administering nasal mupirocin ointment.

Although controversial, some health care facilities have a MRSA-surveillance program in which each patient's nose is swabbed and cultured for MRSA. Staff may also be cultured. All patients with HA-MRSA infection or colonization should be placed on Contact Precautions.

Community-associated MRSA, or CA-MRSA, causes infections in healthy, nonhospitalized people, especially those living in college housing and prisons. It is easily transmitted among family members and can cause serious skin and soft-tissue infections, including abscesses, boils, and blisters. The best way to decrease the incidence of this growing problem is health teaching, including:

- Performing frequent hand hygiene, including using hand sanitizers
- Avoiding close contact with people who have infectious wounds
- Avoiding large crowds
- Avoiding contaminated surfaces
- Using good overall hygiene

Minocycline (Minocin, Apo-Minocycline ✽) and doxycycline (Doryx, Apo-Doxy ✽) are usually effective in treating CA-MRSA.

❓ NCLEX EXAMINATION CHALLENGE

Safe and Effective Care Environment

A client is admitted with a catheter-associated methicillin-resistant *Staphylococcus aureus* (MRSA) infection. Which personal protective equipment is appropriate when providing client care? **Select all that apply.**

A. Mask
B. Gloves
C. Shoe covers
D. Goggles
E. Gown

Vancomycin-Resistant *Enterococcus* (VRE)

Enterococci are bacteria that live in the intestinal tract and are important for digestion. When they move to another area of the body, such as during surgery, they can cause an infection, usually treatable with vancomycin. However, in recent years, many of these infections have become resistant to the drug, and VRE results. Risk factors for this infection include prolonged hospital stays, severe illness, abdominal surgery, enteral nutrition, and immunosuppression. Place patients with VRE infections on Contact Precautions to prevent contamination from body fluids.

Unfortunately, VRE can live on almost any surface for days or weeks and still be able to cause an infection. Contamination of toilet seats, door handles, and other objects is very likely for a lengthy period.

Carbapenem-Resistant *Enterobacteriaceae* (CRE)

Carbapenem antibiotics, most often given for abdominal infections such as peritonitis, have been used extensively for the past 15 years. Examples of this class of antibiotics include imipenem (Cilastin) and meropenem (Merrum IV).

Klebsiella and *Escherichia coli* (*E. coli*) are types of *Enterobacteriaceae* that are located within the intestinal tract. Carbapenem-resistant *Enterobacteriaceae* (CRE) is a family of pathogens that are difficult to treat because they have a high level of resistance to carbapenems due to enzymes that break down the antibiotics. *Klebsiella pneumoniae* (KPC) and New Delhi mettalo-beta-lactamase are examples of these enzymes. Patients who are high risk for CRE include those in intensive care units or nursing homes and patients who are immunosuppressed, including older adults.

To prevent the transmission of this infection, place patients that are high-risk on Contact Precautions. The CDC (2013) also recommends chlorhexidine (2% dilution) bathing to prevent CRE or decrease colonization and other types of infections from MDROs.

OCCUPATIONAL AND ENVIRONMENTAL EXPOSURE TO SOURCES OF INFECTION

The U.S. **Occupational Safety and Health Administration (OSHA)** is a federal agency that protects workers from injury or illness at their place of employment. Unlike the voluntary guidelines developed by the CDC, OSHA regulations are law. Employers can be fined or disciplined for noncompliance with OSHA regulations. The regulation for prevention of exposure to bloodborne pathogens, such as hepatitis B and hepatitis C or the human immune deficiency virus (HIV), is one example of an OSHA regulation.

Reduction of skin and soft-tissue injuries (e.g., needle sticks) is essential to reduce bloodborne pathogen transmission to health care personnel. *OSHA mandates that sharp objects ("sharps") and needles be handled with care.* Many contaminated sharp-object exposures involve nurses. Needleless devices have helped decrease these exposures, especially when caring for patients receiving infusion therapy (see Chapter 13).

Other INFECTION control concerns that nurses and other HCWs have are the possibilities of pandemic influenza or biologic agent exposure. A large outbreak of one of the MDROs is also worrisome, especially if no drug is sensitive enough for successful management. Nurses may fear that they will accidentally bring the infectious agent to their homes and families.

Action Alert

To help prevent the transmission of an MDRO, wear scrubs and change clothes before leaving work. Keep work clothes separate from personal clothes. Take a shower when you get home, if possible, to rid your body of any unwanted pathogens. Be careful not to contaminate equipment that is commonly used, such as your stethoscope.

Another environmental source for infection is animals or insects. For example, *hantaviruses* are caused by exposure to rodent-infected areas such as old sheds or cabins. Lyme disease can be caused by deer ticks (see Chapter 18).

Saliva and excrement from deer mice and rats living in the southwestern part of the United States are the primary sources of hantaviruses. While not a common infection, patients can die from complications such as *hantavirus pulmonary syndrome,* a severe and potentially lethal respiratory disease. Teach patients to avoid exposure to potential hantaviruses by avoiding rodent-infested areas. If infested areas need to be cleaned, teach patients to wear rubber or latex gloves and either a tight-seal negative-pressure respirator or a positive pressure powered air purifying respirator equipped with N100 or P100 filters (Ly, 2013).

PROBLEMS FROM INADEQUATE ANTIMICROBIAL THERAPY

Inadequate antimicrobial therapy may range from an incorrect choice of drug to poor patient adherence. Drug regimen **noncompliance** (deliberate failure to take the drug) or **nonadherence** (accidental failure to take the drug) also contributes to resistant-organism development.

Some diseases such as tuberculosis (TB) have legal sanctions that require that a patient complete treatment. Patients who are at risk for noncompliance or nonadherence with an anti-TB drug regimen may be placed on *directly observed therapy (DOT).* This means that a health care worker must observe and validate patient compliance with the drug regimen. DOT has been very effective at reducing the spread of multidrug-resistant TB.

Serious complications of INFECTION may also result from incomplete or inadequate antibiotic therapy. Local infections that could be cured without complications, such as cellulitis and pneumonia, may progress to abscess formation if appropriate drug therapy is not continued. Although drug therapy does not always prevent abscess, early therapy may prevent or limit the size of an abscess.

In addition to abscess formation, inadequate therapy may lead to systemic spread. If the infection is not resolved or if it is treated with drugs that are ineffective for the offending microorganism, the pathogen may enter the bloodstream (septicemia or bloodstream infection [BSI]). Inadequately treated local infections may also lead to BSI with leukocytosis (increased white blood cell count). In severe or advanced cases, leukopenia (decreased white blood cell count) and life-threatening disseminated intravascular coagulation (DIC) may occur. After pathogens invade the bloodstream, no site is protected from invasion.

BSI may progress to **septic shock,** more accurately called *sepsis-induced distributive shock.* In septic shock, insufficient cardiac output is compounded by hypovolemia. Inadequate blood supply to vital organs leads to hypoxia (lack of oxygen) and organ failure. Chapter 37 describes this type of shock and its management in detail.

❖ PATIENT-CENTERED COLLABORATIVE CARE
◆ Assessment

History. The patient's age, history of tobacco or alcohol use, current illness or disease (e.g., diabetes), past and current drug use (e.g., steroids), and poor nutritional status may place him or her at increased risk for INFECTION. Patients who are immunocompromised as a result of disease or therapies such as chemotherapy and radiation are also at a high risk for infection. Ask the patient about previous vaccinations or immunizations, including the dates of administration.

Ask the patient if he or she has recently been in a hospital or nursing home as a patient or visitor. Inquire about having invasive testing, such as a colonoscopy, or recent surgery. Ask if the patient had an indwelling urinary catheter or IV line. These invasive treatments often are the source of infections.

Determine whether the patient has been exposed to infectious agents. A history of recent exposure to someone with similar clinical symptoms or to contaminated food or water, as well as the time of exposure, assists in identifying a possible source of INFECTION. This information helps determine the incubation period for the disease and thus provides a clue to its cause.

Contact with animals, including pets, may increase exposure to infection. Question the patient about recent animal contact at home or work or in leisure activities (e.g., hiking). Insect bites should be documented.

Obtain a travel history. Travel to areas both within and outside the patient's home country may expose a susceptible person to infectious organisms not encountered in the local community.

A thorough sexual history may reveal behavior associated with an increased risk for sexually transmitted diseases. Obtain a history of IV drug use and a transfusion history to assess the patient's risk for hepatitis B, hepatitis C, and HIV infections.

Identifying the type and location of symptoms may point to affected organ systems. The onset order of symptoms gives clues to the specific problem. Gathering a history of past INFECTION or colonization with multidrug-resistant organisms will help determine which type of Transmission-Based Precautions is needed.

Physical Assessment/Clinical Manifestations. Disorders caused by pathogens vary depending on the INFECTION cause and site. Common clinical manifestations are associated with specific sites of infection. Carefully inspect the skin for symptoms of *local* infection at any site (*pain, swelling, heat, redness, pus*). Wounds can easily become infected because the integrity of the skin is broken.

CONSIDERATIONS FOR OLDER ADULTS
Patient-Centered Care (QSEN)

Fever (generally a temperature above 101° F [38.3° C]), chills, and malaise are primary indicators of a systemic infection. Fever may accompany other noninfectious disorders, and infection can be present without fever, especially in patients who have impaired immunity. The older adult, whose normal temperature may be 1° to 2° lower than the normal temperature in younger adults, may have a fever at 99° F (37.2° C). In most patients with an infection, fever (**hyperthermia**) is a normal immune response that can help destroy the pathogen. Assess the patient for these signs and symptoms, and carefully ask about their history and pattern.

Lymphadenopathy (enlarged lymph nodes), pharyngitis, and GI disturbance (usually diarrhea or vomiting) are often associated with infection. To detect enlargement, palpate the cervical, axillary, and other lymph nodes; examine the throat for redness. Ask about changes in stool and if the patient has had any nausea or vomiting.

Psychosocial Assessment. The patient with an infectious disease often has psychosocial concerns. Delay in diagnosis because of the need to await clinical test results produces anxiety. Assess the patient's and family's level of understanding about various diagnostic procedures and the time required to obtain test results. Plan education on infection risk reduction at a time when they are ready to learn.

Feelings of malaise and fatigue often accompany infection. Assess the patient's current level of activity and the impact of these symptoms on family, occupational, and recreational activities.

The potential spread of INFECTION to others is an additional stress associated with the diagnosis of infection. The patient may curtail family and social interactions for fear of spreading the illness. Determine the patient's and family's understanding of the infection, the mode of transmission, and mechanisms that may limit or prevent transmission. Special precautions, although sometimes necessary for preventing transmission of the organism, can be emotionally difficult for the patient and family.

A number of transmissible infectious diseases, especially those identified with social stigmas (e.g., IV drug abuse), are associated with labeling. The patient may feel socially isolated or have guilt related to behavior that increased the risk for infection. Observe carefully for the patient's reaction to labels and how these feelings further affect socialization.

Laboratory Assessment. The definitive diagnosis of an infectious disease requires identification of a microorganism in the tissues of an infected patient. Direct examination of blood, body fluids, and tissues under a microscope may not yield a definitive identification. However, laboratory assessment usually provides helpful information about organisms, such as shape, motility, and reaction to staining agents. Even when direct microscopy does not provide a conclusive specific diagnosis, often enough information is obtained for starting appropriate antimicrobial therapy.

The best procedure for identifying a microorganism is culture, or isolation of the pathogen by cultivation in tissue cultures or artificial media. Specimens for culture can be obtained from almost any body fluid or tissue. The health care provider usually decides when and where the specimen for culture is taken.

Proper collection and handling of specimens for culture, using Standard Precautions, are essential for obtaining accurate results. Specimens collected must be appropriate for the suspected infection. Be sure that the specimen is of adequate quantity and is freshly obtained and placed in a sterile container to preserve the specimen and microorganism. Label the specimen properly including the date and time it was collected. Follow your agency's policy if you have any questions about how to perform a culture.

After isolation of a microorganism in culture, antimicrobial sensitivity testing is performed to determine the effects of various drugs on that particular microorganism. An agent that is killed by acceptable levels of an antibiotic, for example, is considered sensitive to that drug. An organism that is not killed by tolerable levels of an antibiotic is considered resistant to that

drug. Preliminary results are usually available in 24 to 48 hours, but the final results generally take 72 hours. *Antimicrobial therapy should not begin until after the culture specimen is obtained.*

Rapid cultures or assays are used in ambulatory care settings to provide quicker assessments of infections. The most popular is the rapid antigen detection test for group A streptococci to rule out "strep throat" in patients who present with pharyngitis (sore, inflamed throat). Other examples of newer tests are those for tuberculosis (TB) and influenza ("flu"), discussed in Chapter 31.

A *white blood cell (WBC) count with differential* is often done for the patient with a suspected infection. Five types of leukocytes (white blood cells) are measured as part of the results:

- Neutrophils
- Lymphocytes
- Monocytes
- Eosinophils
- Basophils

In most active infections, especially those caused by bacteria, the total leukocyte count is elevated. Various infections are characterized by changes in the percentages of the different types of leukocytes. The differential count usually shows an increased number of immature neutrophils, or a **shift to the left** ("left shift"). A few infectious diseases, however, such as malaria and infectious mononucleosis, are associated with neutropenia (decreased neutrophils). See Chapter 17 for further discussion.

The *erythrocyte sedimentation rate (ESR)* measures the rate at which red blood cells fall through plasma. This rate is most significantly affected by an increased number of acute-phase reactants, which occurs with inflammation. Thus an elevated ESR (>20 mm/hr) indicates inflammation or infection somewhere in the body. Chronic INFECTION, especially osteomyelitis and chronic abscesses, is commonly associated with an elevated ESR. The ESR is chronically elevated with inflammatory arthritis and other connective tissue diseases as well (see Chapter 18). The effectiveness of therapy is often determined by a decrease in this value.

Serologic testing is performed to identify pathogens by detecting antibodies to the organism. The antibody titer tends to *increase* during the acute phase of infectious diseases such as hepatitis B. The titer *decreases* as the patient improves.

Imaging Assessment. X-ray films may be obtained to determine activity or destruction by an infectious microorganism. Radiologic studies (e.g., chest films, sinus films, joint films, GI studies) are available for diagnosis of infection in a specific body site.

More sophisticated techniques for INFECTION diagnosis include computed tomography (CT) scans and magnetic resonance imaging (MRI). CT and ultrasonography are helpful in assessing for abscesses. CT scans help identify suspected osteomyelitis and fluid collections that point to possible infection. MRI scans provide a cross-sectional assessment for infection.

Another diagnostic tool for the evaluation of a patient with an infectious disease is ultrasonography. This noninvasive procedure is particularly helpful in detecting infection involving the heart valves.

Scanning techniques using radioactive substances such as gallium can determine the presence of inflammation caused by INFECTION. Inflammatory tissue is identified by its increased uptake of the injected radioactive material.

◆ *Analysis*

The priority NANDA-I nursing diagnoses and collaborative problems for patients with an infection or infectious disease include:

1. Hyperthermia related to the immune response triggered by pathogenic invasion (NANDA-I)
2. Social Isolation related to being placed on Transmission-Based Precautions (NANDA-I)

◆ *Planning and Implementation*

Managing Hyperthermia

Planning: Expected Outcomes. Patients with an INFECTION or infectious disease are expected to have a body temperature within normal limits as a result of effective interdisciplinary management.

Interventions. The primary concern is to provide measures to eliminate the underlying cause of fever (also known as *hyperthermia*) and to destroy the causative microorganism. In collaboration with the health care team, nurses use a variety of methods to manage fever.

Drug therapy plays a major role in patient-centered collaborative care of patients with INFECTION. Antimicrobials, also called *anti-infective agents,* are the cornerstone of drug therapy. Antipyretics are used to decrease patient discomfort and reduce fever.

Antibiotics, antiviral agents, and antifungals are common types of antimicrobial drugs that are given for INFECTION, depending on its type. Effective antibiotics are available to treat nearly all bacterial infections, but misuse of antibiotics has contributed to the development of multidrug-resistant organisms (MDROs) discussed earlier in this chapter. A few effective antifungal agents have been developed, but these drugs generally cause more toxicity than antibacterial agents.

Effective antimicrobial therapy requires delivery of an appropriate drug, sufficient dosage, proper administration route, and sufficient therapy duration. These four requirements ensure delivery of a concentration of drug sufficient to inhibit or kill infecting microorganisms. To ensure effectiveness of antibiotic therapy such as vancomycin, health care providers may require serum trough and peak levels be drawn. Specimens for trough levels are drawn about 30 minutes prior to the next scheduled vancomycin dose. Specimens for peak levels are drawn 30 to 60 minutes after medication administration (Rosini & Srivastava, 2013).

Health care providers collaborate on selecting drugs and dosing. Antimicrobials act on susceptible pathogens by:

- Inhibiting cell wall synthesis (e.g., penicillins and cephalosporins)
- Injuring the cytoplasmic membrane (e.g., antifungal agents)
- Inhibiting biosynthesis, or reproduction (e.g., erythromycin and gentamicin)
- Inhibiting nucleic acid synthesis (e.g., actinomycin)

Teach the drug's actions, side effects, and toxic effects to patients and their families. Observe and report side effects and adverse events. These reactions vary according to the specific classification of the drug. Most antibiotics can cause nausea, vomiting, and rashes. Stress the importance of completing the entire course of drug therapy, even if symptoms have improved or disappeared.

Antipyretic drugs, such as acetaminophen (Tylenol, Ace-Tabs ✦), are often given to reduce fever. Because these drugs

TABLE 23-4 Possible Allergic Reactions to Antibiotic Therapy	
• Nausea and/or vomiting • Flushing • Wheezing • Sneezing • Pruritus • Urticaria • Rashes • Maculopapular to exfoliative dermatitis • Vascular eruptions	• Erythema multiforme (Stevens-Johnson syndrome) • Angioneurotic edema • Serum sickness (headache, fever, chills, hives, malaise, conjunctivitis) • Anaphylaxis (laryngeal edema, bronchospasm, hypotension, vascular collapse, cardiac arrest) • Death

> ❗ **NURSING SAFETY PRIORITY** (QSEN)
>
> **Drug Alert**
>
> Before administering an antimicrobial agent, check to see that the patient is not allergic to it (Table 23-4). Be sure to take an accurate allergy history before drug therapy begins to prevent possible life-threatening reactions, such as anaphylaxis!

mask fever, monitoring the course of the disease may be difficult. Therefore, unless the patient is very uncomfortable or if fever presents a significant risk (e.g., in the patient with heart failure, febrile seizures, or head injury), antipyretics are not always prescribed.

Teach patients that they may have waves of sweating after each dose. Sweating may be accompanied by a fall in blood pressure followed by return of fever. These unpleasant side effects of antipyretic therapy can often be alleviated by increasing fluid intake and by regular scheduling of drug administration.

Other interventions to reduce fever may include external cooling and fluid administration. Perform a thorough assessment before and after interventions are implemented.

External cooling by hypothermia blankets or ice bags or packs can be effective mechanisms for reducing a high fever. Alternative cooling methods may be used. Sponging the patient's body with tepid water or applying cool compresses to the skin and pulse points to reduce body temperature is sometimes helpful. *Teach unlicensed assistive personnel (UAP) to observe for and report shivering during any form of external cooling. Shivering may indicate that the patient is being cooled too quickly.*

The use of fans is discouraged because they can disperse airborne- or droplet-transmitted pathogens. Fans can also disturb air balance in negative pressure rooms, making them positive pressure rooms and allowing possible transmission of the agent to those outside the room.

In patients with fever, fluid volume loss is increased from rapid evaporation of body fluids and increased perspiration. As body temperature increases, fluid volume loss increases.

> ❗ **NURSING SAFETY PRIORITY** (QSEN)
>
> **Action Alert**
>
> If fluid volume loss increases, patients may be at risk for dehydration and require additional fluids either orally or IV. Monitor carefully for signs of dehydration, such as increased thirst, decreased skin turgor, dry mucous membranes, and acute confusion, especially in older adults. Increase oral fluid intake and provide IV fluids as prescribed. Chapter 11 discusses interventions for dehydration in detail.

Responding to Feelings of Social Isolation

Planning: Expected Outcomes. The patient with an INFEC-TION or infectious disease who is placed on Transmission-Based Precautions is expected to cope with feelings of isolation and interact with others.

Interventions. Education is the major intervention for meeting this outcome. Teach the patient and family about the mode of transmission of infection and mechanisms that prevent spread to others. Assess coping mechanisms that the patient has used in the past. If he or she is in the hospital, collaborate with the certified hospital chaplain or social worker to help alleviate the patient's stress, anxiety, or depression.

As part of the health care team, ensure that the patient and family understand the disease process and its cause. If necessary, ensure that the patient and family can state specific ways in which precautions will be used in the home after discharge from the hospital.

Because the patient requiring precautions may feel secluded, encourage staff and family members to maintain contact with the patient. Remind them that the pathogen, not the patient, requires special precautions. Encourage family members and friends to visit and to use appropriate infection control measures. Communication by telephone or e-mail is often effective for continuing contact with loved ones. Television, Internet, and handheld mobile devices help bring the outside world into the life of the patient confined to the room.

In the long-term care setting, an outbreak of respiratory or GI INFECTION usually requires limiting visitors, activities, and admissions to the facility. Nurses working in these settings need to be familiar with federal and state regulations regarding managing infections.

Community-Based Care

Patients with infections may be cared for in the home, hospital, nursing home, or ambulatory care setting, depending on the type and severity of the INFECTION. Infections among older adults in nursing homes are common. Residents often have meals together in a communal dining room and participate in group activities. Confused residents may not wash their hands or may enter other resident rooms. Immunizing them against respiratory infections is highly recommended because these illnesses can cause severe complications or death in older adults.

Home Care Management. The patient with an infectious disease such as osteomyelitis may require continued, long-term antibiotic therapy at home or in a long-term care facility. Emphasize the importance of a clean home environment, especially for the patient who continues to have compromised IMMUNITY or who is uniquely susceptible to superinfection (i.e., reinfection or a second infection of the same kind) to reduce the chance of infection. Drugs often need to be refrigerated. Ensure that the patient has access to proper storage facilities, and teach him or her to check for signs of improper storage, such as discoloration of the drug.

Ask about the availability of handwashing facilities in the home, and check that supplies and instructions are provided as needed. Most people do not know how to wash hands correctly. Demonstrate the procedure with the patient and family, and request a repeat demonstration.

Self-Management Education. Explaining the disease and making certain that the patient understands what is causing the illness are the primary purposes of health teaching. Discuss whether the pathogen causing the INFECTION can be spread to others and the modes of transmission.

If the patient has an infectious disease that is potentially transmissible, teach the patient, family, and other home caregivers about precautions. Explain whether any special household cleaning is necessary and, if so, what those special steps include. If syringes with needles are used to administer drug therapy, explain how to dispose safely and legally of needles in the community. Clothing soiled with blood or other body fluids can be washed with bleach or disinfectant (e.g., Lysol). Recommended cleaning measures should be based on actual available equipment and facilities.

For the patient who is discharged to the home setting to complete a course of antimicrobial therapy, the importance of adherence to the planned drug regimen needs to be stressed. Explain the importance of both the timing of doses and the completion of the planned number of days of therapy. Teach the patient (and family as appropriate) how the agents need to be taken (e.g., before meals, with meals, without other agents) and the possible side effects. Side effects include those that are expected (e.g., gastric distress), as well as more severe adverse reactions (e.g., rash, fever, other systemic signs and symptoms). Teach the patient about allergic manifestations and the need to notify a health care provider if an adverse reaction occurs (see Table 23-4). Also discuss what to do if a drug dose is missed (e.g., doubling the dosage, waiting until the next dose time).

Many patients are discharged with an infusion device to continue drug therapy at home or in other inpatient facilities. The patient, family member, or home care nurse administers the drugs. Home care services are often used to teach appropriate administration of drug therapy in the patient's home. Health teaching and wound care may also be needed. These services have proved efficient, effective, psychologically supportive, and less expensive than hospitalization or skilled nursing facilities (SNFs).

The patient is often anxious and fearful that the INFECTION will be transmitted to family members or friends. Teaching the patient and the family ways of preventing the spread of disease allays these fears. Pay careful attention to the patient's and family's concerns. Making concrete suggestions (e.g., "Your wife can wear gloves when changing your dressing") to address specific concerns may reduce these fears.

The patient with an infectious disease associated with lifestyle behaviors, such as sexual activity or IV drug abuse, may have guilt related to the disease. Encourage discussion of feelings associated with the illness, and assist in locating support systems that may help alleviate these feelings, such as clergy or other spiritual or cultural leaders.

Health Care Resources. At times, a patient who has been hospitalized for an infectious disease may not be able to return to the home setting due to lack of caregiver support. In such cases, temporary placement in a SNF may be needed. Document care requirements, patient history of infection or colonization with multidrug-resistant organisms, medication schedules, and personal needs and preferences on transfer forms. Hand-off communication, such as the SBAR, between the two facilities is required to facilitate a smooth transition from the hospital to the intermediate care setting, according to The Joint Commission's National Patient Safety Goals.

TABLE 23-5 Centers for Disease Control and Prevention* Examples of Bioterrorism Agents and General Clinical Management

PATHOGEN OR AGENT AND DISEASE INFORMATION	CLINICAL MANAGEMENT

Anthrax (*Bacillus anthracis*)
Cutaneous: 1-7 days after contact, exposed skin itching, progressing to papular and vesicular lesions, eschar, edema, ulceration, and sloughing. If untreated, may spread to lymph nodes and bloodstream. Fatality 5%-20%.
Inhalation: 48 hr after organism or spore inhalation, flu-like illness with possible brief improvement. 2-4 days from initial symptoms, abrupt onset of severe cardiopulmonary illness (dyspnea, tachycardia, fever, diaphoresis, thoracic edema, shock, and respiratory failure). If antibiotics delayed until onset of cardiopulmonary symptoms, mortality high. May be confused with common upper respiratory infection (URI).
Other forms: Gastrointestinal (GI), meningeal, and sepsis.
	For cutaneous and inhaled anthrax: No person-to-person spread. Contact Precautions are not needed unless patient presents directly from exposure.
	Standard Precautions for:
	  Prescribed wound cleansing and management of lesions
	  Ventilator support for respiratory failure
	    Postmortem care

Botulism (*Clostridium botulinum* and Neurotoxin) Toxin ingestion results in dysphasia, dry mouth, drooping eyelids, and blurred or double vision. Vomiting and constipation or diarrhea may be present initially, extending to symmetric flaccid paralysis in an alert person. Acute bilateral cranial nerve impairment and descending weakness or paralysis follow. Neurologic symptoms after 12-36 hr for foodborne botulism and in 24-72 hr after aerosol exposure. Case fatality up to 10%. Recovery may take months.	Standard Precautions: decontamination of patient is not required. No person-to-person spread. Consider outbreak with suspicion of a single case. Consult with CDC and health departments. Advise careful cleanup and disposal of suspected contaminated food source *after* consultation with health department about any needed laboratory sampling. Interdisciplinary planning for nutrition and rehabilitation support during lengthy neuromuscular and respiratory recovery.

Plague (*Yersinia pestis*)
Lymphatic infection: 2-8 days after bites from fleas of an infected rodent (rarely after infected tissue or body fluid contact), onset of fever and chills, painful lymphadenopathy (or bubo—usually inguinal, axillary, or cervical lymph nodes), headache, GI symptoms, and rapidly progressive weakness. 50%-60% fatality if untreated.
Pneumonic: 1-3 days after aerosolized organism inhalation, fever and chills, productive cough, hemoptysis, rapidly progressive weakness, GI symptoms, and bronchopneumonia. Survival unlikely if not treated within 18 hr of symptom onset.
Other forms: Sepsis with coagulopathy, rarely meningitis.
	Droplet Precautions: required for pneumonic plague (until 72 hr of antibiotic therapy).
	Contact Precautions until decontamination is complete:
	  For any suspected gross contamination. See documentation information listed under Anthrax—above.
	  For prescribed management of bubo(s) if incised to drain.
	Community and other environmental modifications:
	  Apply insecticide to infested environment and pets (to kill fleas).
	  Reduce food and water supply for rodents.
	  Avoid sick or dead animals.

Smallpox (Variola Virus) (Variola Major and Minor) 10-17 days after droplet or airborne virus inhalation or contact with bleeding lesions, onset of severe myalgias, headache, and high fever. 2-3 days later, a papular rash appears on face and spreads to extremities (and palms and soles). The rash quickly (simultaneously) becomes vesicular and then painful and pustular (contrasted to varicella rash that crops and concentrates more on trunk with various stages of macules to vesicles seen at one time). Patients are infectious at onset of rash until scabs separate (3 wk). Historically, variola major kills 20%. May be confused with varicella.	Standard, Contact, and Airborne Precautions for patients with vesicular rash pending diagnosis. Same for varicella and variola. Also, avoid contact with organism while handling contaminated clothes and bedding. Wear protective attire (gloves, gown, and N95 respirator). One case is a public health emergency—highly communicable. Consult CDC and health departments at earliest suspicion. Vaccine does not give reliable lifelong immunity. Previously vaccinated persons are considered susceptible. *Following exposure:* Initiate Airborne Precautions, and observe for unprotected contacts (from days 10-17). Vaccinate within 2-3 days of exposure.

Other Key Points

Assessment: Include account of symptoms, patient's incident (what, where, when, how, others exposed or ill, and officials aware).

Treatment: Antibiotic-resistance possible. Vaccine and postexposure prophylaxis are subject to change. If any of the above diseases are suspected, consult infection control practitioner for coordination with community health officials and CDC about current recommendations and specimen collection. *If bioterrorism suspected,* Federal Bureau of Investigation (FBI) will coordinate evidence collection and delivery.

Multiple exposures planning: Emergency and critical care managers must address availability and acquisition of stocks of medications, vaccines, equipment (e.g., ventilators), and communications with officials, as well as public information needs.

◆ *Evaluation: Outcomes*

Evaluating the care of the patient with an INFECTION or infectious disease on the basis of the identified priority problems is important. The expected outcomes include that the patient:
- Has body temperature and other vital signs within baseline
- Adheres to drug therapy regimen
- Copes with feelings of social isolation

Specific indicators for these outcomes are listed for each priority problem under the Planning and Implementation section (see earlier).

CRITICAL ISSUES: EMERGING INFECTIONS AND GLOBAL BIOTERRORISM

Current concerns related to INFECTION and infection control are the risk for global bioterrorism (Table 23-5), emerging

CLINICAL JUDGMENT CHALLENGE

Evidence-Based Practice; Quality Improvement; Informatics QSEN

The hospital quality improvement (QI) department reports a 25% increase in CRE infections on your surgical intensive care unit during the past month. A unit-based QI team is created to identify possible causes of this increase and strategies for decreasing these infections.

1. What are some possible causes of CRE infections?
2. Using the PICOT format in Chapter 5, develop a clinical question to address the problem.
3. How will your unit QI team begin to answer the clinical question?
4. What data sources might you use?
5. What will you do with the retrieved data?
6. How will you present your findings?

Symptoms of Ebola, which can present from 2 to 21 days after exposure (with an average of 8 to 10 days), include fever greater than 101.5° F, severe headache, muscle pain, weakness, diarrhea, vomiting, abdominal pain, and unexplained hemorrhage (bleeding or bruising) (CDC, 2014). The virus is most commonly spread through exposure to bodily fluids of the infected individual and through needle sticks in which the needle has been contaminated with the virus (CDC, 2014). Recovery from this virus is contingent on appropriate clinical care and the immune response of the patient. Patients who recover from Ebola infection develop antibodies that can last for 10 years (CDC, 2014) (Table 23-7).

With the Dallas Ebola incident, there was reported to be a communication concern within the electronic medical record infectious diseases, and multidrug-resistant organisms (MDROs). As for any pathogen, strict infection control measures can prevent transmission of these microbes to you and your patients. Some of the most serious infections are briefly described here. Table 23-6 lists more emerging infections that may present as problems in the United States and other parts of the world.

The 2014 Ebola epidemic was labeled as the largest in history, with many West African countries affected (CDC, 2014). An epidemic occurs when new cases of a certain disease substantially exceed expectation during a given period. The ongoing struggle with the Ebola virus outbreak in West Africa became a concern within the United States when an individual who flew back from Liberia was diagnosed, although after initial discharge, at a Dallas hospital. That individual later died.

TABLE 23-6   Examples of Global Emerging Infections

Recently Emerging Infections	Older Rapidly Growing Infections
• H1N1 influenza	• Methicillin-resistant *Staphylococcus aureus* (MRSA)
• West Nile virus	• Vancomycin-resistant *Enterococcus* (VRE)
• Avian influenza	• Carbapenem-resistant *Enterobacteriaceae* (CRE)
• Hemorrhagic fevers (e.g., Ebola, Marburg)	• Multidrug-resistant tuberculosis
• Monkeypox	• *Clostridium difficile*
• Bovine spongiform encephalopathy	
• Vancomycin-intermediate *Staphylococcus aureus* (VISA)	
• Vancomycin-resistant *Staphylococcus aureus* (VRSA)	
• *Clostridium difficile* (new strain)	

TABLE 23-7   Care for Patients with Ebola Virus Disease

TRANSMISSION OF DISEASE	PREVENTION OF DISEASE	ASSESSMENT	PATIENT-CENTERED COLLABORATIVE CARE
The primary source of the Ebola virus is most likely contaminated bats or primates (apes and monkeys) in West Africa. Information that is known about transmission includes: • The Ebola virus cannot be transmitted unless a person is sick and has clinical manifestations of the disease. • The Ebola virus is not spread via air, water, or food. • Nurses can help identify people at high risk for having or transmitting the disease by taking a complete history, including asking about travel to West Africa, or exposure to family and friends who have Ebola. • The disease can be transmitted by unprotected contact with people infected with the Ebola virus or with people who have died from Ebola. • Teach patients who recover from Ebola and their partners that the virus is present in semen for up to 3 months. Using a condom may prevent transmission.	Take special training *before* caring for patients with the Ebola virus. Use these precautions: • Avoid direct contact with body fluids (blood, feces, saliva, urine, vomit, and semen). • Use Standard, Contact, and Droplet Precautions, including appropriate PPE. • Isolate patient with Ebola in a single room. • Use dedicated or disposable medical equipment and supplies. • Practice proper sterilization measures.	Clinical manifestations occur 2-21 days after exposure to the Ebola virus. Assess for: • Fever • Severe headache • Muscle pain • Weakness • Fatigue • Diarrhea • Vomiting • Abdominal pain • Unexplained hemorrhage (bleeding and bruising)	No drug therapy or vaccine is yet FDA approved for Ebola. Remember that the virus can enter the body through broken skin or unprotected mucous membranes such as the eyes, nose, and mouth. Supportive care includes: • Intravenous fluid and electrolyte replacement • Oxygen and ventilation support • Blood pressure support • Treatment of other infections • Care and comfort measures • Symptomatic care • Emotional support • Possible end-of-life care

Data from CDC. (2014). *Ebola (Ebola virus disease)*. Accessed in November 2014 from www.cdc.gov/vhf/ebola/index/html.

(EMR) in which the physician was unable to view the nurse's notes and see that the nurse had recorded the patient's recent returne from West Africa. It is of vital importance that the nurse and provider of care be sure to communicate pertinent historical information both verbally and in the EMR so that appropriate interventions for both the individual and the general public can be undertaken immediately.

Pandemic infections, such as influenza, are another threat to the population. As recently as the early 1900s, the "Spanish flu" killed millions of people throughout the world. Health care workers are encouraged to have yearly influenza vaccines to prevent infection with common strains of the virus. The federal government and health care agencies around the United States include the risk for pandemic disease in their disaster planning (see Chapter 10).

Contaminated food is another source of INFECTION. The incidence of foodborne infections has risen in the United States as contaminated fresh spinach, ground beef, and other foods were found to contain *E. coli* 0157:H7. Many illnesses and thousands of recent deaths in the United States have been caused by this infection. Safer food preparation practices and increased monitoring by federal agencies have resulted from demand for public safety.

Another pathogen, *Clostridium difficile (C. difficile)*, is associated with antibiotic therapy use, especially in older adults. Associated problems have led to the development of the diagnosis of C. difficile–associated disease (CDAD) (Grossman & Mager, 2010). A new more virulent strain of this pathogen has developed in the past decade due to the use of fluoroquinolone antibiotics, such as ciprofloxacin (Cipro).

C. difficile is spread by indirect contact with inanimate objects like medical equipment and commodes, and its toxins cause colon dysfunction and cell death from sepsis. CDAD is confirmed by stool culture. Patients who have three or more liquid stools per day for two or more days are suspected of having the infection. Fever and abdominal pain and cramping commonly occur with diarrheal stools. Oral metronidazole (Flagyl) and vancomycin have been the drugs of choice to treat CDAD. However, some patients experience recurrence of infection after treatment with these drugs. A new oral antibacterial drug available for specifically managing *C. difficile* is fidaxomicin (Dificid).

A new controversial treatment for CDAD is fecal bacteriotherapy to transplant stool with normal healthy flora into the infected patient. The donor stool is liquefied with saline, filtered, and administered to the patient with CDAD by nasogastric tube, fecal enema, or colonoscopy. Results of this treatment have been very positive (Meyers, 2011).

In addition to concerns about emerging infections, preparation for and education about *bioterrorism* have been major focuses of the U.S. government since September 11, 2001. In some cases, vaccines are no longer given for biologic agents like smallpox. Many people in the United States have never been vaccinated, and those who had vaccinations many years ago are not guaranteed to have lifelong immunity. Anthrax, usually seen in animals, may be spread to the skin or inhaled. These infections have a high fatality rate in humans. Plague, once seen centuries ago, is one of the biggest threats because the survival rate is low. Vaccines are being researched and stockpiled by the U.S. government for some of the common biologic agents.

NURSING CONCEPTS AND CLINICAL JUDGMENT REVIEW

What might you NOTICE if the patient has INADEQUATE PROTECTION as a result of infection or infectious disease?

- Flushing and sweating
- Localized skin inflammation (redness, warmth, swelling, pain)
- Open wound (draining or non-draining)
- Report of diarrhea or vomiting
- Report of sore throat
- Fatigue
- Rash
- Acute confusion (in older adults)

What should you INTERPRET and how should you RESPOND to a patient with INADEQUATE PROTECTION as a result of infection or infectious disease?

Perform and interpret focused physical assessment findings, including:
- Vital signs
- Skin and/or wound assessment
- Lymph palpation
- Throat inspection

Respond:
- Manage fever if present.
- Take culture of drainage and send to laboratory for analysis.

- Monitor laboratory findings, including complete blood count (CBC) with white blood cell (WBC) differential.
- Place on appropriate Transmission-Based Precautions.
- Teach patients and families about Transmission-Based Precautions and hand hygiene.
- Administer antimicrobial therapy as prescribed.
- Collaborate with the facility's infection control practitioner.
- Teach patients and families about the need to adhere to the drug therapy regimen.
- Follow CDC guidelines and The Joint Commission's National Patient Safety Goals (NPSGs).

On what should you REFLECT?
- Monitor the patient's response to drug therapy.
- Monitor the patient's vital signs for return to baseline.
- Evaluate the patient's and family's knowledge of infection, Transmission-Based Precautions, and drug therapy.
- Monitor the staff's compliance with hand hygiene and personal protective equipment (PPE).
- Evaluate the patient's and family's coping ability.
- Think about what else you might do to make the patient more comfortable.
- Decide whether you need to provide alternative or additional interventions or health teaching.

GET READY FOR THE NCLEX® EXAMINATION!

KEY POINTS

Review these Key Points for each NCLEX Examination Client Needs Category.

Safe and Effective Care Environment

- Handwashing and alcohol-based hand rubs are two methods of hand hygiene (see Chart 23-3).
- The Centers for Disease Control and Prevention (CDC) recommends a ban on artificial fingernails for health care professionals when they are caring for patients at high risk for infection. **Evidence-Based Practice** QSEN
- Infections can be prevented or controlled through hand hygiene, disinfection/sterilization, personal protective equipment (PPE), patient placement, and adequate staffing; proper hand hygiene and gloves are the most important interventions because health care workers' hands are the primary way in which disease is transmitted from patient to patient. **Evidence-Based Practice** QSEN
- Standard Precautions are used with all patients in health care settings, assuming that all body excretions and secretions are potentially infectious (see Table 23-2). **Safety** QSEN
- Airborne Precautions are used for patients who have infections transmitted through the air, such as tuberculosis.
- Droplet Precautions are used for patients who have infections transmitted by droplets, such as influenza and certain types of meningitis.
- Contact Precautions are used for patients who have infections transmitted by direct contact or contact with items in the patient's environment.

Health Promotion and Maintenance

- Health teaching about clinical manifestations of infection and drug therapy is important for the patient with an infection being managed at home; some patients may need health care nursing services for IV antimicrobial therapy.
- Teach patients about antimicrobial therapy and protective measures to prevent infection transmission.
- Teach patients how to avoid community-acquired MRSA by performing frequent hand hygiene and by avoiding crowds and direct contact with others who have infections. **Safety** QSEN

Psychosocial Integrity

- Patients who have Transmission-Based Precautions may feel isolated, anxious, or depressed; they may feel neglected and

dissatisfied with their care. Help patients cope with these feelings through verbalization and collaboration with the health care team. **Teamwork and Collaboration** QSEN

Physiological Integrity

- Patients at the highest risk for infection include older adults, health care professionals at risk for needle sticks, and patients who have diabetes or are immunocompromised. Patients who take long-term steroid therapy or have had invasive procedures or therapies are also at a high risk for infection.
- Multidrug-resistant organisms (MDROs) are the result of the overuse of antibiotic therapy and include methicillin-resistant *Staphylococcus aureus* (MRSA), vancomycin-resistant *Enterococcus* (VRE), and carbapenem-resistant *Enterobacteriaceae* (CRE).
- A biofilm, also called *glycocalyx,* is a complex group of microorganisms that function within a "slimy" gel coating on medical devices, such as urinary catheters, orthopedic implants, and enteral feeding tubes; on parts of the body like the teeth (plaque) and tonsils; and in chronic wounds. Biofilms are difficult to treat, and research is examining methods to manage them to better treat.
- Common clinical manifestations of infections and infectious diseases include fever and lymphadenopathy. If infections are not treated or are inadequately treated, systemic sepsis (septicemia), septic shock, and disseminated intravascular coagulation (DIC) may result.
- A culture is the most definitive way to confirm and identify microorganisms; sensitivity testing determines which antibiotics will destroy the identified microbes.
- The white blood cell differential count usually shows a shift to the left (increased number of immature neutrophils) during active infections.
- Antimicrobials and antipyretics are the most common types of drugs used when infection is accompanied by fever.
- Antipyretics are used only when the fever presents a significant risk or the patient is very uncomfortable, because antipyretics may mask the disease. **Evidence-Based Practice** QSEN
- Critical issues for the next decade include bioterrorism, emerging infectious diseases, and multidrug-resistant organisms (MDROs).

CHAPTER | 24

Assessment of the Skin, Hair, and Nails

Janice Cuzzell and M. Linda Workman

ⓔ http://evolve.elsevier.com/Iggy/

PRIORITY CONCEPTS

- TISSUE INTEGRITY

LEARNING OUTCOMES

Safe and Effective Care Environment
1. Protect hospitalized patients from skin injury and loss of TISSUE INTEGRITY.

Health Promotion and Maintenance
2. Teach all people how to protect the skin from damage and cancer development.

Psychosocial Integrity
3. Reduce the psychological impact for the patient and family regarding the assessment and testing of the integumentary system.

Physiological Integrity
4. Use knowledge of anatomy and physiology to perform a focused assessment of the skin, hair, and nails, incorporating information about genetic risk and age-related changes affecting these structures.

The skin, hair, and nails are the tissues making up the integumentary system. Skin TISSUE INTEGRITY plays a major role in protection. Intact skin has barrier functions, alarm functions, and even combat functions. As shown in Fig. 24-1, the skin protects the body against invasion of pathogenic organisms by providing a first line of defense (the moat), a second line of defense (the castle wall), and even a third line of defense (the knights and soldiers). The normal flora on the surfaces of skin and mucous membranes repels some of the more harmful microorganisms. Specialized cells in the skin engulf foreign substances (antigens) that invade the body when skin TISSUE INTEGRITY is lost and then alert the immune system to the presence of the invader. Localized tissue inflammation and swelling work to contain the invading pathogen until white blood cells can respond and remove this threat.

The skin is the largest organ of the body and, when intact, helps regulate body temperature and maintains fluid and electrolyte balance. Skin changes can provide important information about a person's health and well-being. Emotional stress, systemic disease, some drugs, and skin injury or disease can alter skin function, appearance, and texture.

The skin's sensory function allows the use of touch as an intervention to provide comfort, relieve pain, and communicate caring. Because the skin has many sensory receptors, the patient can report subjective skin sensations that might indicate specific health problems.

ANATOMY AND PHYSIOLOGY REVIEW

Structure of the Skin

The skin has three layers: subcutaneous tissue (fat), dermis, and epidermis (Fig. 24-2). Each layer has unique properties that help the skin maintain its complex functions.

Subcutaneous fat (adipose tissue [fat]) is the innermost layer of the skin, lying over muscle and bone. Fat distribution varies with body area, age, and gender. Fat cells insulate the body and absorb shock, padding internal structures. Blood vessels go through the fatty layer and extend into the dermis, forming capillary networks that supply nutrients and remove wastes.

The dermis (corium) is the layer above the fat layer and contains no skin cells but does contain some protective mast cells and macrophages (see Chapter 17). The dermis is composed of interwoven collagen and elastic fibers that give the skin flexibility and strength.

Collagen, the main component of dermal tissue, is a protein produced by fibroblast cells. Its production increases in areas of tissue injury and helps form scar tissue. Fibroblasts also produce **ground substance,** a lubricant that contributes to skin suppleness and turgor.

Skin elasticity depends on the amount and quality of the dermal elastic fibers. The major component of the elastic fiber is elastin.

The dermis has capillaries and lymph vessels for the exchange of oxygen and heat. It is rich in sensory nerves that transmit the sensations of touch, pressure, temperature, pain, and itch.

The epidermis is the outermost skin layer. It is anchored to the dermis by fingerlike projections (**rete pegs**) that interlock with dermal structures called **dermal papillae.** Less than 1 mm thick, the epidermal layer is the first line of defense between the body and the environment.

The epidermis does not have its own blood supply. Instead it receives nutrients by diffusion from the blood vessels in the dermal layer. Attached to the basement membrane of the epidermis are the basal **keratinocytes**—skin cells that undergo cell division and differentiation to continuously renew skin TISSUE INTEGRITY and maintain optimal barrier function. As basal cells divide, keratinocytes are pushed upward and form the *spinous layer (stratum spinosum).* Together the basal layer and the spinous layer are referred to as the *germinative layer (stratum germinativum),* because these layers are responsible for new skin growth (McCance et al., 2014). The keratinocytes continue to enlarge and flatten as they move upward to form the outermost horny skin layer (**stratum corneum).** When these cells reach the stratum corneum (in 28 to 45 days), they are no longer living cells and are shed from the skin surface. **Keratin,** a protein produced by keratinocytes, makes the horny layer waterproof.

On the palms of the hands and soles of the feet an additional thick layer of epidermis forms known as the *stratum lucidum.* This clear layer of nonliving cells pads and protects the underlying dermal and epidermal structures in these vulnerable areas.

Vitamin D is activated in the epidermis by ultraviolet (UV) light, such as sunlight. Once activated, it is distributed by the blood to the GI tract to promote uptake of dietary calcium.

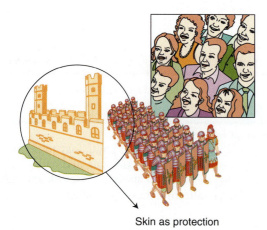

Skin as protection

FIG. 24-1 Role of the skin in the concept of body protection.

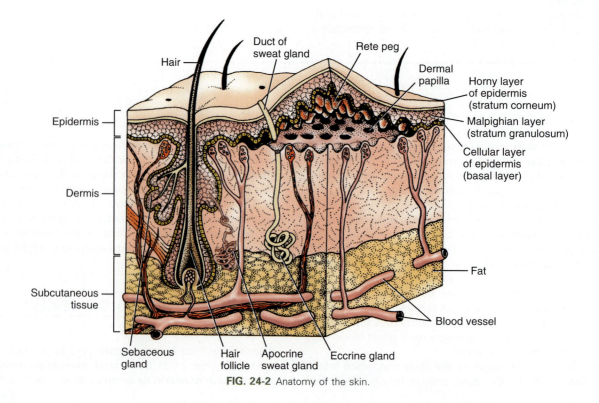

FIG. 24-2 Anatomy of the skin.

Melanocytes are pigment-producing cells found at the basement membrane. These cells give color to the skin and account for the ethnic differences in skin tone. Darker skin tones are not caused by increased numbers of melanocytes; rather, the size of the pigment granules *(melanin)* contained in each cell determines the color. Melanin protects the skin from damage by UV light, which stimulates melanin production. For this reason, people with dark skin are less likely to develop sunburn than lighter-skinned people. Freckles, birthmarks, and age spots are lesions caused by patches of increased melanin production. Melanin production also increases in areas that have endocrine changes or inflammation.

Structure of the Skin Appendages

Hair differs in type and function in various body areas. Hair growth varies with race, gender, age, and genetic predisposition. Individual hairs can differ in both structure and rate of growth, depending on body location.

Hair follicles are located in the dermal layer of the skin but are actually extensions of the epidermal layer (see Fig. 24-2). Within each hair follicle, a round column of keratin forms the hair shaft. Hair color is genetically determined by a person's rate of melanin production.

Hair growth occurs in cycles of a growth phase followed by a resting phase. Growth is dependent on a good blood supply and adequate nutrition. Stressors can alter the growth cycle and result in temporary hair loss. Permanent baldness, such as male pattern baldness, is inherited.

Nails on fingers and toes have cosmetic value and are useful for grasping and scraping. Like hair follicles, the nails are extensions of the keratin-producing epidermal layers of the skin.

The white, crescent-shaped portion of the nail at the lower end of the nail plate is the **lunula** and is where nail keratin is formed and nail growth begins (Fig. 24-3). Nail growth is a continuous but slow process. Fingernail replacement requires 3 to 4 months. Toenail replacement may take up to 12 months.

The cuticle attaches the nail plate to the soft tissue of the nail fold. The nail body is translucent, and the pinkish hue reflects a rich blood supply beneath the nail surface. Nail growth and appearance are often altered during systemic disease or serious illness.

Sebaceous glands are distributed over the entire skin surface except for the palms of the hands and soles of the feet. Most of these glands are connected directly to the hair follicles (see Fig. 24-2).

Sebaceous glands produce **sebum,** a mildly bacteriostatic, fat-containing substance. Sebum lubricates the skin and reduces water loss from the skin surface.

Sweat glands of the skin are of two types: eccrine and apocrine. Eccrine sweat glands arise from the epithelial cells. They are found over the entire skin surface and are not associated with the hair follicle. The odorless, colorless secretions of these glands are important in body temperature regulation. This sweat and the resultant water evaporation can cause the body to lose up to 10 to 12 L of fluid in a single day.

Apocrine sweat glands are in direct contact with the hair follicle and are found mostly in the axillae, nipple, umbilical, and perineal body areas. The interaction of skin bacteria with the secretions of these glands causes body odor.

Functions of the Skin

The skin is a complex organ responsible for the regulation of many body functions throughout the life span (Table 24-1) (McCance et al., 2014). In addition to the skin's protective and regulatory functions, its location on the outside of the body makes it an important way to communicate a patient's state of health and body image.

Skin Changes Associated with Aging

The process of aging begins at birth (Touhy & Jett, 2014). As changes in physiology progress with aging, the skin also undergoes age-related changes in structure and function (Chart 24-1). Figs. 24-4 through 24-8 show age-related skin changes.

FIG. 24-4 Arcus senilis of the iris.

FIG. 24-5 Nail changes: longitudinal ridges and thickening.

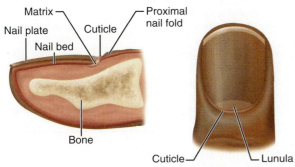

FIG. 24-3 Anatomy of the nail.

Matrix — Proximal nail fold
Nail plate   Cuticle
Nail bed
Bone
Cuticle — Lunula

TABLE 24-1 Functions of the Skin

EPIDERMIS	DERMIS	SUBCUTANEOUS TISSUE
Protection		
Keratin provides protection from injury by corrosive materials	Provides cells for wound healing	Mechanical shock absorber
Inhibits proliferation of microorganisms because of dry external surface	Provides mechanical strength: Collagen fibers	Energy reserve
Mechanical strength through intercellular bonds	Elastic fibers Ground substance Sensory nerve receptors signal skin injury and inflammation	Insulation
Homeostasis (Water Balance)		
Low permeability to water and electrolytes prevents systemic dehydration and electrolyte loss	Lymphatic and vascular tissues respond to inflammation, injury, and infection	No real function in water balance
Temperature Regulation		
Eccrine sweat glands allow dissipation of heat through evaporation of sweat secreted onto the skin surface	Cutaneous vasculature promotes or inhibits heat loss from the skin surface	Fat cells insulate and assist in retention of body heat
Sensory Organ		
Transmits a variety of sensations through the neuroreceptor system	Has many nerve receptors for relaying sensations to the brain	Contains large pressure receptors
Vitamin Synthesis		
Allows photoconversion of 7-dehydrocholesterol to active vitamin D	No function	No function
Psychosocial		
Body image alterations occur with many epidermal diseases	Body image alterations occur with many dermal diseases	Body image alterations may result from changes in body fat stores

CHART 24-1 Nursing Focus on the Older Adult

Changes in the Integumentary System Related to Aging

PHYSICAL CHANGES	CLINICAL FINDINGS	NURSING ACTIONS
Epidermis		
Decreased epidermal thickness	Skin transparency and fragility	Handle patients carefully to reduce skin friction and shear. Assess for excessive dryness or moisture. Avoid taping the skin.
Decreased cell division	Delayed wound healing	Avoid skin trauma, and protect open areas.
Decreased epidermal mitotic homeostasis	Skin hyperplasia and skin cancers (especially in sun-exposed areas)	Assess non–sun-exposed areas for baseline skin features. Assess exposed skin areas for sun-induced changes.
Increased epidermal permeability	Increased risk for irritation	Teach patients how to avoid exposure to skin irritants.
Decreased immune system cells	Decreased skin inflammatory response	Do not rely on degree of redness and swelling to correlate with the severity of skin injury or localized infection.
Decreased melanocyte activity	Increased risk for sunburn	Teach patients to wear hats, sunscreen, and protective clothing. Teach patients to avoid sun exposure from 10 AM to 4 PM.
Hyperplasia of melanocyte activity (especially in sun-exposed areas)	Changes in pigmentation (e.g., liver spots, age spots)	Teach patients to keep track of pigmented lesions. Teach them what changes should be evaluated for malignancy.
Decreased vitamin D production	Increased risk for osteomalacia	Urge patients to take a multiple vitamin or a calcium supplement with vitamin D.
Flattening of the dermal-epidermal junction	Increased risk for shearing forces, resulting in blisters, purpura, skin tears, and pressure-related problems	Avoid pulling or dragging patients. Assist patients confined to bed or chairs to change positions at least every 2 hours. Avoid or use care when removing adhesive wound dressings.

CHART 24-1 Nursing Focus on the Older Adult—cont'd

Changes in the Integumentary System Related to Aging

PHYSICAL CHANGES	CLINICAL FINDINGS	NURSING ACTIONS
Dermis		
Decreased dermal blood flow	Increased susceptibility to dry skin	Teach patients to apply moisturizers when the skin is still moist and to avoid agents that promote skin dryness.
Decreased vasomotor responsiveness	Increased risk for heat stroke and hypothermia	Teach patients to dress for the environmental temperatures.
Decreased dermal thickness	Paper-thin, transparent skin with an increased susceptibility to trauma	Handle patients gently, and avoid the use of tape or tight dressings. Use lift sheets when positioning patients.
Degeneration of elastic fibers	Decreased tone and elasticity	Check skin turgor on the forehead or chest.
Benign proliferation of capillaries	Cherry hemangiomas	Teach patients that these are benign.
Reduced number and function of nerve endings	Reduced sensory perception	Tell patients to use bath thermometer and to lower the water heater temperature to prevent scalds.
Subcutaneous Layer		
Thinning subcutaneous layer	Increased risk for hypothermia	Teach patients to dress warmly in cold weather.
	Increased risk for pressure injury	Assist patients confined to bed or chairs to change positions at least every 2 hours.
Hair		
Decreased number of hair follicles and rate of growth	Increased hair thinning	Suggest wearing hats to prevent heat loss in cold weather and to prevent sunburn.
Decreased number of active melanocytes in follicle	Gradual loss of hair color (graying)	Inform patients that hair color loss can occur at any age.
Nails		
Decreased rate of growth	Increased risk for fungal infections	Inspect the nails of all older adults. Teach patients to keep feet clean and dry.
Decreased nail bed blood flow	Longitudinal nail ridges	Use the oral mucosa to assess for cyanosis.
Thickening of the nail	Toenails thicken and may overhang the toes	Use fingernails to assess capillary refill. Cut toenails straight across. Do not use nail appearance alone to assess for a fungal infection. Assess skin next to the nail to determine whether the thick nail is irritating it.
Glands		
Decreased sebum production	Increased size of nasal pores; large comedones	Teach patients not to squeeze the pores or comedones to prevent skin trauma.
Decreased eccrine and apocrine gland activity	Increased susceptibility to dry skin	Urge patients to use soaps with a high fat content. Teach patients to avoid frequent bathing with hot water. Teach patients to apply moisturizers after bathing while skin is moist.
	Decreased perspiration with decreased cooling effect	Do not use sweat production as an indicator of hyperthermia.

FIG. 24-6 Paper-thin, transparent skin with actinic lentigo (liver spots).

Liver spot

FIG. 24-7 Eyelid eversion, deepening of the eye orbit, and "bags" under the eye.

FIG. 24-8 Senile (cherry) angiomas.

Individual differences exist in how quickly and to what degree the skin ages. Although genetic factors, hormonal changes, and disease may change skin appearance over time, chronic sun exposure is the single most important factor leading to degeneration of the skin components.

ASSESSMENT METHODS

Patient History

Take an accurate history from the patient so that skin problems can be readily identified. Chart 24-2 highlights specific questions to ask during a skin assessment.

Demographic data include age, race, occupation, and hobbies or recreational activities. This information can help identify causative or aggravating factors for skin problems. Age is important because many changes in the skin, hair, and nails are normal for the aging process.

Ethnicity can also be important. Some variations in skin appearance are normal for patients of some ethnicities but are abnormal for those of other races or ethnicities.

Information about occupation and hobbies can provide clues to chronic skin exposure to chemicals, irritants, and other substances that can contribute to skin problems.

Socioeconomic status data can help identify environmental factors that might contribute to skin disease. Unhealthy or crowded living conditions promote the spread of contagious skin pathogens. Recent or frequent travel to tropical climates may be a source of unusual skin infections or infestations.

Regardless of skin color or ethnicity, always ask patients about the amount of time spent in the sun and tanning booths and identify skin problems related to sun overexposure. Use this time to teach the patient about the harmful aspects of sun exposure and how to reduce risk. Also determine whether he or she regularly assesses the skin for lesion development or changes.

Skin problems related to poor hygiene are common. Ask about living conditions and bathing practices. Teach people that keeping the skin and hair clean by bathing and shampooing regularly helps maintain the skin's health.

Information about drug use is important because prescribed drugs, over-the-counter (OTC) drugs, herbal preparations or remedies, and tobacco use can cause skin reactions or affect skin function. Ask about any recent use of prescription drugs, OTC drugs (e.g., laxatives, antacids, cold remedies), and herbal preparations or remedies. Determine when each drug was started,

Questions to Obtain an Accurate Nursing History of the Patient with a Skin Problem

Medical-Surgical History
- Do you have any current or previous medical problems?
- Have you undergone any recent or previous surgical procedures?

Family History
- Is there any family tendency toward chronic skin problems?
- Do any members of your immediate family have recent skin problems?

Medication History
- Are you allergic to any drugs? If so, describe the reaction.
- What prescription drugs have you taken recently? When was the drug started? What is the dose or frequency of administration? When was the last dose taken?
- What over-the-counter drugs have you taken recently? When was the drug started? What is the dose or frequency of administration? When was the last dose taken?

Social History
- What is your occupation?
- What recreational activities do you enjoy?
- Have you traveled recently?
- What is your nutrition status?
- Do you use tobacco or recreational drugs or drink alcohol?

Current Health Problem
- When did you first notice the skin problem?
- Where on the body did the problem begin?
- Has the problem gotten better or worse?
- Has a similar skin condition ever occurred before? If so, what was the course and how was it treated?
- Is the problem associated with any itching, burning, stinging, numbness, pain, fever, nausea and vomiting, diarrhea, sore throat, cold, stiff neck, new foods, new soaps or cosmetics, new clothing or bed linens, or stressful situations?
- What seems to make the problem worse?
- What seems to make the problem better?

the dose and frequency of the drug, and the time the last dose was taken. Ask the patient whether skin changes began after starting a new drug. A drug history also helps identify skin changes that result from management of other health problems, such as the changes that occur with long-term steroid or anticoagulant therapy.

Allergies to environmental substances often have skin manifestations. The allergies may be well documented or have a new onset. Ask about the use of any new personal care product (e.g., shaving products, perfumes, soap, shampoo, lotion, makeup, hair gel), laundry detergents and softeners, and home cleaning products. Ask whether the patient wears gloves to avoid direct contact with cleaning solutions. New clothing may contain chemicals that irritate the skin. Noting the body location(s) of the skin problem can help determine its cause.

Nutrition Status

Document the patient's weight, height, body build and fat distribution, and food preferences. Protein deficiencies, vitamin deficiencies, and obesity can increase the risk for skin lesions and delay wound healing. Fat-free diets and chronic alcoholism can lead to vitamin deficiencies and related skin changes. Skin problems such as chronic urticaria and acne may be worsened by certain foods or food additives.

Hydration influences overall skin health, and the skin reflects hydration status. Reduced fluid intake can lead to dry skin. Skin manifestations of severe fluid losses are seen as loose skin that tents when pinched together. Fluid overload with edema can stretch the skin, masking wrinkles and allowing the formation of skin "pits" (i.e., pitting edema) when pressure is applied to it.

Family History and Genetic Risk

Many skin problems (e.g., psoriasis, keloid formation, eczema) have a familial predisposition. Explore any family tendency of chronic skin problems. Ask about immediate family members' current health to identify a transmittable disorder (e.g., ringworm, scabies).

Current Health Problems

Begin by gathering information about skin changes and skin care practices (see Chart 24-2).

If a skin problem is identified, obtain more information about the specific problem, such as:

- When did the patient first notice the rash or skin change?
- Where on the body did the rash begin?
- Has the problem improved or become worse?

If the problem has occurred before, ask the patient to describe the course of the skin lesion and how it was treated. Try to link the problem with manifestations, such as itching, burning, numbness, pain, fever, sore throat, stiff neck, or nausea and vomiting. Ask him or her to identify anything that seems to make the problem better or worse.

Skin Assessment

Inspection

Skin changes may be related to a specific skin disease or reflect a systemic disorder. Use a thorough skin assessment to identify clues about a patient's overall state of health.

A thorough assessment of the skin is best performed with the patient undressed. (Always provide privacy to maintain the patient's dignity.) Incorporate skin examination as a routine part of daily care during the bath or when assisting with hygiene.

Inspect the patient's skin surfaces in a well-lighted room; natural or bright fluorescent lighting makes subtle skin changes more visible. Use a penlight to closely inspect lesions and to illuminate the mouth.

Assess each skin surface systematically, including the scalp, hair, nails, and mucous membranes. Give particular attention to the skinfold areas. The moist, warm environment of skinfolds can harbor organisms, such as yeast or bacteria. Observe and document these features:

- Obvious changes in color and vascularity
- Presence or absence of moisture
- Edema
- Skin lesions
- Skin integrity

Check the cleanliness of the various body areas to determine whether the patient's self-care activities need to be evaluated.

Skin color is affected by blood flow, oxygenation, body temperature, and pigmentation. The wide variation in skin tones requires different techniques for patients who have darker skin.

(See the Cultural Considerations box for tips for assessing patients with darker skin.)

Describe and document changes in skin color by their appearance (Table 24-2). Include in your description whether the changes are general or confined to one body region. Color changes are more visible in the areas of least pigmentation, such as the oral mucosa, sclera, nail beds, and palms and soles. Inspect these areas to help confirm more subtle color changes of general body areas.

Lesions in skin disease are clinically described in terms of primary and secondary lesions (Fig. 24-9). **Primary lesions** are an initial reaction to a problem that alters skin components. **Secondary lesions** are changes in the appearance of the primary lesion. These changes occur with progression of an underlying disease or in response to a topical or systemic therapeutic intervention. For example, acute dermatitis often occurs as primary vesicles with associated **pruritus** (itching). Secondary lesions in the form of crusts occur as the patient scratches, the vesicles are opened, and the exudate dries. With chronic dermatitis, the skin often becomes **lichenified** (thickened) because of the patient's continual rubbing of the area to relieve itching.

Describe lesions by color, size, location, and shape. Note whether they are isolated or are grouped and form a distinct pattern. Table 24-3 defines terms used to describe lesions.

Assess each lesion for these ABCDE features that are associated with skin cancer (The Skin Cancer Foundation, 2014):

- **A**symmetry of shape
- **B**order irregularity
- **C**olor variation within one lesion
- **D**iameter greater than 6 mm
- **E**volving or changing in any feature (shape, size, color, elevation, itching, bleeding, or crusting)

Teach patients these signs, and encourage them to perform skin self-examination on a monthly basis (American Cancer Society, 2014). *A patient who has a lesion with one or more of the ABCDE features should be evaluated by a dermatologist or surgeon.*

In describing location, determine whether lesions are generalized or localized. If the lesions are localized, identify the specific body areas involved. This information is important because some diseases have a specific pattern of skin lesions. For example, involvement of only the sun-exposed areas of the body is important when considering possible causes. Rashes limited to the skinfold areas (e.g., on the axillae, beneath the breasts, in the groin) may reflect problems related to friction, heat, and excessive moisture.

Edema causes the skin to appear shiny, **taut** (tightly stretched), and paler than uninvolved skin. During skin inspection, document the location, distribution, and color of areas of edema.

Skin elasticity is affected by edema. Using moderate pressure, place the tip of a finger against edematous tissue to determine the degree of indentation, or pitting (see Chapter 11).

Moisture content is assessed by noting the thickness and consistency of secretions. Normally, increased moisture in the form of sweat occurs with increased activity or elevated environmental temperatures. Dampness of skinfold areas occurs with reduced air circulation where the skin surfaces touch. Excess moisture can cause impaired TISSUE INTEGRITY with skin breakdown in bedridden and debilitated patients.

Overly dry skin is caused by a dry environment, poor skin lubrication, inadequate fluid intake, and the normal aging process. Dry skin usually has scaling and flaking and may be

TABLE 24-2   Common Alterations in Skin Color

ALTERATION	UNDERLYING CAUSE	LOCATION	SIGNIFICANCE
White (pallor)	Decreased hemoglobin level	Conjunctivae	Anemia
	Decreased blood flow to the skin (vasoconstriction)	Mucous membranes	Shock or blood loss
		Nail beds	Chronic vascular compromise
		Palms and soles	Sudden emotional upset
		Lips	Edema
	Genetically determined defect of the melanocyte (decreased pigmentation)	Generalized	Albinism
	Acquired patchy loss of pigmentation	Localized	Vitiligo, tinea versicolor
Yellow-orange	Increased total serum bilirubin level (jaundice)	Generalized	Hemolysis of red blood cells
		Mucous membranes	Liver disorders
		Sclera	
	Increased serum carotene level (carotenemia)	Perioral	Increased ingestion of carotene-containing foods (carrots)
		Palms and soles	Pregnancy
		Ears and nose	Thyroid deficiency
		Absent in sclera and mucous membranes	Diabetes
	Increased urochrome level	Generalized	Chronic kidney disease (uremia)
		Absent in sclera and mucous membranes	
Red (erythema)	Increased blood flow to the skin (vasodilation)	Generalized	Generalized inflammation (e.g., erythroderma)
		Localized (to area of involvement)	Localized inflammation (e.g., sunburn, cellulitis, trauma, rashes)
		Face, cheeks, nose, upper chest	Fever, increased alcohol intake
		Area of exposure	Exposure to cold
Blue	Increase in deoxygenated blood (cyanosis)	Nail beds	Cardiopulmonary disease
		Mucous membranes	Methemoglobinemia
		Generalized	
	Bleeding from vessels into tissue:		
	Petechiae (1-3 mm)	Localized	Thrombocytopenia
	Ecchymosis (>3 mm)	Localized	Increased blood vessel fragility
Reddish blue	Increased overall amount of hemoglobin	Generalized	Polycythemia vera
	Decreased peripheral circulation	Distal extremities, nose	Inadequate tissue perfusion
Brown	Increased melanin production	Localized (to area of involvement)	Chronic inflammation
		Pressure points, areolae, palmar creases, and genitalia	Exposure to sunlight
			Addison's disease
		Face, areolae, vulva, linea nigra	Pregnancy; oral contraceptives (melasma)
	Café au lait spots (tan-brown patches):		
	<6 spots	Localized	Nonpathogenic
	>6 spots	Generalized	Possible neurofibromatosis
	Melanin and hemosiderin deposits (bronze or grayish tan color)	Distal lower extremities	Chronic venous stasis
		Exposed areas or generalized	Hemochromatosis

TABLE 24-3   Terms Commonly Used to Describe Skin Lesion Configurations

annular Ringlike with raised borders around flat, clear centers of normal skin

circinate Circular

circumscribed Well-defined with sharp borders

clustered Several lesions grouped together

coalesced Lesions that merge with one another and appear confluent

diffuse Widespread, involving most of the body with intervening areas of normal skin; generalized

linear Occurring in a straight line

serpiginous With wavy borders, resembling a snake

universal All areas of the body involved, with no areas of normal-appearing skin

especially marked in areas of limited circulation, such as the feet and lower legs. It is a common problem during the winter months when the air contains less moisture, living in geographic areas with little humidity, and in the hospital environment where humidity is often low.

Vascular changes or markings may be normal or abnormal, depending on the cause. Normal vascular markings include birthmarks, cherry angiomas (see Fig. 24-8), spider angiomas, and venous stars. Bleeding into the skin is abnormal and results in **purpura** (bleeding under the skin that may progress from red to purple to brownish yellow), petechiae, and ecchymosis.

Petechiae are small, reddish purple lesions (<0.5 mm in diameter) that do not fade or blanch when pressure is applied (Fig. 24-10). They often indicate increased capillary fragility. Petechiae of the lower extremities often occur with stasis

Primary lesions

Macules
(such as *freckles, flat moles* or *rubella*) are flat lesions of less than 1 cm in diameter. Their color is different from that of the surrounding skin—most often white, red or brown.

Nodules
(such as *lipomas*) are elevated marble-like lesions more than 1 cm wide and deep.

Patches
(such as *vitiligo* or *café au lait spots*) are macules that are larger than 1 cm in diameter. They may or may not have some surface changes—either slight scale or fine wrinkles.

Cysts
(such as *sebaceous cysts*) are nodules filled with either liquid or semisolid material that can be expressed.

Papules
(such as *warts* or *elevated moles*) are small, firm, elevated lesions less than 1 cm in diameter.

Vesicle
Bulla

Vesicles
(such as in *acute dermatitis*) and **Bullae** (such as *second-degree burns*) are blisters filled with clear fluid. Vesicles are less than 1 cm in diameter, and bullae are more than 1 cm in diameter.

Plaques
(such as in *psoriasis* or *seborrheic keratosis*) are elevated, plateau-like patches more than 1 cm in diameter that do not extend into the lower skin layers.

Pustules
(such as in *acne* and *acute impetigo*) are vesicles filled with cloudy or purulent fluid.

Wheals
(such as *urticaria* and *insect bites*) are elevated, irregularly shaped, transient areas of dermal edema.

Erosions
(such as in *varicella*) are wider than fissures but involve only the epidermis. They are often associated with vesicles, bullae, or pustules.

Secondary lesions

Scales
(such as in *exfoliative dermatitis* and *psoriasis*) are visibly thickened stratum corneum. They appear dry and are usually whitish. They are seen most often with papules and plaques.

Ulcers
(such as *stage 3 pressure sores*) are deep erosions that extend beneath the epidermis and involve the dermis and sometimes the subcutaneous fat.

Crust   Oozing

Crusts and oozing
(such as in *eczema* and *late-stage impetigo*) are composed of dried serum or pus on the surface of the skin, beneath which liquid debris may accumulate. Crusts frequently result from broken vesicles, bullae, or pustules.

Lichenifications
(such as in *chronic dermatitis*) are palpably thickened areas of epidermis with accentuated skin markings. They are caused by chronic rubbing and scratching.

Fissures
(such as in *athlete's foot*) are linear cracks in the epidermis that often extend into the dermis.

Atrophy
(such as *striae* [stretch marks] and *aged skin*) is characterized by thinning of the skin surface with loss of skin markings. The skin is translucent and paper-like. Atrophy involving the dermal layer results in skin depression.

FIG. 24-9 Classification of skin lesions.

FIG. 24-10 Petechiae.

dermatitis, a condition usually seen with chronic venous insufficiency.

Ecchymoses (bruises) are larger areas of hemorrhage. In older adults, bruising is common after minor trauma to the skin. Certain drugs (e.g., aspirin, warfarin, corticosteroids) and low platelet counts lead to easy or excessive bruising. Anticoagulants and decreased numbers of platelets disrupt clotting action, resulting in ecchymosis.

Skin TISSUE INTEGRITY is assessed by first examining areas with actual breaks or open areas. For example, skin tears are a common finding in older people as a result of aging. The thin, fragile skin is easily damaged by friction or shearing forces, especially if bruising is already present. Look for skin tears in these areas:

- Where constricting clothing rubs against the skin
- On the upper extremities, where the skin is grasped when assisting a patient to ambulate or change position
- Where adhesive tapes or dressings have been applied and removed

Check for the presence of multiple abrasions or early pressure-related skin changes. These changes may indicate unrecognized problems in mobility or sensory perception.

Describe breaks in skin TISSUE INTEGRITY by their location, size, color, and distribution and by the presence of drainage or infection. The evaluation of partial-thickness and full-thickness wounds, including objective criteria that describe progress toward healing, is discussed in Chapter 25.

Cleanliness of the skin is evaluated to learn about self-care needs. Inspect the hair, nails, and skin closely for excessive soiling and offensive odor. Depending on a patient's degree of self-care deficit, hard-to-reach areas (e.g., perirectal and inguinal skinfolds, axillae, feet) may be less clean than other skin surface areas. Staining may occur during work or leisure activities.

Patients who have cognitive problems may not pay attention to hygiene measures. Assess the cognition of any patient whose hygiene of the skin, hair, or nails appears inadequate.

Tattoos and piercings can cause or mask skin problems and must be carefully examined. Bruises and rashes may be difficult to see in tattooed areas. Examine newly pierced areas for inflammation or infection. Scars may be present in old tattoos or pierced areas and should be documented. Closely examine any areas where tattoos have been removed. Skin cancer is more likely to occur in these areas.

NCLEX EXAMINATION CHALLENGE
Physiological Integrity

During skin inspection the nurse observes two brown lesions on the older client's upper back. The lesions are large and irregular with a consistently rough texture and a raised border. Which descriptors does the nurse use to document these observations?
A. Annular, macular
B. Confluent, fissured
C. Circumscribed, plaquelike
D. Serpiginous, pustular, linear

Palpation

Skin inspection can be misleading in areas of color changes, tattoos, and piercings. Use palpation to gather additional information about skin lesions, moisture, temperature, texture, and turgor (Table 24-4). Wash hands thoroughly before and after palpating a patient's skin. Use gloves to examine nonintact skin, and use Standard Precautions when skin areas are draining.

Palpation confirms lesion size and whether they are flat or slightly raised. Consistency of larger lesions can vary from soft and pliable to firm and solid. Subtle changes, such as the difference between a fine macular (flat) rash and a papular (raised) rash, are best determined by palpating with your eyes closed. Ask the patient whether skin palpation causes pain or tenderness.

In areas of excess dryness, rub your finger against the skin surface to determine the degree of flaking or scaling. Changes in skin temperature are detected by placing the back of your hand on the skin surface. First, make certain to have warm hands. Cold hands interfere with accurate assessment and are uncomfortable for the patient.

Palpate skin surfaces to assess texture, which differs according to body area and exposure to irritants. For example, areas of long-term sun exposure have a rougher texture than protected skin surfaces. The patient who has repeated exposure to harsh soaps or chemicals may show skin changes related to this exposure. Increased skin thickness from scarring, lichenification, or edema usually decreases elasticity.

Turgor indicates the amount of skin elasticity. Skin turgor can be altered by water content and aging. Gently pinch the patient's skin between your thumb and forefinger, and then release. If skin turgor is normal, the skin immediately returns to its original state when released. Poor skin turgor is seen as "tenting" of the skin, with a gradual return to the original state (see Chapter 11). Loss of elasticity with aging makes the assessment of skin turgor difficult in an older patient.

NURSING SAFETY PRIORITY (QSEN)
Action Alert

To avoid mistaking dehydration for dry skin in an older adult, always assess skin turgor on the forehead or chest.

Hair Assessment

During the skin assessment, inspect and palpate the hair for general appearance, cleanliness, distribution, quantity, and quality. Hair is normally found in an even distribution over most of the body surfaces, with the hair on the scalp, in the pubic region, and in the axillary folds thicker and coarser than

TABLE 24-4   Common Clinical Findings In Skin Palpation

CLINICAL FINDINGS	CAUSE	LOCATION	EXAMPLES OF PREDISPOSING CONDITIONS
Edema			
Localized	Inflammatory response	Area of involvement	Trauma
Dependent or pitting	Fluid and electrolyte imbalance	Ambulatory: dorsum of foot and medial ankle	Congestive heart failure
	Venous and cardiac insufficiency		Kidney disease
		Bedridden: buttocks, sacrum, and lower back	Liver cirrhosis
			Venous thrombosis or stasis
Nonpitting	Endocrine imbalance	Generalized, but more easily seen over the tibia	Hypothyroidism (myxedema)
Moisture			
Increased	Autonomic nervous system stimulation	Face, axillae, skinfolds, palms, and soles	Fever, anxiety, activity
			Hyperthyroidism
Decreased	Dehydration	Buccal mucous membranes with progressive involvement of other skin surfaces	Fluid loss
	Endocrine imbalance		Postmenopausal status
			Hypothyroidism
			Normal aging
Temperature			
Increased	Increased blood flow to the skin	Generalized	Fever, hypermetabolic states
			Neurotrauma
		Localized	Inflammation
Decreased	Decreased blood flow to the skin	Generalized	Impending shock, sepsis, anxiety
			Hypothyroidism
		Localized	Interference with vascular flow
Turgor			
Decreased	Decreased elasticity of the dermis (tenting when pinched)	Abdomen, forehead, or radial aspect of the wrist	Severe dehydration
			Sudden, severe weight loss
			Normal aging
Texture			
Roughness or thickness	Irritation, friction	Pressure points (e.g., soles, palms, elbows)	Calluses
			Chronic eczema
		Localized areas of pruritus	Atopic skin diseases
	Sun damage	Areas of sun exposure	Normal aging
	Excessive collagen production	Localized or generalized	Scleroderma
			Scars and keloids
Softness or smoothness	Endocrine disturbances	Generalized	Hyperthyroidism

hair on the trunk, arms, and legs. Although color and growth patterns vary, sudden changes in hair characteristics may reflect an underlying disease. Check any abnormal findings by obtaining a detailed history of the change.

How well the hair is groomed, including the cleanliness of areas of thicker hair growth, can confirm information about a patient's social history and health care needs. If the patient has intense itching or scratches continually, examine the scalp and pubis for lice and nits (lice eggs). Inspect the scalp for scaling, redness, open areas, crusting, and tenderness.

Dandruff, a collection of patchy or diffuse white or gray scales on the surface of the scalp, is common. The flaking that occurs with dandruff causes many people to mistakenly think the scalp is too dry; however, it is a problem of excessive oil production. Dandruff is a cosmetic problem, but a very oily scalp can induce inflammatory changes with redness and itching. Severe inflammatory dandruff can extend to the eyebrows and the skin of the face and neck. *If severe dandruff is not treated, hair loss can occur.* Teach the patient that dandruff is not caused by dryness and should be treated to prevent hair loss.

Although gradual hair loss occurs with aging, sudden asymmetric or patchy hair loss at any age is of concern. Assess the scalp for hair distribution and thickness, and document variations. Body hair loss, especially on the feet or lower legs, may occur with decreased blood flow to the area and also is a part of aging.

Hirsutism is excessive growth of body hair or hair growth in abnormal body areas. Increased hair growth across the face and chest in women is a sign of hirsutism. It may occur on the face of a woman as part of aging, is one manifestation of hormonal imbalance, and can also occur as a side effect of drug therapy. If hirsutism is present, look for changes in fat distribution and capillary fragility, which can occur in Cushing's disease, and for clitoral enlargement and deepening of the voice, which may indicate ovarian dysfunction.

Nail Assessment

Dystrophic (abnormal-appearing) nails may occur with a serious systemic illness or local skin disease involving the epidermal keratinocytes. Assess the fingernails and toenails for color, shape, thickness, texture, and the presence of lesions.

Many variations in color, texture, and grooming of the nails are influenced by factors unrelated to disease, such as occupation. When assessing the older adult, observe for minor variations associated with the aging process (see Fig. 24-5), such as a gradual thickening of the nail plate, the presence of longitudinal ridges, or a yellowish gray discoloration.

Color of the nail plate depends on nail thickness and transparency, amount of red blood cells, arterial blood flow, and pigment deposits (Table 24-5). Fig. 24-11 shows normal variations in nail color. Changes in color can be caused by chemical damage that occurs with some occupations and with the long-term use of nail polish. Regardless of skin color, the healthy nail blanches (lightens) with pressure.

During examination, the patient's fingers and toes should be free of any surface pressure that interferes with local blood flow or alters the appearance of the digits. To differentiate between color changes from the underlying blood supply and those from pigment deposits, blanch the nail bed to see whether the color changes with pressure. Gently squeeze the end of the finger or toe, exerting downward pressure on the nail bed, and then release the pressure. Color caused by blood flow changes as pressure is applied and returns to the original state when pressure is released. Color caused by pigment deposits remains unchanged.

Nail shape changes may be related to systemic disease. For example, fingernail clubbing occurs with impaired gas exchange. (See Fig. 30-10 in Chapter 30.)

Assess nail shape by examining the curve of the nail plate and surrounding tissue from all angles. Palpate the fingertips to

TABLE 24-5	**Common Alterations in Nail Color**	
ALTERATION	**CLINICAL FINDINGS**	**SIGNIFICANCE**
White	Horizontal white banding or areas of opacity	Chronic liver or kidney disease (hypoalbuminemia)
	Generalized pallor of nail beds	Shock
		Anemia
		Early arteriosclerotic changes (toenails)
		Myocardial infarction
Yellow-brown	Diffuse yellow to brown discoloration	Jaundice
		Peripheral lymphedema
		Bacterial or fungal infections of the nail
		Psoriasis
		Diabetes
		Cardiac failure
		Staining from tobacco, nail polish, or dyes
		Long-term tetracycline therapy
		Normal aging (yellow-gray color)
	Vertical brown banding extending from the proximal nail fold distally	Normal finding in dark-skinned patients
		Nevus or melanoma of nail matrix in light-skinned patients
Red	Thin, dark red vertical lines 1-3 mm long (splinter hemorrhages)	Bacterial endocarditis
		Trichinosis
		Trauma to the nail bed
		Normal finding in some patients
	Red discoloration of the lunula	Cardiac insufficiency
	Dark red nail beds	Polycythemia vera
Blue	Diffuse blue discoloration that blanches with pressure	Respiratory failure
		Methemoglobinuria
		Venous stasis disease (toenails)

FIG. 24-11 A, Diffuse nail pigmentation. **B,** Linear nail pigmentation.

assess for sponginess, tenderness, or edema. Table 24-6 describes common variations in nail shape.

Thickness of the nail plate varies with age, trauma, dermatologic disease, or decreased arterial blood flow. In older patients, look for a "heaped-up" appearance of the toenails, which occurs with fungal infection (*onychomycosis*).

Consistency of the nail is described as hard, soft, or brittle. Nail plates become hard, with thickening. A warm-water soak or lubrication with petroleum jelly is required to soften the nail plates before they can be trimmed. Soft nail plates, which are thin and bend easily with pressure, are associated with malnutrition, chronic arthritis, myxedema, and peripheral neuritis.

Brittle nails can split, as with onychomycosis or advanced psoriasis involving the fingers or toes. Splitting of the nail plate is caused by repeated exposure to water and detergents, which damage the plate over time.

Lesions can occur around, on, within, or under the nail. Separation of the nail plate from the nail bed (*onycholysis*) creates an air pocket beneath the plate. The pocket first appears as a grayish white opacity. The color changes as dirt and keratin collect in the pocket, and the area begins to have a bad odor. This problem occurs with fungal infections and after trauma. Separation of the nail plate may also occur with psoriasis or with prolonged chemical contact.

Inspect the tissue folds around the nail plate for redness, heat, swelling, and tenderness. **Acute paronychia** (inflammation of the skin around the nail) often occurs with a torn cuticle or an ingrown toenail.

Chronic paronychia is common and is an inflammation that persists for months. People at risk for chronic paronychia are those with frequent exposure to water, such as homemakers, bartenders, laundry workers, and nurses.

CULTURAL CONSIDERATIONS
Patient-Centered Care QSEN

Pallor, erythema, cyanosis, and other skin color changes are less visible in patients with naturally dark skin tones. Although physiologic processes are the same for both light-skinned and dark-skinned patients, the amount of skin pigmentation alters how the skin appears in response to physiologic alterations. Different assessment skills are needed to detect the more subtle color changes. Become familiar with the normal appearance of a dark-skinned patient's mucous membranes, nail beds, and skin tone so that variations from baseline can be identified. Chart 24-3 lists assessment techniques to assess skin manifestations in people with dark skin.

TABLE 24-6	**Common Variations In Nail Shape**		
NAIL SHAPE	**CLINICAL FINDINGS**		**SIGNIFICANCE**
Normal	Angle of 160 degrees between the nail plate and the proximal nail fold Nail surface slightly convex Nail base firm when palpated		Normal finding
Clubbing: Early clubbing	Straightening of angle between the nail plate and the proximal nail fold to 180 degrees Nail base spongy when palpated		Hypoxia Lung cancer
Late clubbing	Angle between the nail plate and the proximal nail fold exceeds 180 degrees Nail base visibly edematous and spongy when palpated Enlargement of the soft tissue of the fingertips gives a "drumstick" appearance when viewed from above		Prolonged hypoxia Emphysema Chronic obstructive pulmonary disease Advanced lung cancer Cystic fibrosis Chronic heart disease
Spoon nails (koilonychia): Early koilonychias	Flattening of the nail plate with an increased smoothness of the nail surface		Iron deficiency (with or without anemia) Poorly controlled diabetes >15 yr in duration Local injury
Late koilonychias	Concave curvature of the nail plate		Psoriasis Chemical irritants Developmental abnormality
Beau's grooves	1-mm–wide horizontal depressions in the nail plates caused by growth arrest (involves all nails)		Acute, severe illness Prolonged febrile state Isolated periods of severe malnutrition
Pitting	Small, multiple pits in the nail plate May be associated with plate thickening and onycholysis Most often involves the fingernails (several or all)		Psoriasis Alopecia areata

Assessing Changes in Dark Skin

Cyanosis
- Examine lips and tongue for gray color.
- Examine nail beds, palms, and soles for blue tinge.
- Examine conjunctiva for pallor.

Inflammation
- Compare affected area with nonaffected area for increased warmth.
- Examine the skin of the affected area to determine whether it is shiny or taut or pits with pressure.
- Compare the skin color of affected area with the same area on the opposite side of the body.
- Palpate the affected area and compare it with unaffected area to determine whether texture is different (affected area may feel hard or "woody").

Jaundice
- Check for yellow tinge to oral mucous membranes, especially the hard palate.
- Examine the sclera nearest to the iris rather than the corners of the eye.

Bleeding
- Compare the affected area with the same area on the unaffected body side for swelling or skin darkening.
- If the patient has thrombocytopenia, petechiae may be present on the oral mucosa or conjunctiva.

Skin Assessment Techniques for Patients with Darker Skin

Pallor can be detected in people with dark skin by first inspecting the mucous membranes for an ash-gray color (Jarvis, 2016). If the lips and the nail beds are not heavily pigmented, they appear paler than normal for that patient. Use good lighting to assess for the absence of the underlying red tones that normally give heavily pigmented skin a healthy glow. With decreased blood flow to the skin, brown skin appears yellow-brown and very dark brown skin is ash gray.

Cyanosis can be present when gas exchange is impaired. Examine the lips, tongue, nail beds, conjunctivae, and palms and soles for subtle color changes (Jarvis, 2016). In a patient with cyanosis, the lips and tongue are gray and the palms, soles, conjunctivae, and nail beds have a bluish tinge. To support these findings, assess for other indicators of hypoxia, including tachycardia, hypotension, changes in respiratory rate, decreased breath sounds, and changes in cognition.

Inflammation in dark-skinned patients appears as excessive warmth and changes in skin consistency or texture (Jarvis, 2016). Use the back of your hand to palpate areas of suspected inflammation for increased warmth. With the fingertips, palpate for hardened areas deep in the tissue, which may give the skin a "woody" feel. Inflamed skin is tender and edematous. If edema is extensive, the skin is taut and shiny.

Skin areas where inflammation has recently resolved appear *darker* than the patient's normal skin tone. This change is due to stimulation of the melanocytes during the inflammatory process and to the increased pigment production that continues after inflammation subsides. Deep skin injury with destruction of melanocytes (e.g., deep ulcer, full-thickness burn) may heal with color changes that are *lighter* than the normal skin tone. Chronic inflammatory changes are not tender. Scarred skin feels less supple, especially over the joints. If chronic inflammatory changes are suspected, ask the patient about a history of skin problems in that area.

Jaundice in a patient with dark skin is best assessed by inspecting the oral mucosa, especially the hard palate, for yellow discoloration (Jarvis, 2016). Yellowness of the conjunctivae and adjacent sclera may be misleading because normal deposits of fat produce a yellowish hue that is visible in contrast to the dark skin around the eyes. Examine the sclera closest to the cornea for a more accurate determination of jaundice. The palms and soles of dark-skinned patients may appear yellow if they are calloused even when jaundice is not present.

Skin bleeding with purpuric lesions may not be visible with deep pigmentation. Areas of ecchymoses appear darker than normal skin; they may be tender and easily palpable, depending on whether hematoma is present. Often, the patient relates a history of trauma to the area that confirms the assessment. Petechiae are rarely visible in dark skin and may be seen only in the oral mucosa and conjunctiva.

Psychosocial Assessment

Skin changes, especially of the face, hair, and hands, often affect a person's body image. Encourage the patient to express his or her feelings about a change in appearance. Assess his or her body language for clues indicating a disturbance in self-concept. The avoidance of eye contact or the use of clothing to cover the affected areas suggests concern about appearance. Patients with chronic skin diseases often become socially isolated related to a fear of rejection by others or a belief that the skin problem is contagious.

Skin changes linked to poor hygiene are common among homeless people and among those who have reduced cognitive functioning. Assess the patient's overall appearance for excessive soiling, matted hair, body odor, or other self-care deficits. Confirm unsanitary living conditions by obtaining a social history. Patients may relate similar skin problems among family members, friends, and sexual contacts.

If skin problems related to poor hygiene are identified in older patients, also evaluate any physical limitations that might interfere with grooming. For example, visual or mobility problems can make it difficult for them to see or reach skin surfaces to clean them.

CLINICAL JUDGMENT CHALLENGE

Patient-Centered Care QSEN

A 55-year-old woman who has blonde hair, very light skin, and blue eyes is being seen because she noticed the recent development several light-brown, flat, irregularly shaped spots on her face just below and in front of her right ear. Although these spots do not extend into the surrounding skin, she is concerned about their appearance on her otherwise flawless complexion and is worried that they may be skin cancer. When asked about her sun exposure, she tells you that her only sun exposure is when she plays golf (4 times per week) and that she uses sunscreen on her arms, legs, and neck. She also says she wears a hat with a front brim while playing golf. When you ask about facial skin protection, she tells you that because she wears makeup, she does not use sunscreen on her face.

1. What other assessment data should you obtain?
2. What risk factors does this woman have for skin cancer?
3. Do the facial lesions have any concerning features? If so, which ones?
4. How should you counsel this woman?

Diagnostic Assessment

Laboratory Tests

When a fungal, bacterial, or viral infection of the skin is suspected, confirmation by microscopic examination is necessary. *Always wear gloves (use Standard Precautions) when examining skin that is not intact.*

Cultures for fungal infection are obtained by using a tongue blade and gently scraping scales from skin lesions into a clean container. Collect fingernail clippings and hair in a similar manner. Waiting for culture results can delay treatment of a superficial fungal infection. For this reason, the specimen is also treated with a potassium hydroxide (KOH) solution and examined microscopically. A positive fungal infection shows branched hyphae when viewed under a microscope after treatment with KOH and may eliminate the need for a culture.

For deeper fungal infections, a piece of tissue is obtained for culture. The physician obtains the specimen by punch biopsy (see the following Skin Biopsy section). Check with the laboratory for any specific instructions related to specimen handling.

Cultures for bacterial infection are obtained from intact primary lesions (bullae, vesicles, or pustules), if possible. Express material from the lesion, collect it with a cotton-tipped applicator, and place the material in a bacterial culture medium specified by the laboratory. For intact lesions, *unroofing* (lifting or puncturing of the outer surface) may be needed using a sterile small-gauge needle before the material can be easily expressed. If crusts are present, the nurse or other health care professional removes the crusts with normal saline and then swabs the underlying exudates to obtain a specimen for culture (Cross, 2014).

A biopsy of deep bacterial infections may be needed to obtain a specimen for culture. If bacterial cellulitis is suspected, the physician or advanced practice nurse can inject nonbacteriostatic saline deep into the tissue and then aspirate it back; the aspirant is sent for culture.

Cultures for viral infection are indicated if a herpes virus infection is suspected. A cotton-tipped applicator is used to obtain vesicle fluid from intact lesions. Viral culture specimen tubes must be placed on ice immediately after specimens are obtained and are transported to the laboratory as soon as possible.

The presence of a viral infection can be confirmed by *Tzanck smear* although the exact virus is not identified. A smear is obtained from the base of the lesion and examined under a microscope. The presence of multinucleated giant cells confirms a viral infection.

Other Diagnostic Tests

Other tests for diagnosis of skin problems include biopsy, special noninvasive examination techniques, and skin testing for allergy (discussed in Chapter 20).

Skin Biopsy. A small piece of skin tissue may be obtained for diagnosis or to assess the effectiveness of an intervention. Check with the health care provider to determine the number, location, and type of skin biopsies to be performed. Depending on the size, depth, and location of the skin changes, the physician may perform a punch biopsy, shave biopsy, or scalpel excision (excisional biopsy).

Punch biopsy is the most common technique. A small circular cutting instrument, or "punch," ranging in diameter from 2 to 6 mm, is used. After the site is injected with a local anesthetic, a small plug of tissue is cut and removed. The site may be closed with sutures or may be allowed to heal without suturing.

Shave biopsies remove only the portion of the skin that rises above the surrounding tissue when injected with a local anesthetic. A scalpel or razor blade is moved parallel to the skin surface to remove the tissue specimen. Shave biopsies are usually indicated for superficial or raised lesions. Suturing is not needed.

Excisional biopsy is rarely used for skin problems. When needed, larger or deeper specimens are obtained by deep excision with a scalpel followed by closure with sutures. Excisional biopsies are more uncomfortable than punch or shave biopsies while healing.

Patient Preparation. Explain to the patient what to expect and that a biopsy is a minor procedure with few complications. If a punch or shave biopsy is planned, reassure him or her that only a small amount of skin is removed and scarring is minimal. For an excisional biopsy, tell the patient that a scar similar to that of a healed surgical incision will result.

Procedure. Establish a sterile field, and assemble all needed supplies and instruments. Local anesthesia is provided by local infiltration using a small-gauge (25-gauge) needle to reduce discomfort during injection. Preparation of the biopsy site differs by health care provider preference, but usually the skin is simply wiped with alcohol.

The injection of a local anesthetic agent, which produces a burning or stinging sensation, is uncomfortable. Reassure the patient that the discomfort will subside as the anesthetic takes effect. Talking the patient through the procedure with a quiet voice along with a gentle touch may have a calming effect.

After removal, tissue specimens for pathologic study are placed in 10% formalin for fixation. Specimens for culture are placed in sterile saline solution. Bleeding of the site may be controlled by applying localized pressure, by applying a topical hemostatic agent, or by suturing.

Follow-up Care. After bleeding is controlled and any sutures are placed, the site is covered with an adhesive bandage or a dry gauze dressing. Instruct the patient to keep the dressing dry and in place for at least 8 hours. Teach him or her to clean the site daily after the dressing is removed. Tap water or saline is used to remove any dried blood or crusts. An antibiotic ointment may be prescribed to reduce the risk for infection. The site may be left open or covered for cosmetic reasons or because the site is an area often soiled. Instruct the patient to report any redness or excessive drainage. Sutures are usually removed 7 to 10 days after biopsy.

Wood's Light Examination. A handheld, long-wavelength ultraviolet (black) light or Wood's light may be used during physical examination. Exposure of some skin infections with this light produces a specific color, such as blue-green or red, that can be used to identify the infection. Hypopigmented skin is more prominent when it is viewed under black light, making evaluation of pigment changes in lighter skin easier. This examination is carried out in a darkened room and does not cause discomfort.

Diascopy. Diascopy is a painless technique to eliminate erythema caused by increased blood flow to the skin, thereby easing the inspection of skin lesions. A glass slide or lens is pressed down over the area to be examined, blanching the skin and revealing the shape of the lesions.

NCLEX EXAMINATION CHALLENGE

Safe and Effective Care Environment

What is the most important action the nurse needs to take when obtaining a specimen for a viral culture for a client who has a suspected viral skin infection?

A. Injecting the vesicle with sterile water, aspirating the fluid, adding a preservative to the specimen, and wrapping the container to protect the specimen from light.

B. Using a cotton-tipped applicator, obtain vesicle fluid from the lesion, immediately placing the specimen on ice, and transporting it to the laboratory as soon as possible.

C. Cleaning the area with an antiseptic solution, removing fluid from the center of the blister with a needle, and sending it to the laboratory.

D. Applying a gauze bandage to the area, removing it after one hour, and sending the entire gauze to the laboratory.

NURSING CONCEPTS AND CLINICAL JUDGMENT REVIEW

What might you NOTICE in a patient with adequate TISSUE INTEGRITY and body protection related to skin function?

Vital signs:
- Body temperature within normal range

Physical assessment:
- Skin intact (no rashes, abnormal lesions, open areas, or drainage)
- Skin color normal (no cyanosis, pallor, jaundice, inflammation, or areas of uneven pigmentation)
- Skin texture and elastic turgor normal (no edema, tenting, flaking, scaling, excessive oiliness, or excessive thickening)

- Oral mucous membranes moist and pink
- Nail beds pink with good capillary refill
- Fingertips and nails normal-shaped (no clubbing, nail splitting, nail separation, or increased nail thickness)
- Body hair distributed evenly over the body, no patchy areas of hair loss
- Scalp free from dandruff, no itching

Psychological assessment:
- Patient's eye contact good
- No unusual "hiding" of body areas normally visible in public
- Skin, hair, and nails clean and free of odor

GET READY FOR THE NCLEX® EXAMINATION!

KEY POINTS

Review these Key Points for each NCLEX Examination Client Needs Category

Safe and Effective Care Environment
- Assist all patients with limited mobility to change positions at least every 2 hours. **Safety** QSEN
- Wash your hands before and after touching any areas of impaired skin TISSUE INTEGRITY. **Safety** QSEN
- Use Standard Precautions when providing care to a patient who has areas of impaired skin TISSUE INTEGRITY or skin with an abnormal appearance. **Safety** QSEN
- Use lift sheets when moving patients with fragile skin. **Safety** QSEN
- Position patients who are confined to bed in a way that promotes air circulation to skinfold areas while minimizing pressure over bony prominences.

Health Promotion and Maintenance
- Encourage all patients to reduce sun exposure and exposure to ultraviolet (UV) light. **Patient-Centered Care** QSEN
- Teach patients to examine all skin areas on a monthly basis for new lesions and changes to existing lesions using the

ABCDE method of checking lesions for manifestations of melanoma. **Evidence-Based Practice** QSEN
- Encourage all patients to bathe, shampoo the hair, and keep fingernails clean and trimmed.

Psychosocial Integrity
- Use effective communication when teaching patients and family members about what to expect during tests and procedures to assess skin function and skin disease. **Patient-Centered Care** QSEN
- Explain all procedures, restrictions, drugs, and follow-up care to the patient and family. **Patient-Centered Care** QSEN
- Check the cognitive function of any patient whose hygiene of the skin, hair, and nails appears inadequate.
- Reassure patients who have skin changes that are variations of normal. **Patient-Centered Care** QSEN

Physiological Integrity
- Modify techniques to assess skin changes in patients with dark skin. **Evidence-Based Practice** QSEN
- Document any known specific allergies that have skin manifestations. **Patient-Centered Care** QSEN

- Ask any patient who has started taking a newly prescribed or over-the-counter drug whether he or she has noticed any skin changes that occurred since starting the drug. **Patient-Centered Care** QSEN
- Use proper terminology to communicate skin assessment findings.

- Distinguish between normal variations and abnormal skin manifestations with regard to skin color, texture, warmth, elastic turgor, and moisture.
- Use the ABCDE method of assessing skin lesions for cancer. **Evidence-Based Practice** QSEN

Care of Patients with Skin Problems

Janice Cuzzell and M. Linda Workman

℮ http://evolve.elsevier.com/Iggy/

PRIORITY CONCEPTS

- TISSUE INTEGRITY
- INFECTION
- INFLAMMATION
- CELLULAR REGULATION

LEARNING OUTCOMES

Safe and Effective Care Environment

1. Use principles of infection control to prevent transmission when caring for a patient with a skin INFECTION.
2. Protect hospitalized patients from skin injury, loss of TISSUE INTEGRITY, and INFECTION.

Health Promotion and Maintenance

3. Teach all people how to protect the skin from damage and cancer development.

Psychosocial Integrity

4. Reduce the psychological impact for the patient and family regarding changes in the appearance or function of any part of the integumentary system.

Physiological Integrity

5. Use knowledge of anatomy and physiology to routinely perform a complete assessment of any skin changes, lesions, and open wounds, and document findings.
6. Work with other members of the health care team to help the patient/family experiencing pressure ulcers or other skin problems achieve desired health outcomes.
7. Coordinate nursing interventions for the patient with serious skin problems in the community.

As discussed in Chapter 24, skin TISSUE INTEGRITY helps protect the entire body. Like the wall surrounding a castle, it provides a strong barrier, especially to invasion by harmful microorganisms.

Skin problems are common, especially among older adults. Changes in skin TISSUE INTEGRITY reduce protective function, and the cause of the change is often difficult to determine. In addition to its primary functions, the skin also reflects underlying medical conditions. Thus problems may truly arise in the skin, or they may be a manifestation of systemic disease or injury.

Drugs and other interventions for any health problem can trigger a skin response. Skin problems can interfere with the management of other conditions. Age-related changes and problems caused by immobility, chronic disease, debility, and reduced immune function increase the older patient's risk for skin damage and loss of TISSUE INTEGRITY.

MINOR SKIN IRRITATIONS

PRURITUS

❖ PATHOPHYSIOLOGY

Pruritus (itching) is a distressing condition caused by stimulation of itch-specific nerve fibers. It may or may not occur with skin disease. Physical or chemical agents can directly trigger the nerve fibers or can activate chemical mediators (i.e., histamine), which then act on the itch receptors.

Itching is a subjective condition similar to pain, and severity of the sensation varies among patients. Regardless of the cause, patients often report that itching is worse at night when there are fewer distractions. Other conditions that make itching worse include skin dryness, increased temperature, perspiration, and emotional stress.

❖ PATIENT-CENTERED COLLABORATIVE CARE

The priority nursing interventions focus on increasing patient comfort and preventing skin injury with loss of TISSUE INTEGRITY. Patients usually try to relieve itching by scratching or rubbing the skin, a response that further stimulates the itch receptors and causes the *"itch-scratch-itch"* cycle (McCance et al., 2014). Itching with skin lesions can often be relieved by treatment of the underlying skin disorder with topical or systemic drugs. Systemic diseases, such as liver and venous disorders, can also cause itching without skin lesions. Liver disease often increases the buildup of bilirubin in the skin, which stimulates itch receptors. Pruritus can also be caused by too little or too much blood flow to an area (especially the feet and legs).

Plan care to promote comfort and prevent disruption of skin tissue integrity from vigorous scratching. Because dry skin worsens itching, emphasize interventions to prevent dry skin (Chart 25-1). Encourage patients to keep the fingernails trimmed short, with rough edges filed to reduce damage from scratching and secondary INFECTION. Wearing mittens or splints at night can help prevent scratching during sleep. If the patient cannot perform self-care, teach the family (for home care) and unlicensed assistive personnel (UAP) to trim the patient's fingernails and apply mittens or gloves. Stress the importance of not breaking the skin or digging into nail corners when trimming the nails of patients with diabetes.

A cool sleeping environment and comfort measures (e.g., cool shower, moisturizers) may help promote sleep. Using sleep-promoting herbal teas or sedating antihistamines at bedtime (when the side effect of drowsiness is welcome) may provide an uninterrupted night's sleep. Colloidal oatmeal or tar extract baths may provide temporary relief.

If antihistamines are prescribed, monitor the patient's response so that the dosage can be adjusted as needed. The effectiveness of topical steroid preparations and other topical agents is increased if the drug is applied to slightly damp skin. Using topical drugs under an occlusive dressing increases the dose being delivered. Avoid occluding treated areas unless specifically prescribed by the health care provider.

URTICARIA

Urticaria (hives) is a rash of white or red edematous papules or plaques of various sizes. This problem is usually caused by exposure to allergens, which releases histamine into the skin. Blood vessel dilation and plasma protein leakage lead to formation of lesions or wheals. Some common causes of urticaria include drugs, temperature extremes, foods, INFECTION, diseases, cancer, and insect bites (Schaefer, 2011).

Management focuses on removal of the triggering substance and relief of manifestations. Because the skin reaction is caused by histamine release, antihistamines such as diphenhydramine (Benadryl) are helpful. Teach the patient to avoid overexertion, alcohol consumption, and warm environments, which further dilate blood vessels and make urticaria worse. Alcohol increases sedating effect of antihistamines, increasing the risk for falls.

TRAUMA

❖ PATHOPHYSIOLOGY

Skin trauma can vary from an aseptic surgical incision to a grossly infected, draining pressure ulcer with deep tissue destruction. Injury to the skin starts a series of actions to repair the skin and restore TISSUE INTEGRITY to this protective barrier.

Phases of Wound Healing

Wound healing occurs in three phases: inflammatory phase, proliferative phase, and maturation phase. Table 25-1 lists the key events for each stage of normal wound healing. The length of each phase depends on the type of injury and degree of loss of TISSUE INTEGRITY, the patient's overall health, and whether the wound is healing by first, second, or third intention (Fig. 25-1).

CHART 25-1 Patient and Family Education: Preparing for Self-Management

Prevention of Dry Skin

- Use a room humidifier during the winter months or whenever the furnace is in use.
- Take a complete bath or shower only every other day (wash face, axillae, perineum, and any soiled areas with soap daily).
- Use tepid water.
- Use a superfatted, nonalkaline soap instead of deodorant soap.
- Rinse the soap thoroughly from your skin.
- If you like bath oil, add the oil to the water at the end of the bath.
- Take care to avoid falls; oil makes the tub slippery.
- Pat rather than rub skin surfaces dry.
- Avoid clothing that continuously rubs the skin, such as tight belts, nylon stockings, or pantyhose.
- Maintain a daily fluid intake of 3000 mL unless contraindicated for another medical condition.
- Do not apply rubbing alcohol, astringents, or other drying agents to the skin.
- Avoid caffeine and alcohol ingestion.

TABLE 25-1 Normal Wound Healing

Inflammatory Phase

- Begins at the time of injury or cell death and lasts 3 to 5 days.
- Immediate responses are vasoconstriction and clot formation.
- After 10 minutes, vasodilation occurs with increased capillary permeability and leakage of plasma (and plasma proteins) into the surrounding tissue.
- White blood cells (especially macrophages) migrate into the wound.
- Clinical manifestations of local edema, pain, erythema, and warmth are present.

Proliferative Phase

- Begins about the fourth day after injury and lasts 2 to 4 weeks.
- Fibrin strands form a scaffold or framework.
- Mitotic fibroblast cells migrate into the wound, attach to the framework, divide, and stimulate the secretion of collagen.
- Collagen, together with ground substance, builds tough and inflexible scar tissue.
- Capillaries in areas surrounding the wound form "buds" that grow into new blood vessels.
- Capillary buds and collagen deposits form the "granulation" tissue in the wound, and the wound contracts.
- Epithelial cells grow over the granulation tissue bed.

Maturation Phase

- Begins as early as 3 weeks after injury and may continue for a year or longer.
- Collagen is reorganized to provide greater tensile strength.
- Scar tissue gradually becomes thinner and paler in color.
- The mature scar is firm and inelastic when palpated.

The process of wound healing

▶
Healing
by first
intention

Clean incision

Early suture

"Hairline" scar

An aseptically made wound with minimal tissue destruction and minimal tissue reaction begins to heal as the edges are approximated by close sutures or staples. No open areas or dead spaces are left to serve as potential sites of infection.

▶
Healing by
second
intention
(granulation)
and
contraction

Gaping, irregular wound

Granulation and contraction

Growth of epithelium over scar

An infected or chronic wound or one with tissue damage so extensive that the edges cannot be smoothly approximated is usually left open and allowed to heal from the inside out. The nurse periodically cleans and assesses the wound for healthy tissue production. Scar tissue is extensive, and healing is prolonged.

▶
Healing by
third
intention
(delayed
closure)

Infected wound

Granulation

Closure with wide scar

A potentially infected surgical wound may be left open for several days. If no clinical signs of infection occur, the wound is then closed surgically.

FIG. 25-1 The process of wound healing.

FIG. 25-2 Appearance of a normally healing surgical wound over time. **A,** Appearance at 1 day postoperative. **B,** Appearance at 1 week postoperative. **C,** Appearance at 2 weeks postoperative. **D,** Appearance at 2 months postoperative. **E,** Appearance at 6 months postoperative. **F,** Appearance at 1 year after surgery.

A wound without tissue loss, such as a clean laceration or a surgical incision, can be closed with sutures, staples, or adhesives. The wound edges are brought together with the skin layers lined up in correct anatomic position (**approximated**) and held in place until healing is complete. This type of wound represents healing by **first intention** in which the closed wound eliminates dead space and shortens the phases of tissue repair. INFLAMMATION resolves quickly, and connective tissue repair is minimal, resulting in less remodeling and a thin scar. Fig. 25-2 shows the healing of a surgical incision over time.

Deeper tissue injuries with greater loss of TISSUE INTEGRITY, such as a chronic pressure ulcer or venous stasis ulcer, result in a cavity that requires gradual filling in of the dead space with connective tissue. This represents healing by **second intention** and prolongs the repair process.

Wounds at high risk for INFECTION, such as surgical incisions into a nonsterile body cavity or contaminated traumatic wounds, may be intentionally left open for several days. After **debris** (dead tissues) and exudate have been removed (débrided) and INFLAMMATION has subsided, the wound is closed by first intention. This type of healing represents delayed primary closure (**third intention**) and results in a scar similar to that found in wounds that heal by first intention. Healing can be impaired by many factors (Table 25-2).

Mechanisms of Wound Healing

When skin injury occurs, the body restores TISSUE INTEGRITY through three processes: re-epithelialization, granulation, and wound contraction. The depth of injury and extent of tissue integrity loss determine to what degree each process contributes to wound healing.

Partial-Thickness Wounds. Partial-thickness wounds are superficial with minimal loss of TISSUE INTEGRITY from damage to the epidermis and upper dermal layers. These wounds heal by **re-epithelialization**, the production of new skin cells by undamaged epidermal cells in the basal layer of the dermis, which also lines the hair follicles and sweat glands (Fig. 25-3). Injury is followed immediately by local INFLAMMATION that causes the formation of a fibrin clot and releases growth factors that stimulate epidermal cell division (mitosis). New skin cells move into open spaces on the wound surface where the fibrin clot acts as a frame to guide cell movement. Regrowth across

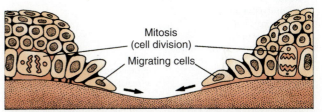

Skin cells at the edge of the wound begin multiplying and migrate toward the center of the wound.

Once advancing epidermal cells from the opposite sides of the wound meet, migration halts.

Epithelial cells continue to divide until the thickness of the new skin layer approaches normal.

FIG. 25-3 Re-epithelialization and wound contraction.

the open area (**resurfacing**) is only one cell layer thick at first. As healing continues, the cell layer thickens, stratifies (forms layers), and produces keratin to resemble normal skin.

In a healthy person, healing of a partial-thickness wound takes about 5 to 7 days. This process is more rapid in skin that is hydrated, well oxygenated, and has few microorganisms.

Full-Thickness Wounds. In deep partial-thickness wounds and full-thickness wounds, loss of TISSUE INTEGRITY and damage extend into the lower layers of the dermis and subcutaneous tissue. As a result, most of the epithelial cells at the base of the wound are destroyed and the wound cannot heal by re-epithelialization alone. Removal of the damaged tissue results

TABLE 25-2 Causes of Impaired Wound Healing

CAUSE	MECHANISM
Altered Inflammatory Response	
Local	
Arteriosclerosis	Reduced local tissue circulation,
Diabetes	resulting in ischemia, impaired
Vasculitis	leukocytic response to
Thrombosis	wounding, and increased
Venous insufficiency	probability of wound infection
Lymphedema	
Pharmacologic vasoconstriction	
Irradiated tissue	
Crush injuries	
Primary closure under tension	
Systemic	
Leukemia	Systemic inhibition of leukocytic
Prolonged administration of	response, resulting in impaired
high-dose anti-inflammatory	host resistance to infection
drugs:	
• Corticosteroids	
• Aspirin	
Impaired Cellular Proliferation	
Local	
Wound infection	Prolonged inflammatory
Foreign body	response, which can result in
Necrotic tissue	low tissue oxygen tension and
Repeated injury or irritation	further tissue destruction
Movement of wound (e.g., across	
a joint)	
Wound desiccation or maceration	
Systemic	
Aging	Impaired cellular proliferation
Chronic stress	and collagen synthesis
Nutritional deficiencies:	Decreased wound contraction
• Calories	
• Protein	
• Vitamins	
• Minerals	
• Water	
Impaired oxygenation:	
• Pulmonary insufficiency	
• Heart failure	
• Hypovolemia	
Cirrhosis	
Uremia	
Prolonged hypothermia	
Coagulation disorders	
Cytotoxic drugs	

in a defect that must be filled with scar tissue (**granulation**) for healing to occur. During the second phase of healing, new blood vessels form at the base of the wound and fibroblast cells begin moving into the wound space. These cells deposit new collagen to replace the lost tissue.

Fibroblasts also begin to pull the wound edges inward along the path of least resistance (**contraction**) (see Fig. 25-3). This causes the wound to decrease in size at a uniform rate of about 0.6 to 0.75 mm/day. Complete wound closure by contraction depends on the mobility of the surrounding skin as tension is applied to it. If tension in the surrounding skin exceeds the force

of wound contraction, healing will be delayed until undamaged epidermal cells at the wound edges can bridge the defect. The bridging of epithelial cells across a large area of granulation tissue results in an unstable barrier rather than near-normal skin. A venous leg ulcer is one example of a skin defect that heals poorly by contraction. Re-epithelialization of these chronic wounds often results in a thin epidermal barrier that is easily re-injured.

The natural healing processes of re-epithelialization, granulation, and contraction can slow down and even stop in the presence of INFECTION, unrelieved pressure, or mechanical obstacles. For example, dead tissue not only supports bacterial growth but also obstructs collagen deposition and wound contraction. Thus thorough wound débridement is needed for healing. In the case of chronic wounds, healing may stop spontaneously without an obvious cause. Also, infection in chronic wounds may not show the expected manifestations. Often the only manifestation is an increase in wound size or failure of the wound to decrease in size. Nonhealing chronic wounds that remain open for extended periods are of particular concern. Although rare, these wounds are at higher risk for evolving into an aggressive malignancy (Marjolin ulcer) (Yu et al., 2013).

CONSIDERATIONS FOR OLDER ADULTS
Patient-Centered Care QSEN

As skin ages, the process of wound healing is less efficient. Re-epithelialization and wound contraction slow, and replacement of connective tissue is reduced. Thus the strength of a healed wound in an older adult is reduced with poor tissue integrity and the area is at greater risk for re-injury. When inadequate nutrition, incontinence, or immobility is present, any wound in an older adult has a high risk for becoming a chronic wound. Although prevention strategies provide the best outcome, aggressive treatment of any degree of loss of skin tissue integrity, no matter how small, should be started as soon as it is discovered in an older adult (Touhy & Jett, 2014).

❖ PATIENT-CENTERED COLLABORATIVE CARE
Collaborative management of skin trauma varies with the depth and type of injury. Interventions always focus on supporting a healing environment, enhancing wound healing, preventing INFECTION, and restoring function to the area.

PRESSURE ULCERS
❖ PATHOPHYSIOLOGY

A **pressure ulcer** (PrU) is a loss of TISSUE INTEGRITY caused when the skin and underlying soft tissue are compressed between a bony prominence and an external surface for an extended period. Although they commonly occur over the sacrum, hips, and ankles, *pressure ulcers can occur on any body surface.* For example, nasal cannula tubing that is too tight can cause pressure ulcers behind the ears or in the nares (Ambutas et al., 2014).

Tissue compression from pressure restricts blood flow to the skin, resulting in reduced tissue perfusion and oxygenation and, eventually, leading to cell death. Ulcers occur most often in people with limited mobility because they cannot change their position to relieve pressure. Patients who cannot feel or communicate the pain that occurs with unrelieved pressure are more likely to develop pressure ulcers. Once formed, these chronic wounds are slow to heal, resulting in increased morbidity and health care costs. Complications include sepsis, kidney failure, infectious arthritis, and osteomyelitis.

Friction and shear are mechanical forces that impair skin TISSUE INTEGRITY and cause skin tears, which set the stage for skin breakdown (LeBlanc & Baronoski, 2014). Excessive skin moisture, such as urinary or fecal incontinence, also increases the risk for skin damage. Nutrition status is an important concern. Protein malnutrition makes normal tissue more prone to breakdown and also delays healing (Posthauer, 2012).

Mechanical Forces

Pressure occurs as a result of gravity. Dependent tissues in contact with a fixed surface experience varying degrees of pressure. Pressure is determined by the amount and distribution of weight exerted at the point of contact and the density of the contacting surface. Excessive or prolonged pressure compresses blood vessels at the point of contact, such as over bony prominences. Pressure occurs when the patient is positioned on a hard surface that does not diffuse the weight, such as when lying on a hard floor for hours after a fall or when remaining in the same position too long. Unrelieved pressure leads to ischemia, INFLAMMATION, and tissue necrosis.

Friction occurs when surfaces rub the skin and irritate or directly pull off epithelial tissue. Such forces are generated when the patient is dragged or pulled across bed linen.

Shearing forces are generated when the skin itself is stationary and the tissues below the skin (e.g., fat, muscle) shift or move (Fig. 25-4). The movement of the deeper tissue layers reduces the blood supply to the skin, leading to skin hypoxia, anoxia, ischemia, INFLAMMATION, and necrosis.

A shear injury usually occurs when a patient is in a wheelchair or in bed in a semi-sitting position and gradually slides downward. The skin over the sacrum may not slide down at the same pace as the deeper tissues, mechanically "shearing" the skin, causing blood vessels to stretch and break. Shearing leads to soft-tissue ischemia and deep tissue injury, even though no external break in skin integrity is observed.

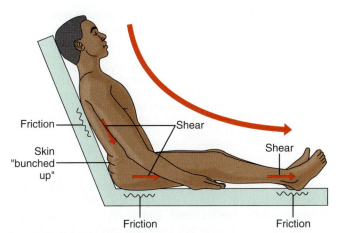

FIG. 25-4 Shearing forces pulling skin layers away from deeper tissue. The skin is "bunched up" against the back of the mattress while the rest of the bone and muscle in the area presses downward on the lower part of the mattress. Blood vessels become kinked, obstructing circulation and leading to tissue death.

Incidence and Prevalence

Pressure ulcer development is a problem found among patients in any care setting, including the home. Although new products are available for prevention and treatment, many hospitalized patients still experience pressure ulcer formation, which contributes significantly to morbidity and mortality in this patient population (Alderden et al., 2011; Lyder et al., 2012).

Health Promotion and Maintenance

Pressure ulcers can be prevented if the risk is recognized and intervention begins early (Chart 25-2) (Ackerman, 2011). Pressure ulcer prevention does not just happen even with conscientious nursing care. Deliberate and consistent interventions, as described in the Quality Improvement box, are needed to prevent hospital-acquired pressure ulcers. Key health care team members for pressure ulcer prevention and management are the certified wound care specialist and the dietitian. Involving unlicensed assistive personnel (UAP) in pressure ulcer prevention also enhances prevention program effectiveness.

A pressure ulcer prevention program consists of two steps: (1) early identification of high-risk patients, and (2) implementation of aggressive intervention for prevention with the use of pressure-relief or pressure-reduction devices. Pressure mapping with a computerized tool that measures pressure distribution during sitting or lying can identify specific body areas at risk for breakdown and can help in planning interventions for patients who are bedridden or wheelchair bound. The map is displayed in colors on the computer screen based on temperature differences. Red indicates areas of greater heat production and increased pressure loads. Blue indicates cooler areas under lower pressure. When used in combination with risk assessment tools, pressure mapping helps identify problem areas before skin changes can be seen and allows for more targeted prevention strategies.

Effective risk identification and prevention measures include patient and caregiver education. Documentation of risk assessment, implementation of prevention measures, and education of all people involved in the care of the patient at risk for pressure ulcer formation are key to the plan's success. Continuing evaluation and risk assessment are critical, especially when the patient's condition changes.

Identification of High-Risk Patients

As suggested by The Joint Commission's National Patient Safety Goals (NPSGs), all patients admitted to a health care facility or home care agency are to be assessed for pressure ulcer risk. The

CHART 25-2 Best Practice for Patient Safety & Quality Care (QSEN)

Preventing Pressure Ulcers

Positioning
- Pad contact surfaces with foam, silicon gel, air pads, or other pressure-relieving pads.
- Do not keep the head of the bed elevated above 30 degrees to prevent shearing.
- Use a lift sheet to move a patient in the bed. Avoid dragging or sliding him or her.
- When positioning a patient on his or her side, do not position directly on the trochanter.
- Re-position an immobile patient at least every 2 hours while in bed and at least every 1 hour while sitting in a chair.
- Do not place a rubber ring or donut under the patient's sacral area.
- When moving an immobile patient from a bed to another surface, use a designated slide board well lubricated with talc or use a mechanical lift.
- Place pillows or foam wedges between two bony surfaces.
- Keep the patient's skin directly off plastic surfaces.
- Keep the patient's heels off the bed surface using bed pillow under ankles.

Nutrition
- Ensure a fluid intake between 2000 and 3000 mL/day.
- Help the patient maintain an adequate intake of protein and calories.

Skin Care
- Perform a daily inspection of the patient's entire skin.
- Document and report any manifestations of skin infection.

- Use moisturizers daily on dry skin, and apply when skin is damp.
- Keep moisture from prolonged contact with skin:
  - Dry areas where two skin surfaces touch, such as the axillae and under the breasts.
  - Place absorbent pads under areas where perspiration collects.
  - Use moisture barriers on skin areas where wound drainage or incontinence occurs.
- ***Do not massage bony prominences.***
- Humidify the room.

Skin Cleaning
- Clean the skin as soon as possible after soiling occurs and at routine intervals.
- Use a mild, heavily fatted soap or gentle commercial cleanser for incontinence.
- Use tepid rather than hot water.
- In the perineal area, use a disposable cleaning cloth that contains a skin barrier agent.
- While cleaning, use the minimum scrubbing force necessary to remove soil.
- Gently pat rather than rub the skin dry.
- Do not use powders or talcs directly on the perineum.
- After cleansing, apply a commercial skin barrier to those areas in frequent contact with urine or feces.

QUALITY IMPROVEMENT (QSEN)

Use of a Team Approach to Prevent Pressure Ulcers

Armour-Burton, T., Fields, W., Outlaw, L., & Deleon, E. (2013). The healthy skin project: Changing nursing practice to prevent and treat hospital-acquired pressure ulcers. *Critical Care Nurse, 33*(3), 32-39.

The incidence of hospital-acquired pressure ulcers, defined as occurring after the first 24 hours following admission, for a 41-bed acute care unit ranged from 0% to 18.92% per quarter for 14 consecutive quarters. Although this unit had a prevention program initially in place, it relied on each patient's primary nurse for ongoing pressure ulcer risk assessment and implementation of prevention practices. This high incidence forced the staff to examine their current pressure ulcer prevention practices and design a sustainable, interdisciplinary "healthy skin project" to improve the outcomes.

Key to the "healthy skin project" was the implementation of a team approach for pressure ulcer prevention assessment and management. In addition to all nurses assigned to the unit, the team now included both a wound-liaison nurse (who has special training but was not a certified wound care nurse) and a registered dietitian. Education for all staff members was started and assessed at regular intervals. A key factor in the success of the program was the involvement of unlicensed assistive personnel (UAP) in the risk assessment and care phases of pressure ulcer prevention. Thus the responsibility of

pressure ulcer prevention shifted from one person, the primary nurse, for each patient to everyone who provided care to each patient. Each patient was assessed for pressure ulcer risk every shift. Those identified at increased risk were started on evidence-based pressure-relieving and skin care algorithmic intervention. During the first 20 quarters of the project's implementation, the pressure ulcer incidence for 17 quarters was 0%. For 3 of the quarters, the incidence was 2.5%, 2.94%, and 3.33% respectively. These data suggest that consistent implementation of evidence-based strategies for pressure ulcer prevention is effective.

Commentary: Implications for Practice and Research

Although a team approach to pressure ulcer prevention is common, this project may be unique by gaining the input and participation of nonprofessional UAPs. These individuals often spend more time with patients while providing direct care, and their observations can contribute to more accurate assessment, which is the first step in pressure ulcer prevention. Research examining the degree to which engaged UAP versus those whose observations are not considered is needed to learn what role UAP may play in the prevention of hospital-acquired pressure ulcers.

use of a risk assessment tool increases the chances of identifying those patients at greater risk for skin breakdown. The Braden scale (Fig. 25-5) is a commonly used valid skin risk assessment tool. Using it helps the nurse assess and document risk categories for pressure ulcer formation (e.g., mental status, activity and mobility, nutritional status, incontinence).

Mental status changes and decreased sensation determine whether the patient is a partner in pressure ulcer prevention.

When the patient understands that turning and shifting of weight prevent tissue damage, the risk for pressure ulcers decreases. Stroke, head injury, organic brain disease, Alzheimer's disease, or other cognitive problems increase the risk for pressure ulcers.

Impaired mobility is a factor in the risk for pressure ulcer formation. Patients who have unimpaired mobility and can respond to pain are at low risk for pressure ulcers. *Regardless of*

Patient's name _____ Evaluator's name _____ Date of assessment _____

Category	1	2	3	4
Sensory perception Ability to respond meaningfully to pressure-related discomfort	**1. Completely limited** Unresponsive to painful stimuli (does not moan, flinch, or grasp) because of diminished level of consciousness or sedation OR limited ability to feel pain over most of body surface	**2. Very limited** Responds only to painful stimuli; cannot communicate discomfort except by moaning or restlessness OR has a sensory impairment that limits the ability to feel pain or discomfort over half of the body	**3. Slightly limited** Responds to verbal commands but cannot always communicate discomfort or need to be turned OR has some sensory impairment that limits ability to feel pain or discomfort in one or two extremities	**4. No impairment** Responds to verbal commands; has no sensory deficit that would limit ability to feel or voice pain or discomfort
Moisture Degree to which skin is exposed to moisture	**1. Constantly moist** Skin is kept moist almost constantly by perspiration, urine; dampness is detected every time the client is moved or turned	**2. Very Moist** Skin is often but not always moist; linen must be changed at least once a shift	**3. Occasionally moist** Skin is occasionally moist, requiring an extra linen change approximately once a day	**4. Rarely moist** Skin is usually dry; linen requires changing only at routine intervals
Activity Degree of physical activity	**1. Bedfast** Confined to bed	**2. Chairfast** Ability to walk severely limited or nonexistent; cannot bear own weight and must be assisted into chair or wheelchair	**3. Walks occasionally** Walks occasionally during the day but for very short distances, with or without assistance; spends the majority of each shift in bed or chair	**4. Walks frequently** Walks outside the room at least twice a day and inside the room at least once every 2 hours during waking hours
Mobility Ability to change or control body position	**1. Completely immobile** Does not make even slight changes in body or extremity position without assistance	**2. Very limited** Makes occasional slight changes in body or extremity position but unable to make frequent or significant changes independently	**3. Slightly limited** Makes frequent though slight changes in body or extremity position independently	**4. No limitations** Makes major and frequent changes in position without assistance
Nutrition Usual food intake pattern	**1. Very poor** Never eats a complete meal; rarely eats more than a third of any food offered; eats two servings or less of protein (meat or dairy products) per day; takes fluids poorly; does not take a liquid dietary supplement OR is NPO or maintained on clear liquids or IV for more than 5 days	**2. Probably inadequate** Rarely eats a complete meal and generally eats only about half of any food offered; protein intake includes only three servings of meat or dairy products per day; occasionally will take a dietary supplement OR receives less than optimal amount of liquid diet or tube feeding	**3. Adequate** Eats over half of most meals; eats a total of four servings of protein (meat, dairy products) each day; occasionally will refuse a meal, but will usually take a supplement if offered OR is receiving tube feeding or total parenteral nutrition, which probably meets most nutritional needs	**4. Excellent** Eats most of every meal; never refuses a meal; usually eats a total of four or more servings of meat and dairy products; occasionally eats between meals; does not require supplementation
Friction and shear	**1. Problem** Requires moderate to maximum assistance in moving; complete lifting without sliding against sheets is impossible; frequently slides down in bed or chair, requiring frequent repositioning with maximum assistance; spasticity, contractures, or agitation leads to almost constant friction	**2. Potential problem** Moves feebly or requires minimum assistance during a move; skin probably slides to some extent against sheets, chair, restraints, or other devices; maintains relatively good position in chair or bed most of the time but occasionally slides down	**3. No apparent problem** Moves in bed and in chair independently and has sufficient muscle strength to lift up completely during move; maintains good position in bed or chair at all times	
				Total score

Scoring system: 15-16 = mild risk, 12-14 = moderate risk, <11 = severe risk

FIG. 25-5 The Braden scale for predicting pressure ulcer risk. *IV,* Intravenous; *NPO,* nothing by mouth.

age, any patient who requires assistance with turning and positioning or who is unable to verbalize discomfort is at higher risk for pressure ulcers. Those confined to bed or a chair also are at higher risk than a patient who requires assistance only with ambulation.

Nutrition status is a critical risk factor for pressure ulcer development and for successful healing (Posthauer, 2012). TISSUE INTEGRITY and wound healing depend on a positive nitrogen balance and adequate serum protein levels. The patient in negative nitrogen balance not only heals more slowly but also is at risk for accelerated tissue destruction. Draining wounds contribute to protein loss and require aggressive intervention.

Nutrition assessment includes laboratory studies; evaluation of weight and weight change; ability of the patient to consume an adequate diet; and the need for vitamin, mineral, or protein supplementation. Serum prealbumin levels are often used to monitor nutrition status. *Nutrition is considered inadequate when the serum prealbumin level is less than 19.5 g/dL, albumin level is less than 3.5 g/dL, or the lymphocyte count is less than 1800/mm³.* Because serum protein levels are affected by a number of other factors, laboratory values are valuable only when supported by additional assessment information. Other indicators of inadequate nutrition include poor daily intake of food and fluids with a weight loss greater than 5% change in 30 days or greater than 10% change in 180 days (Posthauer, 2012).

A positive nitrogen balance requires an intake of 30 to 35 calories per kilogram of body weight daily with a protein intake of 1.25 to 1.5 g/kg/day. Up to 2 g/kg/day of protein may be needed when nutritional deficits are severe or protein loss is ongoing. Vitamin and mineral supplementations are based on the patient's nutrition status. Collaborate with a dietitian for all patients at risk for a pressure ulcer to perform a thorough nutrition assessment and plan interventions for nutrition deficits (National Pressure Ulcer Advisory Panel, European Pressure Ulcer Advisory Panel, & Pan Pacific Pressure Injury Alliance, 2014).

Incontinence results in prolonged contact of the skin with substances that irritate the skin, destroy TISSUE INTEGRITY, and predispose to skin breakdown (e.g., urea, bacteria, yeast, and enzymes in urine and feces). Excessive moisture macerates skin, further increasing the risk for breakdown. Daily inspection of the skin for any areas of redness, maceration, or loss of skin TISSUE INTEGRITY is a major part of pressure ulcer prevention. Maintenance of clean, dry, intact skin also assists in ulcer prevention. Wash the skin with a pH-balanced soap to maintain the normal acid level. Use creams or lotions to lubricate and moisturize the skin. Barrier ointments protect intact skin from urine and feces when incontinence is present. Change absorbent pads or garments immediately after each incontinence episode to avoid prolonged skin contact with urine or feces.

! NURSING SAFETY PRIORITY (QSEN)

Action Alert

Teach all nursing care personnel and family members not to massage reddened skin areas directly or use donut-shaped pillows for pressure relief. These actions can damage capillary beds and increase tissue necrosis.

Pressure-Relieving and Pressure-Reducing Techniques

The cornerstone in the prevention and management of pressure ulcers is maintaining adequate pressure relief so that tissue pressure remains below the **capillary closing pressure**, which is the pressure needed to occlude skin capillary blood flow in a body area. The normal capillary closing pressure ranges from 12 to 32 mm Hg. An effective pressure-relieving device keeps tissue pressure *below* the capillary closing pressure for adequate tissue perfusion and oxygenation. *Most devices have a standardized guaranteed pressure-relief reading; however, these readings do not ensure that capillary blood flow for any given patient is adequate. Observe skin color, TISSUE INTEGRITY, and temperature directly to determine capillary flow adequacy.*

Devices are classified according to whether they relieve pressure or only reduce pressure. They are further classified as *dynamic* or *static.* Dynamic systems alternate inflation and deflation of the device. Static devices made of gel, water, foam, or air are in a constant state of inflation that distributes the patient pressure load over a larger area and reduces the pressure experienced by any particular area.

Pressure-relief/pressure-reduction products are available as specialty beds, mattress replacements, overlays, and assistive devices. Choosing the correct product is important in the success of the prevention plan. These factors are considered in product selection: the patient's ability to move in bed, his or her comfort level, and compatibility of the product with the care setting. Re-evaluate the product in use daily for effectiveness in reducing pressure, providing comfort, and eliminating "bottoming out." Bottoming out occurs when the product is not providing adequate pressure relief and the patient's bony prominences sink into the mattress or cushion.

Pressure-relief devices consistently reduce pressure below capillary closing pressure. These devices are recommended for patients who need:

- Prevention of skin breakdown because they cannot turn (e.g., immobility, loss of sensation)
- Prevention of extension of skin breakdown that has already occurred
- Promotion of healing for breakdown present on several turning surfaces

Pressure-reduction devices lower pressure below that of a standard hospital mattress or chair surface but do not reduce pressure consistently below the capillary closing pressure. These devices are effective for preventing pressure ulcers only when used together with a turning schedule and other skin care measures.

Frequent repositioning of bedbound patients, as described in Chart 25-2, is critical in reducing pressure over bony prominences. A good plan for positioning is the 30-degree rule. This plan ensures that the patient is positioned and propped so that whatever part of the body is elevated is tilted back to no more than a 30-degree angle to the mattress rather than resting directly on a dependent bony prominence. This rule applies to side-lying as well as head-of-bed elevation positions. The patient who requires greater head elevation because of respiratory difficulties should be tilted up above 30 degrees with pillows behind the back to keep pressure off of the sacral/coccyx area. Teach UAP the importance of proper positioning, and demonstrate how to perform it. Also teach family members to use these techniques in the home.

The patient at risk for pressure ulcers in bed is also at risk while sitting. Assess for proper chair cushioning. Collaborate with physical therapists and rehabilitation specialists for selection of these products. Periodically assist high-risk patients who are chair bound to a standing position to promote perfusion and prevent breakdown over the sacral area.

Even with an appropriate mattress or cushion, the patient needs to change or be helped to change positions periodically to prevent loss of skin TISSUE INTEGRITY. Many facilities require turning and positioning every 2 hours. *However, pressure can occur in less time, and the actual turning or repositioning schedule for each patient must be individualized.* When this action is delegated to UAP, teach them the importance of maintaining a repositioning schedule.

Use pillows and other positioning or padding devices to keep heels pressure-free at all times for high-risk patients. Assess heel positioning every 4 hours to ensure that pressure is not redistributed to other high-risk areas, such as the ankles or side of the feet. Check heels even more often when devices that hide the feet (e.g., boots, heel protectors) are used, especially if the patient has a vascular problem. Also check knees and elbows regularly, especially when the patient is in a side-lying position.

❖ **PATIENT-CENTERED COLLABORATIVE CARE**

◆ **Assessment**

History. When a patient already has a pressure ulcer, identify the cause of skin TISSUE INTEGRITY loss, as well as factors that may impair healing. Ask about the circumstances of the skin loss. Patients with chronic pressure ulcers may have a history of delayed healing or recurrence of the ulcer after healing has occurred. Assess for any of these contributing factors:

- Prolonged bedrest
- Immobility
- Incontinence
- Diabetes mellitus
- Inadequate nutrition or hydration
- Decreased sensory perception or cognitive problems
- Peripheral vascular disease

Physical Assessment/Clinical Manifestations. Inspect the entire body, including the back of the head, for areas of skin tissue integrity loss or pressure. Give special attention to bony prominences (e.g., the heels, sacrum, elbows, knees, trochanters, posterior and anterior iliac spines) and areas with excessive moisture. Make sure tubing and other medical devices are not underneath the patient and producing a pressure point. Assess the patient's general appearance for issues related to skin health, such as the proportion of weight to height. Obese patients and thin patients are at increased risk for malnutrition and pressure ulcers. Check overall cleanliness of the skin, hair, and nails. Determine whether any loss of mobility or range of joint motion has occurred. *Do not delegate this assessment to UAP.*

Wound Assessment. The appearance of pressure ulcers changes with the depth of the injury. Chart 25-3 lists the features of the six categories or stages of pressure ulceration, and Fig. 25-6 shows examples.

Assess wounds for location, size, color, extent of tissue involvement, cell types in the wound base and margins, exudate, condition of surrounding tissue, and presence of foreign bodies. Document this initial assessment to serve as a starting point for determining the intervention plan and its effectiveness. How often a wound is assessed is determined by the policies and procedures at the facility or agency. Weekly documented assessment is standard in many long-term care facilities. Daily assessment is needed when the patient is in an acute care setting. *Also assess the wound at each dressing change, comparing the*

CHART 25-3 **Key Features**

Pressure Ulcers

Suspected Deep Tissue Injury
- The intact skin area appears purple or maroon.
- Blood-filled blisters may be present.
- Before the above-listed changes appeared, the tissue in this area may first have been painful.
- Other changes that may have preceded the discoloration include that the area may have felt more firm, boggy, mushy, warmer, or cooler than the surrounding tissue.

Stage 1
- Skin is intact.
- Area, usually over a bony prominence, is red and does not blanch with external pressure.
- For patients with darker skin that does not blanch:
  - Observable pressure-related alteration of intact skin; changes are compared with an adjacent or opposite area and include one or more of these:
    Skin color (darker or lighted than the comparison area)
    Skin temperature (warmth or coolness)
    Tissue consistency (firm or boggy)
    Sensation (pain, itching)
- The ulcer appears as a defined area of persistent redness in lightly pigmented skin, whereas in darker skin tones, the ulcer may appear with persistent red, blue, or purple hues.

Stage 2
- Skin is not intact.
- There is partial-thickness skin loss of the epidermis or dermis.
- Ulcer is superficial and may be characterized as an abrasion, a blister (open or fluid-filled), or a shallow crater.
- Bruising is *not* present.

Stage 3
- Skin loss is full thickness.
- Subcutaneous tissues may be damaged or necrotic.
- Damage extends down to but not through the underlying fascia; bone, tendon, and muscle are *not* exposed.
- The depth can vary with anatomic location; areas of thin skin (e.g., the bridge of the nose) may show only a shallow crater, whereas thicker tissue areas with larger amounts of subcutaneous fat may show a deep, crater-like appearance.
- Undermining and tunneling may or may not be present.

Stage 4
- Skin loss is full thickness with exposed or palpable muscle, tendon, or bone.
- Often includes undermining and tunneling.
- Sinus tracts may develop.
- Slough and eschar are often present on at least part of the wound.

Unstageable
- Skin loss is full thickness, and the base is completely covered with slough or eschar, obscuring the true depth of the wound.

Data from National Pressure Ulcer Advisory Panel, European Pressure Ulcer Advisory Panel, & Pan Pacific Pressure Injury Alliance. (2014). *Prevention and treatment of pressure ulcers: Quick reference guide.* Cambridge Media: Perth, Australia. Retrieved September 2014, from http://www.npuap.org/wp-content/uploads/2014/08/Quick-Reference-Guide-DIGITAL-NPUAP-EPUAP-PPPIA.pdf.

---

existing wound features with those documented previously to determine the current state of healing or deterioration.

For intact areas that are red (in lighter-skinned patients), press firmly with fingers at the center of the area and assess whether the area **blanches** (lightens) with pressure and

FIG. 25-6 Various stages of pressure ulcers. **A,** Stage 1 pressure ulcer. **B,** Stage 2 pressure ulcer. **C,** Stage 3 pressure ulcer. **D,** Stage 4 pressure ulcer. **E,** Unstageable ulcer. **F,** Suspected deep tissue injury.

document the response. An area that blanches with pressure and then returns to normal when pressure is removed indicates color changes related to blood flow rather than to INFLAMMATION or tissue damage. When blanching does not occur with pressure, the redness is often from skin injury. Redness and blanching may be difficult to detect in darker-skinned patients. Look for more subtle differences in the skin color over the pressure point compared with the surrounding area. In addition, compromised skin feels warmer or cooler on palpation.

Record the location and size of the wound first. Wounds are sized by length, width, and depth using millimeters or centimeters. For standardization in documentation, assess the wound as a clock face with the 12 o'clock position in the direction of the patient's head and the 6 o'clock position in the direction of the patient's feet (van Rijswijk, 2013). Using a disposable paper tape measure, always measure the length from the 12 o'clock position to the 6 o'clock position and the width between the 9 o'clock position and the 3 o'clock position. Measure depth as the distance from the deepest portion of the wound base to the skin level. Touch the bottom of the wound with a cotton-tipped applicator or swab and mark the place on the swab that is level with the skin surface to obtain wound depth. Then measure the area of the swab between the tip and the mark. When everyone uses this format, measurement is accurate and progress can be determined.

Inspect the wound margins for **cellulitis** (INFLAMMATION of the skin and subcutaneous tissue) extending beyond the area of injury. Progressive tissue destruction, seen as an increase in the size or depth of the ulcer and increased wound drainage, may indicate an increased risk for INFECTION if proper measures have been taken to relieve pressure.

Inspect the wound for the presence or absence of necrotic tissue. Because of the depth of tissue destruction, a full-thickness pressure ulcer is often covered by a layer of black, gray, or brown collagen called wound **eschar.**

In the early stages of wound healing, the eschar is dry, leathery, and firmly attached to the wound. As the inflammatory phase of wound healing begins and removal of wound debris progresses, the eschar starts to lift and separate from the tissue beneath. This nonliving eschar is a good breeding ground for any bacteria on the skin surface. As bacteria increase, they release enzymes that soften necrotic tissue, which becomes softer and more yellow. With bacterial colonization, wound exudate increases substantially; the color and odor of wound exudate indicate the major organism present. The features of wound exudate are listed in Table 25-3.

Beneath the dead tissue, granulation tissue appears. Early granulation is pale pink, progressing to a beefy red color as it grows and fills the wound. Palpate the wound to determine the granulation texture. Healthy granulation tissue is moist and has a slightly spongy texture. Wounds with a poor arterial blood supply or that have stopped healing appear dry with hard (fibrotic) granulation tissue on palpation. Venous obstruction causes a very moist ulcer surface with a deep reddish purple color from the deoxygenated blood beneath the ulcer surface.

Pressure ulcers may have more tissue destruction than is first seen on inspection. Deep, extensive tissue damage may be present under normal-appearing skin surrounding the wound, with separation of the skin layers from the underlying granulation tissue. This problem is known as **undermining.** Inspect undermined areas for gradual filling with healthy granulations and for wound-healing progress. Palpate the bony prominences

TABLE 25-3	**Types of Wound Exudate**
CHARACTERISTICS	**SIGNIFICANCE**
Serosanguineous Exudate	
Blood-tinged amber fluid consisting of serum and red blood cells	Normal for first 48 hr after injury Sudden increase in amount precedes wound dehiscence in wounds closed by first intention
Purulent Exudate	
Creamy yellow pus	Colonization with *Staphylococcus*
Greenish blue pus causing staining of dressings and accompanied by a "fruity" odor	Colonization with *Pseudomonas*
Beige pus with a "fishy" odor	Colonization with *Proteus*
Brownish pus with a "fecal" odor	Colonization with aerobic coliform and *Bacteroides* (usually occurs after intestinal surgery)

for deep hardening of the surrounding soft tissue, which often occurs with deep tissue ischemia.

After ischemia has occurred, continued pressure over the area increases tissue destruction from the deep tissue layers toward the surface, resulting in the formation of tunnels. This "hidden" wound may have a small opening in the skin with purulent drainage. If such an opening is observed, use a cotton-tipped applicator to probe gently for a much larger tunnel or pocket of necrotic tissue beneath the opening. Additional tunnels may occur along the main wound. Check all wounds for tunneling and, if present, document the location and length of each tunnel.

Psychosocial Assessment. The patient with pressure ulcers may have an altered body image. Many changes in lifestyle are needed for healing. Chronic ulcers are often painful and costly to treat.

Assess the patient's and family's knowledge of the desired treatment outcomes during the healing process, as well as adherence to the prescribed treatment regimen. Also assess the patient's skills in cleaning and dressing the wound. Poor adherence to pressure ulcer care procedures may reflect an inability to cope with the pain, cost, or potential scarring associated with prolonged healing. Depending on the patient's activity level and the ulcer location, family assistance or a home care nurse may be needed to provide pressure ulcer care at home.

Teach the patient and family specific changes in ADLs to relieve pressure and promote healing. Urge increased activity whenever possible to enhance circulation to the affected tissue. Leg position changes may be needed for chronic leg ulcers, depending on whether vascular problems are present. For patients who have arterial insufficiency, keeping the legs and feet in a dependent position helps ensure adequate blood flow to the lower legs. When arterial blood flow is adequate but venous return is impaired, elevation of the legs may be needed for healing. When the patient is bedridden, frequent repositioning to relieve pressure (every 2 hours in bed, every 1 hour in a chair) can be labor intensive. In the home, repositioning, incontinence management, and dressing changes are often needed around the clock, not only increasing patient discomfort but also disrupting family routines and causing added stress.

Laboratory Assessment. An exposed wound is always *contaminated* but is not always *infected. Contamination* is the presence of organisms without any manifestations of infection. Normal immune defenses keep the number of bacteria to a minimum and prevent infection. *Wound* INFECTION is contamination with pathogenic organisms to the degree that organism growth and spread cannot be controlled by the body's immune defenses. Wounds that are red and indurated with moderate to heavy exudate and an odor should be cultured to identify the organism and determine antibiotic sensitivity. *The presence of purulent exudate alone does not indicate an infection because pus forms whenever necrotic tissue liquefies and separates.*

If wounds are extensive, if the patient is severely immunocompromised, or if local blood supply to the wound is impaired, bacterial growth exceeds the body's defenses against invasion into deeper tissues. The result is deep wound INFECTION and eventually bacteremia and sepsis.

Swab cultures are helpful only in identifying the types of bacteria present on the ulcer surface and may not identify bacteria in deeper tissues (Cross, 2014). Wound biopsies allow the numbers of bacteria to be analyzed, but these tests are time consuming, costly, and not always available. Clinical indicators of infection (cellulitis, progressive increase in ulcer size or depth, changes in the quantity and quality of exudate) and systemic signs of bacteremia (e.g., fever, elevated white blood cell [WBC] count) are used to diagnose an INFECTION.

Other Diagnostic Assessments. Additional laboratory studies are performed based on the suspected cause of the wound. For example, noninvasive and invasive arterial blood flow studies are indicated if arterial occlusion is suspected in delayed healing of a pressure ulcer on the heel or ankle. Blood tests to determine nutritional deficiencies (e.g., prealbumin, albumin, total protein) are helpful in managing the debilitated, malnourished patient with a pressure ulcer.

❓ CLINICAL JUDGMENT CHALLENGE

Patient-Centered Care; Evidence-Based Practice QSEN

An 82-year-old woman, who lives alone, fell at home and lay on her right side for 10 hours on a hardwood floor before she was found. Although she broke no bones, she is very sore and does not want to move. She has an open abraded area on her right trochanter. Her other health problems include arthritis, hypertension, type 2 diabetes, osteoporosis, and gastroesophageal reflux disease.

1. Is the open area considered a pressure ulcer? Why or why not?
2. What risk factors does this patient have for pressure ulcer formation?
3. What other body areas should be inspected for possible pressure ulcer formation?
4. How will you handle her request not to move or be moved?

◆ Analysis

The priority NANDA-I nursing diagnoses and collaborative problems for patients with pressure ulcers include:

1. Impaired Tissue Integrity related to vascular insufficiency and trauma (NANDA-I)
2. Potential for wound deterioration related to insufficient wound management

◆ Planning and Implementation

The Concept Map on p. 445 addresses care issues related to patients who have or are at risk for pressure ulcers.

Managing Wounds

Planning: Expected Outcomes. The patient with a pressure ulcer is expected to progress to complete wound healing and not develop new pressure ulcers. Indicators include:

- Presence of granulation, re-epithelialization, and scar tissue formation
- Decreased wound size
- Absence of new pressure ulcers

Interventions. Wound care for pressure ulcers varies according to each patient's needs and the health care provider's preferences. Surgery may be indicated for some patients, whereas a nonsurgical approach to ulcer débridement is preferred for a patient who has adequate defenses but is too ill or debilitated for surgery.

Nonsurgical Management. General interventions for pressure ulcer care are listed in Chart 25-4. Nonsurgical intervention of pressure ulcers is often left to the discretion of the nurse, who coordinates with the health care provider and certified wound care specialist (if available) to select an appropriate method of wound dressing and management. Many agencies have guidelines for wound dressings based on wound size and depth and presence of drainage.

Dressings. A well-designed dressing helps healing by removing surface debris, protecting exposed healthy tissues, and creating a barrier until the ulcer is closed. *For a draining, necrotic ulcer, the dressing must also remove excessive exudate and loose debris without damaging healthy epithelial cells or new granulation tissue. Extensive necrosis and thick eschar require surgical or chemical removal before débridement with dressings can be*

CHART 25-4   Best Practice for Patient Safety & Quality Care QSEN

Wound Management of Pressure Ulcers

- If ulcer is covered, remove old dressings/coverings daily (unless the dressing type is to remain in place until it loosens naturally).
- Measure wound size at greatest length and width using a disposable paper tape measure or, for asymmetric ulcers, by tracing the wound onto a piece of plastic film or sheeting (plastic template) at least weekly or more often if the wound shows signs of deterioration.
- Compare all subsequent measurements against the initial measurement.
- Assess the ulcer for presence of necrotic tissue and amount of exudate.
- Assess and document the condition of the skin surrounding the pressure ulcer in terms of color, temperature, texture, moisture, and appearance.
- Remove or trim loose bits of tissue (may be done by a certified wound care specialist, physical therapist, advanced practice nurse, or other as specified by the agency and the state's nurse practice act).
- Cleanse the ulcer with saline or a prescribed solution (after diluting it as per manufacturer's directions or prescriber's instructions).
- Rinse and dry the ulcer surface.
- In collaboration with the certified wound care specialist, select and apply the dressing materials most appropriate for the volume of wound drainage.
- If possible, avoid positioning the patient on the pressure ulcer.
- Re-position at least every 1 to 2 hours to prevent ulcer extension or generation of additional pressure ulcers.
- Use prescribed pressure-relieving and pressure-reducing devices and techniques as described in Chart 27-2.

CONCEPT MAP

PRESSURE ULCER
- TISSUE INTEGRITY
- INFLAMMATION
- CELLULAR REGULATION
- INFECTION

HISTORY

Older adult Tom McKnight has had a loss of tissue integrity and has developed a stage 3 sacral pressure ulcer (PU) and bilateral stage 1 heel pressure ulcers. These pressure ulcers are due to significant postoperative perfusion issues from cardiac surgery and resulting immobility.

EXPECTED OUTCOMES

Restoration of TISSUE INTEGRITY - demonstrate progress to complete wound healing and no new development of pressure ulcers (evidence of granulation tissue, decreased wound size, absence of new pressure ulcers).

Prevent INFECTION, INFLAMMATION, and wound deterioration - remain free of wound infection or systemic sepsis (indicators: WBC within normal range, negative blood cultures, no purulent drainage, decrease in wound size or depth, and absence of fever).

↑ Planning

PATIENT PROBLEMS

Impaired TISSUE INTEGRITY related to vascular insufficiency and trauma.

Potential for wound deterioration related to insufficient wound management

↑ Data Synthesis

- Prolonged bedrest
- Immobility
- Incontinence
- Inadequate nutrition and dehydration
- Altered mental status (decreased sensory perception, cognitive problems)
- Diabetes mellitus
- Peripheral vascular disease

↑ Risk Factors

Perform and Interpret Physical Assessment → Data Synthesis

- T 100° F; P 92; R 20; BP 130/80
- Stage 3 sacral PU (moderate drainage, no necrotic tissue, red base)
- Stage 1 bilateral heels
- Midsternal chest incision–wound edges approximated, slight redness, tender to touch, no drainage
- Labs - WBC 12,000; albumin 3.0; prealbumin 12 mg/dL

INTERVENTIONS

1 Physical Assessment/Clinical Manifestations

- Identify cause of existing PUs and factors that impair healing: prolonged bedrest, immobility, incontinence, diabetes mellitus, inadequate nutrition or hydration, decreased sensory perception, and peripheral vascular disease. *Identifies risk factors to address for minimizing or eliminating risk of developing impaired TISSUE INTEGRITY.*
- Use an evidence-based risk assessment tool (e.g., Braden) to monitor for risk of skin breakdown. Ensure tubing and other medical devices are not placed underneath the patient to produce a pressure point. *Identifies early risks to develop PU and prevents and maintains TISSUE INTEGRITY.*
- Monitor mental status and vital signs. *Assesses overall condition—confusion can be caused from infection, dehydration, and fluid & electrolyte imbalance.*
- Determine loss of mobility or a decreased range of motion (ROM). *Provides clues about mobility as a risk factor for PUs.*
- Assess wounds at each dressing change; document initial assessment as a starting point for determining the intervention plan and its effectiveness. *Indicates current state of healing or deterioration.*

2 Wound Care Assessment

- Record the location and size of wounds measuring the length, width, and depth. *Accurately measures wounds for evidence of healing and effectiveness of treatment.*
- Elevate the heels off of support surfaces. *Stops the compression of blood vessels that result in ischemia, inflammation, and tissue necrosis.*
- Inspect wounds for necrotic tissue. *Assesses the need for débridement. Dead tissue supports bacterial growth, obstructs collagen deposition, and wound contraction.*
- Coordinate with a WOCN to select the best dressing that promotes an optimal environment for healing. *Promotes evidence-based nursing care to protect new tissue and allow for wound healing.*
- Cleanse the sacral pressure ulcer with normal saline; remove existing dressing using aseptic technique. Use sterile technique for applying new dressings. *Decreases the risk of infection and promotes an environment of moist wound healing.*

3 Nursing Safety Priority: Action Alert!

- Change synthetic dressings when exudate causes the adhesive seal to break and leakage to occur. *Prevents skin maceration around the wound.*

4 Assessment of Infection and Inflammation

- Monitor for signs of INFECTION (cellulitis, progressive increase in ulcer size or depth, changes in quantity and quality of exudate) and systemic signs of bacteremia (fever, elevated WBC count). *Helps prevent the slowing or stopping of wound healing.*
- Inspect wound margins for cellulitis. *Identifies signs of INFLAMMATION extending beyond area of injury which can indicate INFECTION.*
- Use Standard Precautions to care for wounds and dispose of soiled dressings and linens. *Maintains a safe environment to help prevent wound INFECTION and transmission to others.*

5 Reducing Mechanical Forces

- Obtain pressure reduction devices. *Protects against the mechanical forces of pressure, shear, friction, and moisture.*
- Perform daily inspection of the skin, especially bony prominences, skin folds, and perineal area for redness, maceration, or skin breakdown. *Prevents or minimizes mechanical forces that impair TISSUE INTEGRITY.*
- Keep skin clean and dry. *Excessive skin moisture, or urinary or fecal incontinence increases the risk for skin damage and macerates skin.*
- Wash skin with pH-balanced soap, use creams or lotions to lubricate skin, use barrier ointments with incontinence, and change absorbent pads or garments immediately. *Incontinence results in prolonged contact of the skin with irritating substances, destroys TISSUE INTEGRITY, and predisposes to skin breakdown.*

6 Nursing Safety Priority: Action Alert!

- Teach all nursing care personnel and family members not to massage reddened skin areas directly or use donut-shaped pillows for pressure relief. *Prevents damage to capillary beds and decreases risk of tissue necrosis.*

7 Interpretation of Lab Values

- Evaluate WBCs, prealbumin, albumin, and total protein levels. *Indicates signs of infection and protein malnutrition which makes tissue prone to breakdown and delays healing.*

Concept Map by Deanne A. Blach, MSN, RN

TABLE 25-4 Common Dressing Techniques for Wound Débridement

TECHNIQUE	MECHANISM OF ACTION
Wet-to-damp saline-moistened gauze	As with the wet-to-dry technique, necrotic debris is mechanically removed but with less trauma to healing tissue.
Continuous wet gauze	The wound surface is continually bathed with a wetting agent of choice, promoting dilution of viscous exudate and softening of dry eschar.
Topical enzyme preparations	Proteolytic action on thick, adherent eschar causes breakdown of denatured protein and more rapid separation of necrotic tissue.
Moisture-retentive dressing	Spontaneous separation of necrotic tissue is promoted by autolysis.

effective. Different dressing materials help remove debris by **mechanical débridement** (mechanical entrapment and detachment of dead tissue), by **topical chemical débridement** (topical enzyme preparations to loosen necrotic tissue), or by **natural chemical débridement** (promoting self-digestion of dead tissues by naturally occurring bacterial enzymes [*autolysis*]) (Table 25-4).

After all the dead tissue has been removed, protection of exposed healthy tissues is critical to pressure ulcer care. The ideal healing environment is a clean, *slightly* moist ulcer surface with minimal bacterial colonization. Heavy moisture from an excessively draining ulcer or a dressing that is too wet promotes the growth of organisms and causes maceration (mushiness) of healthy tissue. Likewise, if a clean ulcer surface is exposed to air or if highly absorbent dressing materials are used for prolonged periods, overdrying can dehydrate surface cells, form scabs, and convert the wound to a deeper injury. The right balance of moisture is the key to maintaining a healing environment. The type of dressing should change as wound features change with healing (Baranoski & Ayello, 2012).

Assess the ulcer for necrotic tissue and amount of exudate. Coordinate with a wound care specialist to select a dressing material that promotes an optimal environment for healing. For example, a material that does not stick to the wound surface and does not remove new epithelial cells when it is changed is used for protecting new tissue. Depending on the amount of drainage, select either a hydrophobic or a hydrophilic material:

- A **hydrophobic** (nonabsorbent, waterproof) material is useful when the wound has little drainage and needs to be protected from external contamination.
- A **hydrophilic** (absorbent) material draws excessive drainage away from the ulcer surface, preventing maceration.

A variety of synthetic materials with different absorbent properties are available. Unlike cotton gauze dressings, these may be left intact for extended periods. Biologic and synthetic skin substitutes are the newest materials being researched. Although useful, these "smart" dressings may be cost-prohibitive for many patients.

The frequency of dressing changes depends on the amount of necrotic material or exudate. Dry gauze dressings are changed when "strike through" occurs—when the outer layer of the dressing first becomes saturated with exudate. Gauze dressings used for débridement of a wet wound (allowed to become damp and then removed) are changed often enough to take off any loose debris or exudate, usually every 4 to 6 hours.

> **! NURSING SAFETY PRIORITY** (QSEN)
> **Action Alert**
>
> Change synthetic dressings when exudate causes the adhesive seal to break and leakage to occur.

Before reapplying any dressing, gently clean the ulcer surface with saline or another wound cleanser as prescribed. If an antibacterial cleanser is prescribed, dilute the agent to reduce tissue toxicity and then rinse with tap water and dry the surface before applying the dressing.

Physical Therapy. Daily whirlpool treatments along with dressing changes for débridement can help remove dead tissue. The ulcerated area is immersed in or saturated with warm tap water that contains a cleansing agent. Continuous agitation of the water loosens the debris and washes away exudate and debris. During treatment, the ulcer surface is cleansed with a gauze pad. After treatment, the therapist or wound specialist often uses instruments to trim away any obvious bits of dead tissue that are still loosely attached to the ulcer surface.

Drug Therapy. Clean, healthy granulation tissue has a blood supply and is capable of providing white blood cells and antibodies to the ulcer to combat INFECTION. If extensive necrosis is present or if local tissue defenses are impaired, topical antibacterial agents are often needed to control bacterial growth (see Chart 26-5 in Chapter 26 for a list of topical antibacterial agents). Antibiotic use is avoided in the absence of infection to reduce the development of resistant bacterial strains.

Nutrition Therapy. Successful healing of pressure ulcers depends on adequate intake of calories, protein, vitamins, minerals, and water. Nutrition deficiencies are common among chronically ill patients and increase the risk for skin breakdown and delayed wound healing. Severe protein deficiency inhibits healing and impairs host INFECTION defenses.

Coordinate with the dietitian to help the patient eat a well-balanced diet, emphasizing protein, vegetables, fruits, whole grains, and vitamins. Fats also are needed to ensure formation of cell membranes. (See Chapter 60 for interventions to ensure adequate nutrition.) If the patient cannot eat sufficient amounts of food, other types of feedings may be needed to increase protein and caloric intake (see Chapter 60). Vitamin and mineral supplements are also indicated.

New Technologies. For chronic ulcers that remain open for months, new technologies have had some success. These include electrical stimulation, negative pressure wound therapy, hyperbaric oxygen therapy, topical growth factors, and skin substitutes.

Electrical stimulation is the application of a low-voltage current to a wound area to increase blood vessel growth and promote granulation. This treatment is usually performed by a certified wound care specialist. The voltage is delivered in "pulses" that may cause a "tingling" sensation. Usually this technique is performed for 1 hour a day, 5 to 7 days a week. It is not used with patients who have a pacemaker or a wound over the heart.

Negative pressure wound therapy (NPWT) can reduce or even close chronic ulcers by removing fluids or infectious materials from the wound and enhancing granulation. This technique requires that a suction tube be covered by a special sponge and sealed in place. Per manufacturer's instructions, the foam dressing is changed every 48 to 72 hours (or at least 3 times weekly). Continuous low-level negative pressure is applied through the suction tube. Duration of the treatment is determined by the wound's response. It should not be used in areas of skin cancer. Failure of NPWT is often due to the inability to maintain an adequate dressing seal (Rock, 2011).

Current evidence does not support greater effectiveness of NPWT in closing chronic wounds than more traditional methods. Serious bleeding and even deaths have occurred with NPWT, and these devices have received a warning from the Food and Drug Administration (FDA) to exclude high-risk patients from its use. Any patient who is receiving this therapy must be monitored at least every 2 hours for bleeding at or near the wound site.

> **! NURSING SAFETY PRIORITY** (QSEN)
>
> **Critical Rescue**
>
> Do not use a continuous negative pressure wound therapy device with any patient who is on anticoagulant therapy; has reduced tissue health near the wound (e.g., with radiation therapy or poor nutrition); or has any exposed blood vessels, nerves, or organs in the wound area.

Hyperbaric oxygen therapy (HBOT) is the administration of oxygen under high pressure, raising the tissue oxygen concentration. This type of therapy is usually reserved for life- or limb-threatening wounds such as burns, necrotizing infections, brown recluse spider bites, osteomyelitis, and diabetic ulcers. The patient is enclosed in a large chamber and exposed to 100% oxygen at pressures greater than normal atmospheric pressure. Systemic oxygen enhances the ability of white blood cells to kill bacteria and reduce swelling. Treatment usually lasts from 60 to 90 minutes. Smaller topical oxygen delivery devices are also available. These devices are applied directly over an open wound to promote local tissue oxygenation; however, their effectiveness in promoting wound healing requires further study (Woo et al., 2012).

Topical growth factors are normal body substances that stimulate cell movement and growth. These factors are deficient in chronic wounds, and topical application is used to stimulate wound healing. For example, platelet-derived growth factor (PDGF) stimulates the movement of fibroblasts into the wound space. Use of this and other growth factors has been effective for healing of some chronic wounds, but further study is needed (Demidova-Rice et al., 2012b).

Skin substitutes are engineered products that aid in the closure of different types of wounds. These products vary widely in design and application and are used mainly for surgically débrided wounds before reconstruction with grafts or muscle flaps.

Surgical Management. Surgical management of a pressure ulcer includes removal of necrotic tissue and skin grafting or use of muscle flaps to close wounds that do not heal by re-epithelialization and contraction. Not all wounds are candidates for grafting. Those with poor blood flow are unlikely to have successful graft take and heal. The procedures are very similar to the surgical management of burn wounds. See the Surgical Management section of Managing Wound Care on pp. 483–485 of Chapter 26.

Preventing Infection and Wound Deterioration

Planning: Expected Outcomes. The patient with a pressure ulcer is expected to remain free of wound INFECTION or sepsis. Indicators include that the patient will have mild or no:

- White blood cell elevation
- Positive blood culture
- Purulent or malodorous drainage
- Increase in wound size or depth
- Fever

Interventions. Priority nursing interventions focus on preventing wound INFECTION and identifying wound infection early to prevent complications.

Monitoring the ulcer's appearance using objective criteria allows evaluation of the response to treatment and early recognition of INFECTION. If an ulcer shows no progress toward healing within 7 to 10 days or worsens, the treatment plan is re-evaluated. Chart 25-5 outlines objectives of monitoring wounds with and without tissue loss. Patients who are at highest risk for infection are those who are older, have white blood cell (WBC) disorders, are receiving steroid therapy, or have wounds with a compromised blood supply.

Preventing infection and its complications starts with monitoring the ulcer's progress. Routinely check for manifestations of wound INFECTION: increased pain, tenderness, and redness at the wound margins, edema, and purulent and malodorous drainage. Report these changes to the health care provider:

- Sudden deterioration of the ulcer, seen as an increase in the size or depth of the lesion
- Changes in the color or texture of the granulation tissue
- Changes in the quantity, color, or odor of exudate

These changes may occur with or without manifestations of bacteremia, such as fever, an elevated WBC, and positive blood cultures. Use the previously described interventions to prevent the formation of new pressure ulcers and to prevent early-stage ulcers from progressing to deeper wounds (see Chart 25-2).

Maintaining a safe environment can help prevent wound INFECTION. Because of the variety of organisms in the hospital environment, keeping an ulcer totally free of bacteria is impossible. Optimal ulcer management is based on maintaining acceptably low levels of organisms through meticulous wound care and reducing contamination with pathogenic organisms that could lead to sepsis and death. *Teach all personnel to use Standard Precautions and to properly dispose of soiled dressings and linens.*

Community-Based Care

Patients with pressure ulcers may be in acute care, subacute care, long-term care, or home care settings. If pressure ulcer therapy requires hospitalization, most patients are discharged before complete wound closure is achieved. Discharge may be to the home setting or to a long-term care facility, depending on the degree of debilitation and other patient factors.

Home Care Management. Ulcer care in the patient's home is similar to care in the hospital. Most dressing supplies and pressure-relief devices can be obtained at a pharmacy or medical supply store. If ulcer débridement is needed, a handheld shower device or forceful irrigation of the wound with a 35-mL syringe and 19-gauge angiocatheter can be substituted for whirlpool therapy.

CHART 25-5   Best Practice for Patient Safety & Quality Care QSEN

Monitoring the Wound

VARIABLE	FREQUENCY OF ASSESSMENT	RATIONALE
Wounds Without Tissue Loss *Examples* Surgical incisions and clean lacerations closed primarily by sutures or staples		
Observations (using first postoperative dressing change as baseline) Check for the presence or absence of increased: • Localized tenderness • Swelling of the incision line • Erythema of the incision line >1 cm on each side of wound • Localized heat	At least every 24 hr until sutures or staples are removed	To detect cellulitis (bacterial infections)*
Check for the presence or absence of: • Purulent drainage from any portion of the incision site • Localized fluctuance (from fluid accumulation) and tenderness beneath a *portion* of the wound when palpated	At least every 24 hr until sutures or staples are removed	To detect abscess formation related to presence of foreign body (suture material) or deeper wound infection*
Check for the presence or absence of: • Approximation (sealing) of wound edges with or without serosanguineous drainage • Necrosis of skin edges	At least every 24 hr until sutures or staples are removed	To detect potential for wound dehiscence
Wounds with Tissue Loss *Examples* Partial- or full-thickness skin loss caused by pressure necrosis, vascular disease, trauma, etc., and allowed to heal by secondary intention		
Observations **Wound Size** Measure wound size at greatest length and width using a disposable paper tape measure or, for asymmetric ulcers, by tracing the wound onto a piece of plastic film or sheeting (plastic template) Measure depth of full-thickness wounds using cotton-tipped applicator Compare all subsequent measurements against the initial measurement	Once per week	To detect increase in wound size and depth secondary to infectious process
Ulcer Base Check for the presence or absence of: • Necrotic tissue (loose or adherent) • Foul odor from wound when dressing is changed Note the frequency of dressing changes or dressing reinforcements owing to drainage	At least every 24 hr	To detect the need for débridement or the response to treatment (necrotic tissue) and to detect local wound infection (frequent dressing changes and foul odor)
Wound Margins Check for the presence or absence of: • Erythema and swelling extending outward >1 cm from wound margins • Increased tenderness at wound margins	At least every 24 hr or at each dressing change	To detect wound infection*
Systemic Response Check for the presence or absence of elevated body temperature or WBCs or positive blood culture	Check temperature daily; if elevated, check WBCs and blood culture	To detect bacteremia

WBCs, White blood cells.

*The wounds of patients who are severely immunosuppressed or those wounds with compromised blood supply may not exhibit a typical inflammatory response to local wound infection.

Many patients cannot change their own dressings because of wound location, distress over an altered body image, or the pain of dressing removal. Others depend on family members or support personnel because of limited physical mobility.

For some patients, drastic changes in daily activities are needed to promote healing. Patients with leg ulcers may need frequent rest periods with leg elevation to avoid or reduce edema. Immobile patients with pressure ulcers require around-the-clock repositioning as often as every 1 to 2 hours to prevent further breakdown, which takes its toll on caregivers. Explain the rationale for activity changes to the patient and family, and explore ways of coping with these changes.

Some patients may need to continue the use of special beds or mattress overlays at home. Although these items can be expensive, home use can keep the patient out of more-costly health care settings. Consider both the space and power supply when choosing a pressure-relief device for home use. Coordinate with the case manager to work with the insurance company in providing these important aids for quality patient care.

Self-Management Education. Before the patient is discharged, have the patient or caregiver demonstrate competence in removing the dressing, cleaning the wound, and applying the dressing. When choosing a dressing to be used at home, consider the patient's or caregiver's ability to apply the dressing properly. If the patient's finances are limited, address the cost of the dressing material. At times, the more expensive dressing materials that require less frequent changing may be preferred. Explain the manifestations of wound INFECTION, and remind the patient and family to report their presence to the health care provider or wound care clinic.

Encourage the patient to eat a balanced diet, including high-protein snacks. Discuss diet preferences with the patient and consult a dietitian as needed to design a food plan to promote wound healing. Vitamin and mineral supplements may be needed to prevent or treat deficiencies. If the patient is incontinent, emphasize the need to keep the skin clean and dry. If bowel and bladder training are not possible, discuss the use of absorbent underpads, briefs, and topical moisture barrier creams and ointments as methods to reduce skin exposure to urine and feces.

Health Care Resources. A home care nurse may be needed to follow wound progress after discharge. As indicated by The Joint Commission's NPSGs, the hospital nurse provides details of ulcer size and appearance and any special wound care needs in a hand-off report to the home care nurse, who can then accurately judge changes in ulcer appearance. Chart 25-6 is a guideline for a focused assessment of the patient with pressure ulcers.

To help decrease the cost of treatment, emphasize proper use of dressing materials. Clean tap water and nonsterile supplies are used for home management of chronic wounds and are less costly than sterile products. Stress the importance of properly cleaning reused items and of handwashing before touching any supplies.

The patient with activity restrictions may need daily assistance from a home care aide. Collaborate with a physical therapist or occupational therapist to help the patient and family continue rehabilitation efforts in the home.

◆ Evaluation: Outcomes

Evaluate the care of the patient with a pressure ulcer on the basis of the identified priority patient problems. The expected outcomes include that the patient will:

> ### CHART 25-6   Home Care Assessment
>
> **The Patient at Risk for Pressure Ulcers**
>
> Assess cardiovascular status:
> - Presence or absence of peripheral edema
> - Hand-vein filling in the dependent position
> - Neck-vein filling in the recumbent and sitting positions
> - Weight gain or loss
>
> Assess cognition and mental status:
> - Level of consciousness
> - Orientation to time, place, and person
> - Can the patient accurately read a seven-word sentence containing words of three syllables or fewer?
>
> Assess condition of skin:
> - Assess general skin cleanliness
> - Observe all skin areas, paying particular attention to bony prominences and those areas in greatest contact with the bed and other firm surfaces
> - Measure and record any areas of redness or loss of integrity
> - If possible, photograph areas of concern
> - Note the presence or absence of skin tenting over the sternum or the forehead
> - Note the moistness of skin and mucous membranes
> - If wounds are present, remove dressings (noting condition of dressings), cleanse the wound, and compare with previous notations of wound condition:
>   - Presence, amount, and nature of exudate
>   - Use a disposable paper tape measure to measure wound diameter and depth
>   - Amount (%) and type of necrotic tissue
>   - Presence of granulation/epithelium
>   - Presence or absence of cellulitis
>   - Presence or absence of odor
>
> Take the patient's temperature.
>
> Assess the patient's understanding of illness and compliance with treatment:
> - Manifestations to report to health care provider
> - Drug therapy plan (correct timing and dose)
> - Ambulation or positioning schedule
> - Dressing changes/skin care
> - Nutrition modifications (24-hour diet recall)
>
> Assess the patient's nutritional status:
> - Change in muscle mass
> - Lackluster nails, sparse hair
> - Recent weight loss of more than 5% of usual weight
> - Impaired oral intake
> - Difficulty swallowing
> - Generalized edema

- Experience progress toward wound healing by second intention as evidenced by granulation, epithelialization, and reduction or resolution of wound size
- Re-establish skin TISSUE INTEGRITY and restore skin barrier function
- Remain INFECTION free

Specific indicators for these outcomes are listed for each priority patient problem under the Planning and Implementation section (see earlier).

COMMON INFECTIONS

❖ PATHOPHYSIOLOGY

Skin INFECTION can be bacterial, viral, or fungal. Chart 25-7 lists key features and common locations of each type.

CHART 25-7   Key Features

Common Skin Infections

CLINICAL MANIFESTATIONS	DISTRIBUTION
Bacterial Infections	
Folliculitis	
Isolated erythematous pustules occur singly or in groups; hairs grow from centers of many of the lesions.	Areas of hair-bearing skin, especially buttocks, thighs, beard area, and scalp
Occasional papules are present.	
There is little or no associated discomfort.	
There is no residual scarring.	
Furuncle	
Small, tender, erythematous nodules become pus filled and more tender over time.	Areas of hair-bearing skin, especially buttocks, thighs, abdomen, posterior neck regions, and axillae
Lesions may be single or multiple and also recurrent.	
Regional lymphadenopathy is sometimes present; fever is rare.	
Occasional scarring results.	
Cellulitis	
Localized area of inflammation may enlarge rapidly if not treated.	Lower legs, areas of persistent lymphedema, and areas of skin trauma (e.g., leg ulcer, puncture wound)
Redness, warmth, edema, tenderness, and pain are present.	
On rare occasions, blisters are present.	
Cellulitis is often accompanied by lymphadenopathy and fever.	
Viral Infections	
Herpes Simplex	
Grouped vesicles are present on an erythematous base.	Type 1 classically on the face and type 2 on the genitalia, but either may develop in any area where inoculation has occurred; recurrent infections occur repeatedly in the same skin area
Vesicles evolve to pustules, which rupture, weep, and crust.	
Older lesions may appear as punched-out, shallow erosions with well-defined borders.	
Lesions are associated with itching, stinging, or pain.	
Secondary bacterial infection with necrosis is possible in immunocompromised patients.	
Herpes Zoster (Varicella Zoster)	
Lesions are similar in appearance to herpes simplex and also progress with weeping and crusting.	Anterior or posterior trunk following involved dermatome; face, sometimes involving trigeminal nerve and eye
Grouped lesions present unilaterally along a segment of skin following the pathway of a spinal or cranial nerve (dermatomal distribution).	
Eruption is preceded by deep pain and itching.	
Postherpetic neuralgia is common in older adults.	
Secondary infection with necrosis is possible in immunocompromised patients.	
Fungal Infections	
Dermatophytosis	
Annular or serpiginous patches are present with elevated borders, scaling, and central clearing.	Anywhere on the body
Itching is common.	
Lesions may be single or multiple.	
Candidiasis	
Erythematous macular eruption occurs with isolated pustules or papules at the border (satellite lesions).	Skinfold areas: perineal and perianal region, axillae, beneath breasts, and between the fingers; under wet or occlusive dressings
Candidiasis is associated with burning and itching.	Lesions possibly present on the oral or vaginal mucous membranes
Oral lesions (thrush) appear as creamy white plaques on an inflamed mucous membrane.	
Cracks or fissures at the corners of the mouth may be present.	

Bacterial Infections

Bacterial skin lesions usually start at the hair follicle, where bacteria easily collect and grow in the warm, moist environment. **Folliculitis** is a superficial INFECTION involving only the upper portion of the follicle and is often caused by *Staphylococcus*. The rash is raised and red and usually shows small pustules. **Furuncles** (boils) are also caused by *Staphylococcus*, but the infection is much deeper in the follicle (Fig. 25-7). This larger, sore-looking, raised bump may or may not have a pustular

"head" at its point. Cellulitis often occurs as a generalized infection with either *Staphylococcus* or *Streptococcus* and involves the deeper connective tissue.

Minor skin trauma usually occurs before the appearance of folliculitis and furuncles and may contribute to the development of cellulitis. Patients may spread the INFECTION to other parts of their bodies by scratching or rubbing the skin with fingernails. Furuncles most often occur in areas of heat and moisture, such as in the hair-bearing skinfold areas. Cellulitis

FIG. 25-7 A furuncle.

FIG. 25-8 Herpes zoster (shingles).

can occur as a result of secondary bacterial infection of an open wound, or it may be unrelated to skin trauma.

A common skin problem is INFECTION with methicillin-resistant *Staphylococcus aureus* (MRSA). This infection can range from mild folliculitis to extensive furuncles. It is easily spread to other body areas and to other people by direct contact with infected skin and by contact with clothing, linens, athletic equipment, and other objects used by a person with MRSA. The infection does not respond to cleansing with antibacterial soaps or most types of topical and many oral antibiotic therapies. If MRSA infects a wound or enters the bloodstream, deep wound infection, sepsis, organ damage, and death can occur. The incidence is highest among adults living in communal environments, such as dormitories or prisons, and among patients in hospitals or other health care settings. (See Chapter 23 for a more detailed MRSA discussion.)

Viral Infections

Herpes simplex virus (HSV) INFECTION is the most common viral infection of adult skin and has two types. Type 1 (HSV-1) infections cause the classic recurring cold sore. The severity of the disease increases with age and is worse when the patient is immunosuppressed. Genital herpes, caused by type 2 infection (HSV-2), is also recurrent (see Chapter 74).

After the first INFECTION, the virus remains in a dormant state in the nerve ganglia and the patient has no manifestations. Reactivation stimulates the virus to travel down sensory nerves to the skin, where lesions reappear. Recurrence of HSV infection in healthy people is triggered by stressors, such as dry lips, sunburn, trauma, fever, menses, and fatigue. The virus can also be spread by contact between an actively infected person and a susceptible host. *Autoinoculation*, or transfer of either viral type from one part of the body to another, is also possible.

The time span between episodes and the severity of each attack vary. Outbreaks of oral herpes simplex usually last 3 to 10 days. The patient may have tingling or burning of the lip before any lesion is evident. The patient sheds virus and is contagious for the first 3 to 5 days.

The clinical picture of HSV-1 INFECTION is isolated or grouped painful vesicles on a red base. The infection can occur anywhere on the skin and may be spread by respiratory droplets or by direct contact with an active lesion or virus-containing fluid (e.g., saliva).

Herpetic whitlow is a form of herpes simplex that occurs on the fingertips of health care personnel who come into contact with viral secretions. It can be spread easily to patients and can become severe in immunosuppressed patients.

Herpes zoster (shingles) is INFECTION caused by reactivation of the varicella-zoster virus (VZV) in patients who have previously had chickenpox. The dormant virus resides in the dorsal root ganglia of sensory nerves. Multiple lesions occur in a segmental distribution on the skin area innervated by the infected nerve (Fig. 25-8). Herpes zoster eruptions usually occur after several days of discomfort, which may vary from minor irritation and itching to severe, deep pain. The eruption usually lasts several weeks. Postherpetic neuralgia (severe pain persisting after the lesions have resolved) is common in older patients. Early diagnosis of shingles and prompt treatment with antiviral drugs help decrease the duration and severity of postherpetic neuralgia.

Herpes zoster occurs most often in older people or in anyone who is immunosuppressed for any reason. The disorder can be accompanied by fever and malaise. *It is contagious to people who have not previously had chickenpox and have not been vaccinated against the disease.* Keeping patients with fluid-filled blisters separated from other patients until the lesions have crusted reduces the risk for transmitting the virus to others. Complications include full-thickness skin necrosis, Bell's palsy, or eye INFECTION, and scarring if the virus is introduced into the eye.

Fungal Infections

Dermatophyte infections, especially superficial INFECTIONS, differ in lesion appearance, body location, and species of the organism. The term *tinea* is used to describe dermatophytoses; this term is then followed by the location description. For example *tinea pedis* involves the foot (athlete's foot), *tinea manus* involves the hands, *tinea cruris* involves the groin (jock itch), *tinea capitis* involves the head, and *tinea corporis* involves the rest of the body (ringworm).

Depending on the species, dermatophytes live mainly in the soil, on animals, and on humans. Superficial INFECTION can start only when the infecting organism comes in contact with impaired skin in a susceptible host. Infections are spread by direct contact with infected humans or animals. Some infections, such as tinea capitis and tinea corporis, can be transmitted by inanimate objects. For example, tinea capitis can be spread by sharing contaminated combs, hats, pillowcases, and other objects with people who have poor personal hygiene.

Candida albicans, also known as *yeast infection*, is a common fungal INFECTION of skin and mucous membranes. The organism is present almost everywhere and easily grows in a warm, moist environment. Risk factors for this infection include immunosuppression, long-term antibiotic therapy, diabetes mellitus, and obesity.

Infected skin has a moist, red, irritated appearance with itching and burning. Common areas for infection are the perineum, vagina, axillae, under the breasts, and in the mouth (where it is known as *thrush* or *oral candidiasis*).

Prevention is aimed at keeping skinfold areas clean and dry. Turning patients and positioning to enhance airflow also aid in prevention. When the INFECTION is present, meticulous cleanliness and the use of topical antifungal agents are needed.

Health Promotion and Maintenance

Preventing skin INFECTION, especially bacterial and fungal infections, involves avoiding the offending organism and practicing good hygiene to remove the organism before infection can occur. *Handwashing and not sharing personal items with others are the best ways to avoid contact with these organisms, including MRSA.* Chart 25-8 lists strategies to teach patients and family members to prevent infection spread to other body areas and to other people.

For older adults who have had chickenpox and are, therefore, at risk for shingles (herpes zoster), the vaccine *Zostavax* is available to prevent VZV reactivation and shingles. The Centers for Disease Control and Prevention (CDC) recommends the

---

CHART 25-8   Patient and Family Education: Preparing for Self-Management

Preventing the Spread of MRSA

- Avoid close contact with others, including participation in contact sports, until the infection has cleared.
- Take all prescribed antibiotics exactly as prescribed for the entire time prescribed.
- Keep the infected skin area covered with clean, dry bandages.
- Change the bandage whenever drainage seeps through it.
- Place soiled bandages in a plastic bag, and seal it closed before placing it in the regular trash.
- Wash your hands with soap and warm water before and after touching the infected area or handling the bandages.
- Shower (rather than bathe) daily, using an antibacterial soap.
- Wash all uninfected skin areas before washing the infected area, or use a fresh washcloth to wash the uninfected areas.
- Use each washcloth only once before laundering, and avoid using bath sponges or puffs.
- Sleep in a separate bed from others until the infection is cleared.
- Avoid sitting on or using upholstered furniture.
- Do not share clothing, washcloths, towels, athletic equipment, shavers or razors, or any other personal items.
- Clean surfaces that may have come into contact with your infected skin, drainage, or used bandages (e.g., bathroom counters, shower/bath stalls, toilet seats) with household disinfectant or bleach water mixed daily (1 tablespoon of liquid bleach to 1 quart of water).
- Wash all soiled clothing and linens with hot water and laundry detergent. Dry clothing either in a hot dryer or outside on a clothesline in the sun.
- Urge family members and close friends to shower daily with an antibacterial soap.
- If another person assists you in changing the bandages, make certain he or she uses disposable gloves, pulls them off inside out when finished, places them with the soiled bandages in a sealed bag, and washes his or her hands thoroughly.

MRSA, Methicillin-resistant *Staphylococcus aureus.*

---

vaccine for anyone older than 50 years who has a healthy immune system. This one-time subcutaneous injection significantly reduces the incidence of shingles. Cost remains a factor in vaccination, and few insurance carriers currently include this coverage.

! NURSING SAFETY PRIORITY (QSEN)
Drug Alert

Zostavax is a live viral vaccine and should not be used in patients with severe immunosuppression because of the risk for viral dissemination. Always check with the prescriber before giving any live vaccines to severely immune compromised patients or those receiving biologic agents for autoimmune disease.

❖ PATIENT-CENTERED COLLABORATIVE CARE

◆ Assessment

History. Concentrate on risk factors for each type of INFECTION. If the location and appearance of lesions suggest a bacterial infection, ask about a recent history of skin trauma or recent staphylococcal or streptococcal infections. Assess living conditions, home sanitation, personal hygiene habits, and leisure or sport activities. Ask whether fever and malaise are also present.

Lesions appearing on the lips, in the mouth, or in the genital region are more likely to be a possible viral infection. Ask about:

- A history of similar lesions in the same location
- Presence of burning, tingling, or pain
- Recent stress factors that preceded the outbreak
- Recent contact with an infected person

Information that the same type of lesions has occurred before is important in helping differentiate viral from bacterial lesions. Ask whether the patient has had chickenpox in the past and about a history of shingles. Also ask whether he or she has received the shingles vaccination *Zostavax.*

Obtain information about a probable dermatophyte INFECTION based on lesion location. If tinea corporis or tinea capitis is present, assess the social and home factors that may contribute to infection, such as direct contact with an infected person, poor personal hygiene, or frequent contact with animals. If tinea cruris and tinea pedis are suspected, ask about the type and frequency of athletic activities.

Physical Assessment/Clinical Manifestations. Because most skin infections are contagious, take precautions to prevent the spread of INFECTION when performing a physical assessment. See Chart 25-7 for a listing of the manifestations of common skin infections.

Laboratory Assessment. When pustules are present in bacterial INFECTIONS, the infecting organism is confirmed by swab culture of the purulent material. Blood cultures may be helpful if fever and malaise are present. Various cultures and other techniques are used to identify viral and fungal infections (see Chapter 24).

◆ Interventions

Most skin INFECTIONS heal well with nonsurgical management. Surgery may be required when an infectious agent is present in deep tissue layers. *Priority nursing interventions focus on patient and family education to prevent infection spread to other body areas or to other people* (see Chart 25-8). Meticulous skin care is needed for prevention of infection spread. In some instances, drug therapy is needed.

Skin care with proper cleansing is the most effective intervention to prevent INFECTION *spread.* Teach patients with bacterial infections to bathe daily with an antibacterial soap and to not squeeze any pustules or crusts. Teach them to gently remove crusts before applying topical drugs so that the drugs can be more easily absorbed. Teach the patient to apply warm compresses to furuncles or areas of cellulitis to increase comfort. Most superficial skin infections resolve more quickly if the involved skin dries between treatments. Excessive moisture, especially if occluded by dressings, clothing, or bedding, promotes organism growth. Position bedridden patients for optimal air circulation to the area, and avoid occlusive dressings or garments.

Transmission-Based Precautions may be needed to reduce the INFECTION spread to other people. For most superficial bacterial infections, proper handwashing prevents cross-contamination. However, when hospitalized patients are colonized with antibiotic-resistant *Staphylococcus,* strict adherence to isolation procedures is necessary.

Of the dermatophyte INFECTIONS, tinea capitis, tinea corporis, and tinea pedis are most easily transmitted to others. Teach patients to avoid sharing personal items, such as hairbrushes, articles of clothing, or footwear. Repeated infections transmitted by dogs or cats indicate that the pet also needs to be treated.

Drug therapy for superficial INFECTION involves topical agents. Mild bacterial infections of the skin usually resolve with topical antibacterial treatment. Patients with extensive infections, especially if fever or lymphadenopathy is present, require systemic antibiotic therapy. The most common systemic drugs used for bacterial skin infections are the penicillins and cephalosporins. For those who are allergic to drugs from these classes, tetracyclines, macrolides, or aminoglycoside antibiotics may be used. For patients infected with MRSA or other drug-resistant organisms, drug therapy may involve IV vancomycin or oral linezolid or clindamycin.

Acyclovir (Zovirax), valacyclovir (Valtrex), or famciclovir (Famvir) is used for the treatment of viral INFECTIONS. Topical treatment decreases the numbers of active viruses on the skin surface and reduces pain in herpetic infections and localized lesions in immunocompromised patients during an initial outbreak. Topical treatment is of little benefit in recurrent infection. IV administration is limited to severe primary infections, immunosuppressed patients with manifestations of systemic infection, and recurrent outbreaks.

Topical antifungal agents are used for patients with dermatophyte or yeast INFECTIONS at least twice a day until the lesions have cleared. To prevent recurrence, therapy is usually continued for 1 to 2 weeks after clearing. In some instances, antifungal powders may also help suppress fungal growth. For widespread or resistant fungal infections, systemic antifungal agents, such as ketoconazole (Nizoral), are given.

CUTANEOUS ANTHRAX

Cutaneous anthrax is an INFECTION caused by the spores of the bacterium *Bacillus anthracis.* In the United States, the most common risk factor is contact with an infected animal. Those most at risk for cutaneous anthrax include farm workers, veterinarians, and tannery and wool workers. This organism has now become a tool for terrorism.

? NCLEX EXAMINATION CHALLENGE

Health Promotion and Maintenance

Which statement made by a client with a furuncle in the groin indicates to the nurse that teaching about the care needed for this problem has been effective?
A. "I will wear tight jeans to keep the infection from spreading to other areas."
B. "I will shower with an antibacterial soap before applying the topical ointment."
C. "I will squeeze the lesion until it opens so I can remove all the pus and other material."
D. "I will shave the area around the lesion and apply cortisone cream to reduce the inflammation."

! NURSING SAFETY PRIORITY (QSEN)

Action Alert

Consider the possibility of bioterrorism whenever lesions consistent with cutaneous anthrax appear in patients who do not have a history of exposure to infected animals.

The INFECTION can be confined to the skin, or it may be systemic. At first a raised vesicle appears on an exposed body area such as the head or arms (Fig. 25-9). The lesion may itch and often resembles an insect bite. Within a few days, the center of the vesicle becomes hemorrhagic and sinks inward, starting an area of necrosis and ulceration. The tissue around the wound swells and can become very edematous. With necrosis, an eschar forms (see Fig. 25-9). The two features that distinguish anthrax lesions from insect bites or other skin lesions are that it is painless and that eschar forms regardless of treatment. Patients may have only one lesion, or there may be multiple lesions, usually in the same body area.

Some patients develop systemic manifestations with cutaneous anthrax. The area becomes edematous and tender. Fever, chills, and enlarged lymph nodes may be present.

Diagnosis is made based on lesion features, a positive culture, or the presence of anthrax antibodies in the patient's blood. Cultures are obtained from patients who have a fever.

Oral antibiotics for 60 days are indicated for patients who have no edema or systemic manifestations and whose lesions are not located on the head or neck. The antibiotics of choice are ciprofloxacin (Cipro) or doxycycline (Doryx, Vibramycin). For patients who have a fever, have lesions on the head or neck, are pregnant, or have extensive edema, antibiotics are given IV and then followed by an oral course of 60 days.

PARASITIC DISORDERS

Parasitic skin disorders occur most often in patients with poor hygiene and in those who are homeless. Examine any patient who shows obvious signs of a self-care deficit for contagious parasitic infections.

Pediculosis

Pediculosis is a lice infestation: *pediculosis capitis* (head lice), *pediculosis corporis* (body lice), and *pediculosis pubis* (pubic, or crab, lice). Human lice are oval and 2 to 4 mm long. The female louse lays many eggs *(nits)* at the hair shaft base in hair-bearing areas.

FIG. 25-9 Cutaneous anthrax. Note ulcer with vesicular ring, induration, and erythema (**A**). As eschar forms, induration lessens, surrounding desquamation occurs, but erythema persists (**B**).

The most common manifestation of pediculosis is itching (pruritus). Excoriation from scratching also may be present. Some parasites may carry disease (e.g., typhus).

Pediculosis capitis occurs more often in people with longer hair. Scalp itching from parasite bites is intense. A secondary INFECTION may also be present from scratching.

Because the louse is difficult to see, examine the scalp for visible white flecks of the nits attached to the hair shaft near the scalp. Matting and crusting of the scalp and a foul odor indicate a probable secondary INFECTION.

Pediculosis corporis is caused by lice that live and lay eggs in the seams of clothing. The parasites also cause itching. The only visible sign of infestation may be excoriations on the trunk, abdomen, or extremities.

Pediculosis pubis causes intense itching of the vulvar or perirectal region. Pubic lice are more compact and crablike in appearance than body lice and can be contracted from infested bed linens or during sexual intercourse with an infected person. Although these lice are usually found in the genital region, they can also infest the axillae, the eyelashes, and the chest.

The treatment of pediculosis is chemical killing of the parasites with topical sprays, creams, and shampoos. Agents used include permethrin (Elimite), lindane (Bio-Well, Kwell, Kwellada), or topical malathion (Ovide, Prioderm). Oral agents may also be used, such as ivermectin (Stromectol). In the case of pediculosis capitis, areas where the patient's head has rested (e.g., on pillows or chair backs) are also treated. Clothing and bed linens should be washed in hot water with detergent or dry-cleaned. The use of a fine-tooth comb helps remove nits but does not cure the INFECTION. For any louse infestation, social contacts are treated when possible.

Scabies

Scabies is a contagious skin INFECTION caused by mite infestations. It is transmitted by close contact with an infested person or infested bedding. Infestation is common among patients with poor hygiene or crowded living conditions. The scabies mite is carried by pets and is found among homeless people and institutionalized older patients. Health care personnel are at risk for contracting scabies from contact with an infected patient or his or her bed linen.

Scabies is manifested by curved or linear ridges in the skin (Fig. 25-10). The itching is very intense, and patients often report that the itching becomes unbearable at night.

FIG. 25-10 Scabies. Note the horizontal lines indicating burrowing of the organism under the skin.

The visible horizontal white skin ridges are formed by burrowing of the mite into the outer skin layers. Examine the skin between the fingers and on the palms and inner aspects of the wrists, where these ridges are most common. A hypersensitivity reaction to the mite results in excoriated erythematous papules, pustules, and crusted lesions on the elbows, nipples, lower abdomen, buttocks, and thighs and in the axillary folds. Males can have lesions on the penis.

Infestation is confirmed by taking a scraping of a lesion and examining it under the microscope for mites and eggs. Close contacts also should be examined for possible infestation.

Treatment involves the use of scabicides, such as permethrin (Acticin), lindane (Kwell, Kildane, Scabene, Thionex), malathion (Ovide), or benzyl benzoate (Ascabiol). Laundering clothes and personal items with hot water and detergent is sufficient to eliminate the mites.

Bedbugs

A common parasite is the bedbug, *Cimex lectularius*. Infestations are increasingly common as a result of travel and resistance to pesticides. This pest does not live on humans; however, it feeds on human blood. The bite causes an itchy discomfort. The most common mode of infestation is carrying the "hitch-hiking" bug home from an infested environment such as a hotel room. This problem is not related to socioeconomic level or to a lack of cleanliness.

The adult bedbug is about the size, shape, and color of an apple seed. After feeding, it may double in size and have a red or black color. The insect bites a human host at night and sucks blood for 3 to 10 minutes. The bite area resembles a mosquito or flea bite with a raised bite mark surrounded by a wheal. The degree of itching and redness is related to how allergic the person is to the insect's saliva. All body areas are susceptible, and one insect can bite multiple times, resulting in clusters of bite marks.

Management of the patient with bedbug bites is symptomatic for discomfort from itching, usually with topical antihistamines. When the discomfort is more widespread or the allergic reaction is severe, systemic antihistamines or corticosteroids may be used. Because humans do not harbor the insect, the usual topical insecticides are not needed.

Bedbugs can live anywhere, hiding in cracks and crevices. They can live and lay their eggs in soft upholstery or in wooden crevices. Eradicating the infestation and preventing re-infestations require considerable effort and can be frustrating. Often the home environment needs the extensive eradication efforts of a licensed professional pest control company with experience in the management of bedbugs (Barnes & Murray, 2013).

COMMON INFLAMMATIONS

❖ PATHOPHYSIOLOGY

Skin INFLAMMATION can have many nonspecific manifestations, including severe itching, lesions with indistinct borders, and different distribution patterns. The cause may not be identified. Rashes from inflammation can evolve from acute to chronic conditions.

Most skin INFLAMMATIONS are related to allergic immune responses. The responses may be triggered by external skin exposure to allergens or by internal exposure to allergens and irritants. The result is tissue destruction or skin changes induced by the immune system. (A more detailed description of these immune mechanisms is presented in Chapter 17.)

The specific cause of skin INFLAMMATION is not always known. When this is the case, the catch-all diagnosis of *nonspecific eczematous dermatitis,* or *eczema,* is often used.

Contact dermatitis is an acute or chronic rash caused by direct contact with either an irritant or an allergen. Irritants cause a toxic injury to the skin. Allergens result in a cell-mediated immune reaction in the skin.

Atopic dermatitis is a chronic rash that occurs with allergies and atopic skin disease. It is made worse by dry or irritated skin, food allergies, chemicals, or stress. (Atopic reactions are described in Chapter 20.)

❖ PATIENT-CENTERED COLLABORATIVE CARE

Because all skin eruptions from INFLAMMATION appear similar, personal data are needed to identify the cause. Inflammatory skin problems differ from eczematous dermatitis in chronicity, lesion distribution, and associated manifestations. Chart 25-9

CHART 25-9 Key Features	
Common Inflammatory Skin Conditions	
CLINICAL MANIFESTATIONS	**DISTRIBUTION**
Nonspecific Eczematous Dermatitis Evolution of lesions from vesicles to weeping papules and plaques. Lichenification occurs in chronic disease. Oozing, crusting, fissuring, excoriation, or scaling may be present. Itching is common.	Anywhere on the body; localized eczema commonly involves the hands or feet.
Contact Dermatitis Localized eczematous eruption with well-defined, geometric margins that are consistent with contact by an irritant or allergen. Usually seen in the acute form, but may become chronic if exposure is repeated. Allergy to plants (e.g., poison ivy or oak) classically occurs as linear streaks of vesicles or papules.	Cosmetic/perfume allergy: head and neck. Hair product allergy: scalp. Shoe/rubber allergy: dorsum of feet. Nickel allergy: earlobes. Mouthwash/toothpaste allergy: perioral region. Airborne contact allergy (e.g., paint, ragweed): generalized.
Atopic Dermatitis Hallmark in adults is lichenification with scaling and excoriation. Extremely itchy. Face involvement is seen as dry skin with mild to moderate erythema, perioral pallor, and skinfolds beneath the eyes (Dennie-Morgan lines). Associated with linear markings on the palms.	Face, neck, upper chest, and antecubital and popliteal fossae.
Drug Eruption Bright red erythematous macules and papules are found. Skin blisters in extreme cases. Lesions tend to be confluent in large areas. Moderately itchy. Fever is rare. Dehydration and hypothermia can occur with extensive involvement. Condition clears only after offending drug has been discontinued.	Generalized. Involvement begins on trunk, proceeds distally (legs are the last to be involved).

lists the manifestations of many types of inflammatory skin conditions.

If the cause of the rash is identified, avoidance therapy is used to reverse the reaction and clear the rash. For example, if a new soap for handwashing causes contact dermatitis of the hands, teach the patient to avoid that substance. Even when the cause is unclear, certain irritants may worsen the rash and increase discomfort. Additional interventions promote comfort through suppression of INFLAMMATION.

Steroid therapy with topical, intralesional, or systemic steroids is prescribed to suppress INFLAMMATION. Because a side effect of oral corticosteroids (e.g., prednisone) is adrenal suppression, patients receiving long-term systemic therapy must taper their drug dosages rather than stop them abruptly.

Remember that corticosteroids never cure the INFLAMMATION. During active disease, these drugs reduce manifestations and relieve discomfort. Moisten dressings with warm tap water and place them over topical steroids for short periods to increase absorption. Avoid applying topical steroids under occlusive dressings unless prescribed by the health care provider.

❗ NURSING SAFETY PRIORITY (QSEN)

Drug Alert

Caution patients not to apply topical corticosteroids to potentially infected skin lesions anywhere on the body, but especially on the face. These agents suppress the local immune response and can worsen the infection.

Avoid applying oil-based ointments and pastes to the sweaty skinfold areas to prevent blocking of pores and folliculitis. Water-soluble creams are better for these areas. Lotions and gels prevent matting of the hair and are more appropriate for the scalp and other hairy areas. Thick, stiff ointments or pastes (e.g. zinc oxide pastes) are applied to localized areas because they cling to the skin where applied and resist spreading to uninvolved skin.

Antihistamines provide some relief of itching but may not keep the patient totally comfortable. The sedative effects of these drugs may be better tolerated if most of the daily dose is taken near bedtime. Teach patients to avoid driving or operating heavy machinery if these drugs are taken during the day.

Comfort measures such as cool, moist compresses and lukewarm baths with bath additives have a soothing effect, decrease INFLAMMATION, and help débride crusts and scales. Colloidal oatmeal, tar extracts, cornstarch, or oils added to baths may relieve itching.

PSORIASIS

❖ PATHOPHYSIOLOGY

Psoriasis is a chronic, autoimmune disorder affecting the skin with exacerbations and remissions. It results from overstimulation of the immune system (Langerhans' cells) in the skin that activates T-lymphocytes. These cells then target the keratinocytes, causing increased cell division (because some degree of CELLULAR REGULATION is lost) and plaque formation. Even though psoriasis cannot be cured, patients can often achieve control of manifestations with proper management.

Psoriasis lesions are scaled with underlying dermal INFLAMMATION from an abnormality in the growth of epidermal cells. Normally, basal cells take about 28 days to reach the outermost layer where they are shed. In a person with psoriasis, the rate of cell division is speeded up so that cells are shed every 4 to 5 days.

🧬 GENETIC/GENOMIC CONSIDERATIONS

Patient-Centered Care (QSEN)

A genetic predisposition is associated with psoriasis as indicated by the fact that when one identical (monozygotic) twin develops the disease, the second twin also develops the disease about 70% of the time. Variations in many gene sequences, labeled *PSORS1* through *PSORS13*, influence the development of this autoimmune disorder. It is likely that different variations of these gene loci also influence individual patient responses to therapy. Always ask about a family history of the disorder when assessing the patient with psoriasis (Online Mendelian Inheritance in Man [OMIM], 2014b).

Many environmental factors lead to outbreaks and influence the severity of manifestations, but these vary from person to person. Triggering factors may be local or systemic. A psoriatic lesion may appear after skin trauma (Koebner's phenomenon, in which a previously injured area is more susceptible to development of cancer or chronic skin problems) such as surgery, sunburn, or excoriation.

Patients with psoriasis often improve with more exposure to sunlight. Systemic factors that can aggravate the disease include INFECTION (severe streptococcal throat infection, *Candida* infection, upper respiratory infections), hormonal changes (e.g., puberty, menopause), stress, drugs (lithium, beta-blocking agents, indomethacin), obesity, and the presence of other diseases.

Some patients with psoriasis also develop debilitating *psoriatic arthritis*. This arthritis may lead to severe joint changes similar to those seen in rheumatoid arthritis and indicates that psoriasis is a systemic disorder (McCance et al., 2014). See Chapter 18 for more discussion of arthritis.

❖ PATIENT-CENTERED COLLABORATIVE CARE

◆ Assessment

History. Ask the patient about any family history of psoriasis, including the age at onset, a description of the disease progression, and the pattern of recurrences. Have the patient describe the current flare-up of psoriasis, including whether the onset was gradual or sudden, where the lesions first appeared, whether there have been any changes in severity over time, and whether fever and itching are present. Explore possible precipitating factors, and ask about the effectiveness of any previous interventions.

Physical Assessment/Clinical Manifestations. The appearance of psoriasis and its course vary among patients. Typically during flare-ups of the disease, lesions thicken and extend into new body areas. As psoriasis responds to treatment, lesions become thinner with less scaling.

Psoriasis vulgaris is the most common type of psoriasis, with thick, reddened papules or plaques covered by silvery white scales (Fig. 25-11). Borders between the lesions and normal skin are sharply defined. Patches are less red and moister in skinfold areas. Lesions are usually present in the same areas on both sides of the body (bilateral distribution). Common sites include the scalp, elbows, trunk, knees, sacrum, and outside surfaces of the limbs. Facial skin is rarely affected. The patient may have only a few lesions, or the entire skin surface may be affected.

Exfoliative psoriasis (erythrodermic psoriasis) is an explosively eruptive and inflammatory form with generalized erythema and scaling but no obvious lesions. Fluid loss with this severe inflammatory reaction can lead to dehydration and hypothermia or hyperthermia.

Palmoplantar pustulosis (PPP) is a type of psoriasis that forms pustules on the palms of the hands and soles of the feet along with reddened hyperkeratotic plaques. The course of the disease is cyclic, with new outbreaks of pustules occurring after older lesions have resolved. PPP is difficult to treat, and patients often have social and physical problems.

◆ Interventions

The three different approaches to therapy are based on the extent of disease, the patient's distress, and the response of the psoriasis to treatment. Patients must understand that no cure

FIG. 25-11 A, Psoriasis vulgaris in a white patient. **B,** Psoriasis vulgaris in a patient with dark skin.

for psoriasis exists yet. Therapy is aimed at reducing cell proliferation and INFLAMMATION. *Priority nursing strategies include teaching the patient about the disease and its treatment and providing emotional support for the changes in body image often experienced with psoriasis.*

Topical Therapy. The topical agents used to treat psoriasis are topical steroids, topical tar and anthralin preparations, and ultraviolet (UV) light.

Corticosteroids have anti-inflammatory actions. When applied to psoriatic lesions, corticosteroids suppress cell division. The effectiveness of a topical steroid depends on its potency and ability to be absorbed into the skin. The more potent agents are used as therapy for patients with psoriasis.

Teach patients to enhance the skin penetration of these drugs by applying the steroid directly to the skin. When prescribed, using warm, moist dressings and an occlusive outer wrap of plastic (film, gloves, booties, or similar garments) may enhance absorption.

Tar preparations applied to the skin suppress cell division from impaired CELLULAR REGULATION and reduce INFLAMMATION. These drugs are available as solutions, ointments, lotions, gels, and shampoos. The ointments are messy, cause staining, and have an unpleasant odor.

Topical therapy with anthralin (Anthraforte❦, Drithocreme, Lasan), a hydrocarbon similar in action to tar, also relieves chronic psoriasis. These drugs can be used alone or in combination with coal tar baths and UV light.

Teach the patient to apply the high-potency anthralin, suspended in a stiff paste, to each lesion for short periods (not exceeding 2 hours). The drug is a strong irritant and can cause chemical burns. Remind the patient to check for local tissue reaction and to take care to prevent this drug from coming into contact with uninvolved skin.

Other topical therapies can be effective for many patients with mild to moderate psoriasis. These drugs include calcipotriene (Dovonex), a synthetic form of vitamin D that regulates skin cell division, and tazarotene (Avage, Tazorac), a derivative of vitamin A that slows cell division and reduces inflammatory responses. In some cases, calcitriol (Vectical ointment) has been helpful but is quite expensive.

Light Therapy. Ultraviolet (UV) radiation is a physical agent commonly used as a topical therapy in many skin conditions, including psoriasis. Ultraviolet B (UVB) light, which produces more energy, is responsible for the obvious biologic effects of

---

! NURSING SAFETY PRIORITY (QSEN)

Drug Alert

Tazorac is **teratogenic** (can cause birth defects) even when used topically. Teach sexually active women of childbearing age using this drug to adhere to strict contraceptive measures.

---

the sun, such as burning. Although the sun is an inexpensive source of UV radiation, better availability and intensity control occur with the use of artificial light sources. These sources include lamps or cabinets containing UV tubes. *The use of commercial tanning beds is not recommended for the patient with psoriasis.*

Ultraviolet therapy is limited by exposure time and effects on the surrounding normal skin. The time of exposure is gradually increased to achieve a mild suntan effect without burning or tenderness. The patient's skin pigmentation determines the exposure times. Because of the extremely high intensity of most artificial UVB light sources, therapy is measured in seconds of exposure and patients must wear eye protection during treatment. Narrow band UVB light therapy, although intense, can shorten the time to effectiveness and reduce the number of exposures needed to maintain the response.

Light therapy with lasers can be effective in controlling mild to moderate psoriasis. Laser sources, whether administered in a continuous or pulsed exposure, allow for better focus on the lesions and reduce exposure to the surrounding normal skin.

Teach patients to inspect the skin carefully each day for signs of overexposure. If tenderness on palpation occurs and severe erythema or blister formation develops, notify the health care provider before therapy is resumed.

Psoralen and ultraviolet A (UVA) (PUVA) therapy involves the ingestion of a photosensitizing agent (psoralen) 2 hours before exposure to UVA light. Therapy sessions are limited to 2 or 3 times a week and are not given on consecutive days. Exposure is gradually increased until tanning occurs. Dosages are adjusted according to the erythema reaction of normal skin as well as the response of psoriatic lesions.

Teach the patient to check for redness with edema and tenderness. If these are present, treatment must be interrupted until they subside. Because psoralen is a strong photosensitizer, patients must wear dark glasses during treatment and for the rest of the day.

Systemic Therapy. Systemic agents are used when psoriasis does not respond to topical therapies. The most commonly used drugs are oral vitamin A derivatives—retinoids. These drugs include acitretin (Soriatane) and bexarotene (Targretin).

! NURSING SAFETY PRIORITY (QSEN)

Drug Alert

Both acitretin and bexarotene are teratogenic. Teach sexually active women of childbearing age using this drug to adhere to strict contraceptive measures.

A variety of biologic (immunomodulating) agents that alter the immune response and prevent overstimulation of keratinocytes from impaired CELLULAR REGULATION are now being used to manage moderate to severe plaque psoriasis. These agents may be prescribed when other drugs are not effective and when psoriatic arthritis is also present. Most of these drugs are given by intravenous infusion, intramuscular injection, or subcutaneous injection. All of these agents induce some degree of immunosuppression, and patients are at an increased risk for serious infection.

! NURSING SAFETY PRIORITY (QSEN)

Drug Alert

Instruct patients to discontinue the biologic agent and notify the health care provider immediately if manifestations of INFECTION occur.

Biologics currently approved for the treatment of psoriasis are listed in Chart 25-10. These drugs should NOT be used by patients who are pregnant or breast-feeding.

Other less commonly used systemic drugs for the patient whose disease is resistant to topical therapy include methotrexate (Folex, Mexate), cyclosporine (Sandimmune), and azathioprine (Imuran). The many health risks associated with these therapies must be considered along with the potential benefits, especially in older adults (Wong & Woo, 2012).

Emotional Support. Often patients' self-esteem suffers because of the presence of skin lesions. Encourage the patient and family members to express their feelings about having an incurable skin problem that can alter appearance. Support

groups for people with psoriasis are available in many communities. Urge patients and families to consider participating in these groups.

The use of touch takes on an added significance for patients with psoriasis. For example, shake the patient's hand during an introduction or place a hand on the patient's shoulder when explaining a procedure. *Do not wear gloves during these social interactions. Touch, more than any other gesture, communicates acceptance of the person and the skin problem.*

? NCLEX EXAMINATION CHALLENGE

Health Promotion and Maintenance

Which precaution is most important for the nurse to teach the 32-year-old female client prescribed topical tazarotene (Tazorac) cream for psoriasis?
A. Apply a dressing over the site with each application.
B. Stop the drug use when psoriasis manifestations decrease.
C. Report symptoms of infection to the prescriber immediately.
D. Adhere to strict contraceptive measures while using the drug.

SKIN CANCER

❖ PATHOPHYSIOLOGY

Any skin cancer occurs as a result of failure of CELLULAR REGULATION over cell division. (See Chapter 21 for a discussion of the general mechanisms leading to changes in cellular regulation and cancer development.) *Overexposure to sunlight is the major cause of skin cancer, although other factors also are associated.* Because sun damage is an age-related skin finding, screening for suspicious lesions is an important part of physical assessment of the older adult. The most common skin cancers are actinic or solar keratosis, squamous cell carcinoma, basal cell carcinoma, and melanoma. Table 25-5 describes common skin cancers. A biopsy of suspicious lesions is necessary to determine whether a skin lesion is malignant.

Etiology and Genetic Risk

Actinic keratoses are premalignant lesions of the cells of the epidermis. These lesions are common in people with chronically sun-damaged skin. Progression to squamous cell carcinoma may occur if lesions are untreated.

Squamous cell carcinomas are cancers of the epidermis. They can invade locally and are potentially metastatic (Fig. 25-12). Chronic skin damage from repeated injury or irritation also

---

CHART 25-10 Common Examples of Drug Therapy

Plaque Psoriasis

AGENT	ROUTE	DOSE	FREQUENCY
adalimumab (Humira)	Subcutaneous	Loading dose: 80 mg Maintenance dose: 40 mg	Loading dose followed by maintenance dose every other week starting 1 week after the loading dose.
alefacept (Amevive)	Intramuscular	15 mg	Once a week for 12 weeks followed by a 12-week drug-free interval. Cycle may be repeated based on response.
etanercept (Enbrel)	Subcutaneous	50 mg	Twice weekly for 3 months followed by once-a-week injections.
infliximab (Remicade)	Intravenous	5 mg/kg	Infusions at 0, 2, and 6 weeks, then every 8 weeks.
ustekinumab (Stelara)	Subcutaneous	90 mg	Initial dose 90 mg; second dose 4 weeks later Maintenance injections of 90 mg subcutaneously every 12 weeks starting at week 16 after initial dose.

TABLE 25-5 Common Skin Cancers

CLINICAL MANIFESTATIONS	DISTRIBUTION	COURSE
Actinic Keratosis (Premalignant)		
Small (1-10 mm) macule or papule with dry, rough, adherent yellow or brown scale Base may be erythematous Associated with yellow, wrinkled, weather-beaten skin Thick, indurated keratoses more likely to be malignant	Cheeks, temples, forehead, ears, neck, backs of hands, and forearms	May disappear spontaneously or reappear after treatment. Slow progression to squamous cell carcinoma is possible.
Squamous Cell Carcinoma		
Firm, nodular lesion topped with a crust or with a central area of ulceration Indurated margins Fixation to underlying tissue with deep invasion	Sun-exposed areas, especially head, neck, and lower lip Sites of chronic irritation or injury (e.g., scars, irradiated skin, burns, leg ulcers)	Rapid invasion with metastasis via the lymphatics occurs in 10% of cases. Larger tumors are more prone to metastasis.
Basal Cell Carcinoma		
Pearly papule with a central crater and rolled, waxy borders Telangiectasias and pigment flecks visible on close inspection	Sun-exposed areas, especially head, neck, and central portion of face	Metastasis is rare. May cause local tissue destruction. 50% recurrence rate related to inadequate treatment.
Melanoma		
Irregularly shaped, pigmented papule or plaque Variegated colors, with red, white, and blue tones	Can occur anywhere on the body, especially where nevi (moles) or birthmarks are evident Commonly found on upper back and lower legs Soles of feet and palms in dark-skinned people	Horizontal growth phase followed by vertical growth phase. Rapid invasion and metastasis with high morbidity and mortality.

FIG. 25-12 Squamous cell carcinoma.

FIG. 25-13 Basal cell carcinoma.

predisposes to this malignancy. Chronic wounds that remain open for long periods are also at increased risk for malignant transformation to cancer.

Basal cell carcinomas arise from the basal cell layer of the epidermis (Fig. 25-13). Early lesions often go unnoticed, and although metastasis is rare, underlying tissue destruction can occur. Genetic predisposition and chronic irritation are risk factors; however, UV exposure is the most common cause.

Melanomas are pigmented cancers arising in the melanin-producing epidermal cells (Fig. 25-14). Most often they start as the benign growth of a **nevus** (mole) (Skin Cancer Foundation, 2014). Normal nevi have regular, well-defined borders and are uniform in color, ranging from light colors to dark brown. The lesion's surface may be rough or smooth. Nevi with irregular or spreading borders and those with multiple colors are abnormal. Other suspicious features include sudden changes in lesion size and reports of itching or bleeding.

Risk factors include genetic predisposition, excessive exposure to UV light, and the presence of one or more precursor

FIG. 25-14 Melanoma.

lesions that resemble unusual moles. *This skin cancer is highly metastatic, and a person's survival depends on early diagnosis and treatment.*

GENETIC/GENOMIC CONSIDERATIONS
Patient-Centered Care QSEN

Genetic mutations in the *CDKN2A* and *CDK4* have been identified for some cases of familial melanoma. These mutations in a suppressor gene result in loss of cellular regulation for cell growth. Other genetic considerations for melanoma are that some specific mutations in the genes of the actual tumor cells increase the response of these cells to targeted therapy. All melanomas should be tested for mutations of the *BRAF* and *KIT* genes (OMIM, 2014a). Always ask patients who have a diagnosed melanoma whether any other family members have ever had this disease.

Incidence and Prevalence

The incidence of skin cancer is highest among light-skinned races and people older than 60 years (American Cancer Society [ACS], 2014). Skin cancer occurs more often among those who work outdoors, live at higher altitudes or lower latitudes, or spend much time sunbathing. Occupational exposure to arsenic or other chemical carcinogens also increases risk. The incidence of melanoma has increased during the past 30 years, accounting for 4% to 5% of all cancers, although the death rate from melanoma is decreasing (ACS, 2014).

Health Promotion and Maintenance

The most effective prevention strategy for skin cancer is avoiding or reducing skin exposure to sunlight. However, even when people understand the cause of skin cancer and the seriousness of the disease, preventive behaviors are not always practiced. Common prevention practices are listed in Chart 25-11. *Teach all people to avoid tanning beds and salons.*

Secondary prevention (early detection) is critical to survival with melanoma. Teach all people to be aware of their skin markings. Keeping a total body spot and lesion map can provide baseline information about suspicious new lesions and help identify changes in existing lesions. Once a map is made, the person should systematically inspect his or her body monthly for new lesions and for changes in any existing lesions by performing thorough *skin self-examination (SSE)*. Some people find taking pictures of their skin on a regular basis makes identifying changes easier. Teach everyone to evaluate all skin lesions using the ABCDE guide for melanoma (see Chapter 24) and to consult his or her health care provider to examine any lesion having unusual features. When lesions, such as moles, are present, they should be monitored yearly by a dermatologist or other health care professional.

❖ PATIENT-CENTERED COLLABORATIVE CARE

◆ Assessment

In addition to age and race, ask the patient about any family history of skin cancer and any past surgery for removal of skin growths. Recent changes in the size, color, or sensation of any mole, birthmark, wart, or scar are also significant. Ask about which geographic regions the patient has lived in and where he or she currently resides. Obtain information about occupational and recreational activities in relation to sun exposure, as well as any occupational history of exposure to chemical

---

CHART 25-11 **Patient and Family Education: Preparing for Self-Management**

Prevention of Skin Cancer

- Avoid sun exposure between 11 AM and 3 PM.
- Use sunscreens with the appropriate skin protection factor for your skin type.
- Wear a hat, opaque clothing, and sunglasses when you are out in the sun.
- Keep a "body map" of your skin spots, scars, and lesions to detect when changes have occurred.
- Examine your body monthly for possibly cancerous or precancerous lesions.
- Seek medical advice if you note any of these:
  - A change in the color of a lesion, especially if it darkens or shows evidence of spreading
  - A change in the size of a lesion, especially rapid growth
  - A change in the shape of a lesion, such as a sharp border becoming irregular or a flat lesion becoming raised
  - Redness or swelling of the skin around a lesion
  - A change in sensation, especially itching or increased tenderness of a lesion
  - A change in the character of a lesion, such as oozing, crusting, bleeding, or scaling

---

carcinogens (e.g., arsenic, coal tar, pitch, radioactive waste, radium). Ask whether any skin lesions are repeatedly irritated by the rubbing of clothing.

Skin that has been injured previously is at greater risk for cancer development, an effect known as *Koebner's phenomenon.* Ask the patient if he or she has ever experienced a severe skin injury that resulted in a scar. Examine all scarred skin areas for the presence of potentially cancerous lesions. A biopsy may be required to rule out cancer in a chronic open wound that fails to close with proper treatment.

Skin cancers vary in their appearance and distribution. Although most skin cancers appear in sun-exposed areas of the body, inspect the entire skin surface and any unusual lesions, particularly moles, warts, birthmarks, and scars. Also examine hair-bearing areas of the body, such as the scalp and genitalia. Palpate lesions to determine surface texture. Document the location, size, color, and features of all lesions and any reports of tenderness or itching. Use the ABCDE method of evaluating all lesions for possible melanoma (see Chapter 24).

◆ Interventions

Surgical and nonsurgical interventions are combined for the effective management of skin cancer. Treatment is determined by the size and severity of the malignancy, the location of the lesion, and the age and general health of the patient.

Surgical Management. Surgical intervention is needed to manage any type of skin cancer. It can range from local removal of small lesions to massive excision of large areas of the skin and underlying tissue for treatment of melanoma. Surgical types for skin cancer include:

- Cryosurgery—cell destruction by the local application of liquid nitrogen (−200° C) to isolated lesions, causing cell death and tissue destruction.
- Curettage and electrodesiccation—removal of cancerous cells with the use of a dermal curette to scrape away cancerous tissue, followed by the application of an electric probe to destroy remaining tumor tissue.

- Excisional biopsy—total surgical removal of small lesions for pathologic examination.
- Mohs' surgery—a specialized form of excision usually for basal and squamous cell carcinomas. Tissue is sectioned horizontally in layers, and each layer is examined histologically to determine the presence of residual tumor cells.
- Wide excision—deep skin resection often involving removal of full-thickness skin in the area of the lesion. Depending on tumor depth, subcutaneous tissues and lymph nodes may also be removed.

Nonsurgical Management. *Drug therapy* may involve topical or systemic chemotherapy, biotherapy, or targeted therapy. Topical chemotherapy with 5-fluorouracil cream is used for treatment of multiple actinic keratoses or for widespread superficial basal cell carcinoma that would require several surgical procedures to eradicate. Therapy is continued for several weeks, and the treated areas become increasingly tender and inflamed as the lesions crust, ooze, and erode. Prepare the patient for an unsightly appearance during therapy, and reassure him or her that the cosmetic result will be positive.

Systemic chemotherapeutic agents are used in the treatment of locally advanced or metastatic squamous cell skin cancer. These include a platinum based-agent (Cisplatin or Carboplatin), 5-fluorouracil, and cetuximab (Erbitux). A new drug approved for locally advanced or metastatic basal cell skin cancer is vismodegib (Erivedge).

Biotherapy with interferon, monoclonal antibodies, and targeted therapy are now accepted treatment for melanoma after surgical removal. Interferon is used for melanomas that are at stage III or higher. The patient is first started on high-dose IV interferon infusions daily for 5 days per week for 4 weeks. Maintenance doses, given subcutaneously, are then continued 3 times per week for 1 year. The patient must learn to self-inject the drug.

Monoclonal antibody therapy with ipilimumab (Yervoy), a drug that targets the *CTLA4* (cytotoxic T-lymphocyte associated antigen 4) receptor and blocks it, leads to greater T-cell lymphocyte activity. (T-cells are a type of lymphocyte that can stimulate antitumor immune responses.) The side effects of this drug include significant INFLAMMATION in many tissues, including the pituitary gland, liver, skin, GI tract, and nervous system. Some of the side effects can be life threatening (Rubin, 2012).

Targeted therapy is available for melanomas with specific mutations in the *BRAF* gene. Normally, the *BRAF* gene is involved in CELLULAR REGULATION of growth. Mutations in this gene allow melanoma to grow and metastasize. When melanoma cells are positive for a specific *BRAF* mutation *(V600E)*, the cells respond to the drug *vemurafenib* (Zelboraf). The drug inhibits an enzyme important in signaling cell division and prevents melanoma cell division. This oral drug interacts with a variety of other drugs, and allergic reactions are common.

Radiation therapy for skin cancer is limited to older patients with large, deeply invasive basal cell tumors and to those who are poor risks for surgery. Melanoma is relatively resistant to radiation therapy.

OTHER SKIN DISORDERS

Toxic Epidermal Necrolysis

Toxic epidermal necrolysis (TEN) is a rare acute drug reaction of the skin resulting in diffuse erythema and large blister

formation. Mucous membranes are often involved, and systemic toxicity is evident. The most common causative drugs are chemotherapy agents, sulfonamides, pyrazolones, barbiturates, and antibiotics. Removal of the drug is usually followed by gradual healing in 2 to 3 weeks, with widespread peeling of the epidermis.

This problem can occur at any age and as a result of almost any drug therapy. However, older patients with cancer who are receiving chemotherapy, some targeted therapies, and immunotherapy are at greatest risk. Other precipitating factors include stem cell transplantation and neutropenia-induced INFECTIONS.

The drug thought to be causing a toxic reaction is discontinued, and management focuses on systemic support and prevention of secondary INFECTION. Patients are often admitted to burn units, where fluid and electrolyte balance, caloric intake, and hypothermia can be closely monitored. Topical antibacterial drugs are used to suppress bacterial growth until healing occurs.

Stevens-Johnson Syndrome

Stevens-Johnson syndrome is often a drug-induced skin reaction caused by an immunologic mechanism, similar to toxic epidermal necrolysis. The disorder may be mild with only skin involvement, or it may be severe and systemic. The skin lesions are widely distributed, including mucous membranes, and varied in appearance (Fig. 25-15). The patient has a mix of

FIG. 25-15 Stevens-Johnson syndrome.

vesicles, erosions, and crusts. With severe involvement, the patient may have respiratory problems, excessive fluid loss, kidney failure, and blindness (Cooper, 2012).

Removal of the offending drug is critical. Mild forms of the disorder are usually self-limiting in 10 to 14 days unless the episode was triggered by a bacterial INFECTION. Then, antibiotics are needed. Severe problems require high doses of steroids to suppress the INFLAMMATION. Supportive care may include fluid replacement, mechanical ventilation, and even renal replacement therapy.

PLASTIC SURGERY

◆ Assessment

The two main types of plastic surgery are aesthetic and reconstructive. **Aesthetic plastic surgery** is cosmetic, with the aim of altering a person's physical appearance. This intervention is sought by those who are unsatisfied with their body image. These procedures are considered elective surgery and are not covered by insurance. **Reconstructive plastic surgery** is the correction or improvement of functional defects that have occurred

TABLE 25-6	Common Plastic Surgery Procedures		
DESCRIPTION	**INDICATIONS**	**COMPLICATIONS**	
Blepharoplasty			
Excision of bulging fat and redundant skin of the periorbital area with primary closure	Bags under the eyes	Hematoma Ectropion Corneal injury Visual loss (rare) Wound infection (rare)	
Breast Augmentation (Augmentation Mammoplasty)			
Insertion of synthetic breast-shaped implants through a skin incision	Inadequate breast volume or contour	Hematoma or hemorrhage Wound infection (with gram-positive organisms) Phlebitis	
Breast Reduction (Reduction Mammoplasty)			
Excision of excessive breast tissue and skin with primary closure	Hypertrophy of breast tissue caused by elevated hormone levels, endocrine abnormalities, or obesity Weight of large breasts can contribute to back pain	Hematoma or hemorrhage Nipple, areola, and skin flap necrosis Wound infection Fat necrosis Wound dehiscence	
Dermabrasion			
Abrasive removal of the facial epidermis and portion of the dermis followed by healing by second intention	Moderate to severe acne scar Deep wrinkling Multiple actinic keratoses Hyperpigmentation (postinflammatory or after the use of estrogens)	Hypertrophic scarring Altered skin pigmentation Acne flare Wound infection (rare)	
Rhinoplasty			
Removal of excessive cartilage and tissue from the nose with correction of septal defects if indicated	Disproportionate anatomy Post-traumatic nasal deformity Difficulty breathing through the nose	Hematoma or hemorrhage Ecchymosis and edema (temporary) Wound infection (with gram-positive organisms) Septal perforation Minor skin irritation	
Rhytidectomy (Facelift)			
Removal of excess skin and tissue from the face at the level of the hairline followed by primary closure	Excessive wrinkling or sagging of facial skin	Hematoma or hemorrhage Facial nerve damage (temporary or permanent) Wound infection Ecchymosis and edema (temporary) Skin necrosis Hair loss	
Liposuction (Suction Lipectomy)			
Removal of subcutaneous fat from localized areas of accumulation such as the hips, abdomen, neck, and arms	Disproportionate distribution of adipose tissue	Hematoma Severe pain Infection Emboli Sagging of skin (if skin is not elastic enough to contract after fat removal)	

as a result of congenital problems or trauma and scarring (e.g., skin and joint contractures from burn wounds) or from other types of therapy (e.g., mastectomy for breast cancer therapy). These interventions are sought by patients who cannot perform ADLs as a result of an anatomic problem; the cost is often covered by insurance.

Regardless of whether a person is having reconstructive surgery or cosmetic surgery, body image and sense of self are always involved. These feelings may evoke emotional responses in the person, including shame, anger, resentment, and desperation. Use a sensitive, nonjudgmental approach when interacting with the person having or considering plastic surgery. It is important to avoid being directive or expressing your own opinions. Often a patient who asks the nurse "Do you think I need this surgery?" is not comfortable with his or her decision.

Address the patient's expectations of plastic surgery. Often people who seek plastic surgery have unrealistic expectations. The patient with minor deformities who is seeking perfection is sure to be disappointed. The patient who wants a procedure mainly to please a partner is also a poor candidate.

◆ Interventions

Many techniques to improve skin and general appearance without surgery are available. Superficial techniques for skin enhancement include chemical peels, laser resurfacing, and dermabrasion to remove or reduce small scars, fine lines, and other irregular skin surfaces. Dermal filling involves injecting substances to change the contour of a feature or an area. Generally, these fillers replace the collagen lost from the skin through aging. Injection with nerve paralyzing agents (e.g., Botulinum Toxin Type A) can improve appearance temporarily by relaxing muscles beneath the skin surface, which smoothes out some wrinkles and grooves.

Depending on the planned intervention, surgery is performed either in the ambulatory care setting with the patient under local anesthesia or in the hospital. The types and complications of common cosmetic procedures are listed in Table 25-6.

All plastic and reconstructive surgeries have a risk for complications and failure, especially bleeding, infection, and skin reattachment problems. Procedures vary depending on the location, purpose, and extent of reconstruction.

General care after surgery focuses on monitoring for typical postoperative complications (see Chapter 16). Pressure dressings may be applied at the time of surgery and left in place for several days to control hemorrhage and edema formation. Monitor dressings for bright red bleeding, and monitor changes in vital signs and level of consciousness. Positioning varies with the specific procedure performed and the surgeon's preference.

Monitor for wound INFECTION and progress toward healing. Of particular concern are any areas of skin necrosis or eschar formation near the operative site—a complication from excessive tension on the suture line as a result of edema and blood vessel obstruction. See Chart 25-5 for a listing of wound monitoring criteria. Regardless of the planned procedure, inform the patient to expect edema and discoloration of the operative site. Swelling and bruising alter the facial features and may not resolve for several weeks after surgery. The final results of surgery will not be visible until healing is complete—usually 6 months to a year or longer after surgery.

NURSING CONCEPTS AND CLINICAL JUDGMENT REVIEW

What might you NOTICE if the patient is experiencing inadequate protection as a result of loss of skin TISSUE INTEGRITY?
- Open skin areas
- Possible presence of drainage
- Sensation changes in or around the area (patient reports pain, itching, or tightness)

What should you INTERPRET and how should you RESPOND to a patient experiencing inadequate protection as a result of loss of skin TISSUE INTEGRITY?

Perform and interpret physical assessment, including:
- Assessing the wound for pain, size, depth, drainage, and presence of infection
- Assessing the skin immediately surrounding the wound for redness and swelling
- Monitoring oxygen saturation by pulse oximetry in the affected extremity (if the open area is on an extremity)
- Assessing the patient for risk factors for wound development (pressure, shear, immobility, reduced cognition, poor nutrition, advanced age, incontinence)
- Assessing the rest of the patient's skin (especially over bony prominences, between skinfolds, in the perineal area)

Respond by:
- Documenting wound features
- Cleansing the wound (obtaining cultures, if within agency policy)
- Dressing the wound if drainage is present
- Planning a turning or repositioning schedule
- Teaching UAP or family how to relieve/reduce pressure
- Collaborating with the certified wound care specialist and dietitian

On what should you REFLECT?
- Observe the patient for evidence of restored skin integrity (see Chapter 24).
- Think about what may have precipitated this loss of skin tissue integrity and what steps could be taken to either prevent a similar problem or identify it earlier.
- Think about what additional resources could improve the nursing response to this situation.

GET READY FOR THE NCLEX® EXAMINATION!

KEY POINTS

Review these Key Points for each NCLEX Examination Client Needs Category.

Safe and Effective Care Environment

- Wash your hands before and after touching any skin lesions. **Safety** QSEN
- Use Standard Precautions when providing care to a patient who has any areas of nonintact skin. **Safety** QSEN
- Ensure that the skin of incontinent patients is kept clean and dry. **Evidence-Based Practice** QSEN
- Assist all patients with limited mobility to change positions at least every 2 hours while awake. **Evidence-Based Practice** QSEN
- Use a structured approach (e.g., Braden scale or other validated tool) to evaluate the pressure ulcer risk for all patients on admission and regularly thereafter. **Evidence-Based Practice** QSEN
- Be proactive in the use of pressure-relieving devices for any patient who is identified to be at risk for pressure ulcer formation (i.e., requires prolonged bedrest, is an older adult, has some degree of immobility, is incontinent, has some degree of malnutrition, is dehydrated, has decreased sensory perception, or has an altered mental state).
- Use a lift sheet or mechanical lift to move immobilized older patients rather than pulling or dragging them across bed linens. **Safety** QSEN

Health Promotion and Maintenance

- Teach the patient with mobility problems and his or her caregivers how to reduce and relieve skin pressure in the home environment. **Patient-Centered Care** QSEN
- Encourage all patients to reduce sun exposure and exposure to ultraviolet (UV) light. **Patient-Centered Care** QSEN
- Teach patients how to examine all skin areas on a monthly basis for new lesions and changes to existing lesions. They should keep a record or "body map" of skin lesions. **Patient-Centered Care** QSEN
- Teach patients who have skin scarring from a previous skin injury to examine this area at least monthly for changes related to cancer development or chronic skin conditions. **Patient-Centered Care** QSEN
- Urge all patients to bathe, shampoo the hair, and keep fingernails clean and trimmed on a regular basis.
- Teach patients with infected skin lesions or infestations how to limit transmission to others in the home or community.
- Teach all patients the ABCDE method of evaluating a lesion for melanoma. **Patient-Centered Care** QSEN
- Assess the ability of the patient with a skin problem to see and reach the affected area and care for the problem. **Patient-Centered Care** QSEN

Psychosocial Integrity

- Assess the patient's and family's feelings about a chronic skin condition or visible scar. **Patient-Centered Care** QSEN

- Support the patient and family in coping with changes in skin integrity and in body image. **Patient-Centered Care** QSEN
- Encourage the patient with a visible wound or other skin problem to participate in the care of the wound.
- Assess and manage the patient's pain. **Patient-Centered Care** QSEN
- Allow the patient the opportunity to express feelings about a change in body image as a result of changes in the skin, hair, or nails. **Patient-Centered Care** QSEN
- Explain all procedures, restrictions, drugs, and follow-up care to the patient and family.
- Touch the patient who has skin problems to show acceptance. **Patient-Centered Care** QSEN

Physiological Integrity

- Keep skin well hydrated to promote TISSUE INTEGRITY. **Evidence-Based Practice** QSEN
- Use appropriate risk assessment tools to perform a focused skin assessment and re-assessment to determine risk for pressure ulcer development and adequacy of the skin's protective functions. **Safety** QSEN
- Keep skinfold areas clean and dry. **Evidence-Based Practice** QSEN
- Ask any patient who has started taking a newly prescribed drug if he or she has noticed whether any skin changes have occurred since starting the drug. **Patient-Centered Care** QSEN
- Avoid massaging or vigorously rubbing any area of the skin that is reddened or has been subjected to pressure. **Evidence-Based Practice** QSEN
- Encourage patients with itching to avoid scratching the skin.
- Teach patients to avoid using over-the-counter cortisone preparations on skin lesions until the cause has been identified. **Patient-Centered Care** QSEN
- Teach patients who have a skin infection how to avoid spreading the infection to other parts of their own bodies and to other people. **Safety** QSEN
- Evaluate any open skin area on a patient daily for size, depth, exudate, presence of infection, and indicators of healing. **Patient-Centered Care** QSEN
- Differentiate the manifestations for these pressure ulcer categories: stage I through stage IV, unstageable ulcers, and suspected deep tissue injury. **Evidence-Based Practice** QSEN
- Evaluate wounds for size, depth, presence of infection, and indications of healing. **Patient-Centered Care** QSEN
- Supervise skin care delegated to licensed practical nurses/licensed vocational nurses (LPNs/LVNs) or unlicensed assistive personnel (UAP). **Safety** QSEN
- Urge patients with chronic skin problems, especially those that alter appearance, to become involved in a community support group.

Care of Patients with Burns

Tammy Coffee

PRIORITY CONCEPTS

- TISSUE INTEGRITY
- INFECTION
- PAIN
- FLUID AND ELECTROLYTE BALANCE

- PERFUSION
- NUTRITION
- MOBILITY

LEARNING OUTCOMES

Safe and Effective Care Environment

1. Apply the principles of INFECTION prevention to protect burn patients with open wounds.

Health Promotion and Maintenance

2. Teach everyone fire prevention strategies.

Psychosocial Integrity

3. Reduce the psychosocial impact of burn injury for the patient and family.

Physiological Integrity

4. Ensure optimal PAIN control for the patient with a burn injury.

5. Work with all members of the health care team to help the patient and family experiencing a burn injury achieve desired health outcomes.
6. Prioritize nursing care for the patient during the resuscitation phase of burn injury.
7. Prioritize nursing care for the patient during the acute phase of burn injury.
8. Coordinate care for the patient during the rehabilitation phase of burn injury.

Burns are complex injuries with loss of TISSUE INTEGRITY that cause patients to develop many physiologic, metabolic, and psychological changes. These injuries can range from a "sunburn" to major injuries involving all layers of the skin. When the skin is injured, the function of many body systems is changed. The burn patient needs comprehensive care for weeks to months to survive the injury, reduce complications, and return to his or her best functional status. For best care and patient outcomes, nurses coordinate the activities of an interdisciplinary team of health care providers.

PATHOPHYSIOLOGY OF BURN INJURY

The tissue destruction caused by a burn injury leads to local and systemic problems that affect FLUID AND ELECTROLYTE BALANCE and lead to protein losses, sepsis, and changes in metabolic, endocrine, respiratory, cardiac, hematologic, and immune functioning. The extent of problems is related to age, general health, extent of injury, depth of injury, and the specific body area injured. Even after healing, the burn injury may cause late complications such as contracture formation and scarring. Thus care priorities are the prevention of INFECTION and closure of the burn wound. A lack of or delay in wound healing is a key factor for all systemic problems and a major cause of disability and death among patients who are burned.

Skin Changes Resulting from Burn Injury
Anatomic Changes

The skin is the largest organ of the body (see Chapter 24). Each of its two major layers, the epidermis and the dermis, has several sublayers. The epidermis is the outer layer of skin. It can grow back after a burn injury because the epidermal cells surrounding sweat and oil glands and hair follicles extend into dermal tissue and regrow to heal partial-thickness wounds. Together, the sweat and oil glands and the hair follicles are the *dermal appendages,* which vary in depth in different body areas. The sweat and oil glands in the palm of the hand and the sole of the foot, for example, extend deep into the dermis. This allows for healing of deep burns in these areas. The epidermis has no blood vessels, and nutrients must diffuse from the second layer of skin, the dermis.

TABLE 26-1	Classification of Burn Depth				
CHARACTERISTIC	SUPERFICIAL	SUPERFICIAL PARTIAL-THICKNESS	DEEP PARTIAL-THICKNESS	FULL-THICKNESS	DEEP FULL-THICKNESS
Color	Pink to red	Pink to red	Red to white	Black, brown, yellow, white, red	Black
Edema	Mild	Mild to moderate	Moderate	Severe	Absent
Pain	Yes	Yes	Yes	Yes and no	Absent
Blisters	No	Yes	Rare	No	No
Eschar	No	No	Yes, soft and dry	Yes, hard and inelastic	Yes, hard and inelastic
Healing time	3-6 days	About 2 wk	2-6 wk	Weeks to months	Weeks to months
Grafts required	No	No	Can be used if healing is prolonged	Yes	Yes
Example	Sunburn, flash burns	Scalds, flames, brief contact with hot objects	Scalds; flames; prolonged contact with hot objects, tar, grease, chemicals	Scalds; flames; prolonged contact with hot objects, tar, grease, chemicals, electricity	Flames, electricity, grease, tar, chemicals

The dermis is thicker than the epidermis and is made up of collagen, fibrous connective tissue, and elastic fibers. Within the dermis are the blood vessels, sensory nerves, hair follicles, lymph vessels, sebaceous glands, and sweat glands.

When burn injury occurs, skin can regrow as long as parts of the dermis are present. When the entire dermal layer is burned, all cells and dermal appendages are destroyed and the skin can no longer restore itself. The subcutaneous tissue lies below the dermis and is separated from the dermis by the basement membrane, a thin, noncellular protein surface. With deep burns, the subcutaneous tissues may be damaged, leaving bones, tendons, and muscles exposed.

Functional Changes

The skin has many functions when TISSUE INTEGRITY is intact (see Table 24-1 in Chapter 24). It is a protective barrier against injury and microbial invasion. Burns break this barrier, greatly increasing the risk for INFECTION.

The skin helps maintain the delicate FLUID AND ELECTROLYTE BALANCE essential for life. After a burn injury, massive FLUID loss occurs through excessive evaporation. The rate of evaporation is in proportion to the total body surface area (TBSA) burned and the depth of injury.

The skin is an excretory organ through sweating. Full-thickness burns destroy the sweat glands, reducing excretory ability.

The sensations of PAIN, pressure, temperature, and touch are triggered on the skin in normal daily activities, which allows a person to react to changes in the environment. *All burn injuries are painful.* With partial-thickness burns, nerve endings are exposed, increasing sensitivity and PAIN. With full-thickness burns, nerve endings are completely destroyed. At first, these wounds may not transmit sensation except at wound edges. Despite this destruction, patients often have dull or pressure-type of pain in these areas.

Skin exposed to sunlight activates vitamin D. Partial-thickness burns reduce the activation of vitamin D, and this function is lost completely in areas of full-thickness burns.

The internal body temperature remains within a narrow range (about 84.2° to 109.4°F [29° to 43°C]) compared with the temperatures of the external environment. Skin TISSUE INTEGRITY is important in maintaining normal body temperature. Circulating blood in the skin both provides and dissipates heat efficiently. When heat is applied to the skin, the temperature under the dermis rises rapidly. As soon as the heat source is removed, compensatory processes quickly return the area to a normal temperature. If the heat source is not removed or if it is applied at a rate that exceeds the skin's capacity to dissipate it, cells are destroyed.

Physical identity is partly determined by the skin's cosmetic quality, which contributes to each person's unique appearance. A patient who sustains a major burn often develops reduced self-image and other psychosocial problems as a result of a change in appearance.

Depth of Burn Injury

The severity of a burn is determined by how much of the body surface area is involved and the depth of the burn. The degree of TISSUE INTEGRITY loss is related to the agent causing the burn and to the temperature of the heat source, as well as to how long the skin is exposed to it.

Differences in skin thickness in various parts of the body also affect burn depth. In areas where the skin is thin (e.g., eyelids, ears, nose, genitalia, tops of the hands and feet, fingers, and toes), a short exposure to high temperatures causes a deep burn injury. The skin is thinner in older adults (Touhy & Jett, 2014), which increases their risk for greater burn severity, even at lower temperatures of shorter duration.

Burn wounds are classified as superficial-thickness wounds, partial-thickness wounds, full-thickness wounds, and deep full-thickness wounds. The partial-thickness wounds are further divided into superficial and deep subgroups. Table 26-1 lists the differences of these burns.

Burns also are described as minor, moderate, or major depending on the depth, extent, and location of injury (Table 26-2). Fig. 26-1 shows the tissue layers involved with different depths of injury.

TABLE 26-2	Classification of Burn Injury and Burn Center Referral Criteria
CHARACTERISTICS	**COMMENTS**
Minor Burns	
Partial-thickness burns less than 10% TBSA	Patients in this category should receive emergency care at the scene and be taken to a hospital emergency department. A special expertise hospital or designated burn center is usually not necessary.
Full-thickness burns less than 2% TBSA	
No burns of eyes, ears, face, hands, feet, or perineum	
No electrical burns	
No inhalation injury	
No complicated additional injury	
Patient is younger than 60 years and has no chronic cardiac, pulmonary, or endocrine disorder	
Moderate Burns	
Partial-thickness burns 15%-25% TBSA	Patients in this category should receive emergency care at the scene and be transferred either to a special expertise hospital or to a designated burn center.
Full-thickness burns 2%-10% TBSA	
No burns of eyes, ears, face, hands, feet, or perineum	
No electrical burns	
No inhalation injury	
No complicated additional injury	
Patient is younger than 60 years and has no chronic cardiac, pulmonary, or endocrine disorder	
Major Burns	
Partial-thickness burns greater than 25% TBSA	Patients who meet *any one* of the criteria for a major burn should receive emergency care at the nearest emergency department and then be transferred to a designated burn center as soon as possible.
Full-thickness burns greater than 10% TBSA	
Any burn involving the eyes, ears, face, hands, feet, perineum	
Electrical injury	
Inhalation injury	
Patient is older than 60 years	
Burn complicated with other injuries (e.g., fractures)	
Patient has cardiac, pulmonary, or other chronic metabolic disorders	

TBSA, Total body surface area.

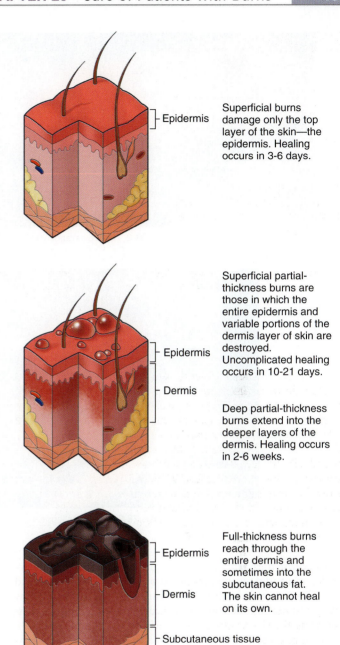

FIG. 26-1 The tissues involved in burns of various depths.

Superficial burns damage only the top layer of the skin—the epidermis. Healing occurs in 3-6 days.

Superficial partial-thickness burns are those in which the entire epidermis and variable portions of the dermis layer of skin are destroyed. Uncomplicated healing occurs in 10-21 days.

Deep partial-thickness burns extend into the deeper layers of the dermis. Healing occurs in 2-6 weeks.

Full-thickness burns reach through the entire dermis and sometimes into the subcutaneous fat. The skin cannot heal on its own.

Superficial-Thickness Wounds. Superficial-thickness wounds have the least damage because the epidermis is the only part of the skin that is injured. The epithelial cells and basement membrane, needed for total regrowth, remain present.

These wounds are caused by prolonged exposure to low-intensity heat (e.g., sunburn) or short (flash) exposure to high-intensity heat. Redness with mild edema, PAIN, and increased sensitivity to heat occurs as a result. **Desquamation** (peeling of dead skin) occurs 2 to 3 days after the burn. The area heals rapidly in 3 to 6 days without a scar or other complication.

Partial-Thickness Wounds. A partial-thickness wound involves TISSUE INTEGRITY loss of the entire epidermis and varying depths of the dermis. Depending on the amount of dermal tissue damaged, partial-thickness wounds are further subdivided into superficial partial-thickness and deep partial-thickness injuries.

Superficial partial-thickness wounds are caused by injury to the upper third of the dermis, leaving a good blood supply. These wounds are pink and moist and **blanch** (lighten) when

pressure is applied (Fig. 26-2). The small vessels bringing blood to this area are injured, resulting in the leakage of large amounts of plasma, which in turn lifts the heat-destroyed epidermis, causing blister formation. The blisters continue to increase in size after the burn as cell and protein breakdown occur. Small blisters are often left intact if they are not located over a joint. Large blisters usually are opened and débrided to promote healing.

Superficial partial-thickness wounds increase PAIN sensation. Nerve endings are exposed, and any stimulation (touch or temperature change) causes intense pain. With standard care, these burns heal in 10 to 21 days with no scar, but some minor pigment changes may occur.

Deep partial-thickness wounds extend deeper into the skin dermis, and fewer healthy cells remain. Blisters usually do not

FIG. 26-2 The typical appearance of a superficial partial-thickness burn injury.

FIG. 26-3 The typical appearance of a deep partial-thickness burn injury.

form because the dead tissue layer is thick, sticks to the underlying dermis, and does not readily lift off the surface. The wound surface is red and dry with white areas in deeper parts (dry because fewer blood vessels are patent). When pressure is applied to the burn, it blanches slowly or not at all (Fig. 26-3). Edema is moderate, and PAIN is less than with superficial burns because more of the nerve endings have been destroyed.

Blood flow to these areas is reduced, and progression to deeper injury can occur from hypoxia and ischemia. Adequate hydration, nutrients, and oxygen are needed for regrowth of skin cells and prevention of conversion to deeper burns. These wounds can convert to full-thickness wounds when tissue damage increases with INFECTION, hypoxia, or ischemia. Deep partial-thickness wounds generally heal in 2 to 6 weeks, but scar formation results. Surgical intervention with skin grafting can reduce healing time.

Full-Thickness Wounds. A full-thickness wound occurs with destruction of the entire epidermis and dermis, leaving no skin cells to repopulate (Fig. 26-4). This wound does not regrow, and areas not closed by wound contraction (see Chapter 25) require grafting.

The full-thickness burn has a hard, dry, leathery *eschar* that forms from coagulated particles of destroyed skin. *The eschar is dead tissue; it must slough off or be removed from the wound before healing can occur.* These thick particles often stick to the lower tissue layers, making eschar removal difficult. Edema is

FIG. 26-4 The typical appearance of a full-thickness burn injury.

severe under the eschar in a full-thickness wound. When the injury is **circumferential** (completely surrounds an extremity or the chest), blood flow and chest movement for breathing may be reduced by tight eschar. **Escharotomies** (incisions through the eschar) or **fasciotomies** (incisions through eschar and fascia) may be needed to relieve pressure and allow normal blood flow and breathing. (See p. 478 of the Surgical Management discussion in the Preventing Hypovolemic Shock and Inadequate Oxygenation section.)

A full-thickness burn may be waxy white, deep red, yellow, brown, or black. Thrombosed and heat-coagulated blood vessels may be seen beneath the surface of the burn and leave the burned tissue without a blood supply. Sensation is reduced or absent because of nerve ending destruction. Healing time depends on establishing a good blood supply in the injured areas. This process can range from weeks to months.

Deep Full-Thickness Wounds. Deep full-thickness wounds extend beyond the skin and damage muscle, bone, and tendons. These burns occur with flame, electrical, or chemical injuries. The wound is blackened and depressed, and sensation is completely absent (Fig. 26-5). All full-thickness burns need early excision and grafting. Grafting decreases PAIN and length of stay and hastens recovery. Amputation may be needed when an extremity is involved.

Vascular Changes Resulting from Burn Injuries

Circulation to the burned skin is disrupted immediately after injury by blood vessel occlusion. Macrophages in damaged tissues release chemicals that at first cause blood vessel constriction. Blood vessel thrombosis may occur, causing necrosis, which can lead to deeper injuries in these areas.

Fluid shift occurs after initial vasoconstriction as a result of blood vessels near the burn dilating and leaking FLUIDS into the interstitial space (Fig. 26-6). This fluid shift, also known as *third spacing* or *capillary leak syndrome,* is a continuous leak of plasma from the vascular space into the interstitial space. The impaired FLUID AND ELECTROLYTE BALANCE leads to loss of plasma fluids and proteins, which decreases blood volume and blood pressure (McCance et al., 2014). Leakage of fluid and electrolytes from the vascular space continues, causing extensive edema, even in areas that were not burned. Fluid shift, with

FIG. 26-5 The typical appearance of a deep full-thickness burn injury.

excessive weight gain, occurs in the first 12 hours after the burn and can continue for 24 to 36 hours.

The amount of fluid shifted depends on the extent and severity of injury. Capillary leak occurs in both burned and unburned areas when tissue damage is extensive (i.e., more than 25% total body surface area [TBSA]). Edema develops as plasma and ELECTROLYTES escape into the interstitial space. The proteins now in the interstitial space increase the movement of *fluids* out from the vascular space.

Profound disruptions of FLUID AND ELECTROLYTE BALANCE and acid-base balance occur as a result of the fluid shift and cell damage. These imbalances often include hypovolemia, metabolic acidosis, **hyperkalemia** (high blood potassium level), and **hyponatremia** (low blood sodium level). Hyperkalemia occurs as a result of direct cell injury that releases large amounts of cellular potassium. Sodium is retained by the body as a result of the endocrine response to stress. Aldosterone secretion increases, leading to increased sodium reabsorption by the kidney. This sodium, however, quickly passes into the interstitial spaces of the burned area with the fluid shift. Thus, despite the increased amount of sodium in the body, most of the sodium is trapped in the interstitial space and a sodium deficit occurs in the blood. **Hemoconcentration** (elevated blood osmolarity, hematocrit, and hemoglobin) develops from vascular dehydration. This problem increases blood viscosity, reducing blood flow and increasing tissue hypoxia.

Fluid remobilization starts at about 24 hours after injury, when the capillary leak stops. The diuretic stage begins at about 48 to 72 hours after the burn injury as capillary membrane integrity returns and edema fluid shifts from the interstitial spaces into the intravascular space. Blood volume increases, leading to increased kidney blood flow and diuresis unless kidney damage has occurred. Body weight returns to normal over the next few days as edema subsides.

During this phase, hyponatremia develops because of increased kidney sodium excretion and the loss of sodium from wounds. **Hypokalemia** (low blood potassium level) results from potassium moving back into the cells and also being excreted in urine. Anemia often develops as a result of hemodilution, but it is generally not severe enough to require blood transfusions. Transfusions are needed only if the patient's hematocrit is less than 20% to 25% and the patient has manifestations of hypoxia. Protein continues to be lost from the wounds. Metabolic acidosis is possible because of the loss of bicarbonate in the urine and the increased rate of metabolism.

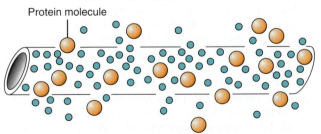

NORMAL BLOOD CAPILLARY
Water molecule

POSTBURN BLOOD CAPILLARY
Protein molecule

Water is the smallest molecule that can pass through the capillary pores.

Permeability is drastically increased, which allows large molecules such as proteins to pass through the capillary pores easily.

FIG. 26-6 The capillary response to burn injury (early phase). This response is also known as *capillary leak syndrome.*

Cardiac Changes Resulting from Burn Injury

Heart rate increases and cardiac output decreases because of the initial fluid shifts and hypovolemia that occur after a burn injury. Cardiac output may remain low until 18 to 36 hours after the burn injury. Cardiac output improves with fluid resuscitation and reaches normal levels before plasma volume is restored completely. Proper fluid resuscitation and support with oxygen prevent further complications.

Pulmonary Changes Resulting from Burn Injury

Direct injury to the lung from contact with flames rarely occurs. Rather, respiratory problems are caused by superheated air, steam, toxic fumes, or smoke. *Such problems are a major cause of death in patients with burns and are most likely to occur when the burn takes place indoors.* Respiratory failure with burn injuries can result from airway edema during fluid resuscitation, pulmonary capillary leak, chest burns that restrict chest movement, and carbon monoxide poisoning.

Respiratory damage from an inhalation injury can occur in the upper and major airways and the lung tissue. The upper airway is affected when inhaled smoke or irritants cause edema and obstruct the trachea. Heat can reach the upper airway, causing an inflammatory response that leads to edema of the mouth and throat with the potential of airway obstruction.

Chemicals and toxic gases produced during combustion can cause airway injury. The ciliated membranes lining the trachea normally trap foreign materials. Smoke and gases slow this activity, allowing particles to enter the bronchi. The lining of the trachea and bronchi may slough 48 to 72 hours after injury and obstruct the lower airways.

Lung tissue injuries result from toxic irritant damage to the alveoli and capillaries. Leaking capillaries cause alveolar edema, which can occur immediately or up to a week after the injury. The *fluid* that diffuses into the lung tissue spaces contains proteins that form fibrinous membranes and lead to respiratory distress. Progressive pulmonary failure develops, leading to acute pulmonary insufficiency and INFECTION.

Gastrointestinal Changes Resulting from Burn Injury

The fluid shifts and decreased cardiac output that occur after injury decrease blood flow to the GI tract. Gastric mucosal TISSUE INTEGRITY and motility are impaired. The sympathetic nervous system stress response increases secretion of epinephrine and norepinephrine, which inhibit GI motility and further reduce blood flow to the area. Peristalsis decreases, and a paralytic ileus may develop. Secretions and gases collect in the GI tract, causing abdominal distention.

Curling's ulcer (acute gastroduodenal ulcer that occurs with the stress of severe injury) may develop within 24 hours after a severe burn injury because of reduced GI blood flow and mucosal damage (McCance et al., 2014). The mucus lining the stomach normally protects the tissue from the hydrogen ions secreted into the stomach. With decreased gastric mucus production and increased hydrogen ion production, ulcers may develop. This complication is now less common because of the use of H_2 histamine blockers, proton pump inhibitors, drugs that protect GI tissues, and early enteral feeding.

Metabolic Changes Resulting from Burn Injury

A serious burn injury greatly increases metabolism by increasing secretion of catecholamines, antidiuretic hormone, aldosterone, and cortisol. With this hypermetabolism, the patient's oxygen use and calorie needs are high.

The catecholamines activate the stress response. The increased production (and loss) of heat breaks down protein and fat (*catabolism*), rapidly uses glucose and calories, and increases urine nitrogen loss. The heat and water lost from the burn also increase metabolic rate and calorie needs. Depending on the extent of injury, the patient's calorie needs double or triple normal energy needs. These increased rates peak 4 to 12 days after the burn and can remain elevated for months until all wounds are closed.

The hypermetabolic condition also increases core body temperature. The patient loses heat through the burned areas. Core body temperature increases as a response to the adjustment in temperature regulation by the hypothalamus, resulting in a low-grade fever.

Immunologic Changes Resulting from Burn Injury

Burn injury disrupts or destroys the protective skin TISSUE INTEGRITY, increasing the risk for INFECTION. The injury activates the inflammatory response and often suppresses all types of immune functions. Antibiotic therapy and other interventions for burns further reduce immune function.

Compensatory Responses to Burn Injury

Any injury is a stressor and can disrupt homeostasis. Two compensatory (adaptive) responses have immediate benefit: the inflammatory response and the sympathetic nervous system stress response. Together these responses cause changes that result in many of the manifestations seen in the first 2 to 3 days after a burn injury.

Inflammatory compensation is helpful by triggering healing in the injured tissues and also is responsible for the serious problems that occur with the fluid shift. This compensation causes blood vessels to leak fluid into the interstitial space and white blood cells to release chemicals that trigger local tissue reactions. These responses cause the massive fluid shift, edema, and hypovolemia that are seen in the resuscitation phase (first 24 to 48 hours) after a burn injury. The extent of the inflammatory response depends on the burn severity. Chapter 17 explains inflammation and the inflammatory responses in detail.

Sympathetic nervous system compensation is the stress response that occurs when any physical stressors are present. Changes caused by sympathetic compensation are most evident in the cardiovascular, respiratory, and GI systems. Fig. 26-7 shows the results of sympathetic nervous system stimulation.

Etiology of Burn Injury

Burn injuries are caused by dry heat (flame), moist heat (scald), contact with hot or rough surfaces, chemicals, electricity, and ionizing radiation. The cause of the injury affects both the prognosis and the treatment.

Dry heat injuries are caused by open flame in house fires and explosions. Explosions usually result in flash burns because they produce a brief exposure to very high temperatures.

Moist heat (scald) injuries are caused by contact with hot liquids or steam. Scald injuries are more common among older adults than younger adults. Hot liquid spills usually burn the upper, front areas of the body. Immersion scald injuries usually involve the lower body.

Contact burns occur when hot metal, tar, or grease contacts the skin, often leading to a full-thickness injury. Hot metal

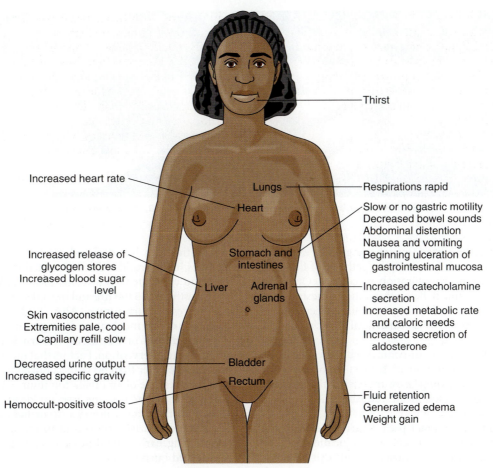

Thirst

Increased heart rate

Lungs

Heart

Respirations rapid

Slow or no gastric motility
Decreased bowel sounds
Abdominal distention
Nausea and vomiting
Beginning ulceration of
gastrointestinal mucosa

Increased release of
glycogen stores
Increased blood sugar
level

Stomach and
intestines

Liver

Adrenal
glands

Increased catecholamine
secretion
Increased metabolic rate
and caloric needs
Increased secretion of
aldosterone

Skin vasoconstricted
Extremities pale, cool
Capillary refill slow

Decreased urine output
Increased specific gravity

Bladder

Rectum

Hemoccult-positive stools

Fluid retention
Generalized edema
Weight gain

FIG. 26-7 The physiologic actions of the sympathetic nervous system compensatory responses to burn injury (early phase).

injuries occur when a body part contacts a hot surface, such as a space heater or iron. They also can occur in industrial settings from molten metals. Tar and asphalt temperatures usually are greater than 400°F, and deep injuries occur within seconds when the skin is immersed in or splashed with them. Hot grease injuries from cooking are usually deep because of the high temperature of the grease.

Chemical burns occur in home or industrial accidents or as the result of assault. Injury occurs when chemicals directly contact the skin and epithelial tissues or are ingested. The severity of the injury depends on the duration of contact, the concentration of the chemical, the amount of tissue exposed, and the action of the chemical.

Alkalis found in oven cleaners, fertilizers, drain cleaners, and heavy industrial cleaners damage the tissues by causing the skin and its proteins to liquefy. This allows for deeper spread of the chemical and more severe burns. Acids found in bathroom cleaners, rust removers, pool chemicals, and industrial drain cleaners damage TISSUE INTEGRITY by coagulating cells and skin proteins, which can limit the depth of tissue damage. Chemical disinfectants and gasoline are easily absorbed through the skin and have toxic effects on the kidneys and liver.

Electrical injuries are burns occurring when an electrical current enters the body (Fig. 26-8). These injuries have been called the "grand masquerader" of burns because the surface injuries may look small but the associated internal injuries can be huge. Tissue injury from electrical trauma results from

Arc burn
(in axilla)

Current

Electrical wire

Entrance wounds
(contact site)

Exit wound (contact site)

FIG. 26-8 The mechanism of electrical injury: currents passing through the body follow the path of least resistance to the ground.

FIG. 26-9 Electrical contact sites. **A,** Possible entrance site. **B,** Possible exit site.

electrical energy being converted to heat energy. The extent of injury depends on the type of current, the pathway of flow, the local tissue resistance, and the duration of contact. Once the current penetrates the skin, it flows throughout the involved body part generating heat and damaging tissues. Deep muscle injury may be present even when superficial muscles appear normal or uninjured.

The longer the electricity is in contact with the body, the greater the damage. The duration of contact is increased by tetanic contractions of the strong flexor muscles in the forearm, which can prevent the person from releasing the electrical source.

It is difficult to know the exact path a current takes in the body. The course of flow is defined by the locations of the "contact sites," which are the entrance and exit wounds (Fig. 26-9). At first, the wounds may not be obvious. The path of the injury may involve many internal organs between the two contact sites.

Burn injuries from electricity can occur as *thermal burns, flash burns,* or *true electrical injury.* Thermal burns occur when clothes ignite from heat or flames produced by electrical sparks. External burn injuries can occur when the electrical current jumps, or "arcs," between two body surfaces. These injuries usually are severe and deep. True electrical injury occurs when direct contact is made with an electrical source. Internal damage results and can be devastating. Damage starts on the inside and goes out; deep-tissue destruction may not be apparent immediately after injury. Organs in the path of the current may become ischemic and necrotic.

Radiation injuries occur when people are exposed to large doses of radioactive material. The most common type of tissue injury from radiation exposure occurs with therapeutic radiation. This injury is usually minor and rarely causes extensive skin damage.

Radiation exposure is more serious in industrial settings where radioactive energy is produced or used. Injury severity depends on the type of radiation, distance from the source, duration of exposure, absorbed dose, and depth of penetration into the body. Chapter 22 discusses potential tissue damage from alpha, beta, and gamma radiation.

Incidence and Prevalence of Burn Injury

Fires and burns are the fifth most common cause of unintentional injury deaths in the United States and the third leading cause of fatal home injuries (American Burn Association [ABA], 2012). Although the number of fatalities and injuries caused by

residential fires has declined gradually over the past several decades, many residential fire-related deaths remain preventable and continue to pose a significant public health problem.

An estimated 3400 fire and burn deaths occur each year from all sources of burn injury (ABA, 2012). Most deaths occur at the scene of the incident or during transport.

The number of deaths from burn injuries decreases with appropriate intervention. Factors that increase the risk for death include age older than 60 years, a burn greater than 40% TBSA, and the presence of an inhalation injury. When a patient has all three of these factors, the risk for death is very high. Better outcomes from burn injuries occur because of vigorous fluid resuscitation, early burn wound excision, improved critical care monitoring, early enteral NUTRITION, antibiotics, and the use of specialized burn centers.

HEALTH PROMOTION AND MAINTENANCE

Minor burns are common, and prevention involves planning and awareness. Teach all people to assess how hot the water is before bathing, showering, or immersing a body part in it. Hot water tanks should be set below 140° F (60° C). Reinforce the use of potholders when taking food from ovens. Stress the importance of never adding a flammable substance (e.g., gasoline, kerosene, alcohol, lighter fluid, charcoal starter) to an open flame. Suggest the use of sunscreen agents and protective clothing to avoid sunburn.

Teach people to reduce the risk for house fires by never smoking in bed, avoiding smoking when drinking alcohol or taking drugs that induce sleep, and keeping matches and lighters out of the reach of children or people who are cognitively impaired. When space heaters are used, stress the importance of keeping clothing, bedding, and other flammable objects away from them. Remind people to keep the screens and doors closed on the fronts of fireplaces and to have chimneys swept each year. Also remind patients using home oxygen not to smoke or have open flames in a room where oxygen is in use (Murabit & Tredget, 2012).

Leaving a burning building is critical to prevent injury or death. Teach all people to use home smoke detectors and carbon monoxide detectors and to ensure these are in good working order. The number of detectors needed depends on the size of the home. Recommendations are that each bedroom has a separate smoke detector, there should be at least one detector in the hallway of each story, and at least one detector is needed for the kitchen, each stairwell, and each home entrance. Teach everyone to develop a planned escape route with alternatives for when a main route is blocked by fire. Reinforce that no one should ever re-enter a burning building to retrieve belongings.

RESUSCITATION PHASE OF BURN INJURY

Events within the first hour after injury can make the difference between life and death for the patient with a burn injury. Immediate care focuses on maintaining an open airway, ensuring adequate breathing and circulation, limiting the extent of injury, and maintaining the function of vital organs. Chart 26-1 outlines the emergency management of a burn injury.

The **resuscitation phase** is the first phase of a burn injury. It begins at the onset of injury and continues for about 24 to 48 hours. During this phase, the injury is evaluated and the immediate problems of FLUID imbalance (loss), edema, and reduced blood flow are assessed. The priorities for management during this period are to (1) secure the airway, (2) support circulation and organ PERFUSION by fluid replacement, (3) keep the patient comfortable with analgesics, (4) prevent INFECTION through careful wound care, (5) maintain body temperature, and (6) provide emotional support.

CHART 26-1   Best Practice for Patient Safety & Quality Care QSEN

Emergency Management of Burns

General Management for All Types of Burns
- Assess for airway patency.
- Administer oxygen as needed.
- Cover the patient with a blanket.
- Keep the patient on NPO status.
- Elevate the extremities if no fractures are obvious.
- Obtain vital signs.
- Initiate an IV line, and begin fluid replacement.
- Administer tetanus toxoid for prophylaxis.
- Perform a head-to-toe assessment.

Specific Management
Flame Burns
- Smother the flames.
- Remove smoldering clothing and all metal objects.

Chemical Burns
- If dry chemicals are present on skin or clothing, DO NOT WET THEM.
- Brush off any dry chemicals present on the skin or clothing.
- Remove the patient's clothing.
- Ascertain the type of chemical causing the burn.
- Do not attempt to neutralize the chemical unless it has been positively identified and the appropriate neutralizing agent is available.

Electrical Burns
- At the scene, separate the patient from the electrical current.
- Smother any flames that are present.
- Initiate cardiopulmonary resuscitation.
- Obtain an electrocardiogram (ECG).

Radiation Burns
- Remove the patient from the radiation source.
- If the patient has been exposed to radiation from an unsealed source, remove his or her clothing (using tongs or lead protective gloves).
- If the patient has radioactive particles on the skin, send him or her to the nearest designated radiation decontamination center.
- Help the patient bathe or shower.

❖ PATIENT-CENTERED COLLABORATIVE CARE

◆ Assessment

History. Knowledge of circumstances surrounding the burn injury is valuable in planning the management of a burn patient. If possible, obtain information directly from the patient. If this is not possible, ask family members or witnesses to the event. Ask about the circumstances of the injury, the time and place of injury, and the source and cause of injury. Asked detailed questions about how the burn occurred and the events occurring from the time of injury until help arrived. Also obtain demographic data, health history (including pre-existing illness), drug use, any additional injuries, and PAIN information.

Demographic data include age, weight, and height. The rate of serious complications and death from burn injuries is increased among adults older than 50 years. Chart 26-2 lists the age-related differences in older adults' responses to a burn injury. The patient's preburn weight is used to calculate fluid rates, energy requirements, and drug doses. This weight is the *dry weight*, because it is the patient's weight before edema forms. Calculations based on a weight obtained after fluid replacement is started are not accurate. Height is important in determining total body surface area (TBSA), which is used to calculate NUTRITION needs.

A health history, including any pre-existing illnesses, must be known for appropriate management. Obtain specific information about the patient's history of cardiac or kidney problems, chronic alcoholism, substance abuse, and diabetes mellitus; any of these problems influence fluid resuscitation. The stress of a burn can make a mild disease process worsen. Obtain a drug history that includes allergies, current drugs, and immunization status from the patient or family. Determine the dose and time the last drug was taken. Ask whether the patient smokes or drinks alcohol daily; these factors influence treatment plans and responses.

Other injuries may occur at the time of the burn. Such injuries increase the risk for complications or death. Determine whether additional injuries such as fractures, chest injuries, and abdominal trauma are causing PAIN or discomfort.

Physical Assessment/Clinical Manifestations. Physical assessment findings in the resuscitation phase differ greatly from findings later in the course of the injury. Use a systematic approach to ensure that no problem is missed. Assessment of the respiratory system is most critical to prevent life-threatening complications.

Respiratory Assessment. Patients with major burn injuries and those with inhalation injury are at risk for respiratory problems. Respiratory manifestations common with a burn injury are listed in Table 26-3. *Thus continuous airway assessment is a nursing priority.*

Direct Airway Injury. The degree of inhalation damage depends on the fire source, temperature, environment, and types of toxic gases generated. Ask about the source of the fire, duration of exposure, and whether the fire was in an enclosed space. Inspect the mouth, nose, and pharynx. Burns of the lips, face, ears, neck, eyelids, eyebrows, and eyelashes are strong indicators that an inhalation injury may be present. Burns inside the mouth and singed nasal hairs also indicate possible inhalation injury. Black particles of carbon in the nose, mouth, and sputum; edema of the nasal septum; and a "smoky" smell to the patient's breath indicate smoke inhalation.

CHART 26-2 **Nursing Focus on the Older Adult**

Age-Related Changes Increasing Complications from Burn Injury

AGE-RELATED CHANGES	COMPLICATIONS AND NURSING CONSIDERATIONS
Thinner skin, sensory impairment, decreased mobility	Sensory impairment and decreased mobility increase the risk for burn injury. Thinner skin increases the depth of injury even when the exposure to the cause of injury is of shorter duration.
Slower healing time	Longer time with open areas results in a greater risk for infection, metabolic derangements, and loss of function from contracture formation and scar tissue.
More likely to have cardiac impairments	Limits the aggressiveness of fluid resuscitation. Increases the risk for shock and acute kidney injury (AKI).
Reduced inflammatory and immune responses	Increases the risk for infection and sepsis. Patient may not have a fever when infection is present.
Reduced thoracic and pulmonary compliance	Increased risk for atelectasis, hypoxia, and other pulmonary complications.
More likely to have pre-existing medical conditions such as diabetes mellitus, kidney impairment, or pulmonary impairment	Any of these disorders compromise vital organ function and can interfere with fluid resuscitation efforts or other treatments.

TABLE 26-3 **Factors Determining Inhalation Injury or Airway Obstruction**

- Patients who were injured in a closed space
- Patients with extensive burns or with burns of the face
- Intra-oral charcoal, especially on teeth and gums
- Patients who were unconscious at the time of injury
- Patients with singed scalp hair, nasal hairs, eyelids, or eyelashes
- Patients who are coughing up carbonaceous sputum
- Changes in voice such as hoarseness or brassy cough
- Use of accessory muscles or stridor
- Poor oxygenation or ventilation
- Edema, erythema, and ulceration of airway mucosa
- Wheezing, bronchospasm

A change in respiratory pattern may indicate a pulmonary injury. The patient may:
- Become progressively hoarse
- Develop a brassy cough
- Drool or have difficulty swallowing
- Produce sounds on exhalation that include audible wheezes, crowing, and stridor

Any of these changes may mean the patient is about to lose his or her airway.

⚠ NURSING SAFETY PRIORITY (QSEN)

Critical Rescue

For a burn patient in the resuscitation phase who is hoarse, has a brassy cough, drools or has difficulty swallowing, or produces an audible breath sound on exhalation, immediately apply oxygen and notify the Rapid Response Team.

Upper airway edema and inhalation injury are most common in the trachea and mainstem bronchi. Auscultation of these areas may reveal wheezes, which indicate partial obstruction. *Patients with severe inhalation injuries may have such rapid obstruction that, within a short time, they cannot force air through the narrowed airways. As a result, the wheezing sounds disappear. This finding indicates impending airway obstruction and demands immediate intubation.* Many patients are intubated when an inhalation injury is first suspected rather than waiting until obstruction makes intubation difficult or impossible.

Carbon Monoxide Poisoning. Carbon monoxide (CO) is one of the leading causes of death from a fire. It is a colorless, odorless, tasteless gas released in the process of combustion. Inhalation injury is a risk for carbon monoxide poisoning (Alharbi et al., 2012).

CO is rapidly transported across the lung membrane and binds tightly to hemoglobin in place of oxygen to form carboxyhemoglobin (COHb), which impairs oxygen unloading at the tissue level. Even though the oxygen-carrying capacity of the hemoglobin is reduced, the blood gas value of partial pressure of arterial oxygen (Pao_2) is normal (Laing, 2013). The vasodilating action of carbon monoxide causes the "cherry red" color (or at least the absence of cyanosis) in these patients. Manifestations vary with the concentration of COHb (Table 26-4).

Thermal (Heat) Injury. Except for steam inhalation, aspiration of scalding liquid, or explosion of flammable gases under pressure, thermal burns to the respiratory tract are usually limited to the upper airway above the glottis (nasopharynx, oropharynx, and larynx). *Heat damage of the pharynx is often severe enough to produce edema and upper airway obstruction, especially epiglottitis. The problem can occur any time during resuscitation. In the unresuscitated patient, supraglottic edema may be delayed because of the dehydration that occurs with hypovolemia. During fluid resuscitation, however, the tissues rehydrate and then swell. When it is known that the upper airways were exposed to heat, intubation may be performed as an early intervention before obstruction occurs.*

Inhaled steam can injure the lower respiratory tract down to the major bronchioles. Ulcerations, redness, and edema of the mouth and epiglottis occur first, with rapid swelling leading to upper airway obstruction. Stridor, hoarseness, and shortness of breath result.

TABLE 26-4 Physiologic Effects of Carbon Monoxide Poisoning

CARBON MONOXIDE LEVEL	PHYSIOLOGIC EFFECTS
1%-10% (normal)	Increased threshold to visual stimuli Increased blood flow to vital organs
11%-20% (mild poisoning)	Headache Decreased cerebral function Decreased visual acuity Slight breathlessness
21%-40% (moderate poisoning)	Headache Tinnitus Nausea Drowsiness Vertigo Altered mental state Confusion Stupor Irritability Decreased blood pressure, increased and irregular heart rate Depressed ST segment on ECG and dysrhythmias Pale to reddish purple skin
41%-60% (severe poisoning)	Coma Convulsions Cardiopulmonary instability
61%-80% (fatal poisoning)	Death

ECG, Electrocardiogram.

! NURSING SAFETY PRIORITY (QSEN)

Action Alert

When intubation has not been performed in a patient whose upper airways were exposed to heat or toxic gases, continually assess the upper airway for recognition of edema and obstruction.

Smoke Poisoning. Smoke poisoning, or chemical injury from the inhalation of combustion by-products, is a common type of inhalation injury. Toxic by-products are produced when plastics or home furnishings are burned. The products impair respiratory cell function.

Pulmonary Fluid Overload. Pulmonary edema can occur even when the lung tissues have not been damaged directly. Other damaged tissues release such large amounts of inflammatory mediators causing capillary leak that even lung capillaries leak FLUID into the pulmonary tissue spaces.

Circulatory overload from fluid resuscitation may cause congestive heart failure. This problem creates high pressure within pulmonary blood vessels that pushes fluid into the lung tissue spaces. Excess lung tissue fluid makes gas exchange difficult. *The patient is short of breath and has dyspnea in the supine position. Crackles are heard on auscultation.*

! NURSING SAFETY PRIORITY (QSEN)

Critical Rescue

When manifestations of pulmonary edema are present, elevate the head of the bed to at least 45 degrees, apply oxygen, and notify the burn team or the Rapid Response Team.

External Factors. Patients with burn injuries also may have breathing problems from external factors, such as tight eschar from deep circumferential chest burns. The eschar either restricts chest movement or compresses structures in the neck and throat so that airflow is impaired. Inspect the patient's chest hourly for ease of respiration, amount of chest movement, rate of breathing, and effort. If the patient is being mechanically ventilated, increased airway pressures may indicate the need for an escharotomy. Use continuous pulse oximetry to assess breathing effectiveness in maintaining blood oxygen levels.

? NCLEX EXAMINATION CHALLENGE

Physiological Integrity

For which type of burn injury is it most important for the nurse to assess the client for a respiratory injury?
A. Hot liquid scald burn
B. Liquid chemical burn
C. Electrical burn
D. Dry heat burn

Cardiovascular Assessment. Changes in the cardiovascular system begin immediately after the burn injury and include shock as a result of disrupted FLUID AND ELECTROLYTE BALANCE. *Hypovolemia shock is a common cause of death in the resuscitation phase in patients with serious injuries.* See Chapter 37 for discussion of shock.

At first, cardiac manifestations are from hypovolemia and decreased cardiac output. Monitor the degree of edema, and assess cardiac status by measuring central and peripheral pulses, blood pressure, capillary refill, and pulse oximetry. Noninvasive blood pressure readings are inaccurate in patients with large burns of the upper extremities, and invasive blood pressure monitoring may be needed. At first, the patient has tachycardia, decreased blood pressure, and decreased peripheral pulses. Peripheral capillary refill is slow or absent as blood flow decreases. With fluid resuscitation, peripheral edema increases, as does the patient's weight.

Electrocardiographic (ECG) changes can indicate damage to the heart as a result of electrical burn injuries or stress that induces a myocardial infarction. Obtain baseline ECG tracings at the time of admission, and continue the ECG monitoring throughout the resuscitation phase. Compare current ECG tracings with the initial tracings to assess whether the patient is experiencing new-onset conduction abnormalities from the burn injury or the fluid resuscitation.

Kidney/Urinary Assessment. Changes in kidney function with burn injury are related to decreased blood flow and to cellular debris. During the fluid shift, blood flow to the kidney may not be adequate for filtration. As a result, urine output is greatly decreased compared with IV fluid intake. The urine is very concentrated and has a high specific gravity.

Other substances may be present in the blood that flows through the kidney. Destroyed red blood cells release hemoglobin and potassium. When muscle damage occurs from a major burn or electrical injury, *myoglobin* is released from damaged muscle and circulates to the kidney. Most damaged cells release proteins that form uric acid. All of these large molecules in the blood may precipitate in the kidney tubular system. A "sludge" then forms that blocks kidney blood and urine flow and may cause kidney failure.

Assess kidney function by accurately measuring urine output hourly and comparing this value with fluid intake. Urine output is decreased during the first 24 hours of the resuscitation phase. Fluid resuscitation is provided at the rate needed to maintain urine output at 30 to 50 mL per hour or 0.5 mL/kg/hr. Assess response to fluid resuscitation by measuring urine specific gravity, blood urea nitrogen (BUN), serum creatinine, and serum sodium levels in addition to hourly urine output. Examine the urine for color, odor, and the presence of particles or foam.

Skin Assessment. Assess the skin to determine the size and depth of burn injury. The size of the injury is first estimated in comparison with the *total body surface area (TBSA)*. For example, a burn that involves 40% of the TBSA is a 40% burn. The size of the injury is important not only for diagnosis and prognosis but also for calculating drug doses, fluid replacement volumes, and caloric needs.

Inspect the skin TISSUE INTEGRITY to identify injured areas and changes in color and appearance. Except with electrical burns, this initial size assessment usually can be made accurately with specific assessment tools and charts.

The most rapid method for calculating the size of a burn injury in adult patients whose weights are in normal proportion to their heights is the *rule of nines* (Fig. 26-10). With this method, the body is divided into areas that are multiples of 9%. It is useful at the site of injury, but more accurate evaluations using other methods are made in the burn unit.

Because specific treatments are related to the depth of the burn injury, initial assessment of the skin includes estimations of burn depth. Criteria for depth of injury are based on appearance and associated characteristics (see Depth of Burn Injury section, p. 466).

Accurate evaluation of burn depth is performed using thermography, vital dyes, indocyanine green (ICG) video

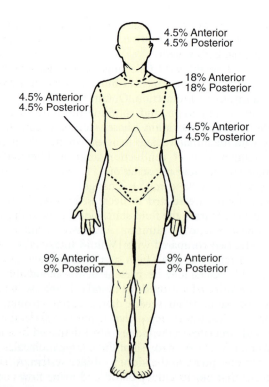

FIG. 26-10 The rule of nines for estimating burn percentage.

4.5% Anterior
4.5% Posterior

18% Anterior
18% Posterior

4.5% Anterior
4.5% Posterior

4.5% Anterior
4.5% Posterior

9% Anterior
9% Posterior

9% Anterior
9% Posterior

angiography, and laser Doppler imaging (LDI) that provide precise measurement of the amount of PERFUSION of the injured tissue. ICG and LDI are the most accurate of the three methods. LDI is used more frequently because it is relatively accurate, less invasive, and faster than the other methods (Park et al., 2013).

Gastrointestinal Assessment. Although the GI tract usually is not directly injured, changes in function occur in all burn patients. The decreased blood flow and sympathetic stimulation reduce GI motility and promote development of a paralytic ileus. Bowel sounds are usually reduced or absent in a patient with severe burns. Other indications of a paralytic ileus include nausea, vomiting, and abdominal distention. Patients with burns of 25% TBSA or who are intubated generally require a nasogastric (NG) tube inserted to prevent aspiration and remove gastric secretions. Assess the tube for placement and patency after insertion. Examine each stool and vomitus for gross blood or other material that indicates partially digested blood ("coffee ground"–appearing crumbs). Test for the presence of occult blood on any vomit or stool.

Laboratory Assessment. Certain changes in laboratory test values are found in different phases of postburn recovery and reflect tissue damage or compensatory responses. However, other changes in specific laboratory findings may suggest complications.

During the resuscitation phase and before the start of fluid resuscitation, blood analysis reflects the fluid shift and direct tissue damage. Baseline laboratory test values and early postburn expected changes are listed in Chart 26-3.

Changes in the total white blood cell (WBC) count and differential reflect immune function and inflammatory responses to the burn injury. The burn patient's total WBC count, especially the neutrophil percentage, first rises and then drops rapidly, with a "left shift" (see Chapter 17) as the immune system becomes unable to sustain its defenses. If sepsis occurs, the total WBC count may be as low as 2000 cells/mm^3.

Other laboratory tests that provide useful information about the burn patient's status include urine electrolyte assays, urine cultures, liver enzyme studies, and clotting studies. Drug and alcohol screens are obtained if drug or alcohol intoxication is suspected.

🌐 CULTURAL CONSIDERATIONS

Patient-Centered Care QSEN

For African-American patients, a sickle cell preparation is performed if sickle status is unknown. The trauma of a burn injury can trigger a sickle cell crisis in patients who have the disease and in those who carry the trait.

Imaging Assessment. Standard x-rays and scans do not provide direct assessment data about the burn wound. These assessments are not performed unless other trauma is suspected.

Other Diagnostic Assessment. Specific diagnostic studies are performed when deep organ trauma is suspected. Such studies include renal scans, computed tomography (CT), ultrasonography, bronchoscopy, and magnetic resonance imaging (MRI). When burn injuries involve the eye, an ophthalmic evaluation is performed to detect corneal damage (see Chapters 46 and 47 for specific eye and vision evaluation procedures).

CHART 26-3 Laboratory Profile

Burn Assessment During the Resuscitation Phase

TEST	NORMAL RANGE FOR ADULTS	SIGNIFICANCE OF ABNORMAL FINDINGS
Serum Studies		
Hemoglobin	12-16 g/dL (women) 14-18 g/dL (men)	Elevated as a result of fluid volume loss
Hematocrit	37%-47% (women) 42%-52% (men)	Elevated as a result of fluid volume loss
Urea nitrogen	10-20 mg/dL	Elevated as a result of fluid volume loss
Glucose	70-110 mg/dL	Elevated as a result of the stress response and altered uptake across injured tissues
Electrolytes		
Sodium	136-145 mEq/L (mmol/L)	Decreased; sodium is trapped in edema fluid and lost through plasma leakage
Potassium	3.5-5.0 mEq/L (mmol/L)	Elevated as a result of disruption of the sodium-potassium pump, tissue destruction, and red blood cell hemolysis
Chloride	98-106 mEq/L (mmol/L)	Elevated as a result of fluid volume loss and reabsorption of chloride in urine
Arterial Blood Gas Studies		
PaO_2	80-100 mm Hg	Slightly decreased
$PaCO_2$	35-45 mm Hg	Slightly increased from respiratory injury
pH	7.35-7.45	Low as a result of metabolic acidosis
Carboxyhemoglobin	0%-10%	Elevated as a result of inhalation of smoke and carbon monoxide
Other		
Total protein	6.4-8.3 g/dL	Low; protein exudate is lost through the wound
Albumin	3.5-5.0 g/dL	Low; protein is lost through the wound and through vascular membranes because of increased permeability

Data from Pagana, K., & Pagana, T. (2014). *Mosby's manual of diagnostic and laboratory tests* (5th ed). St. Louis: Mosby.

◆ **Analysis**

The priority NANDA-I nursing diagnoses and collaborative problems for patients with burn injuries in the resuscitation phase who have sustained a burn injury greater than 25% of the TBSA include:

1. Potential for inadequate oxygenation related to upper airway edema, pulmonary edema, airway obstruction, or pneumonia
2. Risk for Shock related to increase in capillary permeability, active fluid volume loss, electrolyte imbalance, and inadequate fluid resuscitation (NANDA-I)
3. Potential for organ ischemia (brain, heart, kidney, gastrointestinal) related to hypovolemia and hypotension
4. Pain (Acute and Chronic) related to tissue injury, damaged or exposed nerve endings, débridement, dressing changes, invasive procedures, and donor sites (NANDA-I)
5. Potential for acute respiratory distress syndrome (ARDS) related to inhalation injury

◆ **Planning and Implementation**

Supporting Oxygenation

Planning: Expected Outcomes. With proper intervention, the patient is expected to maintain a patent airway and have adequate oxygenation. Indicators include that the patient should have either normal or nearly normal oxygen saturation, PaO_2, $PaCO_2$, and arterial pH.

Interventions. Nursing and medical interventions are used to support normal pulmonary function and prevent the pulmonary problems that can result from lung injury or from fluid overload and heart failure. (Even young, healthy people can develop fluid overload and heart failure.) Specific management plans depend on the cause of the problem and the status of the respiratory tract. *Thus a priority nursing intervention is monitoring the patient's respiratory status.*

Nonsurgical Management. Interventions include airway maintenance, promotion of ventilation, monitoring gas exchange, oxygen therapy, drug therapy, positioning, and deep breathing.

Airway maintenance begins at the burn scene in an unconscious patient and may involve only a chin-lift or a head-tilt maneuver. *Remember that upper airway edema becomes pronounced 8 to 12 hours after the beginning of fluid resuscitation. Then patients often require nasal or oral intubation if crowing, stridor, or dyspnea is present.*

A bronchoscopy is performed to examine the vocal cords and airways of patients at risk for obstruction. Patients with severe smoke inhalation or poisoning may require a bronchoscopy on admission and routinely thereafter for examination of the respiratory tract, deep suctioning of the lungs, and removal of sloughing necrotic tissue. Assess the endotracheal tube hourly to ensure patency and location in intubated patients.

Other causes of airway obstruction are excessive secretions and sloughed tissue from damaged lungs. Suction as indicated based on clinical assessment. Vigorous endotracheal or nasotracheal tube suctioning is performed after chest physiotherapy and aerosol treatments. Patients report that deep endotracheal suctioning is extremely painful. Therefore suctioning the endotracheal tube often requires increased analgesia or sedation.

Promoting ventilation includes ensuring that skeletal muscle movement of the chest is adequate for ventilation. Chest movement can be restricted by eschar and by tight dressings that cover the neck, chest, and abdomen. Observe the patient for ease of respiratory movements, and loosen tight dressings as needed to assist with ventilation.

Monitor for gas exchange by using laboratory tests (e.g., arterial blood gas, carboxyhemoglobin levels) and by assessing for cyanosis, disorientation, and increased pulse rate. Additional monitoring may include chest x-ray findings, pulmonary artery catheter pressures, and central venous pressure measurement.

Cyanide poisoning may occur in patients burned in house fires. An elevated plasma lactate level is one indicator of cyanide toxicity even in patients who do not have severe burns.

Oxygen therapy with humidified oxygen by facemask, cannula, or hood is used to manage any breathing impairment in the burn patient. Arterial oxygenation less than 60 mm Hg is an indication for intubation and mechanical ventilation. Keep emergency airway equipment near the bedside. This equipment includes oxygen, masks, cannulas, manual resuscitation bags, laryngoscope, endotracheal tubes, and equipment for tracheostomy. Chapter 32 addresses specific nursing actions for patients during mechanical ventilation.

Drug therapy with antibiotics is used when pneumonia or other pulmonary INFECTIONS impair breathing. Drug selection is based on known culture and sensitivity reports or on the specific organisms common to that burn unit.

Patients with pulmonary edema and any degree of heart failure may receive beta blockers to improve left ventricular function and prevent or treat pulmonary edema. Diuretics, a mainstay of therapy for pulmonary edema from other causes, may or may not be used in the resuscitation phase, depending on the patient's blood volume and kidney function.

When a patient's activity during mechanical ventilation severely compromises respiratory mechanics, it may be necessary to use a paralytic drug, such as atracurium (Tracrium) or vecuronium (Norcuron). Paralytic drugs remove all breathing control from the patient, making mechanical ventilation easier. *These drugs do not prevent the patient from seeing and hearing or from experiencing fear, PAIN, and loss of control. Any patient receiving neuromuscular blockade drugs must also receive drugs for sedation, analgesia, and antianxiety unless clinically contraindicated.*

> ⚠ **NURSING SAFETY PRIORITY** (QSEN)
>
> **Critical Rescue**
>
> As required by The Joint Commission's National Patient Safety Goals, ensure that all alarms are operative on ventilators. Check patients who are receiving neuromuscular blockage frequently, because they cannot call for help if they become extubated accidentally.

Positioning and deep breathing can improve breathing and oxygenation. Turn the patient frequently, and assist him or her out of bed to a chair as much as possible. Teach the patient to use coughing and deep-breathing exercises. Urge him or her to use incentive spirometry hourly while awake. Chest physiotherapy may be helpful to mobilize lung secretions.

Surgical Management. A tracheotomy may be needed when long-term intubation is expected. This procedure increases the risk for INFECTION in burn patients even more than in nonburned patients. Emergency tracheotomies are performed when an airway becomes occluded and oral or nasal intubation cannot be achieved.

Other surgical procedures for improving the burn patient's oxygenation include inserting chest tubes and performing an escharotomy. Chest tubes are used to re-expand the lung when a pneumothorax or hemothorax has occurred (see Chapter 32). Tight eschar on the neck, chest, or abdomen can restrict respiratory movement. Escharotomies (described on p. 479) can relieve this restriction and permit greater respiratory movement.

Preventing Hypovolemic Shock and Inadequate Oxygenation

Planning: Expected Outcomes. With appropriate intervention, the patient is expected to have blood pressure and tissue oxygenation restored to normal. Indicators include these vital signs and assessment parameters:

- Blood pressure at or near the patient's normal range
- Palpable peripheral pulses (or heard with Doppler) in all extremities
- Oxygen saturation, partial pressure of arterial oxygen (Pao_2), partial pressure of arterial carbon dioxide ($Paco_2$), and arterial pH at or near the normal ranges

Interventions. Interventions focus on increasing blood fluid volume, supporting compensation, and preventing complications. Nonsurgical management is often sufficient for achieving these aims. Surgical management may be needed for full-thickness burns.

Nonsurgical Management. FLUID volume and tissue blood flow (PERFUSION) are restored through IV fluid therapy and drug therapy. Priority nursing interventions are carrying out fluid resuscitation and monitoring for indications of effectiveness or complications.

Rapid infusion of IV fluids, known as *fluid resuscitation,* is needed to maintain sufficient blood volume for normal cardiac output, mean arterial pressure, and tissue oxygenation. Chart 26-4 lists best practices for fluid resuscitation. There are many formulas for calculating IV fluid needs, but the most commonly used one for adult patients is the Parkland Formula (4 mL/kg/%TBSA burn of crystalloid solution). Although the types and amounts of electrolytes, crystalloids, and colloids vary, the purpose of any formula is to prevent shock by maintaining blood fluid volume.

Resuscitation for a severe burn requires large FLUID loads in a short time to maintain blood flow to vital organs. All common formulas recommend that half of the calculated fluid volume for 24 hours be given in the first 8 hours after injury. The other half is given over the next 16 hours for a total of 24 hours (Culleiton & Simko, 2013b). Fluid boluses are avoided because they increase capillary pressure and worsen edema. In the second 24-hour period after a burn injury, the volume and content of the IV fluids are based on the patient's specific FLUID AND ELECTROLYTE BALANCE needs and his or her response to treatment. This resuscitation involves hourly infusion volumes that are greatly in excess of the 125 mL to 150 mL per hour common infusion rates.

FLUID replacement formulas are calculated from the time of injury and not from the time of arrival at the hospital. For example, if a burn injury occurred at 8 AM but the patient was not admitted to the hospital until 10 AM, the first 8-hour period would be completed at 4 PM (8 hours after the injury). Thus if resuscitation was delayed by 2 hours until admission to the hospital, calculated fluids would need to be given over the next 6-hour period rather than an 8-hour period. Burn resuscitation formulas are guides. The patient's response to therapy determines exact fluid requirements.

CHART 26-4 Best Practice for Patient Safety & Quality Care (QSEN)

Fluid Resuscitation of the Burn Patient

- Initiate and maintain at least one large-bore IV in an area of intact skin (if possible).
- Coordinate with physicians to determine the appropriate fluid type and total volume to be infused during the first 24 hours postburn.
- Administer one half of the total 24-hour prescribed volume within the first 8 hours postburn and the remaining volume over the next 16 hours.
- Assess IV access site, infusion rate, and infused volume at least hourly.
- Monitor these vital signs at least hourly:
  - Blood pressure
  - Pulse rate
  - Respiratory rate
  - Breath sounds
  - Voice quality (if not intubated)
  - Oxygen saturation
  - End-tidal carbon dioxide levels
- Assess urine output at least hourly:
  - Volume
  - Color
  - Specific gravity
  - Character
  - Presence of protein
- Assess for fluid overload:
  - Formation of dependent edema
  - Engorged neck veins
  - Rapid, thready pulse
  - Presence of lung crackles or wheezes on auscultation
- Measure additional body fluid output hourly.

blood flow to other vital organs (especially the heart, lungs, and brain) and greatly increases the risk for severe hypovolemic shock. Therefore diuretics are not generally used to improve urine output for burn patients. An exception is the patient with an electrical burn injury. In electrical burns, muscle and deep-tissue damage release the large protein *myoglobin*, which precipitates in and obstructs the renal tubules. Although the diuretic *mannitol* (Osmitrol) is often used in this situation, it should always be given after adequate urine output has been established.

CONSIDERATIONS FOR OLDER ADULTS

Patient-Centered Care (QSEN)

In older patients, especially those with cardiac disease, a complicating factor in fluid resuscitation may be heart failure or myocardial infarction. Drugs that increase cardiac output (e.g., dopamine [Intropin]) or that strengthen the force of myocardial contraction may be used along with fluid therapy. Assess the cardiac status of older adults at least every hour during fluid resuscitation.

The management of extensive burns requires a large-bore central venous catheter so that massive fluid loads can be given. Peripheral lines are less useful.

Monitoring patient responses is critical to determine the adequacy of resuscitation for hydration and blood PERFUSION of the brain, heart, and kidneys. Urine output is the most common and most sensitive noninvasive assessment parameter for cardiac output and tissue perfusion. *Regardless of the total amount of fluid calculated as needed for the patient, the amount of fluid given depends on how much IV fluid per hour is needed to maintain the hourly urine output at 0.5 mL/kg (about 30 mL/hr).* Adjustment of the IV fluid rate on the basis of urine output plus serum electrolyte values is known as the *titration* of fluid. In burns larger than 35% TBSA, the use of invasive cardiac and pulmonary function monitoring may be needed in addition to urine output and vital signs to guide resuscitation.

Burn patients can develop severe hypovolemic shock and need invasive cardiac monitoring. Vital parameters such as central venous pressure, pulmonary artery pressures, and cardiac output are obtained on an hourly to continuous basis.

Monitor the ECG activity of patients who have sustained large burns. Compare current ECG findings with those obtained on admission.

Drug therapy for shock prevention in burn patients is different from that for the heart failure patient. A common mistake in management is giving diuretics to increase urine output rather than changing the amount and rate of fluid infused. *Diuretics do not increase cardiac output; they actually decrease circulating volume and cardiac output by pulling fluid from the circulating blood volume to enhance diuresis.* This effect reduces

Surgical Management. The surgical procedure for the treatment of inadequate tissue PERFUSION is *escharotomy.* An incision through the burn eschar relieves pressure caused by the constricting force of fluid buildup under circumferential burns on the extremity or chest and improves circulation. If the pressure is not relieved, arterial compression can occur with a loss of blood flow to the extremity, leading to ischemia and possible necrosis. Incisions are made along the length of the extremity and extend into the subcutaneous tissue, relieving the tourniquet effect of the eschar (Figs. 26-5 and 26-11). If tissue pressure remains elevated after escharotomy, a *fasciotomy* (a deeper incision extending through the fascia) may be needed.

Managing Pain. The PAIN with burn injuries is both chronic and acute. Many factors contribute to burn pain and may be altered to reduce pain perception. Accurate assessment of the patient's pain before and during procedures is an essential part of pain management.

Planning: Expected Outcomes. The patient's PAIN level is expected to be alleviated or reduced. Indicators include that the patient should rarely demonstrate these behaviors:

- Reporting PAIN
- Moaning and crying
- Making facial expressions of PAIN
- Losing his or her appetite

Interventions. PAIN management is tailored to the patient's tolerance for pain, coping mechanisms, and physical status. *The priority nursing actions include continually assessing the patient's pain level, using appropriate pain-reducing strategies, and preventing complications.*

FIG. 26-11 Escharotomy to release circumferential burn eschar and improve circulation to a distal extremity. **A,** Tight circumferential eschar restricting swelling as edema forms in the tissue beneath the eschar. Edema compresses blood vessels, which inhibits blood flow to the distal extremity. **B,** An escharotomy incision allows outward swelling of edematous tissues. The restricted blood flow to the distal extremity is relieved. **C,** An anterior axillary incision is made bilaterally to relieve respiratory distress.

Nonsurgical Management. Interventions for the patient having PAIN include drug therapy, complementary therapy measures, and environmental manipulation.

Drug therapy for PAIN usually requires opioid analgesics (e.g., morphine sulfate, hydromorphone [Dilaudid], fentanyl) and non-opioid analgesics. Although these drugs may provide adequate pain relief when no procedures are being performed, they rarely offer more than moderate relief during painful procedures. They may depress respiratory function and reduce intestinal motility. Thus nonpharmacologic interventions also are needed for the burn patient.

During the resuscitation phase, the IV route is used for giving opioid drugs because of problems with absorption from the muscle and stomach (Culleiton & Simko, 2013c). When given IM or subcutaneously, these drugs remain in the tissue spaces and do not relieve PAIN. In addition, when edema is present, all the doses are rapidly absorbed at once when the fluid shift is resolving. This delayed but rapid absorption can result in lethal blood levels of opioids.

> ! **NURSING SAFETY PRIORITY** (QSEN)
>
> *Drug Alert*
>
> Give opioid drugs for pain only by the intravenous route during the resuscitation phase to prevent delayed rapid absorption leading to lethal blood levels.

Anesthetic agents, such as ketamine (Ketalar) and nitrous oxide, also reduce PAIN. Use strict protocols when giving these agents to prevent serious complications.

Complementary and alternative therapy measures for PAIN reduction include relaxation techniques, meditative breathing, guided imagery, music therapy, massage, and healing or therapeutic touch. Hypnosis and autohypnosis can be used by lucid, cooperative patients under the direction of trained therapists. Therapeutic touch, acupuncture, and acupressure are used to a limited extent for burn patients; the results are variable. Active music interventions for distraction have been useful in reducing patients' perceptions of pain and anxiety.

Environmental changes, such as providing a quiet environment, using nonpainful tactile stimulation, and increasing the patient's control, can increase comfort. Sleep deprivation increases patients' discomfort. Increasing sleep or rest time in a quiet environment helps reduce the adverse effects of sleep deprivation, replenishes hormone stores, helps prevent critical care unit psychosis, and restores the diurnal effects of endorphins. Coordinate with the health care team to ensure that procedures are performed during the patient's waking hours.

Tactile stimulation can reduce PAIN. Help the patient change positions every 2 hours to reduce pressure on any specific area, improve circulation to painful areas, and ease pain. Massage nonburn areas to reduce pain transmission and stimulate endorphin release. Apply heat and maintain warm room temperatures to prevent shivering.

To reduce anxiety and increase feelings of confidence and independence, encourage the patient to participate in PAIN control measures. For example, make a contract with him or her that specifies how long a painful procedure will last. This helps patients deal with the pain for that particular period. Patient-controlled analgesia (PCA) also reduces pain. Important issues and techniques for the best use of PCA include giving an initial bolus of 5 to 10 mg of morphine (or equivalent drug), increasing the PCA dose as needed to achieve pain relief, and planning for a change in dosing regimen at night (e.g., giving a bolus dose at bedtime). See Chapter 3 for a detailed discussion of combination drug therapy for pain management.

Surgical Management. Early surgical excision of the burn wound is used in many burn centers (see the Surgical Excision section on p. 484). Early excision under anesthesia reduces the PAIN from daily débridement at the bedside or during hydrotherapy.

Preventing Acute Respiratory Distress Syndrome

Planning: Expected Outcome. The patient with a burn injury is expected to:

- Not experience acute respiratory distress
- Have arterial blood gases (ABGs) within normal limits
- Maintain normal lung compliance

Interventions. Patients who develop acute respiratory distress syndrome (ARDS) from burn injuries require thorough assessments and interventions. Interventions focus on increasing lung compliance and improving partial pressure of arterial oxygen (Pao_2) levels. The priority nursing care actions are coordinating respiratory therapy strategies and monitoring the patient's response to these interventions.

In collaboration with the physician and respiratory therapist, give positive end-expiratory pressure (PEEP) to provide a continuous positive pressure in the airways and alveoli. This procedure enhances the diffusion of oxygen across the alveolar-capillary membrane. PEEP can be combined with intermittent mandatory volume (IMV) to enhance its effectiveness.

Assess and document the patient's response so that needed ventilator changes can be made. Monitor pulse oximetry and ABG levels to assess changes in respiratory status.

! NURSING SAFETY PRIORITY QSEN

Critical Rescue

Document and immediately report any signs of respiratory distress or change in respiratory patterns to the burn team and the respiratory therapist.

Neuromuscular blocking drugs (atracurium) can be used in patients receiving mechanical ventilation to reduce oxygen consumption (see the discussion of specific nursing care in the Supporting Oxygenation section, pp. 477-478).

ACUTE PHASE OF BURN INJURY

The acute phase of burn injury begins about 36 to 48 hours after injury, when the fluid shift resolves, and lasts until wound closure is complete. During this phase, the nurse coordinates interdisciplinary care that is directed toward continued assessment and maintenance of the cardiovascular and respiratory systems, as well as toward GI and NUTRITION status, burn wound care, PAIN control, and psychosocial interventions.

❖ PATIENT-CENTERED COLLABORATIVE CARE

◆ Assessment

Physical Assessment/Clinical Manifestations

Cardiopulmonary Assessment. *In the acute phase of burn injury, the priority nursing interventions are to assess the cardiovascular and respiratory systems to maintain these systems and to identify or prevent complications.* At this time, the patient may develop pneumonia that can result in respiratory failure requiring mechanical ventilation. Although cardiovascular problems related to the fluid shift should be resolved, the patient is at risk for INFECTION and sepsis, which affect cardiovascular function.

Neuroendocrine Assessment. The increased metabolic demands placed on the body after a severe burn injury can severely deplete NUTRITION stores. Weigh the patient daily without dressings or splints, and compare it with his or her preburn weight. A 2% loss of body weight indicates a mild deficit. A 10% or more weight loss requires the evaluation and modification of calorie intake. For very accurate calorie requirements, indirect calorimetry may be used. This method assesses energy expenditure by measuring oxygen consumption and carbon dioxide production. Measurements are taken while the patient is at rest—usually at least 30 minutes after the most recent dressing changes or other stressful procedures. Indirect calorimetry may be performed on admission to a burn center and then weekly until the wounds are closed.

Immune Assessment. The patient with a burn injury is at risk for INFECTION because of open wounds and reduced immune function. *Burn wound sepsis is a serious complication of burn injury, and infection is the leading cause of death during the acute phase of recovery.* Continually assess the patient for manifestations of local and systemic infections (Table 26-5), including changes in wound appearance, changes in neurologic and GI function, and subtle changes in vital signs. Monitor for manifestations of gram-positive, gram-negative, and fungal infections (Table 26-6). Enforce meticulous handwashing by all care personnel.

Musculoskeletal Assessment. Patients with a burn injury are at risk for musculoskeletal and MOBILITY problems as a result of other injuries, immobility, healing processes, and treatment. The musculoskeletal status is evaluated on admission and throughout the postburn period. Assess active and passive range of motion for all joints, including the neck. Give special attention to joints in the burn area. Ranges and limitations are documented for future reference.

◆ Analysis

During the acute phase of the burn injury, the patient may have initial problems that extend into the acute phase and may develop new problems.

The priority NANDA-I nursing diagnoses and collaborative problems for patients with burn injuries greater than 25% TBSA in the acute phase of recovery include:

1. Wound care management related to burn injury, skin grafting procedures, and immobilization
2. Risk for Infection related to open burn wounds, the presence of multiple invasive catheters, reduced immune function, and poor nutrition (NANDA-I)
3. Excessive weight loss related to increased metabolic rate, reduced calorie intake, and increased urinary nitrogen losses
4. Impaired Mobility: Physical related to open burn wounds, pain, and scars and contractures (NANDA-I)
5. Reduced self-image related to trauma, changes in physical appearance and lifestyle, and alterations in sensory and motor function

◆ Planning and Implementation

Managing Wound Care

Planning: Expected Outcomes. With appropriate intervention, the burn patient is expected to have no wound extension and have wounds healed. Indicators include that the patient:

- Has presence of granulation, re-epithelialization, and scar tissue formation
- Has decreased wound size
- Has no new wounds

Interventions. Interventions focus on preserving skin TISSUE INTEGRITY, enhancing burn wound healing, and preventing complications.

Nonsurgical Management. Nonsurgical burn wound management involves removing exudates and necrotic tissue, cleaning the area, stimulating granulation and revascularization, and applying dressings. Restoring skin TISSUE INTEGRITY, whether by natural healing or grafting, starts with the removal of eschar and other cellular debris from the burn wound. This removal is called **débridement**, and can be performed nonsurgically through mechanical or enzymatic actions that separate eschar over time. The purpose is to prepare the wound for grafting and wound closure by a natural process. *Priority nursing interventions include assessing the wound, providing wound care, and preventing infection and other complications.*

Mechanical Débridement. Burn wounds are débrided and cleaned 1 or 2 times each day during **hydrotherapy** (the application of water for treatment). Nurses, unlicensed assistive personnel (UAP), and physical therapists perform hydrotherapy daily to débride and examine the wounds. Hydrotherapy is performed by showering the patient on a special shower table or washing only small areas of the wound at the bedside. Showering enhances wound inspection and allows water temperature

TABLE 26-5	Local and Systemic Indicators of Infection
Local Indicators	**Systemic Indicators**
• Conversion of a partial-thickness injury to a full-thickness injury	• Altered level of consciousness
• Ulceration of healthy skin at the burn site	• Changes in vital signs (tachycardia, tachypnea, temperature instability, hypotension)
• Erythematous, nodular lesions in uninvolved skin and vesicular lesions in healed skin	• Increased fluid requirements for maintenance of a normal urine output
• Edema of healthy skin surrounding the burn wound	• Hemodynamic instability
• Excessive burn wound drainage	• Oliguria
• Pale, boggy, dry, or crusted granulation tissue	• GI dysfunction (diarrhea, vomiting, abdominal distention, paralytic ileus)
• Sloughing of grafts	• Hyperglycemia
• Wound breakdown after closure	• Thrombocytopenia
• Odor	• Change in total white blood cell count (above normal or below normal)
	• Metabolic acidosis
	• Hypoxemia

TABLE 26-6	Indications of Sepsis Caused by Different Organisms		
MANIFESTATIONS	**GRAM-POSITIVE**	**GRAM-NEGATIVE**	**FUNGAL**
Onset	Insidious, 2-6 days	Rapid, 12-36 hr	Delayed
Cognition	Severe disorientation and lethargy	Mild disorientation	Mild disorientation
Ileus	Severe	Severe	Mild
Diarrhea	Rare	Severe	Occasional
Temperature	Fever	Hypothermia	Fever
Hypotension	Late	Early	Late
White blood cell count	Neutrophilia	Neutropenia	Neutrophilia
Platelets	Normal	Low	Low

to be kept constant. Immersion of the patient in a tub or whirlpool is no longer performed because it increases the risk for INFECTION.

Nurses and skilled technicians use forceps and scissors to remove loose, dead tissue during hydrotherapy. At most burn units, small blisters are left intact because they are a protective barrier that promotes wound healing. Larger blisters are opened. Washcloths or gauze sponges are used to débride soft, "cheesy" eschar. Wash burn areas thoroughly and gently with mild soap or detergent and water. Then rinse these areas with room-temperature water.

Enzymatic Débridement. Enzymatic débridement can occur naturally by autolysis or artificially by the application of exogenous agents. **Autolysis** is the disintegration of tissue by the action of the patient's own cellular enzymes. This process is seldom used alone in North America for larger burns because it is slow and prolongs the hospital stay, increasing the risk for INFECTION.

Topical enzyme agents, such as collagenase (Santyl), are used for rapid wound débridement. When these agents are applied to the burn wound in a once-a-day dressing change, the enzymes digest collagen in necrotic tissues.

Dressing the Burn Wound. After burn wounds are cleaned and débrided, topical antibiotics are reapplied to prevent INFECTION. Some type of dressing is then applied to the burn wound. Burn dressings include standard wound dressings, biologic dressings, synthetic dressings, and artificial skin.

Standard Wound Dressings. Standard dressings are multiple layers of gauze applied over the topical agents on the wound. The number of gauze layers depends on:
- Depth of the injury
- Amount of drainage expected
- Area injured
- Patient's MOBILITY
- Frequency of dressing changes

The gauze layers are held in place with roller-type gauze bandages applied in a distal to proximal direction or with circular net fabrics. Cover gauze dressings on the patient's extremities with elastic wraps, especially if the patient is ambulatory. Dressings are generally changed and are reapplied every 12 to 24 hours after thoroughly cleaning the areas.

Biologic Dressings. Biologic dressings are often used for temporary wound coverage and closure. These dressings are skin or membranes obtained from human tissue donors (homograft or allograft) or animals (heterograft or xenograft). When applied over open wounds, a biologic dressing adheres and promotes healing or prepares the wound for permanent skin graft coverage.

Various biologic materials are used in healing partial-thickness and granulating full-thickness wounds that are clean and free of eschar. The type of biologic dressing selected depends on the type of wound to be covered and the availability of the material.

Homografts, also called *allografts,* are human skin obtained from a cadaver and provided through a skin bank. Disadvantages to the use of homografts are the high costs and the risk for transmitting a bloodborne infection.

Heterografts, also called *xenografts,* are skin obtained from another species. Pigskin (porcine) is the most common heterograft and is compatible with human skin. Pigskin is assessed daily for adherence and need for replacement. Fig. 26-12 shows a small burn covered with a porcine dressing.

FIG. 26-12 Burn wound covered with a porcine dressing.

Cultured skin can be grown from a small specimen of epidermal cells from an unburned area of the patient's body. The cells are grown in a laboratory to produce cell sheets that can be grafted on the patient to generate a permanent skin surface. The length of time for culturing and growing the skin is long, and the cell sheets are fragile. This process is very costly.

Artificial skin is a substance with two layers—a Silastic epidermis and a porous dermis made from beef collagen and shark cartilage. After the artificial skin is applied to a clean, excised wound surface, fibroblasts move into the collagen portion and create a structure similar to normal dermis. The artificial dermis slowly dissolves and is replaced with blood vessels and connective tissue (*neodermis*). The neodermis supports a standard autograft placed over it when the Silastic layer is removed.

Biosynthetic Wound Dressings. Biosynthetic wound dressings are a combination of biosynthetic and synthetic materials. Biobrane is commonly used and effective in the treatment of clean superficial partial-thickness burns such as scalds, as a covering for meshed autografts, and as a donor site dressing. It is made up of a nylon fabric that is partially embedded into a silicone film. Collagen is incorporated into both the silicone and the nylon components. The nylon fabric comes into contact with the wound surface and adheres to it until epithelialization has occurred. The porous silicone film allows exudates to pass through.

Synthetic Dressings. Synthetic dressings are made of solid silicone and plastic membranes. They are applied directly to the surface of a prepared wound and remain in place until they fall off or are removed. Many of these dressings are transparent or translucent, and the wound can be inspected without removing the dressing. PAIN is reduced at the site because these agents also prevent contact of the wound's nerve endings with air. These dressings also are used to cover donor sites where skin was obtained for autografting.

Transparent film is the dressing commonly used for the care of donor site wounds (Fig. 26-13). This dressing type promotes faster healing with low INFECTION rates, minimal PAIN, and reduced cost.

Surgical Management. Grafting is used for wound closure when full-thickness injuries cannot close and when natural healing would result in loss of joint function, an unacceptable cosmetic appearance, or a high potential for wound recurrence. Successful skin grafting requires a clean and granulating or freshly excised wound bed. Partial-thickness (split-thickness) or full-thickness strips of skin are removed from the donor area, transferred to the ulcer, and sutured or stapled in place. Full-thickness free grafts and myocutaneous flaps are used to cover deep, massive ulcers or ulcers in which vital structures, such as bone or tendon, are exposed.

Surgical management of burn wounds involves excision and wound covering. Surgical excision is performed early in the postburn period. Autografting by taking an area of the patient's healthy skin with intact TISSUE INTEGRITY and transplanting it to an excised burn wound may be performed throughout the acute phase when wounds are ready and donor sites are available. Early grafting reduces the time patients are at risk for INFECTION and sepsis.

FIG. 26-13 Donor sites covered with dressings. **A,** Transparent dressing. **B,** Xeroform dressing.

Surgical Excision. Surgical excision is a common treatment for full-thickness and deep partial-thickness wounds. The patient is taken to the operating room within the first 5 days after injury and again as needed until all wounds are closed permanently.

The surgeon excises the burn wound usually by removing very thin layers of the necrotic burn surface until bleeding tissue is encountered. (Bleeding indicates that a bed of healthy dermis or subcutaneous fat has been reached.) For very deep burns, the surgeon cuts away the wound to the level of superficial fascia. Blood loss is minimal, and grafting is usually successful.

Wound Covering. Permanent skin coverage for large full-thickness injuries occurs by applying an autograft. Skin for an autograft is taken from the patient's body. The surgeon removes a piece of skin from a remote unburned area of the body and transplants it to cover the burn wound. Skin grafts are generally of split thickness, and a partial-thickness injury is formed at the site of surgical removal (the *donor site*). Grafts are placed either on a clean granulated bed or over an area from which dead tissue has just been removed.

Patients with larger burns may have only 5% to 20% of the skin surface available to use for covering the 80% to 95% burned area. Coverage for these wounds may require either repeated skin removal from the same donor site (with time allowed between harvests for healing) or meshing of the split-thickness skin grafts (Fig. 26-14). This technique allows a small graft to be stretched to cover a larger area. Healing time is slower for a meshed graft because the skin must fill in open meshed areas (interstices), as well as attach to the granulation bed.

After surgery, graft sites are immobilized with bulky cotton pressure dressings for 3 to 5 days to allow vascularization, or "take," of the newly grafted skin. Do not disturb the dressing, and encourage elevation and complete rest of the grafted area to allow blood vessels to connect the graft with the wound bed. Any activity that might cause movement of the dressing against the body and separation of the graft from the wound is prohibited.

After dressings are removed, monitor the graft for indications of failure to vascularize, nonadherence to the wound, or graft necrosis. A dusky color or sharp line of color change suggests inadequate venous or lymphatic drainage. Other techniques to monitor trends of blood flow in the graft, depending on the graft's location, include pulse oximetry, laser

FIG. 26-14 The typical appearance of meshed autografts. **A,** Appearance of meshed autograft at application. **B,** Appearance of meshed autograft after healing.

Doppler imaging, ultrasonography, and transcutaneous oxygen determination.

Grafts and donor sites on posterior body surfaces present special problems. For the graft to become fully vascularized or for the donor sites to dry, the patient must be immobilized in a side-lying or prone position for 7 to 10 days.

An alternative to this positioning is the use of special low-pressure or air-fluidized beds, such as the Clinitron bed or KinAir bed, which not only reduce ischemia of the graft while the patient is supine but also help prevent breakdown of intact skin.

Minimizing Infection. Burn wound INFECTION occurs through auto-contamination, in which the patient's own normal flora overgrows and invades other body areas; and cross-contamination, in which organisms from other people or environments are transferred to the patient.

Planning: Expected Outcomes. The patient is expected to remain free from INFECTION and not develop sepsis. Indicators are that the patient has only mild or none of these manifestations:

- Foul-smelling discharge
- Fever
- Blood culture colonization
- Wound site colonization
- White blood cell count elevation

Interventions. Interventions focus on preventing INFECTION and removing infected tissue.

Nonsurgical Management. Priority nursing interventions include using principles of INFECTION *control to prevent transmission, providing a safe environment, and monitoring for early detection of infection.* Drug therapy, isolation therapy, and environmental management are strategies for preventing and managing infection.

Drug Therapy for Infection Prevention. Burn wound conditions promote the growth of *Clostridium tetani,* and all burn patients are at risk for this deadly INFECTION. Tetanus toxoid, 0.5 mL given IM, enhances immunity to *C. tetani* and is routinely given on admission. Administration of tetanus immune globulin (human) (HyperTet) is recommended when the patient's tetanus immunization status is not known.

Topical antimicrobial drugs are used for INFECTION prevention in burn wounds. Chart 26-5 lists commonly used agents. The expected outcome of this therapy is to reduce bacterial growth in the wound and prevent sepsis. A variety of agents can be used. Some topicals come in a form of ointments and creams (e.g., silver sulfadiazine, Sulfamylon, bacitracin) and need to be applied once or twice daily (Silverstein et al., 2011). Other products such as Acticoat, Mepilex Ag, and Aquacel Ag contain antimicrobials, which release over a period of several days and can be left on the wound for up to 7 days, thus eliminating the need for daily dressing changes.

Drug Therapy for Treatment of Infection. Systemic antibiotics are used when burn patients have symptoms of an actual INFECTION, including septicemia. Broad-spectrum antibiotics are given until the results of blood cultures and sensitivity status are available. At that time, antibiotics that are effective against the specific organism(s) causing the infection are used. Often burn patients require a higher dose of these drugs to maintain effective blood levels. Peak and trough blood levels may be used to determine treatment effectiveness and risk for toxicity.

Providing a Safe Environment. Providing a safe environment can include isolation therapy, which is used in some burn centers in the belief that it reduces cross-contamination. More often, it involves coordinating all members of the health care team in the use of asepsis and monitoring for early recognition of actual infection. Proper and consistent handwashing is the most effective technique for preventing INFECTION transmission.

Use of asepsis requires all health care personnel to wear gloves during all contact with open wounds. The use of sterile versus clean gloves for routine wound care varies by agency and is a matter of debate. Regardless of sterility, change gloves when handling wounds on different areas of the body and between handling old and new dressings.

The equipment on burn units is not shared among patients. Disposable items (e.g., pillows, dishes) are used as much as possible. Assign any equipment used in daily routine care (e.g., blood pressure cuffs, stethoscopes) to each patient for the duration of his or her stay. Daily cleaning of the equipment and general housekeeping are essential for INFECTION control. All other equipment must be cleaned after use on one patient and before use on another. Because *Pseudomonas* has been found in plants, the presence of plants and flowers is prohibited. Some burn units do not permit patients to eat raw foods (e.g., salads, fruit, pepper) to reduce exposure to organisms. Rugs and upholstered articles harbor organisms, and their use is restricted.

Visitors are restricted when the patient is immunosuppressed. Ill people, small children, and other patients should not come into direct contact with the burn patient. Some burn units recommend that all visitors wear protective clothing (gowns, gloves, masks, and shoe and hair covers) in the burn patient's room, but no data support the effectiveness of this approach.

Early detection involves careful monitoring of the burn wounds at each dressing change. Examine all wounds for these manifestations of INFECTION:

- Pervasive odor
- Color changes—focal, dark red, brown discoloration in the eschar
- Change in texture
- Purulent drainage
- Exudate
- Sloughing grafts
- Redness of wound edges extending to nonburned skin

Laboratory cultures and biopsies are recommended. Quantitative biopsies of the eschar and granulation tissue are performed routinely to monitor the growth of organisms.

Surgical Management. Infected burn wounds with colony counts at or near 10^5 colonies per gram of tissue may be life threatening, even with antibiotic therapy. Surgical excision of the wound may be needed to control these infections.

❓ NCLEX EXAMINATION CHALLENGE
Safe and Effective Care Environment

Which action by the nurse changing the dressings on the client who has burns on the right arm, the left arm, and the upper chest is most effective at preventing auto-contamination?
A. Changing gloves after cleaning and dressing one wound area before cleaning and dressing the next wound area.
B. Using sterile gloves to remove the old dressings and changing to fresh sterile gloves before applying the new dressings.
C. Ensuring that the blood pressure cuff used on another client is thoroughly cleaned before using it on this client.
D. Warning the client's family not to bring fresh fruits and vegetables or house plants into the client's environment.

CHART 26-5   Common Examples of Drug Therapy

Burn Wounds

TOPICAL DRUG	ACTION	INTERVENTIONS
Silver sulfadiazine (Silvadene, Thermazene)	Adheres to bacterial cell membranes inhibiting DNA synthesis and bacterial replication	Watch for allergic reaction causing a drop in white blood cell count. Do not use if reaction to sulfonamide has occurred. Use on deep partial-thickness or full-thickness wounds. Monitor wounds for infection.
Collagenase (Santyl) with polysporin powder	Digests collagen in necrotic tissue	Apply once a day. Use on partial-thickness wounds with eschar. Monitor wounds for infection. May be used with barrier dressing such as Xeroform.
Mafenide acetate (Sulfamylon)	Bacteriostatic action against many gram-positive and gram-negative organisms	Premedicate for pain before application. Monitor blood gas and serum electrolyte levels. Monitor wounds for infection.
Nitrofurazone (Furacin)	Wide-spectrum antibacterial agent	Observe closely for signs of allergic reaction and evidence of superinfection.
Gentamicin sulfate (Garamycin, Gentamar)	Aminoglycoside antibacterial that inhibits bacterial protein synthesis and results in bactericidal responses	Nephrotoxic; monitor kidney function closely, especially changes in serum creatinine and blood urea nitrogen. Ototoxic; monitor hearing weekly.
Polymyxin B-bacitracin (Poly-Bac, Polysporin)	Inhibits bacterial cell wall synthesis and destroys bacterial membranes, leading to bacterial killing effects	Apply every 2-8 hours to keep area moist.
Acticoat	Releases antimicrobial silver ions when moistened with sterile water	Do not use with oil-based products or other antimicrobials. Do not use for any patient with a known sensitivity to any of the components of this drug. May dry out and adhere to wound surface; soak off to remove.
PolyMem	Dressing material containing silver granules that suppress bacterial growth	Normally leave in place for 7 days. Remove earlier if exudate is visible through outer membrane. Use on partial-thickness wounds and on donor sites. Cover with a secondary dressing. Monitor wounds for infection.
Aquacel Ag	Dressing material that releases ionic silver in a controlled manner as exudate is absorbed into dressing to support wound healing	Use on partial-thickness wounds and on donor-sites. Cover with a secondary dressing. Do not use for patients who have allergic reactions to the dressing or any of its components. Moisten with sterile water or normal saline to ease removal. Do not use with oil-based products.
Mepilex Ag	Dressing material containing silver ions that begin to inactivate wound pathogens within 30 minutes of application	Do not use along with oxidizing agents such as hydrogen peroxide. Cover with secondary dressing. May be used with partial-thickness burns, full-thickness burns, skin grafts, and donor-sites.

Minimizing Weight Loss

Planning: Expected Outcomes. The patient is expected to maintain adequate nutrient intake for meeting the body's calorie needs. Indicators include that the patient should have mild or no deviations from the normal ranges for:

- Weight/height ratio
- Food intake
- Hematocrit and hemoglobin
- Serum albumin and prealbumin
- Blood glucose

Interventions. Interventions include calculating the patient's calorie needs and providing an adequate daily source of calories and nutrients that the patient can ingest. Coordinate with a registered dietitian to meet the expected outcomes regarding the patient's NUTRITION status. Therapy begins with calculating the patient's current daily calorie needs. Several formulas and charts are used for this calculation. Nutrition requirements for a patient with a large burn area can exceed 5000 kcal/day. Not meeting this need leads to very rapid weight loss (Williams et al., 2011). In addition to a high-calorie intake, a diet high in protein is needed for wound healing. Work with the dietitian and the patient to plan additions to standard nutrition patterns.

Oral diet therapy may be delayed for several days after the injury until the GI tract is motile. Nasoduodenal tube feedings are often started soon after admission. Beginning enteral feedings early helps decrease weight loss, gut atrophy, bacterial translocation, and sepsis. This type of supplement prevents NUTRITION deficits in severely burned patients.

Encourage patients who can eat solid foods to ingest as many calories as possible. Consider the patient's preferences with diet planning and food selection. Encourage patients to request food whenever they feel they can eat, not just according to the hospital's standard meal schedule. Offer frequent high-calorie,

CHART 26-6 Best Practice for Patient Safety & Quality Care QSEN

Positioning to Prevent Contractures

AFFECTED BODY PART	POSITION OF FUNCTION	INTERVENTION
Head and neck	Hyperextension	No pillow. Place a towel roll under the patient's neck or shoulder. Neck splint.
Posterior neck	Flexion	Have patient turn the head from side to side.
Upper chest and chest	Shoulder retraction	Place patient in supine position. Place a folded towel under the spine, between the scapulae.
Lateral trunk	Flexion to uninvolved side	Place patient supine with arm on the affected side up over the head.
Anterior shoulder	Abduction and external rotation	Maintain the upper arm at 90 degrees of abduction from the lateral aspect of the trunk.
Posterior shoulder	Slight flexion and interior rotation	Keep the arm slightly behind the midline.
Axilla	Abduction with 10- to 15-degree forward flexion and external rotation	Support the abducted arm with suspension from IV pole or bedside table. Axilla splint.
Elbow	Extension and supination	Keep the joint in the extended position.
Wrist	30 to 45 degrees of extension	Use a splint.
Fingers		
MP joints	70 to 90 degrees of flexion	Use a splint.
PIP and DIP joints	Extension	Use a splint.
Ankle	90 degrees of dorsiflexion	Use a padded footboard or splint with heels free of pressure.
Legs	15 to 20 degrees of abduction	Place small pillow between legs.
Hip	Extension and neutral rotation	Place patient supine with lower extremity extended. Use trochanter roll. Use foam wedge along lateral aspect of thigh.

DIP, Distal interphalangeal; MP, metatarsophalangeal; PIP, proximal interphalangeal.

high-protein supplemental feedings. Keep an accurate calorie count for foods and beverages that are actually ingested by the patient.

Patients who cannot swallow but who have adequate gastric motility may meet calorie and NUTRITION needs through enteral tube feedings (see Chapter 60). Parenteral nutrition may be used when the GI tract is not functional or when the patient's nutrition needs cannot be met by oral and enteral feeding. This method is used as a last resort because it is invasive and can lead to infectious and metabolic complications.

Maintaining Mobility

Planning: Expected Outcomes. The patient with a burn injury is expected to maintain or regain an optimal MOBILITY. Indicators include that the patient has minimal limitations in these actions:

- Muscle movement
- Joint MOBILITY
- Walking
- Self-positioning

Interventions. Interventions focus on maintaining or achieving the patient's preburn range of joint motion and MOBILITY and preventing contracture formation.

Nonsurgical Management. Nonsurgical management includes the nursing interventions of positioning, range-of-motion exercises, ambulation, and pressure dressings.

Positioning is critical for patients with burn injuries because the position of comfort for the patient is often one of joint flexion, which leads to contracture development. Maintain the patient in a neutral body position with minimal flexion. Best practices for preventing contractures are listed in Chart 26-6. Splints and other devices may be used to maintain good positioning of the hands, elbows, knees, neck, and axillae.

Range-of-motion exercises to maintain MOBILITY are performed actively at least 3 times a day. If the patient cannot move a joint actively, perform passive range-of-motion exercises. Give burned hands special attention. Urge the patient to perform active range-of-motion exercises for the hand, thumb, and fingers every hour while he or she is awake.

Ambulation is started as soon as possible after the fluid shifts have resolved because it maintains MOBILITY, inhibits bone density loss, strengthens muscles, stimulates immune function, promotes ventilation, and prevents many complications. Patients with attached equipment (IV catheters, nasogastric tubes, ECG leads, extensive dressings) can ambulate with preparation and assistance. This activity is performed 2 or 3 times a day and progresses in length each time.

Compression dressings are applied after grafts heal to help prevent contractures and tight hypertrophic scars, which can inhibit MOBILITY. They also inhibit venous stasis and edema in areas with decreased lymph flow. Compression dressings may be elastic wraps or specially designed, custom-fitted, elasticized clothing that provides continuous pressure. Fig. 26-15 shows such a garment. For best effectiveness, pressure garments must be worn at least 23 hours a day, every day, until the scar tissue

FIG. 26-15 A patient wearing full-body compression garments.

is mature (12 to 24 months). They can be uncomfortable with itchiness and increased warmth. Reinforce to the patient and family that wearing pressure garments is beneficial in saving mobility and reducing scarring.

Surgical Management. Surgical management restores MOBIL- ITY rather than prevents immobility. Surgical release of contrac- tures is commonly performed in the neck, axilla, elbow flexion areas, and hand. Specific surgical procedures vary for each patient.

Nursing responsibilities include interventions to prevent contractures from re-forming, as well as the care of new grafts and suture lines. Constantly reinforce the need for the patient to adhere to exercise and splinting regimens to prevent the recurrence of joint immobility.

Supporting Positive Self-Image

Planning: Expected Outcomes. After intervention, the patient with a burn injury is expected to have a positive percep- tion of his or her own appearance, body functions, and self- worth. Indicators include that the patient should consistently demonstrate these behaviors:

- Willingness to touch the affected body part
- Adjustment to changes in body function
- Willingness to use strategies to enhance appearance and function
- Successful progression through the grieving process
- Use of support systems

Interventions. Nonsurgical and surgical interventions can assist patients who have self-image problems as a result of burn injury.

Nonsurgical Management. Understanding the stages of grief is helpful in managing care for the patient with burns. Assess which stage of grief the patient is currently experiencing, and help interpret his or her behaviors. The patient often is unaware of or is confused by his or her feelings. Reassure the patient that feelings of grief, loss, anxiety, anger, fear, and guilt are normal. The patient may be grieving the loss of body parts, appearance, role identity, social identity, and family members. Coordinate

with other health care team members (e.g., psychologist/ psychiatrist, social worker, clergy or religious leader) to address these issues.

Accept the physical and psychological features of the patient. Present patients and families with realistic expected outcomes for the patient's functional capacity and physical appearance. Provide information sessions and counseling for the family to identify patterns of support. Facilitate the patient's use of these systems and the development of new support systems. Make referrals to support groups. Evaluate the effectiveness and use of support resources throughout the course of recovery.

Engaging in decision making and independent activities fosters feelings of self-worth. Plan and encourage the patient's active participation in care activities. Assist family members to understand that it is more beneficial for the patient to perform these activities than to have them performed by someone else. Urge families to include the patient in family decision making to the same degree that he or she participated in this process before the injury.

Surgical Management. Reconstructive and cosmetic surgery can be performed many years after the burn injury. Restoring function and improving appearance through surgical tech- niques often promote the patient's positive self-image and self-worth. Many patients have unrealistic expectations of reconstructive surgery and envision an appearance identical or equal in quality to the preburn state. Teach the patient and family about expected cosmetic outcomes.

REHABILITATIVE PHASE OF BURN INJURY

Although rehabilitation efforts are started at the time of admis- sion, the technical rehabilitative phase begins with wound closure and ends when the patient achieves his or her highest level of functioning. The emphasis is on the psychosocial adjust- ment of the patient, the prevention of scars and contractures, and the resumption of preburn activity, including resuming work, family, and social roles. This phase may take years or even last a lifetime as patients adjust to permanent limitations (Dahl et al., 2012).

❖ *PATIENT-CENTERED COLLABORATIVE CARE*

Although attention is placed first on the physical interventions for the burn injury, psychological care is equally important. Continue to provide psychosocial support to the patient and family throughout hospitalization and in the rehabilitative phase.

Obtaining information from the patient and family aids in the assessment and diagnosis of psychological problems and directs management. Explore the patient's feelings about the burn injury. It is extremely difficult for patients to concentrate on the many tasks before them when obstacles such as guilt and grief are in the forefront.

Ask whether there is a history of psychological problems. To assist with a future plan of care, assess and document the type of coping mechanisms the patient has used successfully during times of stress. Also assess the patient's family unit and the history of interaction. Consider cultural and ethnic factors when planning psychosocial interventions.

Throughout the hospitalization, the patient progresses through a variety of stages and exhibits many feelings, including denial, regression, and anger. Assess the patient's feelings at each stage so appropriate plans of care can be implemented.

TABLE 26-7 Needs to Address Before Discharge of the Patient with Burns

- Early patient assessment
- Financial assessment
- Evaluation of family resources
- Weekly discharge planning meeting
- Psychological referral
- Patient and family teaching (home care)
- Designation of principal learners (specific family members or significant others who will help with care)
- Development of teaching plan
- Training for wound care
- Rehabilitation referral
- Home assessment (on-site visit)
- Medical equipment
- Public health nursing referral
- Evaluation of community resources
- Visit to referral agency
- Re-entry programs for school or work environment
- Long-term care placement
- Environmental interventions
- Auditory testing
- Speech therapy
- Prosthetic rehabilitation

Community-Based Care

Discharge planning for the patient with a burn injury begins at admission to the hospital or burn center. The interdisciplinary team meets regularly to evaluate the progress of each discipline and help the patient reach mutually established discharge outcomes. Table 26-7 lists common discharge needs of the patient with burns.

Psychosocial Preparation. During the recovery period and for some time after discharge, patients with severe burn injuries often have psychological problems that require intervention. Such problems include post-traumatic stress disorder, sexual dysfunction, and severe depression. Assistance is coordinated with the patient, family, and health care team. Psychosocial assistance is best provided by a professional counselor with experience in helping burn patients.

One specific area to address with the patient is the reaction of others to the sight of healing wounds and disfiguring scars. Patients with facial burns are especially subjected to stares and other negative reactions from the public. Visits from friends and short public appearances before discharge may help the patient begin adjusting to this problem. Community reintegration programs can assist the psychosocial and physical recovery of the patient with serious burns.

Home Care Management. The patient with severe burns is discharged from the acute care setting when serious complications are resolved and minimal wound areas remain open. During the first weeks at home, the patient usually needs at least daily wound care, physical therapy, NUTRITION support, symptom management, and drug therapy.

Although the patient usually views going home positively, the problems of physical care and the psychological stresses from changes in appearance, role, function, and lifestyle may overwhelm the patient and family. Successful discharge depends on extensive planning and preparation of the patient, family, and home environment through education and the involvement of appropriate support agencies and services.

Preparation for discharge includes assessment of the family and home care situation from physical and social perspectives. Consider the needs of the patient when evaluating the home for cleanliness; access to bathing facilities, electricity, and running water; stairways; number of occupants; temperature control; and safety. If the burn injuries occurred in a house fire, a new residence may need to be established.

Self-Management Education. Education about burn care and living with the consequences of burn injuries begins when the patient is admitted to the hospital or burn center. A weekly plan for patient education is outlined; a positive outcome is progression toward independence for the patient and family. Critical for this outcome is teaching patients and family members to perform such care tasks as dressing changes. Allow patients and family members to first observe dressing changes, then to assist in performing the changes, and then to change the dressings independently under your supervision.

Before discharge, all people who will be involved in the patient's home care participate in discharge planning and teaching sessions. In addition to details about dressing changes, explain:
- Indications of INFECTION
- Drug regimens
- Proper use of prosthetic and positioning devices
- Correct application and care of pressure garments
- Comfort measures to reduce pruritus
- Dates for follow-up appointments

Health Care Resources. The health care team evaluates the family's capacity and willingness to assist in caring for the patient after discharge. A visiting nurse or case manager with extensive experience in providing burn care can assist the family with care problems arising at home. This nurse can help the family determine what special equipment, supplies, or services will be needed. The frequency of home visits depends on the patient's condition and the ability of family members to function as care providers. The home care nurse may need a brief visit to the patient while in the hospital and may need to observe burn wound care.

The home care of a patient after a serious burn often involves daily physical therapy and rehabilitation sessions at special centers. Address and resolve transportation problems before the patient is discharged.

When rehabilitation is prolonged, the patient may be discharged to a rehabilitation facility. Consult with the rehabilitation team, and provide copies of the care and teaching plans used with the patient.

◆ Evaluation: Outcomes

Evaluate the care of the patient with a burn injury on the basis of the identified priority patient problems. The expected outcomes include that the patient should:
- Maintain adequate oxygenation and circulation to all vital organs
- Maintain a patent airway
- Have cardiac output restored to normal
- Have PAIN alleviated or reduced
- Experience no further loss of skin TISSUE INTEGRITY
- Have wounds healed without complications
- Remain free from INFECTION
- Not experience sepsis
- Maintain an adequate NUTRITION for meeting the body's calorie needs
- Regain and maintain an optimal ability to move purposefully
- Have a positive perception of his or her own appearance and body functions

Specific indicators for these outcomes are listed for each priority patient problem in the Planning and Implementation section (see earlier).

NURSING CONCEPTS AND CLINICAL JUDGMENT REVIEW

What might you NOTICE if the patient is experiencing INFECTION as a result of a problem of protection from a burn injury?
- Change in burn wound, including:
  Pervasive odor
  Color changes—focal, dark red, brown discoloration in the eschar
  Change in texture
  Purulent drainage
  Exudate
  Sloughing grafts
  Redness of wound edges extending to nonburned skin
- Elevated temperature
- Change in sensation in burn wound
- Change in cognition or level of consciousness

What should you INTERPRET and how should you RESPOND to a patient experiencing INFECTION as a result of a problem of protection from a burn injury?

Perform and interpret physical assessment, including:
- Taking vital signs, especially temperature
- Checking for change in cognitive status or level of consciousness

- Assessing burn wound for changes in appearance or amount/type of exudate

Interpret laboratory values:
- Elevated white blood cell count
- Positive burn wound cultures
- Positive blood cultures

Respond by:
- Documenting indicators of infection
- Notifying health care professional
- Implementing appropriate infection protocols
- Assisting the patient and family to understand the rationale for infection protocols

On what should you REFLECT?
- Observe patient for evidence of response to antimicrobial therapy and infection protocols.
- Determine whether the infection occurred by auto-contamination or cross-contamination.
- Think about what staff and patient teaching focus could help reduce the occurrence of a wound infection in the future.

GET READY FOR THE NCLEX® EXAMINATION!

KEY POINTS

Review these Key Points for each NCLEX Client Needs Category.

Safe and Effective Care Environment
- Use strict aseptic technique when caring for patients who have open burn wounds to prevent INFECTION. **Safety** `QSEN`
- Monitor the patient's vital signs at least every 8 hours for indications of wound INFECTION or sepsis. (For patients with greater than 25% TBSA burn, monitor vital signs more frequently.) **Safety** `QSEN`
- Assess burn wounds at least daily for indicators of INFECTION. **Safety** `QSEN`
- Give prescribed opioid analgesics by the IV route during the resuscitation phase of burn recovery. **Safety** `QSEN`

Health Promotion and Maintenance
- Encourage all people to have and maintain home smoke and carbon monoxide detectors.
- Warn patients who smoke about not smoking in bed or in rooms where home oxygen is in use and not smoking when taking any substance that induces sedation (drugs or alcohol). **Safety** `QSEN`
- Instruct patients who have reduced sensation in hands or feet to use a bath thermometer to check water temperature before bathing. **Safety** `QSEN`
- Teach patients to avoid exposing burned skin to the sun or to temperature extremes. **Patient-Centered Care** `QSEN`
- Instruct everyone to set hot water tank temperatures to the manufacturer's recommendations. **Safety** `QSEN`

Psychosocial Integrity
- Allow patients time to grieve over a change in body image. **Patient-Centered Care** `QSEN`
- Reassure patients that PAIN will be managed effectively. **Patient-Centered Care** `QSEN`
- Explain all procedures to the patient and family.
- Assess the patient's and family's use of coping strategies related to burn injury, treatment, possible role changes, and possible outcomes. **Patient-Centered Care** `QSEN`
- Support the patient and family in coping with permanent changes in appearance and function. **Patient-Centered Care** `QSEN`
- Encourage the burn patient with wounds and scars to participate in self-care. **Patient-Centered Care** `QSEN`
- Allow patients who have lost family members, homes, or jobs time to grieve for these losses.

Physiological Integrity
- Assess the burn patient's airway and adequacy of breathing before assessing any other body system. **Safety** `QSEN`
- Keep an endotracheal kit or tracheostomy kit at the bedside of any patient with facial burns, burns inside the mouth, singed nasal hairs, or a "smoky" smell to the breath. **Safety** `QSEN`
- Notify the Rapid Response Team immediately if the patient with an inhalation injury becomes more breathless or audible wheezes disappear. **Safety** `QSEN`
- Give analgesics, sedatives, and antianxiety drugs to patients receiving paralytic drugs during mechanical ventilation. **Patient-Centered Care** `QSEN`

- Give half of the fluid volume calculated for the first 24 hours after burn injury in the first 8 hours postburn. **Evidence-Based Practice** **QSEN**
- Use laboratory data and clinical manifestations to determine the effectiveness of fluid resuscitation during the resuscitation phase of burn injury. **Evidence-Based Practice** **QSEN**
- Encourage the patient to actively participate in PAIN control measures. **Patient-Centered Care** **QSEN**
- Position patients to prevent contractures and promote joint function. **Evidence-Based Practice** **QSEN**

- Assist patients to ambulate several times each day as soon as the fluid shifts have resolved.
- Coordinate with the registered dietitian to meet the nutrition needs for the patient during the acute phase of burn injury. **Teamwork and Collaboration** **QSEN**
- Evaluate the patient's wound healing during the acute phase of burn injury. **Patient-Centered Care** **QSEN**
- Use appropriate positioning and range-of-motion interventions for prevention of MOBILITY problems in the patient with burns. **Patient-Centered Care** **QSEN**

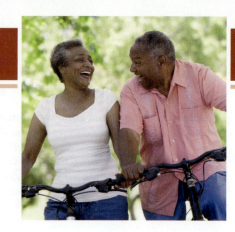

Oxygenation

Meeting the body's need for oxygenation is dependent on the concepts of GAS EXCHANGE and PERFUSION (Giddens, 2013). All cells and tissues need oxygen to live and function. Some cells, such as brain cells and heart muscle cells, are very dependent on oxygen. Without oxygen, brain cells stop functioning and die in about 5 to 10 minutes. Other cells, such as skin cells, can live and function for many hours with low oxygen levels or even without oxygen. Skeletal muscle cells can survive for hours with low levels of oxygen but cannot function for very long without it.

The source of the oxygen for all body cells is the air we breathe into our lungs. The process of GAS EXCHANGE first occurs in the alveoli of lungs. The carbon dioxide generated in body cells as a result of metabolism diffuses from the blood into the alveoli where it is exhaled down its concentration gradient into atmospheric air. At the same time, atmospheric oxygen is inhaled into the alveoli where it then moves down its concentration gradient into capillary blood. These steps compose alveolar or pulmonary GAS EXCHANGE even though the exchange is not equal (not a one-for-one exchange between oxygen molecules and carbon dioxide molecules). Delivery of oxygen to the cells and tissues, PERFUSION, requires the pumping mechanism of the heart and the oxygen-carrying mechanism of the hemoglobin in red blood cells. Once PERFUSION delivers oxygen to the tissues, a second GAS EXCHANGE takes place with oxygen moving from capillary blood into cells at the same time that carbon dioxide leaves the cells and enters capillary blood.

In health, the need of body tissues for oxygen is balanced by the body's GAS EXCHANGE and PERFUSION systems (Fig. 1). When oxygen needs increase, such as during mild to moderate exercise, oxygen intake through the respiratory system and pulmonary GAS EXCHANGE increase to compensate (or adjust) and keep tissue oxygen PERFUSION in balance with cellular oxygen need (Fig. 2).

When oxygen need increases as a result of heavy exercise or an illness in which metabolism is increased (and the person has a fever), all GAS EXCHANGE and PERFUSION systems must adjust by increasing their activity to match the increased oxygen need. When this compensation is perfect, the increased rate and depth of respiration, along with the increased heart rate and blood pressure, keep oxygenation in balance with oxygen need (Fig. 3).

FIG. 3

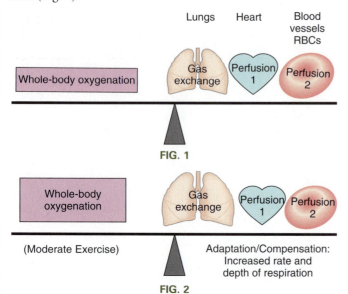

FIG. 1

FIG. 2

Some health problems reduce the body's ability to compensate when oxygen need is greater than basic (basal) levels. For example, in a person who has asthma, the lungs may be able to take in enough oxygen to meet basic oxygen needs but cannot adjust or compensate when a greater oxygen intake is needed, such as during mild to moderate exercise (Fig. 4). In this situation, the heart and blood need to compensate *more* to increase delivery of the set amount of oxygen taken in (Fig. 5).

In another situation, when the person has a cardiac problem and the heart rate alone cannot increase oxygen delivery during mild to moderate exercise (Fig. 6), his or her respiratory rate would have to increase more than usual to keep oxygen delivery in balance with oxygen need.

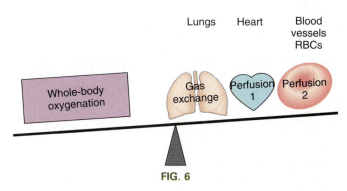

FIG. 6

What happens when any part of the oxygen intake (GAS EXCHANGE) or delivery systems (PERFUSION) has a problem that interferes with ensuring that the cells have enough oxygen? Consider a person with pneumonia who has great difficulty with pulmonary GAS EXCHANGE to the point that the body's basic oxygen need is not met. Even though the oxygen need is at a basic level, the need is unbalanced compared with pulmonary GAS EXCHANGE and oxygen PERFUSION. The person's compensation mechanisms are working (respiratory rate is increased, heart rate is increased) but are not completely effective. How could balance be restored? Interventions are needed to support the body's compensation efforts to restore balance.

The best way is to eliminate the pneumonia, which could take days even with proper drug therapy. Other ways involve (1) reducing oxygen need to the lowest possible level by having the patient rest and (2) improving pulmonary GAS EXCHANGE by increasing the percentage of oxygen in the air that he or she breathes (oxygen therapy) (Fig. 7).

Lungs   Heart   Blood vessels RBCs

Whole-body oxygenation — Gas exchange — Perfusion 1 — Perfusion 2

FIG. 4

Whole-body oxygenation — Gas exchange — Perfusion 1 — Perfusion 2

Adaptation/Compensation: Increased heart rate and increased RBCs (and Hgb)

FIG. 5

Intervention: Oxygen administration reduces the amount of compensation needed by heart and RBCs to maintain tissue oxygenation

Adaptation/Compensation: Increased heart rate and increased RBCs (and Hgb)

FIG. 7

27 | CHAPTER

Assessment of the Respiratory System

Harry Rees

 http://evolve.elsevier.com/Iggy/

PRIORITY CONCEPTS

- GAS EXCHANGE
- PERFUSION

LEARNING OUTCOMES

Health Promotion and Maintenance

1. Teach all people measures to take to protect the respiratory system, including the avoidance of tobacco use.

Psychosocial Integrity

2. Reduce the psychological impact for the patient and family regarding the assessment and testing of the respiratory system with regard to GAS EXCHANGE and PERFUSION.

Physiological Integrity

3. Perform a focused assessment of respiratory function, incorporating information about genetic risk and age-related changes affecting respiratory function.
4. Coordinate appropriate care for patients after invasive and noninvasive testing of respiratory function.

Oxygen (O$_2$) is an essential nutrient for all cells to live and perform their specific jobs. Oxygen intake with GAS EXCHANGE and PERFUSION depends on the respiratory system because the source of the oxygen for all body cells is the air we breathe (Fig. 27-1). This system includes the upper airways, lungs, lower airways, and alveolar air sacs. Air with oxygen enters the nose and mouth and moves through the airways or respiratory tubes (trachea, bronchi, bronchioles) and into the air sacs (alveoli) of the lungs. Once in the air sacs, the oxygen from the air moves into the blood so that it can be carried to all tissues and organs. Carbon dioxide (CO$_2$), the waste gas created in the tissues, moves from the blood into the lungs so it can be exhaled. All systems depend on adequate oxygen intake with GAS EXCHANGE for tissue PERFUSION. Any respiratory problem affects total body health and well-being.

HEALTH PROMOTION AND MAINTENANCE

Lung and breathing problems are common causes of death in North America (McCance et al., 2014). Some respiratory problems are chronic, and the patient has physical and lifestyle limitations. Many acute health problems, medical therapies, and surgeries adversely affect respiratory function temporarily or permanently. Exposure to inhalation irritants, especially to tobacco smoke, is the most common cause of chronic respiratory problems and physical limitations. In addition, cigarette smoking is a modifiable factor that greatly increases the risk for cardiovascular disease, stroke, and many types of cancer. Three compounds in cigarette smoke that have been implicated in the development of these serious diseases are tar, nicotine, and carbon monoxide. In the years after a patient has stopped smoking, his or her risk for respiratory-related disorders decreases significantly. Therefore assessing smoking habits, actively promoting smoking cessation, determining exposure to other inhalation irritants, and teaching people to protect the respiratory system are important nursing functions.

Assessing smoking habits begins by determining whether the patient is a current smoker or has ever smoked. The smoking history includes the number of cigarettes smoked daily, the duration of the smoking habit, and the age of the patient when smoking started even for patients who are not current smokers. Record the smoking history in **pack-years**, which is the number

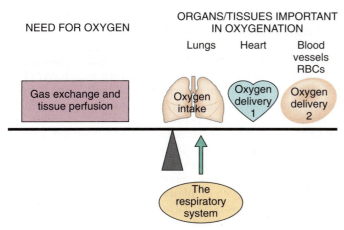

NEED FOR OXYGEN

ORGANS/TISSUES IMPORTANT IN OXYGENATION

FIG. 27-1 Role of the respiratory system in the concepts of gas exchange and tissue perfusion. *RBCs,* Red blood cells.

of packs per day multiplied by the number of years the patient has smoked.

Be sure to ask those who do not currently smoke whether and to what extent they are exposed to the smoke of others. This passive smoking has two origins: direct exposure to smoke by being in the same environment with a person(s) who is actively smoking *(secondhand smoke [SHS]);* and indirect exposure from smoke that clings to hair and clothing *(thirdhand smoke).* Both types of passive smoking contribute to health problems, especially when exposure occurs in small, confined spaces and is chronic.

Another category of cigarette smoking, particularly among younger adults, is *social smoking.* This term is used to describe people who claim to smoke cigarettes only in the presence of others, borrow rather than purchase cigarettes, prefer the company of nonsmokers, and do not smoke for stress relief (Butler et al., 2012). Often the social smoker does not consider himself or herself to be a smoker and must be asked specifically, "Do you ever smoke in social situations?" Although this type of smoking is intermittent, it can still have an adverse effect on respiratory and cardiovascular health and may lead to nicotine addiction.

Hookah or water pipe smoking is becoming more popular in North America. The highest incidence is among young people. Studies have determined that the exposure to inhaled toxins is as great or greater than with cigarette smoking. Although many cities have instituted smoking bans, water pipe smoking may be exempt, raising concerns for secondhand smoke exposure (Fiala et al., 2012).

E-cigarettes have emerged as an alternative to traditional cigarettes and are used as a method of quitting smoking. The cartridges within an e-cigarette, as well as the vapors produced, may contain nicotine or other toxins. Thus the safety for the user or the bystander has not been established. E-cigarettes are not currently an approved method of smoking cessation (Riker et al., 2012).

Promoting smoking cessation is a sensitive and sometimes uncomfortable issue for nurses and other health care professionals to approach with patients who smoke. However, this opportunity for a "teachable moment" may be the beginning support a patient needs to be successful in this healthful pursuit. Many acute care settings now have automatic smoking-cessation protocols that attach to the patient's electronic medical record

as soon as an active smoking history is recorded. The Centers for Medicare and Medicaid Services (CMS) no longer requires smoking cessation as part of their Core Measures. However, The Joint Commission requires documentation of screening for tobacco use and that a tobacco treatment program was offered or provided, as part of their quality measures.

Ask about the patient's desire to quit, past attempts to quit, and the methods used. Determine nicotine dependence by asking questions such as:

- How soon after you wake up in the morning do you smoke?
- Do you wake up in the middle of your sleep time to smoke?
- Do you find it difficult not to smoke in places where smoking is prohibited?
- Do you smoke when you are ill?

A variety of drug therapies are available over the counter and by prescription to help those addicted to nicotine to modify their behavior and stop smoking. Over-the-counter nicotine replacement therapies (NRTs) include nicotine-releasing transdermal patches, gums, and lozenges. Prescribed NRT products include nasal sprays and inhalers. NRT products have a success rate of smoking cessation between 50% and 70% (Grief, 2011). They have been shown to have the highest success rates when used in association with a smoking-cessation program. Chart 27-1 lists suggestions for you to use in providing support to the person interested in stopping cigarette smoking.

! NURSING SAFETY PRIORITY QSEN
Drug Alert

Teach people using drugs for nicotine replacement therapy that smoking while taking these drugs greatly increases circulating nicotine levels and the risk for stroke or heart attack.

Additional drug therapy for smoking cessation includes the oral drugs *bupropion* (Zyban) and *varenicline* (Chantix). Bupropion encourages smoking cessation by decreasing cravings and withdrawal manifestations as well as reducing the depression associated with nicotine withdrawal symptoms. Varenicline interferes with the nicotine receptors. This promotes smoking cessation by reducing the pleasure derived from nicotine and by reducing the manifestations of nicotine withdrawal.

CULTURAL CONSIDERATIONS
Patient-Centered Care (QSEN)

The prevalence of smoking remains higher among African Americans, blue-collar workers, and less-educated people than in the overall population of the United States. Smoking prevalence is highest among Northern Plains American Indians and Alaskan Natives. Development of culturally appropriate smoking-cessation programs as well as research examining barriers to cessation in these populations may help reduce this disparity.

CHART 27-1 Patient and Family Education: Preparing for Self-Management
Smoking Cessation

- Make a list of the reasons you want to stop smoking (e.g., your health and the health of those around you, saving money, social reasons).
- Set a date to stop smoking, and keep it. Decide whether you are going to begin to cut down on the amount you smoke or are going to stop "cold turkey." Whatever way you decide to do it, keep this important date!
- Ask for help from those around you. Find someone who wants to quit smoking and "buddy up" for support. Look for assistance in your community, such as formal smoking-cessation programs, counselors, and certified acupuncture specialists or hypnotists.
- Consult your health care provider about nicotine replacement therapy (e.g., patch, gum) or other pharmacologic therapy to assist in smoking cessation.
- Remove ashtrays and lighters from your view.
- Talk to yourself! Remind yourself of all the reasons you want to quit.
- Think of a way to reward yourself with the money you save from not smoking for a year.
- Avoid places that might tempt you to smoke. If you are used to having a cigarette after meals, get up from the table as soon as you are finished eating. Think of new things to do at times when you used to smoke (e.g., taking a walk, exercising, calling a friend).
- Find activities that keep your hands busy: needlework, painting, gardening, even holding a pencil.
- Take five deep breaths of clean, fresh air through your nose and out your mouth if you feel the urge to smoke.
- Keep plenty of healthy, low-calorie snacks, such as fruits and vegetables, on hand to nibble on. Try sugarless gum or mints as a substitute for tobacco.
- Drink at least eight glasses of water each day.
- Begin an exercise program with the approval of your health care provider. Be aware of the positive, healthy changes in your body since you stopped smoking.
- List the many reasons why you are glad that you quit. Keep the list handy as a reminder of the positive things you are doing for yourself.
- If you have a cigarette, think about what the conditions were that caused you to light it. Try and think of a strategy to avoid that (or those) conditions.
- Don't beat yourself up for backsliding; just face the next day as a new day.
- Think of each day without tobacco as a major accomplishment. It is!!

NURSING SAFETY PRIORITY (QSEN)
Drug Alert

Both bupropion and varenicline carry a black box warning that use of these drugs can cause manic behavior and hallucinations. These drugs also may unmask serious mental health issues. Teach the patient prescribed either of these drugs and their families to report any change in behavior or thought processes to the prescriber immediately.

Assessing exposure to inhalation irritants should be part of any health assessment. Usually this information is obtained as part of the demographic history, which includes the patient's current and past geographic living area, occupation, home conditions, and hobbies. Geographic areas with high levels of air pollution contribute to respiratory problems. Exposures to dust, particles, chemicals, gases, or toxic fumes can occur in the workplace, making work history information important. Ask about the exact dates of employment and a brief job description. Exposure to industrial dusts of any type or to the chemicals found in smoke and fumes may cause breathing disorders. Bakers, coalminers, stone masons, cotton handlers, woodworkers, welders, potters, plastic and rubber manufacturers, printers, asbestos workers, farm workers, and steel foundry workers are at risk for breathing problems.

Ask about home conditions, such as the type of heat used (e.g., gas heater, wood-burning stove, fireplace, kerosene heater). Determine exposure to irritants (e.g., fumes, chemicals, animals, birds, air pollutants). Ask about hobbies such as painting, ceramics, model airplanes, refinishing furniture, or woodworking, which may expose the patient to harmful chemicals.

Protecting the respiratory system starts with making people aware of the sources of inhalation irritants. Teach people who live in areas with high levels of air pollution to remain indoors with windows closed on days when air quality is poor and not to engage in heavy physical activity. Teach people who have workplace or home exposure to inhalation irritants to wear masks during these exposures and to ensure the area is well ventilated.

ANATOMY AND PHYSIOLOGY REVIEW

The purpose of breathing is to ensure GAS EXCHANGE. This process has two parts: (1) oxygenation for tissue PERFUSION so that cells have enough oxygen to metabolize and generate energy; and (2) removal of carbon dioxide, the waste product of metabolism. The respiratory system also influences acid-base balance, speech, sense of smell, fluid balance, and temperature control. The lungs are also an excretory organ because they can also break down some toxins and eliminate them from the body during exhalation.

Upper Respiratory Tract

The upper airways include the nose, the sinuses, the pharynx, and the larynx (Fig. 27-2).

Nose and Sinuses

The nose is the organ of smell, with receptors from cranial nerve I *(olfactory)* located in the upper areas. The nose is rigid with a bony upper portion and a cartilaginous lower portion that can move to some extent. The septum divides the nose into two cavities that are lined with mucous membranes that have a rich blood supply. The anterior nares are the external openings into the nasal cavities. The posterior nares are openings from the nasal cavity into the throat.

The turbinates are three bones that protrude into the nasal cavities from the internal portion of the nose (see Fig. 27-2). Turbinates increase the total surface area for filtering, heating, and humidifying inspired air before it passes into the nasopharynx. Inspired air is humidified by the mucous membrane and is warmed by heat from the vascular network.

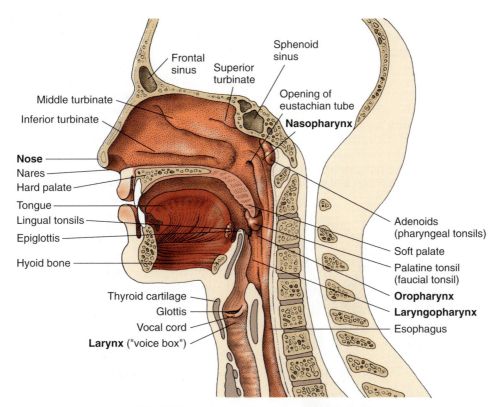

FIG. 27-2 Structures of the upper respiratory tract.

The paranasal sinuses are air-filled cavities within the bones that surround the nasal passages (Fig. 27-3). Lined with ciliated membrane, the sinuses provide resonance during speech, decrease the weight of the skull, and act as shock absorbers in the event of facial trauma.

Pharynx

The pharynx, or throat, is a passageway for both the respiratory and digestive tracts. It is located behind the oral and nasal cavities. The throat is divided into the nasopharynx, the oropharynx, and the laryngopharynx (see Fig. 27-2).

The nasopharynx is located behind the nose, above the soft palate. It contains the adenoids and the opening of the eustachian tube. The adenoids trap organisms that enter the nose or mouth. The eustachian tubes connect the nasopharynx with the middle ears and open during swallowing to equalize pressure within the middle ear.

The oropharynx is located behind the mouth, below the nasopharynx. It extends from the soft palate to the base of the tongue and is used for breathing and swallowing. The *palatine tonsils*, which are part of the immune system, are located on the sides of the oropharynx and protect against invading organisms.

The laryngopharynx is the area located behind the larynx from the base of the tongue to the esophagus. It is the dividing point between the larynx and the esophagus.

Larynx

The **larynx** is the "voice box" and is located above the trachea, just below the throat at the base of the tongue. It is composed of several cartilages (Fig. 27-4). The *thyroid cartilage* is the largest and is commonly called the "Adam's apple." The *cricoid*

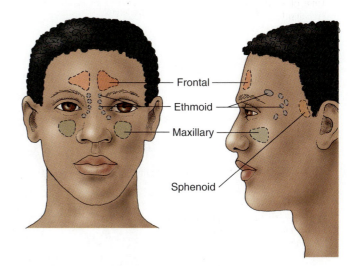

FIG. 27-3 The paranasal sinuses.

cartilage, which contains the vocal cords, lies below the thyroid cartilage. The *cricothyroid membrane* is located below the level of the vocal cords and joins the thyroid and cricoid cartilages. This site is used in an emergency for access to the lower airways. In this procedure, called a *cricothyroidotomy*, an opening is made between the thyroid and cricoid cartilage and results in a tracheostomy. The two *arytenoid* cartilages work with the thyroid cartilage in vocal cord movement.

Inside the larynx are two pairs of vocal cords: the false vocal cords and the true vocal cords. The glottis is the opening between the true vocal cords (Fig. 27-5). The epiglottis is a small, elastic structure attached along one edge to the top of the larynx. It prevents food from entering the trachea (aspiration) by closing over the glottis during swallowing. The epiglottis opens during breathing and coughing.

Lower Respiratory Tract
Airways
The lower airways are the trachea; two mainstem bronchi; lobar, segmental, and subsegmental bronchi; bronchioles; alveolar ducts; and alveoli (Fig. 27-6). The lower respiratory tract *(tracheobronchial tree)* consists of muscle, cartilage, and elastic tissues forming branching tubes. These tubes decrease in size from the trachea to the respiratory bronchioles and allow gases to move to and from the lungs. GAS EXCHANGE takes place in the lung tissue between the alveoli and the lung capillaries, not in the airways.

The trachea is in front of the esophagus. It branches into the right and left mainstem bronchi at the *carina* junction. The trachea contains 6 to 10 C-shaped rings of cartilage. The open portion of the C is the back portion of the trachea and shares a wall with the esophagus.

The mainstem bronchi, or primary bronchi, begin at the carina and contain the same tissues as the trachea. The right bronchus is slightly wider, shorter, and more vertical than the left bronchus and can more easily be accidentally intubated when an endotracheal tube is passed. Also, when a foreign object is aspirated from the throat, it usually enters the right bronchus.

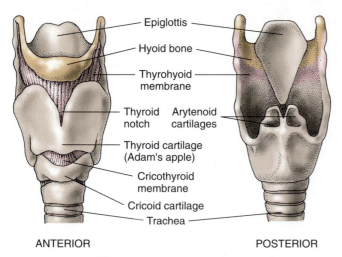

FIG. 27-4 Structures of the larynx.

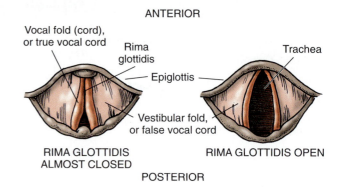

FIG. 27-5 Detail of the glottis (two vocal folds and the intervening space, the rima glottidis).

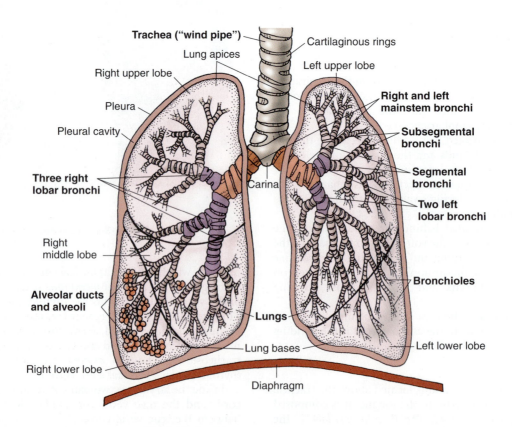

FIG. 27-6 Structures of the lower respiratory tract.

The mainstem bronchi branch into the secondary (lobar) bronchi that enter each of the five lobes of the two lungs. Each lobar bronchus branches into progressively smaller divisions. The cartilage rings of these lobar bronchi are complete and resist collapse. The bronchi are lined with a ciliated, mucus-secreting membrane that moves particles away from the lower airways.

The bronchioles branch from the secondary bronchi and divide into smaller and smaller tubes, which are the terminal and respiratory bronchioles (Fig. 27-7). These tubes have a small diameter, have no cartilage, and depend entirely on the elastic recoil of the lung to remain open.

Alveolar ducts branch from the respiratory bronchioles and resemble a bunch of grapes. Alveolar sacs arise from these ducts and contain groups of alveoli, which are the basic units of GAS EXCHANGE (see Fig. 27-7). A pair of healthy adult lungs has about 290 million alveoli, which are surrounded by lung capillaries. These numerous small alveoli normally make a large surface area for GAS EXCHANGE (about the size of a tennis court). Acinus is a term for the structural unit consisting of a respiratory bronchiole, an alveolar duct, and an alveolar sac.

The alveolar walls have cells called *type II pneumocytes* that secrete **surfactant,** a fatty protein that reduces surface tension in the alveoli. Without surfactant, **atelectasis** (alveolar collapse) occurs, reducing GAS EXCHANGE because the alveolar surface area is reduced.

Lungs

The lungs are elastic, cone-shaped organs located in the pleural cavity in the chest. The apex (top) of each lung extends above the clavicle; the base (bottom) of each lung lies just above the diaphragm. The lungs are composed of millions of alveoli and their related ducts, bronchioles, and bronchi. The right lung, which is larger and wider than the left, is divided into three lobes: upper, middle, and lower. The left lung is divided into only two lobes. About 60% to 65% of lung function occurs in the right lung. Any problem with the right lung interferes with

GAS EXCHANGE and PERFUSION to a greater degree than a problem in the left lung.

The **pleura** is a continuous smooth membrane with two surfaces that totally enclose the lungs. The parietal pleura lines the inside of the chest cavity and the upper surface of the diaphragm. The visceral pleura covers the lung surfaces. These surfaces are lubricated by a thin fluid that allows the surfaces to glide across each other smoothly during breathing.

Blood flow in the lungs occurs through two separate systems: bronchial and pulmonary. The bronchial system carries the blood needed to oxygenate lung tissues. These arteries are part of systemic circulation and do not participate in gas exchange.

The pulmonary circulation is a highly vascular capillary network. Oxygen-poor blood travels from the right ventricle of the heart into the pulmonary artery. This artery eventually branches into arterioles to form capillary networks that are meshed around and through the alveoli—the site of GAS EXCHANGE (see Fig. 27-7). Freshly oxygenated blood travels from the capillaries to the pulmonary veins and then to the left atrium. From the left atrium, oxygenated blood flows into the left ventricle, where it is pumped throughout the systemic circulation.

Accessory Muscles of Respiration

Breathing occurs through changes in the size of and pressure within the chest cavity. Contraction and relaxation of chest muscles (and the diaphragm) cause changes in the size and pressure of the chest cavity. At times, back and abdominal muscles are used in addition to chest muscles when the work of breathing is increased.

Oxygen Delivery and the Oxygen-Hemoglobin Dissociation Curve

Oxygen delivery to the tissues requires the binding of oxygen to hemoglobin in red blood cells. Each molecule of hemoglobin can bind four oxygen molecules, which fills (*saturates*) all of its binding sites. Each red blood cell normally has hundreds of thousands of hemoglobin molecules. When blood passes through the lung alveoli, where oxygen concentration is the greatest, oxygen diffuses from the alveoli into red blood cells and binds to all those hemoglobin molecules. This oxygen-rich blood then goes to the left side of the heart and is pumped out into systemic circulation. In tissues away from the source of oxygen, hemoglobin unloads (**dissociates**) the oxygen molecules and delivers them to the tissues. Fig. 27-8 shows the oxygen-hemoglobin dissociation curve.

Tissue oxygen delivery through dissociation or unloading from hemoglobin is based on tissues' need for oxygen. The curve in Fig. 27-8 shows that the rate of this unloading changes depending on how much oxygen is already in the tissues. When blood perfuses tissues in which the oxygen levels are high, as indicated in the upper right-hand corner of the figure, hemoglobin binds oxygen very tightly and little oxygen is unloaded or dissociated from the hemoglobin into the tissues. This prevents oxygen delivery from being wasted by unloading it where it is not needed. When blood perfuses tissues in which oxygen levels are very low, as indicated in the lower left-hand corner of Fig. 27-8, hemoglobin binds oxygen less tightly and will rapidly and easily unload its remaining oxygen to provide these tissues with needed oxygen. So, how rapidly and easily hemoglobin dissociates oxygen to the tissues changes depending on oxygen need. The S-shaped curve indicates that it is harder for oxygen

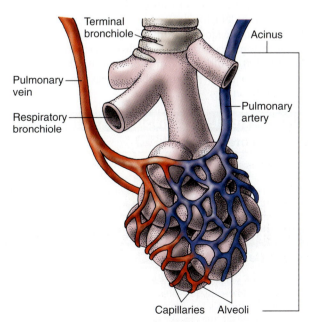

FIG. 27-7 The terminal bronchioles and the acinus.

FIG. 27-8 The oxygen-hemoglobin dissociation curve. P_{50}, The partial pressure of O_2 at which hemoglobin is 50% saturated; PO_2, oxygen partial pressure.

to dissociate from hemoglobin in tissues that are well-oxygenated and much easier in tissues that are "starving" for oxygen.

The curve in Fig. 27-8 indicates that, on average, 50% of hemoglobin molecules have completely dissociated their oxygen molecules when blood perfuses tissues that have an oxygen tension (concentration) of 26 mm Hg. This is considered a "normal" point at which 50% of hemoglobin molecules are no longer saturated with oxygen.

When the need for oxygen is greater in tissues, this curve shifts to the *right*, which means the hemoglobin will dissociate oxygen faster even when the tissue oxygen tension levels are greater than 26 mm Hg. Conditions that shift the curve to the right include increased tissue temperature, increased tissue carbon dioxide concentration, and decreased tissue pH (acidosis). This means that it is easier for hemoglobin to unload oxygen to these tissues because they need it to support the higher metabolism and is a tissue protection that increases oxygen delivery to the tissues that need it the most.

When tissues have less need of oxygen because they are metabolizing more slowly than usual, the oxygen-hemoglobin dissociation curve shifts to the *left*, which means that the tissue oxygen tension level has to be even *lower* for hemoglobin to unload oxygen. Tissue conditions that cause a shift to the left include decreased tissue temperature, decreased carbon dioxide levels, decreased glucose breakdown products, and a higher tissue pH (alkalosis). This action prevents wasting oxygen delivery to tissues that are not using the oxygen they already have.

A clinical example of how these actions are helpful is one in which a person is having a myocardial infarction (heart attack). Blood flow to the area is reduced and the heart muscle is metabolizing under hypoxic conditions, which creates more carbon dioxide in the tissue and acidosis. As a result, the hemoglobin that reaches this hypoxic tissue unloads more oxygen at a faster rate to prevent ischemia and cardiac muscle cell death. What if this person believes he or she is having indigestion, which can have similar manifestations, and tries to correct the problem by taking in large amounts of bicarbonate-based antacids? The antacids increase the pH in the blood and all tissues, shifting the oxygen-hemoglobin dissociation curve to the left. As a result, the hypoxic cardiac muscle cells receive even less oxygen and more of them die.

Respiratory Changes Associated with Aging

The respiratory changes that occur with aging are described in Chart 27-2. Many additional respiratory changes in older patients result from heredity and a lifetime of exposure to environmental pollutants (e.g., cigarette smoke, bacteria, industrial fumes and irritants).

Respiratory disease is a major cause of illness and chronic disability in older patients. Although respiratory function normally declines with age, there is usually no problem keeping pace with the demands of ordinary activity. The sedentary older adult, however, often feels breathless during exercise (Touhy & Jett, 2014).

It is difficult to determine which respiratory changes in older adults are related to normal aging and which changes are caused by respiratory disease or exposure to pollutants. Age-related changes in the muscles and the cardiac and vascular system also may cause abnormal breathing, even if the lungs are normal.

❓ NCLEX EXAMINATION CHALLENGE

Physiological Integrity

What is the effect of age-related decreased skeletal muscle strength on the effectiveness of gas exchange?
A. Reduced gas exchange as a result of decreased alveolar surface
B. Reduced gas exchange as a result of longer relaxation of bronchiolar smooth muscles
C. Reduced gas exchange as a result of decreased changes in pressures of the chest cavity
D. Reduced gas exchange as a result of failure of pulmonary circulation to fully perfuse lung tissue

ASSESSMENT METHODS

Patient History

Obtaining accurate information from the patient is important for identifying the type and severity of breathing problems. Age, gender, and race can affect the physical and diagnostic findings related to breathing (Jarvis, 2016). Many of the diagnostic studies for respiratory disorders (e.g., pulmonary function tests) use these data for determining predicted normal values. As described in the Health Promotion and Maintenance section, explore the home, community, and workplace for environmental factors that could cause or worsen lung disease. Use this opportunity to teach patients about measures to protect the respiratory system.

GENDER HEALTH CONSIDERATIONS

Patient-Centered Care QSEN

Women, especially smokers, have greater bronchial responsiveness (i.e., bronchial hyperreactivity) and larger airways than men. This factor increases the risk for a more rapid decline in lung function as a woman ages, especially in women who were or are smokers.

🌐 CULTURAL CONSIDERATIONS

Patient-Centered Care QSEN

Compared with white people, black people and others with dark skin usually show a lower oxygen saturation (3% to 5% lower) as measured by pulse oximetry; this results from deeper coloration of the nail bed and does not reflect true oxygen status.

CHART 27-2 Nursing Focus on the Older Adult
Changes in the Respiratory System Related to Aging

PHYSIOLOGIC CHANGE	NURSING INTERVENTIONS	RATIONALES
Alveoli Alveolar surface area decreases. Diffusion capacity decreases. Elastic recoil decreases. Bronchioles and alveolar ducts dilate. Ability to cough decreases. Airways close early.	Encourage vigorous pulmonary hygiene (i.e., encourage patient to turn, cough, and deep breathe) and to use incentive spirometry, especially if he or she is confined to bed or has had surgery. Encourage upright position.	Potential for mechanical or infectious respiratory complications is increased in these situations. The upright position minimizes ventilation-perfusion mismatching.
Lungs Residual volume increases. Vital capacity decreases. Efficiency of oxygen and carbon dioxide exchange decreases. Elasticity decreases.	Include inspection, palpation, percussion, and auscultation in lung assessments. Help patient actively maintain health and fitness. Assess patient's respirations for abnormal breathing patterns. Encourage frequent oral hygiene.	Inspection, palpation, percussion, and auscultation are needed to detect normal age-related changes. Health and fitness help keep losses in respiratory functioning to a minimum. Periodic breathing patterns (e.g., Cheyne-Stokes) can occur. Oral hygiene aids in the removal of secretions.
Pharynx and Larynx Muscles atrophy. Vocal cords become slack. Laryngeal muscles lose elasticity, and airways lose cartilage.	Have face-to-face conversations with patient when possible.	Patient's voice may be soft and difficult to understand.
Pulmonary Vasculature Vascular resistance to blood flow through pulmonary vascular system increases. Pulmonary capillary blood volume decreases. Risk for hypoxia increases.	Assess patient's level of consciousness and cognition.	Patient can become confused during acute respiratory conditions.
Exercise Tolerance Body's response to hypoxia and hypercarbia decreases.	Assess for subtle manifestations of hypoxia.	Early assessment helps prevent complications.
Muscle Strength Respiratory muscle strength, especially the diaphragm and the intercostals, decreases.	Encourage pulmonary hygiene, and help patient actively maintain health and fitness.	Regular pulmonary hygiene and overall fitness help maintain maximal functioning of the respiratory system and prevent illness.
Susceptibility to Infection Effectiveness of the cilia decreases. Immunoglobulin A decreases. Alveolar macrophages are altered.	Encourage pulmonary hygiene, and help patient actively maintain health and fitness.	Regular pulmonary hygiene and overall fitness help maintain maximal functioning of the respiratory system and prevent illness.
Chest Wall Anteroposterior diameter increases. Thorax becomes shorter. Progressive kyphoscoliosis occurs. Chest wall compliance (elasticity) decreases. Mobility of chest wall may decrease. Osteoporosis is possible, leading to chest wall abnormalities.	Discuss the normal changes of aging. Discuss the need for increased rest periods during exercise. Encourage adequate calcium intake (especially during a woman's premenopause phase).	Patients may be anxious because they must work harder to breathe. Older patients have less tolerance for exercise. Calcium intake helps prevent osteoporosis by building bone in younger patients.

Ask patients about their respiratory history (Table 27-1), including smoking history, drug use, travel, and area of residence. Document the smoking history in pack-years.

Drug use, both prescribed drugs and illicit drugs, can affect lung function. Some drugs affect the lungs when taken systemically. Ask about drugs taken for breathing problems and about drugs taken for other conditions. For example, a cough can be a side effect of some antihypertensive drugs (angiotensin-converting enzyme [ACE] inhibitors and angiotensin receptor blockers [ARBs]). Determine which over-the-counter drugs (e.g., cough syrups, antihistamines, decongestants, inhalants) the patient is using. Also assess the use of complementary and alternative therapies. Ask about past drug use. Some drugs for other conditions can cause permanent changes in lung

TABLE 27-1 Important Aspects to Assess in A Respiratory System History	

• Smoking history
• Childhood illnesses:
  • Asthma
  • Pneumonia
  • Communicable diseases
  • Hay fever
  • Allergies
  • Eczema
  • Frequent colds
  • Croup
  • Cystic fibrosis
• Adult illnesses:
  • Pneumonia
  • Sinusitis
  • Tuberculosis
  • HIV and AIDS
  • Lung disease such as emphysema and sarcoidosis
  • Diabetes
  • Hypertension
  • Heart disease
	• Influenza, pneumococcal (Pneumovax), and BCG vaccinations
	• Surgeries of the upper or lower respiratory system
	• Injuries to the upper or lower respiratory system
	• Hospitalizations
	• Date of last chest x-ray, pulmonary function test, tuberculin test, or other diagnostic tests and results
	• Recent weight loss
	• Night sweats
	• Sleep disturbances
	• Lung disease and condition of family members
	• Geographic areas of recent travel
	• Occupation and leisure activities

AIDS, Acquired immune deficiency syndrome; *BCG,* bacille Calmette-Guérin; *HIV,* human immune deficiency virus.

function. For example, patients may have pulmonary fibrosis if they received bleomycin (Blenoxane) as chemotherapy for cancer or amiodarone (Cordarone) for cardiac problems. Marijuana and illicit drugs, such as cocaine, are often inhaled and can affect lung function.

Allergies to foods, dust, molds, pollen, bee stings, trees, grass, animal dander and saliva, or drugs can affect breathing. Ask the patient to describe specific allergic responses. For example, does he or she wheeze, have trouble breathing, cough, sneeze, or have rhinitis after exposure to the allergen? Has he or she ever been treated for an allergic response? If the patient has allergies, ask about the specific cause, treatment, and the response to treatment.

> **! NURSING SAFETY PRIORITY (QSEN)**
> **Action Alert**
>
> Document any known allergies and the specific type of allergic response in a prominent place in the patient's medical record.

Travel and geographic area of residence may reveal possible exposure to certain diseases. For example, *histoplasmosis,* a fungal disease caused by inhalation of contaminated dust, is found in the central parts of the United States and Canada. *Coccidioidomycosis* is found mostly in the western and southwestern parts of the United States, in Mexico, and in portions of Central America, as is *Hantavirus.*

Nutrition Status

Assess the patient's diet history and nutrition status to determine allergic reactions to certain foods or preservatives. Manifestations range from rhinitis, chest tightness, weakness, dyspnea (shortness of breath), urticaria, and severe wheezing to loss of consciousness. Ask about usual food intake and whether any breathing problems occur with eating.

Family History and Genetic Risk

Obtain a family history to assess for respiratory disorders that have a genetic component, such as cystic fibrosis, some lung cancers, and emphysema. Patients with asthma often have a family history of allergy. Ask about a history of infectious disease, such as tuberculosis, because family members may have similar environmental exposures.

Current Health Problems

Whether the breathing problem is acute or chronic, the current health problem usually includes cough, sputum production, chest pain, and shortness of breath at rest or on exertion. Explore the current illness in chronologic order. Ask about the onset of the problem, how long it lasts, the location of the problem, how often it occurs, whether the problem has become worse over time, what manifestations occur with it, which actions or interventions provide relief and which ones make it worse, and what treatments have been used.

Cough is a sign of lung disease. Ask the patient how long the cough has been present and whether it occurs at a specific time of day (e.g., on awakening in the morning) or in relation to any physical activity. Ask whether the cough produces sputum or is dry, tickling, or hacking.

Sputum production is an important manifestation associated with coughing. Check the color, consistency, odor, and amount of sputum.

Describe the consistency of sputum as thin, thick, watery, or frothy. Smokers with chronic bronchitis have mucoid sputum. Excessive pink, frothy sputum is common with pulmonary edema. Bacterial pneumonia often produces rust-colored sputum, and foul-smelling sputum often occurs with a lung abscess. Hemoptysis (blood in the sputum) is most often seen in patients with chronic bronchitis or lung cancer. Grossly bloody sputum may occur with tuberculosis, pulmonary infarction, lung cancer, or lung abscess.

Ask the patient to quantify sputum by describing its volume in terms such as teaspoon, tablespoon, and cup. Normally, the lungs can produce up to 90 mL of sputum per day.

Chest pain can occur with other health problems as well as with lung problems. A detailed description of chest pain helps distinguish its cause. Ask the patient whether the pain is continuous or made worse by coughing, deep breathing, or swallowing. Cardiac pain is usually intense and "crushing" and may radiate to the arm, shoulder, or neck. Pulmonary pain varies depending on the cause and most often feels like something is "rubbing" inside. The pain may appear only on deep inhalation or be present at the end of inhalation and the end of exhalation. Pulmonary pain is not made worse by touching or pressing over the area.

Dyspnea (difficulty in breathing or breathlessness) is a subjective perception and varies among patients (Baker et al., 2013). A patient's feeling of dyspnea may not be consistent with the severity of the problem. Determine the type of onset (slow or abrupt); the duration; relieving factors (position changes, drug use, activity cessation); and whether wheezing or stridor occurs with dyspnea.

Try to quantify dyspnea by asking whether this manifestation interferes with ADLs and, if so, how severely. For example, does dyspnea occur after walking one block or climbing one flight of stairs? Table 27-2 classifies dyspnea with changes in ADL performance.

TABLE 27-2 Correlation of Dyspnea Classification with Performance of ADLs

CLASSIFICATION	ADLs KEY
Class I: No significant restrictions in normal activity. Employable. Dyspnea occurs only on more-than-normal or strenuous exertion.	4: No breathlessness, normal.
Class II: Independent in essential ADLs but restricted in some other activities. Dyspneic on climbing stairs or on walking on an incline but not on level walking. Employable only for sedentary job or under special circumstances.	3: Satisfactory, mild breathlessness. Complete performance is possible without pause or assistance but not entirely normal.
Class III: Dyspnea commonly occurs during usual activities, such as showering or dressing, but the patient can manage without assistance from others. Not dyspneic at rest; can walk for more than a city block at own pace but cannot keep up with others of own age. May stop to catch breath partway up a flight of stairs. Is probably not employable in any occupation.	2: Fair, moderate breathlessness. Must stop during activity. Complete performance is possible without assistance, but performance may be too debilitating or time consuming.
Class IV: Dyspnea produces dependence on help in some essential ADLs such as dressing and bathing. Not usually dyspneic at rest. Dyspneic on minimal exertion; must pause on climbing one flight, walking more than 100 yards, or dressing. Often restricted to home if lives alone. Has minimal or no activities outside of home.	1: Poor, marked breathlessness. Incomplete performance; assistance is necessary.
Class V: Entirely restricted to home and often limited to bed or chair. Dyspneic at rest. Dependent on help for most needs.	0: Performance not indicated or recommended; too difficult.

ADLs, Activities of daily living.

Ask about **orthopnea**, which is a shortness of breath occurring when lying down and is relieved by sitting up. Assess for paroxysmal nocturnal dyspnea (PND), which awakens the patient from sleep with the feeling of an inability to breathe. PND also occurs while lying flat and is relieved by sitting up. It often occurs with chronic lung disease and left-sided heart failure.

Physical Assessment
Assessment of the Nose and Sinuses

Inspect the patient's external nose for deformities or polyps, and inspect the nares for symmetry of size and shape. To observe the interior nose, ask the patient to tilt the head back ·for a penlight examination. The experienced nurse may use a nasal speculum and nasopharyngeal mirror for a more thorough inspection of the nasal cavity.

Inspect for color, swelling, drainage, and bleeding. The mucous membrane of the nose normally appears redder than the oral mucosa, but it is pale, engorged, and bluish gray in patients with allergic rhinitis. Check the nasal septum for bleeding, perforation, or deviation. Septal deviation is common and appears as an S shape, tilting toward one side or the other. A perforated septum is present if the light shines through the perforation into the opposite side; this condition is often found in cocaine users. Nasal polyps are pale, shiny, gelatinous lumps or "bags" attached to the turbinates. Block one naris at a time to check how well air moves through the unblocked side.

? NCLEX EXAMINATION CHALLENGE
Physiological Integrity

For which problem does the nurse assess the client who cannot breathe through the nose because of a severe septal deviation?
A. Dry respiratory tract membranes
B. Frequent episodes of tonsillitis
C. Development of nasal polyps
D. Difficulty swallowing

Assessment of the Pharynx, Trachea, and Larynx

Assessment of the pharynx begins with inspection of the mouth. To examine the posterior pharynx, use a tongue depressor to press down one side of the tongue at a time (to avoid stimulating the gag reflex). As the patient says "ah," observe the rise and fall of the soft palate and inspect for color and symmetry, drainage, edema or ulceration, and enlarged tonsils.

Inspect the neck for symmetry, alignment, masses, swelling, bruises, and the use of accessory neck muscles in breathing. Palpate lymph nodes for size, shape, mobility with palpation, consistency, and tenderness.

Gently palpate the trachea for position, mobility, tenderness, and masses. The trachea should be in the midline. Many lung disorders cause the trachea to deviate from the midline. Tension pneumothorax, large pleural effusion, mediastinal mass, and neck tumors push the trachea *away* from the affected area. Pneumonectomy, fibrosis, and atelectasis pull it *toward* the affected area.

The larynx is usually examined by a specialist with a laryngoscope. An abnormal voice, especially hoarseness, may be heard when there are problems of the larynx.

Assessment of the Lungs and Thorax

Inspection. Inspect the front and back of the thorax with the patient sitting up. Normal landmarks of the chest front (anterior) and back (posterior) are shown in Fig. 27-9. The patient should be undressed to the waist. Observe the chest, and compare one side with the other. Work from the top (apex) and move downward toward the base, going from side to side, while inspecting for discoloration, scars, lesions, masses, and spinal curvatures. Assessing from side to side allows you to compare the findings for each lung at the same level (Jarvis, 2016).

Observe the rate, rhythm, and depth of inspirations as well as the symmetry of chest movement. Impaired movement or unequal expansion may indicate disease. Observe the type of breathing (e.g., pursed-lip or diaphragmatic breathing) and the use of accessory muscles.

Examine the shape of the patient's chest, and compare the anteroposterior (AP or front-to-back) diameter with the lateral (side-to-side) diameter. This ratio normally is about 1:1.5, depending on body build. The ratio increases to 1:1 in patients

FIG. 27-9 Anterior and posterior chest landmarks.

with emphysema, which results in the typical barrel-chest appearance.

Normally the ribs slope downward. Patients with air trapping in the lungs caused by emphysema have ribs that are more horizontal. Observe or palpate the distance between the ribs *(intercostal space)*. This distance is usually one finger-breadth (2 centimeters). The distance increases in disorders that cause air trapping, such as emphysema. Observe for retraction of muscle between the ribs and at the sternal notch. Retractions are areas that get sucked inward when the patient inhales. This does not occur during normal respiratory effort. Retractions may occur when the patient is working hard to inhale around an obstruction.

Palpation. Palpate the chest after inspection to assess respiratory movement symmetry and observable abnormalities. Palpation also can help identify areas of tenderness and check vocal or tactile **fremitus** (vibration).

Assess chest expansion by placing your thumbs on the patient's spine at the level of the ninth ribs and extending the fingers sideways around the rib cage. As the patient inhales, both sides of the chest should move upward and outward together in one symmetric movement and move your thumbs apart. On exhalation, the thumbs should come back together as they return to the midline. Unequal expansion may be a result of pain, trauma, or air in the pleural cavity. Respiratory lag or slowed movement on one side indicates a pulmonary problem (Jarvis, 2016).

Palpate any abnormalities found on inspection (e.g., masses, lesions, swelling). Also palpate for tenderness, especially if the patient reports pain. Crepitus (air trapped in and under the skin, also known as *subcutaneous emphysema*) is felt as a crackling sensation beneath the fingertips. Document this finding and report it to the health care provider when it occurs around a wound site or a tracheostomy site or if a pneumothorax is suspected.

FIG. 27-10 Percussion technique.

Tactile (vocal) fremitus is a vibration of the chest wall produced when the patient speaks. This vibration can be felt on the chest wall. Fremitus is decreased if the transmission of sound waves from the larynx to the chest wall is slowed, such as when the pleural space is filled with air (pneumothorax) or fluid (**pleural effusion**) or when the bronchus is obstructed. Fremitus is increased with pneumonia and lung abscesses because the increased density of the chest enhances transmission of the vibrations.

Percussion. Use percussion to assess for pulmonary resonance, the boundaries of organs, and diaphragmatic excursion. Percussion involves tapping the chest wall, which sets the underlying tissues into motion and produces audible sounds (Fig. 27-10). This action produces five different sounds that help determine whether the lung tissue contains air or fluid or is solid (Table 27-3).

TABLE 27-3	**Characteristics of the Five Percussion Notes**				
NOTE	**PITCH**	**INTENSITY**	**QUALITY**	**DURATION**	**FINDINGS**
Resonance	Low	Moderate to loud	Hollow	Long	Resonance is characteristic of normal lung tissue.
Hyperresonance	Higher than resonance	Very loud	Booming	Longer than resonance	Hyperresonance indicates the presence of trapped air, so it is commonly heard over an emphysematous or asthmatic lung and occasionally over a pneumothorax.
Flatness	High	Soft	Extreme dullness	Short	An example location is the sternum. Flatness percussed over the lung fields may indicate a massive pleural effusion.
Dullness	Medium	Medium	Thudlike	Medium	Example locations are over the liver and the kidneys. Dullness can be percussed over an atelectatic lung or a consolidated lung.
Tympany	High	Loud	Musical, drumlike	Short	Examples are the cheek filled with air and the abdomen distended with air. Over the lung, a tympanic note usually indicates a large pneumothorax.

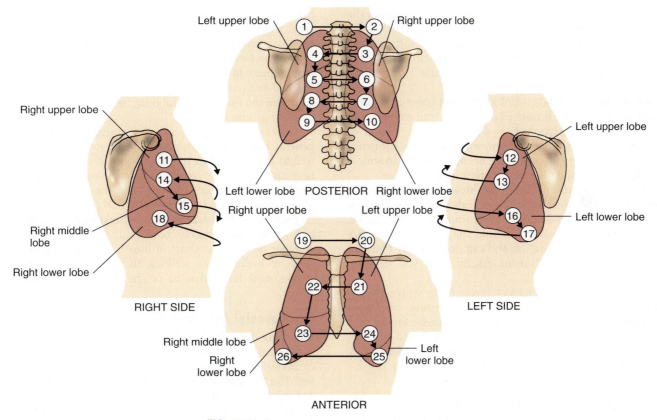

FIG. 27-11 Sequence for percussion and auscultation.

Auscultation. Auscultation includes listening with a stethoscope for normal breath sounds, abnormal (*adventitious*) sounds, and voice sounds. This technique provides information about the flow of air through the trachea and lungs and helps identify fluid, mucus, or obstruction in the respiratory system.

Begin auscultation with the patient sitting in an upright position. With the stethoscope pressed firmly against the chest wall (clothing can muffle sounds), instruct the patient to breathe slowly and deeply through an open mouth. (Breathing through the nose sets up turbulent sounds that are transmitted to the lungs.) Use a systematic approach, beginning at the lung apices and moving from side to side down through the intercostal spaces to the lung bases (Fig. 27-11). Avoid listening over bony structures. Listen to a full respiratory cycle, noting the quality and intensity of the breath sounds.

Normal breath sounds are produced as air vibrates while moving through the passages from the larynx to the alveoli. Breath sounds are identified by their location, intensity, pitch, and duration within the respiratory cycle (e.g., early or late inspiration and expiration). Normal breath sounds are known

TABLE 27-4   **Characteristics of Normal Breath Sounds**

	PITCH	AMPLITUDE	DURATION	QUALITY	NORMAL LOCATION
Bronchial (tubular, tracheal)	High	Loud	Inspiration < expiration	Harsh, hollow, tubular, blowing	Trachea and larynx
Bronchovesicular	Moderate	Moderate	Inspiration = expiration	Mixed	Over major bronchi where fewer alveoli are located; posterior, between scapulae (especially on right); anterior, around upper sternum in first and second intercostal spaces
Vesicular	Low	Soft	Inspiration > expiration	Rustling, like the sound of the wind in the trees	Over peripheral lung fields where air flows through smaller bronchioles and alveoli

From Jarvis, C. (2016). *Physical examination and health assessment* (7th ed.). St. Louis: Saunders.

as "bronchial" or "tubular" (harsh hollow sounds heard over the trachea and mainstem bronchi), "bronchovesicular" (heard over the branching bronchi), and "vesicular" (soft rustling sounds heard in lung tissue over small bronchioles) (Table 27-4). Describe these sounds as *normal, increased, diminished,* or *absent.*

Bronchial breath sounds heard at the lung edges are abnormal and occur when the bronchial sounds are transmitted to an area of increased density, such as with atelectasis, tumor, or pneumonia. When heard in an abnormal location, bronchovesicular breath sounds may indicate normal aging or an abnormality such as consolidation and chronic airway disease.

Adventitious sounds are additional breath sounds superimposed on normal sounds, and they indicate pathologic changes in the lung. Table 27-5 describes adventitious sounds: crackle, wheeze, rhonchus, and pleural friction rub. These sounds vary in pitch, intensity, and duration and can occur in any phase of the respiratory cycle. Document exactly what you hear on auscultation.

Voice sounds (vocal resonance) through the normally air-filled lung are muffled and unclear because sound vibrations travel poorly through air. These sounds become louder and more distinct when the sound travels through a solid tissue or liquid. The presence of pneumonia, atelectasis, pleural effusion, tumor, or abscess causes increased vocal resonance.

❓ NCLEX EXAMINATION CHALLENGE

Physiological Integrity

When auscultating the client's breath sounds, the nurse hears soft rustling sounds at the lung edges. What is the nurse's best action?
A. Listen again with the bell of the stethoscope rather than the diaphragm.
B. Ask the client to cough and spit out any collected mucus.
C. Document the finding as the only action.
D. Notify the health care provider.

Other Indicators of Respiratory Adequacy

Assess other indicators of respiratory adequacy, because GAS EXCHANGE affects all body systems. Some indicators (e.g.,

cyanosis) reflect immediate gas exchange and PERFUSION problems. Other changes (e.g., clubbing, weight loss) reflect long-term oxygenation problems.

Skin and mucous membrane changes (e.g., pallor, cyanosis) may indicate inadequate GAS EXCHANGE and PERFUSION. Assess the nail beds and the mucous membranes of the oral cavity. Examine the fingers for clubbing (see Fig. 30-10), which indicates long-term hypoxia.

General appearance includes muscle development and general body build. Long-term respiratory problems lead to weight loss and a loss of general muscle mass. Arms and legs may appear thin or poorly muscled. Neck and chest muscles may be hypertrophied, especially in the patient with chronic obstructive pulmonary disease (COPD) (McCance et al., 2014).

Endurance decreases whenever breathing is inadequate for GAS EXCHANGE. Observe how easily the patient moves and whether he or she is short of breath while resting or becomes short of breath when walking 10 to 20 steps. As the patient speaks, note how often he or she pauses for breath between words.

Psychosocial Assessment

Breathing difficulty from any cause often induces anxiety. The patient may be anxious because of reduced oxygen to the brain or because the sensation of not getting enough air is frightening. The thought of having a serious respiratory problem, such as lung cancer, can also induce anxiety. Encourage the patient to express his or her feelings and fears about manifestations and their possible meaning.

Assess those aspects of the patient's lifestyle that either can affect respiratory function or are affected by it. Some respiratory problems may become worse with stress. Ask about current life stresses and usual coping mechanisms.

Chronic respiratory disease may cause changes in family roles or relationships, social isolation, financial problems, and unemployment or disability. Discuss coping mechanisms to assess the patient's reaction to these stressors and identify strengths. For example, the patient may react to stress with dependence on family members, withdrawal, or failure to adhere to interventions. Assist the patient to identify available support systems.

TABLE 27-5   Characteristics of Adventitious Breath Sounds

ADVENTITIOUS SOUND	CHARACTER	ASSOCIATION
Fine crackles Fine rales High-pitched rales	Popping, discontinuous sounds caused by air moving into previously deflated airways; sounds like hair being rolled between fingers near the ear "Velcro" sounds late in inspiration usually associated with restrictive disorders	Asbestosis Atelectasis Interstitial fibrosis Bronchitis Pneumonia Chronic pulmonary diseases
Coarse crackles Low-pitched crackles	Lower-pitched, coarse, rattling sounds caused by fluid or secretions in large airways; likely to change with coughing or suctioning	Bronchitis Pneumonia Tumors Pulmonary edema
Wheeze	Squeaky, musical, continuous sounds associated with air rushing through narrowed airways; may be heard without a stethoscope Arise from the small airways Usually do not clear with coughing	Inflammation Bronchospasm Edema Secretions Pulmonary vessel engorgement (as in cardiac "asthma")
Rhonchus (rhonchi)	Lower-pitched, coarse, continuous snoring sounds Arise from the large airways	Thick, tenacious secretions Sputum production Obstruction by foreign body Tumors
Pleural friction rub	Loud, rough, grating, scratching sounds caused by the inflamed surfaces of the pleura rubbing together; often associated with pain on deep inspirations Heard in lateral lung fields	Pleurisy Tuberculosis Pulmonary infarction Pneumonia Lung cancer

? CLINICAL JUDGMENT CHALLENGE

Patient-Centered-Care; Teamwork and Collaboration QSEN

The patient is a 68-year-old man who has had shortness of breath (SOB) for the past 2 to 3 days. His past medical history includes a 40–pack-year smoking history, COPD, and heart failure. He reports that he became concerned when he woke from sleep because he could not breathe. Your physical assessment reveals crackles in the lower lobes bilaterally. His oxygen saturation (SpO$_2$) is 84% without supplemental oxygen.

1. What are some areas of focus to assess as part of this patient's current history?
2. Whom should you contact and why?
3. What are some factors that may affect gas exchange for this patient?
4. What additional referrals might be appropriate for this patient?

Diagnostic Assessment

Laboratory Assessment

Several laboratory tests (Chart 27-3) are useful in assessing respiratory problems. A red blood cell (RBC) count provides data about the transport of oxygen. Hemoglobin, found in RBCs, transports oxygen to the tissues. A deficiency of hemoglobin could cause hypoxemia.

Arterial blood gas (ABG) analysis assesses GAS EXCHANGE and PERFUSION as oxygenation (partial pressure of arterial oxygen [Pao$_2$]), alveolar ventilation (partial pressure of arterial carbon dioxide [Paco$_2$]), and acid-base balance. Blood gas studies provide information for monitoring treatment results, adjusting oxygen therapy, and evaluating the patient's responses (Barnette & Kautz, 2013). See Chapter 12 for more details on blood gas analysis.

Sputum specimens can help identify organisms or abnormal cells. Sputum culture and sensitivity analyses identify bacterial infection and determine which specific antibiotics will be most effective. Cytologic examination can identify cancer cells. Allergic conditions may be identified by cytologic testing. Eosinophils and Curschmann's spirals (a mucus form) are often found by cytologic study in patients with allergic asthma.

Imaging Assessment

Chest x-rays with digital images are used for patients with pulmonary problems to evaluate the status of the chest and to provide a baseline for comparison with future changes. These chest x-rays are performed from **posteroanterior** (PA; back to front) and left lateral (LL) positions.

Chest x-rays are used to assess lung pathology such as with pneumonia, atelectasis, pneumothorax, and tumor. They also can detect pleural fluid and the placement of an endotracheal tube or other invasive catheters. A computer-enhanced image can be adjusted to emphasize a specific area. These images have limitations, however, and may appear normal, even when severe chronic bronchitis, asthma, or emphysema is present.

Sinus and facial x-rays are used to assess fluid levels in the sinus cavities to assist in the diagnosis of acute or chronic sinusitis.

Computed tomography (CT) assesses soft tissues with consecutive cross-sectional views of the entire chest. This type of imaging can verify the identity of a suspicious lesion or clot. Often CT scans require a contrast agent injected IV to enhance the visibility of structures such as tumors, blood vessels, and heart chambers. These scans assist in making a diagnosis. Your role in this diagnostic test is to provide information to the patient and to determine whether the patient has any sensitivity to the contrast material. Ask the patient whether he or she has a known allergy to iodine or shellfish. In addition, IV contrast

CHART 27-3 Laboratory Profile

Respiratory Assessment

TEST	NORMAL RANGE FOR ADULTS	SIGNIFICANCE OF ABNORMAL FINDINGS
Blood Studies		
Complete Blood Count		
Red blood cells	*Females:* 4.2-5.4 million/mm^3 *Males:* 4.7-6.1 million/mm^3	*Elevated levels* (polycythemia) often related to the excessive production of erythropoietin in response to a chronic hypoxic state, as in COPD, and from living at a high altitude. *Decreased levels* indicate possible anemia, hemorrhage, or hemolysis.
Hemoglobin, total	*Females:* 12-16 g/dL, or 7.4-9.9 mmol/L *Males:* 14-18 g/dL, or 8.7-11.2 mmol/L	Same as for red blood cells.
Hematocrit	*Females:* 37%-47%, or 0.37-0.47 SI units *Males:* 42%-52%, or 0.42-0.52 SI units	Same as for red blood cells.
White blood cell count (leukocyte count, WBC count)	*Total:* 5,000-10,000/mm^3	*Elevations* indicate possible acute infections or inflammations. *Decreased levels* may indicate an overwhelming infection, an autoimmune disorder, or immunosuppressant therapy.
Differential White Blood Cell (Leukocyte) Count		
Neutrophils	2500-8000/mm^3, or 55%-70% of total	*Elevations* indicate possible acute bacterial infection (pneumonia), COPD, or inflammatory conditions (smoking). *Decreased levels* indicate possible viral disease (influenza).
Eosinophils	50-500/mm^3, or 1%-4% of total	*Elevations* indicate possible COPD, asthma, or allergies. *Decreased levels* indicate pyogenic infections.
Basophils	25-100/mm^3, or 0.5%-1% of total	*Elevations* indicate possible inflammation; seen in chronic sinusitis, hypersensitivity reactions. *Decreased levels* may be seen in an acute infection.
Lymphocytes	1000-4000/mm^3, or 20%-40% of total	*Elevations* indicate possible viral infection, pertussis, and infectious mononucleosis. *Decreased levels* may be seen during corticosteroid therapy.
Monocytes	100-700/mm^3, or 2%-8% of total	*Elevations:* see Lymphocytes; also may indicate active tuberculosis. *Decreased levels:* see Lymphocytes.
Arterial Blood Gases		
Pao$_2$	80-100 mm Hg *Older adults:* values may be lower	*Elevations* indicate possible excessive oxygen administration. *Decreased levels* indicate possible COPD, asthma, chronic bronchitis, cancer of the bronchi and lungs, cystic fibrosis, respiratory distress syndrome, anemias, atelectasis, or any other cause of hypoxia.
Paco$_2$	35-45 mm Hg	*Elevations* indicate possible COPD, asthma, pneumonia, anesthesia effects, or use of opioids (respiratory acidosis). *Decreased levels* indicate hyperventilation/respiratory alkalosis.
pH	*Up to 60 yr:* 7.35-7.45 *60-90 yr:* 7.31-7.42 *>90 yr:* 7.26-7.43	*Elevations* indicate metabolic or respiratory alkalosis. *Decreased levels* indicate metabolic or respiratory acidosis.
HCO$_3$	21-28 mEq/L	*Elevations* indicate possible respiratory acidosis as compensation for a primary metabolic alkalosis. *Decreased levels* indicate possible respiratory alkalosis as compensation for a primary metabolic acidosis.
Spo$_2$	95%-100% *Older adults:* values may be slightly lower	*Decreased levels* indicate possible impaired ability of hemoglobin to release oxygen to tissues.

COPD, Chronic obstructive pulmonary disease; *HCO$_3$,* bicarbonate ion; *Paco$_2$,* partial pressure of arterial carbon dioxide; *Pao$_2$,* partial pressure of arterial oxygen; *Spo$_2$,* peripheral oxygen saturation.

material can be nephrotoxic. Ask about his or her kidney function and whether he or she takes drugs for type 2 diabetes. If the patient usually takes metformin, the drug is stopped at least 24 hours before contrast dye is used and is not restarted until adequate kidney function has been established (see Chapter 64).

Other Noninvasive Diagnostic Assessment

Pulse Oximetry. Pulse oximetry identifies hemoglobin saturation with oxygen. Usually hemoglobin is almost 100% saturated with oxygen in superficial tissues. The pulse oximeter uses a wave of infrared light and a sensor placed on the patient's finger, toe, nose, earlobe, or forehead (Fig. 27-12). Ideal normal pulse oximetry values are 95% to 100%. Normal values are a little lower in older patients and in patients with dark skin. To avoid confusion with the Pao$_2$ values from arterial blood gases, pulse oximetry readings are recorded as the Spo$_2$ (peripheral arterial oxygen saturation) or Sao$_2$.

Pulse oximetry can detect desaturation before manifestations (e.g., dusky skin, pale mucosa, pale or blue nail beds) occur. Causes for low readings include patient movement, hypothermia, decreased peripheral blood flow, ambient light (sunlight, infrared lamps), decreased hemoglobin, edema, and

FIG. 27-12 A typical pulse oximeter.

fingernail polish. When patients have any degree of impaired peripheral blood flow, the most accurate place to test oxygen saturation is on the forehead. Covering the sensor with a fingertip cut from a glove or changing its position may help accuracy if too much ambient light is present.

Results lower than 91% (and certainly below 86%) are an emergency and require immediate assessment and treatment. When the SpO_2 is below 85%, body tissues have a difficult time becoming oxygenated. An SpO_2 lower than 70% is usually life threatening, but in some cases, values below 80% may be life threatening. Pulse oximetry is less accurate at lower values.

Capnometry and Capnography. Capnometry and capnography are methods that measure the amount of carbon dioxide present in exhaled air, which is an indirect measurement of arterial carbon dioxide levels. These noninvasive tests measure the partial-pressure of end-tidal carbon dioxide ($PETCO_2$, also known as $ETCO_2$) levels in both intubated patients and those breathing spontaneously. With capnometry, the exhaled air sample is tested with a sensor that changes the CO_2 level into a color or number for analysis. With capnography, the CO_2 level is graphed as a specific waveform along with a number. These methods provide information about CO_2 production, pulmonary perfusion, alveolar ventilation, respiratory patterns, ventilator effectiveness, and possible rebreathing of exhaled air (Carlisle, 2014).

The normal value of the partial pressure of end-tidal carbon dioxide ($PETCO_2$) ranges between 20 and 40 mm Hg. Changes in $PETCO_2$ reflect changes in breathing effectiveness and GAS EXCHANGE. These changes occur before hypoxia can be detected using pulse oximetry. The use of both pulse oximetry and $PETCO_2$ for patients at risk for respiratory problems can provide information to direct early intervention (Carlisle, 2014).

Conditions that increase $PETCO_2$ above normal levels are those that reflect inadequate GAS EXCHANGE or an increase in cellular metabolism, both of which increase production of carbon dioxide (CO_2). Conditions of inadequate gas exchange include hypoventilation, partial airway obstruction, and rebreathing exhaled air. Conditions that increase cellular metabolism include fever, acidosis, and heavy exercise.

Conditions that decrease $PETCO_2$ below normal levels are those that reflect poor pulmonary ventilation, such as pulmonary embolism, apnea, total airway obstruction, and tracheal extubation. Other causes of low $PETCO_2$ include hyperventilation not based on oxygen need in which CO_2 is "blown off" faster than it is generated in the tissues.

Pulmonary Function Tests. Pulmonary function tests (PFTs) assess lung function and breathing problems. These tests measure lung volumes and capacities, flow rates, diffusion capacity, GAS EXCHANGE, airway resistance, and distribution of ventilation. The results are interpreted by comparing the patient's data with expected findings for age, gender, race, height, weight, and smoking status.

The PFTs are useful in screening patients for lung disease even before the onset of manifestations. Repeated testing over time provides data that may be used to guide management (e.g., changes in lung function can support a decision to continue, change, or discontinue a specific therapy). Testing before surgery may identify patients at risk for lung complications after surgery. The most common reason for performing PFTs is to determine the cause of dyspnea. When performed while the patient exercises, PFTs help determine whether dyspnea is caused by lung or cardiac dysfunction or by muscle weakness.

Patient Preparation. Explain the purpose of the tests, and advise the patient not to smoke for 6 to 8 hours before testing. Depending on the reasons for testing, bronchodilator drugs may be withheld for 4 to 6 hours before the test. The patient with breathing problems often fears further breathlessness and is anxious before these "breathing" tests. Help reduce anxiety by describing what will happen during and after the testing.

Procedure. PFTs can be performed at the bedside or in the respiratory laboratory by a respiratory therapist or respiratory technician. The patient is asked to breathe through the mouth only. A nose clip may be used to prevent air from escaping. The patient performs different breathing maneuvers while measurements are obtained. Table 27-6 describes the most commonly used PFTs and their uses.

Follow-up Care. Because many breathing maneuvers are performed during PFTs, assess the patient for increased dyspnea or bronchospasm after these studies. Document any drugs given during testing.

Exercise Testing. Exercise increases metabolism and increases gas transport because energy is used. Exercise testing assesses the patient's ability to work and perform ADLs, differentiates reasons for exercise limitation, evaluates disease influence on exercise capacity, and determines whether supplemental oxygen is needed during exercise. These tests are performed on a treadmill or bicycle or by a self-paced 12-minute walking test. Exercise in the patient with normal pulmonary function is limited by circulatory factors, whereas exercise in the pulmonary patient is limited by breathing capacity, GAS EXCHANGE compromise, or both. Explain exercise testing, and assure the patient that he or she will be closely monitored by trained professionals throughout the test.

Skin Tests. Skin tests are used with other diagnostic data to identify various infectious diseases (e.g., tuberculosis), viral diseases (e.g., mononucleosis, mumps), and fungal diseases (e.g., coccidioidomycosis, histoplasmosis). Allergies and the status of the immune system also can be checked through skin testing. (See Chapters 17 and 20 for further discussion of these tests.)

Other Invasive Diagnostic Assessment

Endoscopic Examinations. Endoscopic studies to assess breathing problems include bronchoscopy, laryngoscopy, and mediastinoscopy. With *laryngoscopy,* a tube for visualization is

TABLE 27-6 Characteristics and Purposes of Pulmonary Function Tests

TEST	PURPOSE
FVC (forced vital capacity) records the maximum amount of air that can be exhaled as quickly as possible after maximum inspiration.	Indicates respiratory muscle strength and ventilatory reserve. Reduced in obstructive and restrictive diseases.
FEV$_1$ (forced expiratory volume in 1 sec) records the maximum amount of air that can be exhaled in the first second of expiration.	Is effort dependent and declines normally with age. It is reduced in certain obstructive and restrictive disorders.
FEV$_1$/FVC is the ratio of expiratory volume in 1 sec to FVC.	Indicates obstruction to airflow. This ratio is the hallmark of obstructive pulmonary disease. It is normal or increased in restrictive disease.
FEF$_{25\%-75\%}$ records the forced expiratory flow over the 25%-75% volume (middle half) of the FVC.	This measure provides a more sensitive index of obstruction in the smaller airways.
FRC (functional residual capacity) is the amount of air remaining in the lungs after normal expiration. FRC test requires use of the helium dilution, nitrogen washout, or body plethysmography technique.	Increased FRC indicates hyperinflation or air trapping, often from obstructive pulmonary disease. FRC is normal or decreased in restrictive pulmonary diseases.
TLC (total lung capacity) is the amount of air in the lungs at the end of maximum inhalation.	Increased TLC indicates air trapping from obstructive pulmonary disease. Decreased TLC indicates restrictive disease.
RV (residual volume) is the amount of air remaining in the lungs at the end of a full, forced exhalation.	RV is increased in obstructive pulmonary disease such as emphysema.
DLCO (diffusion capacity of the lung for carbon monoxide) reflects the surface area of the alveolocapillary membrane. The patient inhales a small amount of CO, holds for 10 sec, and then exhales. The amount inhaled is compared with the amount exhaled.	Is reduced whenever the alveolocapillary membrane is diminished (emphysema, pulmonary hypertension, and pulmonary fibrosis). It is increased with exercise and in conditions such as polycythemia and congestive heart disease.

inserted into the larynx to assess the function of the vocal cords, remove foreign bodies caught in the larynx, or obtain tissue samples for biopsy or culture. A *mediastinoscopy* is the insertion of a flexible tube through the chest wall just above the sternum into the area between the lungs. It is performed in the operating room with the patient under general anesthesia to examine for the presence of tumors and to obtain tissue samples for biopsy or culture. Most complications are related to the anesthetic agents and bleeding. The most common procedure is the bronchoscopy.

A bronchoscopy is the insertion of a tube in the airways, usually as far as the secondary bronchi, to view airway structures and obtain tissue samples for biopsy or culture. It is used to diagnose and manage pulmonary diseases. Rigid bronchoscopy usually requires general anesthesia in the operating room. Flexible bronchoscopy can be performed in the intensive care unit (ICU) with low-dose sedation. A flexible bronchoscopy is used to evaluate the airway and to assist with placing or changing an endotracheal tube, collecting specimens, and diagnosing infections. It is often used for lung cancer staging and removal of secretions that are not cleared with normal suctioning procedures. Stents can be placed during bronchoscopy to open up strictures in the trachea and bronchus.

Patient Preparation. Explain the procedure to the patient, and verify that consent for the procedure was obtained. Expected outcomes, risks, and benefits of the procedure must be discussed with the patient by the health care provider performing the procedure. Document patient allergies. Other tests before the procedure may include a complete blood count, platelet count, prothrombin time, electrolytes, and chest x-ray. The patient should be NPO for 4 to 8 hours before the procedure to reduce the risk for aspiration. Premedication with one of the benzodiazepines may be used to provide both sedation and amnesia. Opioids may also be used.

> **! NURSING SAFETY PRIORITY (QSEN)**
> *Critical Rescue*
>
> In accordance with The Joint Commission's National Patient Safety Goals, verify the patient's identity with *two* types of identifiers (name and at least one person-specific number such as birth date, medical record number, or Social Security number) before a bronchoscopy.

Benzocaine spray as a topical anesthetic to numb the oropharynx is used cautiously, if at all. This agent may induce a condition called methemoglobinemia, which is the conversion of normal hemoglobin to methemoglobin (Wesley, 2014). Methemoglobin is an altered iron state that does not carry oxygen, resulting in tissue hypoxia. Other topical anesthetic sprays, such as lidocaine, appear less likely to induce this problem.

The normal blood level of methemoglobin is less than 1%. When this level increases, tissue GAS EXCHANGE is reduced. Cyanosis occurs with methemoglobin levels between 10% and 20%, and death can occur when levels reach 50% to 70%. Suspect methemoglobinemia if a patient becomes cyanotic after receiving a topical anesthetic, if he or she does not respond to supplemental oxygen, and if blood is a characteristic chocolate-brown in color. It can be reversed with oxygen and IV injection of 1% methylene blue (1 to 2 mg/kg).

> **! NURSING SAFETY PRIORITY (QSEN)**
> *Critical Rescue*
>
> Notify the Rapid Response Team if the patient has any manifestations of methemoglobinemia (cyanosis unresponsive to oxygen therapy, chocolate-brown–colored blood) after the use of benzocaine topical anesthetic.

Procedure. The procedure can be done in a bronchoscopy suite or at the ICU bedside. The bronchoscope is inserted through either the naris or the oropharynx. Maintain IV access, and continuously monitor the patient's pulse, blood pressure, respiratory rate, and oxygen saturation. Apply supplemental oxygen.

Follow-up Care. Monitor the patient until the effects of the sedation have resolved and a gag reflex has returned. Continue to monitor vital signs, including oxygen saturation, and assess breath sounds every 15 minutes for the first 2 hours. Also assess for potential complications, including bleeding, infection, or hypoxemia.

Thoracentesis. Thoracentesis is the needle aspiration of pleural fluid or air from the pleural space for diagnostic or management purposes. Microscopic examination of the pleural fluid helps in making a diagnosis. Pleural fluid may be drained to relieve blood vessel or lung compression and the respiratory distress caused by cancer, empyema, pleurisy, or tuberculosis. Drugs can also be instilled into the pleural space during thoracentesis.

Patient Preparation. Patient preparation is essential before thoracentesis to ensure cooperation during the procedure and to prevent complications. Tell the patient to expect a stinging sensation from the local anesthetic agent and a feeling of pressure when the needle is pushed through the posterior chest. Stress the importance of not moving, coughing, or deep breathing during the procedure to avoid puncture of the pleura or lung.

Ask the patient about any allergy to local anesthetic agents. Verify that the patient has signed an informed consent. The entire chest or back is exposed, and the hair on the skin over the aspiration site is clipped if necessary. The site depends on the volume and location of the fluid.

Fig. 27-13 shows the best position for thoracentesis, which widens the spaces between the ribs and permits easy access to the pleural fluid. Properly position and physically support the patient during the procedure. Use pillows to make the patient comfortable and to provide physical support. When the sitting position is used for the procedure, stand in front of the patient to prevent the table from moving and the patient from falling.

Procedure. Thoracentesis is often performed at the bedside by a nurse practitioner or a physician, although CT or ultrasound may be used to guide it. The person performing the procedure and any assistants wear goggles and masks to prevent accidental eye or oral splash exposure to the pleural fluid. After the skin is prepped, a local anesthetic is injected into the selected site. Keep the patient informed of the procedure while observing for shock, pain, nausea, pallor, diaphoresis, cyanosis, tachypnea, and dyspnea.

The short 18- to 25-gauge thoracentesis needle (with an attached syringe) is advanced into the pleural space. Fluid in the pleural space is slowly aspirated with gentle suction. A vacuum collection bottle may be needed to remove larger volumes of fluid. To prevent re-expansion pulmonary edema, usually no more than 1000 mL of fluid is removed at one time. If a biopsy is performed, a second, larger needle with a cutting edge and collection chamber is used. After the needle is withdrawn, pressure is applied to the puncture site and a sterile dressing is applied. In some cases, pigtail drain catheters may be left in place to a waterseal drainage system, rather than doing a thoracentesis aspiration on a recurring basis.

Follow-up Care. After thoracentesis, a chest x-ray is performed to rule out possible pneumothorax and **mediastinal shift** (shift of central thoracic structures toward one side). Monitor vital signs, and listen to the lungs for absent or reduced sounds on the affected side. Check the puncture site and dressing for leakage or bleeding. Assess for complications, such as reaccumulation of fluid in the pleural space, subcutaneous emphysema, infection, and tension pneumothorax. Urge the patient to breathe deeply to promote lung expansion. Document the procedure, including the patient's response; the volume and character of the fluid removed; any specimens sent to the laboratory; the location of the puncture site; and respiratory assessment findings before, during, and after the procedure.

Teach the patient about the manifestations of a **pneumothorax** (partial or complete collapse of the lung), which can occur within the first 24 hours after a thoracentesis. Manifestations include:

- Pain on the affected side that is worse at the end of inhalation and the end of exhalation
- Rapid heart rate
- Rapid, shallow respirations
- A feeling of air hunger
- Prominence of the affected side that does not move in and out with respiratory effort
- Trachea slanted more to the unaffected side instead of being in the center of the neck
- New onset of "nagging" cough
- Cyanosis

Instruct the patient to go to the nearest emergency department immediately if these manifestations occur.

Lung Biopsy. A lung biopsy is performed to obtain tissue for histologic analysis, culture, or cytologic examination. The samples are used to make a definite diagnosis of inflammation, cancer, infection, or lung disease. There are several types of lung biopsies. The site and extent of the lesion determine which one is used. Transbronchial biopsy (TBB) and transbronchial needle aspiration (TBNA) are performed during bronchoscopy. Transthoracic needle aspiration is performed through the skin (percutaneous) for areas that cannot be reached by bronchoscopy.

Patient Preparation. The patient may worry about the outcome of the biopsy and may associate the term *biopsy* with *cancer*. Explain what to expect before and after the procedure, and explore the patient's feelings. An analgesic or sedative may be prescribed before the procedure. Inform the patient

FIG. 27-13 Position for thoracentesis.

undergoing percutaneous biopsy that discomfort is reduced with a local anesthetic agent but that pressure may be felt during needle insertion and tissue aspiration. Open lung biopsy is performed in the operating room with the patient under general anesthesia, and the usual preparations before surgery apply (see Chapter 14).

Procedure. Percutaneous lung biopsy is usually performed in the radiology department after an informed consent has been obtained. Fluoroscopy or CT is often used to visualize the area and guide the procedure. The patient is usually placed in the side-lying position, depending on the location of the lesion. The skin is cleansed with an antiseptic agent, and a local anesthetic is given. Under sterile conditions, a spinal-type needle is inserted through the skin into the desired area and tissue is obtained for microscopic examination. Apply a dressing after the procedure. A CT scan or chest x-ray must follow the biopsy to confirm there is no pneumothorax.

An open lung biopsy is performed in the operating room. The patient undergoes a thoracotomy in which lung tissue is exposed and appropriate tissue specimens are taken. A chest tube is placed to remove air and fluid so the lung can re-inflate, and then the chest is closed.

Follow-up Care. Monitor the patient's vital signs and breath sounds at least every 4 hours for 24 hours, and assess for signs of respiratory distress (e.g., dyspnea, pallor, diaphoresis, tachypnea). Pneumothorax is a serious complication of needle biopsy and open lung biopsy. Report reduced or absent breath sounds immediately. Monitor for hemoptysis (which may be scant and transient) or, in rare cases, for frank bleeding from vascular or lung trauma.

 CLINICAL JUDGMENT CHALLENGE

Safety; Patient-Centered Care; Teamwork and Collaboration QSEN

Your patient is the 68-year-old man from the previous *Clinical Judgment Challenge* who had shortness of breath (SOB) for the past 2 to 3 days. His clinical condition deteriorated further, requiring intubation. The health care provider orders a CT scan of the chest.
1. What are your responsibilities when preparing the patient for the CT scan?
2. Why is it important to monitor your patient using capnography?
3. A large fluid collection on the left side is found during the CT scan, and a thoracentesis is planned. What are your responsibilities in preparing for and assisting with this procedure?
4. Your patient was extubated after the left thoracentesis. Within 12 hours he again develops respiratory distress, decreased breath sounds, and a trachea that appears deviated to the right. What is your assessment?

NURSING CONCEPTS AND CLINICAL JUDGMENT REVIEW

What might you NOTICE in a patient with adequate GAS EXCHANGE and tissue PERFUSION related to respiratory function?

Vital signs:
- Respiratory rate and heart rate within normal range
- Oxygen saturation of 95% or higher

Physical assessment:
- Able to speak a sentence of 12 words without stopping for breath
- Able to walk and talk without stopping for breath
- Skin color normal (no cyanosis or pallor)
- Oral mucous membrane and nail beds pink with rapid capillary refill
- Fingertips and nails normal shape, no clubbing
- Anterior to posterior diameter of chest about two-thirds the size of the lateral diameter
- Space between each rib no larger than the breadth of the patient's finger

- Usually breathes in through the nose and out through the mouth or nose
- Breathing quiet
- Air movement heard (with a stethoscope) in all lobes of both lungs
- Sputum production minimal, clear or white
- Muscle development even with no muscle loss on arms and legs
- Weight proportionate to height; does not appear underweight

Psychological assessment:
- Oriented and not confused
- Energy level good, can engage in desired work, recreational, and personal activities

Laboratory assessment:
- Red blood cell, hemoglobin, hematocrit, and white blood cell levels within normal limits for age and gender

GET READY FOR THE NCLEX® EXAMINATION!

KEY POINTS

Review these Key Points for each NCLEX Client Needs Category.

Health Promotion and Maintenance

- Assess any patient's geographic, home, occupational, and recreational exposure to inhalation irritants. **Patient-Centered Care** QSEN
- Encourage all people to use masks and adequate ventilation when exposed to inhalation irritants.
- Promote smoking cessation for people who smoke. **Patient-Centered Care** QSEN
- Support the person who chooses to stop smoking by assisting him or her to decide about drug therapy for smoking cessation and finding an appropriate smoking-cessation program. **Patient-Centered Care** QSEN

Psychosocial Integrity

- Allow the patient the opportunity to express fear or anxiety about tests of respiratory function or about a potential change in respiratory function. **Patient-Centered Care** QSEN
- Teach patients and family members about what to expect during tests and procedures to assess respiratory function and respiratory disease. **Patient-Centered Care** QSEN

Physiological Integrity

- Ask the patient about respiratory problems in any other members of the family, because some problems have a genetic component. **Patient-Centered Care** QSEN

- Ask the patient about current and past drug use (prescribed, over-the-counter, and illicit), and evaluate drug use for potential lung damage.
- Calculate the pack-year smoking history for the patient who smokes or who has ever smoked cigarettes. **Patient-Centered Care** QSEN
- Use concepts of anatomy and appropriate psychomotor skills to apply respiratory assessment techniques correctly.
- Distinguish between normal and abnormal (adventitious) breath sounds.
- Interpret arterial blood gas values to assess the patient's respiratory status.
- Assess the degree to which breathing problems interfere with the patient's ability to perform ADLs. **Patient-Centered Care** QSEN
- Document any known specific allergies that have respiratory manifestations. **Patient-Centered Care** QSEN
- Assess the airway and breathing effectiveness for any patient who has shortness of breath or any change in mental status. **Evidence-Based Practice** QSEN
- Assess the patient's respiratory status every 15 minutes for at least the first 2 hours after undergoing an endoscopic test for respiratory disorders. **Patient-Centered Care** QSEN
- Explain nursing care needs for the patient after bronchoscopy or open lung biopsy.

28 | CHAPTER

Care of Patients Requiring Oxygen Therapy or Tracheostomy

Harry Rees

 http://evolve.elsevier.com/Iggy/

PRIORITY CONCEPTS

- GAS EXCHANGE
- PERFUSION

LEARNING OUTCOMES

Safe and Effective Care Environment

1. Act as a patient advocate for patients receiving oxygen or who have tracheostomies.
2. Protect the patient receiving oxygen or who has a tracheostomy from injury and infection.

Health Promotion and Maintenance

3. Teach the patient and family how to avoid injury and complications related to oxygen therapy or tracheostomy in the home.

Psychosocial Integrity

4. Reduce the psychological impact of oxygen therapy or tracheostomy for the patient and family.

5. Work with other members of the health care team to ensure that patient values, preferences, and expressed needs related to a tracheostomy and oxygen therapy are respected.

Physiological Integrity

6. Apply knowledge of anatomy and physiology to perform a focused respiratory assessment and re-assessment to determine adequacy of GAS EXCHANGE, oxygenation, and tissue PERFUSION for the patient receiving oxygen therapy or who has a tracheostomy.
7. Use appropriate techniques to administer prescribed oxygen therapy.
8. Use appropriate techniques to provide tracheostomy care.

Oxygen (O_2) is an essential element that serves as a nutrient for all cells to live and perform their specific jobs. For cells to receive oxygen, GAS EXCHANGE must occur first in the lungs and then at the tissue level with PERFUSION of oxygenated blood. These processes rely on three systems—the respiratory system, the cardiovascular system, and the hematologic system—to work together to ensure sufficient oxygen for cell survival and proper function (see Fig. 27-1). Gas exchange with oxygenation and tissue perfusion needs can go unmet as a result of many problems with the lungs. When a respiratory problem interferes with adequate gas exchange, both the cardiac system and the hematologic system adjust (compensate) and work harder to restore balance and maintain oxygenation and tissue perfusion (Fig. 28-1) (McCance et al., 2014). Oxygen therapy through various delivery systems, including tracheostomy, can help improve gas exchange and tissue perfusion and reduce the burden on the cardiovascular and hematologic systems.

OXYGEN THERAPY

Oxygen (O_2) is a gas used as a drug for relief of **hypoxemia** (low levels of oxygen in the blood) and **hypoxia** (decreased tissue oxygenation). The oxygen content of atmospheric air is about 21%. Oxygen therapy is prescribed for both acute and chronic breathing problems when the oxygen needs of the patient cannot be met by atmospheric or "room air" alone. Indications for use include decreased partial pressure of arterial oxygen (Pao_2) levels or decreased arterial oxygen saturation (Sao_2). Non-respiratory conditions, such as heart failure, sepsis, fever, some poisons, and decreased hemoglobin levels or poor hemoglobin quality, can affect GAS EXCHANGE and oxygenation and are indications for oxygen therapy. These conditions increase oxygen demand, decrease the oxygen-carrying capability of the blood, or decrease cardiac output.

The purpose of oxygen therapy is to use the lowest *fraction of inspired oxygen (Fio₂)* to have an acceptable blood oxygen level without causing harmful side effects. *Although oxygen improves the Pao₂ level, it does not cure the problem or stop the disease process.* Most patients with hypoxia require an oxygen flow of 2 to 4 L/min via nasal cannula or up to 40% via Venturi mask to achieve an oxygen saturation of at least 95%. For a patient who is hypoxemic and has chronic **hypercarbia** (increased partial pressure of arterial carbon dioxide [$Paco_2$] levels), the Fio_2 delivered should be titrated to correct the

NORMAL TISSUE OXYGEN NEEDS AND PROBLEMS OF
OXYGEN INTAKE WITH NORMAL OXYGEN DELIVERY

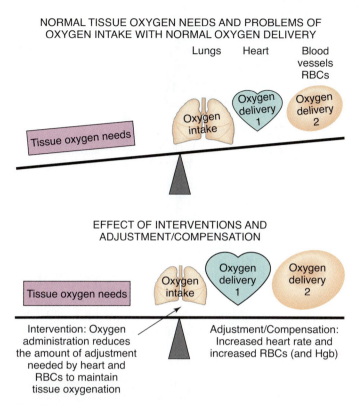

EFFECT OF INTERVENTIONS AND
ADJUSTMENT/COMPENSATION

Intervention: Oxygen administration reduces the amount of adjustment needed by heart and RBCs to maintain tissue oxygenation

Adjustment/Compensation: Increased heart rate and increased RBCs (and Hgb)

FIG. 28-1 Restoration of adequate oxygenation and tissue perfusion by oxygen delivery adjustments and oxygen therapy when respiratory problems interfere with meeting tissue oxygen needs. *Hgb,* Hemoglobin, *RBCs,* red blood cells.

CHART 28-1 Best Practice for Patient Safety & Quality Care (QSEN)

Oxygen Therapy

- Check the health care provider's prescription with the type of delivery system and liter flow or percentage of oxygen actually in use.
- Obtain a prescription for humidification if oxygen is being delivered at 4 L/min or more.
- Be sure the oxygen and humidification equipment are functioning properly.
- Check the skin around the patient's ears, back of the neck, and face every 4 to 8 hours for pressure points and signs of irritation.
- Ensure that mouth care is provided every 8 hours and as needed; assess nasal and oral mucous membranes for cracks or other signs of dryness.
- Pad the elastic band and change its position frequently to prevent skin breakdown.
- Pad tubing in areas that put pressure on the skin.
- Cleanse the cannula or mask by rinsing with clear, warm water every 4 to 8 hours or as needed.
- Cleanse skin under the tubing, straps, and mask every 4 to 8 hours or as needed.
- Lubricate the patient's nostrils, face, and lips with non-petroleum cream to relieve the drying effects of oxygen.
- Position the tubing so it does not pull on the patient's face, nose, or artificial airway.
- Ensure that there is no smoking and that no candles or matches are lit in the immediate area.
- Assess and document the patient's response to oxygen therapy.
- Ensure that the patient has an adequate oxygen source during any periods of transport.
- Provide the patient with ongoing teaching and reassurance to enhance his or her adherence with oxygen therapy.

---

hypoxemia to achieve generally acceptable oxygenation saturations in the range of 88% to 92% (Abdo & Heunks, 2012).

❖ PATIENT-CENTERED COLLABORATIVE CARE

◆ Assessment

Arterial blood gas (ABG) analysis is the best measure for determining the need for oxygen therapy and for evaluating its effects. Oxygen need is also determined by noninvasive monitoring, such as pulse oximetry and capnography (Carlisle, 2014).

◆ Interventions

Before starting oxygen therapy and while caring for a patient receiving oxygen therapy, you must be knowledgeable about oxygen hazards and complications. Know the rationale and the expected outcome related to oxygen therapy for each patient receiving oxygen. Chart 28-1 lists best practices for patients using oxygen therapy.

Hazards and Complications of Oxygen Therapy

Combustion. Oxygen itself does not burn, but it enhances combustion so that fire burns better in the presence of oxygen. For example, when the oxygen content of the air around a lighted cigarette is nearly 50%, the entire cigarette flames up and can catch items nearby on fire (Murabit & Tredget, 2012). Open fires, even small ones like candles or cigarettes, should not be in the same room during oxygen therapy. Take precautions during oxygen delivery, including posting a sign on the door of the patient's room. Smoking is prohibited in the patient's room, including at home, when oxygen is in use.

All electrical equipment in rooms where oxygen is in use must have grounded plugs and be plugged into grounded outlets to prevent fires from electrical arcing sparks. Frayed cords must be repaired because they can cause a spark that can ignite a flame. Flammable solutions (containing high concentrations of alcohol or oil) are not used in rooms in which oxygen is in use. (This does not include alcohol-based hand rubs.)

Oxygen-Induced Hypoventilation. For many years, oxygen was thought to induce hypoventilation in the patient with chronic lung disease who also had carbon dioxide retention (**hypercarbia**). As a result, nurses and physicians were reluctant to administer oxygen to these hypoxic patients, leading to serious problems and even deaths related to inadequate GAS EXCHANGE and PERFUSION. More recent research disproves the hypoxic drive theory and has found that patients with chronic lung disease are at risk for oxygen-induced hypercapnia but not for severely reduced respiratory effort (Makic et al., 2013). Therefore oxygen therapy is prescribed at the lowest liter flow needed to manage hypoxemia (Mac Sweeney et al., 2011). A system that delivers more precise oxygen levels (e.g., a Venturi mask) is preferred. However, some patients with chronic lung disease may not tolerate a facemask. Monitor the patient's response to therapy closely to ensure adequate gas exchange and correction of hypoxemia. Parameters to monitor include the level of consciousness, respiratory pattern and rate, and pulse oximetry. Remember, untreated or inadequately treated hypoxemia is a threat to life for any person with a breathing problem.

Oxygen Toxicity. Oxygen toxicity is related to the concentration of oxygen delivered, duration of oxygen therapy, and degree of lung disease present. In general, an oxygen level greater than 50% given continuously for more than 24 to 48 hours may damage the lungs.

The causes and manifestations of lung injury from oxygen toxicity are the same as those for acute respiratory distress syndrome (ARDS) (see Chapter 32). Initial problems include dyspnea, nonproductive cough, chest pain beneath the sternum, GI upset, and crackles on auscultation. As exposure to high levels of oxygen continues, the problems become more severe with decreased vital capacity, decreased compliance, and hypoxemia. With prolonged exposure to high oxygen levels, atelectasis, pulmonary edema, hemorrhage, and hyaline membrane formation may result. Surviving this critical condition depends on correcting the underlying disease process and decreasing the oxygen amount delivered.

The toxic effects of oxygen are difficult to manage, making prevention a priority. The lowest level of oxygen needed to maintain GAS EXCHANGE and oxygenation and prevent oxygen toxicity is prescribed. Closely monitor arterial blood gases (ABGs) during oxygen therapy, and notify the health care provider when Pao_2 levels become greater than 90 mm Hg. Also monitor the prescribed oxygen level and length of therapy to identify patients at higher risk. High oxygen levels are avoided unless absolutely necessary. The use of noninvasive positive airway pressure techniques with oxygen or the use of mechanical ventilation (see Chapter 32) may reduce the amount of oxygen needed. As soon as the patient's condition allows, the prescribed amount of oxygen is decreased.

Absorptive Atelectasis. Normally, nitrogen in the air maintains patent airways and alveoli. Making up 79% of room air, nitrogen prevents alveolar collapse. When high oxygen levels are delivered, nitrogen is diluted, oxygen diffuses from the alveoli into the blood, and the alveoli collapse. Collapsed alveoli cause atelectasis (called *absorptive atelectasis*), which is detected as crackles and decreased breath sounds on auscultation.

> ### ! NURSING SAFETY PRIORITY (QSEN)
> **Action Alert**
>
> Monitor the patient receiving high levels of oxygen closely for indications of absorptive atelectasis (new onset of crackles and decreased breath sounds) every 1 to 2 hours when oxygen therapy is started and as often as needed thereafter.

Drying of the Mucous Membranes. When the prescribed oxygen flow rate is higher than 4 L/min, humidify the delivery system (Fig. 28-2). Ensure that oxygen bubbles through the water in the humidifier.

Oxygen can also be humidified via a large-volume jet nebulizer in mist form (aerosol). A heated nebulizer raises the humidity even more and is used for oxygen delivery through an artificial airway. Usually the upper airway passages warm the air during breathing, but these passages are bypassed with an artificial airway, such as an endotracheal tube.

For the patient to receive properly humidified oxygen, the humidifier or nebulizer must have a sufficient amount of sterile water and the flow rate must be adequate. Condensation often forms in the tubing. Remove this condensation as it collects by disconnecting the tubing and emptying the water. Minimize the time the tubing is disconnected because the patient does not

FIG. 28-2 A bubble humidifier bottle used with oxygen therapy.

receive oxygen during this period. Some humidifiers and nebulizers have a water trap that hangs from the tubing so that the condensation can be drained without disconnecting. Check the water level and change the humidifier as needed.

> ### ! NURSING SAFETY PRIORITY (QSEN)
> **Action Alert**
>
> To prevent bacterial contamination of the oxygen delivery system, never drain the fluid from the water trap back into the humidifier or nebulizer.

Infection. The humidifier or nebulizer may be a source of bacteria, especially if it is heated. Oxygen delivery equipment such as cannulas and masks can also harbor organisms. Change equipment as per agency policy, which ranges from every 24 hours for humidification systems to every 7 days or whenever necessary for cannulas and masks.

> ### ? NCLEX EXAMINATION CHALLENGE
> **Physiological Integrity**
>
> Which manifestations in a client receiving oxygen therapy at 60% for more than 24 hours alert the nurse to the possibility of oxygen toxicity?
> A. Oxygen saturation greater than 100%
> B. Decreased rate and depth of respiration
> C. Wheezing on inhalation and exhalation
> D. Discomfort or pain under the sternum

Oxygen Delivery Systems. Oxygen can be delivered by many systems. Regardless of the type of delivery system used, it is important to understand its indications, advantages, and disadvantages. Use the equipment properly, and ensure appropriate equipment maintenance. Consult a respiratory therapist whenever there is a question or concern about an oxygen delivery system.

The type of delivery system used depends on:
- Oxygen concentration required by the patient
- Oxygen concentration achieved by a delivery system
- Importance of accuracy and control of the oxygen concentration

TABLE 28-1 Comparison of Low-Flow Oxygen Delivery Systems

FiO_2 DELIVERED	NURSING INTERVENTIONS	RATIONALES
Nasal Cannula 24%-40% FiO_2 at 1-6 L/min ≈24% at 1 L/min ≈28% at 2 L/min ≈32% at 3 L/min ≈36% at 4 L/min ≈40% at 5 L/min ≈44% at 6 L/min	Ensure that prongs are in the nares properly. Apply water-soluble jelly to nares PRN. Assess the patency of the nostrils. Assess the patient for changes in respiratory rate and depth.	A poorly fitting nasal cannula leads to hypoxemia and skin breakdown. This substance prevents mucosal irritation related to the drying effect of oxygen; promotes comfort. Congestion or a deviated septum prevents effective delivery of oxygen through the nares. The respiratory pattern affects the amount of oxygen delivered. A different delivery system may be needed.
Simple Facemask 40%-60% FiO_2 at 5-8 L/min; flow rate must be set at least at 5 L/min to flush mask of carbon dioxide ≈40% at 5 L/min ≈45%-50% at 6 L/min ≈55%-60% at 8 L/min	Be sure mask fits securely over nose and mouth. Assess skin and provide skin care to the area covered by the mask. Monitor the patient closely for risk for aspiration. Provide emotional support to the patient who feels claustrophobic. Suggest to the health care provider to switch the patient from a mask to the nasal cannula during eating.	A poorly fitting mask reduces the FiO_2 delivered. Pressure and moisture under the mask may cause skin breakdown. The mask limits the patient's ability to clear the mouth, especially if vomiting occurs. Emotional support decreases anxiety, which contributes to a claustrophobic feeling. Use of the cannula prevents hypoxemia during eating.
Partial Rebreather Mask 60%-75% at 6-11 L/min, a liter flow rate high enough to maintain reservoir bag two-thirds full during inspiration and expiration	Make sure that the reservoir does not twist or kink, which results in a deflated bag. Adjust the flow rate to keep the reservoir bag inflated.	Deflation results in decreased oxygen delivered and increases the rebreathing of exhaled air. The flow rate is adjusted to meet the pattern of the patient.
Non-Rebreather Mask 80%-95% FiO_2 at a liter flow high enough to maintain reservoir bag two-thirds full	Interventions as for partial rebreather mask; this patient requires close monitoring. Make sure that valves and rubber flaps are patent, functional, and not stuck. Remove mucus or saliva. Closely assess the patient on increased FiO_2 via non-rebreather mask. Intubation is the only way to provide more precise FiO_2.	Rationales as for partial rebreather mask. Monitoring ensures proper functioning and prevents harm. Valves should open during expiration and close during inhalation to prevent dramatic decrease in FiO_2. Suffocation can occur if the reservoir bag kinks or if the oxygen source disconnects. The patient may require intubation.

FiO_2, Fraction of inspired oxygen.

- Patient comfort
- Importance of humidity
- Patient mobility

Oxygen delivery systems are classified by the rate of oxygen delivery into either low-flow systems or high-flow systems. Low-flow systems have a low fraction of inspired oxygen (FiO_2) and therefore do not provide enough oxygen to meet the total oxygen need and air volume of the patient. So, part of the tidal volume is supplied by the patient as he or she breathes room air. The total level of oxygen inspired depends on the respiratory rate and tidal volume. High-flow systems have a flow rate that meets the entire oxygen need and tidal volume regardless of the patient's breathing pattern. These systems are used for critically ill patients and when delivery of precise levels of oxygen is needed.

If the patient needs a mask but is able to eat, request a prescription for a nasal cannula to be used at mealtimes only. Reapply the mask after the meal is completed. To increase mobility, up to 50 feet of connecting tubing can be used with connecting pieces.

Low-Flow Oxygen Delivery Systems. Low-flow systems include the nasal cannula, simple facemask, partial rebreather mask, and non-rebreather mask (Table 28-1). These systems are inexpensive, easy to use, and fairly comfortable, but the amount of oxygen delivered varies and depends on the patient's breathing pattern. The oxygen is diluted with room air (21% oxygen), which lowers the amount actually inspired.

Nasal Cannula. The nasal cannula (prongs) (Fig. 28-3), is used at flow rates of 1 to 6 L/min. Oxygen concentrations of 24% (at 1 L/min) to 44% (at 6 L/min) can be achieved. Flow rates greater than 6 L/min do not increase gas exchange because the anatomic dead space (places where air flows but the structures are too thick for gas exchange) is full. Also, high flow rates increase mucosal irritation.

The nasal cannula is often used for chronic lung disease and for any patient needing long-term oxygen therapy. Place the

FIG. 28-3 A nasal cannula (prongs).

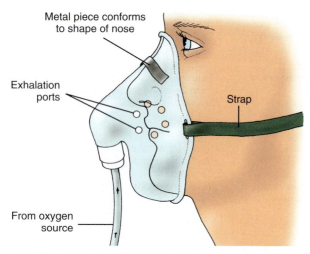

FIG. 28-4 A simple facemask used to deliver oxygen.

FIG. 28-5 A partial rebreather mask.

FIG. 28-6 A non-rebreather mask.

nasal prongs in the nostrils, with the openings facing the patient, following the natural anatomic curve of the nares.

Facemasks. Facemasks can deliver a wide range of oxygen flow rates and concentrations.

Simple facemasks are used to deliver oxygen concentrations of 40% to 60% for short-term oxygen therapy or in an emergency (Fig. 28-4). A minimum flow rate of 5 L/min is needed to prevent the rebreathing of exhaled air. Ensure that the mask fits well to maintain inspired oxygen levels. Care for the skin under the mask and strap to prevent skin breakdown (Ambutas et al., 2014).

Partial rebreather masks provide oxygen concentrations of 60% to 75% with flow rates of 6 to 11 L/min. It is a mask with a reservoir bag but no flaps (Fig. 28-5). With each breath, the patient rebreathes one third of the exhaled tidal volume, which is high in oxygen and increases the fraction of inspired oxygen (Fio_2). For best oxygen delivery, be sure that the bag remains slightly inflated at the end of inspiration. If needed, call the respiratory therapist for assistance.

Non-rebreather masks provide the highest oxygen level of the low-flow systems and can deliver an Fio_2 greater than 90%,

depending on the patient's breathing pattern. This mask is often used with patients whose respiratory status is unstable and who may require intubation.

The non-rebreather mask has a one-way valve between the mask and the reservoir and usually has two flaps over the exhalation ports (Fig. 28-6). The valve allows the patient to draw all needed oxygen from the reservoir bag, and the flaps

TABLE 28-2	Comparison of High-Flow Oxygen Delivery Systems	
FiO₂ DELIVERED	**NURSING INTERVENTIONS**	**RATIONALES**
Venturi Mask (Venti Mask)		
24%-50% FiO₂ with flow rates as recommended by the manufacturer, usually 4-10 L/min; provides high humidity	Perform constant surveillance to ensure an accurate flow rate for the specific FiO₂.	An accurate flow rate ensures FiO₂ delivery.
	Keep the orifice for the Venturi adaptor open and uncovered.	If the Venturi orifice is covered, the adaptor does not function and oxygen delivery varies.
	Provide a mask that fits snugly and tubing that is free of kinks.	FiO₂ is altered if kinking occurs or if the mask fits poorly.
	Assess the patient for dry mucous membranes.	Comfort measures may be indicated.
	Change to a nasal cannula during mealtime.	Oxygen is a drug that needs to be given continuously.
Aerosol Mask, Face Tent, Tracheostomy Collar		
24%-100% FiO₂ with flow rates of at least 10 L/min; provides high humidity	Assess that aerosol mist escapes from the vents of the delivery system during inspiration and expiration.	Humidification should be delivered to the patient.
	Empty condensation from the tubing.	Emptying prevents the patient from being lavaged with water, promotes an adequate flow rate, and ensures a continued prescribed FiO₂.
	Change the aerosol water container as needed.	Adequate humidification is ensured only when there is sufficient water in the canister.
T-Piece		
24%-100% FiO₂ with flow rates of at least 10 L/min; provides high humidity	Empty condensation from the tubing.	Condensation interferes with flow rate delivery of FiO₂ and may drain into the tracheostomy if not emptied.
	Keep the exhalation port open and uncovered.	If the port is occluded, the patient can suffocate.
	Position the T-piece so that it does not pull on the tracheostomy or endotracheal tube.	The weight of the T-piece pulls on the tracheostomy and causes pain or erosion of skin at the insertion site.
	Make sure the humidifier creates enough mist. A mist should be seen during inspiration and expiration.	An adequate flow rate is needed to meet the inspiration effort of the patient. If not, the patient will be "air-hungry."

FiO₂, Fraction of inspired oxygen.

prevent room air from entering through the exhalation ports (which would dilute the oxygen concentration). During exhalation, air leaves through these exhalation ports while the one-way valve prevents exhaled air from re-entering the reservoir bag. The flow rate is kept high (10 to 15 L/min) to keep the bag inflated during inhalation. Assess for this safety feature at least hourly.

> **⚠ NURSING SAFETY PRIORITY** (QSEN)
>
> *Critical Rescue*
>
> Ensure that the valve and flaps on a non-rebreather mask are intact and functional during each breath. If the oxygen source should fail or be depleted when both flaps are in place, the patient would not be able to inhale room air.

High-Flow Oxygen Delivery Systems. High-flow systems (Table 28-2) include the Venturi mask, aerosol mask, face tent, tracheostomy collar, and T-piece. These devices deliver an accurate oxygen level when properly fitted, with oxygen concentrations from 24% to 100% at 8 to 15 L/min.

Venturi masks (Venti masks) deliver the most accurate oxygen concentration without intubation. It works by pulling in a proportional amount of room air for each liter flow of oxygen. An adaptor is located between the bottom of the mask and the oxygen source (Fig. 28-7). Adaptors with holes of different sizes allow specific amounts of air to mix with the oxygen, resulting in more precise delivery of oxygen. Each adaptor requires a different flow rate. For example, to deliver 24% of oxygen, the flow rate must be 4 L/min. Another type of Venturi

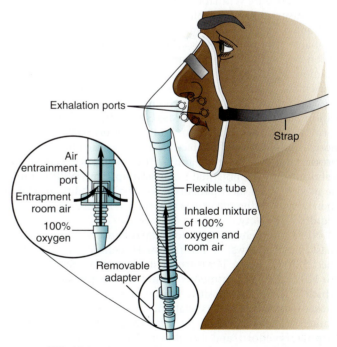

FIG. 28-7 A Venturi mask for precise oxygen delivery.

mask has one adaptor with a dial that is used to select the amount of oxygen desired. Humidification is not needed with the Venturi mask.

Other high-flow systems include the face tent, aerosol mask, tracheostomy collar, and T-piece. They are often used to provide

Flexible tubing from oxygen source

T-piece adapter

Reservoir tube

15-mm adapter

Endotracheal tube

FIG. 28-8 A T-piece apparatus for attachment to an endotracheal or tracheostomy tube.

FIG. 28-9 Nasal continuous positive airway pressure (CPAP).

high humidity with oxygen delivery. A dial on the humidity source regulates the delivered oxygen level. A face tent fits over the chin, with the top extending halfway across the face. The oxygen level delivered varies, but the face tent, instead of a tight-fitting mask, is useful for patients who have facial trauma or burns. An aerosol mask is used when high humidity is needed. The tracheostomy collar is used to deliver high humidity and the desired oxygen to the patient with a tracheostomy. A special adaptor, called the *T-piece,* is used to deliver any desired Fio$_2$ to the patient with a tracheostomy, laryngectomy, or endotracheal tube (Fig. 28-8). Adjust the flow rate so that the aerosol appears on the exhalation side of the T-piece.

Noninvasive Positive-Pressure Ventilation. Noninvasive positive-pressure ventilation (NPPV) is a technique using positive pressure to keep alveoli open and improve GAS EXCHANGE without the need for airway intubation. It is now being used to manage dyspnea, hypercarbia, and acute exacerbations of chronic obstructive pulmonary disease (COPD), cardiogenic pulmonary edema, and acute asthma attacks. Although NPPV prevents the complications associated with intubation, including ventilator-associated pneumonia (VAP), risks and complications are associated with it. Masks must fit tightly in order to form a proper seal, which can lead to skin breakdown over the nose or other areas of the face. Leaks can cause uncomfortable pressure around the eyes, and gastric insufflation can lead to vomiting and the potential for aspiration. Thus NPPV should be used only on alert patients who have the ability to protect their airway, although a nasogastric (NG) tube may still be required for safety.

NPPV can deliver oxygen or may use just room air. A nasal mask, nasal pillows, or full-face mask delivery system allows mechanical delivery. The three most common modes of delivery for NPPV are (1) continuous positive airway pressure (CPAP), which delivers a set positive airway pressure throughout each cycle of inhalation and exhalation; (2) volume-limited or flow-limited, which delivers a set tidal volume with the patient's inspiratory effort; and (3) pressure-limited, which includes pressure support, pressure control, and bi-level positive airway pressure (BiPAP), which cycles different pressures at inspiration and at expiration.

For BiPAP, a cycling machine delivers a set inspiratory positive airway pressure each time the patient begins to inspire. As he or she begins to exhale, the machine delivers a lower set end-expiratory pressure. Together, these two pressures improve tidal volume, can reduce respiratory rate, and may relieve dyspnea.

For CPAP, the effect is to open collapsed alveoli. Patients who may benefit from this form of oxygen or air delivery include those with atelectasis after surgery or cardiac-induced pulmonary edema or those with COPD. It is not beneficial for patients with respiratory failure following extubation. NPPV is also being used in palliative care for alleviating dyspnea, including for those patients with "do-not-intubate" orders. However, this practice is controversial. The Society of Critical Care Medicine (SCCM) recommends that goals of therapy and expected outcomes be discussed with the patient and family before initiating therapy.

NPPV is used for sleep apnea. The effect is to hold open the upper airways (Fig. 28-9). Patients using CPAP or BiPAP at home to manage sleep apnea often bring their home equipment to the hospital. They are familiar with their own machines and feel more comfortable using their own masks. The reasons for using NPPV still exist when the patient enters the hospital, and with some problems, there may be a greater need for them to continue NPPV while hospitalized.

The number of patients using NPPV therapy is increasing, and they are often cared for outside of the ICU setting. Nurses caring for the patient with NPPV must be knowledgeable about the equipment, the technique, and the potential complications. Adequate respiratory therapy support also is needed to safely manage a patient receiving NPPV.

Transtracheal Oxygen Therapy. Transtracheal oxygen (TTO) is a long-term method of delivering oxygen directly into the lungs. A small, flexible catheter is passed into the trachea through a small incision with the patient under local anesthesia. TTO avoids the irritation from nasal prongs and is less visible. A TTO team provides patient education, including the purpose of TTO and care of the catheter. Flow rates are prescribed for rest and for activity. A flow rate also is prescribed for the nasal cannula, which is used when the TTO catheter is being cleaned. Most patients using this delivery method have a 55% reduction in required oxygen flow at rest and a 30% decrease with activity.

❓ CLINICAL JUDGMENT CHALLENGE

Patient-Centered Care; Teamwork and Collaboration; Evidence-Based Practice **QSEN**

Your patient is an 81-year-old male with end-stage COPD who is admitted with pneumonia and COPD exacerbation. He has a 60–pack-year smoking history and has been hospitalized many times over the past year for respiratory distress. The admitting provider orders an arterial blood gas (ABG). The patient is not using supplemental oxygen.

1. Based on your understanding of his disease process (see Chapter 30), would you expect this patient to have normal or altered ABG values, especially carbon dioxide ($PaCO_2$) level?
2. The results of the ABG indicate hypoxemia (PaO_2 of 40 mm Hg). Should you provide your patient with supplemental oxygen? Why or why not? If so, how much and which method would be best?
3. What areas will be the focus of your assessment and documentation? Provide a rationale for your choice(s).
4. Your patient has continually increasing oxygen requirements. He is now wearing a simple mask, and one of your colleagues would like to switch to a non-rebreather mask to deliver 100% oxygen. What are other good options for this patient?

FIG. 28-10 Small E size oxygen tank (cylinder) for portability.

Community-Based Care

Home Care Management. The patient must be stable before home oxygen is considered. For Medicare to cover the cost of home oxygen therapy, the patient must have severe hypoxemia defined as a partial pressure of arterial oxygen (PaO_2) level of less than 55 mm Hg or an arterial oxygen saturation (SpO_2) of less than 88% on room air and at rest. The criteria vary when hypoxemia is caused by nonpulmonary problems or when oxygen is needed only at night or with exercise.

Self-Management Education. When home oxygen therapy is prescribed, begin a teaching plan about oxygen therapy. The nurse or respiratory therapist teaches the patient about the equipment needed for home oxygen therapy and the safety aspects of using and maintaining the equipment. Equipment may include the oxygen source, delivery devices, and humidity sources. Work with the discharge planner to help the patient select a durable medical equipment (DME) company to deliver oxygen equipment and select a community health nursing agency for follow-up care in the home. Re-evaluation of the need for oxygen therapy occurs on a periodic basis.

While providing discharge planning and teaching, be sensitive to the patient's emotional adjustment to oxygen therapy. Encourage the patient to share feelings and concerns. He or she may be concerned about social acceptance. Help him or her realize that adherence to oxygen therapy is important for being able to participate in ADLs and other events that bring enjoyment.

Home Care Preparation. Home oxygen therapy is provided in one of three ways: compressed gas in a tank or a cylinder, liquid oxygen in a reservoir, or an oxygen concentrator. Compressed gas in an oxygen tank (green) is the most often used oxygen source. The large H cylinder may be used as a stationary source, and the small E tank is available for transporting the patient (Fig. 28-10). Smaller cylinders are available for the patient to carry. Teach the patient and family to check the gauge daily to assess the amount of oxygen left in the tank. As a safety precaution, the tanks must always be in a stand or rack. A tank that is accidentally knocked over could

FIG. 28-11 Portable liquid oxygen.

suddenly decompress and move around in an uncontrolled manner.

Liquid oxygen for home use is oxygen gas that has been liquefied. A concentrated amount of oxygen is available in a lightweight and easy-to-carry container similar to a Thermos bottle (Fig. 28-11). This portable tank is filled from a large stationary liquid vessel. Liquid oxygen lasts longer than gaseous oxygen; however, it is expensive and the oxygen evaporates if it is not used continuously.

The **oxygen concentrator** or *oxygen extractor* is a machine that removes nitrogen from room air, increasing oxygen levels to more than 90%. This device is the least expensive system and does not need to be filled. It is often used in the home as a stationary system. A smaller version that can plug into DC electrical outlets can be rented for longer car or boat trips. Liquid oxygen and E tanks are used for short trips.

Regardless of the type of oxygen delivery system used, review safety issues with the patient and all family members.

? **NCLEX EXAMINATION CHALLENGE**
Health Promotion and Maintenance

For which activity does the nurse teach the client who is receiving oxygen by a transtracheal oxygen (TTO) delivery system to switch to a nasal cannula oxygen delivery system?
A. Eating a meal
B. Sleeping at night
C. Cleaning the catheter
D. Performing mouth care

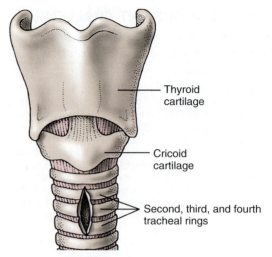

FIG. 28-12 A vertical tracheal incision for a tracheostomy.

TRACHEOSTOMY

Tracheotomy is the surgical incision into the trachea to create an airway. **Tracheostomy** is the tracheal *stoma* (opening) that results from the tracheotomy. A tracheotomy can be an emergency procedure or a scheduled surgery. Tracheostomies can be temporary or permanent. Some indications for tracheostomy include acute airway obstruction, the need for airway protection, laryngeal or facial trauma or burns, and airway involvement during head or neck surgery. Tracheostomies also are used for prolonged unconsciousness, paralysis, or the inability to be weaned from mechanical ventilation. With temporary tracheostomies, the nurse is key in evaluating patient readiness for progression toward decannulation (removal of the tracheostomy tube) (Morris et al., 2014).

❖ PATIENT-CENTERED COLLABORATIVE CARE

◆ Analysis

The priority NANDA-I nursing diagnoses and collaborative problems for patients requiring tracheostomy include:
- Impaired Gas Exchange related to weak chest muscles, obstruction, or other physical problems that interfere with ventilation and diffusion of gases (NANDA-I)
- Impaired Verbal Communication related to tracheostomy or intubation (NANDA-I)
- Imbalanced Nutrition: Less Than Body Requirements related to presence of endotracheal tube (NANDA-I)
- Potential for infection related to invasive procedures or problems with the normal protective mechanisms of the respiratory tract
- Damaged oral mucosa related to mechanical factors (endotracheal tube)

◆ Interventions

Preoperative Care. The care for the patient having a tracheotomy is similar to that for a laryngectomy (see Chapter 29). Focus on his or her knowledge deficits through teaching, and discuss tracheostomy care, communication, and speech.

Operative Procedures. Initially, the neck is extended and an endotracheal (ET) tube is placed by the anesthesia provider to maintain the airway. Incisions are made through the neck and the tracheal rings to enter the trachea (Fig. 28-12). The types of incisions and techniques vary, depending on the surgeon's preference and the reason for the surgery.

After the trachea is entered, the ET tube is removed while the tracheostomy tube is inserted. The tracheostomy tube is secured in place with sutures and tracheostomy ties or Velcro tube holders. A chest x-ray determines proper placement of the tube.

Postoperative Care. Immediately after surgery, focus care on ensuring a patent airway. Confirm the presence of bilateral breath sounds. Perform a respiratory assessment at least hourly. Assess the patient for complications from the procedure.

Complications. Major complications can arise after surgery. Table 28-3 lists manifestations, management, and prevention of complications of tracheostomy.

Tube obstruction can occur as a result of secretions or by cuff displacement. Indicators include difficulty breathing; noisy respirations; difficulty inserting a suction catheter; thick, dry secretions; and unexplained peak pressures (if a mechanical ventilator is in use). Assess the patient at least hourly for tube patency. Prevent obstruction by helping the patient cough and deep breathe, providing inner cannula care, humidifying oxygen, and suctioning. If tube obstruction occurs as a result of cuff prolapse over the end of the tracheostomy tube, the health care provider repositions or replaces the tube.

Tube dislodgement and accidental decannulation can occur when the tube is not secure. Prevent this problem by securing the tube in place to reduce movement and traction from the tubing or from accidental pulling by the patient. *Tube dislodgment in the first 72 hours after surgery is an emergency because the tracheostomy tract has not matured and replacement is difficult. The tube may end up in the subcutaneous tissue instead of in the trachea (also referred to as "false passage"). The patient will not be able to be ventilated.* Obese patients or those with short, large necks may be particularly difficult to recannulate if the tracheostomy tube is dislodged.

TABLE 28-3 Complications of Tracheostomy

COMPLICATIONS AND DESCRIPTION	MANIFESTATIONS	MANAGEMENT	PREVENTION
Tracheomalacia: constant pressure exerted by the cuff causes tracheal dilation and erosion of cartilage.	An increased amount of air is required in the cuff to maintain the seal. A larger tracheostomy tube is required to prevent an air leak at the stoma. Food particles are seen in tracheal secretions. The patient does not receive the set tidal volume on the ventilator.	No special management is needed unless bleeding occurs.	Use an uncuffed tube as soon as possible. Monitor cuff pressure and air volumes closely, and detect changes.
Tracheal stenosis: narrowed tracheal lumen is due to scar formation from irritation of tracheal mucosa by the cuff.	Stenosis is usually seen after the cuff is deflated or the tracheostomy tube is removed. The patient has increased coughing, inability to expectorate secretions, or difficulty in breathing or talking.	Tracheal dilation or surgical intervention is used.	Prevent pulling of and traction on the tracheostomy tube. Properly secure the tube in the midline position. Maintain proper cuff pressure. Minimize oronasal intubation time.
Tracheoesophageal fistula (TEF): excessive cuff pressure causes erosion of the posterior wall of the trachea. A hole is created between the trachea and the anterior esophagus. The patient at highest risk also has a nasogastric tube present.	Similar to tracheomalacia: Food particles are seen in tracheal secretions. Increased air in cuff is needed to achieve a seal. The patient has increased coughing and choking while eating. The patient does not receive the set tidal volume on the ventilator.	Manually administer oxygen by mask to prevent hypoxemia. Use a small, soft feeding tube instead of a nasogastric tube for tube feedings. A gastrostomy or jejunostomy may be performed by the physician. Monitor the patient with a nasogastric tube closely; assess for TEF and aspiration.	Maintain cuff pressure. Monitor the amount of air needed for inflation, and detect changes. Progress to a deflated cuff or cuffless tube as soon as possible.
Trachea–innominate artery fistula: a malpositioned tube causes its distal tip to push against the lateral wall of the tracheostomy. Continued pressure causes necrosis and erosion of the innominate artery. **This is a medical emergency.**	The tracheostomy tube pulsates in synchrony with the heartbeat. There is heavy bleeding from the stoma. This is a life-threatening complication.	Remove the tracheostomy tube immediately. Apply direct pressure to the innominate artery at the stoma site. Prepare the patient for immediate surgical repair.	Correct the tube size, length, and midline position. Prevent pulling or tugging on the tracheostomy tube. Immediately notify the physician of the pulsating tube.

⚠ **NURSING SAFETY PRIORITY** (QSEN)

Critical Rescue

If the tube is dislodged on an immature tracheostomy, ventilate the patient using a manual resuscitation bag and facemask while another nurse calls the Rapid Response Team.

For safety, ensure that a tracheostomy tube of the same type (including an obturator) and size (or one size smaller) is at the bedside at all times, along with a tracheostomy insertion tray. If decannulation occurs after 72 hours, extend the patient's neck and open the tissues of the stoma with a curved Kelly clamp to secure the airway. With the obturator inserted into the tracheostomy tube, quickly and gently replace the tube and remove the obturator. Check for airflow through the tube and for bilateral breath sounds. *If you cannot secure the airway, notify a more experienced nurse, respiratory therapist, or physician for assistance. Ventilate with a bag-valve mask. If the patient is in distress, call the Rapid Response Team for help.* To minimize tube dislodgment problems, many institutions have developed policies for patients with new tracheostomies and those identified at high risk (i.e., obese patients or those identified by the surgeon or anesthesiologist as high risk). One policy is to have a "difficult airway" cart available for these high-risk patients.

Pneumothorax (air in the chest cavity) can develop during the tracheotomy procedure if the chest cavity is entered. Chest x-rays after placement are used to assess for pneumothorax.

Subcutaneous emphysema occurs when there is an opening or tear in the trachea and air escapes into the fresh tissue planes of the neck. Air can progress throughout the chest and other tissues into the face. Inspect and palpate for air under the skin around the new tracheostomy.

⚠ **NURSING SAFETY PRIORITY** (QSEN)

Critical Rescue

If the skin around a new tracheostomy is puffy and you can feel a crackling sensation when pressing on this skin, notify the physician immediately.

Bleeding in small amounts from the tracheotomy incision is expected for the first few days, but constant oozing is abnormal. Wrap gauze around the tube and pack gauze gently into the wound to apply pressure to the bleeding sites.

Infection can occur at any time. In the hospital, use sterile technique to prevent infection during suctioning and tracheostomy care. Assess the stoma site at least once every 8 hours for purulent drainage, redness, pain, or swelling. Tracheostomy dressings may be used to keep the stoma clean and dry. These dressings resemble a 4 × 4 gauze pad with an area removed to fit around the tube. If tracheostomy dressings are not available, fold standard sterile 4 × 4s to fit around the tube. *Do not cut the dressing because small bits of gauze could then be aspirated*

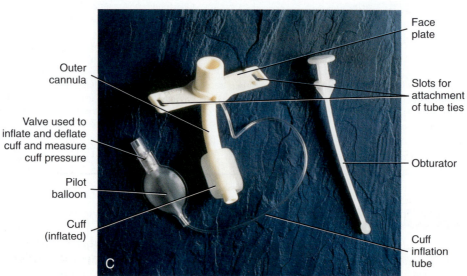

FIG. 28-13 Tracheostomy tubes. **A,** Dual-lumen cuffed tracheostomy tube with disposable inner cannula. **B,** Dual-lumen cuffed fenestrated tracheostomy tube. **C,** Single-lumen cannula cuffed tracheostomy tube.

through the tube. Change these dressings often because moist dressings provide a medium for bacterial growth. Careful wound care prevents most local infections.

Tracheostomy Tubes. Many types of tracheostomy tubes are available (Fig. 28-13). The one chosen depends on the needs of the patient. Tracheostomy tubes are available in many sizes and are made of plastic or metal. Most tubes in use today are disposable. A tracheostomy tube may have a cuff and may have an inner cannula. For patients receiving mechanical ventilation, a cuffed tube is used. A noncuffed tube is used when mechanical ventilation is not required.

For tubes with a reusable inner cannula, inspect, suction, and clean the inner cannula. During the first 24 hours after surgery, perform cannula care as often as needed, perhaps every 30 to 60 minutes. Thereafter, care is determined by the patient's needs and agency policy. In planning for self-care, teach the patient to remove the inner cannula and check for cleanliness. Also instruct him or her about suctioning and tracheostomy cleaning.

Because breathing and swallowing move the tube, a cuffed tube does not protect against aspiration. Having a cuffed tube inflated may give a false sense of security that aspiration cannot occur during feeding or mouth care. In addition, the pilot balloon does not reflect whether the correct amount of air is present in the cuff.

A fenestrated tube functions in many different ways. When the inner cannula is in place, the fenestration is closed and this tube works like a double-lumen tube. With the inner cannula removed and the plug or stopper locked in place, air can pass through the fenestration, around the tube, and up through the natural airway so that the patient can cough and speak. If the patient has trouble with these actions, he or she should be evaluated for proper tube placement, patency, size, and fenestration. *Do not cap the tube until the problem is identified and corrected.*

A fenestrated tube may or may not have a cuff. With a cuff, some air flows through the natural airway when the patient is not being mechanically ventilated.

Action Alert

Always deflate the cuff before capping the tube with the decannulation cap; otherwise, the patient has no airway.

Patients with metal tracheostomy tubes scheduled for magnetic resonance imaging (MRI) need to change to a plastic tube. Metal tubes could be dislodged or heat up with exposure to the magnetic field during the scan.

Care Issues for the Patient with a Tracheostomy

Preventing Tissue Damage. Tissue damage can occur at the point where the inflated cuff presses against the tracheal mucosa. Mucosal ischemia occurs when the pressure exerted by the cuff on the mucosa exceeds the capillary perfusion pressure. To reduce the risk for tracheal damage, keep the cuff pressure between 14 and 20 mm Hg or 20 and 30 cm H_2O (ideally, 25 cm H_2O or less) (Sole et al., 2011).

Most cuffs use a high volume of air while keeping low pressure on the tracheal mucosa. Inflate the cuff to form a seal between the trachea and the cuff with the least amount of pressure. If the cuff cannot be inflated to seal well enough, a larger-diameter tube may be needed. A pressure cuff inflator can be used to inflate the cuff to a specified pressure or to check the cuff pressure (Fig. 28-14).

Check the cuff pressure at least once during each shift, especially with the minimal leak technique, and keep the pressure at 14 to 20 mm Hg or 20 to 30 cm H_2O. In rare situations, the cuff pressure is increased to maintain ventilator volumes when peak pressures are greater than 50 mm Hg (65 cm H_2O) and positive end-expiratory pressure (PEEP) is greater than 10 mm Hg (14 cm H_2O). High PEEP values can deflate the cuff over time, and more air may need to be added to maintain a proper seal. Manufacturers have guidelines for the specific volumes for each cuff size. Most cuffs are adequately inflated with less than 10 mL of air.

Although a high cuff pressure alone causes tracheal damage, other factors contribute to the risk for damage (Makic et al.,

2013). The patient who is malnourished, dehydrated, hypoxic, older, or receiving corticosteroids is at risk for greater tissue damage. Tube friction and movement damage the mucosa and lead to tracheal stenosis. Reduce local airway damage by maintaining proper cuff pressures, stabilizing the tube, suctioning only when needed, and preventing malnutrition, dehydration, and hypoxia.

Ensuring Air Warming and Humidification. The tracheostomy tube bypasses the nose and mouth, which normally humidify and warm the inspired air. If humidification and warming are not adequate, tracheal damage can occur. Thick, dried secretions can occlude the airways.

To prevent these complications, humidify the air as prescribed. Continually assess for a fine mist emerging from the tracheostomy collar or T-piece during ventilation. To increase the amount of humidity delivered, a warming device can be attached to the water source with a temperature probe in the tubing circuit. Monitor the circuit temperature hourly by feeling the tubing and by checking the probe. Ensure adequate hydration, which also helps liquefy secretions. Increasing the flow rate at the flowmeter increases the amount of delivered humidity.

Action Alert

Keep the temperature of the air entering a tracheostomy between 98.6° and 100.4°F (37° and 38°C) and never exceed 104°F (40°C).

Suctioning. Suctioning maintains a patent airway and promotes GAS EXCHANGE by removing secretions when the patient cannot cough adequately. Chart 28-2 lists best practices for

FIG. 28-14 An aneroid pressure manometer for cuff inflation and measuring cuff pressures.

CHART 28-2 Best Practice for Patient Safety & Quality Care (QSEN)

Suctioning the Artificial Airway

1. Assess the need for suctioning (routine unnecessary suctioning causes mucosal damage, bleeding, and bronchospasm).
2. Wash hands. Don protective eyewear. Maintain Standard Precautions.
3. Explain to the patient that sensations such as shortness of breath and coughing are to be expected but that any discomfort will be very brief.
4. Check the suction source. Occlude the suction source, and adjust the pressure dial to between 80 and 120 mm Hg to prevent hypoxemia and trauma to the mucosa.
5. Set up a sterile field.
6. Preoxygenate the patient with 100% oxygen for 30 seconds to 3 minutes (at least three hyperinflations) to prevent hypoxemia. Keep hyperinflations synchronized with inhalation.
7. Quickly insert the suction catheter until resistance is met. *Do not apply suction during insertion.*
8. Withdraw the catheter 0.4 to 0.8 inch (1 to 2 cm), and begin to apply suction. Apply suction and use a twirling motion of the catheter during withdrawal. *Never suction longer than 10 to 15 seconds.*
9. Hyperoxygenate for 1 to 5 minutes or until the patient's baseline heart rate and oxygen saturation are within normal limits.
10. Repeat as needed for up to three total suction passes.
11. Suction mouth as needed, and provide mouth care.
12. Remove gloves, and wash hands.
13. Describe secretions, and document patient's responses.

suctioning. Assess the patient's need for suctioning (e.g., audible or noisy secretions; crackles or wheezes heard on auscultation; restlessness; increased pulse or respiratory rates; or mucus present in the artificial airway). Other indications include patient requests for suctioning or an increase in the peak airway pressure on the ventilator.

Deep endotracheal suctioning is painful. Some unconscious or noncommunicative patients still feel pain, and this should be kept in mind during the suctioning procedure (see the Evidence-Based Practice box). At the very least, provide verbal acknowledgment of the discomfort and reassurance of when the procedure will end.

EVIDENCE-BASED PRACTICE QSEN

How Do You Know When Suctioning is Painful to a Patient?

Rahu, M., Grap, M., Cohn, J., Munro, C., Lyon, D., & Sessler, C. (2013). Facial expression as an indicator of pain in critically ill intubated adults during endotracheal suctioning. *American Journal of Critical Care, 22*(5), 412-422.

Endotracheal suctioning is often painful, and patients may require pain medication before the procedure. Patients who are not able to communicate may still feel pain during the procedure, but often this is not addressed. The investigators sought to determine whether pain in noncommunicative critically ill patients during endotracheal suctioning could be discerned by changes in facial expression.

Fifty noncommunicative patients who had endotracheal tubes were video recorded during rest phases in which no treatments or procedures were being performed and during periods of endotracheal suctioning. The video-recorded facial changes were coded using the Facial Action Coding System of the Behavioral Pain Scale. A total of 14 different facial expressions were present during suctioning that were seldom seen during rest phases. Five of the 14 accounted for 71% of the variance from expected responses as measured in stepwise multivariate analysis. These expression changes were brow raised, brow lowered, nose wrinkling, head turned right or left, and head turned up. The investigators suggest that such changes in upper facial expressions in noncommunicative critically ill patients could be used as a valid alternative to self-reports of procedural pain.

Level of Evidence: 3

The results of this quasi-experimental study in which patients served as their own controls provide significant evidence that non-communicative critically ill patients feel pain during the suctioning procedure. The use of video-recording and the observer software analysis of facial changes strengthened the study by reducing observer bias and providing opportunity for re-examination. The Facial Action Coding System (FACS) is an established and reliable instrument useful for assessing behavioral responses to pain. The statistical analysis methods used were appropriate for the study design.

Commentary: Implications for Practice and Research

This study is important in that it was conducted under real clinical conditions using a variety of noncommunicative and intubated patients. The results indicate that the FACS could be used to standardize pain evaluation in this patient population. Additional research with larger sample sizes are needed to determine whether the instruments could be used to quantify the pain experienced by noncommunicative patients so that appropriate pain-relieving measures could be instituted. Although some limitations were present in this study, the nature of the question and the patient population do not lend themselves to randomized controlled clinical trials.

Suctioning is often performed through an artificial airway, but the nose or mouth also can be used. Suctioning of both routes is routine for the patient with retained secretions.

Suctioning through the nose has similar complications as suctioning through an artificial airway and can be painful. Slow, careful placement of the catheter following the nasopharyngeal anatomy reduces pain and trauma. Placing a nasopharyngeal airway and suctioning through it can prevent trauma to the nasal mucosa. Advance the catheter through the nasopharynx and into the laryngopharynx while the patient receives oxygen by mask or nasal cannula. Once the catheter enters the larynx, the patient may cough. On inhalation, insert the catheter into the trachea. If needed, disconnect the catheter from suction and attach it to an oxygen source so that the patient receives oxygen via the catheter.

Suctioning can cause hypoxia, mucosal trauma, infection, vagal stimulation, bronchospasm, and cardiac dysrhythmias.

Hypoxia can be caused by these factors in the patient with a tracheostomy:
- Ineffective oxygenation before, during, and after suctioning
- Use of a catheter that is too large for the artificial airway
- Prolonged suctioning time
- Excessive suction pressure
- Too frequent suctioning

Prevent hypoxia by hyperoxygenating the patient with 100% oxygen using a manual resuscitation bag attached to an oxygen source. Instruct the patient to take deep breaths 3 or 4 times with the existing oxygen delivery system before suctioning. Monitor the heart rate or use a pulse oximeter while suctioning to assess tolerance of the procedure. Assess for hypoxia (e.g., increased heart rate and blood pressure, oxygen desaturation, cyanosis, restlessness, anxiety, dysrhythmias). Oxygen saturation below 90% by pulse oximetry indicates hypoxemia. If hypoxia occurs, stop the suctioning procedure. Using the 100% oxygen delivery system, reoxygenate the patient until baseline parameters return.

Use a correct-size catheter to reduce the risk for hypoxia and still remove secretions effectively. The size should not exceed half of the size of the tracheal lumen. The standard catheter size for an adult is 12 Fr or 14 Fr.

Tissue trauma results from frequent suctioning, prolonged suctioning, excessive suction pressure, and non-rotation of the catheter. Prevent trauma to the mucosa by suctioning only when needed and lubricating the catheter with sterile water or saline before insertion. *Apply suction only during catheter withdrawal.* Use a twirling motion during withdrawal to prevent grabbing of the mucosa.

Apply suction for only 10 to 15 seconds. Estimate this time frame by holding your own breath and counting to 10 or 15 during suctioning. At the end of the 15 seconds, stop suctioning. Longer suctioning can cause alveolar collapse (*suction atelectasis*).

Infection is possible because each catheter pass introduces bacteria into the trachea. In the hospital, use sterile technique for suctioning and for all suctioning equipment (e.g., suction catheters, gloves, saline or water). Suction the mouth or nose *after* suctioning the artificial airway. Clean technique is used at home because the number of virulent organisms in the home environment is lower than in the hospital.

Action Alert

> Never use oral suction equipment for suctioning an artificial airway, because this can introduce oral bacteria into the lungs.

Vagal stimulation and bronchospasm are possible during suctioning. Vagal stimulation results in bradycardia, hypotension, heart block, ventricular tachycardia, or other dysrhythmias. *If vagal stimulation occurs, stop suctioning immediately and oxygenate the patient manually with 100% oxygen.* Bronchospasm may occur when the catheter passes into the airway. The patient may need a bronchodilator to relieve bronchospasm and respiratory distress. The hypoxia caused by suctioning can stimulate a variety of cardiac dysrhythmias. If the patient has cardiac monitoring in place, check the monitor during suctioning.

? **NCLEX EXAMINATION CHALLENGE**
Safe and Effective Care Environment

> During nasotracheal suctioning, the client's heart rate changes from 78 beats/min to 48 beats/min. What is the nurse's best first action?
> A. Immediately stop suctioning
> B. Gently pinch the client's cheek
> C. Administer oxygen by mask at 2 L/min
> D. Document the change as the only action

Providing Tracheostomy Care. Tracheostomy care keeps the tube free of secretions, maintains a patent airway, and provides wound care. It is performed whether or not the patient can clear secretions. Perform tracheostomy care according to agency policy, usually every 8 hours and as needed. Chart 28-3 outlines best practices for tracheostomy care.

Before tracheostomy care, assess the patient as described in Chart 28-4. The need for suctioning and tracheostomy care is determined by the secretions, the specific disorder, the ability of the patient to cough, the need for mechanical ventilation, and wound care. Using a penlight, inspect the inner lumen of a single-lumen tube to assess for secretions.

Secure tracheostomy tubes in place using either twill tape ties or commercial tube holders. Both devices require changing when soiled or at least daily to keep them clean, to prevent infection, and to assess for skin irritation under the ties. A properly secured tie or holder allows space for only one finger to be placed between the tie or holder and the neck (Morris et al., 2013). Tube movement causes irritation and coughing and may lead to decannulation. Keeping the tube secure while changing the ties or holder to prevent accidental decannulation is critical. Include the patient in tracheostomy care as a step toward self-care. Fig. 28-15 shows correct placement of a tracheostomy dressing.

! **NURSING SAFETY PRIORITY** (QSEN)
Critical Rescue

> Prevent decannulation during tracheostomy care by keeping the old ties or holder on the tube while applying new ties or holder or by keeping a hand on the tube until it is securely stable. (This is best performed with the assistance of another person.)

CHART 28-3 Best Practice for Patient Safety & Quality Care (QSEN)
Tracheostomy Care

1. Assemble the necessary equipment.
2. Wash hands. Maintain Standard Precautions.
3. Suction the tracheostomy tube if necessary.
4. Remove old dressings and excess secretions.
5. Set up a sterile field.
6. Remove and clean the inner cannula. Use half-strength hydrogen peroxide to clean the cannula and sterile saline to rinse it. If the inner cannula is disposable, remove the cannula and replace it with a new one.
7. Clean the stoma site and then the tracheostomy plate with half-strength hydrogen peroxide followed by sterile saline. Ensure that none of the solutions enters the tracheostomy.
8. Change tracheostomy ties if they are soiled. Secure new ties in place before removing soiled ones to prevent accidental decannulation. If a knot is needed, tie a square knot that is visible on the side of the neck. Only one finger should be able to be placed between the tie tape and the neck.
9. Wash hands.
10. Document the type and amount of secretions and the general condition of the stoma and surrounding skin. Document the patient's response to the procedure and any teaching or learning that occurred.

CHART 28-4 Focused Assessment
The Patient with a Tracheostomy

- Note the quality, pattern, and rate of breathing:
  - Within patient's baseline?
    Tachypnea can indicate hypoxia.
    Dyspnea can indicate secretions in the airway.
- Assess for any cyanosis, especially around the lips, which could indicate hypoxia.
- Check the patient's pulse oximetry reading.
- If oxygen is prescribed, is the patient receiving the correct amount, with the correct equipment and humidification?
- Assess the tracheostomy site:
  - Note the color, consistency, and amount of secretions in the tube or externally.
  - If the tracheostomy is sutured in place, is there any redness, swelling, or drainage from suture sites?
  - If the tracheostomy is secured with ties, what is the condition of the ties? Are they moist with secretions or perspiration? Are the secretions dried on the ties? Is the tie secure?
  - Assess the condition of the skin around the tracheostomy and neck. Be sure to check underneath the neck for secretions that may have drained to the back. Check for any skin breakdown related to pressure from the ties or related to excess secretions.
  - Assess behind the faceplate for the size of the space between the outer cannula and the patient's tissue. Are any secretions collected in this area?
- If the tube is cuffed, check cuff pressure.
- Auscultate the lungs.
- Are a second (emergency) tracheostomy tube and obturator available?

Providing Bronchial and Oral Hygiene. Bronchial hygiene promotes a patent airway and prevents infection. Turn and reposition the patient every 1 to 2 hours, support out-of-bed activities, and encourage ambulation to promote lung expansion and GAS EXCHANGE and help remove secretions. Coughing and deep breathing, combined with the chest percussion, vibration, and postural drainage, promote pulmonary hygiene (see Chapter 30).

FIG. 28-15 Placement of tracheostomy gauze dressing and Velcro tracheostomy tube holder.

Good oral hygiene keeps the airway patent, prevents bacterial overgrowth, and promotes comfort. Avoid using glycerin swabs or mouthwash that contains alcohol for oral care because these products dry the mouth, change its pH, and promote bacterial growth. Instead, use a sponge tooth cleaner or soft-bristle toothbrush moistened in water for mouth care. Hydrogen peroxide solutions can help remove crusted matter but may break down healing tissue and should be used only with a physician's prescription. Help the patient rinse his or her mouth with normal saline every 4 hours while awake or as often as he or she desires.

Examine the mouth for open areas or dental problems. Ulcers and infections are treated medically. Apply lip balm or water-soluble jelly to prevent cracked lips and promote comfort. Mouth care helps promote oral health, comfort, and aesthetic appearance. Offering an opportunity for the patient or family member to perform mouth care allows participation in care and increases self-esteem.

Oral secretions can move down the trachea and collect above the inflated cuff of the endotracheal tube. When the cuff is deflated, the secretions can move into the lungs. Some endotracheal tubes have an extra lumen open to the area above the cuff, which allows suctioning of the airway above the cuff before deflating and reduces the risk for aspiration.

Ensuring Nutrition. Swallowing can be a major problem for the patient with a tracheostomy tube in place. In a normal swallow, the larynx lifts and moves forward to prevent the entering of food and saliva. The tracheostomy tube sometimes tethers the larynx in place, making it unable to move effectively. The result is difficulty in swallowing. Also, when the tracheostomy tube cuff is inflated, it can balloon backwards and interfere with food passage through the esophagus because the wall separating the back of the trachea and the front of the esophagus is thin.

Instruct the patient to keep the head of the bed elevated for at least 30 minutes after eating. Chart 28-5 outlines best practices to prevent aspiration during swallowing.

Maintaining Communication. The patient can speak when there is a cuffless tube, when a fenestrated tracheostomy tube is in place, and when the fenestrated tube is capped or covered. Until natural speech is feasible, teach him or her and the family about other communication means. A writing tablet, a board with pictures and letters, communication "flash cards" on a ring, hand signals, and a computer, as well as a call light within reach, are used to promote communication and decrease frustration from not being able to speak or be understood. Phrase questions

for "yes" or "no" answers to help the patient respond easily. Move the patient closer to the nurses' station, and mark the central call light system to indicate that he or she cannot speak.

The inability to talk is a stressor for the patient. Helping communication is an important nursing action and is required by The Joint Commission's National Patient Safety Goals (NPSGs). When the patient can tolerate cuff deflation, he or she places a finger over the tracheostomy tube on exhalation, forcing air up through the larynx and mouth and allowing speech.

A device to facilitate speech for the patient with a tracheostomy is a one-way valve that fits over the tube and replaces the need for finger occlusion. The valve allows him or her to breathe in through the tracheostomy tube. On exhalation, the valve closes so that air is forced through the vocal cords, allowing speech. For this valve to assist in speech, the patient must not be connected to a ventilator, must have the cuff deflated, and must be able to breathe around the tube. Some valves have a port for supplemental oxygen without impairing the ability to speak.

Supporting Psychosocial Needs and Self-Image. Addressing psychological concerns is an important aspect of caring for patients recovering from a tracheostomy. Always keep in mind the emotional impact of an artificial airway. Acknowledge the patient's frustration with communication, and allow sufficient time for communication. When speaking to him or her, use a normal tone of voice because hearing and comprehension are not altered by the presence of a tube.

The patient may have a change in self-image because of the presence of a stoma or artificial airway, speech changes, a change in the method of eating, or difficulty with speech. Help the patient set realistic goals, starting with involvement in self-care.

Work with the family to ease the patient into a more normal social environment. Provide encouragement and positive reinforcement while demonstrating acceptance and caring behaviors. Assess the family for the need for counseling.

After surgery, the patient may feel shy and socially isolated. He or she can wear loose-fitting shirts, decorative collars, or scarves to cover the tracheostomy tube.

Weaning. Weaning the patient from a tracheostomy tube entails a gradual decrease in the tube size and ultimate removal of the tube. Carefully monitor this process, especially after each change. The physician or advanced practice nurse performs the steps in the process.

First, the cuff is deflated as soon as the patient can manage secretions and does not need mechanical ventilation. This change allows him or her to breathe through the tube and through the upper airway. Next, the tube is changed to an uncuffed tube. If this is tolerated, the size of the tube is gradually decreased. When a small fenestrated tube is placed, the tube is capped so that all air passes through the upper airway and the fenestra, with none passing through the tube. Assess the patient to ensure adequate airflow around the tube when it is capped. The tube may be removed after he or she tolerates more than 24 hours of capping. Place a dry dressing over the stoma (which gradually heals on its own).

Another device used for the transition from tracheostomy to natural breathing is a *tracheostomy button*. The button maintains stoma patency and assists spontaneous breathing. The Kistner tracheostomy tube and Olympic tracheostomy button are examples of this type of device. To function, the button must fit properly. A disadvantage is the possibility of decannulation—the tube can dislodge from the trachea but remain in the neck tissues.

Community-Based Care

By the time of discharge, the patient should be able to provide self-care, which may include tracheostomy care, nutrition care, suctioning, and communication. Although education begins before surgery, most self-care is taught in the hospital. Teach the patient and family how to care for the tracheostomy tube. Review airway care, including cleaning and signs of infection. Teach clean suction technique, and review the plan of care.

Instruct the patient to use a shower shield over the tracheostomy tube when bathing to prevent water from entering the airway. Teach him or her to cover the airway loosely with a small cotton cloth to protect it during the day. Covering the opening filters the air entering the stoma, keeps humidity in the airway, and enhances appearance. Attractive coverings are available as cotton scarves, decorative collars, and jewelry.

Teach the patient to increase humidity in the home. Tell the patient to continue using the method of communication that began in the hospital and to wear a medical alert bracelet that identifies the inability to speak.

The health care team assesses specific discharge needs and makes referrals to home care agencies and durable medical equipment companies (for suction equipment and tracheostomy supplies). Follow-up visits occur early after discharge, and the home care nurse also is an important resource for the patient and family. This nurse initiates and coordinates the services of dietitians, nurses, speech and language pathologists, and social workers. He or she informs the patient and family of community resources that can offer support and friendship.

? CLINICAL JUDGMENT CHALLENGE

Safety; Patient-Centered Care QSEN

Your patient is a 41-year-old woman with a significant closed head injury (CHI) from a motor vehicle crash (MVC). She is not anticipated to be able to be weaned from the ventilator, and the physicians have asked the patient's family for permission to create a tracheostomy. The family is concerned that the patient will not be able to speak again.

1. What is your response?
2. What are some possible concerns for patient care in the immediate postoperative period?
3. What can you do to minimize tracheal damage?
4. The patient's family is concerned that the tracheostomy will be permanent and they are worried about her image. How do you respond?

CONSIDERATIONS FOR OLDER ADULTS

Patient-Centered Care QSEN

Self-managing tracheostomy care and oxygen therapy can be difficult for the older patient who has vision problems or difficulty with upper arm movement. Teach him or her to use magnifying lenses or glasses to ensure the proper setting on the oxygen gauge. Assess his or her ability to reach and manipulate the tracheostomy. If possible, work with a family member who can provide assistance during tracheostomy care.

NURSING CONCEPTS AND CLINICAL JUDGMENT REVIEW

What might you NOTICE if the patient is experiencing inadequate GAS EXCHANGE with oxygenation and tissue PERFUSION as a result of respiratory problems?

- Respirations rapid and shallow
- Respirations noisy
- Cannot speak more than 4 or 5 words without pausing for breath
- Change in cognition, acute confusion
- Decreased oxygen saturation by pulse oximetry
- Skin cyanosis or pallor (lighter-skinned patients)
- Cyanosis or pallor of the lips and oral mucous membranes (in patients of any skin color)
- Tachycardia
- Patient appears to strain to catch breath
- Fatigue

What should you INTERPRET and how should you RESPOND to a patient experiencing inadequate GAS EXCHANGE with oxygenation and tissue PERFUSION as a result of a respiratory problem?

Perform and interpret physical assessment, including:

- Taking vital signs
- Auscultating all lung fields

- Monitoring oxygen saturation by pulse oximetry
- Checking most recent laboratory values for hematocrit, hemoglobin, and ABG levels
- Assessing cognition (Mini-Mental State Examination [MMSE])
- Assessing for the use of accessory muscles
- Assessing for the presence of thick or excessive secretions
- Assessing the patient's ability to cough and clear the airway

Respond by:
- Applying oxygen and assessing the patient's responses to this intervention
- Keeping the patient's head elevated to about 30 degrees

- Suctioning (oral, pharyngeal, endotracheal, tracheostomy), if needed
- Notifying the physician or Rapid Response Team
- Prioritizing and pacing activities to prevent fatigue

On what should you REFLECT?
- Observe the patient for evidence of restored gas exchange (see Chapter 27).
- Think about what may have made the impaired gas exchange worse and what steps could be taken to either prevent a similar episode or identify it earlier.
- Think about what additional resources could improve the nursing response to this situation.

GET READY FOR THE NCLEX® EXAMINATION!

KEY POINTS

Review these Key Points for each NCLEX Examination Client Needs Category.

Safe and Effective Care Environment
- Never allow water condensation in an oxygen delivery system to drain back into the system. **Safety** QSEN
- Use sterile technique when performing endotracheal or tracheal suctioning. **Safety** QSEN
- Inspect the oral mucous membranes each shift for anyone who has an endotracheal tube. **Safety** QSEN
- Keep a tracheostomy tube (and obturator) and tracheostomy insertion tray at the bedside for the first 72 hours after a tracheostomy has been created. **Safety** QSEN
- Never use oral suctioning equipment to suction an artificial airway. **Safety** QSEN
- Use Aspiration Precautions for any patient with an altered level of consciousness or who has an endotracheal tube (see Chart 28-5). **Safety** QSEN
- Verify safe use of appropriate oxygen delivery systems and tracheostomy equipment. **Safety** QSEN

Health Promotion and Maintenance
- Teach the patient and family about home management of oxygen therapy, including the avoidance of smoking or open flames in rooms in which oxygen is being used. **Patient-Centered Care** QSEN
- Teach the patient and family how to perform tracheostomy care (see Chart 28-3). **Patient-Centered Care** QSEN

Psychosocial Integrity
- Provide opportunity for the patient and family to express concerns about a change in breathing status or the possibility of intubation and mechanical ventilation.
- Teach family members ways to communicate with a patient who is intubated or being mechanically ventilated. **Patient-Centered Care** QSEN

- Reassure patients who are intubated that the loss of speech is temporary. **Patient-Centered Care** QSEN
- Encourage patients with permanent tracheostomies to become involved in self-care. **Patient-Centered Care** QSEN

Physiological Integrity
- Apply oxygen to anyone who is hypoxemic. **Evidence-Based Practice** QSEN
- Ensure that oxygen therapy delivered to the patient is humidified appropriately. **Evidence-Based Practice** QSEN
- Monitor arterial blood gases (ABGs) and oxygen saturation of all patients receiving oxygen therapy. **Evidence-Based Practice** QSEN
- Assess the skin under the mask and under the plastic tubing every shift for patients receiving oxygen by mask. **Patient-Centered Care** QSEN
- Assess the skin of the nares and under the elastic band every shift for patients receiving oxygen by nasal cannula. **Patient-Centered Care** QSEN
- Observe any patient receiving oxygen at greater than a 50% concentration for early manifestations of oxygen toxicity (i.e. dyspnea, nonproductive cough, chest pain, GI upset). **Patient-Centered Care** QSEN
- Use a manual resuscitation bag to ventilate the patient if the tracheostomy tube has dislodged or become decannulated. **Safety** QSEN
- Assess the new tracheostomy stoma site at least once per shift for purulent drainage, redness, pain, and swelling as indicators of infection. **Evidence-Based Practice** QSEN
- Keep the tracheal cuff pressure between 14 and 20 mm Hg to prevent tissue injury. **Safety** QSEN

CHAPTER 29

Care of Patients with Noninfectious Upper Respiratory Problems

M. Linda Workman

 http://evolve.elsevier.com/Iggy/

PRIORITY CONCEPTS

- GAS EXCHANGE
- CELLULAR REGULATION

LEARNING OUTCOMES

Safe and Effective Care Environment

1. Protect patients with upper respiratory problems from hypoxia, injury, infection, and impairment in GAS EXCHANGE.

Health Promotion and Maintenance

2. Teach all people measures to take to protect the upper respiratory system from damage and cancer (loss of CELLULAR REGULATION), including the avoidance of known environmental causative agents.
3. Teach the patient and family how to manage a chronic lower respiratory disorder and avoid injury and complications in the home.

Psychosocial Integrity

4. Reduce the psychological impact for the patient and family experiencing an acute or chronic upper respiratory problem.
5. Work with other members of the health care team to ensure that values, preferences, and expressed needs of patients experiencing upper respiratory problems and reduced GAS EXCHANGE are respected.

Physiological Integrity

6. Assess and re-assess the manifestations of patients being managed for an upper respiratory problem.
7. Use laboratory data and clinical manifestations to prioritize nursing care for the patient who has an acute or chronic upper respiratory problem.
8. Prioritize nursing care needs of a patient after a nasoseptoplasty.
9. Prioritize the nursing care needs of the patient and family experiencing head and neck cancer.
10. Work with other health care professionals who help the patient and family experiencing a chronic upper respiratory problem achieve desired health outcomes.
11. Coordinate nursing interventions for the patient with a chronic upper respiratory problem in the community.

The nose, sinuses, oropharynx, larynx, and trachea are the upper airway structures. They are important for GAS EXCHANGE and perfusion by providing the entrance site for air. Problems of the upper airways, especially the larynx and trachea, can interfere with oxygen delivery. Patients with upper respiratory problems are found in the community and in all health care settings. *The nursing priority with disorders of the upper respiratory tract is to promote gas exchange by ensuring a patent airway.*

DISORDERS OF THE NOSE AND SINUSES

FRACTURE OF THE NOSE

❖ PATHOPHYSIOLOGY

Nasal fractures often result from injuries received during falls, sports activities, car crashes, or physical assaults and can interfere with GAS EXCHANGE. If the bone or cartilage is not displaced and no complications are present, treatment may not be needed. Displacement of either the bone or cartilage, however, can cause airway obstruction or cosmetic deformity and is a potential source of infection.

❖ PATIENT-CENTERED COLLABORATIVE CARE

◆ Assessment

Document any nasal problem, including deviation, malaligned nasal bridge, a change in nasal breathing, crackling of the skin *(crepitus)* on palpation, bruising, and pain. Blood or clear fluid (cerebrospinal fluid [CSF]) rarely drains from one or both nares as a result of a simple nasal fracture and, if present, indicates a serious injury (e.g., skull fracture). CSF can be differentiated from normal nasal secretions because CSF contains glucose that will test positive with a dipstick test for glucose. When CSF dries on a piece of filter paper, a yellow "halo" appears as a ring at the dried edge of the fluid. X-rays are not always useful in the diagnosis of simple nasal fractures.

◆ Interventions

The health care provider performs a simple closed reduction (moving the bones by palpation to realign them) of the nasal fracture using local or general anesthesia within the first 24 hours after injury. After 24 hours, the fracture is more difficult to reduce because of edema and scar formation. Then reduction may be delayed for several days until edema is gone. Simple closed fractures may not need surgical intervention. Management focuses on pain relief and cold compresses to decrease swelling.

Rhinoplasty. Reduction and surgery may be needed for severe fractures or for those that do not heal properly. Rhinoplasty is a surgical reconstruction of the nose. It can be performed to repair a fractured nose and also can be performed to change the shape of the nose. The patient returns from surgery with packing in both nostrils, which prevents bleeding and provides support for the reconstructed nose. As long as the packing is in place, the patient cannot breathe through the nose. A "moustache" dressing (or drip pad), often a folded 2 × 2 gauze pad, is usually placed under the nose (Fig. 29-1). A splint or cast may cover the nose for better alignment and protection. Change or teach the patient to change the drip pad as necessary.

After surgery, observe for edema and bleeding. Check vital signs every 4 hours until the patient is discharged. The patient with uncomplicated rhinoplasty is discharged the day of surgery. Instruct him or her and the family about the routine care described below.

> ### ! NURSING SAFETY PRIORITY (QSEN)
>
> **Action Alert**
>
> Assessing how often the patient swallows after nasal surgery is a priority because repeated swallowing may indicate posterior nasal bleeding. Use a penlight to examine the throat for bleeding, and notify the surgeon if bleeding is present.

FIG. 29-1 Immediate postoperative appearance of a patient who has undergone rhinoplasty. Note the splint and gauze drip pad (moustache dressing).

Instruct the patient to stay in a semi-Fowler's position and to move slowly. Suggest that he or she rests and uses cool compresses on the nose, eyes, and face to help reduce swelling and bruising. If a general anesthetic was used, soft foods can be eaten once the patient is alert and the gag reflex has returned. Urge the patient to drink at least 2500 mL/day.

To prevent bleeding, teach the patient to limit Valsalva maneuvers (e.g., forceful coughing or straining during a bowel movement), not to sniff upward or blow the nose, and not to sneeze with the mouth closed for the first few days after the packing is removed. Instruct the patient to avoid aspirin and other NSAIDs to prevent bleeding. Antibiotics may be prescribed to prevent infection. Recommend the use of a humidifier to prevent mucosal drying. Explain that edema lasts for weeks and that the final surgical result will be evident in 6 to 12 months.

Nasoseptoplasty. Nasoseptoplasty, or submucous resection (SMR), may be needed to straighten a deviated septum when chronic "stuffy" nose, snoring, sinusitis, or discomfort occurs. Slight nasal septum deviation causes no manifestations. Major deviations may obstruct the nasal passages or interfere with airflow and sinus drainage. The deviated section of cartilage and bone is removed or reshaped as an ambulatory surgical procedure. Nursing care is similar to that for a rhinoplasty.

EPISTAXIS

❖ PATHOPHYSIOLOGY

Epistaxis (nosebleed) is a common problem because of the many capillaries within the nose. Nosebleeds occur as a result of trauma, hypertension, blood dyscrasia (e.g., leukemia), inflammation, tumor, decreased humidity, nose blowing, nose picking, chronic cocaine use, and procedures such as nasogastric suctioning. Older adults tend to bleed most often from the posterior portion of the nose.

❖ PATIENT-CENTERED COLLABORATIVE CARE

The patient often reports that the bleeding started after sneezing or blowing the nose. Document the amount and color of the blood, and take vital signs. Ask the patient about the number, duration, and causes of previous bleeding episodes.

Chart 29-1 lists the best practices for emergency care of the patient with a nosebleed. An additional intervention for use at

---

> ### CHART 29-1 Best Practice for Patient Safety & Quality Care (QSEN)
>
> **Emergency Care of a Patient with an Anterior Nosebleed**
>
> - Maintain Standard Precautions or Body Substance Precautions.
> - Position the patient upright and leaning forward to prevent blood from entering the stomach and possible aspiration.
> - Reassure the patient and attempt to keep him or her quiet to reduce anxiety and blood pressure.
> - Apply direct lateral pressure to the nose for 10 minutes, and apply ice or cool compresses to the nose and face if possible.
> - If nasal packing is necessary, loosely pack both nares with gauze or nasal tampons.
> - To prevent rebleeding from dislodging clots, instruct the patient to not blow the nose for 24 hours after the bleeding stops.
> - Seek medical assistance if these measures are ineffective or if the bleeding occurs frequently.

home or in the emergency department is a special nasal plug that contains an agent to promote blood clotting (sold by HemCon). The plug expands on contact with blood and compresses mucosal blood vessels.

Medical attention is needed if the nosebleed does not respond to these interventions. In such cases, the affected capillaries may be cauterized with silver nitrate or electrocautery and the nose packed. Anterior packing controls bleeding from the anterior nasal cavity.

Posterior nasal bleeding is an emergency because it cannot be easily reached and the patient may lose a lot of blood quickly (Vacca & Poirier, 2013). Posterior packing, epistaxis catheters (nasal pressure tubes), or a gel tampon is used to stop bleeding that originates in the posterior nasal region. With packing, the health care provider positions a large gauze pack in the posterior nasal cavity above the throat, threads the attached string through the nose, and tapes it to the patient's cheek to prevent pack movement. Epistaxis catheters look like very short (about 6 inches) urinary catheters (Fig. 29-2, *A*). These tubes have an exterior balloon along the tube length in addition to an anchoring balloon on the end. Placement of posterior packing or pressure tubes is uncomfortable, and the airway may be obstructed and GAS EXCHANGE impaired if the pack slips. Fig. 29-2, *B*, shows a patient with tubes in place for a posterior nasal bleed.

Observe the patient for respiratory distress and for tolerance of the packing or tubes. Humidity, oxygen, bedrest, and antibiotics may be prescribed. Opioid drugs may be prescribed for pain. Assess patients receiving opioids at least hourly for gag and cough reflexes. Use pulse oximetry to monitor for hypoxemia. The tubes or packing is usually removed after 1 to 3 days.

For posterior bleeds that do not respond to packing or tubes, additional options include cauterizing the blood vessels, ligating the vessels, or performing an embolization of the bleeding artery with interventional radiology. Potential complications of embolization include facial pain, necrosis of skin or nasal mucosa, facial nerve paralysis, and blindness (Poetker, 2013).

After the tubes or packing is removed, teach the patient and family these interventions to use at home for comfort and safety:

- Petroleum jelly can be applied sparingly to the nares for lubrication and comfort. (Excessive application could cause inhalation of the jelly into the lungs and increase the risk for pneumonia.)
- Nasal saline sprays and humidification add moisture and prevent rebleeding.
- Avoid vigorous nose blowing, the use of aspirin or other NSAIDs, and strenuous activities such as heavy lifting for at least 1 month.

CANCER OF THE NOSE AND SINUSES

Tumors of the nasal cavities and sinuses are rare, the result of loss of CELLULAR REGULATION, and may be either benign or malignant. This type of cancer is more common among people with chronic exposure to wood dusts, dusts from textiles, leather dusts, flour, nickel and chromium dust, mustard gas, and radium. Cigarette smoking along with these exposures increases the risk (American Cancer Society [ACS], 2014).

The onset of sinus cancer is slow, and manifestations resemble sinusitis. These include persistent nasal obstruction, drainage, bloody discharge, and pain that persists after treatment of sinusitis. Lymph node enlargement often occurs on the side with tumor mass. Tumor location is identified with x-ray, CT, or MRI. A biopsy is performed to confirm the diagnosis.

Surgical removal of all or part of the tumor is the main treatment for nasopharyngeal cancers. It is usually combined with radiation therapy, especially intensity modulated radiation therapy (IMRT) (see Chapter 22). Chemotherapy may be used in conjunction with surgery and radiation for some tumors. Problems after surgery include a change in body image or speech and altered nutrition, especially when the maxilla and floor of the nose are involved in the surgery. Patients often also have changes in taste and smell.

Provide general postoperative care (see Chapter 16), including maintaining a patent airway, monitoring for hemorrhage,

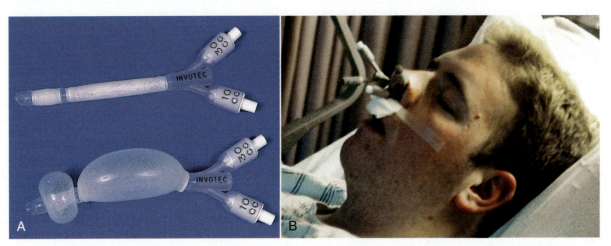

FIG. 29-2 A, The Ultra-Stat epistaxis catheter. **B,** Patient with epistaxis catheters in place to control a posterior nasal bleed.

providing wound care, assessing nutrition status, and performing tracheostomy care (if needed). (See Chapter 28 for tracheostomy care.) Perform careful mouth and sinus cavity care with saline irrigations using an electronic irrigation system (e.g., Waterpik, Sonicare) or a syringe. Assess the patient for pain and infection. Collaborate with the dietitian to help the patient make food selections that promote healing.

FACIAL TRAUMA

❖ PATHOPHYSIOLOGY

Facial trauma is described by the specific bones (e.g., mandibular, maxillary, orbital, nasal fractures) and the side of the face involved. Mandibular (lower jaw) fractures are the most common. *Le Fort I* is a nasoethmoid complex fracture. *Le Fort II* is a maxillary *and* nasoethmoid complex fracture. *Le Fort III* combines I and II plus an orbital-zygoma fracture, called "craniofacial disjunction" because the midface has no connection to the skull. The rich facial blood supply results in extensive bleeding and bruising.

❖ PATIENT-CENTERED COLLABORATIVE CARE

◆ Assessment

The priority action when caring for a patient with facial trauma is airway assessment for GAS EXCHANGE. Manifestations of airway obstruction are stridor, shortness of breath, dyspnea, anxiety, restlessness, hypoxia, **hypercarbia** (elevated blood levels of carbon dioxide), decreased oxygen saturation, cyanosis, and loss of consciousness. After establishing the airway, assess the site of trauma for bleeding and possible fractures. Check for soft-tissue edema, facial asymmetry, pain, or leakage of spinal fluid through the ears or nose, indicating a skull fracture. Assess vision and eye movement because orbital and maxillary fractures can entrap the eye nerves and muscles. Check behind the ears (mastoid area) for extensive bruising, known as the "battle sign," which is often associated with skull fracture and brain trauma. Because facial trauma can occur with spinal trauma and skull fractures, cranial CT, facial series, and cervical spine x-rays are obtained.

◆ Interventions

The priority action is to establish and maintain an airway for adequate GAS EXCHANGE. Anticipate the need for emergency intubation, **tracheotomy** (surgical incision into the trachea to create an airway), or **cricothyroidotomy** (creation of a temporary airway by making a small opening in the throat between the thyroid cartilage and the cricoid cartilage). Care at first focuses on establishing an airway, controlling hemorrhage, and assessing for the extent of injury. If shock is present, fluid resuscitation and identification of bleeding sites are started immediately.

Time is critical in stabilizing the patient who has head and neck trauma. Early response and treatment by special services (e.g., trauma team, maxillofacial surgeon, general surgeon, otolaryngologist, plastic surgeon, dentist) optimize the patient's recovery.

Stabilizing the fractured jaw allows the teeth to heal in proper alignment and involves **fixed occlusion** (wiring the jaws together with the mouth in a closed position). The patient remains in fixed occlusion for 6 to 10 weeks. Treatment delay, tooth infection, or poor oral care may cause jaw bone infection. This condition may then require surgical removal of dead tissue, IV antibiotic therapy, and a longer period with the jaws in a fixed position.

Extensive jaw fractures may require open reduction with internal fixation (ORIF) procedures. Compression plates and reconstruction plates with screws may be applied. Plates may be made of stainless steel, titanium, or Vitallium. If the mandibular fracture is repaired with titanium plates, the plates are permanent and do not interfere with MRI studies.

Facial fractures may be repaired with microplating surgical systems that involve bone substitutes. These shaping plates hold the bone fragments in place until new bone growth occurs. Bone cells grow into the bone substitute and re-matrix into a stable bone support. The plates may remain in place permanently or may be removed after healing.

Other fixation methods include the use of resorbable devices (plates and screws) to hold tissues in place. These devices are made from a plastic-like material that retains its integrity for about 8 weeks and then slowly biodegrades. With inner maxillary fixation (IMF), the bones are realigned and then wired in place with the bite closed. Nondisplaced aligned fractures can be repaired in a clinic or office using local dental anesthesia. General anesthesia is used to repair displaced or complex fractures or fractures that occur with other facial bone fractures.

After surgery, teach the patient about oral care with an irrigating device, such as a Waterpik or Sonicare. If the patient has inner maxillary fixation, teach self-management with wires in place, including a dental liquid diet. If the patient vomits, watch for aspiration because of the patient's inability to open the jaws to allow ejection of the emesis. Teach him or her how to cut the wires if vomiting occurs to maintain GAS EXCHANGE. If the wires are cut, instruct the patient to return to the surgeon for rewiring as soon as possible to reinstitute fixation.

> **❗ NURSING SAFETY PRIORITY** (QSEN)
>
> **Action Alert**
>
> Instruct the patient to keep wire cutters with him or her at all times to prevent aspiration if vomiting occurs.

Nutrition is important and difficult for a patient with fractures because of oral fixation, pain, and surgery. Collaborate with the dietitian for patient teaching and support.

OBSTRUCTIVE SLEEP APNEA

❖ PATHOPHYSIOLOGY

Obstructive sleep apnea (OSA) is a breathing disruption during sleep that lasts at least 10 seconds and occurs a minimum of 5 times in an hour. The most common cause of sleep apnea is upper airway obstruction by the soft palate or tongue. Factors that contribute to sleep apnea include obesity, a large uvula, a short neck, smoking, enlarged tonsils or adenoids, and oropharyngeal edema.

During sleep, the muscles relax and the tongue and neck structures are displaced. As a result, the upper airway is obstructed but chest movement is unimpaired. The apnea impairs GAS EXCHANGE and increases blood carbon dioxide levels and decreases the pH. These blood gas changes stimulate neural centers. The sleeper awakens after 10 seconds or longer of apnea and corrects the obstruction, and respiration resumes. After he or she goes back to sleep, the cycle begins again, sometimes as often as every 5 minutes.

This cyclic pattern of disrupted sleep prevents the deep sleep needed for best rest. Thus the person may have excessive daytime sleepiness, an inability to concentrate, and irritability. The long-term effects of OSA include increased risk for hypertension, stroke, neurocognitive deficits, weight gain, diabetes, and pulmonary and cardiovascular disease (Woidtke, 2013).

❖ *PATIENT-CENTERED COLLABORATIVE CARE*

◆ *Assessment*

Patients are often unaware that they have sleep apnea. The disorder should be suspected for any person who has persistent daytime sleepiness or reports "waking up tired," particularly if he or she also snores heavily. Other manifestations include irritability and personality changes. Sleep apnea may be verified by family members who observe the problem when the person sleeps. A complete assessment is performed when excessive daytime sleepiness is a problem.

A beginning assessment includes having the patient complete the Epworth Sleepiness Scale (ESS) (Simmons & Pruitt, 2012). The patient is asked to score his or her likelihood of falling asleep during eight common activities or scenarios. Each is self-scored from 0 to 3. Those patients who score 18 or above are considered at risk for severe sleep apnea.

The most accurate test for sleep apnea is an overnight sleep study. In this study, the patient is directly observed while wearing a variety of monitoring equipment to evaluate depth of sleep, type of sleep, respiratory effort, oxygen saturation, and muscle movement. Monitoring devices include an electroencephalograph (EEG), an electrocardiograph (ECG), a pulse oximeter, and an electromyograph (EMG). Home-based sleep studies also are available but often not covered by insurance (Carlucci et al., 2013).

◆ *Interventions*

A change in sleeping position or weight loss may correct mild sleep apnea and improve GAS EXCHANGE. Position-fixing devices may prevent subluxation of the tongue and neck structures and reduce obstruction. Severe sleep apnea requires additional methods to prevent obstruction.

A common method to prevent airway collapse is the use of noninvasive positive-pressure ventilation (NPPV) to hold open the upper airways. A nasal mask or full-face mask delivery system allows mechanical delivery of either bi-level positive airway pressure (BiPAP), autotitrating positive airway pressure (APAP), or nasal continuous positive airway pressure (CPAP). With BiPAP, a machine delivers a set inspiratory positive airway pressure at the beginning of each breath. As the patient begins to exhale, the machine delivers a lower end-expiratory pressure. These two pressures hold open the upper airways. With APAP, the machine adjusts continuously, resetting the pressure throughout the breathing cycle to meet the patient's needs. Nasal CPAP delivers a set positive airway pressure continuously during each cycle of inhalation and exhalation. For any positive-pressure ventilation delivered through a facemask during sleep, a small electric compressor is required. Proper fit of the mask over the nose and mouth or just over the nose is key to successful treatment (see Fig. 28-9 in Chapter 28). Although noisy, these methods are accepted by most patients after an adjustment period.

One drug has been approved to help manage the daytime sleepiness associated with sleep apnea. Modafinil (Attenace, Provigil) is helpful for patients who have *narcolepsy* (uncontrolled daytime sleep) from sleep apnea by promoting daytime wakefulness. This drug does *not* treat the cause of sleep apnea. Sleep-inducing sedatives also are not considered first-line therapy.

Surgical intervention may involve a simple adenoidectomy, uvulectomy, or remodeling of the entire posterior oropharynx (uvulopalatopharyngoplasty [UPP]). Both conventional and laser surgeries are used for this purpose. A tracheostomy may be needed for very severe sleep apnea that is not relieved by more moderate interventions.

DISORDERS OF THE LARYNX

VOCAL CORD PARALYSIS

Vocal fold (cord) paralysis may result from injury, trauma, or diseases that affect the larynx, laryngeal nerves, or vagus nerve. Prolonged intubation with an endotracheal (ET) tube may cause temporary or permanent paralysis. Paralysis may occur in patients with neurologic disorders or with conditions that damage either the vagus nerve or the laryngeal nerves. Paralysis of both vocal cords may result from injury, brainstem stroke, or total thyroidectomy.

Vocal fold paralysis may affect both cords or only one. When only one vocal cord is involved (most common), the airway remains patent but the voice is affected. Manifestations of open bilateral vocal cord paralysis include hoarseness; a breathy, weak voice; and aspiration of food. *Bilateral closed vocal cord paralysis causes airway obstruction and is an emergency if the manifestations are severe and the patient cannot compensate. Stridor is the major manifestation.*

Securing an airway is the main intervention. Place the patient in a high-Fowler's position to aid in breathing and proper alignment of airway structures. Assess for airway obstruction.

❗ NURSING SAFETY PRIORITY (QSEN)

Critical Rescue

Immediately notify the Rapid Response Team if dyspnea with stridor occurs. Emergency endotracheal intubation or tracheotomy may be needed.

Various surgical procedures can improve the voice. One simple procedure for open vocal cord paralysis involves injecting polytef (Teflon) into the affected cord so it enlarges toward the unaffected cord. This technique improves closure during speaking and eating.

The patient with open cord paralysis is at risk for aspiration because the airway is open during swallowing. Teach him or her to hold the breath during swallowing to allow the larynx to rise, close, and push food back into the esophagus during swallowing. Teach the patient to tuck the chin down and tilt the forehead forward during swallowing. Indications of aspiration include immediate coughing on swallowing of liquids or solids, a "wet"-sounding voice, and "tearing up" or watery eyes on swallowing. Chest x-rays are used to diagnose aspiration pneumonia.

LARYNGEAL TRAUMA

Laryngeal trauma occurs with a crushing or direct blow injury, fracture, or prolonged endotracheal intubation. Manifestations include difficulty breathing (dyspnea), inability to produce sound (aphonia), hoarseness, and subcutaneous emphysema (air present in the subcutaneous tissue). Bleeding from the airway (hemoptysis) may occur, depending on the location of the trauma. The health care provider performs a direct visual examination of the larynx by laryngoscopy or fiberoptic laryngoscopy to determine the extent of the injury.

Management of patients with laryngeal injuries consists of assessing the effectiveness of GAS EXCHANGE and monitoring vital signs (including respiratory status and pulse oximetry) every 15 to 30 minutes. *Maintaining a patent airway is a priority.* Apply oxygen and humidification as prescribed to maintain adequate oxygen saturation. Manifestations of respiratory difficulty include tachypnea, nasal flaring, anxiety, sternal retraction, shortness of breath, restlessness, decreased oxygen saturation, decreased level of consciousness, and stridor.

> **! NURSING SAFETY PRIORITY (QSEN)**
> *Critical Rescue*
>
> If the patient has respiratory difficulty, stay with him or her and instruct other trauma team members or the Rapid Response Team to prepare for an emergency intubation or tracheotomy.

Surgical intervention is needed for lacerations of the mucous membranes, cartilage exposure, and cord paralysis. Laryngeal repair is performed as soon as possible to prevent laryngeal stenosis and to cover any exposed cartilage. An artificial airway may be needed.

OTHER UPPER AIRWAY DISORDERS

UPPER AIRWAY OBSTRUCTION

❖ PATHOPHYSIOLOGY

Upper airway obstruction is a life-threatening emergency in which airflow through nose, mouth, pharynx, or larynx is interrupted and GAS EXCHANGE is impaired. Early recognition is essential to prevent complications, including respiratory arrest. Causes of upper airway obstruction include:

- Tongue edema (surgery, trauma, angioedema as an allergic response to a drug)
- Tongue occlusion (e.g., loss of gag reflex, loss of muscle tone, unconsciousness, coma)
- Laryngeal edema
- Peritonsillar and pharyngeal abscess
- Head and neck cancer
- Thick secretions
- Stroke and cerebral edema
- Smoke inhalation edema
- Facial, tracheal, or laryngeal trauma
- Foreign-body aspiration
- Burns of the head or neck area
- Anaphylaxis

One preventable cause of airway obstruction leading to asphyxiation is inspissated (thickly crusted) oral and nasopharyngeal secretions. In this condition, poor oral hygiene leads to

thickening and hardening of secretions that can completely block the airway and lead to death. Proper nursing care can eliminate this cause of airway obstruction. Patients at highest risk are those with an altered mental status and level of consciousness, are dehydrated, are unable to communicate, are unable to cough effectively, or are at risk for aspiration.

> **! NURSE SAFETY PRIORITY (QSEN)**
> *Action Alert*
>
> Assess the oral care needs of the patient with risk factors for inspissated secretions daily. Ensure that whoever provides oral care understands the importance and the correct techniques for preventing secretion buildup and airway obstruction.

❖ PATIENT-CENTERED COLLABORATIVE CARE

◆ Assessment

Airway obstruction is frightening, and prompt care is essential to prevent a partial obstruction from progressing to a complete obstruction. Partial obstruction produces general manifestations such as diaphoresis, tachycardia, and elevated blood pressure. Persistent or unexplained manifestations must be evaluated even though vague. Diagnostic procedures include chest or neck x-rays, laryngoscopic examination, and computed tomography.

Observe for hypoxia and hypercarbia, restlessness, increasing anxiety, sternal retractions, a "seesawing" chest, abdominal movements, or a feeling of impending doom from air hunger. Use pulse oximetry or end-tidal carbon dioxide (ETCO₂ or PETCO₂) for ongoing monitoring of GAS EXCHANGE. Continually assess for stridor, cyanosis, and changes in level of consciousness.

◆ Interventions

Assess for the cause of the obstruction. When the obstruction is due to the tongue falling back or excessive secretions, slightly extend the patient's head and neck and insert a nasal or an oral airway. Suction to remove obstructing secretions. If the obstruction is caused by a foreign body, perform abdominal thrusts (Fig. 29-3).

Upper airway obstruction may require emergency procedures such as cricothyroidotomy, endotracheal intubation, or tracheotomy to improve GAS EXCHANGE. Direct laryngoscopy may be performed before or with these procedures to determine the cause of obstruction or to remove foreign bodies.

Cricothyroidotomy is an emergency procedure performed by emergency medical personnel as a stab wound at the cricothyroid membrane between the thyroid cartilage and the cricoid cartilage (see Fig. 27-4 in Chapter 27). Any hollow tube—but preferably a tracheostomy tube—can be placed through the opening to hold this airway open until a tracheotomy can be performed. This procedure is used when it is the *only* way to secure an airway. Another emergency procedure to bypass an obstruction is the insertion of a 14-gauge needle directly into the cricoid space to allow airflow into and out of the lungs.

Endotracheal intubation is performed by inserting a tube into the trachea via the nose (nasotracheal) or mouth (orotracheal) by a physician, anesthesia provider, or other specially trained personnel.

Tracheotomy is a surgical procedure and takes about 5 to 10 minutes to perform. It is best performed in the operating room

With the conscious victim standing or sitting, place your fist between the victim's lower rib cage and navel. Wrap the palm of your hand around your fist. A quick inward, upward thrust expels the air remaining in the victim's lungs, and with it the foreign body. If the first thrust is unsuccessful, repeat several thrusts in rapid succession until the foreign body is expelled or until the victim loses consciousness.

With the unconscious victim lying supine, straddle the victim's thighs. Place one hand on top of the other as shown, with the heel of the bottom hand just above the victim's navel. Quickly thrust inward and upward, toward the victim's head.

FIG. 29-3 The abdominal thrust maneuver (formerly known as the *Heimlich maneuver*) for relief of upper airway obstruction caused by a foreign body.

(OR) with the patient under local or general anesthesia but can be performed at the bedside. Local anesthesia is used if there is concern that the airway will be lost during the induction of anesthesia. A tracheotomy is reserved for the patient who cannot be easily intubated with an endotracheal tube. An emergency tracheotomy can establish an airway in less than 2 minutes. See Chapter 28 for a discussion of care of the patient with a tracheotomy.

Patients receiving mechanical ventilation for upper airway obstruction or respiratory failure may require a tracheostomy after 7 or more days of continuous intubation. In such cases, a tracheotomy is performed to prevent laryngeal injury by the endotracheal tube.

💡 NCLEX EXAMINATION CHALLENGE

Physiological Integrity

The client is a woman with severe angioedema and tongue swelling from exposure to seafood. She has stridor, and her oxygen saturation is 70%. For which type of respiratory support does the nurse prepare?
A. Nasal BiPAP
B. Tracheotomy
C. Cricothyroidotomy
D. Endotracheal intubation

NECK TRAUMA

Neck injuries may be caused by any weapon or trauma. The patient with neck trauma may have other injuries, including cardiovascular, respiratory, intestinal, and neurologic damage. The final outcome of this type of injury depends on initial assessment and care. Consult a critical care textbook and see Chapter 43 for more detailed information.

The priority nursing care for a patient with neck trauma is assessing for and maintaining a patent airway. After airway patency is ensured, assess for bleeding or impending shock.

Perform a neurologic assessment for mental status, sensory level, and motor function. Injury to the carotid artery may result in death, stroke, or paralysis from disruption of blood flow to the brain (see Chapter 41). A carotid angiogram may be needed to rule out vascular injuries.

Esophagus injury may occur with neck trauma. Assess for chest pain and tenderness, oral bleeding, and **crepitus** (crackling sounds when palpating the skin). A barium or meglumine diatrizoate (Gastrografin) swallow may be needed to rule out an esophageal perforation injury.

Cervical spine injuries often occur at the same time as a neck injury (see Chapter 43). Obstruction can occur as a result of the initial injury or from swelling after surgery to repair the injury. Health care personnel must take great care not to make these injuries worse by causing neck movement while establishing the airway using the jaw-thrust maneuver. Prepare to assist in emergency intubation, cricothyrotomy, or tracheotomy to establish a patent airway. Interventions for patients in shock are detailed in Chapter 37.

HEAD AND NECK CANCER

❖ *PATHOPHYSIOLOGY*

Head and neck cancer can disrupt breathing (GAS EXCHANGE), eating, facial appearance, self-image, speech, and communication. This form of cancer can be devastating, even when cured. The care needs for patients with these problems are complex, requiring a coordinated and comprehensive team approach.

Head and neck cancers are usually squamous cell carcinomas. These slow-growing tumors are curable when treated early. The prognosis for those who have more advanced disease at diagnosis depends on the extent and location of the tumors. Untreated cancer of the head and neck is a fatal disease within 2 years of diagnosis (ACS, 2014).

The cancer begins as a loss of CELLULAR REGULATION when the mucosa is chronically irritated and becomes tougher and thicker (*squamous metaplasia*). At the same time, genes controlling cell growth are damaged, allowing excessive growth of these abnormal cells, which eventually become malignant. These lesions may then be seen as white, patchy lesions (leukoplakia) or red, velvety patches (erythroplakia).

Head and neck cancer first spreads (metastasizes) into nearby structures, such as lymph nodes, muscle, and bone. Later spread is systemic to distant sites, usually to the lungs or liver.

The cancer type and stage are determined by cellular analysis. Earlier-stage cancers are described as *carcinoma in situ* and *well differentiated*. Without treatment, cancers progress to be *moderately differentiated* and, finally, *poorly differentiated*. Most head and neck cancers arise from the mucous membrane and skin, but they also can start from salivary glands, the thyroid, or other structures. Treatment is based on tumor cell type and degree of spread at diagnosis.

Etiology. The two most important risk factors for head and neck cancer are tobacco and alcohol use, especially in combination. Other risk factors include voice abuse, chronic laryngitis, exposure to chemicals or dusts, poor oral hygiene, long-term or severe gastroesophageal reflux disease, and oral infection with the human papillomavirus (ACS, 2014).

Incidence and Prevalence. The frequency of head and neck carcinoma is increasing in North America. About 60,000 new cases of oral, pharyngeal, and laryngeal cancers are diagnosed each year and account for more than 13,000 deaths per year (ACS, 2014; Canadian Cancer Society, 2014). They affect men twice as often as women and are most common in people older than 60 years.

❖ PATIENT-CENTERED COLLABORATIVE CARE

◆ Assessment

History. The patient may have difficulty speaking because of hoarseness, shortness of breath, tumor bulk, and pain. Pace the interview to avoid tiring the patient.

Ask about tobacco and alcohol use, history of acute or chronic laryngitis or pharyngitis, oral sores, and lumps in the neck. Calculate the patient's pack-years of smoking history (see Chapter 27). Ask about alcohol intake (how many drinks per day and for how many years). Also ask about exposure to pollutants.

Assess problems related to risk factors. For example, nutrition may be poor because of alcohol intake and impaired liver function. Assess dietary habits and any weight loss. Ask about any chronic lung disease, which may have an impact on GAS EXCHANGE.

Physical Assessment/Clinical Manifestations. Table 29-1 lists the warning signs of head and neck cancer. With laryngeal cancer, painless hoarseness may occur because of tumor size and an inability of the vocal cords to come together for normal speech. Vocal cord lesions form early in laryngeal cancer. Any person who has a history of hoarseness, mouth sores, or a lump in the neck for 3 to 4 weeks should be evaluated for laryngeal cancer.

Inspect the head and neck for symmetry and the presence of lumps or lesions. An advanced practice nurse or physician may perform a laryngeal examination using a laryngeal mirror or fiberoptic laryngoscope. The neck is palpated to assess for enlarged lymph nodes.

Psychosocial Assessment. Often the patient with head and neck cancer has a long-standing history of tobacco or alcohol use or both. Assess the adequacy of support systems and coping mechanisms. Document social and family support because the patient often needs extensive assistance at home after treatment. Collaborate with a social worker as needed. Assess the level of education or literacy of the patient and family to plan teaching before and after surgery.

Document any family history of cancer, as well as the patient's age, gender, occupation, and ability to perform ADLs. Ask the patient whether his or her occupation requires continual oral communication. Job retraining may be needed if treatment affects speech.

Laboratory Assessment. Diagnostic tests include a complete blood cell count, bleeding times, urinalysis, and blood chemistries. The patient with chronic alcoholism may have low protein and albumin levels from poor nutrition. Liver and kidney function tests are performed to rule out cancer spread and to evaluate the patient's ability to metabolize drugs and chemotherapy agents.

Imaging Assessment. Many types of imaging studies, including x-rays of the skull, sinuses, neck, and chest, are useful in diagnosing cancer spread, other tumors, and the extent of tumor invasion. Computed tomography (CT), with or without contrast medium, helps evaluate the tumor's exact location. Magnetic resonance imaging (MRI) can help differentiate normal from diseased tissue.

The brain, bone, and liver are evaluated with nuclear imaging, bone scans, single-photon emission computerized tomography (SPECT) scans, and positron emission tomography (PET) scans. These tests locate additional tumor sites.

Other Diagnostic Assessment. Other helpful tests include direct and indirect laryngoscopy, tumor mapping, and biopsy. *Panendoscopy* (laryngoscopy, nasopharyngoscopy, esophagoscopy, and bronchoscopy) is performed with general anesthesia to define the extent of the tumor. Tumor-mapping biopsies are performed to identify tumor location. Biopsy tissues taken at the time of the panendoscopy confirm the diagnosis, tumor type, cell features, location, and stage (see Chapter 21).

TABLE 29-1	Warning Signs of Head and Neck Cancer

- Pain
- Lump in the mouth, throat, or neck
- Difficulty swallowing
- Color changes in the mouth or tongue to red, white, gray, dark brown, or black
- Oral lesion or sore that does not heal in 2 weeks
- Persistent or unexplained oral bleeding
- Numbness of the mouth, lips, or face
- Change in the fit of dentures
- Burning sensation when drinking citrus juices or hot liquids
- Persistent, unilateral ear pain
- Hoarseness or change in voice quality
- Persistent or recurrent sore throat
- Shortness of breath
- Anorexia and weight loss

Health Promotion and Maintenance

The 62-year-old client whose brother was just diagnosed with head and neck cancer asks the nurse what he could do to reduce his risk for also developing this cancer. What is the nurse's best response?

A. "Because head and neck cancer has a strong hereditary component, participating in screening twice yearly is critical for you."

B. "Always wear sunscreen with a 50% or greater protection factor whenever you are outdoors."

C. "Avoid shouting and singing to prevent stress to your vocal cords and larynx."

D. "Stop smoking, and drink alcohol only in moderation."

◆ Analysis

The priority NANDA-I nursing diagnoses and collaborative problems for patients with head and neck cancer include:

1. Potential for respiratory obstruction
2. Risk for Aspiration related to edema, anatomic changes, or altered protective reflexes (NANDA-I)
3. Anxiety related to threat of death, change in role status, or change in economic status (NANDA-I)
4. Reduced self-concept related to tumor and treatment modalities

◆ Planning and Implementation

Preventing Respiratory Obstruction. Without treatment, head and neck cancers grow, obstruct the airway, and prevent GAS EXCHANGE leading to death. Airway obstruction also can occur as a complication of treatment modalities.

Planning: Expected Outcomes. The patient with head and neck cancer is expected to attain and maintain adequate GAS EXCHANGE and tissue oxygenation. Indicators include:

- Arterial blood gas values within the normal range
- Rate and depth of respiration within the normal range
- Pulse oximetry within the normal range

Interventions. The focus of treatment is to remove or eradicate the cancer while preserving as much normal function as possible. The physician presents the available treatment options. Surgery, radiation, chemotherapy, or biotherapy may be used alone or in combination. Considerations for treatment options include the patient's physical condition, nutrition status, and age; the effects of the tumor on body function; and the patient's personal choice. Treatment for laryngeal cancer may range from radiation therapy (for a small specific area or tumor) to total laryngopharyngectomy with bilateral neck dissections followed by radiation therapy, depending on the extent and location of the lesion. Voice-conservation procedures are used only if they do not risk incomplete removal of the tumor. Nursing care focuses on the patient's total needs, including preoperative preparation, optimal in-hospital care, discharge planning and teaching, and extensive outpatient rehabilitation.

Nonsurgical Management. Monitor GAS EXCHANGE and the respiratory system by assessing respiratory rate, breath sounds, pulse oximetry, and arterial blood gas values. Airway obstruction can occur from tumor growth, edema, or both. Teach the patient to use the Fowler's and semi-Fowler's positions for best gas exchange. Sitting upright in a reclining chair may promote more comfortable breathing. Chapters 3 and 7 provide additional information on palliation and pain control for patients

who elect not to have therapy and for those whose therapy has not been effective.

Radiation therapy for treatment of small cancers in specific locations has a cure rate of at least 80%. Standard therapy uses 5000 to 7500 rad (radiation absorbed dose), usually over 6 weeks and in daily or twice-daily doses. Intensity modulated radiotherapy (IMRT) is being used increasingly to provide higher doses directly to the tumor with less damage to surrounding normal tissues. Radiation may be used alone or, more often, in combination with surgery and chemotherapy (see Chapter 22). It can be performed before or after surgery. Most patients have hoarseness, dysphagia, skin problems, and dry mouth for a few weeks after radiation therapy.

Hoarseness may become worse during therapy. Reassure the patient that voice improves within 4 to 6 weeks after completion of radiation therapy. Urge the patient to use voice rest and alternative means of communication until the effects of radiation therapy have passed.

Most patients have a sore throat and difficulty swallowing during radiation therapy to the neck. Gargling with saline or sucking ice may decrease discomfort. Mouthwashes and throat sprays containing a local anesthetic agent such as lidocaine or diphenhydramine can provide temporary relief. Analgesic drugs may be prescribed.

The skin at the site of irradiation becomes red and tender and may peel during therapy. Instruct the patient to avoid exposing this area to sun, heat, cold, and abrasive actions such as shaving. Teach the patient to wear protective clothing made of soft cotton and to wash this area gently daily with a mild soap, such as Dove (Mannix et al., 2012). Using appropriate skin care products (approved by the radiation-oncology department) can reduce the intensity of skin reactions.

If the salivary glands are in the irradiation path, the mouth becomes dry (**xerostomia**). This side effect is long-term and may be permanent. Some of the problems from reduced saliva include increased risk for dental caries, increased risk for oral infections, halitosis (bad breath), and taste changes. Fluoride gel trays and nightly fluoride treatments can reduce the incidence of tooth deterioration. The trays can be worn during radiation therapy to prevent radiation scatter from the beam deflecting off existing metal inside the mouth. Although there is no cure for xerostomia, interventions can help reduce the discomfort. Heavy fluid intake, particularly water, and humidification can help ease the discomfort. Some patients benefit from the use of artificial saliva, such as Salivart; moisturizing sprays or gels, such as Mouth Kote; or saliva stimulants, such as Salagen and cevimeline (cholinergic drugs).

Chemotherapy can be used alone or in addition to surgery or radiation for head and neck cancer. Often, chemotherapy and radiation therapy *(chemoradiation)* are used at the same time. Although the exact drugs used may vary, depending on cancer cell features, most chemotherapy regimens for head and neck cancers include cisplatin (National Comprehensive Cancer Network, 2013). The oral cavity effects of radiation are intensified with concurrent chemotherapy. These can be uncomfortable, and patients often request breaks in the treatment regimen. However, these breaks in treatment do affect the outcome of treatment and should be avoided. Intense patient education before treatment and support during treatment can improve patient adherence to the treatment plan (Mason et al., 2013). Chapter 22 discusses the general care needs of patients receiving chemotherapy.

Biotherapy in the form of epidermal growth factor receptor inhibitors (EGFRIs) may be effective for patients whose cancers overexpress the receptor. Currently, the drug approved for this purpose is cetuximab (Erbitux). Although it is a targeted therapy, this drug blocks EGFRs in normal tissues as well as those in the tumor. As a result, severe skin reactions are common and difficult for the patient (Boucher et al., 2011).

Surgical Management. Tumor size, node number, and metastasis location (TNM classification) determines the type of surgery needed for the specific head and neck cancer (see Chapter 21). Very small, early-stage tumors may be removed by laser therapy or photodynamic therapy; however, few head and neck tumors are found at this stage and most require extensive traditional surgery. Reconstruction is also determined by the tumor size and amount of tissue to be resected and reconstructed. Surgical procedures for head and neck cancers include laryngectomy (total and partial), tracheotomy, and oropharyngeal cancer resections. The major types of surgery for laryngeal cancer include cord stripping, removal of a vocal cord (**cordectomy**), partial laryngectomy, and total laryngectomy. If cancer is in the lymph nodes in the neck, the surgeon performs a nodal neck dissection along with removal of the primary tumor ("radical neck").

Preoperative Care. Teach the patient and family about the tumor. The surgeon explains the surgical procedure and obtains informed consent. Discuss and interpret the implications of such consent with the patient and family.

Explain about self-management of the airway, suctioning, pain-control methods, the critical care environment (including ventilators and critical care routines), nutrition support, feeding tubes, and plans for discharge. The patient will need to learn new methods of speech, at least during the time that mechanical ventilation is used and, depending on surgery type, perhaps forever. Help him or her prepare for this change before surgery and to practice the use of the selected form of communication (see Chart 29-2 and the discussion of Maintaining Communication in Chapter 28). Determine the communication method preferred by the patient.

A team approach for planning care and rehabilitation is critical for the best outcome. The team includes nurses, physicians, speech and language pathologists, social workers, dietitians, respiratory therapists, and occupational and physical therapists. These professionals help evaluate and prepare the patient who has head and neck cancer. Chapter 14 describes general preoperative assessment and education.

Operative Procedures. Table 29-2 lists specific information about the various surgical procedures for laryngeal cancer. Hemilaryngectomy (vertical or horizontal) and supraglottic laryngectomy are types of partial voice-conservation laryngectomies.

To protect the airway, a tracheostomy is needed. With a partial laryngectomy, the tracheostomy is usually temporary. With a total laryngectomy, the upper airway is separated from the throat and esophagus and a permanent laryngectomy stoma in the neck is created.

Neck dissection includes the removal of lymph nodes, the sternocleidomastoid muscle, the jugular vein, the 11th cranial nerve, and surrounding soft tissue. Shoulder drop is expected after extensive surgery. Physical therapy can help the patient ease the shoulder drop by using other muscle groups.

Postoperative Care. Head and neck surgery often lasts 8 hours or longer. Usually the patient spends the immediate period after

---

CHART 29-2 Best Practice for Patient Safety & Quality Care QSEN

Communicating with a Patient Who Is Unable to Speak

- Assess the patient's reading skills and cognition.
- Determine in what language (languages) the patient is most fluent.
- Collaborate with a speech and language pathologist.
- If the patient requires vision-enhancing devices or hearing-enhancing devices, be sure these are available and in use.
- Provide the patient with a variety of techniques to practice before verbal skills are lost to determine with which one(s) the patient feels most comfortable. These may include:
  - Alphabet board
  - Picture board
  - Paper and pencil
  - Magic Slate
  - Hand signals/gestures
  - Computer with e-triloquist program
  - Programmable speech-generating devices (text-to-speech communication aid)
- Reinforce to the patient the technique for esophageal speech presented by the speech and language pathologist, and provide the time for practice.
- Use a normal tone of voice to talk with the patient (unless hearing is a pre-existing problem, a change in the ability to speak does not interfere with the patient's ability to hear).
- Ensure that the call-light board at the nurses' station indicates a non-speaking patient.
- Teach the patient to make noise to indicate immediate attention is needed at the bedside when he or she signals by call light. Such noises can include tapping the siderail with a spoon, making clicking noises with the tongue, using a bell, or working a noisemaker. Be sure that whatever method is selected is listed on the call-light board.
- When face-to-face with the patient:
  - Phrase questions in a "yes" or "no" format.
  - Watch the patient's face for indications of understanding or the lack of it.
  - Listen attentively to any sound the patient makes.
- If writing is selected as the method to communicate, assess whether the patient is right-handed or left-handed and ensure appropriate writing materials are within reach. Use the other arm for IV placement.
- Ensure the preferred method of communication is documented in the patient record and is communicated to all care providers.
- Encourage the family to work with the patient in the use of the selected method.
- Provide praise and encouragement.
- Do not avoid talking with the patient.
- Allow the patient to set the pace for communication.

---

surgery in the surgical intensive care unit. Monitor airway patency, vital signs, hemodynamic status, and comfort level. Monitor for hemorrhage and other general complications of anesthesia and surgery (see Chapter 16). Take vital signs hourly for the first 24 hours and then according to agency policy until the patient is stable. After the patient is transferred from the critical care unit, monitor vital signs every 4 hours or according to agency policy.

Complications after surgery include airway obstruction, hemorrhage, wound breakdown, and tumor recurrence. *The first priorities after head and neck surgery are airway maintenance and GAS EXCHANGE.* Other priorities are wound, flap, and reconstructive tissue care; pain management; nutrition; and psychological adjustment, including speech and language therapy.

TABLE 29-2 Surgical Procedures for Laryngeal Cancer and their Effect on Voice Quality

PROCEDURE	DESCRIPTION	RESULTING VOICE QUALITY
Laser surgery	Tumor reduced or destroyed by laser beam through laryngoscope	Normal/hoarse
Transoral cordectomy	Tumor (early lesion) resected through laryngoscope	Normal/hoarse (high cure rate)
Laryngofissure	No cord removed (early lesion)	Normal (high cure rate)
Supraglottic partial laryngectomy	Hyoid bone, false cords, and epiglottis removed Neck dissection on affected side performed if nodes involved	Normal/hoarse
Hemilaryngectomy or vertical laryngectomy	One true cord, one false cord, and one half of thyroid cartilage removed	Hoarse
Total laryngectomy	Entire larynx, hyoid bone, strap muscles, one or two tracheal rings removed Nodal neck dissection if nodes involved	No natural voice

Airway Maintenance and Gas Exchange. Immediately after surgery, the patient may need ventilatory assistance. Most patients wean easily from the ventilator after this type of surgery because the thoracic and abdominal cavities are not entered. During weaning, the patient usually uses a tracheostomy collar (over the artificial airway or open stoma) with oxygen and humidity to help move mucus secretions. Secretions may remain blood-tinged for 1 to 2 days. Use Standard Precautions, and report any increase in bleeding to the surgeon. Humidity helps remove crusts and prevents obstruction of the tube with secretions. A laryngectomy tube is used for patients who have undergone a *total laryngectomy* and need an appliance to prevent scar tissue shrinkage of the skin-tracheal border. This tube is similar to a tracheostomy tube but is shorter and wider with a larger lumen. Laryngectomy tube care is similar to tracheostomy tube care (see Chapter 28) except that the patient can change the laryngectomy tube daily or as needed. A laryngectomy button is similar to a laryngectomy tube but is softer, has a single lumen, and is very short. A button is comfortable for the patient, is easily removed for cleaning, and is available in various sizes for a custom fit. Provide alternative communication techniques because the patient cannot speak.

Coughing and deep breathing are usually effective in clearing secretions. Instruct the patient how to cough and deep breathe to clear secretions.

Oral secretions can be suctioned by the alert patient using a Yankauer or tonsillar suction or a soft red latex catheter. Teach the patient to suction *away* from the surgical side to prevent opening the wound. Using a table mirror helps the patient see the area more clearly. Provide a clean environment for the catheter.

Stoma care after a total laryngectomy is a combination of wound care and airway care. Inspect the stoma with a flashlight. Clean the suture line with sterile saline (or a prescribed solution) to prevent secretions from forming crusts and obstructing the airway. Perform suture line care every 1 to 2 hours during the first few days after surgery and then every 4 hours. The mucosa of the stoma and trachea should be bright and shiny and without crusts, similar to the appearance of the oral mucosa.

Wound, Flap, and Reconstructive Tissue Care. Tissue "flaps" may be used to close the wound and improve appearance. Flaps are skin, subcutaneous tissue, and sometimes muscle, taken from other body areas used for reconstruction after head and neck resection. After neck dissection, the surgeon places a split-thickness skin graft (STSG) over the exposed carotid artery before covering it with skin flaps or reconstructive flaps.

The first 24 hours after surgery are critical. Evaluate all grafts and flaps hourly for the first 72 hours. Monitor capillary refill, color, drainage, and Doppler activity of the major blood vessel to the area. Report changes to the surgeon immediately because surgical intervention may be needed. Position the patient so that the surgical flaps are not dependent.

Hemorrhage. Hemorrhage is a possible complication after any surgery, but it is uncommon with laryngectomy. The surgeon often places a closed surgical drain in the neck area to collect blood and drainage for about 72 hours after surgery. The drain also helps maintain the position of the reconstructed skin flaps. Any drain obstruction or equipment malfunction may cause a buildup of blood or fluid under the flaps that can impair blood flow and result in flap failure. A sudden stoppage of drainage may indicate drain obstruction by a clot. Monitor and record the amount and character of drainage. Check the patency and functioning of the drainage system. Report any drain malfunction or change in flap appearance to the surgeon. Depending on the surgeon's preference and the agency's policy, you may need to empty the drainage container or "milk" the drain.

Wound Breakdown. Wound breakdown is a complication caused by poor nutrition, a long smoking history, alcohol use, wound contamination, and radiation therapy before surgery. Manage wound breakdown with packing and local care as prescribed to keep the wound clean and to stimulate the growth of healthy granulation tissue. Wounds may be extensive, and the carotid artery may be exposed. Split-thickness skin grafts often are placed over the carotid artery for protection in the event of wound dehiscence. As the wound heals, granulation tissue covers the artery and prevents rupture. If granulation is slow and the carotid artery is at risk, another surgical flap may be made to cover the artery and close the wound.

When the carotid artery ruptures, large amounts of bright red blood spurt quickly. It is also possible for the carotid artery to have a small leak, with continuous oozing of bright red blood. Usually, a small leak leads to a complete rupture within a short time.

! NURSING SAFETY PRIORITY (QSEN)

Critical Rescue

If a carotid artery leak is suspected, call the Rapid Response Team and *do not touch the area because additional pressure could cause an immediate rupture.* If the carotid artery ruptures because of drying or infection, immediately place constant pressure over the site and secure the airway. Maintain direct manual, continuous pressure on the carotid artery, and immediately transport the patient to the operating room for carotid resection. Do not leave the patient. Carotid artery rupture has a high risk for stroke and death.

Pain Management. Pain is caused by the surgical cutting or manipulation of tissue and by nerve compression. Pain should be controlled, and the patient should still be able to participate in his or her care. Morphine (Statex ✤) often is given IV by a patient-controlled analgesia (PCA) pump for the first 1 to 2 days after surgery. As the patient progresses, liquid opioid analgesics can be given by feeding tube. Oral drugs for pain and discomfort are started only after the patient can tolerate oral intake. After discharge, the patient still requires pain management, especially if he or she is receiving radiation therapy. An adjunct to the pain regimen may be liquid NSAIDs along with opioid analgesics. Tricyclic antidepressants may also be used for the lancinating pain of nerve-root involvement.

Nutrition. Many patients with head and neck cancer have taste changes and some degree of malnutrition before cancer treatment begins (Ardilio, 2011; McLaughlin, 2013). All patients are at risk for malnutrition during treatment for head and neck cancer. A nasogastric, gastrostomy, or jejunostomy tube is placed during surgery for nutrition support while the head and neck heal. After the intestinal tract is motile, nutrients can be given via the feeding tube. The nutrition support team or dietitian assesses the patient before surgery and is available for consultation after surgery. Replacement of calories, protein, and water loss is calculated carefully for each patient (Ardilio, 2011).

The feeding tube usually remains in place for 7 to 10 days after surgery. Before removing the tube, assess the patient's ability to swallow if nutrition is to be given by mouth. Aspiration *cannot* occur after a total laryngectomy because the airway is completely separated from the esophagus. Stay with the patient during the first few swallowing attempts. Swallowing may be uncomfortable at first, and analgesics may be needed.

Speech and Language Rehabilitation. The patient's voice quality and speech are altered after surgery. Although this problem has enormous effects on the patient's ability to maintain social interactions, continue employment, and maintain a desired quality of life, it is often poorly addressed while he or she is hospitalized. Working with him or her and the family toward developing an acceptable communication method during the inpatient period is essential for a satisfactory outcome (Happ et al., 2011).

Together with the speech and language pathologist (SLP), discuss the principles of speech therapy with the patient and family early in the course of the treatment plan (see Chart 29-2). Voice and speech differences depend on the type of surgical resection (see Table 29-2). Speech production varies with patient practice, amount of tissue removed, and radiation effects, but the speech can be very understandable. Patients have reported ongoing difficulties with speech and communication to be the most distressing problem for months to years after head and neck cancer therapy (Fletcher et al., 2012; Haisfield-Wolfe et al., 2012).

The speech rehabilitation plan for patients who have a total laryngectomy at first consists of writing, using a picture board, or using a computer. The patient then uses an artificial larynx and may eventually learn esophageal speech. For success, the patient needs encouragement and support from the SLP, hospital team, and family while relearning to speak. This process can be time consuming and requires concentration each time the patient speaks. Having a **laryngectomee** (a person who has had a laryngectomy) from one of the local self-help organizations visit the patient and family is often

Listener

Speaker using Electro-Larynx

FIG. 29-4 An Electro-Larynx to generate speech after a laryngectomy.

beneficial. The International Association of Laryngectomees is very supportive, as is the American Cancer Society (ACS) Visitor Program.

Esophageal speech is attempted by most patients who have a total laryngectomy. Sound can be produced this way by "burping" the air swallowed or injected into the esophageal pharynx and shaping the words in the mouth. The voice produced is a monotone; it cannot be raised or lowered and carries no pitch. If patients do not have adequate hearing, esophageal speech will be difficult because they need to use their mouth to shape the words as they hear them. Hearing-impaired patients may need hearing aids.

Mechanical devices, called *electrolarynges,* may be used for communication. Most are battery-powered devices placed against the side of the neck or cheek (Fig. 29-4). The air inside the mouth and throat is vibrated, and the patient moves his or her lips and tongue as usual. The quality of speech generated with mechanical devices is robot-like.

Tracheoesophageal puncture (TEP) (formerly call a *fistula*) may be used if esophageal speech is ineffective and if the patient meets strict criteria. A small surgical puncture is created between the trachea and the esophagus using a special catheter. After the puncture heals, a silicone prosthesis (e.g., the Blom-Singer prosthesis or the Panje Voice Button) is inserted in place of the catheter. The patient covers the stoma and the opening of the prosthesis with a finger or with a special valve to divert air from the lungs, through the trachea, into the esophagus, and out of the mouth where lip and tongue movement produces speech.

Surgical Procedures for Other Head and Neck Cancers. The major types of surgeries for other head and neck cancers are called *composite resections.* These resections are a combination of surgical procedures, including partial or total glossectomies (tongue removal), partial mandibulectomies (jaw removal), and, if needed, nodal neck dissections. Tracheostomy may be planned to provide an adequate airway. (See Chapter 53 for more information about oral cancer.)

Tracheotomy. A **tracheotomy** is a surgical incision into the trachea for the purpose of establishing an airway (tracheostomy). It can be performed as an emergency procedure or as a scheduled surgical procedure. A tracheostomy can be temporary or permanent. Chapter 28 discusses the nursing care of a patient with a tracheostomy.

Preventing Aspiration

Planning: Expected Outcomes. The patient with head and neck cancer is expected to not aspirate food, gastric contents, or oral secretions into the lungs. Indicators include that the patient often or consistently demonstrates these behaviors:

- Positions self upright for eating or drinking
- Selects foods according to swallowing ability
- Chooses liquids and foods of proper consistency

Interventions. The surgical changes in the upper respiratory tract and altered swallowing mechanisms increase the patient's risk for aspiration. Aspiration can result in pneumonia, weight loss, and prolonged hospitalization. Chart 29-3 lists actions for aspiration prevention.

A nasogastric (NG) feeding tube may further increase the risk for aspiration because it keeps the lower esophageal sphincter partially open. The one exception is the patient who has undergone a total laryngectomy. In these cases, the airway is separated from the esophagus, making aspiration impossible and the patient is *not* at risk. Most patients who need enteral feeding supplementation have a percutaneous endoscopic gastrostomy (PEG) tube placed rather than an NG tube. See Chapter 60 for care of patients receiving enteral nutrition by NG or PEG tube.

A dynamic swallow study, such as a barium swallow under fluoroscopy, evaluates a patient's ability to protect the airway from aspiration and helps determine the appropriate method of swallow rehabilitation. In many cases, enteral feedings are used either because of the patient's inability to swallow or because of continued aspiration risk.

Swallowing can be a major problem for the patient who has a tracheostomy tube. Swallowing can be normal if the cranial nerves and anatomic structures are intact. In a normal swallow, the larynx rises and moves forward to protect itself from the passing stream of food and saliva. The tracheostomy tube sometimes fixes the larynx in place, resulting in difficulty swallowing.

An inflated tracheostomy tube cuff can balloon backward into the esophagus and interfere with the passage of food. The wall between the posterior trachea and the esophagus is very thin, which allows this pushing action. The patient who is cognitively intact may adapt to eating normal food when the tracheostomy tube is small and the cuff is not inflated.

The patient who has had a partial vertical or supraglottic laryngectomy *must* be observed for aspiration. It is critical to teach the patient to use alternate methods of swallowing without aspirating. The "supraglottic" method of swallowing is especially effective after a partial laryngectomy or base-of-tongue resection (Chart 29-4). To reinforce teaching and learning, place a chart in the patient's room detailing the steps. A dynamic swallow study is performed to guide rehabilitation for swallowing and to evaluate the patient's ability to protect the airway.

Minimizing Anxiety

Planning: Expected Outcomes. The patient with head and neck cancer is expected to have decreased anxiety. Indicators include that the patient often or consistently demonstrates:

- Verbalization of reduced anxiety
- Absence of distress, irritability, and facial tension
- Effective use of coping strategies

Interventions. Conferences with the physician, clinical nurse specialist, dietitian, speech and language pathologist, physical therapist, psychologist, social worker, and general nursing staff may be beneficial. Explore the reason for anxiety (e.g., fear of the unknown, lack of teaching, fear of pain, fear of death, loss of control, uncertainty). The patient and family often benefit from further information. Before the patient is scheduled for surgery (and while still at home), home care nurses or community-sponsored programs, such as the ACS, may be able to decrease fears about the disease process and surgical interventions.

Give prescribed antianxiety drugs, such as diazepam (Valium, Meval ✦), with caution because of the risk for respiratory depression and because some of these drugs are eliminated slowly. Shorter-duration drugs, such as lorazepam (Ativan), may have fewer respiratory side effects. The location of the tumor and the presence of other lung disease may cause some

---

CHART 29-3 Best Practice for Patient Safety & Quality Care (QSEN)

Prevention of Aspiration During Swallowing

- Avoid serving meals when the patient is fatigued.
- Provide smaller and more frequent meals.
- Provide adequate time; do not "hurry" the patient.
- Provide close supervision if the patient is self-feeding.
- Keep emergency suctioning equipment close at hand.
- Avoid water and other "thin" liquids.
- Thicken liquids.
- Avoid foods that generate thin liquids during the chewing process, such as fruit.
- Position the patient in the most upright position possible.
- When possible, completely (or at least partially) deflate the tube cuff during meals.
- Suction after initial cuff deflation to clear the airway and allow maximum comfort during the meal.
- Feed each bite or encourage the patient to take each bite slowly.
- Encourage the patient to "dry swallow" after each bite to clear residue from the throat.
- Avoid consecutive swallows by cup or straw.
- Provide controlled small volumes of liquids, using a spoon.
- Encourage the patient to "tuck" his or her chin down and move the forehead forward while swallowing.
- Allow the patient to indicate when he or she is ready for the next bite.
- If the patient coughs, stop the feeding until the patient indicates the airway has been cleared.
- Continuously monitor tolerance to oral food intake by assessing respiratory rate, ease, pulse oximetry, and heart rate.

CHART 29-4 Patient and Family Education: Preparing for Self-Management

The Supraglottic Method of Swallowing

1. Place yourself in an upright, preferably out-of-bed, position.
2. Clear your throat.
3. Take a deep breath.
4. Place $\frac{1}{2}$ to 1 teaspoon of food into your mouth.
5. Hold your breath, or "bear down" (Valsalva maneuver).
6. Swallow twice.
7. Release your breath, and clear your throat.
8. Swallow twice again.
9. Breathe normally.

This method exaggerates the normal protective mechanisms of cessation of respiration during the swallow. The double swallow attempts to clear food that may be pooling in the pharynx, vallecula, and piriform sinuses. This method is used only after a dynamic radiographic swallow study has demonstrated that it is appropriate and safe for the patient.

degree of airway obstruction. For anxiety in these patients, drug therapy may include lorazepam (Ativan, Novo-Lorazem ✦) rather than a sedating agent.

Supporting Self-Concept

Planning: Expected Outcomes. The patient with head and neck cancer is expected to accept body image changes. Indicators include that the patient often or consistently demonstrates:

- Willingness to touch and care for the affected body part
- Willingness to use strategies to enhance appearance
- Interaction with visitors, staff, and family members

Interventions. The patient with head and neck cancer usually has a change in self-concept and self-image resulting from functional and psychological issues. Common functional issues include the presence of a stoma or artificial airway, speech changes, and a change in the method of eating. Psychological issues often include guilt, regret, and uncertainty. He or she may not be able to speak at all or may have permanent speech deficits. Help the patient set realistic goals, starting with involvement in self-care. Teach the patient alternative communication methods so he or she can communicate in the hospital and after discharge (Fletcher et al., 2012; Suzuki, 2012).

Teach the family to ease the patient into a normal social environment. Use positive reinforcement and encouragement while demonstrating acceptance and caring behaviors. The family also may benefit from counseling sessions while the patient is still in the hospital.

After surgery, the patient may feel socially isolated because of the change in voice and facial appearance. Loose-fitting, high-collar shirts or sweaters, scarves, and jewelry can be worn to cover the laryngectomy stoma, tracheostomy tube, and other changes related to surgery. Cosmetics may aid in covering disfigurement. Most surgeons try to place the incisions in the natural skinfold lines if doing so does not pose a risk for cancer recurrence.

Community-Based Care

If no complications occur, the patient is usually discharged home or to an extended-care facility within 2 weeks. At the time of discharge, he or she or a family member should be able to perform tracheostomy or stoma care and participate in nutrition, wound care, and communication methods.

The patient and family may feel more secure about discharge with a referral to support groups or a community health agency familiar with the care of patients recovering from head and neck cancer. Coordinate the efforts of the health care team in assessing the specific discharge needs and making the appropriate referrals to home care agencies. Dietitians, nurses, physical therapists, speech and language pathologists, and social workers may be needed. Coordinate the scheduling for chemotherapy or radiation therapy with the patient and family.

Home Care Management. Extensive home care preparation is needed after a laryngectomy for cancer. The convalescent period is long, and airway management is complicated. The patient or family must be able to take an active role in care.

General cleanliness of the home is assessed by the home care nurse or case manager. For the patient with severe respiratory problems, home changes to allow for one-floor living may be needed. Increased humidity is needed. A humidifier add-on to a forced-air furnace can be obtained, or a room humidifier or vaporizer may be used. Be sure to stress that meticulous

---

CHART 29-5 Home Care Assessment

Patients After Laryngectomy

Assess respiratory status:
- Observe rate and depth of respiration.
- Auscultate lungs.
- Check patency of airway.
- Examine the tracheostomy drainage for amount, color, and character.
- Examine nail beds and mucous membranes for evidence of cyanosis.
- Obtain a pulse oximetry reading.

Assess condition of wound:
- Remove dressings (noting condition of dressings).
- Cleanse the wound.
- Compare with previous notations of wound condition:
  - Presence, amount, and nature of exudate
  - Presence/absence of cellulitis
  - Presence/absence of odor

Assess patient's psychosocial status:
- Ask the patient about passing the time, visitors, and trips outside the house.
- Observe whether the patient communicates responses directly or whether a family member speaks for the patient.
- Observe patient and family member interactions.
- Determine what method of communication the patient has selected, and observe the patient's skill with it.
- Observe whether the patient is wearing pajamas or is dressed in street clothes.

Take the patient's temperature at each home care visit.

Assess the patient's understanding of illness and adherence to treatment:
- Manifestations to report to the health care provider
- Medication plan (correct timing and dose)
- Ambulation or positioning schedule
- Dressing changes/skin care
- Diet modifications (24-hour diet recall)
- Skill in tracheostomy or dressing care

Assess patient's nutrition status:
- Change in muscle mass
- Lackluster nails/sparse hair
- Recent weight loss greater than 10% of usual weight
- Impaired oral intake
- Difficulty swallowing
- Generalized edema

---

cleaning of these items is needed to prevent spread of mold or other sources of infection.

A home care nurse often is involved with care after discharge and is an important resource for the patient and family. This nurse assesses the patient and home situation for problems in self-care, complications, adjustment, and adherence to the medical regimen. Chart 29-5 lists assessment areas for the patient in the home after a laryngectomy. This nurse reinforces health care teaching, self-care teaching, and smoking-cessation regimens.

Self-Management Education. Education begins before surgery, and most self-care is taught in the hospital. Teach the patient and family how to care for the stoma or tracheostomy or laryngectomy tube, depending on the type of surgery performed. Review incision and airway care, including cleaning and inspecting for signs of infection. Chart 29-6 lists self-care actions for the patient after laryngeal cancer surgery. Many of these actions also apply to any surgery for head and neck cancer.

> **CHART 29-6 Patient and Family Education: Preparing for Self-Management**
>
> ### Home Laryngectomy Care
>
> - Avoid swimming, and use care when showering or shaving.
> - Lean slightly forward and cover the stoma when coughing or sneezing.
> - Wear a stoma guard or loose clothing to cover the stoma.
> - Clean the stoma with mild soap and water. Lubricate the stoma with a non–oil-based ointment as needed.
> - Increase humidity by using saline in the stoma as instructed, a bedside humidifier, pans of water, and houseplants.
> - Obtain and wear a MedicAlert bracelet and emergency care card for life-threatening situations.

Stoma care teaching is focused on protection. Use a plastic head-and-neck cut-away model or create one from Styrofoam to use as an accurate aid for teaching about the anatomic changes resulting from surgery (Zeien, 2011). Instruct the patient to use a shower shield over the tube or stoma when bathing to prevent water from entering the airway. Teach men who use electric shavers to cover the stoma while shaving to keep hair from falling into it. Suggest that the patient wear a protective cover or stoma guard to protect the stoma during the day. For those with permanent stomas after laryngectomy or for those with permanent tracheostomies, covering the opening has two benefits: (1) to filter the air entering the stoma while keeping humidity in the airway; and (2) to enhance aesthetic appearance. Attractive coverings are available in the form of scarves, crocheted collars, and jewelry.

Instruct the patient how to increase humidity in the home. Stress the importance of keeping well hydrated to prevent secretions from thickening.

Communication involves having the patient continue the selected communication method that began in the hospital. Instruct him or her to wear a medical alert (MedicAlert) bracelet and carry a special identification card. For patients with a laryngectomy, this card is available from the local chapters of the International Association of Laryngectomees. The card instructs the reader about providing an emergency airway or resuscitating someone who has a stoma.

Smoking cessation is a difficult but important issue after head and neck cancer surgery. Stress that smoking cessation can reduce the risk for developing other cancers and can increase the rate of healing from surgery. See Chapter 27 for a detailed discussion about smoking cessation.

Psychosocial Preparation. The many changes resulting from a laryngectomy influence physical, social, and emotional functioning. Patients may perceive changes in their quality of life. Begin preparing the patient and family by scheduling a visit from a person who has adjusted to these changes.

The patient with a permanent stoma, tracheostomy tube, NG or PEG tube, and wounds has an altered body image. Stress the importance of returning to as normal a lifestyle as possible. Most patients can resume many of their usual activities within 4 to 6 weeks after surgery. A longer time is needed after a combination of radiation therapy and surgery and for those patients who also have other chronic diseases. The patient may be frustrated at times while trying to adjust to the many changes resulting from treatment of head and neck cancer.

The patient with a total laryngectomy cannot produce sounds during laughing and crying. Mucus secretions may appear unexpectedly when these emotions arise or when coughing or sneezing occurs. The mucus can be embarrassing, and the patient needs to be prepared to cover the stoma with a handkerchief or gauze. The patient who has undergone composite resections has difficulty with speech *and* swallowing. He or she may need to deal with tracheostomy and feeding tubes in public places.

Health Care Resources. Inform the patient and family of community organizations (e.g., ACS) and local laryngectomee clubs, which can offer support, information, and friendships. When the patient has problems paying for health care services, equipment, and prescriptions, a visiting nurse agency and social worker may be helpful in locating available resources.

In many areas, the local unit of the ACS or Canadian Cancer Society can help provide dressing materials and nutritional supplements to patients in need. These organizations may also provide transportation to and from follow-up visits or radiation therapy.

> **❓ CLINICAL JUDGMENT CHALLENGE**
>
> ### Patient-Centered Care; Evidence-Based Practice; Teamwork and Collaboration QSEN
>
> A patient who had a supraglottic partial laryngectomy with a right-sided radical neck dissection 4 weeks ago is now receiving radiation therapy. He has lost 24 pounds since his surgery, which makes him 15 pounds less than his ideal weight. He tells you that he has no appetite and that what food he does eat "has no taste." In addition, although he expresses that he is glad to be alive, he does not want friends to visit because it takes so much energy to interact with them. He also says that he can no longer play the piano because of difficulty moving his right arm and shoulder.
>
> 1. What factors are contributing to his fatigue?
> 2. Is the weight loss a concern? If so, what should you do about it?
> 3. Should you further press the issue of not wanting to visit with friends? Why or why not?
> 4. What other health care professionals or resources would be appropriate at this time?

◆ **Evaluation: Outcomes**

Evaluate the care of the patient with head and neck cancer based on the identified priority patient problems. The expected outcomes are that the patient:

- Maintains a patent airway
- Performs self-care of the artificial airway and wound
- Performs ADLs independently or with minimal assistance
- Attains or maintains adequate nutrition
- Does not aspirate gastric contents or food
- Engages in desired social interactions

Specific indicators for these outcomes are listed for priority patient problems in the Planning and Implementation section (see earlier).

NURSING CONCEPTS AND CLINICAL JUDGMENT REVIEW

What might you NOTICE if the patient is experiencing inadequate GAS EXCHANGE as a result of upper airway problems?
- Voice changes (nasal quality if the problem is above the palate, "breathy" or "whispery" if the problem is in the larynx or trachea)
- Snoring or mouth breathing
- Change in cognition or level of consciousness or acute confusion
- Decreased oxygen saturation by pulse oximetry
- Skin cyanosis or pallor (lighter-skinned patients)
- Cyanosis or pallor of the lips and oral mucous membranes (patients of any skin color)
- Tachycardia and dysrhythmia

What should you INTERPRET and how should you RESPOND to a patient experiencing inadequate GAS EXCHANGE as a result of an upper airway respiratory problem?

Perform and interpret physical assessment, including:
- Taking vital signs
- Monitoring oxygen saturation by pulse oximetry
- Assessing for the presence of thick or excessive secretions
- Assessing the patient's ability to cough and clear the airway

- Assessing nasal drainage and sputum for color and blood
- Checking most recent laboratory values for white blood cell and arterial blood gas (ABG) levels
- Assessing cognition
- Assessing hydration status

Respond by:
- Suctioning (oral, pharyngeal, endotracheal, tracheostomy), if needed
- Applying oxygen, and assessing the patient's responses to this intervention
- Keeping the patient's head elevated to about 30 degrees
- Notifying physician or Rapid Response Team
- Ensuring venous access

On what should you REFLECT?
- Observe patient for evidence of restored oxygenation (see Chapter 27).
- Think about what may have precipitated this episode and what steps could be taken to either prevent a similar episode or identify it earlier.
- Think about what additional resources could improve the nursing response to this situation.

GET READY FOR THE NCLEX® EXAMINATION!

KEY POINTS

Review these Key Points for each NCLEX Examination Client Needs Category.

Safe and Effective Care Environment
- Use sterile technique when performing endotracheal or tracheal suctioning. **Safety** QSEN
- Use Standard Precautions when caring for a patient with epistaxis. **Safety** QSEN
- Supervise care delegated to licensed practical nurses/licensed vocational nurses (LPNs/LVNs) or nursing assistants to patients who have risk factors for airway obstruction.
- Act as a patient advocate for patients who have tracheostomies or other issues that impair communication.

Health Promotion and Maintenance
- Assess the patient for risk factors for head and neck cancer.
- Encourage people who smoke to quit smoking or using tobacco in any way. **Patient-Centered Care** QSEN
- Encourage people who use alcohol to reduce their intake of alcoholic beverages.
- Use Aspiration Precautions for any patient with an altered level of consciousness or who has an endotracheal tube (see Chart 29-3). **Safety** QSEN
- Teach the patient and family how to perform tracheostomy care (see Chart 28-3 in Chapter 28). **Patient-Centered Care** QSEN
- Teach patients who have had radiation therapy to the oral cavity to have dental examinations at least every 6 months. **Patient-Centered Care** QSEN

- Teach the patient and family about home management of a laryngectomy stoma or tracheostomy. **Patient-Centered Care** QSEN

Psychosocial Integrity
- Allow the patient and family members the opportunity to express fear or anxiety regarding a cancer diagnosis or a change in breathing status.
- Teach family members ways to communicate with a patient who cannot speak after surgery for head and neck cancer. **Patient-Centered Care** QSEN
- Encourage patients with permanent tracheostomies or laryngectomies to become involved in self-care and to look at the wound and touch the affected area. **Patient-Centered Care** QSEN
- Allow the patient and family to grieve the loss of function and change in body image. **Patient-Centered Care** QSEN
- Allow time to communicate with the patient who has voice loss. **Patient-Centered Care** QSEN
- Refer patients and families to local chapters of the ACS or the Canadian Cancer Society after surgery for head and neck cancer.

Physiological Integrity
- Assess the airway patency of any patient who experiences facial or nasal trauma. **Safety** QSEN
- Perform a focused upper respiratory assessment and re-assessment to determine adequacy of GAS EXCHANGE and tissue perfusion. **Patient-Centered Care** QSEN

- Notify the Rapid Response Team when a patient experiences a posterior nasal bleed. **Safety** QSEN
- Check the airway and packing at least every hour for a patient who has posterior nasal packing placed after nasal surgery or posterior epistaxis. **Evidence-Based Practice** QSEN
- Instruct patients who have had mandibular immobilization or fixation after a mandibular fracture to keep wire cutters with them at all times. **Safety** QSEN
- Apply oxygen to any patient who develops stridor. **Safety** QSEN
- Use a manual resuscitation bag to ventilate the patient if the tracheostomy tube has dislodged or been decannulated. **Safety** QSEN

- Assess the new tracheostomy stoma site at least once per shift for purulent drainage, redness, pain, and swelling, as indicators of infection. **Safety** QSEN
- Keep the tracheal cuff pressure between 14 and 20 mm Hg to prevent tissue injury. **Evidence-Based Practice** QSEN
- Apply knowledge of anatomy to prevent aspiration in a patient with a tracheostomy. **Evidence-Based Practice** QSEN
- Use correct technique to suction via a tracheostomy or laryngectomy tube. **Evidence-Based Practice** QSEN
- Collaborate with physicians, speech and language pathologists, social workers, dietitians, respiratory therapists, and occupational and physical therapists to provide optimal care for the patient experiencing head and neck cancer. **Teamwork and Collaboration** QSEN

Care of Patients with Noninfectious Lower Respiratory Problems

M. Linda Workman

 http://evolve.elsevier.com/Iggy/

PRIORITY CONCEPTS

- Gas Exchange
- Perfusion
- Inflammation
- Cellular Regulation

LEARNING OUTCOMES

Safe and Effective Care Environment

1. Ensure safe oxygen delivery to promote GAS EXCHANGE.
2. Protect patients with lower respiratory problems from injury or infection.

Health Promotion and Maintenance

3. Teach all people measures to take to protect the respiratory system from damage and cancer, including the avoidance of known environmental causative agents.
4. Teach the patient and family how to manage a chronic lower respiratory disorder and avoid injury and complications in the home.
5. Use assessment information to identify people at increased genetic risk for a respiratory disease that affects GAS EXCHANGE and PERFUSION.

Psychosocial Integrity

6. Reduce the psychological impact for the patient and family experiencing a chronic lower respiratory problem.

7. Work with other members of the health care team to ensure that values, preferences, and expressed needs of patients experiencing lower respiratory problems are respected.

Physiological Integrity

8. Assess and re-assess the manifestations of patients being managed for a lower respiratory problem.
9. Use laboratory data and clinical manifestations to prioritize nursing care for the patient who has an acute or chronic lower respiratory problem.
10. Collaborate with other health care professionals who help patients and families experiencing a chronic lower respiratory problem achieve desired health outcomes.
11. Coordinate nursing interventions for the patient with a chronic lower respiratory problem in the community.
12. Prioritize nursing care for the patient with chest tubes.

The alveoli and the smallest airways are sites for direct GAS EXCHANGE. Any problem of these tissues reduces gas exchange and interferes with PERFUSION. Many lower airway problems are chronic and progressive, requiring changes in lifestyle, especially for older adults. Chart 30-1 lists nursing issues for the older patient with a respiratory problem.

Chronic airflow limitation (CAL) is a group of chronic lung diseases that includes asthma, chronic bronchitis, and pulmonary emphysema. More than 10% of American adults suffer from some form of CAL, and many have moderate to severe disability from it (Centers for Disease Control and Prevention [CDC], 2012). Although CAL problems are not all reversible, good management can help maintain adequate GAS EXCHANGE and improve overall health.

ASTHMA

❖ PATHOPHYSIOLOGY

Asthma is often a chronic condition in which reversible airflow obstruction in the airways occurs intermittently (Fig. 30-1). Airway obstruction occurs by INFLAMMATION and by airway tissue sensitivity (hyperresponsiveness) that leads to bronchoconstriction. Inflammation obstructs the airway **lumens** (i.e., the insides) (Fig. 30-2). Airway hyperresponsiveness and constriction of bronchial smooth muscle narrow the airways from the outside. Airway inflammation and sensitivity can trigger bronchiolar constriction, and many people with asthma have both problems. Severe airway obstruction impairs GAS EXCHANGE and can be fatal. At least 3400 deaths from acute asthma occur in the United States each year (CDC, 2014a).

Etiology and Genetic Risk

Although asthma is classified into types based on what triggers the attacks, the effect on GAS EXCHANGE is the same. INFLAMMATION of the mucous membranes lining the airways is a key event in triggering an asthma attack. It occurs in response to the presence of specific allergens; general irritants such as cold air, dry air, or fine airborne particles; microorganisms; and aspirin and other NSAIDs. Increased airway sensitivity (hyperresponsiveness) can occur with exercise, with an upper respiratory illness, and for unknown reasons.

When asthma is well controlled, the airway changes are temporary and reversible. With poor control, chronic INFLAMMATION can lead to airway damage and altered CELLULAR REGULATION with enlargement of the bronchial epithelial cells

In **asthma**, the airways overreact to common stimuli with bronchospasm, edematous swelling of the mucous membranes, and copious production of thick, tenacious mucus by abundant hypertrophied mucous glands. Airway obstruction is usually intermittent.

Centriacinar or **centrilobular emphysema** affects the respiratory bronchioles most severely. It is usually more severe in the upper lung.

In **emphysema**, lung proteases collapse the walls of bronchioles and alveolar air sacs. As these walls collapse, the bronchioles and alveoli transform from a number of small elastic structures with great air-exchanging surface area into fewer, larger, inelastic structures with little surface area. Air is trapped in these distal structures, especially during forced expiration such as coughing, and the lungs hyperinflate. The trapped air stagnates and can no longer supply needed oxygen to the nearby capillaries.

In **chronic bronchitis**, infection or bronchial irritants cause increased secretions, edema, bronchospasm, and impaired mucociliary clearance. Inflammation of the bronchial walls causes them to thicken. This thickening, together with excessive mucus, blocks the airways and hinders gas exchange.

Panacinar or **panlobular** emphysema affects the entire acinar unit. It is usually more severe in the lower lung.

FIG. 30-1 The pathophysiology of chronic airflow limitation (CAL).

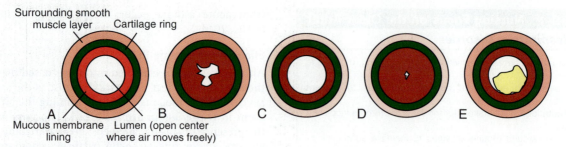

FIG. 30-2 Causes of narrowed airways. **A,** Cross section of a small airway showing the tissue layers. **B,** Mucosal swelling. **C,** Constriction of smooth muscle. **D,** Mucosal swelling and constriction of smooth muscle. **E,** Mucus plug.

GENETIC/GENOMIC CONSIDERATIONS

Patient-Centered Care QSEN

Results of genome-wide association studies (GWAS) indicate that more than 50 gene variations are associated with asthma, although asthma is a multifactorial disorder with both genetic and environmental input required for expression (Beery & Workman, 2012; Online Mendelian Inheritance in Man [OMIM], 2013b). Some variations have a greater influence for asthma expression within certain racial or ethnic groups. Also, genetic variation in the gene that controls the synthesis and activity of beta-adrenergic receptors has an impact on drug therapy for asthma. Patients who have a mutation in this gene do not respond as expected to beta agonist drugs and need an altered therapy plan. Teaching these patients about why their drug therapies are different from standard recommendations is a nursing responsibility that can assist with therapy adherence.

and changes in the bronchial smooth muscle. When asthma attacks are frequent, even exposure to low levels of the triggering agent or event may stimulate an attack.

Inflammation triggers asthma for some people when allergens bind to specific antibodies (especially immunoglobulin E [IgE]). These antibodies are attached to tissue *mast cells* and white blood cells (WBCs) called *basophils,* which are filled with chemicals that can start local inflammatory responses (see Chapters 17 and 20). Some chemicals, such as histamine, start an immediate inflammatory response, which can be blocked by drugs like diphenhydramine (Benadryl). Others, such as leukotriene and eotaxin, are slower and cause later, prolonged inflammatory responses, which can be blocked by drugs like montelukast (Singulair), zafirlukast (Accolate), and zileuton (Zyflo). Chemicals also attract more WBCs (eosinophils, macrophages, basophils) to the area, which then continue the responses of blood vessel dilation and capillary leak, leading to mucous membrane swelling and increased mucus production (McCance et al., 2014). These responses narrow the lumens even more, which then interferes with airflow and GAS EXCHANGE. INFLAMMATION can also occur through general irritation rather than allergic responses.

Bronchospasm is a narrowing of the bronchial tubes by constriction of the smooth muscle around and within the bronchial walls. It can occur when small amounts of pollutants or respiratory viruses stimulate nerve fibers, causing constriction of bronchial smooth muscle. If an inflammatory response is stimulated at the same time, the chemicals released during INFLAMMATION also trigger constriction. Severe bronchospasm alone,

especially in smaller bronchioles, can profoundly limit airflow to the alveoli and greatly reduce GAS EXCHANGE.

Aspirin and other NSAIDs can trigger asthma in some people, although this response is not a true allergy. It results from increased production of leukotriene when aspirin or NSAIDs suppress other inflammatory pathways.

Gastroesophageal reflux disease (GERD) can trigger asthma in some people, who then have more asthma manifestations at night (Global Initiative for Asthma [GINA], 2014). GERD allows highly acidic stomach contents to enter the airway and make the pre-existing tissue sensitivity worse.

Incidence and Prevalence

Asthma can occur at any age. About half of adults with asthma also had the disease in childhood. Asthma affects nearly 20.8 million adults in the United States and Canada (CDC, 2012). It is more common in urban settings than in rural settings.

CONSIDERATIONS FOR OLDER ADULTS

Patient-Centered Care QSEN

Asthma occurs as a new disorder in about 3% of people older than 55 years. Another 3% of people older than 60 years have asthma as a continuing chronic disorder (CDC, 2012). Lung and airway changes as a part of aging make any breathing problem more serious in the older adult. One problem related to aging is a decrease in the sensitivity of beta-adrenergic receptors. When stimulated, these receptors relax smooth muscle and cause bronchodilation. As these receptors become less sensitive, they no longer respond as quickly or as strongly to agonists (epinephrine, dopamine) and beta-adrenergic drugs, which are often used as rescue therapy during an acute asthma attack. Thus teaching older patients how to avoid asthma attacks and to correctly use preventive drug therapy is a nursing priority.

❖ *PATIENT-CENTERED COLLABORATIVE CARE*

◆ *Assessment*

Asthma is classified on the basis of how well controlled the manifestations are, as well as on the patient's response to asthma drugs. These classes are the basis for current asthma therapy (Charts 30-2 and 30-3).

History. The patient with asthma usually has a pattern of intermittent episodes of **dyspnea** (shortness of breath), chest tightness, coughing, wheezing, and increased mucus production. Ask whether the manifestations occur continuously, seasonally, in association with specific activities or exposures, or more frequently at night. Some patients have manifestations for

---

CHART 30-2 **Key Features**

Levels of Asthma Control

CHARACTERISTIC	CONTROLLED (ALL OF THESE CHARACTERISTICS MUST BE PRESENT)	PARTLY CONTROLLED (THE PRESENCE OF ANY ONE OF THESE CHARACTERISTICS IS CONSIDERED PARTLY CONTROLLED)	UNCONTROLLED (THE PRESENCE OF THREE OR MORE CHARACTERISTICS FROM THE PARTLY CONTROLLED LIST IS CONSIDERED UNCONTROLLED ASTHMA)
Daytime manifestations	Manifestations occur twice per week or less	Manifestations occur more than twice per week	
Activity limitations	None	Any	
Nighttime manifestations	None	Any	
Reliever drug use	Reliever used twice per week or less	Reliever used more than twice per week	
PEF or FEV$_1$	Normal	Less than 80% of predicted or established personal best	
Treatment action	Find and maintain lowest step level that controls manifestations	Increase step until manifestations are controlled on a regular basis and then reduce step to the lowest step level that consistently controls manifestations	Increase step (step up) until control is reached and maintained

FEV$_1$, Forced expiratory volume in the first second; *PEF,* peak expiratory flow.

CHART 30-3 **Key Features**

The Step System for Medication Use in Asthma Control

STEP 1	STEP 2	STEP 3	STEP 4	STEP 5
As-needed rapid-acting beta$_2$ agonist (relief inhaler)	As-needed rapid-acting beta$_2$ agonist (relief inhaler)	As-needed rapid-acting beta$_2$ agonist (relief inhaler)	As-needed rapid-acting beta$_2$ agonist (relief inhaler)	As-needed rapid-acting beta$_2$ agonist (relief inhaler)
No daily drugs needed	Daily treatment involves the use of *one* of these two options:	Daily treatment involves the use of *one* of these four options:	Daily treatment involves the use of the Step 3 option that provided the best degree of control and was well tolerated along with one or more of these two options:	Daily treatment involves the use of the Step 4 option(s) that provided the best degree of control and was well tolerated along with either of these two options:
	Low-dose ICS*	Low-dose ICS *and* long-acting beta$_2$ agonist	Medium-dose or high-dose ICS *and* long-acting beta$_2$ agonist	Oral glucocorticosteroid (lowest dose)
	Leukotriene modifier†	Medium-dose or high-dose ICS Low-dose ICS and leukotriene modifier Low-dose ICS and sustained-release theophylline	Leukotriene modifier and sustained-release theophylline	Anti-IgE‡ treatment

Data compiled from Global Initiative for Asthma (GINA). (2014). Pocket guide for asthma management and prevention. Retrieved June 2014, from www.ginasthma.org/Guidelines/guidelines-resources.html.
*ICS = Inhaled corticosteroid.
†Leukotriene modifier = Leukotriene receptor antagonist or leukotriene synthesis inhibitor.
‡IgE = Immunoglobulin E.

---

4 to 8 weeks after a cold or other upper respiratory infection. The patient with atopic (allergic) asthma often has other allergic problems such as rhinitis, skin rash, or pruritus. Ask whether any family members have asthma or respiratory problems. Ask about current or previous smoking habits. If the patient smokes, use this opportunity to teach him or her about smoking cessation (see Chart 27-1 in Chapter 27). Wheezing in nonsmokers is important in the diagnosis of asthma.

Physical Assessment/Clinical Manifestations. The patient with mild to moderate asthma may have no manifestations between asthma attacks. During an acute episode, common manifestations are an audible wheeze and increased respiratory rate. At first, the wheeze is louder on exhalation. When INFLAMMATION occurs with asthma, coughing may increase.

The patient may use accessory muscles to help breathe during an attack. Observe for muscle retraction at the sternum and the suprasternal notch and between the ribs. The patient with long-standing, severe asthma may have a "barrel chest," caused by air trapping (Fig. 30-3). The anteroposterior (AP) diameter (diameter between the front and the back of the chest)

FIG. 30-3 A, Normal adult. The thorax has an oval shape with an anteroposterior-to-transverse diameter of 1 : 1.5 or 5 : 7. **B,** Barrel chest. Note equal anteroposterior-to-transverse diameter and that ribs are horizontal instead of the normal downward slope. This is associated with chronic obstructive pulmonary disease and severe asthma as a result of hyperinflation of the lungs.

increases with air trapping, giving the chest a rounded rather than an oval shape. The normal chest is about 1.5 times as wide as it is deep. In severe, chronic asthma, the AP diameter may equal or exceed the lateral diameter. Compare the AP diameter of the chest with the lateral diameter. Chronic air trapping also flattens the diaphragm and increases the space between the ribs.

Along with an audible wheeze, the breathing cycle is longer with prolonged exhalation and requires more effort. The patient may be unable to speak more than a few words between breaths. Hypoxia occurs with severe attacks. Pulse oximetry shows **hypoxemia** (poor blood oxygen levels). Examine the oral mucosa and nail beds for cyanosis. Other indicators of hypoxemia include changes in the level of cognition or consciousness and tachycardia.

Laboratory Assessment. Laboratory tests can determine asthma type and the degree of breathing impairment. Arterial blood gas (ABG) levels show the effectiveness of GAS EXCHANGE (see Chapter 12 for discussion of ABGs). The arterial oxygen level (Pao_2) may decrease during an asthma attack. Early in the attack, the arterial carbon dioxide level ($Paco_2$) may be decreased as the patient increases the breathing rate and depth. Later in an asthma episode, $Paco_2$ rises, indicating carbon dioxide retention. Allergic asthma often occurs with elevated serum eosinophil counts and immunoglobulin E (IgE) levels. The sputum

may contain eosinophils and mucus plugs with shed epithelial cells (Curschmann's spirals).

Pulmonary Function Tests. The most accurate tests for measuring airflow in asthma are the pulmonary function tests (PFTs) using spirometry (O'Laughlen & Rance, 2012). Baseline PFTs are obtained for all patients diagnosed with asthma. The most important PFTs for a patient with asthma are the forced vital capacity (FVC), the forced expiratory volume in the first second (FEV_1), and the peak expiratory flow (PEF), sometimes called *peak expiratory rate flow (PERF)*. Definitions of PFTs are listed in Chapter 27. A decrease in either the FEV_1 or the PEF (PERF) of 15% to 20% below the expected value for age, gender, and size is common for the patient with asthma. Asthma is diagnosed when these values increase by 12% or more after treatment with bronchodilators. Airway responsiveness is tested by measuring the PEF and FEV_1 before and after the patient inhales the drug *methacholine,* which induces bronchospasm in susceptible people.

◆ Interventions

The purposes of asthma therapy are to control and prevent episodes, improve airflow and GAS EXCHANGE, and relieve manifestations. Asthma is best controlled when the patient is an active partner in the management plan (Pruitt, 2011). Priority nursing actions focus on patient education about implementation of the personal asthma action plan, which includes drug therapy and lifestyle management strategies to assist the patient in understanding his or her disease and its management (GINA, 2014).

Self-Management Education. Asthma often has intermittent overt manifestations. With guided self-care, patients can co-manage this disease, increasing symptom-free periods and decreasing the number and severity of attacks (Pruitt, 2011). Good management decreases hospital admissions and increases participation in patient-chosen work and leisure activities. Self-care requires extensive education for the patient to be able to self-assess respiratory status, self-manage (by adjusting the frequency and dosage of prescribed drugs), and know when to consult the health care provider.

Ideally, a personal asthma action plan is developed by the health care provider and the patient. The plan is tailored to meet the patient's personal triggers, asthma manifestations, and drug responses. It includes:
- The prescribed daily controller drug(s) schedule and prescribed reliever drug directions
- Patient-specific daily asthma control assessment questions
  - Directions for adjusting the daily controller drug schedule
  - When to contact the health care provider (in addition to regularly scheduled visits)
  - What emergency actions to take when asthma is not responding to controller and reliever drugs

Teach the patient to assess asthma severity at least daily with a peak flow meter (Fig. 30-4) and to adjust drugs according to his or her personal asthma action plan to manage INFLAMMATION and bronchospasms to prevent or relieve manifestations. Chart 30-4 describes the correct method to use the peak flow meter. The patient first establishes a baseline or "personal best" peak expiratory flow (PEF) by measuring his or her PEF twice daily for 2 to 3 weeks when asthma is well controlled and recording the results. This way, the patient will know when his or her peak flow is reduced to the point that more drugs are needed or that

FIG. 30-4 A typical peak flowmeter. This model will show faster exhalation rates in *green*, reduced exhalation rates in *yellow,* and seriously reduced exhalation rates in *red.*

CHART 30-4 Patient and Family Education: Preparing for Self-Management

Using a Peak Flow Meter

- Set the peak flowmeter at zero.
- Use a standing position, without leaning or supporting yourself on anything, if possible.
- Take as deep a breath as you can.
- Place the mouthpiece of the meter in your mouth, taking care to wrap your lips tightly around it.
- Blow your breath out through the mouthpiece as hard and as fast as you are able. (If you cough, sneeze, or have any type of interruption while you exhale, reset the meter and perform the test again.)
- Reset and perform the test two additional times.
- The highest reading of the three is your current peak flow rate.
- Keep a record or graph of your peak flow rates and examine these for trends.

---

emergency assistance is needed. When the patient has established a "personal best," all other readings are compared with this value. Some meters are color-coded to help the patient interpret the results. Green zone readings are at least 80% of or above the "personal best." This is the ideal range for asthma control and indicates that no increases in drug therapy are needed. Yellow is a range between 50% and 80% of personal best. When a patient has a reading in this range, he or she needs to use the prescribed reliever drug. Within a few minutes after using the reliever drug, another PEF reading should be made to determine whether the reliever drug is working. *Frequent readings in the yellow zone or increasing use of reliever drugs indicates the need to reassess the asthma plan for the need to change controller drugs.* Red is a range below 50% of the patient's personal best, indicating serious respiratory obstruction.

⚠ NURSING SAFETY PRIORITY ⬢QSEN

Action Alert

Teach the patient that if a red zone reading occurs when using the peak flowmeter to immediately use the reliever drugs and seek emergency help.

CHART 30-5 Patient and Family Education: Preparing for Self-Management

Asthma Management

- Avoid potential environmental asthma triggers, such as smoke, fireplaces, dust, mold, and weather changes of warm to cold.
- Avoid drugs that trigger your asthma (e.g., aspirin, NSAIDs, beta blockers).
- Avoid food that has been prepared with monosodium glutamate (MSG) or metabisulfite.
- If you have exercise-induced asthma, use your bronchodilator inhaler 30 minutes before exercise to prevent or reduce bronchospasm.
- Be sure you know the proper technique and correct sequence when you use metered dose inhalers.
- Get adequate rest and sleep.
- Reduce stress and anxiety; learn relaxation techniques; adopt coping mechanisms that have worked for you in the past.
- Wash all bedding with hot water to destroy dust mites.
- Monitor your peak expiratory flow rates with a flow meter at least twice daily.
- Seek immediate emergency care if you experience any of these:
  - Gray or blue fingertips or lips
  - Difficulty breathing, walking, or talking
  - Retractions of the neck, chest, or ribs
  - Nasal flaring
  - Failure of drugs to control worsening symptoms
  - Peak expiratory rate flow (PERF) declining steadily after treatment, or a flow rate 50% below your usual flow rate

---

Teach the patient to keep a symptom and intervention diary to learn specific triggers of asthma, early cues for impending attacks, and personal response to drugs. Stress the importance of proper use of his or her personal asthma action plan for any severity of asthma. Chart 30-5 lists areas to emphasize when teaching the patient with asthma.

Drug Therapy. Pharmacologic management of adults with asthma is based on the step category for severity and treatment (see Charts 30-2 and 30-3) (GINA, 2014). **Control therapy drugs** are drugs used to reduce airway sensitivity (responsiveness) to prevent asthma attacks from occurring. *They are used every day, regardless of symptoms.* **Reliever drugs** (also called "rescue drugs") are those used to actually stop an attack once it has started. Some patients may need drug therapy only during an asthma episode. For others, daily drugs are needed to keep asthma episodic rather than a more frequent problem. This therapy involves the use of bronchodilators and various drug types to reduce INFLAMMATION. Some drugs reduce the asthma response, and other drugs actually prevent the response. Combination drugs are two agents from different classes combined together for better response. Chart 30-6 lists the most common preferred drugs in each class for control and relief therapy of asthma. The actions, interventions, and rationales for most drugs within a single class are similar although drug dosages may differ. Be sure to consult a pharmacology text or drug handbook for more information on a specific drug.

Bronchodilators. Bronchodilators cause bronchiolar smooth muscle relaxation. They have no effect on INFLAMMATION. Thus when a patient with asthma has airflow obstruction by both bronchospasm and inflammation, at least two types of drug therapy are needed. Some bronchodilators work by stimulating the beta$_2$-adrenergic receptors on bronchial smooth muscle in the same way that the hormones *epinephrine* and *norepinephrine* do; others work by blocking the parasympathetic nervous

CHART 30-6 Common Examples of Drug Therapy
Asthma Prevention and Treatment

DRUG/USUAL DOSAGE	NURSING INTERVENTIONS	RATIONALE
Bronchodilators Cause bronchodilation through relaxing bronchiolar smooth muscle by binding to and activating pulmonary beta$_2$ receptors.		
Short-Acting Beta$_2$ Agonist (SABA) Primary use is a fast-acting reliever (rescue) drug to be used either during an asthma attack or just before engaging in activity that usually triggers an attack.		
Albuterol (Proventil, Ventolin) 1-2 inhalations every 4-6 hr (90 mcg/inhaled dose)	Teach patients to carry drug with them at all times.	The drug can stop or reduce life-threatening bronchoconstriction, which can occur anytime.
	Teach patient to monitor heart rate.	Excessive use causes systemic symptoms, especially tachycardia.
	When taking this drug with other inhaled drugs, teach patient to use this drug at least 5 minutes before the other inhaled drugs.	The bronchodilation effect of the drug allows better penetration of the other inhaled drugs.
	Teach patient the correct technique for using the MDI or DPI.	Correct technique is essential to getting the drug to the site of action.
Long-Acting Beta$_2$ Agonist (LABA) Causes bronchodilation through relaxing bronchiolar smooth muscle by binding to and activating pulmonary beta$_2$ receptors. Onset of action is slow with a long duration. Primary use is prevention of an asthma attack.		
Salmeterol (Serevent) 2 inhalations every 12 hr (25 mcg/inhalation with MDI) (50 mcg/inhalation with DPI)	Teach patient to shake inhaler (MDI) well before using.	Drug separates easily.
	Teach patient to not use this drug as a reliever drug.	Drug has slow onset of action and does not relieve symptoms.
	Teach patient the correct technique for using the MDI or DPI.	Correct technique is essential to getting the drug to the site of action.
Indacaterol (Arcapta Neohaler) 1 inhalation daily (75 mcg/inhalation with DPI) (COPD only)	Same as for salmeterol.	Same as for salmeterol.
Cholinergic Antagonist Causes bronchodilation by inhibiting the parasympathetic nervous system, allowing the sympathetic system to dominate, releasing norepinephrine that activates beta$_2$ receptors. Purpose is to both relieve and prevent asthma.		
Ipratropium (Atrovent, Apo-Ipravent) 2-4 inhalations 4-6 times daily (18 mcg/inhalation)	If patient is to use this as a reliever drug, teach him or her to carry it at all times.	The drug can stop or reduce life-threatening bronchoconstriction, which can occur anytime.
	Teach patient to shake MDI well before using.	Drug separates easily.
	Teach patient to increase daily fluid intake.	Drug causes mouth dryness.
	Teach patient to observe for and report blurred vision, eye pain, headache, nausea, palpitations, tremors, inability to sleep.	These are systemic symptoms of overdose and require intervention.
	Teach patient the correct technique for using the MDI or DPI.	Correct technique is essential to getting the drug to the site of action.
Anti-inflammatories All of these drugs help improve bronchiolar airflow by decreasing the inflammatory response of the mucous membranes in the airways. *They do not cause bronchodilation.*		
Corticosteroids Disrupt production pathways of inflammatory mediators. The main purpose is to prevent an asthma attack caused by inflammation or allergies (controller drug).		
Fluticasone (Flovent) 50 mcg by MDI twice daily; 100-250 mcg by DPI daily	Teach patient to use the drug daily, even when no symptoms are present.	Maximum effectiveness requires continued use for 48-72 hr and depends on regular use.
	Teach patient to use good mouth care and to check mouth daily for lesions or drainage.	Drug reduces local immunity and increases the risk for local infections, especially *Candida albicans* (yeast).
	Teach patient to not use this drug as a reliever drug.	Drug has slow onset of action and does not relieve symptoms.
	Teach patient the correct technique for using the MDI or DPI.	Correct technique is essential to getting the drug to the site of action.
Prednisone (Deltasone, Predone) 1-40 mg orally daily	Teach patient about expected side effects.	Knowing the side effects to expect reduces anxiety.
	Teach patient to avoid anyone who has an upper respiratory infection.	Drug reduces all protective inflammatory responses, increasing the risk for infection.
	Teach patient to avoid activities that lead to injury.	Blood vessels become more fragile, leading to bruising and petechiae.
	Teach patient to take drug with food.	Food helps reduce the drug side effect of GI ulceration.
	Teach patient not to suddenly stop taking the drug for any reason.	The drug suppresses adrenal production of corticosteroids, which are essential for life.

CHART 30-6 Common Examples of Drug Therapy—cont'd

Asthma Prevention and Treatment

DRUG/USUAL DOSAGE	NURSING INTERVENTIONS	RATIONALE
Cromone Stabilizes the membranes of mast cells and prevents the release of inflammatory mediators. Purpose is to prevent asthma attack triggered by inflammation or allergens.		
Nedocromil (Tilade) 4 mg by MDI every 6 hr	Teach patient to use the drug daily, even when no symptoms are present.	Drug has slow onset of action for asthma prevention and is most effective when taken consistently.
	Teach patient to not use this drug as a reliever drug.	Drug does not relieve or reverse symptoms.
	Teach patient the correct technique for using the MDI.	Correct technique is essential to getting the drug to the site of action.
Leukotriene Modifier Blocks the leukotriene receptor, preventing the inflammatory mediator from stimulating inflammation. Purpose is to prevent asthma attack triggered by inflammation or allergens.		
Montelukast (Singulair) 10 mg orally daily	Teach patient to use the drug daily, even when no symptoms are present.	Drug has slow onset of action for asthma prevention and is most effective when taken consistently.
	Teach patient not to decrease the dose of or stop taking any other asthma drugs unless instructed by the health care professional.	This drug is for long-term asthma control and does not replace other drugs, especially corticosteroids and reliever (rescue) drugs.

Data from Global Initiative for Asthma (GINA). (2014). *Pocket guide for asthma management and prevention.* Retrieved June 2014, from www.ginasthma.org/Guidelines/guidelines-resources.html; Global Initiative for Chronic Obstructive Lung Disease (GOLD). (2014). *Global strategy for the diagnosis, management, and prevention of chronic obstructive pulmonary disease.* Retrieved June 2014, from www.goldcopd.org/.
COPD, Chronic obstructive pulmonary disease; *DPI,* dry powder inhaler; *MDI,* metered dose inhaler.

system. Bronchodilators include beta$_2$ agonists and cholinergic antagonists.

Beta$_2$ agonists bind to the beta$_2$-adrenergic receptors and cause an increase in smooth muscle relaxation. Short-acting beta$_2$ agonists (SABAs) provide rapid but short-term relief. These inhaled drugs are most useful when an attack begins (as relief) or as premedication when the patient is about to begin an activity that is likely to induce an attack (GINA, 2014). Such agents include albuterol (Proventil, Ventolin), bitolterol (Tornalate), levalbuterol (Xopenex), pirbuterol (Maxair), and terbutaline (Brethaire). Teach the patient the correct technique for using an inhaled drug with a metered dose inhaler (MDI) (Chart 30-7). Fig. 30-5 shows a patient using a "spacer" with an MDI. Spacer use increases the amount of drug that is delivered to the lungs. Chart 30-8 describes the proper care and use of a dry powder inhaler (DPI).

! NURSING SAFETY PRIORITY (QSEN)

Action Alert

Teach the patient with asthma to always carry the relief drug inhaler with him or her and to ensure that enough drug remains in the inhaler to provide a quick dose when needed.

Dry powder inhalers indicate the amount of remaining drug. Some aerosol inhalers (MDIs) have meters that indicate the number of doses left in the canister, and others do not. It is recommended that the patient count the number of doses as they are used; however, many patients have difficulty keeping the dose count accurate.

Long-acting beta$_2$ agonists (LABAs) are also delivered by inhaler directly to the site of action—the bronchioles. Proper use of the long-acting agonists can decrease the need to use reliever drugs as often. Unlike short-acting agonists, long-acting drugs need time to build up an effect but the effects are longer lasting. Thus these drugs are useful in preventing an asthma

CHART 30-7 Patient and Family Education: Preparing for Self-Management

How to Use an Inhaler Correctly*

With a Spacer (Preferred Technique)
1. Before each use, remove the caps from the inhaler and the spacer.
2. Insert the mouthpiece of the inhaler into the non-mouthpiece end of the spacer.
3. Shake the whole unit vigorously 3 or 4 times.
4. Place the mouthpiece into your mouth, over your tongue, and seal your lips tightly around it.
5. Press down firmly on the canister of the inhaler to release one dose of medication into the spacer.
6. Breathe in slowly and deeply. If the spacer makes a whistling sound, you are breathing in too rapidly.
7. Remove the mouthpiece from your mouth, and, keeping your lips closed, hold your breath for at least 10 seconds and then breathe out slowly.
8. Wait at least 1 minute between puffs.
9. Replace the caps on the inhaler and the spacer.
10. At least once a day, clean the plastic case and cap of the inhaler by thoroughly rinsing in warm, running tap water; at least once a week, clean the spacer in the same manner.

Without a Spacer
1. Before each use, remove the cap and shake the inhaler according to the instructions in the package insert.
2. Tilt your head back slightly, and breathe out fully.
3. Open your mouth, and place the mouthpiece 1 to 2 inches away.
4. As you begin to breathe in deeply through your mouth, press down firmly on the canister of the inhaler to release one dose of medication.
5. Continue to breathe in slowly and deeply (usually over 5-7 sec).
6. Hold your breath for at least 10 seconds to allow the medication to reach deep into the lungs, and then breathe out slowly.
7. Wait at least 1 minute between puffs.
8. Replace the cap on the inhaler.
9. At least once a day, remove the canister and clean the plastic case and cap of the inhaler by thoroughly rinsing in warm, running tap water.

*Avoid spraying in the direction of the eyes.

FIG. 30-5 Patient using an aerosol metered dose inhaler with a spacer.

CHART 30-8 Patient and Family Education: Preparing for Self-Management

How to Use a Dry Powder Inhaler (DPI)

For Inhalers Requiring Loading
- First load the drug by:
  - Turning the device to the next dose of drug, *or*
  - Inserting the capsule into the device, *or*
  - Inserting the disk or compartment into the device

After Loading the Drug and for Inhalers That Do Not Require Drug Loading
- Read your doctor's instructions for how fast you should breathe for your particular inhaler.
- Place your lips over the mouthpiece, and breathe in forcefully (there is no propellant in the inhaler; only your breath pulls the drug in).
- Remove the inhaler from your mouth as soon as you have breathed in.
- *Never exhale (breathe out) into your inhaler.* Your breath will moisten the powder, causing it to clump and not be delivered accurately.
- *Never wash or place the inhaler in water.*
- *Never shake your inhaler.*
- Keep your inhaler in a dry place at room temperature.
- If the inhaler is preloaded, discard the inhaler after it is empty.
- Because the drug is a dry powder and there is no propellant, you may not feel, smell, or taste it as you inhale.

---

attack but have no value during an acute attack. Therefore teach patients not to use LABAs alone to relieve them during an attack or when wheezing is getting worse but, instead, to use a SABA. Examples of LABAs include formoterol (Foradil) and salmeterol (Serevent). *These drugs should never be prescribed as the **only** drug therapy for asthma. Teach the patient to use these control drugs daily as prescribed, even when no manifestations are present.*

Cholinergic antagonists, also called *anticholinergic drugs,* are similar to atropine and block the parasympathetic nervous system. This action results in increased bronchodilation and decreased pulmonary secretions. The most common drug in this class is ipratropium (Atrovent), which is used as an inhalant. Most cholinergic antagonists are short acting and must be used several times a day, although long-acting agents such as tiotropium (Spiriva) are available for use once a day.

Xanthines, such as theophylline and aminophylline, are used only when other types of management are ineffective. These drugs are given systemically, and the dosage that is effective is close to the dosage that produces many dangerous side effects. Blood levels must be monitored closely to ensure the drug level is within the therapeutic range.

Anti-Inflammatory Agents. Anti-inflammatory agents decrease INFLAMMATION in the airways. Those used as inhalants have fewer systemic side effects than those taken systemically.

Corticosteroids decrease inflammation in many ways, including by reducing the production of inflammatory chemicals. Inhaled corticosteroids (ICSs) can be helpful in controlling asthma manifestations. High-potency steroid inhalers, such as fluticasone (Flovent), budesonide (Pulmicort), and mometasone (Asmanex), may be used once per day for maintenance. Systemic corticosteroids, because of severe side effects, are avoided for mild to moderate intermittent asthma and are used on a short-term basis for moderate asthma. For some patients with severe asthma, daily oral corticosteroids may be needed. *Both inhaled corticosteroids and those taken orally are controller drugs. They are not effective in reversing symptoms during an asthma attack and should not be used as reliever drugs. Teach patients to take corticosteroids on a scheduled basis, even when no manifestations are present.*

Cromones, both those that are inhaled and those that are taken orally, are useful as *controller* asthma therapy when taken on a scheduled basis. These agents reduce airway INFLAMMATION by either inhibiting the release of inflammatory chemicals (nedocromil [Tilade]) or preventing mast cell membranes from opening when an allergen binds to IgE (cromolyn sodium [Intal]). *Thus these drugs help prevent asthma attacks but are not effective in reversing symptoms during an asthma attack and should not be used alone as relief drugs.*

Leukotriene modifiers are oral drugs that work in several ways to control asthma when taken on a scheduled basis. Montelukast (Singulair) and zafirlukast (Accolate) block the leukotriene receptor. Zileuton (Zyflo) prevents leukotriene synthesis. *These drugs do not reverse symptoms during an asthma attack and should not be used alone as relief drugs.*

Exercise/Activity. Regular exercise is a recommended part of asthma therapy to maintain cardiac health, strengthen muscles, and promote GAS EXCHANGE and PERFUSION. Teach patients to examine the conditions that trigger an attack and adjust the exercise routine as needed. Some may need to use an inhaled SABA before beginning activity. For others, adjusting the environment may be needed (e.g., changing from outdoor ice-skating in cold, dry air to indoor ice-skating).

Oxygen Therapy. Supplemental oxygen by mask or nasal cannula is often used during an acute asthma attack. High flow delivery may be needed when bronchospasms are severe and limit flow of oxygen through the bronchiole tubes. Heliox, a mixture of helium and oxygen (often 50% helium and 50% oxygen), can help improve oxygen delivery to the alveoli. This gas mixture is lower in density than oxygen alone or room air and flows even when airway resistance is high.

! NURSING SAFETY PRIORITY (QSEN)
Action Alert

Ensure that no open flames (e.g., cigarette smoking, fireplaces, burning candles) or other combustion hazards are in rooms where oxygen is in use.

Status Asthmaticus. Status asthmaticus is a severe, life-threatening acute episode of airway obstruction that intensifies once it begins and often does not respond to usual therapy. The patient arrives in the emergency department with extremely labored breathing and wheezing. Use of accessory muscles for breathing and distention of neck veins are observed. *If the condition is not reversed, the patient may develop pneumothorax and cardiac or respiratory arrest.* IV fluids, potent systemic bronchodilators, steroids, epinephrine, and oxygen are given immediately to reverse the condition. Prepare for emergency intubation. Sudden absence of wheezing indicates complete airway obstruction and requires a tracheotomy. When breathing improves, management is similar to that for any patient with asthma.

🔍 NCLEX EXAMINATION CHALLENGE

Safe and Effective Care Environment

Which parameter indicates to the nurse that the short-acting beta-adrenergic agonist the client took 5 minutes ago for an acute asthma attack is effective?
A. SpO₂ decrease from 85% to 78%
B. Peak expiratory flow rate increase from 50% to 70%
C. The obvious use of accessory muscles during inhalation and exhalation
D. Active bubbling in the humidifier chamber of the oxygen delivery system

---

CHRONIC OBSTRUCTIVE PULMONARY DISEASE

❖ PATHOPHYSIOLOGY

Chronic obstructive pulmonary diseases (COPD) include emphysema and chronic bronchitis. Although these are separate disorders with different pathologic processes, many patients with emphysema also have chronic bronchitis at the same time (Fig. 30-6).

Emphysema. The two major changes that occur with emphysema are loss of lung elasticity and hyperinflation of the lung (see Fig. 30-1). These changes result in dyspnea and the need for an increased respiratory rate.

In the healthy lung, enzymes called *proteases* are present to destroy and eliminate particulates and organisms inhaled during breathing. If these proteases are present in higher-than-normal levels, they damage the alveoli and the small airways by breaking down elastin. Over time, alveolar sacs lose their elasticity and the small airways collapse or narrow. Some alveoli are

destroyed, and others become large and flabby, with less area for GAS EXCHANGE.

An increased amount of air is trapped in the lungs. Causes of air trapping are loss of elastic recoil in the alveolar walls, overstretching and enlargement of the alveoli into air-filled spaces called *bullae,* and collapse of small bronchioles. These changes greatly increase the work of breathing. The hyperinflated lung flattens the diaphragm (Fig. 30-7), weakening the effectiveness of this muscle. As a result, the patient with emphysema needs to use accessory muscles in the neck, chest wall, and abdomen to inhale and exhale. This increased effort increases the need for oxygen, making the patient have an "air hunger" sensation. Inhalation starts before exhalation is completed, resulting in an uncoordinated breathing pattern.

GAS EXCHANGE is affected by the increased work of breathing and the loss of alveolar tissue. Although some alveoli enlarge, the curves of alveolar walls decrease and less surface area is available for gas exchange. Often the patient adjusts by increasing the respiratory rate, so arterial blood gas (ABG) values may not show gas exchange problems until the patient has advanced disease. Then carbon dioxide is produced faster than it can be eliminated, resulting in carbon dioxide retention and chronic respiratory acidosis (see Chapter 12). The patient with late-stage emphysema also has a low arterial oxygen (Pao₂) level because it is difficult for oxygen to move from diseased alveoli into the blood.

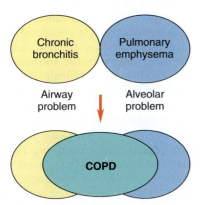

FIG. 30-6 The interaction of chronic bronchitis and emphysema in chronic obstructive pulmonary disease (COPD).

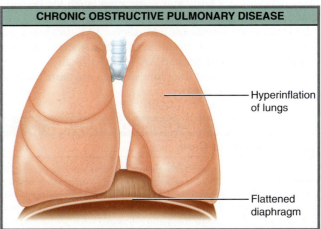

FIG. 30-7 Diaphragm shape and lung inflation in the normal patient and in the patient with chronic airflow limitation (CAL), especially chronic obstructive pulmonary disease (COPD).

Emphysema is classified as *panlobular, centrilobular,* or *paraseptal* depending on the pattern of destruction and dilation of the gas-exchanging units (acini) (see Fig. 30-1). Each type can occur alone or in combination in the same lung. Most are associated with smoking or chronic exposure to other inhaled particles such as wood smoke and biomass fuels (Global Initiative for Chronic Obstructive Lung Disease [GOLD], 2014).

Chronic Bronchitis. Bronchitis is an INFLAMMATION of the bronchi and bronchioles caused by exposure to irritants, especially cigarette smoke. The irritant triggers inflammation, vasodilation, mucosal edema, congestion, and bronchospasm. Bronchitis affects only the airways, not the alveoli.

Chronic INFLAMMATION increases the number and size of mucus glands, which produce large amounts of thick mucus. The bronchial walls thicken and impair airflow. This thickening, along with excessive mucus, blocks some of the smaller airways and narrows larger ones. Mucus provides a breeding ground for organisms and leads to chronic infection.

Chronic bronchitis impairs airflow and GAS EXCHANGE because mucus plugs and infection narrow the airways. As a result, the PaO_2 level decreases (hypoxemia) and the arterial carbon dioxide ($PaCO_2$) level increases (respiratory acidosis).

Etiology and Genetic Risk. *Cigarette smoking* is the greatest risk factor for COPD. The patient with a 20–pack-year history or longer often has early-stage COPD with changes in pulmonary function tests (PFTs).

The inhaled smoke triggers the release of excessive proteases in the lungs. These enzymes break down elastin, the major component of alveoli. By impairing the action of cilia, smoking also inhibits the cilia from clearing the bronchi of mucus, cellular debris, and fluid.

Alpha1-antitrypsin deficiency is a less common but important risk factor for COPD. The enzyme *alpha1-antitrypsin* (AAT) is normally present in the lungs. AAT inhibits excessive protease activity so that the proteases only break down inhaled pollutants and organisms and do not damage lung structures.

The production of normal amounts of AAT depends on the inheritance of a pair of normal gene alleles for this protein. The AAT gene is recessive. Thus if one of the pair of alleles is faulty and the other allele is normal, the person makes enough AAT to prevent COPD unless there is significant exposure to cigarette smoke or other inhalation irritants. This person, however, is a carrier for AAT deficiency. When both alleles are faulty, COPD develops at a fairly young age even when the person is not exposed to cigarette smoke or other irritants.

About 100,000 Americans have severe AAT deficiency, and many more have mild to moderate deficiencies (Beery & Workman, 2012). Although an AAT deficiency also can cause problems in the skin and liver, lung diseases are more common (Kessenich & Bacher, 2014).

GENETIC/GENOMIC CONSIDERATIONS

Patient-Centered Care QSEN

The gene for AAT has many known variations, and some increase the risk for emphysema. Different variations result in different levels of AAT deficiency and is a reason why the disease is more severe for some people than for others. The most serious variation for emphysema risk is the Z mutation, although others also increase the risk but to a lesser degree. Table 30-1 shows the most common AAT mutations increasing the risk for emphysema. Urge patients who have any ATT deficiency to avoid smoking and other environmental pollutants.

TABLE 30-1 **Characteristics Associated with the Most Common Alpha1-Antitrypsin Gene Mutations**

MUTATION GENOTYPE	LEVEL OF SERUM ALPHA1-ANTITRYPSIN (% OF NORMAL)	DISEASE SEVERITY
M/S	80%	No detectable disease
S/S	50%-60%	Minimal to no disease expression
M/Z	50%-55%	Minimal to no disease expression
S/Z	30%-35%	Pulmonary disease, early age
Z/Z	10%-15%	Severe COPD, extrapulmonary involvement

From Workman, M.L., & Winkelman, C. (2008). Genetic influences in common respiratory disorders. *Critical Care Nursing Clinics of North America, 20*(2), 171-189. *COPD,* Chronic obstructive pulmonary disease.

In addition to genetic and environmental factors, asthma also appears to be a risk factor for COPD. The incidence of COPD is reported to be 12 times greater among adults with asthma compared with adults without asthma after adjusting for smoking history (GOLD, 2014).

Incidence and Prevalence. The prevalence of chronic bronchitis and emphysema in the United States has been estimated at about 15.8 million, and more than 10% of nursing home residents have COPD (CDC, 2014b). COPD is the fourth leading cause of morbidity and mortality in the United States (GOLD, 2014).

Complications. COPD affects GAS EXCHANGE and the oxygenation of all tissues. Complications include hypoxemia, acidosis, respiratory infection, cardiac failure, dysrhythmias, and respiratory failure.

Hypoxemia and acidosis occur because the patient with COPD has reduced GAS EXCHANGE, leading to decreased oxygenation and increased carbon dioxide levels. These problems reduce cellular function.

Respiratory infection risk increases because of the increased mucus and poor oxygenation. Bacterial infections are common and make COPD manifestations worse by increasing INFLAMMATION and mucus production and inducing more bronchospasm. Airflow becomes even more limited, the work of breathing increases, and dyspnea results.

Cardiac failure, especially cor pulmonale (right-sided heart failure caused by pulmonary disease), occurs with bronchitis or emphysema. Air trapping, airway collapse, and stiff alveolar walls increase the lung tissue pressure and narrow lung blood vessels, making blood flow more difficult. The increased pressure creates a heavy workload on the right side of the heart, which pumps blood into the lungs. To pump blood through the narrowed vessels, the right side of the heart generates high pressures. In response to this heavy workload, the right chambers of the heart enlarge and thicken, causing right-sided heart failure with backup of blood into the general venous system. Chart 30-9 lists key features of cor pulmonale.

Cardiac dysrhythmias are common in patients with COPD. They result from hypoxemia (from decreased oxygen to the heart muscle), other cardiac disease, drug effects, or acidosis.

CHART 30-9   Key Features

Cor Pulmonale

- Hypoxia and hypoxemia
- Increasing dyspnea
- Fatigue
- Enlarged and tender liver
- Warm, cyanotic hands and feet, with bounding pulses
- Cyanotic lips
- Distended neck veins
- Right ventricular enlargement (hypertrophy)
- Visible pulsations below the sternum
- GI disturbances, such as nausea or anorexia
- Dependent edema
- Metabolic and respiratory acidosis
- Pulmonary hypertension

FIG. 30-8 Orthopnea positions that patients with chronic obstructive pulmonary disease (COPD) often assume to ease the work of breathing.

Health Promotion and Maintenance

The incidence and severity of COPD would be greatly reduced by smoking cessation. Urge all people who smoke to quit smoking. Chart 27-1 in Chapter 27 provides tips to teach people about smoking cessation. Also, as described in Chapter 27, teach all people specific actions to take to avoid exposure to other inhalation irritants.

❖ PATIENT-CENTERED COLLABORATIVE CARE

The Concept Map addresses assessment and nursing care issues related to COPD.

◆ Assessment

History. Ask about risk factors such as age, gender, and occupational history. COPD is seen more often in older men. Some types of emphysema occur in families, especially those with alpha₁-antitrypsin (AAT) deficiency.

Obtain a thorough smoking history, because tobacco use is a major risk factor. Ask about the length of time the patient has smoked and the number of packs smoked daily. Use these data to determine the pack-year smoking history.

Ask the patient to describe the breathing problems, and assess whether he or she has any difficulty breathing while talking. Does he or she speak in complete sentences, or is it necessary to take a breath between every one or two words? Ask about the presence, duration, or worsening of wheezing, coughing, and shortness of breath. Determine what activities trigger these problems. Assess any cough, and ask whether sputum is clear or colored and how much is produced each day. Ask about the time of day when sputum production is greatest. Smokers often have a productive cough when they get up in the morning; nonsmokers generally do not.

Ask the patient to compare the activity level and shortness of breath now with those of a month ago and a year ago. Ask about any difficulty with eating and sleeping. Many patients sleep in a semi-sitting position because breathlessness is worse when lying down (orthopnea). Ask about usual daily activities and any difficulty with bathing, dressing, or sexual activity. Document this assessment to personalize the intervention plan.

Weigh the patient, and compare this weight with previous weights. Unplanned weight loss is likely when COPD severity increases, because the work of breathing increases metabolic needs. Dyspnea and mucus production often result in poor food intake and inadequate nutrition. Ask the patient to recall a typical day's meals and fluid intake. When heart failure is present with COPD, general edema with weight gain may occur.

Physical Assessment/Clinical Manifestations. General appearance can provide clues about respiratory status and energy level. Observe weight in proportion to height, posture, mobility, muscle mass, and overall hygiene. The patient with increasingly severe COPD is thin, with loss of muscle mass in the extremities, although the neck muscles may be enlarged. He or she tends to be slow moving and slightly stooped. The person often sits in a forward-bending posture with the arms held forward, a position known as the *orthopneic* or *tripod position* (Fig. 30-8). When dyspnea becomes severe, activity intolerance may be so great that bathing and general grooming are neglected.

Respiratory changes occur as a result of obstruction, changes in chest size, and fatigue. Inspect the chest and assess the breathing rate and pattern. The patient with respiratory muscle fatigue breathes with rapid, shallow respirations and may have an abnormal breathing pattern in which the abdominal wall is sucked in during inspiration or may use accessory muscles in the abdomen or neck. During an acute exacerbation, the respiratory rate could be as high as 40 to 50 breaths/min and requires immediate medical attention. As respiratory muscles become fatigued, respiratory movement is jerky and appears uncoordinated.

Check the patient's chest for retractions and for asymmetric chest expansion. The patient with emphysema has limited diaphragmatic movement (excursion) because the diaphragm is flattened and below its usual resting state. Chest vibration (fremitus) is often decreased and the chest sounds hyperresonant on percussion because of trapped air.

Auscultate the chest to assess the depth of inspiration and any abnormal breath sounds. Wheezes and other abnormal sounds often occur on inspiration and expiration, although crackles are usually not present. Reduced breath sounds are common, especially with emphysema. Note the pitch and location of the sound and the point in the respiratory cycle at which the sound is heard. A silent chest may indicate serious airflow obstruction or pneumothorax.

CONCEPT MAP

COPD
- GAS EXCHANGE
- PERFUSION
- INFLAMMATION
- CELLULAR REGULATION

EXPECTED OUTCOMES

- Attain and maintain GAS EXCHANGE at usual baseline level: SpO₂ at least 88%, no cyanosis, maintain cognitive orientation, cough and clear secretions effectively, and maintain respiratory rate and rhythm appropriate to activity level.
- Achieve and maintain body weight within 10% of ideal: maintain appropriate weight/height ratio, maintain serum albumin or prealbumin within normal range.
- Have decreased anxiety, identify contributory factors, and perform activities to decrease or eliminate anxiety.
- Increase activity to an acceptable level: maintain baseline SpO₂ with activity, perform ADLs with no or minimal assistance, perform selected activities with minimal dyspnea or tachycardia, participate in family, work, or social activities as desired.
- Avoid serious respiratory infection: describe clinical manifestations, monitoring procedures, preventative strategies, and seek medical assistance when manifestations of respiratory infection appear.

HISTORY

Nick Williams, age 66, is a long-time smoker admitted with an exacerbation of COPD. He reports shortness of breath and a productive cough with thick yellow sputum.

Physical Assessment →

ASSESSMENT DATA

ABGs–pH 7.31; PaO₂ 66; PaCO₂ 59; HCO₃⁻ 26. Bilateral wheezing, dyspnea and tachypnea 28/min, O₂ sat 86%, T 100.6° F, HR 104; BP 140/88; use of accessory muscles; productive cough, thick yellow sputum; digital clubbing; barrel-shaped chest; skin cool and dry. No peripheral edema.

Data Synthesis →

PATIENT PROBLEMS

- Hypoxemia with hypercapnia
- Weight loss related to dyspnea, excessive secretions, anorexia, and fatigue
- Anxiety related to dyspnea, a change in health status, and situational crisis
- Activity Intolerance
- Potential for pneumonia or other respiratory infections

Planning →

INTERVENTIONS

1. History Assessment

- Assess ability to perform ADLs. *Good management maintains adequate GAS EXCHANGE and improves overall health.*
- Trend and monitor weight. *Monitors for unplanned weight loss when work of breathing increases metabolic needs.*
- Ask patient to recall a typical day's meals and fluid intake. *Evaluates for inadequate nutrition.*

2. Physical Assessment

- Observe weight/height proportion, posture, mobility, muscle mass, and overall hygiene. *Provides clues about GAS EXCHANGE and energy level.*
- Inspect chest size and shape; assess breath sounds, respiratory rate, pattern, depth of inspiration, presence of retractions, asymmetry of chest expansion, cyanosis and sputum production. *Determines state of respiratory distress and whether chronic symptoms are present.*
- Assess degree of dyspnea using VADS, cyanosis, delayed capillary refill, and finger clubbing. *Indicates decreased arterial oxygen levels.*
- Assess heart rate & rhythm, dependent edema or other signs and symptoms of right heart failure. *Indicates cardiac changes related to COPD-associated anatomic changes.*
- Examine nail beds and oral mucous membranes. *Indicates adequacy of GAS EXCHANGE and oxygenation of all tissues.*

3. Nursing Priority – Improving GAS EXCHANGE

- Teach patient to participate in COPD management: airway maintenance, breathing techniques, positioning, effective coughing, oxygen therapy, exercise conditioning, suctioning, hydration, use of a vibratory positive pressure device, and adhering to prescribed drug therapy. *Promotes airway maintenance to improve GAS EXCHANGE.*
- Consult with Registered Dietitian for nutritional assessment. Monitor weight and serum prealbumin levels. *Prevents loss of muscle mass and strength, lung elasticity, and alveolar-capillary surface area, which reduce GAS EXCHANGE.*
- Assist patient with strategies to manage anxiety. *Keeps patient calm during acute dyspneic episodes.*
- Assist with ADLs. Encourage patient to self-pace activities, note skin color changes, pulse rate and regularity, O₂ saturation and work of breathing, supplemental low dose O₂ for high energy activities. *Helps to manage chronic fatigue.*
- Teach patient to avoid crowds and get pneumonia and influenza vaccines. *Prevents risk for respiratory tract infections.*

4. Laboratory Assessment

- Review ABG values and monitor pulse oximetry. *Assesses changes in respiratory status and gauges treatment response to identify abnormal GAS EXCHANGE.*
- Obtain sputum samples for culture & sensitivity and white blood cell count. *Evaluates for infections and helps identify necessary treatment.*
- Review hemoglobin & hematocrit. Assess electrolytes. *Assesses for polycythemia. Evaluates for acidosis. Low electrolyte levels reduce muscle strength.*

5. Drug Therapy

- Teach patient about drug management and correct techniques for inhaler use. *Helps ensure patient receives full dose of inhaled medication and ensures correct sequence is done.*

6. Psychosocial Assessment

- Assess patient's home environment, interests, hobbies, and potential factors that contribute to respiratory infections. *Helps prevent isolation due to fatigue or embarrassment from coughing and excessive sputum production.*
- Explore economic impact of disease on patient. *Evaluates patient ability to purchase and take drugs correctly.*
- Encourage the expression of concerns about lifestyle, disease progression, and use of support groups. *Urges patient to participate in a full life, and reduces anxiety and fear from feelings of breathlessness.*

Concept Map by Deanne A. Blach, MSN, RN

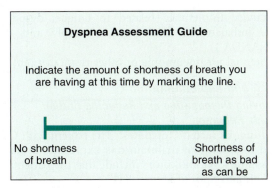

Dyspnea Assessment Guide

Indicate the amount of shortness of breath you
are having at this time by marking the line.

No shortness
of breath

Shortness of
breath as bad
as can be

FIG. 30-9 A visual analog scale to assess dyspnea.

FIG. 30-10 Late digital clubbing *(on left)* compared with a normal digit *(on right).*

Assess the degree of dyspnea using a Visual Analog Dyspnea Scale (VADS), which is a straight line with verbal anchors at the beginning and end of a 100-mm line (Fig. 30-9). Ask the patient to place a mark on the line to indicate his or her perceived breathing difficulty. Document the response, and use this scale to determine the therapy effectiveness and pace the patient's activities.

Examine the patient's chest for the presence of a "barrel chest" (see Fig. 30-3). With a barrel chest, the ratio between the anteroposterior (AP) diameter of the chest and its lateral diameter is 1:1 rather than the normal ratio of 1:1.5, as a result of lung overinflation and diaphragm flattening.

The patient with chronic bronchitis often has a cyanotic, or blue-tinged, dusky appearance and has excessive sputum production. Assess for cyanosis, delayed capillary refill, and finger clubbing (Fig. 30-10), which indicate chronically decreased arterial oxygen levels.

Cardiac changes occur as a result of the anatomic changes associated with COPD. Assess the patient's heart rate and rhythm. Check for swelling of the feet and ankles (dependent edema) or other manifestations of right-sided heart failure. Examine nail beds and oral mucous membranes. In late-stage emphysema the patient may have pallor or cyanosis and is usually underweight.

Psychosocial Assessment. COPD affects all aspects of a person's life. The patient may be isolated because dyspnea causes fatigue or because of embarrassment from coughing and excessive sputum production.

Ask the patient about interests and hobbies to assess whether socialization has decreased or whether hobbies cause exposure to irritants. Ask about home conditions for exposure to smoke or crowded living conditions that promote transmission of respiratory infections.

Economic status may be affected by the disease through changes in income and health insurance coverage. Drugs,

especially the metered dose inhalers (MDIs) and dry powder inhalers (DPIs), are expensive, and many patients with limited incomes may use them only during exacerbations and not as prescribed on a scheduled basis.

Anxiety and fear from feelings of breathlessness may reduce the patient's ability to participate in a full life. Work, family, social, and sexual roles can be affected. Encourage the patient and family to express their feelings about the limitations on lifestyle and disease progression. Assess their use of support groups and community services.

Laboratory Assessment. Arterial blood gas (ABG) values identify abnormal GAS EXCHANGE, oxygenation, ventilation, and acid-base status. Compare repeated ABG values to assess changes in respiratory status. Once baseline ABG values are obtained, pulse oximetry can gauge treatment response. As COPD worsens, the amount of oxygen in the blood decreases (**hypoxemia**) and the amount of carbon dioxide increases (**hypercarbia**). Chronic respiratory acidosis (increased arterial carbon dioxide [$Paco_2$]) then results; metabolic alkalosis (increased arterial bicarbonate) occurs as compensation by kidney retention of bicarbonate. This change is seen on ABGs as an elevation of HCO_3^- although pH remains lower than normal. Not all patients with COPD are CO_2 retainers, even when hypoxemia is present, because CO_2 diffuses more easily across lung membranes than does oxygen. Hypercarbia is a problem in advanced emphysema (because the alveoli are affected) rather than in bronchitis (wherein the airways are affected). For more detailed information about acidosis, see Chapter 12.

Sputum samples are obtained for culture from hospitalized patients with an acute respiratory infection. The infection is treated on the basis of manifestations and the common bacterial organisms in the local community. A WBC count helps confirm the presence of infection.

Other blood tests include hemoglobin and hematocrit to determine *polycythemia* (a compensatory increase in red blood cells [RBCs] and iron in the chronically hypoxic patient). Serum electrolyte levels are examined because acidosis can change electrolyte values. Low phosphate, potassium, calcium, and magnesium levels reduce muscle strength. In patients with a family history of COPD, serum AAT levels may be drawn.

Imaging Assessment. Chest x-rays are used to rule out other lung diseases and to check the progress of patients with respiratory infections or chronic disease. With advanced emphysema, chest x-rays show hyperinflation and a flattened diaphragm.

Other Diagnostic Assessments. COPD is classified from mild to very severe on the basis of manifestations and pulmonary function test (PFT) changes (Table 30-2; see Table 27-6 in Chapter 27). Airflow rates and lung volume measurements help distinguish airway disease (obstructive diseases) from interstitial lung disease (restrictive diseases). PFTs determine lung volumes, flow volume curves, and diffusion capacity. Each test is performed before and after the patient inhales a bronchodilator agent. Encourage the patient to express his or her feelings about testing and the potential impact of the results. Explain the preparations for the procedures (if any), whether pain or discomfort will be involved, and any needed follow-up care.

The lung volumes measured for COPD are vital capacity (VC), residual volume (RV), forced expiratory volume (FEV), and total lung capacity (TLC). Although all volumes and

TABLE 30-2 Gold Classification of COPD Severity

STAGE	MANIFESTATIONS	PULMONARY FUNCTION TEST RESULTS
0 (At risk)	±Chronic cough ±Chronic sputum production	Normal
1 (Mild)	+Chronic cough ±Sputum production	FEV_1/FVC <70% FEV_1 ≥80% of predicted
2 (Moderate)	±Dyspnea ±Chronic cough ±Sputum production	FEV_1/FVC <70% FEV_1 <80% but at least 50% of predicted
3 (Severe)	+Dyspnea +Chronic cough +Sputum production	FEV_1/FVC <70% FEV_1 <50% but at least 30% of predicted
4 (Very severe)	++Dyspnea ++Chronic cough ++Sputum production	FEV_1/FVC <70% FEV_1 <30% of predicted

Data from Global Initiative for Chronic Obstructive Lung Disease (GOLD). (2014). *Global strategy for the diagnosis, management, and prevention of chronic obstructive pulmonary disease.* Retrieved June 2014, from www.goldcopd.org/.
FEV_1, Volume of air blown out as hard and fast as possible during the first second of the most forceful exhalation after the greatest full inhalation; *FVC*, functional vital capacity.

capacities change to some degree in COPD, the RV is most affected, with increases reflecting the trapped, stale air remaining in the lungs.

A diagnosis of COPD is based mostly on the FEV_1 (the FEV in the first second of exhalation). FEV_1 can also be expressed as a percentage of the forced vital capacity (FVC). As the disease progresses, the ratio of FEV_1 to FVC becomes smaller (Smith & Tasota, 2011).

The diffusion test measures how well a test gas (carbon monoxide) diffuses across the alveolar-capillary membrane and combines with hemoglobin. In emphysema, alveolar wall destruction decreases the large surface area for diffusion of gas into the blood, leading to a decreased diffusion capacity. In bronchitis alone, the diffusion capacity is usually normal.

The patient with COPD has decreased oxygen saturation, often much lower than 90%. Changes in Spo_2 below the patient's usual saturation require medical attention.

Peak expiratory flow meters are used to monitor the effectiveness of drug therapy to relieve obstruction. Peak flow rates increase as obstruction resolves. Teach the patient to self-monitor the peak expiratory flow rates at home and adjust drugs as needed.

◆ **Analysis**

The priority NANDA-I nursing diagnoses and collaborative problems for patients with chronic obstructive pulmonary disease (COPD) include:

1. Hypoxemia with hypercapnia related to alveolar-capillary membrane changes, reduced airway size, ventilatory muscle fatigue, excessive mucus production, airway obstruction, diaphragm flattening, fatigue, and decreased energy
2. Weight loss related to dyspnea, excessive secretions, anorexia, and fatigue
3. Anxiety related to dyspnea, a change in health status, and situational crisis (NANDA-I)

4. Activity Intolerance related to fatigue, dyspnea, and an imbalance between oxygen supply and demand (NANDA-I)
5. Potential for pneumonia or other respiratory infections

◆ **Planning and Implementation**

Improving Oxygenation and Reducing Carbon Dioxide Retention

Planning: Expected Outcomes. The patient with COPD is expected to attain and maintain GAS EXCHANGE at his or her usual baseline level. Indicators include that the patient:
- Maintains Spo_2 of at least 88%
- Remains free from cyanosis
- Maintains cognitive orientation
- Coughs and clears secretions effectively
- Maintains a respiratory rate and rhythm appropriate to his or her activity level

Interventions. Most patients with COPD use nonsurgical management to improve or maintain GAS EXCHANGE. Surgical management requires that the patient meet strict criteria.

Nonsurgical Management. Nursing management for patients with COPD focuses on airway maintenance, monitoring, breathing techniques, positioning, effective coughing, oxygen therapy, exercise conditioning, suctioning, hydration, and use of a vibratory positive-pressure device. A nursing priority is to teach the patient how to be a partner in COPD management by participating in therapies to improve GAS EXCHANGE and by adhering to prescribed drug therapy.

Before any intervention, assess the breathing rate, rhythm, depth, and use of accessory muscles. The accessory muscles are less efficient than the diaphragm, and the work of breathing increases. Determine whether any factors are contributing to the increased work of breathing, such as respiratory infection. *Airway maintenance is the most important focus of interventions to improve* GAS EXCHANGE.

Monitoring. Monitoring for changes in respiratory status is key to providing prompt interventions to reduce complications. Assess the hospitalized patient with COPD at least every 2 hours, even when the purpose of hospitalization is not COPD management. Apply prescribed oxygen, assess the patient's response to therapy, and prevent complications.

If the patient's condition worsens, more aggressive therapy is needed. Noninvasive ventilation (NIV) may be useful for patients with stable, very severe COPD and daytime hypercapnia (GOLD, 2014). Intubation and mechanical ventilation may be needed for patients in respiratory failure.

Breathing Techniques. Diaphragmatic or abdominal and pursed-lip breathing may be helpful for managing dyspneic episodes. Teach the patient to use these techniques, shown in Chart 30-10, during all activities to reduce the amount of stale air in the lungs and manage dyspnea. Teach these techniques when the patient has less dyspnea.

In diaphragmatic breathing, the patient consciously increases movement of the diaphragm. Lying on the back allows the abdomen to relax. Breathing through pursed lips creates mild resistance, which prolongs exhalation and increases airway pressure. This technique delays airway compression and reduces air trapping. Pursed-lip breathing can be used during diaphragmatic or abdominal breathing.

Positioning. Placing the patient in an upright position with the head of the bed elevated can help alleviate dyspnea by increasing chest expansion and keeping the diaphragm in the

CHART 30-10 Patient and Family Education: Preparing for Self-Management

Breathing Exercises

Diaphragmatic or Abdominal Breathing

- If you can do so comfortably, lie on your back with your knees bent. If you cannot lie comfortably, perform this exercise while sitting in a chair.
- Place your hands or a book on your abdomen to create resistance.
- Begin breathing from your abdomen while keeping your chest still. You can tell if you are breathing correctly if your hands or the book rises and falls accordingly.

Pursed-Lip Breathing

- Close your mouth, and breathe in through your nose.
- Purse your lips as you would to whistle. Breathe out slowly through your mouth, without puffing out your cheeks. Spend at least twice the amount of time it took you to breathe in.
- Use your abdominal muscles to squeeze out every bit of air you can.
- Remember to use pursed-lip breathing during any physical activity. Always inhale before beginning the activity and exhale while performing the activity. Never hold your breath.

In

Out

proper position to contract. This position conserves energy by supporting the patient's arms and upper body. Assist the patient who can tolerate sitting in a chair out of bed for 1-hour periods 2 or 3 times a day. This position also helps move secretions.

Effective Coughing. Coughing effectively can improve GAS EXCHANGE by helping increase airflow in the larger airways. The patient with COPD often has difficulty with removal of secretions, which results in poor gas exchange and oxygenation. Excessive mucus also increases the risk for respiratory infections.

Controlled coughing is helpful in removing excessive mucus. Teach the patient to cough on arising in the morning to eliminate mucus that collected during the night. Coughing to clear mucus before mealtimes may make meals more pleasant. Coughing before bedtime may help clear lungs for a less interrupted night's sleep.

For effective coughing, teach the patient to sit in a chair or on the side of a bed with feet placed firmly on the floor. Instruct him or her to turn the shoulders inward and to bend the head slightly downward, hugging a pillow against the stomach. The patient then takes a few breaths, attempting to exhale more fully. After the third to fifth breath (in through the nose, out through pursed lips), instruct him or her to take a deeper breath and bend forward slowly while coughing 2 or 3 times ("mini-coughs") from the same breath. On return to a sitting position, the patient takes a comfortably deep breath. The entire coughing procedure is repeated at least twice.

Oxygen Therapy. Oxygen is prescribed for relief of hypoxemia and hypoxia. The need for oxygen therapy and its effectiveness can be determined by arterial blood gas (ABG) values and oxygen saturation by pulse oximetry. The patient with COPD may need an oxygen flow of 2 to 4 L/min via nasal cannula or up to 40% via Venturi mask. Ensure that there are no open flames or other combustion hazards in rooms in which oxygen is in use. More information on oxygen therapy is found in Chapter 28.

In the past, the patient with COPD was thought to be at risk for extreme hypoventilation with oxygen therapy because of a decreased drive to breathe as blood oxygen levels rose. However, this concern has not been shown to be evidence-based and has been responsible for ineffective management of hypoxia in patients with COPD. All hypoxic patients, even those with COPD and hypercarbia, should receive oxygen therapy at rates appropriate to reduce hypoxia and bring SpO_2 levels up between 88% and 92% (Abdo & Heunks, 2012; Burt & Corbridge, 2013; Makic et al., 2013).

Drug Therapy. Drugs used to manage COPD are the same drugs as for asthma and include beta-adrenergic agents, cholinergic antagonists, xanthines, corticosteroids, and cromones (see Chart 30-6). The focus is on long-term control therapy with longer-acting drugs, such as arformoterol (Brovana), indacaterol (Arcapta Neohaler), tiotropium (Spiriva), aclidinium bromide (Tudorza Pressair), and the combination drug fluticasone furoate/vilanterol (BREO ELLIPTA). The patient with COPD is more likely to be taking systemic agents (in addition to inhaled drugs) than is the patient with asthma. An additional drug class for COPD is the mucolytics, which thin the thick secretions, making them easier to cough up and expel. Nebulizer treatments with normal saline or with a mucolytic agent such as acetylcysteine (Mucosil, Mucomyst ✦) or dornase alfa (Pulmozyme) and normal saline help thin secretions. Guaifenesin (Organidin, Naldecon Senior EX) is a systemic mucolytic that is taken orally. A combination of guaifenesin and dextromethorphan (Mucinex DM) also raises the cough threshold.

Stepped therapy, which adds drugs as COPD progresses, is recommended for patients with chronic bronchitis or emphysema, although the patient's response to drug therapy is the best indicator of when drugs or their dosages need changing. Ideally, the patient notices changes and participates in management strategies. Teach patients and family members the correct techniques for using inhalers and to care for them properly.

Many inhalers for COPD drug therapy are dry powder inhalers. These often require having the patient "load in" each dose. The steps for this process involve opening the inhaler's capsule chamber, removing the dry powder capsule from a separate blister pack, placing the capsule in the chamber, closing the inhaler until it clicks and punctures the capsule, and then using the inhaler. Often the patient with severe COPD is older, has muscle weakness, has poor manual dexterity, and may have some problems with cognition. All of these issues can be barriers to proper use of a DPI inhaler for COPD management (Lareau & Hodder, 2012).

FIG. 30-11 The FLUTTER® flutter valve mucus clearance device, a type of vibratory positive-pressure device.

? NCLEX EXAMINATION CHALLENGE

Health Promotion and Maintenance

A client with chronic obstructive pulmonary disease (COPD) prescribed a long-acting inhaled beta₂ agonist reports hating the inhaler and asks why the drug can't be taken as a pill. What is the nurse's best response?
A. "Drugs taken by inhaler work more slowly and remain in the system longer."
B. "Drugs taken by inhaler have no side effects and are less expensive."
C. "Drugs taken by mouth are more expensive because they must be sterile."
D. "Drugs taken by mouth have systemic side effects and are harder to control."

Exercise Conditioning. Exercise for conditioning and pulmonary rehabilitation can improve function and endurance in patients with COPD. Patients often respond to the dyspnea of COPD by limiting their activity, even basic ADLs. Over time, the muscles used in breathing weaken, resulting in increased dyspnea with lower activity levels.

Pulmonary rehabilitation involves education and exercise training to prevent muscle deconditioning. Each patient's exercise program is personalized to reflect his or her current limitations and planned outcomes. The simplest plan involves having the patient walk (indoors or outdoors) daily at a self-paced rate until manifestations limit further walking, followed by a rest period, and then continue walking until 20 minutes of actual walking has been accomplished. As the time during rest periods decreases, the patient can add 5 more minutes of walking time. Teach patients whose manifestations are severe to modify the exercise by using a walker with wheels or, if needed, to use oxygen while exercising. Remind patients that the exercise needs to be performed at least 2 or 3 times weekly for best improvement. Formal pulmonary rehabilitation programs can be beneficial even for patients who are severely impaired.

Additional exercise techniques to retrain ventilatory muscles include isocapneic hyperventilation and resistive breathing. Isocapneic hyperventilation, in which the patient hyperventilates into a machine that controls the levels of oxygen and carbon dioxide, increases endurance. In resistive breathing, the patient breathes against a set resistance. Resistive breathing increases respiratory muscle strength and endurance.

Suctioning. Perform suctioning only when needed—not on a routine schedule. For the patient with a weak cough, weak pulmonary muscles, and inability to expectorate effectively, perform nasotracheal suctioning. Assess the patient for dyspnea, tachycardia, and dysrhythmias during the procedure. Assess for

improved breath sounds after suctioning. Suctioning is discussed in detail in Chapter 28.

Hydration. Maintaining hydration may thin the thick, tenacious (sticky) secretions, making them easier to remove by coughing. Unless hydration needs to be avoided for other health problems, teach the patient with COPD to drink at least 2 to 3 L/day. Humidifiers may be useful for those living in a dry climate or those who use dry heat during the winter.

Vibratory Positive Expiratory Pressure Device. The use of a vibratory positive expiratory pressure device can help patients remove airway secretions. The device is a small, handheld plastic pipe with a short, fat stem and a perforated lid over the bowl (Fig. 30-11). A movable steel ball is inside the bowl. The patient inhales deeply and then exhales through the device, causing the ball to move and set up vibrations that are transmitted to the chest and airways. The vibrations loosen secretions and allow them to be coughed out more easily.

Surgical Management. Lung transplantation and lung reduction surgery can improve GAS EXCHANGE in the patient with COPD. Transplantation is a relatively rare procedure because of cost and the scarce availability of donor lungs. The more common surgical procedure for patients with emphysema is lung reduction surgery.

The purpose of lung reduction surgery is to improve GAS EXCHANGE through removal of hyperinflated lung tissues that are filled with stagnant air containing little, if any, oxygen. Instead, the level of carbon dioxide is the same as that in the capillary and no gas exchange occurs. Successful lung reduction results in increased forced expiratory volume and decreased total lung capacity and residual volume. Activity tolerance increases, and oxygen therapy may no longer be needed.

Preoperative Care. Patients who are selected for this procedure have end-stage emphysema, minimal chronic bronchitis, and stable cardiac function. They also must be ambulatory; not ventilator dependent; free of pulmonary fibrosis, asthma, or cancer; and not have smoked for at least 6 months. The patient must be rehabilitated to the stage that he or she is able to walk, without stopping, for 30 minutes at 1 mile/hr and maintain a 90% or better oxygen saturation level.

In addition to standard preoperative testing, tests to determine the location of greatest lung hyperinflation and poorest lung blood flow are performed. These tests include pulmonary plethysmography, gas dilution, and perfusion scans.

Operative Procedures. Usually lung reduction is performed on both lungs, most often by the minimally invasive surgical technique of video-assisted thoracoscopic surgery (VATS) or through bronchoscopy (GOLD, 2014). Each lung is deflated separately and examined for color and texture differences. Normal lung tissue darkens to purple or gray when deflated and becomes more dense or rubbery in texture. Hyperinflated areas do not deflate and remain pink with a spongy texture. The surgeon removes as much of this tissue as possible.

Postoperative Care. After lung reduction surgery, the patient needs close monitoring for continuing respiratory problems as well as for usual postoperative complications. Bronchodilator and mucolytic therapies are maintained. Pulmonary hygiene includes incentive spirometry 10 times per hour while awake, chest physiotherapy starting on the first day after surgery, and hourly pulmonary assessment.

Preventing Weight Loss

Planning: Expected Outcomes. The patient with COPD is expected to achieve and maintain a body weight within 10% of ideal. Indicators include that the patient:

- Maintains an appropriate weight/height ratio
- Maintains serum albumin or prealbumin within the normal range

Interventions. The patient with COPD often has food intolerance, nausea, *early satiety* (feeling too "full" to eat), poor appetite, and meal-related dyspnea. The increased work of breathing raises calorie and protein needs, which can lead to protein-calorie malnutrition. Malnourished patients lose muscle mass and strength, lung elasticity, and alveolar-capillary surface area, all of which reduce GAS EXCHANGE.

Identify patients at risk for or who have this complication, and request that a registered dietitian perform a nutrition assessment. Monitor weight and other indicators of nutrition, such as serum prealbumin levels.

Dyspnea management is needed because shortness of breath interferes with eating. Teach the patient to plan the biggest meal of the day for the time when he or she is most hungry and well rested. Four to six small meals a day may be preferred to three larger ones. Remind patients to use pursed-lip and abdominal breathing and to use the prescribed bronchodilator 30 minutes before the meal to reduce bronchospasm.

Food selection can help prevent weight loss. Abdominal bloating and a feeling of fullness often prevent the patient from eating a complete meal. Collaborate with the dietitian to teach about foods that are easy to chew and not gas-forming. Advise the patient to avoid dry foods that stimulate coughing and caffeine-containing drinks that increase urine output and may lead to dehydration.

Urge the patient to eat high-calorie, high-protein foods. Dietary supplements, such as Pulmocare, provide nutrition with reduced carbon dioxide production. If early satiety is a problem, advise him or her to avoid drinking fluids before and during the meal and to eat smaller, more frequent meals.

Minimizing Anxiety

Planning: Expected Outcomes. The patient with COPD is expected to have decreased anxiety. Indicators include that the patient consistently demonstrates these behaviors:

- Identifies factors that contribute to anxiety
- Identifies activities to decrease anxiety
- States anxiety is reduced or absent

Interventions. Patients with COPD become anxious during acute dyspneic episodes, especially when excessive secretions are present. Anxiety also may cause dyspnea.

Help the patient understand that anxiety can increase dyspnea, and have a plan for dealing with anxiety. Together with the patient, develop a written plan that states exactly what he or she should do if symptoms flare. Having a plan provides confidence and control in knowing what to do, which

often helps reduce anxiety. Stress the use of pursed-lip and diaphragmatic breathing techniques during periods of anxiety or panic.

Family, friends, and support groups can be helpful. Recommend professional counseling, if needed, as a positive suggestion. Stress that talking with a counselor can help identify techniques to maintain control over dyspnea and panic.

Explore other approaches to help the patient control dyspneic episodes and panic attacks, such as progressive relaxation, hypnosis therapy, and biofeedback. For some patients, antianxiety drug therapy may be needed for severe anxiety.

Improving Activity Tolerance

Planning: Expected Outcomes. The patient with COPD is expected to increase activity to a level acceptable to him or her. Indicators include that the patient:

- Maintains his or her baseline Spo_2 with activity
- Performs ADLs with no or minimal assistance
- Performs selected activities with minimal dyspnea or tachycardia
- Participates in family, work, or social activities as desired

Interventions. The patient with COPD often has chronic fatigue. During acute exacerbations, he or she may need extensive help with the ADLs of eating, bathing, and grooming. As the acute problem resolves, encourage the patient to pace activities and perform as much self-care as possible. Teach him or her to not rush through morning activities, because rushing increases dyspnea, fatigue, and hypoxemia. As activity gradually increases, assess the patient's response by noting skin color changes, pulse rate and regularity, oxygen saturation, and work of breathing. Suggest the use of oxygen during periods of high energy use, such as bathing or walking.

Energy conservation is the planning and pacing of activities for best tolerance and minimum discomfort. Ask the patient to describe a typical daily schedule. Help him or her divide each activity into its smaller parts to determine whether that task can be performed in a different way or at a different time. Teach about planning and pacing daily activities with rest periods between activities. Help the patient develop a chart outlining the day's activities and planned rest periods.

Encourage the patient to avoid working with the arms raised. Activities involving the arms decrease exercise tolerance because the accessory muscles are used to stabilize the arms and shoulders rather than to assist breathing. Many activities involving the arms can be done sitting at a table leaning on the elbows. Teach the patient to adjust work heights to reduce back strain and fatigue. Remind him or her to keep arm motions smooth and flowing to prevent jerky motions that waste energy. Work with the occupational therapist to teach about the use of adaptive tools for housework, such as long-handled dustpans, sponges, and dusters, to reduce bending and reaching.

Suggest organizing work spaces so that items used most often are within easy reach. Measures such as dividing laundry or groceries into small parcels that can be handled easily, using disposable plates to save washing time, and letting dishes dry in the rack also conserve energy. Teach the patient to not talk when engaged in other activities that require energy, such as walking. In addition, teach him or her to avoid breath-holding while performing any activity.

Preventing Respiratory Infection

Planning: Expected Outcomes. The patient with COPD is expected to avoid serious respiratory infection. Indicators include that the patient consistently demonstrates these behaviors:

- Describes clinical manifestations of respiratory infection
- Describes respiratory infection–monitoring procedures
- Uses prevention activities such as pneumonia and influenza vaccination and crowd avoidance
- Seeks medical assistance when manifestations of respiratory infection first appear

Interventions. Pneumonia is a common complication of COPD, especially among older adults. Patients who have excessive secretions or who have artificial airways are at increased risk for respiratory tract infections. Teach patients to avoid crowds, and stress the importance of receiving a pneumonia vaccination and a yearly influenza vaccine.

Community-Based Care

Home Care Management. Most patients with COPD are managed in the ambulatory care setting and cared for at home. When pneumonia or a severe exacerbation develops, the patient often returns home after hospitalization. For those with advanced disease, 24-hour care may be needed for ADLs and for monitoring. If home care is not possible, placement in a long-term care setting may be needed.

Patients with hypoxemia may use oxygen at home either as needed or continually. Continuous, long-term oxygen therapy can reverse tissue hypoxia and improve cognition and well-being. For more information on home oxygen therapy, see Chapter 28.

Collaborate with the case manager to obtain the equipment needed for care at home. Patient needs may include oxygen therapy, a hospital-type bed, a nebulizer, a tub transfer bench, and scheduled visits from a home care nurse for monitoring and evaluation.

The patient with COPD faces a lifelong disease with remissions and exacerbations. Explain to the patient and family that he or she may have periods of anxiety, depression, and ineffective coping. The person who was a smoker may also have self-directed anger.

Financial concerns often increase anxiety. The disease may worsen to the point that the patient cannot work, requiring disability benefits to help ease the financial burden. Medicare or other health insurers may help pay for home oxygen therapy and nebulizer treatments. Coordinate with the social worker or case manager to help the patient make the needed arrangements.

Self-Management Education. Patients with COPD need to know as much about the disease as possible so that they can better manage it and themselves. Patients and families should be able to discuss drug therapy, manifestations of infection, avoidance of respiratory irritants, the nutrition therapy regimen, and activity progression. Instruct them to identify and avoid stressors that can worsen the disease.

Reinforce the techniques of pursed-lip breathing, diaphragmatic breathing, positioning, relaxation therapy, energy conservation, and coughing and deep breathing. Teaching about all of the needed topics may require coordination with the home care or clinic staff.

Health Care Resources. Provide appropriate referrals as needed. Home care visits may be needed especially when home oxygen therapy is first prescribed. Chart 30-11 lists assessment areas for the patient with COPD at home. Referral to assistance programs, such as Meals on Wheels, can be helpful. Provide a

---

CHART 30-11 **Home Care Assessment**

The Patient with Chronic Obstructive Pulmonary Disease

Assess respiratory status and adequacy of ventilation.
- Measure rate, depth, and rhythm of respirations.
- Examine mucous membranes and nail beds for evidence of hypoxia.
- Determine use of accessory muscles.
- Examine chest and abdomen for paradoxical breathing.
- Count number of words patient can speak between breaths.
- Determine need and use of supplemental oxygen. (How many liters per minute is the patient using?)
- Determine level of consciousness and presence/absence of confusion.
- Auscultate lungs for abnormal breath sounds.
- Measure oxygen saturation by pulse oximetry.
- Determine sputum production, color, and amount.
- Ask about activity level.
- Observe general hygiene.
- Measure body temperature.

Assess cardiac status.
- Measure rate, quality, and rhythm of pulse.
- Check dependent areas for edema.
- Check neck veins for distention with the patient in a sitting position.
- Measure capillary refill.

Assess nutritional status.
- Check weight maintenance, loss, or gain.
- Determine food and fluid intake.
- Determine use of nutritional supplements.
- Observe general condition of the skin.
- Assess patient's and caregiver's adherence and understanding of illness and treatment, including:
  — Correct use of supplemental oxygen
  — Correct use of inhalers
  — Drug schedule and side effects
  — Manifestations to report to the health care provider indicating the need for acute care
  — Increasing severity of resting dyspnea
  — Increasing severity of usual manifestations
  — Development of new manifestations associated with poor oxygenation
  — Respiratory infection
  — Failure to obtain the usual degree of relief with prescribed therapies
  — Unusual change in condition
  — Use of pursed-lip and diaphragmatic breathing techniques
  — Scheduling of rest periods and priority activities
  — Participation in rehabilitation activities

---

list of support groups, as well as Better Breather clubs sponsored by the American Lung Association. If the patient wants to quit smoking, make the appropriate referrals.

◆ Evaluation: Outcomes

Evaluate the care of the patient with COPD based on the identified priority patient problems. The expected outcomes of care are that the patient should:

- Attain and maintain GAS EXCHANGE at a level within his or her chronic baseline values
- Achieve an effective breathing pattern that decreases the work of breathing
- Maintain a patent airway
- Achieve and maintain a body weight within 10% of his or her ideal weight

- Have decreased anxiety
- Increase activity to a level acceptable to him or her
- Avoid serious respiratory infections

Specific indicators for these outcomes are listed for each priority patient problem under the Planning and Implementation section (see earlier).

💡 CLINICAL JUDGMENT CHALLENGE

Patient-Centered Care; Safety **QSEN**

The patient is a 64-year-old man with COPD who lives with his wife of 35 years. He retired 2 years ago when his disease interfered with his job as a carpenter. He also quit smoking about a year ago. Since then, his disease has remained stable; however, he now reports that he thinks his wife is preparing for widowhood by taking over all the home chores that he always performed (including driving and bill paying), limiting his interaction with friends, and making all decisions. He is angry and depressed. Routine assessment with pulmonary function testing show his FEV_1 to be 40% of his predicted value, which is an improvement over the 32% value of FEV_1 last year.

1. What severity classification is his COPD? Provide a rationale for your choice.
2. How should you respond to his statement about the wife probably preparing for widowhood?
3. Should he continue to drive and pay bills? Why or why not?
4. What psychosocial assessment of this patient and his situation should you make?
5. Should you include the wife in any part of this discussion? Why or why not?

CYSTIC FIBROSIS

❖ PATHOPHYSIOLOGY

Cystic fibrosis (CF) is a genetic disease that affects many organs and lethally impairs lung function. Although this disorder is present from birth and usually is first seen in early childhood, almost half of all people with cystic fibrosis in the United States are adults (Cystic Fibrosis Foundation, 2014).

The underlying problem of CF is blocked chloride transport in the cell membranes (Beery & Workman, 2012). Poor chloride transport causes the formation of mucus that has little water content and is thick. The thick, sticky mucus causes problems in the lungs, pancreas, liver, salivary glands, and testes. The mucus plugs up the airways in the lungs and the glandular tissues in nonpulmonary organs, causing atrophy and organ dysfunction. Nonpulmonary problems include pancreatic insufficiency, malnutrition, intestinal obstruction, poor growth, male sterility, and cirrhosis of the liver. Additional problems of CF in young adults include osteoporosis and diabetes mellitus. Respiratory failure is the main cause of death. Improved management has increased life expectancy even among those with severe disease to about 37 years (Cystic Fibrosis Foundation, 2014).

The pulmonary problems of CF result from the constant presence of thick, sticky mucus and are the most serious complications of the disease. The mucus narrows airways, reducing airflow and interfering with GAS EXCHANGE and oxygenation. The constant presence of mucus results in chronic respiratory tract infections, chronic bronchitis, and chronic dilation of the bronchioles (bronchiectasis). Lung abscesses are common. Over time, the bronchioles distend and have increased numbers (hyperplasia) and increased size (hypertrophy) of mucus-producing cells. Complications include pneumothorax, arterial erosion and hemorrhage, and respiratory failure.

CF is most common among white people, and about 4% are carriers. It is rare among African Americans and Asians. Males and females are affected equally.

GENETIC/GENOMIC CONSIDERATIONS

Patient-Centered Care **QSEN**

CF is an autosomal recessive disorder in which both gene alleles must be mutated for the disease to be expressed. The CF gene (*CTFR*: cystic fibrosis transmembrane conductance regulator) produces a protein that controls chloride movement across cell membranes. The severity of CF varies greatly; however, life expectancy is always considerably reduced, with an average of 37 years. People with one mutated allele are carriers and have few or no symptoms of CF but can pass the abnormal allele on to their children. More than 1700 different mutations have been identified (OMIM, 2013c). The inheritance of different mutations is responsible for variation in disease severity. Help patients understand why their manifestations may be more or less severe than others with the disease, even within the same family.

❖ PATIENT-CENTERED COLLABORATIVE CARE

◆ Assessment

Usually, but not always, cystic fibrosis (CF) is diagnosed in childhood. The major diagnostic test is sweat chloride analysis (Pagana & Pagana, 2014). The sweat chloride test is positive for CF when the chloride level in the sweat ranges between 60 and 200 mEq/L (mmol/L), compared with the normal value of 5 to 35 mEq/L. Genetic testing can be performed to determine which specific mutation a person may have. Different mutations result in different degrees of disease severity.

Nonpulmonary manifestations include abdominal distention, gastroesophageal reflux, rectal prolapse, foul-smelling stools, and **steatorrhea** (excessive fat in stools). The patient is often malnourished and has many vitamin deficiencies, especially of the fat-soluble vitamins (e.g., vitamins A, D, E, K). As pancreatic function decreases, diabetes mellitus develops with loss of insulin production. The adult with severe CF is usually smaller and thinner than average.

Pulmonary manifestations caused by CF are progressive. Respiratory infections are frequent or chronic with exacerbations. Patients usually have chest congestion, limited exercise tolerance, cough, sputum production, use of accessory muscles, and decreased pulmonary function (especially forced vital capacity [FVC] and forced expiratory volume in the first second of exhalation [FEV_1]). Chest x-rays show infiltrate and an increased anteroposterior (AP) diameter.

During an acute exacerbation or when the disease progresses to end stage, the patient has increased chest congestion, reduced activity tolerance, increased crackles, increased cough, increased sputum production (often with hemoptysis), and severe dyspnea with fatigue. Arterial blood gas (ABG) studies show acidosis (low pH), greatly reduced arterial oxygen (Pao_2) levels, increased arterial carbon dioxide ($Paco_2$) levels, and increased bicarbonate levels.

With infection, the patient has fever, an elevated white blood cell count, and decreased oxygen saturation. Other

FIG. 30-12 Inflatable chest physiotherapy vest for high-frequency chest wall oscillation (HFCWO).

manifestations of infection include tachypnea, tachycardia, intercostal retractions, weight loss, and increased fatigue.

◆ **Interventions**

The patient with CF needs daily therapy to slow disease progress and enhance GAS EXCHANGE. There is no cure for CF.

Nonsurgical Management. The management of the patient with CF is complex and lifelong. Nutrition management focuses on weight maintenance, vitamin supplementation, diabetes management, and pancreatic enzyme replacement. Pulmonary management focuses on preventive maintenance and management of exacerbations. Priority nursing interventions focus on teaching about drug therapy, infection prevention, pulmonary hygiene, nutrition, and vitamin supplementation.

Preventive/maintenance therapy involves the use of positive expiratory pressure, active cycle breathing technique, and an individualized exercise program. Daily chest physiotherapy with postural drainage is beneficial for the patient with CF (Fig. 30-12). This therapy uses chest percussion, chest vibration, and dependent drainage to loosen secretions and promote drainage. Increasingly the use of a chest physiotherapy (CPT) vest is recommended (Neufeld & Keith, 2012). This system uses an inflatable vest that rapidly fills and deflates, gently compressing and releasing the chest wall up to 25 times per second, a process called high-frequency chest wall oscillation (HFCWO). The action creates mini-coughs that dislodge mucus from the bronchial walls, increase mobilization, and move it toward central airways where it can be removed by coughing or suctioning. HFCWO also thins secretions, making them easier to clear. Pulmonary function tests are monitored regularly. Daily drugs include bronchodilators, anti-inflammatories, mucolytics, and antibiotics.

Exacerbation therapy is needed when the patient with CF has increased chest congestion, reduced activity tolerance, increased or new-onset crackles, and at least a 10% decrease in FEV_1. Other exacerbation manifestations include increased sputum production with bloody or purulent sputum, increased coughing, decreased appetite, weight loss, fatigue, decreased Spo_2, and chest muscle retractions. Often infection is present, with fever, increased lung infiltrate on x-ray, and an elevated white blood cell count.

Every attempt is made to avoid mechanical ventilation for the patient with CF. Bi-level positive airway pressure (BiPAP) may be a part of daily therapy for the patient with advanced

disease (Neufeld & Keith, 2012). Management focuses on airway clearance, increased GAS EXCHANGE, and antibiotic therapy. Supplemental oxygen is prescribed on the basis of Spo_2 levels. Heliox delivery of 50% oxygen and 50% helium may improve gas exchange and oxygen saturation. The respiratory therapist initiates airway clearance techniques 4 times a day. Bronchodilator and mucolytic therapies are intensified. Steroidal agents are started or increased.

Depending on the severity of the exacerbation, a 10- to 14-day course of oral antibiotics may be prescribed. For severe exacerbation, aerosolized tobramycin may be prescribed. If antibiotics are not effective or if the exacerbation is very severe, IV antibiotics are used—usually an aminoglycoside, such as tobramycin and colistin, or meropenem (Merrem).

A serious bacterial infection for patients with CF is *Burkholderia cepacia.* The organism lives in the respiratory tracts of patients with CF and is often resistant to antibiotic therapy. It is spread by casual contact from one CF patient to another. For this reason, the Cystic Fibrosis Foundation bans infected patients from participating in any foundation-sponsored events. It is also possible for *B. cepacia* to be transmitted to a CF patient during clinic and hospital visits; thus special infection control measures that limit close contact between people with CF are needed. These measures include separating infected CF patients from noninfected CF patients on hospital units and seeing them in the clinic on different days. Strict CF Foundation–approved procedures are used to clean clinic rooms and respiratory therapy equipment. Drug therapy for this infection usually includes co-trimoxazole (a combination of trimethoprim and sulfamethoxazole [Bactrim, Septra]) along with the usual drugs used for exacerbation therapy.

Teach patients about protecting themselves by avoiding direct contact of bodily fluids such as saliva and sputum. Teach them to not routinely shake hands or kiss people in social settings. Handwashing is critical because the organism also can be acquired indirectly from contaminated surfaces, such as sinks and tissues.

As life span increases for patients with CF, other problems, such as bronchiole bleeding from lung arteries, may develop. Interventional radiology may be needed to embolize the bleeding arterial branches. Patients with CF may undergo this procedure repeatedly to control hemoptysis. See Chapter 36 for information on interventional radiology vascular procedures.

Other problems that occur with CF over time include severe gastroesophageal reflux disease (GERD), osteoporosis, and sensory hearing loss. Osteoporosis increases the risk for bone fractures.

Gene therapy for CF is available for use in patients with specific gene mutations (Nakano & Tluczek, 2014). A new drug, ivacaftor (Kalydeco) has been found to be of value to patients with CF who have any one of the following specific mutations in the *CFTR* gene: G551D, G1244E, G1349D, G178R, G551S, S1251N, S1255P, S549N, or S549R. In patients with any of these mutations, the oral drug specifically targets and potentiates the CFTR channel opening so this transporter can move chloride ions across the cell membrane. This action reduces sodium and fluid absorption so that mucus is less thick and sticky. This drug has no effect in patients whose *CFTR* gene does not have any of these mutations. The most common adverse effect of the drug is an elevation of liver enzymes.

Surgical Management. The surgical management of the patient with CF involves lung and/or pancreatic transplantation. The patient has reduced manifestations but is at continuing risk for lethal pulmonary infections, especially with anti-rejection drug therapy. Transplantation may extend life for some years, depending on other factors, but transplant rejection rate is high among this population, possibly caused by poor intestinal absorption of anti-rejection drugs.

Fewer lung transplants are performed compared with transplantation of other solid organs because of the scarcity of available lungs. Also, many of the people who could benefit from lung transplantation have serious problems in other organs that make this procedure even more dangerous.

Lung transplant procedures include two lobes or a single lung transplantation, as well as double-lung transplantation. The type of procedure is determined by the patient's overall condition and the life expectancy after transplantation. Usually the patient with CF has a bilateral lobe transplant from either a cadaver donor or living-related donor.

Preoperative Care. Many factors are considered before lung transplantation surgery. Recipient and donor criteria vary from one program to another, but some criteria are universal.

Recipient criteria for the patient with CF include that he or she must have severe, irreversible lung damage and still be well enough to survive the surgery. Age at transplantation is considered on an individual basis. Common exclusion criteria include a cancer diagnosis, systemic infection, human immune deficiency virus (HIV)/acquired immune deficiency syndrome (AIDS), and irreversible heart, kidney, or liver damage/disease.

Donor criteria, regardless of whether the lung tissue is obtained from a cadaver or from a living-related donor, include that the donor be infection free and cancer free, have healthy lung tissue, be a close tissue match with the recipient, and have the same blood type as the recipient. When the donor is living-related, additional criteria include an age restriction, healthy organs, and no previous chest surgery. *The two nursing priorities before surgery are teaching the patient the expected regimen of pulmonary hygiene to be used in the period immediately after surgery and assisting the patient in a pulmonary muscle strengthening/conditioning regimen.*

Operative Procedures. The patient may or may not need to be placed on cardiopulmonary bypass, depending on the exact procedure. Those having single-lung or lobe transplantation usually do not need bypass; those having double-lung transplantation usually do.

The most common incision used for lung transplantation is a transverse thoracotomy ("clamshell"). The diseased lung or lungs are removed. The new lobes, lung, or lungs are placed in the chest cavity with proper connections made to the trachea, bronchi, and blood vessels. Usually lung transplantation surgery is completed within 4 to 6 hours.

Postoperative Care. The patient is intubated for at least 48 hours, and chest tubes and arterial lines are in place. The care needed is the same as that for any thoracic surgery.

Major problem areas after lung transplantation are bleeding, infection, and transplant rejection. The patient usually remains in the ICU for several days after transplantation. Postoperative chest physiotherapy often is performed with high-frequency chest wall oscillation (HFCWO) at this time (Esguerra-Gonzalez et al., 2013).

Anti-rejection drug regimens must be started immediately after surgery, which increases the risk for infection. Combination therapy with the anti-rejection drugs, described in Chapter 17, is used for the rest of the patient's life. Corticosteroids are avoided in the first 10 to 14 days after surgery because of their negative impact on the healing process.

PULMONARY ARTERIAL HYPERTENSION

❖ PATHOPHYSIOLOGY

General pulmonary hypertension can occur as a complication of other lung disorders. Primary pulmonary arterial hypertension (PAH) (also known as *idiopathic pulmonary hypertension*) occurs in the absence of other lung disorders, and its cause is unknown; however, exposure to some drugs, such as fenfluramine/phentermine (Pondimin or "Fen-Phen") or dasatinib (Sprycel), increases the risk (World Health Organization [WHO], 2011). The disorder is rare and occurs mostly in women between the ages of 20 and 40 years (McCance et al., 2014). The familial PAH form appears to be transmitted in an autosomal dominant pattern with reduced penetrance (OMIM, 2013d).

The pathologic problem in PAH is blood vessel constriction with increasing vascular resistance in the lung. Pulmonary blood pressure rises and blood flow decreases through the lungs, leading to poor PERFUSION and GAS EXCHANGE with hypoxemia. Eventually, the right side of the heart fails *(cor pulmonale)* from the continuous workload of pumping against the high pulmonary pressures. Without treatment, death usually occurs within 2 years after diagnosis.

⚕ GENETIC/GENOMIC CONSIDERATIONS

Patient-Centered Care QSEN

About 50% of patients with pulmonary arterial hypertension have a genetic mutation in the *BMPR2* gene, which codes for a growth factor receptor (Weber et al., 2011). Excessive activation of this receptor allows increased growth of arterial smooth muscle in the lungs, making these arteries thicker. Many more people have mutations in this gene than have PAH. It is thought that these mutations increase the susceptibility to PAH when other, often unknown, environmental factors also are present. Mutations in other genes, such as the *PPH1* gene and the *SMAD9* gene, are also associated with thickening of lung arteries and increased risk for PAH (OMIM, 2013d).

Often PAH is not diagnosed until late in the disease process when the lungs and heart have already been significantly damaged. Teach people, especially women, who have a first-degree relative (parent or sibling) with PAH to have regular health checks and to consult a health care provider whenever pulmonary problems are present.

TABLE 30-3 Severity Classification for Primary Pulmonary Arterial Hypertension

CLASS	MANIFESTATIONS
I	Pulmonary hypertension diagnosed by pulmonary function tests and right-sided cardiac catheterization No limitation of physical activity Moderate physical activity does not induce dyspnea, fatigue, chest pain, or light-headedness
II	No manifestations at rest Mild to moderate physical activity induces dyspnea, fatigue, chest pain, or light-headedness
III	No or slight manifestations at rest Mild (less than ordinary) activity induces dyspnea, fatigue, chest pain, or light-headedness
IV	Dyspnea and fatigue present at rest Unable to carry out any level of physical activity without manifestations Manifestations of right-sided heart failure apparent (dependent edema, engorged neck veins, enlarged liver)

❖ PATIENT-CENTERED COLLABORATIVE CARE

◆ Assessment

The most common early manifestations are dyspnea and fatigue in an otherwise healthy adult. Some patients also have angina-like chest pain. Table 30-3 lists the classification of PAH.

Diagnosis is made from the results of right-sided heart catheterization showing elevated pulmonary pressures. Other test results suggesting PAH include abnormal ventilation-perfusion scans, pulmonary function tests (PFTs) showing reduced functional pulmonary volumes with reduced diffusion capacity, and computed tomography (CT).

◆ Interventions

Drug therapy can reduce pulmonary pressures and slow the development of cor pulmonale by dilating pulmonary vessels and preventing clot formation. Warfarin (Coumadin) is taken daily to achieve an international normalized ratio (INR) of 1.5 to 2.0. Calcium channel blockers have been used to dilate blood vessels. The two classes of drugs that have been shown to be most effective in the treatment of PAH are the endothelin-receptor antagonists and the prostacyclin agents.

Endothelin-receptor agonists, such as bosentan (Tracleer), induce blood vessel relaxation and decrease pulmonary arterial pressure. These agents, however, cause general vessel dilation and some degree of hypotension. A new endothelin receptor antagonist drug, macitentan (Opsumit), has been approved for management of adults with PAH. This oral drug is taken as a 10-mg tablet once daily, with or without food. Teach patients to take the drug with a glass of water, and teach them not to break, chew, or crush the tablet.

Because macitentan can cause birth defects, its use is contraindicated for women who are pregnant or breastfeeding. Instruct women who are sexually active and within childbearing age to use at least two reliable methods of contraception while taking this drug. In addition, the drug can harm the liver, and patients should avoid drinking alcoholic beverages while taking it.

Natural and synthetic prostacyclin agents provide the best specific dilation of pulmonary blood vessels. Continuous

QUALITY IMPROVEMENT (QSEN)
Continuous Prostacyclin Therapy Error Prevention

Kingman, M., & Chin, K. (2013). Safety recommendations for administering intravenous prostacyclins in the hospital. *Critical Care Nurse, 33*(5), 32-34, 36-41.

Intravenous prostacyclin drugs are most widely prescribed for management of pulmonary arterial hypertension. These drugs are categorized as *high risk* and have some unique issues, one of which is that the patient receives them by continuous infusion 24 hours daily, 7 days a week. In the hospital setting, administration of these drugs is associated with a high error rate. Two of the most common errors were flushing the dedicated prostacyclin infusion line and administering the wrong brand of prostacyclin. Because patient lives depend on continuous and correct infusion of prostacyclins, leading experts in the field were asked to generate recommendations for IV administration to reduce the error rate.

In addition to many standard recommendations for reducing drug errors, two unique ones were developed. The first involved safety strategies for ensuring the dedicated line is not flushed. The second unique recommendation involved including the patient in the administration of the prostacyclins. Most patients have been responsible for self-administration of the drug in the community setting and have been highly trained to do so correctly. Thus the recommendation is that the patient should be included in the administration (while in the hospital setting) to the "fullest extent possible," as an expert on drug administration and trouble-shooting.

Commentary: Implications for Practice and Research

This expert-generated set of recommendations for drug administration safety is a departure from the usual quality improvement (QI) project that is either unit-based or institution-based. It represents the next step in the QI process of standardizing procedures for an identified population-based problem across multiple institutions. Because it is a beginning project using a descriptive design rather than a randomized clinical trial, it was reasonable to first determine the justification for a practice change. A randomized clinical trial approach should be the next step in establishing the evidence to support a specific process or procedure to reduce drug administration errors.

infusion of epoprostenol (Flolan, Veletri) or treprostinil (Remodulin) through a small IV pump reduces pulmonary pressures and increases lung blood flow (Fuentes et al., 2012). Treprostinil also can be delivered by continuous subcutaneous infusion. These continuous infusions of prostacyclin drugs can be performed by the patient at home and in other settings. These drugs also are continued when the patient is hospitalized for any reason. The unusual continuous infusion, the need to keep an IV line dedicated strictly to prostacyclin infusion, and the varied dosages of the different brands of prostacyclins contribute to a high drug error rate for administration of this drug. See the Quality Improvement box for some recommendations to reduce this error rate.

The prostacyclin agents iloprost (Ilomedin, Ventavis) and treprostinil (Tyvaso) can be delivered by inhalation (Poms & Kingman, 2011). A drug given along with prostacyclins is sildenafil (Revatio, Viagra) administered orally or IV.

While most patients with PAH need to stay on prostacyclin drugs until lung transplantation or disease progression to death, a small percentage of patients have been successfully weaned off prostacyclin drug therapy. These patients are maintained on oral bosentan, sildenafil, and warfarin therapy (Demerouti et al., 2013). The uncertain outcome of treatment and the serious nature of the disorder have been reported to increase the levels of depression and anxiety in patients diagnosed with PAH (Roberts-Collins et al., 2013).

Another critical priority is helping the patient receiving IV prostacyclin agents prevent sepsis. The central line IV setup provides an access for organisms to directly enter the bloodstream. Teach the patient to use strict aseptic technique in all aspects of using the drug delivery system. Also teach him or her to notify the pulmonologist at the first manifestation of any infection.

When the heart has undergone hypertrophy and cardiac output has fallen, the patient may be started on a regimen of digoxin (Lanoxin) and diuretics. Oxygen therapy is used when dyspnea is uncomfortable. This therapy improves function and reduces manifestations but does not cure PAH.

Surgical management of PAH involves lung transplantation. When cor pulmonale also is present, the patient may need a combined heart-lung transplantation. It is not known whether the process of pulmonary vasoconstriction can begin again in the transplanted lungs or if this is a "cure."

INTERSTITIAL PULMONARY DISEASES

The category of interstitial pulmonary diseases contains a variety of lung disorders, also called *fibrotic lung diseases,* that have some features in common. All affect the alveoli, blood vessels, and surrounding support tissue of the lungs rather than the airways. Thus these disorders are restrictive (preventing good expansion and recoil of the gas exchange unit), not obstructive. With restrictive disease, the lung tissues thicken, causing reduced GAS EXCHANGE and "stiff" lungs that do not expand well. Air trapping does not occur, and the patient does not develop a "barrel chest." Often the onset of these disorders is slow, and dyspnea is the most common manifestation.

SARCOIDOSIS
❖ PATHOPHYSIOLOGY

Sarcoidosis is a disease of INFLAMMATION of unknown cause that can affect any organ, but the lung is involved most often. It develops over time with noncancerous inflammatory growths called granulomas forming in the lungs.

Pulmonary sarcoidosis involves autoimmune responses in which the normally protective T-lymphocytes increase and cause damaging actions in the alveolar cells. No single cause for T-lymphocyte activation has been identified, although infection and genetic predisposition may play a role. Alveolar inflammation (alveolitis) occurs from the presence of immune cells in the alveoli. Chronic INFLAMMATION causes fibrosis (scar tissue formation) in the lungs. The fibrosis reduces lung compliance (elasticity) and GAS EXCHANGE. Cor

pulmonale (right-sided cardiac failure) is often present because the heart can no longer pump effectively against the stiff, fibrotic lung.

The disease affects young adults. Manifestations include enlarged lymph nodes in the hilar area of the lungs, lung infiltrate on chest x-ray, skin lesions, and eye lesions. The first indication of disease may be an abnormal chest x-ray in an otherwise healthy patient. Common manifestations include cough, dyspnea, hemoptysis, and chest discomfort. In many patients, the illness resolves permanently. Others have progressive pulmonary fibrosis and severe systemic disease.

❖ PATIENT-CENTERED COLLABORATIVE CARE

Sarcoidosis is suspected in the patient who has a cough, dyspnea, and an abnormal chest x-ray but is otherwise asymptomatic. Other conditions to rule out before diagnosing sarcoidosis are lung infections and cancer. Bronchoscopy with biopsy may help diagnose this disorder (see Chapter 27).

Sarcoidosis is staged on the basis of x-ray findings. Higher stages have greater damage and more widespread disease. Pulmonary function studies often show a restrictive pattern of decreased lung volumes and impaired diffusing capacity. Irreversible lung changes occur in a small percentage of patients. Patients who have severe restrictive disease may develop pulmonary hypertension.

The focus of therapy is to reduce manifestations and prevent fibrosis. Management varies. If the patient is asymptomatic and has normal pulmonary function, no treatment is given. Decreased total lung capacity (TLC), diffusing capacity, or forced vital capacity (FVC); involvement of other organs; and hypercalcemia are indicators for treatment.

Corticosteroids are the main type of therapy. Dosages vary from 40 to 60 mg daily with tapering doses over 6 to 8 weeks, to a maintenance dose of 10 to 15 mg daily for 6 months. Further therapy may continue over 12 months. Drugs under study for management of this disease include thalidomide (Thalomid), infliximab (Remicade), and adalimumab (Humira). Follow-up and monitoring include assessment of symptom severity, pulmonary function studies, chest x-rays, a complete blood count, serum creatinine, serum calcium, and urinalysis. Teach the patient and family about side effects of steroid therapy, the need to avoid infection, and energy conservation strategies (see discussion of activity intolerance, p. 565 in the Chronic Obstructive Pulmonary Disease section).

IDIOPATHIC PULMONARY FIBROSIS
❖ PATHOPHYSIOLOGY

Idiopathic pulmonary fibrosis is a common restrictive lung disease. The patient usually is an older adult with a history of cigarette smoking, chronic exposure to inhalation irritants, or exposure to the drugs *amiodarone* (Cordarone) or *ambrisentan* (Letairis, Volibris) (WHO, 2012). Most patients have progressive disease with few remission periods. Even with proper treatment, most patients usually survive less than 5 years after diagnosis.

Pulmonary fibrosis is an example of excessive wound healing with loss of CELLULAR REGULATION. Once lung injury occurs, inflammation begins tissue repair. The INFLAMMATION continues beyond normal healing time, causing fibrosis and scarring. These changes thicken alveolar tissues, making GAS EXCHANGE difficult.

❖ *PATIENT-CENTERED COLLABORATIVE CARE*

The onset is slow, with early manifestations of mild dyspnea on exertion. Pulmonary function tests show decreased forced vital capacity (FVC). High resolution computed tomography (HRCT) shows a "honeycomb" pattern in affected lung tissue (Lewis & Scullion, 2012). As the fibrosis progresses, the patient becomes more dyspneic and hypoxemia becomes severe. Eventually, he or she needs high levels of oxygen and often is still hypoxemic. Respirations are rapid and shallow.

Therapy focuses on slowing the fibrotic process and managing dyspnea. Corticosteroids and other immunosuppressants are the mainstays of therapy. Immunosuppressant drugs include cytotoxic drugs such as cyclophosphamide (Cytoxan, Neosar, Procytox ❖), azathioprine (Imuran), chlorambucil (Leukeran), or methotrexate (Folex). These drugs have many side effects, including increased infection risk, nausea, and lung and liver damage, and have shown limited benefit. New studies using the combination therapy of corticosteroids, azathioprine, interferon gamma 1b, and *N*-acetylcysteine show promise of slowing disease progression. Early clinical trials using drugs that help improve CELLULAR REGULATION, such as those that belong to the class of mitogen-activated protein kinases inhibitors (MAPKIs), are being conducted. Starting any drug therapy early is critical, even though not all patients respond to therapy. Even among those who have a response to therapy, the disease eventually continues to progress and leads to death by respiratory failure. Lung transplantation is a curative therapy; however, the selection criteria, cost, and availability of organs make this option unlikely for most patients.

The patient and family need support and help with community resources after diagnosis. Nursing care focuses on assisting the patient and family in understanding the disease process and maintaining hope for control of the fibrosis (Lewis & Scullion, 2012). It is important to prevent respiratory infections. Teach the patient and family about the manifestations of infection and to avoid respiratory irritants, crowds, and people who are ill.

Home oxygen is needed by the time the patient has dyspnea because significant fibrosis has already occurred and GAS EXCHANGE is reduced. Teach about oxygen use as a continuous therapy. Fatigue is a major problem. Teach the patient and family about energy conservation measures (see discussion of activity intolerance on p. 565 in the Chronic Obstructive Pulmonary Disease section). These measures and rest help reduce the work of breathing and oxygen consumption. Encourage the patient to pace activities and accept assistance as needed.

In the later stages of the disease, the focus is to reduce the sensation of dyspnea. This is often accomplished with the use of oral, parenteral, or nebulized morphine. Provide information about hospice, which supports and coordinates resources to meet the needs of the patient and family when the prognosis for survival is less than 6 months (see Chapter 7).

OCCUPATIONAL PULMONARY DISEASE

❖ *PATHOPHYSIOLOGY*

Exposure to occupational or environmental fumes, dust, vapors, gases, bacterial or fungal antigens, and allergens can result in a variety of respiratory disorders. Depending on the degree, frequency, and intensity of exposure and on the specific disease, patients may have acute reversible effects or chronic lung disease. All occupational pulmonary diseases are made worse by cigarette smoking; thus smoking-cessation efforts are very important.

Many occupational diseases have an onset of manifestations long after the initial exposure to the offending agent. The patient's personal history can provide clues about the presence and cause of occupational pulmonary diseases such as occupational asthma, pneumoconiosis, diffuse interstitial fibrosis, and extrinsic allergic alveolitis. Chart 30-12 lists the key features of these disorders.

❖ *PATIENT-CENTERED COLLABORATIVE CARE*

Consider an occupational cause for patients with new-onset asthma or dyspnea. Ask about occupational exposure and onset of manifestations because there may or may not be a latency period between exposure and development of manifestations. Determine whether manifestations are acute or chronic. Ask about the use of inhalation protection and about cigarette smoking (see Chapter 27).

The patient who develops occupational asthma should be removed from the site of exposure, transferred to a job without exposure, and treated with asthma drugs. Nursing care is similar to the care for asthma not caused by the workplace environment. Refer the patient to a social worker, who provides information regarding compensation and pensions.

Nursing interventions for patients with occupational lung restrictive disease are the same as for those with emphysema. Hypoxemic patients require supplemental oxygen. In addition, respiratory therapies to promote sputum clearance are essential.

BRONCHIOLITIS OBLITERANS ORGANIZING PNEUMONIA

❖ *PATHOPHYSIOLOGY*

Bronchiolitis obliterans organizing pneumonia (BOOP) is an INFLAMMATION that reduces CELL REGULATION and allows connective tissue plugs to form in the lower airways and the tissue between the alveoli. Inflammation in the lumen triggers white blood cell clumping with uncontrolled fibroblast growth that occludes and eventually obliterates these airways and leads to restricted lung volume with decreased vital capacity. BOOP is not a true pneumonia, but the manifestations resemble respiratory infection.

The cause of BOOP is not known although many personal and environmental conditions are associated with it. Suggested triggers include infectious organisms, drugs (chemotherapy agents, certain antibiotics [sulfa-based drugs, cephalosporins, amphotericin B], antiseizure drugs, cocaine, and amiodarone), or the presence of a connective tissue disorder, such as rheumatoid arthritis or systemic lupus erythematosus. It is also associated with chest radiotherapy for breast or lung cancer.

BOOP is most common in people between ages 30 and 60 years and affects both genders. It is not associated with cigarette smoking. Depending on how fast the problem progresses and the degree to which it interferes with GAS EXCHANGE, BOOP can lead to death.

❖ *PATIENT-CENTERED COLLABORATIVE CARE*

An event or condition triggers excessive INFLAMMATION in the lumens of lower airways, causing dyspnea, fever, mild cough,

CHART 30-12 Key Features
Common Occupational Pulmonary Diseases

DISEASE AND CATEGORY	CAUSES AND MANIFESTATIONS
Occupational Asthmas	
Latency (allergic) asthma	Airway narrowing related only to workplace exposures Atopic allergic response to industrial irritants Develops after a period of exposure (from several weeks to several years) Characterized by airflow limitation Usually resolves when exposure ceases Obstructive disease
Irritant-induced asthma	Manifestations appear only in the workplace First onset usually occurs within 24 hours of exposure Common irritants are chlorine, ammonia, and phosgene Characterized by sloughing of epithelium, thickening of the basement membranes, and mucosal inflammation Early manifestations include cough, wheeze, and dyspnea High exposures can lead to pulmonary edema, ARDS, and death Most tissue changes are permanent Obstructive and restrictive disease
Pneumoconiosis	
Silicosis	Chronic fibrosis from long-term inhalation of silica dust Found among people working in mines, stone quarries, and foundries. Also found in people working in these industries: glass making, pottery, sandblasting, tile and brick making, soap and polishes, and manufacture of filters Characterized by nodule formation between alveoli leading to fibrosis Manifestations include dyspnea on exertion, fatigue, weight loss, reduced lung volume, and upper lobe fibrosis Restrictive disease
Coal Miner's Disease (Black Lung Disease)	Massive deposits of coal dust in the lungs leading to diffuse fibrosis Develops earlier among miners who smoke Early manifestations are similar to bronchitis Emphysema is a late development Restrictive disease
Diffuse Interstitial Fibrosis	
Asbestosis	Occurs among people who work in asbestos mines, building construction/remodeling, and shipyards Characterized by diffuse pleural thickening and diaphragmatic calcification Restrictive disease
Talcosis	Occurs among people who work in industries that manufacture paint, ceramics, roofing materials, cosmetics, and rubber goods Restrictive disease
Berylliosis	Occurs among people who work in industries in which metal is heated (steel mills, welding) or metal is machined, creating dust Has a genetic component for increased susceptibility to disease after beryllium exposure Restrictive disease
Extrinsic Allergic Alveolitis	
"Farmer's Lung" "Bird Fancier's Lung" "Machine Operator's Lung"	Hypersensitivity pneumonitis as an immunologic response to inhaling dust or chemical that contains bacterial or fungal antigens Characterized by formation of granulomas with central necrosis in the alveoli and surrounding blood vessels Restrictive disease

ARDS, Acute respiratory distress syndrome.

flu-like symptoms, and crackles on auscultation. In some patients, the problem resolves spontaneously. In others, it can rapidly progress to death within days. Usually manifestations are present for weeks or months and do not improve with antibiotic therapy.

Diagnosis of BOOP is difficult because manifestations are similar to many other respiratory problems. Chest x-rays and CT scans may show pulmonary tissue changes that only suggest BOOP, not confirm it. Biopsy with histologic findings is needed to confirm a BOOP diagnosis.

The most effective treatment for BOOP is corticosteroid therapy. A short course of the drug for acute disease can reduce manifestations, and the patient may never have a relapse. For those patients with more severe disease and those with any type of additional health problem, a year of corticosteroid therapy may be needed. In this population, BOOP is more of a chronic disease with some degree of permanent restrictive disease. Exacerbations can occur.

LUNG CANCER

❖ PATHOPHYSIOLOGY

Lung cancer is a leading cause of cancer-related deaths worldwide. In North America, more deaths from lung cancer occur each year than from prostate cancer, breast cancer, and colon cancer combined. The American Cancer Society estimates that more than 228,000 new cases of lung cancer are diagnosed each year and that more than 160,000 deaths occur each year from it (American Cancer Society [ACS], 2014). The overall 5-year survival for all patients with lung cancer is only 16%. This poor long-term survival is because most lung cancers are diagnosed at a late stage, when metastasis is present. Only 15% of patients have small tumors and localized disease at the time of diagnosis. The 5-year survival rate for this population is 52% (ACS, 2014).

Despite many advances in cancer treatment, the prognosis for lung cancer remains poor unless the tumor can be removed completely by surgery. Treatment often focuses on relieving symptoms (palliation) rather than cure because of metastasis.

Most primary lung cancers arise as a result of failure of CELLULAR REGULATION in the bronchial epithelium. These cancers are collectively called *bronchogenic carcinomas*. Lung cancers are classified as small cell lung cancer (SCLC) and non–small cell lung cancer (NSCLC). Chapter 21 discusses the general mechanisms and processes of cancer development.

Metastasis (spread) of lung cancer occurs by direct extension, through the blood, and by invading lymph glands and vessels. Tumors in the bronchial tubes can grow and obstruct the bronchus partially or completely. Tumors in other areas of lung tissue can grow so large that they can compress and obstruct the airway. Compression of the alveoli, nerves, blood vessels, and lymph vessels can occur and also interfere with GAS EXCHANGE. Lung cancer can spread to the lung lymph nodes, distant lymph nodes, and other tissues including bone, liver, brain, and adrenal glands.

Additional manifestations, known as *paraneoplastic syndromes*, complicate certain lung cancers. The paraneoplastic syndromes are caused by hormones secreted by tumor cells and occur most commonly with SCLC. Table 30-4 lists the endocrine paraneoplastic syndromes that may occur with lung cancer.

Staging of lung cancer is performed to assess the size and extent of the disease. These factors are related to survival. Lung cancer staging is based on the TNM system (T, primary **t**umor; N, number of regional lymph **n**odes; M, distant **m**etastasis). See Table 21-5 in Chapter 21 for a cancer staging system. Higher numbers represent later stages and less chance for cure or long-term survival.

Incidence and Prevalence

Lung cancers occur as a result of repeated exposure to inhaled substances that cause chronic tissue irritation or INFLAMMATION interfering with CELLULAR REGULATION of cell growth. Cigarette smoking is the major risk factor and is responsible for 85% of all lung cancer deaths (ACS, 2014). The risk for lung cancer is directly related to the total exposure to cigarette smoke as determined by the number of years of smoking and number of packs of cigarettes smoked per day (pack-years). Pipe and cigar smoking also increase risk. The incidence of lung cancer decreases when smoking stops but remains higher than among people who have never smoked.

Etiology and Genetic Risk

Nonsmokers exposed to "passive," or "secondhand," smoke also have a greater risk for lung cancer than do nonsmokers who are minimally exposed to cigarette smoke. See Chapter 27 for a discussion of passive smoking risks.

Other risk factors include chronic exposure to asbestos, beryllium, chromium, coal distillates, cobalt, iron oxide, mustard gas, petroleum distillates, radiation, tar, nickel, and uranium (Held-Warmkessel & Schiech, 2014). Air pollution with hydrocarbons also increases the risk for lung cancer.

GENETIC/GENOMIC CONSIDERATIONS
Patient-Centered Care QSEN

Lung cancer development varies among people with similar smoking histories, suggesting that genetic factors can influence susceptibility. Genome-wide association studies have found specific variations in a variety of genes that increase the susceptibility to lung cancer development (OMIM, 2013a). Differences in a gene that regulates cell division, the *Tp53* gene, may be the most important genetic susceptibility link for lung cancer development. Mutations in the alleles of this gene are known to increase the susceptibility to a wide variety of cancers both with and without exposure to environmental risks, including lung cancer development among smokers and nonsmokers. Help patients understand that lung cancer susceptibility varies by genetic issues as well as by exposure to carcinogens.

Health Promotion and Maintenance

Primary prevention for lung cancer is directed at reducing tobacco smoking. Chapter 27 discusses strategies for assisting people to reduce smoking and means to protect lungs from other exposures to inhalation irritants linked to lung cancer development.

Secondary prevention by early detection involves screening of people at high risk for lung cancer development. Annual CT scans can detect cancers at stage I, when cure is probable and long-term survival (longer than 5 years) is very likely (ACS, 2014; Lehto, 2014).

❖ PATIENT-CENTERED COLLABORATIVE CARE

◆ Assessment

History. Ask the patient about risk factors, including smoking, hazards in the workplace, and warning signals (Table 30-5). Calculate the pack-year smoking history as described in Chapter 27.

Ask about the presence of lung cancer manifestations, such as hoarseness, cough, sputum production, hemoptysis, shortness of breath, or change in endurance. Assessing for and

TABLE 30-4	**Endocrine Paraneoplastic Syndromes Associated with Lung Cancer**
ECTOPIC HORMONE	**MANIFESTATION**
Adrenocorticotropic hormone (ACTH)	Cushing's syndrome
Antidiuretic hormone	Syndrome of inappropriate antidiuretic hormone (SIADH) Weight gain General edema Dilution of serum electrolytes
Follicle-stimulating hormone (FSH)	Gynecomastia
Parathyroid hormone	Hypercalcemia
Ectopic insulin	Hypoglycemia

TABLE 30-5	**Warning Signals Associated with Lung Cancer**
• Hoarseness • Change in respiratory pattern • Persistent cough or change in cough • Blood-streaked sputum • Rust-colored or purulent sputum • Frank hemoptysis • Chest pain or chest tightness • Shoulder, arm, or chest wall pain	• Recurring episodes of pleural effusion, pneumonia, or bronchitis • Dyspnea • Fever associated with one or two other signs • Wheezing • Weight loss • Clubbing of the fingers

documenting these manifestations provide information about the extent of nursing care and teaching the patient needs now and can be used later to determine therapy effectiveness. Many manifestations are common and may have been present for years. Ask the patient to describe any recent changes in manifestations or if position affects them.

Assess for chest pain or discomfort, which can occur at any stage of tumor development. Chest pain may be localized or on just one side and can range from mild to severe. Ask about any sensation of fullness, tightness, or pressure in the chest, which may suggest obstruction. A piercing chest pain or pleuritic pain may occur on inspiration. Pain radiating to the arm results from tumor invasion of nerve plexuses in advanced disease.

Physical Assessment/Clinical Manifestations—Pulmonary. Manifestations of lung cancer are often nonspecific and appear late in the disease. Specific manifestations depend on tumor location. Chills, fever, and cough may be related to pneumonitis or bronchitis that occurs with obstruction. Assess sputum quantity and character. Blood-tinged sputum may occur with bleeding from a tumor. Hemoptysis is a later finding in the course of the disease. If infection or necrosis is present, sputum may be purulent and copious.

Breathing may be labored or painful. Obstructive breathing may occur as prolonged exhalation alternating with periods of shallow breathing. Rapid, shallow breathing occurs with pleuritic chest pain and an elevated diaphragm. Look for and document abnormal retractions, the use of accessory muscles, flared nares, stridor, and asymmetric diaphragmatic movement on inspiration. Dyspnea and wheezing may be present with airway obstruction. Ask about the level of dyspnea at rest, with activity, and in the supine position. Determine how much the dyspnea interferes with the patient's participation in ADLs, work, recreational activities, and family responsibilities. Ask him or her to compare participation in activities during the past week with that of a month ago and a year ago.

Areas of tenderness or masses may be felt when palpating the chest wall. Increased vibrations felt on the chest wall (**fremitus**) indicate areas of the lung where airspaces are replaced with tumor or fluid. Fremitus is decreased or absent when the bronchus is obstructed. The trachea may be displaced from midline if a mass is present in the area.

Lung areas with masses sound dull or flat rather than hollow or resonant on chest percussion. Breath sounds may change with the presence of a tumor. Wheezes indicate partial obstruction of airflow in passages narrowed by tumors. Decreased or absent breath sounds indicate complete obstruction of an airway by a tumor or fluid. Increased loudness or sound intensity of the voice while listening to breath sounds indicates increased density of lung tissue from tumor compression. A pleural friction rub may be heard when INFLAMMATION also is present.

Physical Assessment/Clinical Manifestations—Nonpulmonary. Many other systems can be affected by lung cancer and have changes at the time of diagnosis. Heart sounds may be muffled by a tumor or fluid around the heart (*cardiac tamponade*). Dysrhythmias may occur as a result of hypoxemia or direct pressure of the tumor on the heart. Cyanosis of the lips and fingertips or clubbing of the fingers may be present (see Fig. 30-10).

Bones lose density with tumor invasion and break easily. The patient may have bone pain or pathologic fractures. Handle him or her carefully. Thin bones can fracture with little pressure and without trauma. Even heavy coughing can break a rib.

Late manifestations of lung cancer usually include fatigue, weight loss, anorexia, dysphagia, and nausea and vomiting. Superior vena cava syndrome may result from tumor pressure in or around the vena cava. This syndrome is an emergency (see Chapter 22) and requires immediate intervention. The patient may have confusion or personality changes from brain metastasis. Bowel and bladder tone or function may be affected by tumor spread to the spine and spinal cord, which also can change gait.

Psychosocial Assessment. The poor prognosis for lung cancer has made it a much-feared disease. Dyspnea and pain add to the patient's fear and anxiety. The patient with a history of cigarette smoking may feel guilt and shame. Convey acceptance, and interact with the patient in a nonjudgmental way. Encourage the patient and family to express their feelings about the possible diagnosis of lung cancer.

Diagnostic Assessment. The diagnosis of lung cancer is made by examination of cancer cells. Cytologic testing of early-morning sputum specimens may identify tumor cells; however, cancer cells may not be present in the sputum. When pleural effusion is present, fluid is obtained by thoracentesis for cytology.

Most commonly, lung lesions are first identified on chest x-rays. CT examinations are then used to identify the lesions more clearly and to guide biopsy procedures.

A thoracoscopy to directly view lung tissue may be performed through a video-assisted thoracoscope entering the chest cavity via small incisions through the chest wall. Spread to mediastinal lymph nodes is assessed with a mediastinoscopy through a small chest incision.

Other diagnostic studies may be needed to determine how widely the cancer has spread. Such tests include needle biopsy of lymph nodes, direct surgical biopsy, and thoracentesis with pleural biopsy. MRI and radionuclide scans of the liver, spleen, brain, and bone help determine the location of metastatic tumors. Pulmonary function tests (PFTs) and arterial blood gas (ABG) analysis help determine the overall respiratory status. Positron emission tomography (PET) scanning is becoming the most thorough way to locate metastases. Together, these tests help determine the extent of the cancer and the best methods to treat it.

◆ **Interventions for Cure**

Interventions for the patient with lung cancer can have the purposes of curing the disease, increasing survival time, and enhancing quality of life through palliation. Both nonsurgical and surgical interventions are used to achieve these purposes. Some patients with lung cancer may undergo interventions for all three purposes at different stages in the disease process. Cure is most likely for patients who undergo treatment for stage I or II disease. Cure is rare for patients who undergo treatment for stage III or IV disease, although survival time is increasing.

Nonsurgical Management. *Chemotherapy* is often the treatment of choice for lung cancers, especially small cell lung cancer (SCLC). It may be used alone or as adjuvant therapy in combination with surgery for non–small cell lung cancer (NSCLC). The exact combination of drugs used depends on the response of the tumor and the overall health of the patient; however, most include platinum-based agents.

Side effects that occur with chemotherapy for lung cancer include chemotherapy-induced nausea and vomiting (CINV), alopecia (hair loss), open sores on mucous membranes (mucositis), immunosuppression with neutropenia, anemia, thrombocytopenia (decreased numbers of platelets), and peripheral neuropathy. Consult Chapter 22 for a thorough discussion of the nursing care needs for patients who have these side effects.

Immunosuppression with neutropenia, which greatly increases the risk for infection, is the major dose-limiting side effect of chemotherapy for lung cancer. It can be managed by the use of growth factors to stimulate bone marrow production of immune system cells. Teach the patient and family about precautions to take to reduce the patient's chances of developing an infection (see Chart 22-4 in Chapter 22). (See Chapter 22 for more information about chemotherapy and associated nursing care.)

Targeted therapy is now becoming common in the treatment of lung cancer. These agents take advantage of one or more differences in cancer cell growth or metabolism that is either not present or only slightly present in normal cells. Agents used as targeted therapies often are antibodies that work to disrupt cancer cell division in one of several ways. Some of these drugs "target" and block growth factor receptors, such as the epithelial growth factor receptor inhibitors (EGFRIs) or the vascular endothelial growth factor receptor inhibitors (VEGFRIs). When a lung cancer cell's growth depends on having the growth factors bind to their specific receptors, blocking the receptors may slow cancer cell growth. Agents most often used, along with other therapy, for targeted therapy of certain types of non–small cell lung cancer are erlotinib (Tarceva), bevacizumab (Avastin), and crizotinib (Xalkori) (Cagle & Chirieac, 2012).

Radiation therapy can be an effective treatment for locally advanced lung cancers confined to the chest. Best results are seen when radiation is used in addition to surgery or chemotherapy. Radiation may be performed before surgery to shrink the tumor and make resection easier.

Usually radiation therapy for lung cancer is performed daily for a 5- to 6-week period. Only the areas thought to have cancer are positioned in the radiation path. The immediate side effects of this treatment are skin irritation and peeling, fatigue, nausea, and taste changes. Some patients have esophagitis during therapy, making nutrition more difficult. Collaborate with a dietitian to teach patients to eat foods that are soft, bland, and high in calories. Suggest that the patient drink liquid nutrition supplements between meals to maintain weight and energy levels.

Skin care in the radiation-treated area can be difficult. Because skin in the radiation path is more sensitive to sun damage, advise patients to avoid direct skin exposure to the sun during treatment and for at least 1 year after radiation is completed. See Chapter 22 for other nursing care issues associated with radiation therapy.

Photodynamic therapy (PDT) may be used to remove small bronchial tumors when they are accessible by bronchoscopy. The patient is first injected with an agent that sensitizes cells to light. This drug enters all cells but leaves normal cells more rapidly than cancer cells. Usually, within 48 to 72 hours, most of the drug has collected in high concentrations in cancer cells. At this time, the patient goes to the operating room where, under anesthesia and intubation, a laser light is focused on the tumor. The light activates a chemical reaction within those cells retaining the sensitizing drug that induces irreversible cell damage. Some cells die and slough immediately; others continue to slough for several days.

When PDT is used in the airways, the patient usually requires a stay in the ICU for airway management. The sloughing tissue can block the airway as can airway edema from the inflammatory response of the tissues. In addition, the patient is at risk for bronchial hemorrhage, fistula formation, and hemoptysis. Patients who have undergone bronchial PDT are very sensitive to light for days to weeks after treatment.

Surgical Management. Surgery is the main treatment for stage I and stage II NSCLC. Total tumor removal may result in a cure. If complete resection is not possible, the surgeon removes the bulk of the tumor. The specific surgery depends on the stage of the cancer and the patient's overall health. Lung cancer surgery may involve removal of the tumor only, removal of a lung segment, removal of a lobe (lobectomy), or removal of the entire lung (pneumonectomy). These procedures can be performed by open thoracotomy or by thoracoscopy with minimally invasive surgery in select patients.

Preoperative Care. The focus of nursing care before surgery is to relieve anxiety and promote the patient's participation (see Chapter 14 for routine preoperative care). Encourage the patient to express fears and concerns, reinforce the surgeon's explanation of the procedure, and provide education related to what is expected after surgery. Teach about the probable location of the surgical incision or thoracoscopy openings, shoulder exercises, and the chest tube and drainage system (except after pneumonectomy).

Operative Procedures. Three types of incisions can be made depending on the location of the cancer: posterolateral, anterolateral, and median sternotomy (Fig. 30-13). The incisions are large and are held open with retractors during surgery, contributing to pain after surgery.

Surgery may consist of a lobectomy, pneumonectomy, segmental resection, or wedge resection. A segmental resection is a lung resection that includes the bronchus, pulmonary artery and vein, and tissue of the involved lung segment or segments of a lobe. A wedge resection is removal of the peripheral portion of small, localized areas of disease.

Removal of a lobe or entire lung can be accomplished through video-assisted thoracoscopic surgery (VATS) for select patients. The procedure involves making three small incisions in the chest for placement of the instruments. These same openings are used later for placement of drains and chest tubes. The lung section, lobe, or lung is isolated from its airway, which is surgically closed. The lobe or the lung is closed off from the rest of the lung using a double-stapling technique. The tissue is sealed in a bag to prevent leakage of tumor tissue and possible

FIG. 30-13 Common incision locations for partial or total pneumonectomy.

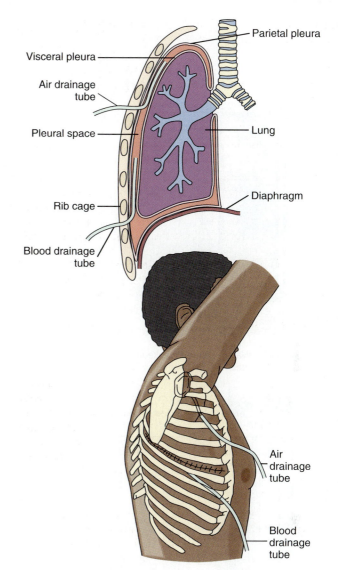

FIG. 30-14 Chest tube placement.

seeding of the cancer and is then removed whole through one of the small incisions.

Postoperative Care. Care after surgery for patients who have undergone thoracotomy (except for pneumonectomy) requires closed–chest drainage to drain air and blood that collect in the pleural space. A **chest tube,** a drain placed in the pleural space, allows lung re-expansion (Fig. 30-14). The chest tube also prevents air and fluid from returning to the chest. The drainage system consists of one or more chest tubes or drains, a collection container placed below the chest level, and a water seal to keep air from entering the chest. The drainage system may be a stationary, disposable, self-contained system (Fig. 30-15) or a smaller, portable, disposable, self-contained system that requires no connection to a vacuum source (Fig. 30-16). The nursing care priorities for the patient with a chest tube are to ensure the integrity of the system, promote comfort, ensure chest tube patency, and prevent complications.

Chest Tube Placement and Care. The tip of the tube used to drain air is placed near the front lung apex (see Fig. 30-14). The tube that drains liquid is placed on the side near the base of the lung. After lung surgery, two tubes, anterior and posterior, are used. The wounds are covered with airtight dressings.

The chest tube is connected by about 6 feet of tubing to a collection device placed below the chest. The tubing allows the patient to turn and move without pulling on the chest tube. Keeping the collection device below the chest allows gravity to drain the pleural space. When two chest tubes are inserted, they are joined by a Y-connector near the patient's body; the 6 feet of tubing is attached to the Y-connector.

Stationary chest tube drainage systems use a water seal mechanism that acts as a one-way valve to prevent air or liquid from moving back into the chest cavity. The Pleur-evac system is a common device using a one-piece disposable plastic unit with three chambers. The three chambers are connected to one another. The tube(s) from the patient is(are) connected to the first chamber in the series of three. This chamber is the drainage collection container. The second chamber is the water seal to prevent air from moving back up the tubing system and into the chest. The third chamber, when suction is applied, is the suction regulator.

In setting up the system, chamber one (nearest to the patient) does not at first have fluid in it. The tubing from the patient

penetrates shallowly into this chamber, as does the tube connecting chamber one with chamber two.

Chamber one collects the fluid draining from the patient. This fluid is measured hourly during the first 24 hours. The fluid in chamber one must never fill to the point that it comes into contact with any tubes! If the tubing from the patient enters the fluid, drainage stops and can lead to a tension pneumothorax.

Chamber two is the water seal that prevents air from re-entering the patient's pleural space. As the trapped air leaves the pleural space, it will pass through chamber one (drainage

---

! NURSING SAFETY PRIORITY (QSEN)

Action Alert

For a water seal chest tube drainage system, 2 cm of water is the minimum needed in the water seal to prevent air from flowing backward into the patient. Check the water level every shift, and add sterile water to this chamber to the level marked on the indicator (specified by the manufacturer of the drainage system).

FIG. 30-15 *Left,* The Pleur-evac drainage system, a commercial three-chamber chest drainage device. *Right,* Schematic of the drainage device.

FIG. 30-16 A portable chest drainage system.

collection chamber) before entering chamber two (the water seal chamber), which should always contain at least 2 cm of water to prevent air from returning to the patient. As trapped air from the patient's pleural space passes through the water seal, which serves as a one-way valve, the water will bubble. Once all the air has been evacuated from the pleural space, bubbling of the water seal stops.

The bubbling of the water in the water seal chamber indicates air drainage from the patient. Bubbling is seen when intrathoracic pressure is greater than atmospheric pressure, such as when the patient exhales, coughs, or sneezes. When the air in the pleural space has been removed, bubbling stops. A blocked or kinked chest tube also can cause bubbling to stop. Excessive bubbling in the water seal chamber (chamber two) may indicate an air leak. The water in the narrow column of the water seal

chamber normally rises 2 to 4 inches during inhalation and falls during exhalation, a process called *tidaling.* An absence of fluctuation may mean that the lung has fully re-expanded or can mean that there is an obstruction in the chest tube (Bauman & Handley, 2011).

Chamber three is the suction control of the system. There are different types of suction, most commonly wet or dry. With wet suction, the fluid level in chamber three is prescribed by the health care provider (usually −20 cm water). The chamber is connected to wall suction, which is turned up until there is gentle bubbling in the chamber. With dry suction, the health care provider prescribes the suction level to be dialed in on the device. When connected to wall suction, the regulator is set to the amount indicated by the device's manufacturer. For either type of suction, the amount of suction in the system is determined not by the wall suction unit but by the chest tube drainage device.

Chart 30-13 summarizes best safety practices when caring for a patient with a water seal chest tube drainage system. Check hourly to ensure the sterility and patency of the drainage system. Tape tubing junctions to prevent accidental disconnections, and keep an occlusive dressing at the chest tube insertion site. Keep sterile gauze at the bedside to cover the insertion site immediately if the chest tube becomes dislodged. Also keep padded clamps at the bedside for use if the drainage system is interrupted. Position the drainage tubing to prevent kinks and large loops of tubing, which can block drainage and prevent lung re-expansion.

Manipulation of the chest tube should be kept to a minimum. Do not vigorously "strip" the chest tube because this can create up to −400 cm of water negative pressure and damage lung tissue. If any tube manipulation is needed, gentle hand-over-hand "milking" of the tube, with stopping between each hand hold, is used to move blood clots and prevent obstruction. Follow surgeon prescriptions, as well as agency policies and guidelines on this action.

Assess the respiratory status and document the amount and type of drainage hourly on the collection chamber. Notify the surgeon if more than 100 mL/hr of drainage occurs. After the

Management of Chest Tube Drainage Systems

Patient

- Ensure that the dressing on the chest around the tube is tight and intact. Depending on agency policy and the surgeon's preference, reinforce or change loose dressings.
- Assess for difficulty breathing.
- Assess breathing effectiveness by pulse oximetry.
- Listen to breath sounds for each lung.
- Check alignment of trachea.
- Check tube insertion site for condition of the skin. Palpate area for puffiness or crackling that may indicate subcutaneous emphysema.
- Observe site for signs of infection (redness, purulent drainage) or excessive bleeding.
- Check to see if tube "eyelets" are visible.
- Assess for pain and its location and intensity, and administer drugs for pain as prescribed.
- Assist patient to deep breathe, cough, perform maximal sustained inhalations, and use incentive spirometry.
- Reposition the patient who reports a "burning" pain in the chest.

Drainage System

- Do not "strip" the chest tube.
- Keep drainage system lower than the level of the patient's chest.
- Keep the chest tube as straight as possible, avoiding kinks and dependent loops.
- Ensure the chest tube is securely taped to the connector and that the connector is taped to the tubing going into the collection chamber.
- Assess bubbling in the water seal chamber; should be gentle bubbling on patient's exhalation, forceful cough, position changes.
- Assess for "tidaling."
- Check water level in the water seal chamber, and keep at the level recommended by the manufacturer.
- Check water level in the suction control chamber, and keep at the level prescribed by the surgeon (unless dry suction system is used).
- Clamp the chest tube only for brief periods to change the drainage system or when checking for air leaks.
- Check and document amount, color, and characteristics of fluid in the collection chamber, as often as needed according to the patient's condition and agency policy.
- Empty collection chamber or change the system before the drainage makes contact with the bottom of the tube.
- When a sample of drainage is needed for culture or other laboratory test, obtain it from the chest tube; after cleansing chest tube, use a 20-gauge (or smaller) needle and draw up specimen into a syringe.

Immediately Notify Physician or Rapid Response Team For:

- Tracheal deviation
- Sudden onset or increased intensity of dyspnea
- Oxygen saturation less than 90%
- Drainage greater than 70 mL/hr
- Visible eyelets on chest tube
- Chest tube falls out of the patient's chest (first, cover the area with dry, sterile gauze)
- Chest tube disconnects from the drainage system (first, put end of tube in a container of sterile water and keep below the level of the patient's chest)
- Drainage in tube stops (in the first 24 hours)

forceful expiration or coughing because air in the chest is being expelled. Continuous bubbling indicates an air leak. Notify the health care provider if bubbling occurs continuously in the water seal chamber. With a prescription, gently apply a padded clamp briefly on the drainage tubing close to the occlusive dressing. If the bubbling stops, the air leak may be at the chest tube insertion site or within the chest, requiring physician intervention. Bubbling that does not stop when a padded clamp is applied indicates that the air leak is between the clamp and the drainage system. Release the clamp as soon as this assessment is made.

Mobile or portable chest tube drainage systems are "dry" chest drainage systems without a water seal to prevent air from re-entering the patient's lung through the chest tube. Instead, these light-weight devices use a dynamic control "flutter" valve that prevents backflow of air. When the patient exhales, air is forced from the chest cavity into the chest tube, under pressure. This pressure forces the soft flutter valve open and air moves into the harder surrounding tube shell (which has a vent for air). Portable units allow the patient to ambulate and go home with chest tubes still in place.

❓ NCLEX EXAMINATION CHALLENGE

Safe and Effective Care Environment

The chest tube of a client 16 hours postoperative from a lobectomy is accidentally pulled out by a portable x-ray machine. What is the nurse's best first action?
- A. Clamp the tubing with padded clamps as close as possible to the insertion site.
- B. Reposition the client on the nonoperative side and support the tube(s) with pillows.
- C. Cover the insertion site with a sterile occlusive dressing and tape down on three sides.
- D. Don sterile gloves and attempt to reinsert the chest tube at the original insertion site.

Pain Management. Most patients have intense pain after an open thoracotomy. Pain is considerably less for the patient after surgery using minimally invasive techniques. However, pain control is needed in either case for patient comfort and to assist him or her to participate in techniques to reduce the risk for complications (see Chapter 16). Give the prescribed drugs for pain, and assess the patient's responses to them. Teach patients using patient-controlled analgesia (PCA) devices to self-administer the drug before pain intensity becomes too severe. Monitor vital signs before and after giving opioid analgesics, especially for the patient who is not being mechanically ventilated. Plan care activities around the timing of analgesia to reduce pain.

Respiratory Management. Immediately after surgery the patient is mechanically ventilated. See Chapter 32 for nursing care of the patient receiving mechanical ventilation.

Once the patient is breathing on his or her own, the priorities are to maintain a patent airway, ensure adequate ventilation, and prevent complications. Assess the patient at least every 2 hours for adequacy of ventilation and GAS EXCHANGE. Check the alignment of the trachea. Assess oxygen saturation and the rate and depth of respiration. Listen to breath sounds in all lobes on the nonoperative side, particularly noting the presence of crackles. Assess the oral mucous membranes for cyanosis and

first 24 hours, assess drainage at least every 8 hours. Usually the drainage in chamber one is not emptied unless it is so full that the fluid is in danger of coming into contact with the chest drainage tube.

Check the water seal chamber for unexpected bubbling created by an air leak in the system. Bubbling is normal during the nail beds for rate of capillary refill. Perform oral suctioning as necessary.

Usually the patient receives oxygen by mask or nasal cannula for the first 2 days after surgery. Warm and humidify the oxygen. Assist the patient to a semi-Fowler's position or up in a chair as soon as possible. Encourage him or her to use the incentive spirometer every hour while awake. If coughing is permitted, help him or her cough by splinting any incision and ensuring that the chest tube does not pull with movement. Ensuring that pain is well managed increases the patient's ability to cough and deep breathe effectively.

Pneumonectomy Care. After pneumonectomy, the pleural cavity on the affected side is an empty space. The surgeon sometimes inserts a clamped chest tube for only a day. Serous fluid collection in the empty space creates adhesions that help reduce mediastinal shift toward the affected side. Closed–chest drainage is not usually used.

Complications of a pneumonectomy include empyema (purulent material in the pleural space) and development of a bronchopleural fistula (an abnormal duct that develops between the bronchial tree and the pleura). Positioning of the patient after pneumonectomy varies according to surgeon preference and the patient's comfort. Some surgeons want the patient placed on the nonoperative side immediately after a pneumonectomy to reduce stress on the bronchial stump incision. Others prefer to place the patient on the operative side to allow fluids to fill in the now empty space.

? CLINICAL JUDGMENT CHALLENGE

Patient-Centered Care; Evidence-Based Practice [QSEN]

The patient is a 60-year-old man who has just been diagnosed with non–small cell lung cancer. He smoked cigarettes for about 25 years starting when he was 16 years old and quit when he was 41 years old. His lung cancer is at stage I in the left lower lobe. He is distraught, saying that he can't die now because he has one child in college and two in high school. He also fears chemotherapy and seems bitter that he quit smoking and got lung cancer anyway. His next statement is: "Why couldn't I get prostate cancer like most men? At least they survive. No one beats lung cancer."
1. What can you tell him about lung cancer survival?
2. What can you tell him about the benefits of having quit smoking?
3. For this cancer stage and type, what is/are the most likely therapy/therapies?
4. What resources could you recommend to help him at this time?

◆ Interventions for Palliation

Oxygen therapy is prescribed when the patient is hypoxemic. Even if the hypoxemia is not severe, humidified oxygen may be prescribed to relieve dyspnea and anxiety. (See Chapter 28 for issues related to home oxygen therapy.)

Drug therapy with bronchodilators and corticosteroids is prescribed for the patient with bronchospasm to decrease bronchospasm, INFLAMMATION, and edema. Mucolytics may help ease removal of thick mucus and sputum. Bacterial infections are treated with antibiotic therapy.

Radiation therapy can help relieve hemoptysis, obstruction of the bronchi and great veins (superior vena cava syndrome), difficulty swallowing from esophageal compression, and pain from bone metastasis. Radiation for palliation uses higher doses for shorter periods. Skin care issues and fatigue are the same as those occurring with radiation therapy for cure.

Thoracentesis is performed when pleural effusion is a problem for the patient with lung cancer. The excess fluid increases dyspnea, discomfort, and the risk for infection. The purpose of treatment is to remove pleural fluid and prevent its formation. Thoracentesis is fluid removal by suction after the placement of a large needle or catheter into the intrapleural space. Fluid removal temporarily relieves hypoxia; however, the fluid can rapidly re-form in the pleural space. When fluid development is continuous and uncomfortable, a continuously draining catheter may be placed into the intrapleural space to collect the fluid.

Dyspnea management is needed because the patient with lung cancer tires easily and is often most comfortable resting in a semi-Fowler's position. Dyspnea is reduced with oxygen, use of a continuous morphine infusion, and positioning for comfort. The severely dyspneic patient may be most comfortable sitting in a lounge chair or reclining chair.

Pain management may be needed to help the patient be as pain-free and comfortable as possible. Pain may be present in the chest or in almost any area when bone metastasis occurs. Perform a complete pain assessment with attention to onset, intensity, quality, duration, and the patient's description of the pain.

Pharmacologic management with opioid drugs as oral, parenteral, or transdermal preparations is needed. Analgesics are most effective when given around the clock. Additional PRN analgesics are used for breakthrough pain. Ongoing evaluation of pain control effectiveness is a primary nursing responsibility.

Hospice care can be beneficial for the patient in the terminal phase of lung cancer. Hospice programs provide support to the terminally ill patient and the family, meet physical and psychosocial needs, adjust the palliative care regimen as needed, make home visits, and provide volunteers for errands and respite care. (See Chapter 7 for a more complete discussion of end-of-life issues.) The American Cancer Society may provide assistance through support groups for patients and families or through the use of equipment, such as a hospital bed or bedside commode. Family members and significant others are heavily burdened at this time. They have many needs and also require much support while performing the caregiver role during this time (Grant et al., 2013).

NURSING CONCEPTS AND CLINICAL JUDGMENT REVIEW

What might you NOTICE if the patient is experiencing inadequate GAS EXCHANGE and tissue PERFUSION as a result of chronic obstructive respiratory problems?
- Respirations rapid and shallow
- Decreased oxygen saturation by pulse oximetry
- Skin cyanosis or pallor (in lighter-skinned patients)
- Cyanosis or pallor of the lips and oral mucous membranes (in patients of any skin color)
- Tachycardia
- Patient appears to work hard to inhale and exhale
- Patient is restless or anxious
- Patient's general appearance is thin relative to height
- Muscles of the neck appear thick
- Arm and leg muscles appear thin
- Fingers are clubbed
- Chest is barrel-shaped
- Ribs are spaced more than a fingerbreadth apart

What should you INTERPRET and how should you RESPOND to a patient experiencing inadequate GAS EXCHANGE and tissue PERFUSION as a result of an acute critical respiratory problem?

Perform and interpret physical assessment, including:
- Taking vital signs
- Auscultating all lung fields
- Monitoring oxygen saturation by pulse oximetry
- Assessing cognition
- Assessing for the presence and characteristics of sputum production
- Assessing the patient's ability to cough and clear the airway

Interpret laboratory values, including:
- Elevated red blood cell count, hematocrit, and hemoglobin
- Elevated white blood cell count
- Arterial blood gas values: pH lower than 7.35; HCO_3^- greater than 24 mEq/L; $Paco_2$ greater than 45 mm Hg; Pao_2 lower than 80 mm Hg

Respond by:
- Assisting the patient to an upright position, with arms resting on a table or armrests
- Performing or assisting the patient to perform chest physiotherapy/pulmonary hygiene
- Prioritizing and pacing activities to prevent fatigue
- Administering prescribed inhaled drugs
- Administering respiratory therapy treatments or collaborating with the respiratory therapist to administer these treatments
- Re-assessing respiratory status after respiratory therapy treatment
- Ensuring a fluid intake of at least 2 liters per day

On what should you REFLECT?
- Observe the patient for evidence of improved oxygenation (see Chapter 27).
- Think about what may have made the patient's dyspnea worse and what steps could be taken to prevent a similar episode.
- Think about what patient education focus could help reduce the intensity of dyspnea in the future.

GET READY FOR THE NCLEX® EXAMINATION!

KEY POINTS

Review these Key Points for each NCLEX Examination Client Needs Category.

Safe and Effective Care Environment
- Ensure there are no open flames or combustion hazards in rooms where oxygen is in use. **Safety** QSEN
- Ensure that oxygen therapy delivered to the patient is humidified. **Safety** QSEN
- Protect the patient with cystic fibrosis from hospital-acquired pulmonary infections. **Safety** QSEN
- Ensure proper function of chest tube drainage equipment. **Safety** QSEN

Health Promotion and Maintenance
- Teach patients who come into contact with inhalation irritants in their workplaces or leisure-time activities to use a mask to avoid respiratory contact with these substances. **Safety** QSEN
- Teach anyone who smokes that smoking increases the risk for development of many pulmonary problems. **Evidence-Based Practice** QSEN

- Teach patients with asthma to develop a management plan based on their identified personal best on peak expiratory rate flow testing. **Patient-Centered Care** QSEN
- Instruct patients with asthma to carry a reliever inhaler with them at all times. **Safety** QSEN
- Encourage all patients older than 50 years and anyone with a respiratory problem to receive a yearly influenza vaccination. **Patient-Centered Care** QSEN
- Teach all patients who smoke the warning signs of lung cancer. **Evidence-Based Practice** QSEN

Psychosocial Integrity
- Encourage the patient and family to express their feelings regarding the diagnosis of a chronic respiratory disease or cancer and about management/treatment regimens.
- Explain all diagnostic procedures, restrictions, and follow-up care to the patient scheduled for tests.
- Help patients use strategies to improve their appearance when alopecia occurs. **Patient-Centered Care** QSEN
- Refer patients and family members to local cancer resources and support groups. **Patient-Centered Care** QSEN

- Ensure that patient preferences are honored whenever possible. **Patient-Centered Care** `QSEN`

Physiological Integrity
- Assess the airway and breathing effectiveness for GAS EXCHANGE for any patient who experiences shortness of breath or any change in mental status. **Evidence-Based Practice** `QSEN`
- Assess the degree to which breathing problems interfere with the patient's ability to perform ADLs, work, and leisure-time activities. **Patient-Centered Care** `QSEN`
- Apply oxygen to anyone who is hypoxemic. **Evidence-Based Practice** `QSEN`

- Monitor arterial blood gases and oxygen saturation of all patients receiving oxygen therapy. **Evidence-Based Practice** `QSEN`
- Teach patients receiving radiation therapy how to care for the skin in the radiation path (see Chart 22-2 in Chapter 22). **Patient-Centered Care** `QSEN`
- Collaborate with respiratory therapists, registered dietitians, and social workers to meet the hospital and home care needs of patients with chronic lower respiratory problems. **Teamwork and Collaboration** `QSEN`

CHAPTER 31

Care of Patients with Infectious Respiratory Problems

Meg Blair

 http://evolve.elsevier.com/Iggy/

PRIORITY CONCEPTS

- GAS EXCHANGE
- INFECTION
- INFLAMMATION

LEARNING OUTCOMES

Safe and Effective Care Environment

1. Apply principles of infection control and disease-containment activities when providing care to patients with respiratory INFECTIONS.
2. Protect patients receiving mechanical ventilation from developing ventilator-associated pneumonia.

Health Promotion and Maintenance

3. Provide information to everyone about preventing respiratory INFECTIONS.
4. Describe techniques for home care of the patient with active tuberculosis.

Psychosocial Integrity

5. Reduce the psychological impact of respiratory INFECTIONS for the patient and family.

Physiological Integrity

6. Identify adults at highest risk for contracting influenza, pneumonia, tuberculosis, and other respiratory INFECTIONS.
7. Perform focused respiratory assessment and re-assessment.
8. Recognize manifestations of infectious respiratory diseases and inadequate GAS EXCHANGE.
9. Implement appropriate interventions for the patient with a respiratory infection to ensure adequate GAS EXCHANGE and oxygenation.

DISORDERS OF THE NOSE AND SINUSES

RHINITIS

❖ PATHOPHYSIOLOGY

Rhinitis, an INFLAMMATION of the nasal mucosa, is a common problem of the nose and often involves the sinuses. It can be caused by INFECTION (viral or bacterial) or contact with allergens. An allergic rhinitis makes the mucous membranes more susceptible to bacterial invasion that may lead to INFECTION.

Allergic rhinitis *(hay fever* or *allergies)* is triggered by hypersensitivity reactions to airborne allergens. Some episodes are "seasonal," recurring at the same time of year (Krouse & Krouse, 2014). *Perennial rhinitis* occurs intermittently with no seasonal pattern or continuously whenever the person is exposed to an offending allergen such as dust, animal dander, wool, or foods (e.g., seafood). Rhinitis also occurs as a "rebound" nasal congestion from overuse of nasal decongestant drops or sprays *(rhinitis medicamentosa)* and chronic nasal inhalation of cocaine.

Acute viral rhinitis (**coryza**, or the common cold) is caused by any of over 200 viruses. It spreads from person to person by droplets from sneezing or coughing and by direct contact. Colds are most contagious in the first 2 to 3 days after symptoms appear. Colds are self-limiting unless a bacterial INFECTION occurs at the same time. Complications occur most often in immunosuppressed people and older adults.

❖ PATIENT-CENTERED COLLABORATIVE CARE

In allergic rhinitis, the presence of the allergen causes a release of histamine and other chemicals from basophils and mast cells in the nasal mucosa. These chemicals bind to blood vessel receptors, causing local blood vessel dilation and capillary leak, leading to local edema and swelling. Manifestations include headache, nasal irritation, sneezing, nasal congestion, **rhinorrhea** (watery drainage from the nose), and itchy, watery eyes.

Viral or bacterial invasion of the nasal passages causes the same local tissue responses as allergic rhinitis. Often the patient also has systemic manifestations, including a sore, dry throat; low-grade fever; and malaise.

Management of the patient with any type of rhinitis focuses on symptom relief and patient education. Teach him or her about correct use of the drug therapy prescribed.

Drug therapy commonly includes antihistamines, decongestants, and intranasal steroid spray (especially for chronic rhinitis). For severe disease, immunotherapy can be used. *Antihistamines, leukotriene inhibitors,* and *mast cell stabilizers* block or reduce the amount of chemical mediators in nasal tissues and prevent local edema and itching. *Decongestants* constrict blood vessels and decrease edema. *Antipyretics* are given if fever is present. *Antibiotics* are prescribed only when a bacterial INFECTION accompanies rhinitis. Rhinitis caused by overuse of nose drops or sprays is treated by discontinuing the drug.

CONSIDERATIONS FOR OLDER ADULTS
Patient-Centered Care QSEN

First-generation antihistamines are included as potentially inappropriate drugs for use in older adults. In this population, the drugs lead to problems with reduced clearance, higher risk for confusion, and anticholinergic effects such as dry mouth and constipation. Common drugs in this category include chlorpheniramine (Chlor-Trimeton), diphenhydramine (Benadryl), and hydroxyzine (Vistaril). Warn the older adult about these side effects.

Supportive therapy can increase the patient's comfort and help prevent spread of the INFECTION. Instruct the patient about the importance of rest (8 to 10 hours a day) and fluid intake of at least 2000 mL/day unless other health problems require fluid restriction. Humidifying the air helps relieve congestion. Humidity can be increased with a room humidifier or by breathing steamy air in the bathroom after running hot shower water. If the condition is caused by allergies, limiting exposure to the offending agent is helpful (see Chapter 20).

Teach patients to reduce the risk for spreading colds by thoroughly washing hands, especially after nose blowing, sneezing, coughing, rubbing the eyes, or touching the face. Other precautions include staying home from work, school, or places where people gather; covering the mouth and nose with a tissue when sneezing or coughing; disposing properly of used tissues immediately; and avoiding close contact with others. Stress the need to avoid close contact with people who are more susceptible to INFECTION, such as older adults, infants, and anyone who has a chronic respiratory problem. An uncomplicated cold typically subsides within 7 to 10 days.

RHINOSINUSITIS
❖ PATHOPHYSIOLOGY

Sinusitis is an INFLAMMATION of the mucous membranes of one or more of the sinuses and is usually associated with rhinitis. The preferred term for this condition is *rhinosinusitis* (Brook, 2013). Other conditions leading to rhinosinusitis include deviated nasal septum, nasal polyps or tumors, inhaled air pollutants or cocaine, facial trauma, and dental INFECTION. Swelling can obstruct the flow of secretions from the sinuses, which may then become infected.

Most episodes of rhinosinusitis are caused by viruses and usually develop in the maxillary and frontal sinuses, although bacterial INFECTIONS also can occur. Complications include cellulitis, abscess, and meningitis.

Diagnosis is made on the basis of the patient's history and manifestations. Other tests for rhinosinusitis include sinus x-rays, endoscopic examination, and computed tomography (CT). Bacterial sinusitis is usually indicated by purulent drainage from one or both nares, sometimes fever, and lack of response to decongestant therapy. Cultures are not usually necessary but may be useful in patients who do not respond to therapy or who develop complications.

❖ PATIENT-CENTERED COLLABORATIVE CARE

Assess for manifestations of rhinosinusitis. Common manifestations include pain over the cheek radiating to the teeth, tenderness to percussion over the sinuses, referred pain to the temple or back of the head, and general facial pain that is worse when bending forward. Additional manifestations that may accompany bacterial INFECTION include purulent nasal drainage with postnasal drip, fever, erythema, swelling, fatigue, dental pain, and ear pressure.

Treatment for bacterial rhinosinusitis includes the use of broad-spectrum antibiotics (e.g., amoxicillin [Amoxil]), analgesics for pain (e.g., acetaminophen [Tylenol, Abenol ♣, Atasol ♣, Panadol]; ibuprofen [Advil]), decongestants (e.g., phenylephrine [Neo-Synephrine]), antipyretics, steam humidification, hot and wet packs over the sinus area, and nasal saline irrigations. In some cases, nasal steroids may be prescribed. Nasal saline irrigation is an inexpensive treatment with few side effects (Thornton et al., 2011). Sleeping with the head of the bed elevated and avoiding cigarette smoke may reduce discomfort. Teach the patient to increase fluid intake unless another medical problem requires fluid restriction. If this treatment plan is not successful (no improvement seen within 48 hours), he or she may need further evaluation. Surgical intervention with endoscopic sinus surgery to relieve obstruction and promote sinus drainage may be needed if nonsurgical management fails to provide relief.

DISORDERS OF THE ORAL PHARYNX AND TONSILS

PHARYNGITIS
❖ PATHOPHYSIOLOGY

Pharyngitis, or "sore throat," is a common INFLAMMATION of the pharyngeal mucous membranes that often occurs with rhinitis and sinusitis. It accounts for up to 40 million office visits each year in the United States (Aung, 2013).

Acute pharyngitis can be caused by bacteria, viruses, other organisms, trauma, irritants, dehydration, and tobacco or alcohol use. A common bacterium causing pharyngitis is group A beta-hemolytic *Streptococcus,* but most adult cases are caused by a virus (Acerra, 2014).

❖ PATIENT-CENTERED COLLABORATIVE CARE
◆ Assessment

The patient with pharyngitis has throat soreness and dryness, throat pain, pain on swallowing (*odynophagia*), difficulty swallowing, and may have fever. Viral and bacterial pharyngitis are often difficult to distinguish on physical assessment. When inspecting a throat infected with either virus or bacteria, mild to severe redness may be seen with or without enlarged tonsils and with or without exudate. Ask about nasal discharge, which varies from thin and watery to thick and purulent. Enlargement of neck lymph nodes occurs with both viral and bacterial pharyngitis.

Bacterial INFECTIONS are often associated with enlarged red tonsils, exudate, petechiae on the soft palate, purulent discharge, and local lymph node enlargement. Chart 31-1 compares the

CHART 31-1 Key Features
Acute Viral and Bacterial Pharyngitis

FEATURE	VIRAL PHARYNGITIS	BACTERIAL PHARYNGITIS
Temperature	Low-grade or no fever	High temperature (>101°F [38.3°C] and usually 102°-104°F [38.9°-40°C])*
Ear manifestations	Retracted or dull tympanic membrane	Retracted or dull tympanic membrane
Throat manifestations	Scant or no tonsillar exudate Slight erythema of pharynx and tonsils	Severe hyperemia of pharyngeal mucosa, tonsils, tongue, and uvula Erythema of tonsils with yellow exudates Petechiae on the soft palate
Neck manifestations	Possible lymphadenopathy	Anterior cervical lymphadenopathy and tenderness
Skin manifestations	No rash	Possible scarlatiniform rash Possible petechiae on chest or abdomen or both
Dysphagia, odynophagia	Present	Present
Other symptoms	No cough Rhinitis Mild hoarseness Headache	No cough Pain on speaking and "hot potato" muffled voice Headache Arthralgia Myalgia
Laboratory data	Complete blood count usually normal White blood cell count usually ≤10,000/mm³ Negative throat culture results	Complete blood count abnormal White blood cell count usually >12,000/mm³* Throat culture results positive for beta-hemolytic *Streptococcus*
Onset	Gradual	Abrupt

*May not be present in adults older than 65 years.

TABLE 31-1 Complications of Group A Streptococcal Infection

- Rheumatic fever
- Acute glomerulonephritis
- Peritonsillar abscess
- Retropharyngeal abscess
- Otitis media
- Sinusitis
- Mastoiditis
- Bronchitis
- Pneumonia
- Scarlet fever

manifestations of viral and bacterial pharyngitis. Viral pharyngitis is contagious for 2 to 3 days. Symptoms usually subside within 3 to 10 days after onset, and the disease is usually self-limiting.

Bacterial pharyngitis caused by group A streptococcal INFECTION can lead to serious complications (Table 31-1), including acute glomerulonephritis and rheumatic fever. Acute glomerulonephritis may occur 7 to 10 days after the acute infection, and rheumatic fever may develop 3 to 5 weeks after the acute infection. Because rheumatic fever is rare, some experts question the need to prescribe antibiotics for all cases of pharyngitis (Acerra, 2014).

Many types of rapid antigen tests (RATs) and screens for group A beta-hemolytic streptococcal antigen are available. These tests vary in specificity and sensitivity, and the results are available in less than 15 minutes. Two common tests are the Gen-Probe and the Optical Immunoassay (OIA).

In some cases, throat cultures can be important in distinguishing viral from a group A beta-hemolytic streptococcal INFECTION. Usually 24 to 48 hours is required for results.

With either RAT or culture methods, it is essential to obtain throat specimens properly for an accurate test result. The organisms are not uniformly distributed throughout the throat and can be missed during swabbing. To obtain a specimen, rub a sterile cotton swab from a throat culture kit first over the right tonsillar area, moving across the right arch, the uvula, and then across the left arch to the left tonsillar area. Remove the swab without touching the patient's teeth, tongue, or gums. Consult with the laboratory for proper handling of the specimen. Send it to the laboratory as quickly as possible.

A complete blood count (CBC) may be performed when pharyngitis is severe or does not improve. Indications for a CBC are high fever, lethargy, or manifestations of complications.

Ask about the patient's recent contacts (within the past 10 days) with people who have been ill. Specifically ask whether he or she has been ill with manifestations of a cold or upper respiratory tract INFECTION recently. Document any history of streptococcal infections, rheumatic fever, valvular heart disease, or penicillin allergy. Ask whether the patient has had a diphtheria immunization.

◆ Interventions

Most sore throats in adults are viral, do not require antibiotic therapy, and respond to supportive interventions. Teach the patient to rest, increase fluid intake, humidify the air, and use analgesics for pain. Gargling several times each day with warm saline and using throat lozenges can increase comfort.

Management of bacterial pharyngitis involves antibiotics and the same supportive care as with viral pharyngitis. For streptococcal INFECTION, an oral penicillin or cephalosporin is prescribed. Drugs from the macrolide class (e.g., azithromycin or erythromycin) are used if the patient is allergic to penicillin.

! NURSING SAFETY PRIORITY (QSEN)
Action Alert

Teach patients with any bacterial INFECTION the importance of completing the entire antibiotic prescription, even when manifestations improve or subside. This action helps eradicate the organism and prevents development of resistant bacterial strains.

The patient should be re-evaluated if there is no improvement in 3 days or if manifestations are still present after completion of the antibiotic course. Any patient whose bacterial pharyngitis does not improve with antibiotics should consider human immune deficiency virus (HIV) testing.

A rare complication of pharyngitis is INFECTION of the epiglottis and supraglottic structures (**epiglottitis**). The epiglottis is a flaplike structure that closes over the trachea during swallowing to prevent aspiration. An inflamed epiglottis can swell and obstruct the airway, inhibiting GAS EXCHANGE and tissue perfusion.

> ⚠️ **NURSING SAFETY PRIORITY** (QSEN)
> **Critical Rescue**
>
> If a patient with pharyngitis develops stridor or other indications of airway obstruction, notify the Rapid Response Team. Teach patients at home to call 911 or go to the nearest emergency department if difficulty breathing, stridor, or drooling occurs.

Teach the patient with bacterial pharyngitis how to take his or her temperature every morning and evening until the INFECTION resolves. He or she is not contagious after 24 hours of effective antibiotic therapy. Family members or close contacts who also have a sore throat should be evaluated.

TONSILLITIS

❖ PATHOPHYSIOLOGY

Tonsillitis is an INFLAMMATION and INFECTION of the tonsils and lymphatic tissues located on each side of the throat. The tonsils are lymphatic tissue shaped like small almonds. They are covered by mucous membranes and have small valleys (*crypts*) across their surface. Tonsils filter organisms and protect the respiratory tract from infection (McCance et al., 2014).

Tonsillitis is a contagious airborne INFECTION that can occur in any age-group but is less common in adults. The disease usually lasts 7 to 10 days and often is caused by bacteria—most commonly *Streptococcus*. Viruses also cause tonsillitis. Chronic tonsillitis may result from an unresolved acute infection or recurrent infections.

❖ PATIENT-CENTERED COLLABORATIVE CARE

Chart 31-2 lists the manifestations of acute tonsillitis. Diagnostic tests often used to rule out other causes of the sore throat and fever include a rapid antigen test (RAT), CBC, throat culture and sensitivity (C&S) studies, and Monospot test. If respiratory manifestations are present, chest x-rays may be needed. The white blood cell (WBC) count usually is elevated in bacterial INFECTIONS and normal in viral infections.

Antibiotics, usually a non-penicillin drug, are prescribed for 7 to 10 days (Shah, 2014b). Nursing priorities include teaching the patient about supportive care and stressing the importance of completing antibiotic therapy. Teach him or her to rest, increase fluid intake, humidify the air, use analgesics for pain, gargle several times each day with warm saline, and use throat lozenges.

Surgical intervention for tonsillitis may be needed for recurrent acute or chronic INFECTIONS, a peritonsillar abscess, and enlarged tonsils or adenoids that obstruct the airway. It is usually performed after the patient has recovered from an acute tonsillitis and no infection is present (except with an acute peritonsillar abscess). The procedure also may involve adenoid removal. A variety of techniques are used to remove tonsils from adults; however, the dissection and snare technique is still

---

CHART 31-2 **Key Features**
Acute Tonsillitis

- Sudden onset of a mild to severe sore throat
- Fever
- Muscle aches
- Chills
- Dysphagia, odynophagia (painful swallowing of food)
- Pain in the ears
- Headache
- Anorexia
- Malaise
- "Hot potato" voice (muffled voice)
- Tonsils visually swollen and red, possibly with pus
- Tonsils may be covered with a white or yellow exudate
- Purulent drainage may be expressed by pressing a tonsil
- Uvula visually edematous or inflamed
- Cervical lymph nodes usually tender and enlarged

---

the most common and is performed under general anesthesia. After surgery, nursing interventions focus on assessing for airway clearance, providing pain relief, and monitoring for excessive bleeding.

PERITONSILLAR ABSCESS

Peritonsillar abscess (PTA) is a complication of acute tonsillitis in which the INFECTION spreads from the tonsil to the surrounding tissue and forms an abscess. The most common cause of PTA is group A beta-hemolytic *Streptococcus*, although they often contain multiple organisms (Shah, 2014a).

Manifestations include a collection of pus behind the tonsil causing one-sided swelling with deviation of the uvula toward the unaffected side. The patient may drool, have severe throat pain radiating to the ear, have a muffled voice, and have difficulty swallowing. He or she may also have a tonic contraction of the muscles of chewing (trismus) and have difficulty breathing. Bad breath is present, and lymph nodes on the affected side are swollen. An ultrasound or a CT scan may be used for diagnosis (Shah, 2014a).

Ambulatory care management with antibiotic therapy and percutaneous needle aspiration and drainage of the abscess is needed. Antibiotics alone are often ineffective. Acute management may include IV opioid analgesics for severe pain and IV steroids to reduce the swelling. *Stress the importance of completing the antibiotic regimen and of coming to the emergency department quickly if manifestations of obstruction (drooling and stridor) appear.* Hospitalization is needed when the airway is endangered or when the INFECTION does not respond to antibiotic therapy. Incision and drainage of the abscess and additional antibiotic therapy may be needed. A tonsillectomy may be performed to prevent recurrence.

DISORDERS OF THE LUNGS

SEASONAL INFLUENZA

❖ PATHOPHYSIOLOGY

Seasonal influenza, or "flu," is a highly contagious acute viral respiratory INFECTION that can occur at any age. Epidemics are common and lead to complications of pneumonia or death, especially in older adults or immunocompromised patients. Between 5% and 20% of the U.S. population develop influenza each year, and up to 49,000 deaths in a single year have been attributed to it (Centers for Disease Control and Prevention

[CDC], 2014b). Hospitalization may be required. Influenza may be caused by one of several virus families, referred to as *A, B,* and *C.*

The patient with influenza often has a rapid onset of severe headache, muscle aches, fever, chills, fatigue, and weakness. Adults are contagious from 24 hours before manifestations occur and up to 5 days after they begin. Sore throat, cough, and watery nasal discharge may follow the initial manifestations for a week or longer. Infection with influenza strain B also can cause nausea, vomiting, and diarrhea (Gould, 2011). Most patients feel fatigued for 1 to 2 weeks after the acute episode has resolved.

Health Promotion and Maintenance

Vaccinations for the prevention of influenza are widely available and are recommended for adults by The Joint Commission's National Patient Safety Goals (NPSGs). The vaccine is changed every year on the basis of which specific viral strains are most likely to pose a problem during the influenza season (i.e., late fall and winter in the Northern Hemisphere). Usually the vaccines contain three or four antigens for the three or four most expected viral strains (trivalent influenza vaccine [TIV]). Influenza vaccinations can be taken as an IM injection (Fluvirin, Fluzone) or as a live attenuated influenza vaccine (LAIV) by intranasal spray (FluMist). The intranasal vaccine is live, and some people develop influenza symptoms after its use. It is recommended only for healthy people up to 49 years of age. Yearly vaccination is recommended for those older than 50 years, people with chronic illness or immune compromise, those living in institutions, people living with or caring for adults with health problems that put them at risk for severe complications of influenza, and health care personnel providing direct care to patients (CDC, 2014b).

Teach the patient who is sick to reduce the risk for spreading the flu by thoroughly washing hands, especially after nose blowing, sneezing, coughing, rubbing the eyes, or touching the face. Other precautions include staying home from work, school, or places where people gather; covering the mouth and nose with a tissue when sneezing or coughing; disposing properly of used tissues immediately; and avoiding close contact with other people. Although handwashing is a good method to prevent transmitting the virus in droplets from sneezing or coughing, many people cannot wash their hands as soon as they have coughed or sneezed. The technique recommended by the CDC for controlling flu spread is to sneeze or cough into the upper sleeve rather than into the hand (CDC, 2010a). (Respiratory droplets on the hands can contaminate surfaces and be transmitted to other people.)

❖ PATIENT-CENTERED COLLABORATIVE CARE

Viral INFECTIONS do not respond to traditional antibiotic therapy. Antiviral agents may be effective for prevention and treatment of some types of influenza. Amantadine (Symmetrel) and rimantadine (Flumadine) have been effective in the prevention and treatment of some strains of influenza A. Ribavirin (Virazole) has been used for severe influenza B. Two drugs that shorten the duration of influenza A and influenza B are zanamivir (Relenza) and oseltamivir (Tamiflu). These drugs prevent viral spread in the respiratory tract by inhibiting a viral enzyme that allows the virus to penetrate respiratory cells. To be effective, they must be taken within 24 to 48 hours after the onset of manifestations. Zanamivir should be used with caution in

patients who have chronic obstructive pulmonary disease (COPD) or asthma and in older adults (Dambaugh, 2012).

Advise the patient to rest for several days and increase fluid intake unless another problem requires fluid restriction. Saline gargles may ease sore throat pain. Antihistamines may reduce the rhinorrhea. Other supportive measures are the same as those for acute rhinitis.

❓ NCLEX EXAMINATION CHALLENGE
Safe and Effective Care Environment

The charge nurse at an assisted-living facility receives report from an emergency department (ED) nurse about one of the resident clients. The client was sent to the ED with a fever, chills, muscle aches, and headache. The ED nurse reports the client's rapid influenza report came back from the laboratory positive for influenza A. What action by the nurse at the assisted-living facility is most appropriate?
A. Prepare to administer antibiotics.
B. Have the resident eat meals in his room.
C. Provide oseltamivir (Tamiflu) to the staff.
D. Arrange a follow-up chest x-ray in 2 weeks.

PANDEMIC INFLUENZA
❖ PATHOPHYSIOLOGY

Many viral INFECTIONS among animals and birds are not usually transmitted to humans. A few notable exceptions have occurred when these animal and bird viruses mutated and became highly infectious to humans. These infections are termed **pandemic** because they have the potential to spread globally. Such pandemics include the 1918 "Spanish" influenza that resulted in 40 million to 100 million deaths worldwide. This virus, the H1N1 strain, also known as "swine flu," mutated and became highly infectious to humans. Most recently, the 2009 H1N1 influenza A resulted in a pandemic infection that spread to 215 countries. In the United States, the number of people infected with this virus during the pandemic is estimated at 61 million, resulting in more than 12,000 deaths (CDC, 2010b). A vaccine was developed in 2009 as a single antigen (monovalent) and was administered separately from the seasonal influenza vaccine. Now the trivalent seasonal vaccine contains the H1N1 antigen.

A new avian virus is the H5N1 strain, known as "avian influenza" or "bird flu," which has infected millions of birds, especially in Asia, and now has started to spread by human-to-human contact. World health officials are concerned that this strain could become a pandemic because humans have no naturally occurring immunity to this virus and it could lead to a worldwide pandemic with very high mortality rates. Another avian strain, H7N9, has appeared in China, resulting in several deaths but has not spread out of that region (CDC, 2014a).

Health Promotion and Maintenance

The prevention of a worldwide influenza pandemic of any virus is the responsibility of everyone. Health officials have been monitoring human outbreaks and testing both wild and domestic bird species throughout the world. A vaccine (Vepacel) is available but is stockpiled and not part of general influenza vaccination. The recommended early approach to disease prevention with H5N1 is early recognition of new cases and the implementation of community and personal quarantine and social-distancing behaviors to reduce exposure to the virus.

Plans for prevention and containment in North America have been developed with the cooperation of most levels of government. When a cluster of cases is discovered in an area, the stockpiled vaccine is to be made available for immunization. Because vaccination with this vaccine is a two-step process with the first IM injection followed 28 days later by a second IM injection, additional prevention measures are needed (Medication Update, 2014; Plosker, 2012).

The antiviral drugs *oseltamivir* (Tamiflu) and *zanamivir* (Relenza) should be widely distributed. These drugs are not likely to prevent the disease but may reduce the severity of the INFECTION and reduce the mortality rate. The infected patients must be cared for in strict isolation. All nonessential public activities in the area should be stopped, including public gatherings of any type, attendance at schools, religious services, shopping, and many types of employment. People should stay home and use the emergency preparedness food, water, and drugs they have stockpiled to last at least 2 weeks (see Chapter 10). Travel to and from this area should be stopped.

Urge all people to pay attention to public health announcements and early warning systems for disease outbreaks. Teach them the importance of starting prevention behaviors immediately upon notification of an outbreak. Teach all people to have a minimum of a 2-week supply of all their prescribed drugs and at least a 2-week supply of nonperishable food and water for each member of the household. They should also have a battery-powered radio (and batteries) to keep informed of updates in an active prevention situation. See Chapter 10 for more information on items to have ready in the home for disaster preparedness. *An influenza pandemic is a disaster, and containing it requires the cooperation of all people.*

❖ PATIENT-CENTERED COLLABORATIVE CARE

The care priorities for the patient with avian or any pandemic influenza are supporting the patient and preventing spread of the disease. Both are equally important. The initial manifestations of avian influenza are similar to other respiratory INFECTIONS—cough, fever, and sore throat. These progress rapidly to shortness of breath and pneumonia. In addition, diarrhea, vomiting, abdominal pain, and bleeding from the nose and gums occur. *Ask any patient with these manifestations if he or she has recently (within the past 10 days) traveled to areas of the world affected by H5N1. If such travel has occurred, coordinate with the health care team to place the patient in an airborne isolation room with negative air pressure. These precautions remain until the diagnosis of H5N1 is ruled out or the threat of contagion is over.* Diagnosis is made based on clinical manifestations and positive testing. The most rapid test currently approved for testing of H5N1 is the AVantage A/H5N1 Flu Test. It can detect a specific protein (NS1), which indicates the presence of H5N1, from nasal or throat swabs in less than 40 minutes.

When providing care to the patient with avian influenza, personal protective equipment is essential. Coordinate the protection activity by ensuring that anyone entering the patient's room for any reason wears a fit-tested respirator or a standard surgical mask. Use other Airborne Precautions and Contact Precautions as described in Chapter 23. Teach others to self-monitor for disease manifestations, especially respiratory INFECTION, for at least a week after the last contact with the patient. Use the antiviral drug *oseltamivir* (Tamiflu) or *zanamivir* (Relenza) within 48 hours of contact with the infected patient. All health care personnel working with patients suspected of having avian influenza should receive the vaccine in the recommended two-step process.

No effective treatment for this INFECTION currently exists. Antibiotics and antiviral drugs cannot kill the virus or prevent its replication. Interventions are supportive to allow the patient's own immune system to fight the infection. Oxygen is given when hypoxia or breathlessness is present. Respiratory treatments to dilate the bronchioles and move respiratory secretions are used. If hypoxemia is not improved with oxygen therapy, intubation and mechanical ventilation may be needed. Antibiotics are used to treat a bacterial pneumonia that may occur with H5N1.

In addition to the need for respiratory support, the patient with H5N1 may have severe diarrhea and need fluid therapy. The Transmission Precautions may prevent the use of a scale to determine fluid needs by weight changes. Monitor the patient's hydration status, and carefully measure intake and output. The type of fluid therapy varies with the patient's cardiovascular status and blood osmolarity. The two most important areas to monitor during rehydration are pulse rate and quality and urine output.

❓ CLINICAL JUDGMENT CHALLENGE
Prioritization, Delegation, and Supervision

The patient is a 67-year-old man with moderate emphysema. He has just been admitted to the medical unit with a diagnosis of shortness of breath related to influenza. In the emergency department he received a chest x-ray and a nebulizer treatment with albuterol. He also had a saline lock placed, and arterial blood gases were sent to the laboratory. Vital signs before transfer were: BP, 158/92; HR, 92; RR, 32; T, 101.4° F.

The health care provider has prescribed:
- Schedule pulmonary function tests
- Obtain admission vital signs
- Tylenol 650 mg orally as needed
- Oxygen at 2 L per nasal cannula
- Nebulizer treatment with albuterol every 6 hours
- Intravenous antibiotic administration
- Use of incentive spirometer hourly
- Blood drawn for culture and sensitivity

1. Which order takes priority at this time? Provide a rationale for your choice.
2. Which action should you delegate to the unlicensed assistive personnel (UAP) who is helping you admit the patient? Provide a rationale for your choice.
3. The patient's SaO$_2$ is 90% on admission. What action would you take at this time? Provide a rationale for your choice.
4. The patient continues to have an elevated temperature (now 102.4° F). Which actions should you delegate to the licensed practical nurse/licensed vocational nurse (LPN/LVN) working with you and why?

PNEUMONIA
❖ PATHOPHYSIOLOGY

Pneumonia is excess fluid in the lungs resulting from an inflammatory process. The INFLAMMATION is triggered by many infectious organisms and by inhalation of irritating agents. The INFLAMMATION occurs in the interstitial spaces, the alveoli, and often the bronchioles. The process begins when organisms penetrate the airway mucosa and multiply in the alveolar spaces. White blood cells (WBCs) migrate to the area of INFECTION, causing local capillary leak, edema, and exudate. These fluids collect in and around the alveoli, and the alveolar walls thicken. Both events seriously reduce GAS EXCHANGE and lead to hypoxemia, interfering with oxygenation and possibly leading to death. Red blood cells (RBCs) and fibrin move into the alveoli, and capillary leak spreads the infection to other areas of the lung. If the organisms move into the bloodstream, septicemia results; if the infection extends into the pleural cavity, **empyema** (a collection of pus in the pleural cavity) results.

The fibrin and edema stiffen the lung, reducing compliance and decreasing the vital capacity. Alveolar collapse (atelectasis) further reduces the ability of the lung to oxygenate the blood moving through it. As a result, arterial oxygen levels fall, causing hypoxemia.

Pneumonia may occur as *lobar pneumonia* with **consolidation** (solidification, lack of air spaces) in a segment or an entire lobe of the lung or as *bronchopneumonia* with diffusely scattered patches around the bronchi. The extent of lung involvement depends on the host defenses. Bacteria multiply quickly in a person whose immune system is compromised. Tissue necrosis results when an abscess forms and perforates the bronchial wall.

Etiology

Pneumonia develops when the immune system cannot overcome the invading organisms. Organisms from the environment, invasive devices, equipment and supplies, staff, or other people can invade the body. Risk factors are listed in Table 31-2. Pneumonia can be caused by bacteria, viruses, mycoplasmas, fungi, rickettsiae, protozoa, and helminths (worms). Noninfectious causes of pneumonia include inhalation of toxic gases, chemical fumes, and smoke and aspiration of water, food, fluid (including saliva), and vomitus (Echevarria & Schwoebel, 2012). Pneumonia can be categorized as community-acquired (CAP), hospital-acquired (HAP), health care–associated (HCAP) or ventilator-associated (VAP) (Table 31-3).

Incidence and Prevalence

In the United States, 2 to 5 million cases of pneumonia occur each year and it is a major cause of death. The incidence is higher among older adults, nursing home residents, hospitalized patients, and those being mechanically ventilated. CAP is more common than HAP and occurs in late fall and winter, often as a complication of influenza.

Health Promotion and Maintenance

Patient education about vaccination is important in the prevention of pneumonia (Chart 31-3). The Joint Commission NPSGs require that nurses especially encourage people older than 65 years and those with a chronic health problem to receive immunization against pneumonia. Antigens from 23 different types of pneumonia organisms are included in the pneumococcal polysaccharide vaccine (PPV23). This vaccine is usually given once; however, some experts believe that older adults and those with chronic health problems could benefit from a second vaccination if more than 5 years has passed since the first vaccination (American Lung Association [ALA], 2010a). Because pneumonia often follows influenza, especially among older adults, urge all people to receive the seasonal influenza vaccination yearly (Scott & Kardos, 2012).

Other prevention techniques include strict handwashing to avoid the spread of organisms and avoiding large gatherings of people during cold and flu season. Teach the patient who has a cold or the flu to see his or her health care provider if fever lasts more than 24 hours, if the problem lasts longer than 1 week, or if manifestations worsen.

Respiratory therapy equipment must be well maintained and decontaminated or changed as recommended. Use sterile water rather than tap water in GI tubes, and institute Aspiration Precautions as indicated, including screening patients for aspiration risk.

VAP is on the rise, but the risk can be reduced with conscientious assessment and meticulous nursing care (Echevarria &

TABLE 31-2 Risk Factors for Pneumonia

Community-Acquired Pneumonia
- Is an older adult
- Has never received the pneumococcal vaccination or received it more than 5 years ago
- Did not receive the influenza vaccine in the previous year
- Has a chronic health problem or other coexisting condition that reduces immune responses
- Has recently been exposed to respiratory viral or influenza infections
- Uses tobacco or alcohol or is exposed to high amounts of secondhand smoke

Health Care–Acquired Pneumonia
- Is an older adult
- Has a chronic lung disease
- Has presence of gram-negative colonization of the mouth, throat, and stomach
- Has an altered level of consciousness
- Has had a recent aspiration event
- Has presence of endotracheal, tracheostomy, or nasogastric tube
- Has poor nutritional status
- Has immunocompromised status (from disease or drug therapy)
- Uses drugs that increase gastric pH (histamine [H₂] blockers, antacids) or alkaline tube feedings
- Is currently receiving mechanical ventilation (ventilator-associated pneumonia [VAP])

CHART 31-3 Patient and Family Education: Preparing for Self-Management

Preventing Pneumonia

- Know whether you are at risk for pneumonia (older than 65 years, have a chronic health problem [especially a respiratory problem], or have limited mobility and are confined to a bed or chair during your waking hours).
- Have the annual influenza vaccine after discussing appropriate timing of the vaccination with your primary health care provider.
- Discuss the pneumococcal vaccine with your primary health care provider, and have the vaccination as recommended.
- Avoid crowded public areas during flu and holiday seasons.
- If you have a mobility problem, cough, turn, move about as much as possible, and perform deep-breathing exercises.
- If you are using respiratory equipment at home, clean the equipment as you have been taught.
- Avoid indoor pollutants, such as dust, secondhand (passive) smoke, and aerosols.
- If you do not smoke, do not start.
- If you smoke, seek professional help on how to stop (or at least decrease) your habit.
- Be sure to get enough rest and sleep on a daily basis.
- Eat a healthy, balanced diet.
- Drink at least 3 liters (quarts) of nonalcoholic fluids each day (unless fluid restrictions are needed because of another health problem).

TABLE 31-3   Differentiation of Types of Pneumonia

TYPE OF PNEUMONIA	DEFINITION	MANAGEMENT CONSIDERATIONS
Community acquired	Contracted outside a health care setting; acquired in the community	Most common bacterial agents: *Streptococcus pneumoniae*, *Haemophilus influenzae* Most common viral agents: influenza, respiratory syncytial virus (RSV) Antibiotics are often empirical based on multiple patient and environmental factors Treatment length: minimum of 5 days Prompt initiation of antibiotics required; in ED setting, first dose given before patient leaves unit for inpatient bed, or within 6 hours of presentation to the ED
Health care associated	Onset/diagnosis of pneumonia occurs <48 hours after admission in patient with specific risk factors: In hospital for >48 hours in the past 90 days Living in nursing home or assisted-living facility Received IV therapy, wound care, antibiotics, chemotherapy in the past 30 days Seen at a hospital or dialysis clinic within the past 30 days	May have multidrug-resistant organisms Hand hygiene is critical
Hospital acquired	Onset/diagnosis of pneumonia >48 hours after admission to hospital	Encourage pulmonary hygiene and progressive ambulation Provide adequate hydration Assess risk for aspiration using an evidence-based tool Monitor for early signs of sepsis Hand hygiene is critical

Ventilator associated	Onset/diagnosis of pneumonia within 48-72 hours after endotracheal intubation	Presence of ET tube increases risk for pneumonia by bypassing protective airway mechanisms and by allowing aspiration of secretions from the oropharynx and stomach; dental plaque also increases risk
		Initiate ventilator bundle order set, including:
		   Elevate HOB at least 30 degrees
		   Daily sedation "vacation" and weaning assessment
		   DVT prophylaxis
		   Oral care regimen
		   Stress ulcer prophylaxis
		   Suctioning; either as needed or continuous subglottal suction
		Hand hygiene is critical

Data from Echevarria, I. & Schwoebel, A. (2012). Development of an intervention model for the prevention of aspiration pneumonia in high-risk patients on a medical-surgical unit. *MEDSURG Nursing, 21*(5), 303-308; Luttenberger, K. (2010). Battling VAP from a new angle. *Nursing2010, 40*(2), 52-55; Roark, D.C. (2012). Working toward perfection on the pneumonia core measure. *Journal of Emergency Nursing, 38,* 127-129; Scott, S. & Kardos, C. (2012). Community-acquired, health care-associated, and ventilator-associated pneumonia: Three variations of a serious disease. *Critical Care Nursing Clinics of North America, 24*(3), 431-441.
DVT, Deep vein thrombosis; *ED,* emergency department; *ET,* endotracheal; *HOB,* head of bed.

Schwoebel, 2012; Roark, 2012; Scott & Kardos, 2012). The preventive care for VAP is discussed in detail in Chapter 32.

> ### ! NURSING SAFETY PRIORITY (QSEN)
> #### Action Alert
> Because pneumonia is a frequent cause of sepsis, use a sepsis screening tool to monitor patients who have pneumonia. For patients with pneumonia, always check oxygen saturation with vital signs.

❖ PATIENT-CENTERED COLLABORATIVE CARE

The Concept Map addresses assessment and nursing care issues related to patients who have pneumonia. The manifestations of pneumonia differ in older patients compared with younger patients.

◆ Assessment

History. Assess for the risk factors for INFECTION (see Table 31-2). Document age; living, work, or school environment; diet, exercise, and sleep routines; swallowing problems; presence of a nasogastrointestinal tube; tobacco and alcohol use; and past and current use of or addiction to "street" drugs. Remember that often aspiration is "silent" with no manifestations. Ask about past respiratory illnesses and whether the patient has been exposed to influenza or pneumonia or has had a recent viral infection. Ask about recent skin rashes, insect bites, and exposure to animals.

If the patient has chronic respiratory problems, ask whether respiratory equipment is used in the home. Assess whether the patient's home cleaning level is adequate to prevent INFECTION. Ask when he or she received the last influenza or pneumococcal vaccine.

Physical Assessment/Clinical Manifestations. Observe the general appearance. Many patients with pneumonia have flushed cheeks and an anxious expression. The patient may have chest pain or discomfort, myalgia, headache, chills, fever, cough, tachycardia, dyspnea, tachypnea, hemoptysis, and sputum production. Severe chest muscle weakness also may be present from sustained coughing.

Observe the patient's breathing pattern, position, and use of accessory muscles. The hypoxic patient may be uncomfortable in a lying position and will sit upright, balancing with the hands

CONCEPT MAP

COMMUNITY-ACQUIRED PNEUMONIA

INFLAMMATION

INFECTION

GAS EXCHANGE

HISTORY

60-year-old Diane Owens is admitted with CA pneumonia. She says, "My chest hurts from coughing so much." She is coughing up thick, green and rust-colored sputum. She is becoming confused and has lost her appetite.

Physical Assessment/Clinical Manifestations →

- Confused.
- T 99.1° F; HR 128; pulse weak; RR 24; BP 96/58 mm Hg
- Cheeks are flushed; fatigued, weak, lethargic; pain present; dyspneic; anxious
- Bilateral crackles and wheezing; fremitus over RLL; dulled percussion; unequal chest expansion on inspiration

Older Adult Considerations ↑

Most common sign/symptom is acute confusion from hypoxia. Other signs/symptoms: weakness, fatigue, lethargy, poor appetite. Fever and cough may be absent. White blood cells may not be elevated until infection is severe. Greatly increased risk for sepsis and death.

Planning →

PATIENT PROBLEMS

- Impaired GAS EXCHANGE related to decreased diffusion at the alveolar-capillary membrane
- Potential for airway obstruction related to excessive tracheobronchial secretions, fatigue, chest discomfort, muscle weakness
- Potential for sepsis related to the presence of microorganisms in a very vascular area

Data Synthesis →

EXPECTED OUTCOMES

Adequate GAS EXCHANGE:
- Maintains patent airway; SaO2 of at least 95% or in patient's normal range
- Maintains cognitive orientation
- Effective cough with absence of chest pain, crackles, or hemoptysis
- Absence of tachycardia or tachypnea, breathing discomfort with speaking, or cyanosis
- Returns to pre-pneumonia health status

INFLAMMATION:
- Absence of wheezing

INFECTION:
- Free from invading organisms in blood and sputum
- WBC and differential within normal limits
- Afebrile

INTERVENTIONS

1. Nursing Priority – Improving GAS EXCHANGE, Eliminating INFECTION
- Deliver oxygen therapy; assist with bronchial hygiene. *Promotes GAS EXCHANGE and oxygenation*
- Administer antibiotics for 5-7 days; reinforce, clarify, and provide information regarding drug therapy. *Helps to rid body of INFECTION and encourages drug compliance.*

2. Providing Safe and Effective Care
- Apply principles of infection control (e.g., hand hygiene, Isolation or Airborne Precautions). *Protects client and health care providers from INFECTION transmission.*

3. Respiratory Assessment
- Perform focused respiratory assessment and re-assessment; observe breathing pattern, position, and use of accessory muscles. *Assesses for respiratory distress.*
- Assess cough and amount, color, consistency; odor produced by sputum. *Assesses for infection and inadequate GAS EXCHANGE.*
- Assess for breath sounds and document wheezes, rhonchi, crackles, and evidence of decreased breath sounds. *Crackles indicate fluid in interstitial and alveolar areas; wheezing indicates INFLAMMATION or exudate in airways; bronchial breath sounds indicate areas of density or consolidation.*

4. Vital Signs Assessment
- Evaluate oxygen saturation and vital sign trends, effectiveness of antibiotics, fluids, and antipyretics. *Monitors for signs of sepsis, hypotension with orthostatic changes; rapid, weak pulse; and dysrhythmias.*

5. Promoting Breathing
- Assist with coughing, deep breathing, and incentive spirometry at least every 2 hours. Encourage alert patient to drink at least 2 L of fluid daily, unless contraindicated. *Promotes removal of secretions, hydration, and ensures adequate GAS EXCHANGE and oxygenation.*
- Monitor intake & output, especially when fever and tachypnea are present. *Monitors for signs of dehydration.*

6. Diagnostic Tests
- Obtain complete blood count with differential, sputum and blood cultures. *Determines whether organisms have invaded the blood and caused sepsis.*
- Determine oxygenation status by arterial blood gas values and pulse oximetry. *Determines baseline PaO2 and PaCO2 and helps identify need for supplemental oxygen.*
- Assess electrolytes, blood urea nitrogen (BUN), and creatinine levels. *Checks for dehydration and kidney function.*
- Review chest x-rays. *Provides early diagnosis in older adults because pneumonia symptoms are often vague.*

7. Minimizing Anxiety
- Assess expressions and general tenseness of facial and shoulder muscles. Listen using calm, slow approach. *Encourages calmness because pain, fatigue, and dyspnea promote anxiety.*

8. Nursing Safety Priority: Action Alert!
Teach the importance of completing the entire course of antibiotic therapy even when symptoms improve or subside. *Helps eradicate organisms and prevents drug resistance.*

Concept Map by Deanne A. Blach, MSN, RN

("tripod position"). Assess the cough and the amount, color, consistency, and odor of sputum produced.

Crackles are heard with auscultation when fluid is in interstitial and alveolar areas, and breath sounds may be diminished. Wheezing may be heard if INFLAMMATION or exudate narrows the airways. Bronchial breath sounds are heard over areas of density or consolidation. Fremitus is increased over areas of pneumonia, and percussion is dulled. Chest expansion may be diminished or unequal on inspiration.

In evaluating vital signs, compare the results with baseline values. The patient with pneumonia is often hypotensive with orthostatic changes as a result of vasodilation and dehydration, especially the older adult. A rapid, weak pulse may indicate hypoxemia, dehydration, or impending sepsis and shock. Dysrhythmias may occur as a result of cardiac tissue hypoxia. Common pneumonia manifestations and their causes are listed in Table 31-4.

Use an evidence-based pneumonia severity scale to assist in determining what treatment site is appropriate for the patient. Two such tools are the Pneumonia Severity Index (PSI) and the CURB-65. The PSI uses four risk categories (demographics, comorbid conditions, physical examination, and selected laboratory values) to determine a score reflective of the severity of the patient's pneumonia, whereas the CURB-65 relies on laboratory values (blood urea nitrogen [BUN], age, respirations, blood pressure, and presence of confusion (Scott & Kardos, 2012).

CONSIDERATIONS FOR OLDER ADULTS

Patient-Centered Care [QSEN]

The older adult with pneumonia has weakness, fatigue, lethargy, confusion, and poor appetite. Fever and cough may be absent, but hypoxemia is often present. The most common manifestation of pneumonia in the older adult patient is acute confusion from hypoxia. The WBC count may not be elevated until the infection is severe. Waiting to treat the disease until more typical manifestations appear greatly increases the risk for sepsis and death (Touhy & Jett, 2014).

Psychosocial Assessment. The patient with pneumonia often has pain, fatigue, and dyspnea, all of which promote anxiety. Assess anxiety by looking at his or her facial expression and general tenseness of facial and shoulder muscles. Listen to the patient carefully, and use a calm approach. Because of airway obstruction and muscle fatigue, the patient with dyspnea speaks in broken sentences. Keep the interview short if severe dyspnea or breathing discomfort is present.

Laboratory Assessment. Sputum is obtained and examined by Gram stain, culture, and sensitivity testing; however, the responsible organism often is not identified. A sputum sample is easily obtained from the patient who can cough into a specimen container. Extremely ill patients may need suctioning to obtain a sputum specimen. In these situations, a specimen is obtained by sputum trap (Fig. 31-1) during suctioning. A CBC is obtained to assess an elevated WBC count, which is a common finding except in older adults. Blood cultures may be performed to determine whether the organism has invaded the blood.

In severely ill patients, arterial blood gases (ABGs) and serum lactate levels may be assessed to determine baseline arterial oxygen and carbon dioxide levels and help identify a need for supplemental oxygen. Serum electrolyte, blood urea nitrogen (BUN), and creatinine levels also are assessed. A high BUN level may occur as a result of dehydration. Hypernatremia (high blood sodium levels) occurs with dehydration.

TABLE 31-4 Pathophysiology of Common Clinical Manifestations of Pneumonia

CLINICAL MANIFESTATION	PATHOPHYSIOLOGY
Increased respiratory rate/dyspnea	Stimulation of chemoreceptors Increased work of breathing as a result of decreased lung compliance Stimulation of J receptors Anxiety Pain
Hypoxemia	Alveolar consolidation Pulmonary capillary shunting
Cough	Fluid accumulation in the receptors of the trachea, bronchi, and bronchioles
Purulent, blood-tinged, or rust-colored sputum	A result of the inflammatory process in which fluid from the pulmonary capillaries and red blood cells moves into the alveoli
Fever	Phagocytes release pyrogens that cause the hypothalamus to increase body temperature
Pleuritic chest discomfort	Inflammation of the parietal pleura causes pain on inspiration

FIG. 31-1 A Lukens tube for collection of sterile sputum/mucus specimens.

Imaging Assessment. Chest x-ray is the most common diagnostic test for pneumonia but may not show changes until 2 or more days after manifestations are present. It usually appears on chest x-ray as an area of increased density. It may involve a lung segment, a lobe, one lung, or both lungs. *In the older adult, the chest x-ray is essential for early diagnosis because pneumonia manifestations are often vague* (Touhy & Jett, 2014).

Other Diagnostic Assessments. Pulse oximetry is used to assess for hypoxemia. Invasive tests such as transtracheal aspiration, bronchoscopy, or direct needle aspiration of the lung may be needed. Thoracentesis is used in patients who have an accompanying pleural effusion.

◆ Analysis

The priority NANDA-I nursing diagnoses and collaborative problems for patients with pneumonia include:
1. Impaired Gas Exchange related to decreased diffusion at the alveolar-capillary membrane (NANDA-I)

2. Potential for airway obstruction related to excessive tracheobronchial secretions, fatigue, chest discomfort, muscle weakness
3. Potential for sepsis related to the presence of microorganisms in a very vascular area

◆ **Planning and Implementation**

Improving Gas Exchange

Planning: Expected Outcomes. The patient with pneumonia is expected to have adequate GAS EXCHANGE and oxygenation. Indicators of adequacy are:
- Maintenance of Sao$_2$ of at least 95% or in the patient's normal range
- Absence of cyanosis
- Maintenance of cognitive orientation

Interventions. Interventions to improve GAS EXCHANGE and oxygenation are similar to those for the patient with chronic airflow limitation (CAL) (see Chapter 30). Nursing priorities include delivery of oxygen therapy and assisting the patient with bronchial hygiene.

Oxygen therapy is usually delivered by nasal cannula or mask unless the hypoxemia does not improve with these devices. The patient who is confused may not tolerate a facemask. Check the skin under the device and under the elastic band, especially around the ears, for areas of redness or skin breakdown. Actions for oxygen therapy are listed in Chart 28-1 in Chapter 28.

Incentive spirometry is used to improve inspiratory muscle action and to prevent or reverse atelectasis (alveolar collapse). Instruct the patient to exhale fully, then place the mouthpiece in his or her mouth, and then take a long, slow, deep breath for 3 to 5 seconds. Evaluate technique, and record the volume of air inspired. Teach the patient to perform 5 to 10 breaths per session every hour while awake.

Preventing Airway Obstruction

Planning: Expected Outcomes. The patient with pneumonia is expected to maintain a patent airway. Indicators are:
- Effective cough
- Absence of pallor or cyanosis
- Absence of crackles and wheezes on auscultation
- Pulse oximetry at or above 95%

Interventions. Interventions to avoid airway obstruction in pneumonia are similar to those for chronic obstructive pulmonary disease (COPD) or asthma. Because of fatigue, muscle weakness, chest discomfort, and excessive secretions, the patient often has difficulty clearing secretions. Help him or her cough and deep breathe at least every 2 hours. The alert patient may use an incentive spirometer to facilitate deep breathing and stimulate coughing. Encourage the alert patient to drink at least 2 liters of fluid daily to prevent dehydration unless another health problem requires fluid restriction. Monitor intake and output, oral mucus membranes, and skin turgor to assess hydration status, especially when fever and tachypnea are present.

Bronchodilators, especially beta$_2$ agonists (see Chart 30-6 in Chapter 30), are prescribed when bronchospasm is present. They are initially given by nebulizer and then by metered dose inhaler. Inhaled or IV steroids are used with acute pneumonia when airway swelling is present. Expectorants such as guaifenesin (Mucinex) may be used.

Preventing Sepsis

Planning: Expected Outcomes. The patient with pneumonia is expected to be free of the invading organism and to return to a pre-pneumonia health status. Indicators are:

- Absence of fever
- Absence of pathogens in blood and sputum cultures
- WBC count and differential within normal limits

Interventions. The key to effective treatment of pneumonia is eradication of the infecting organism. When sepsis occurs with pneumonia, the risk for death is high. Anti-infectives are given for all types of pneumonias except those caused by viruses. Which anti-infective therapy is prescribed is based on how the pneumonia was acquired (i.e., CAP, HAP, or HCAP). The exact drug or drugs and their routes of delivery are determined by the severity of the INFECTION, the organism suspected or identified, and whether the patient has other conditions or factors that increase the risk for complications. Drug therapy choices must reflect the degree of drug resistance in the specific geographic area and in that hospital setting.

The course of anti-infective therapy varies with the drug used and the organism(s) involved. Usually anti-infectives are used for 5 to 7 days for a patient with uncomplicated CAP and up to 21 days for an immunocompromised patient or one with HAP.

Drug resistance is becoming increasingly common, especially for INFECTIONS with *Streptococcus pneumoniae* (drug-resistant *Streptococcus pneumoniae* [DRSP]). It is most common in people older than 65 years and among those who became infected as a result of exposure to young children from a daycare environment.

For pneumonia resulting from aspiration of food or stomach contents, interventions focus on preventing lung damage and treating the INFECTION. Aspiration of acidic stomach contents can cause widespread INFLAMMATION, leading to acute respiratory distress syndrome (ARDS) and permanent lung damage. In these conditions, steroids and NSAIDs are used with antibiotics to reduce the inflammatory response.

🔍 NCLEX EXAMINATION CHALLENGE
Physiological Integrity

A nurse is caring for an 89-year-old client admitted with pneumonia. He has an IV of normal saline running at 100 mL/hr and antibiotics that were initiated in the emergency department 3 hours ago. He has oxygen at 2 liters/nasal cannula. What assessment finding by the nurse indicates that goals for a priority diagnosis have been met for this client?
A. The client is alert and oriented to person, place, and time.
B. Blood pressure is within normal limits and client's baseline.
C. Skin behind the ears demonstrates no redness or irritation.
D. Urine output has been >30 mL/hr per Foley catheter.

Community-Based Care

The patient needs to continue the anti-infective drugs as prescribed. An important nursing role is to reinforce, clarify, and provide information to the patient and family as needed.

Home Care Management. No special changes are needed in the home. If the home has a second story, the patient may prefer to stay on one floor for a few weeks, because stair climbing can be tiring. Toileting needs may be met by using a bedside commode if a bathroom is not located on the level the patient is using. Home care needs depend on the patient's level of fatigue, dyspnea, and family and social support.

CHART 31-4 Focused Assessment

The Patient Recovering from Pneumonia

Ask whether the patient has had any of these:	Assess the patient for:
• New-onset confusion	• Fever
• Chills	• Diaphoresis
• Fever	• Cyanosis, especially around the mouth or conjunctiva
• Persistent cough	• Dyspnea, tachypnea, or tachycardia
• Dyspnea	• Adventitious or abnormal breath sounds
• Wheezing	• Weakness
• Hemoptysis	
• Increased sputum production	
• Chest discomfort	
• Increasing fatigue	
• Any other symptoms that have failed to resolve	

The long recovery phase, especially in the older adult, can be frustrating. Fatigue, weakness, and a residual cough can last for weeks. Some patients fear they will never return to a "normal" level of functioning. Prepare them for the disease course, and offer reassurance that complete recovery will occur. After discharge, a home nursing assessment may be helpful (Chart 31-4).

Self-Management Education. Review all drugs with the patient and family, and emphasize completing anti-infective therapy. Teach the patient to notify the health care provider if chills, fever, persistent cough, dyspnea, wheezing, hemoptysis, increased sputum production, chest discomfort, or increasing fatigue recurs or fails to resolve. Instruct him or her to get plenty of rest and increase activity gradually.

An important aspect of education for the patient and family is the avoidance of upper respiratory tract INFECTIONS and viruses. Teach him or her to avoid crowds (especially in the fall and winter when viruses are prevalent), people who have a cold or flu, and exposure to irritants such as smoke. Stress the importance of following his or her health care provider's recommendations for vaccination against influenza and pneumonia. A balanced diet and adequate fluid intake are essential.

Health Care Resources. Inform patients who smoke that smoking is a risk factor for pneumonia. Provide them with information on local smoking-cessation classes and nicotine replacement options as required by The Joint Commission's NPSGs (see Chapter 27). Provide information booklets on pneumonia, and urge the patient who has not already been vaccinated against influenza or pneumonia to take this preventive measure after the pneumonia has resolved.

! NURSING SAFETY PRIORITY (QSEN)

Drug Alert

Warn the patient using nicotine patches or supplements of the danger of myocardial infarction if smoking is continued while using other forms of nicotine.

◆ Evaluation: Outcomes

Evaluate the care of the patient with pneumonia based on the identified priority patient problems. The expected outcomes are that he or she:

• Attains or maintains adequate GAS EXCHANGE
• Maintains patent airways
• Is free of the invading organism
• Returns to his or her pre-pneumonia health status

Specific indicators for these outcomes are listed for each priority patient problem under the Planning and Implementation section (see earlier).

❓ CLINICAL JUDGMENT CHALLENGE

Evidence-Based Practice; Patient-Centered Care QSEN

The nurse is caring for a frail, older patient in the hospital after surgery to repair a bowel obstruction. The patient has a nasogastric (NG) tube to suction, through which all her scheduled drugs are given, oxygen at 1 liter/nasal cannula at night (home order), an indwelling urinary catheter, and a saline lock. The patient is weak and fatigued, has pain not relieved by IV opioids, and is reluctant to participate in any activities.

1. What risk factors does this patient have for developing pneumonia?
2. What actions does the nurse take to decrease the patient's risk for pneumonia?
3. Two days later, the NG tube is removed and the patient is started on ice chips and other clear liquids. The patient swallows repeatedly when given sips of water. What action does the nurse perform?
4. The nurse does hourly rounds on the patient, and the patient's daughter states, "Something is just not right with mom." What action should the nurse take first? What other actions should the nurse perform?
5. The physician orders a chest x-ray, and the results show pneumonia. What actions by the nurse are most important?

SEVERE ACUTE RESPIRATORY SYNDROME (SARS)

Severe acute respiratory syndrome (SARS) is a respiratory infection first identified in China early in November 2002. The cause of SARS is a new virus from a family of virus types known as *coronaviruses*. This family of viruses causes many forms of the common cold. The new virus, known as *SARS Co-V,* is a mutated form of the coronavirus and is very virulent. It infects cells of the respiratory tract, triggering INFLAMMATION, and stays in the respiratory passageways rather than spreading into the blood.

The virus is easily spread by airborne droplets from infected people through sneezing, coughing, and talking. People at greatest risk for SARS are those in close direct contact with an infected person. The portals of entry are the mucous membranes of the eyes, nose, and mouth.

No new cases of SARS have been reported since 2004. There is no vaccination to prevent the disease, and no known effective treatment exists at this time. If such an outbreak were to occur, the same types of precautions used to prevent INFECTION spread for an avian influenza outbreak, discussed on p. 588, would be used. Patients diagnosed with or suspected of having SARS would be managed with supportive care under strict Airborne and Contact Precautions plus eye protection.

A disease similar in some respects to SARS, and also caused by a coronavirus *(MERS-CoV),* is MERS (Middle East respiratory syndrome). The first U.S. case of MERS, which originates in the Arabian peninsula, appeared in May 2014. Although SARS is considered more infectious, MERS has a higher mortality rate because patients progress to respiratory failure faster with MERS than with SARS, (Barclay, 2013; CDC, 2014d; Todd, 2014).

PULMONARY TUBERCULOSIS
❖ *PATHOPHYSIOLOGY*

Tuberculosis (TB) is a highly communicable disease caused by *Mycobacterium tuberculosis.* It is one of the most common bacterial INFECTIONS worldwide (CDC, 2014c). The organism is transmitted via **aerosolization** (i.e., an airborne route) (Fig. 31-2). When a person with active TB coughs, laughs, sneezes, whistles, or sings, droplets are airborne and may be inhaled by others. Far more people are infected with the bacillus than actually develop active TB.

The bacillus multiplies freely when it reaches a susceptible site (bronchi or alveoli). An exudative response occurs, causing pneumonitis. With the development of acquired immunity, further growth of bacilli is controlled in most initial lesions. These lesions usually resolve and leave little or no residual bacilli. Only a small percentage of people initially infected with the bacillus ever develop active TB.

Cell-mediated immunity develops 2 to 10 weeks after INFECTION and is manifested by a positive reaction to a tuberculin test. The primary infection may be so small that it does not appear on a chest x-ray. The process of infection occurs in this order:

1. The granulomatous INFLAMMATION created by the TB bacillus in the lung becomes surrounded by collagen, fibroblasts, and lymphocytes.

2. **Caseation necrosis,** which is necrotic tissue being turned into a granular mass, occurs in the center of the lesion. If this area shows on x-ray, it is the *primary* lesion.

Areas of caseation then undergo resorption, degeneration, and fibrosis. These necrotic areas may calcify (*calcification*) or liquefy (*liquefaction*). If liquefaction occurs, this material then empties into a bronchus and the evacuated area becomes a cavity (*cavitation*). Bacilli continue to grow in the necrotic cavity wall and spread via lymph channels into new areas of the lung.

A lesion also may progress by direct extension if bacilli multiply rapidly during INFLAMMATION. The lesions may extend through the pleura, resulting in pleural or pericardial effusion. **Miliary** or **hematogenous TB** is the spread of TB throughout the body when a large number of organisms enter the blood. Many tiny nodules scattered throughout the lung are seen on chest x-ray. Other body areas can become infected as a result of this spread.

Initial infection is seen more often in the middle or lower lobes of the lung. The local lymph nodes are infected and enlarged. An asymptomatic period usually follows the primary INFECTION and can last for years or decades before clinical symptoms develop. *An infected person is not infectious to others until manifestations of disease occur.*

Secondary TB is a reactivation of the disease in a previously infected person. It is more likely when defenses are lowered, such as with older adults and people with HIV disease. The upper lobes are the most common site of reactivation.

Etiology

M. tuberculosis is a slow-growing, acid-fast rod transmitted via the airborne route. People most often infected are those having repeated close contact with an infectious person who has not yet been diagnosed with TB. The risk for transmission is reduced after the infectious person has received proper drug therapy for 2 to 3 weeks, clinical improvement occurs, and acid-fast bacilli (AFB) in the sputum are reduced.

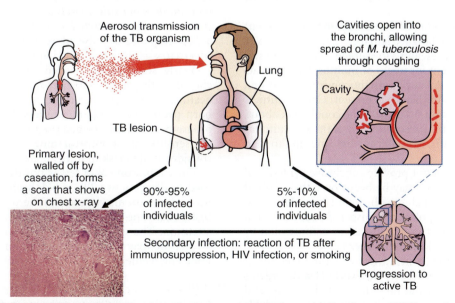

FIG. 31-2 Primary TB infection with progression to secondary infection and active disease. *HIV,* Human immune deficiency virus; *M. tuberculosis, Mycobacterium tuberculosis;* TB, tuberculosis.

Incidence and Prevalence

Worldwide, 8.7 million people were diagnosed and an additional 1.4 million people died from TB in 2012 (WHO, 2014b). The incidence of TB has been steadily decreasing in North America, although increases in incidence are seen in many other countries (ALA, 2010b). In North America, the people who are at greatest risk for development of TB are:

- Those in constant, frequent contact with an untreated person
- Those who have decreased immune function or HIV
- People who live in crowded areas such as long-term care facilities, prisons, homeless shelters, and mental health facilities
- Older homeless people
- Abusers of injection drugs or alcohol
- Lower socioeconomic groups
- Foreign immigrants (especially from Mexico, the Philippines, Vietnam, China, Japan, and Eastern Mediterranean countries [WHO, 2014b])

❖ PATIENT-CENTERED COLLABORATIVE CARE

◆ Assessment

Early detection of TB depends on subjective findings rather than on observable manifestations. TB has a slow onset, and patients are not aware of problems until the disease is advanced. *TB should be considered for any patient with a persistent cough or other manifestations compatible with TB, such as weight loss, anorexia, night sweats, hemoptysis, shortness of breath, fever, or chills.*

History. Assess the patient's past exposure to TB. Ask about his or her country of origin and travel to foreign countries where incidence of TB is high. It is important to ask about the results of any previous tests for TB. Also ask whether the patient has had bacille Calmette-Guérin (BCG) vaccine, which contains attenuated tubercle bacilli. *Anyone who has received BCG vaccine within the previous 10 years will have a positive skin test that can complicate interpretation* (Heavey, 2013). Usually the size of the skin response decreases each year after BCG vaccination. These patients should be evaluated for TB with a chest x-ray or the QuantiFERON-TB Gold test.

Physical Assessment/Clinical Manifestations. The patient with TB has progressive fatigue, lethargy, nausea, anorexia, weight loss, irregular menses, and a low-grade fever. Manifestations may have been present for weeks or months. Night sweats may occur with the fever. A cough with mucopurulent sputum, which may be streaked with blood, is present. Chest tightness and a dull, aching chest pain occur with the cough. Ask about, assess for, and document the presence of any of these manifestations to help with diagnosis, to establish a baseline, and to plan nursing interventions.

Chest examination does not provide conclusive evidence of TB. Dullness with percussion may be heard over the involved lung fields, as may bronchial breath sounds, crackles, and increased transmission of spoken or whispered sounds. Partial obstruction of a bronchus from the disease or compression by lymph nodes may produce localized wheezing.

Diagnostic Assessment. A new rapid test for tuberculosis has been developed and approved by the World Health Organization (2014b). This test is the fully automated nucleic acid amplification (NAA) test for tuberculosis. Results are available in less than 2 hours. Widespread use of this test is recommended

FIG. 31-3 Positive tuberculin skin test with induration.

by the CDC to replace other diagnostic methods for patients who are suspected to have TB.

Blood analysis by an enzyme-linked immunosorbent assay using the QuantiFERON-TB Gold (QFT-G) is a relatively rapid test for the presence of *M. tuberculosis*. Results are ready in 24 hours and are still used in acute care settings to determine whether a symptomatic patient has TB.

Sputum culture confirms the diagnosis. Enhanced TB cultures and automated mycobacterial cultures require 1 to 4 weeks to determine a positive or negative result. After drugs are started, sputum samples are obtained again to determine therapy effectiveness. Cultures are usually negative after 3 months of effective treatment.

The tuberculin test (Mantoux test) is the most commonly used reliable screening test of TB infection. A small amount (0.1 mL) of purified protein derivative (PPD) is placed intradermally in the forearm. An area of **induration** (localized swelling with hardness of soft tissue), not just redness, measuring 10 mm or greater in diameter 48 to 72 hours after injection indicates exposure to and possible INFECTION with TB (Fig. 31-3). If possible, the site is re-evaluated after 72 hours because the incidence of false-negative readings is greater at 48 hours. *A positive reaction does not mean that active disease is present but indicates exposure to TB or the presence of inactive (dormant) disease.* A reaction of 5 mm or greater is considered positive in people with HIV infection. *A reduced skin reaction or a negative skin test does not rule out TB disease or infection of the very old or anyone who is severely immunocompromised.* Failure to have a skin response because of reduced immune function when INFECTION is present is called **anergy**.

Yearly screening is needed for anyone who comes into contact with people who may be infected with TB, including health care workers. Screening is very important for foreign-born people and migrant workers. Participation in screening programs is enhanced when programs are delivered in a culturally sensitive and nonthreatening manner. Urge anyone who is considered high risk to have an annual TB screening test.

Once a person's skin test is positive for TB, a chest x-ray is used to detect active TB or old, healed lesions. Caseation and INFLAMMATION may be seen on the x-ray if the disease is active. Instruct anyone who has manifestations of TB to seek medical attention. The chest x-rays of HIV-infected patients may be normal or may show infiltrates in any lung zone and lymph node enlargement.

◆ Interventions

Combination drug therapy is the most effective method of treating TB and preventing transmission. Active TB is treated with

CHART 31-5 Common Examples of Drug Therapy

First-Line Treatment for Tuberculosis

DRUG/USUAL DOSAGE	PURPOSE/ACTION	NURSING INTERVENTIONS	RATIONALES
Isoniazid (INH) 200-300 mg orally daily or 600-900 mg orally twice each week	Kills actively growing mycobacteria outside the cell and inhibits the growth of dormant bacteria inside macrophages and caseating granulomas.	Teach the patient to take the drug on an empty stomach (1 hour before or 2 hours after meals) and to avoid antacids. Teach the patient to take a daily multiple vitamin that contains the B-complex vitamins while on this drug. Remind the patient to avoid drinking alcoholic beverages while on this drug. Teach the patient to report darkening of the urine, a yellow appearance to the skin or whites of the eyes, and an increased tendency to bruise or bleed.	Food and antacids slow or prevent absorption of the drug from the GI tract. Drug can deplete the body of this vitamin. The drug can cause liver damage. This effect is potentiated by alcohol. These manifestations may indicate liver toxicity or failure.
Rifampin (RIF) 500-600 mg orally daily or twice each week	Kills slower-growing organisms, even those that reside in macrophages and caseating granulomas.	Teach the patient to expect the drug to stain the skin and urine and expect all other secretions to have a reddish orange tinge; also, soft contact lenses will become permanently stained. Teach women using oral contraceptives to use an additional method of contraception while taking this drug and for 1 month after stopping the drug. Remind the patient to avoid drinking alcoholic beverages while on this drug. Teach the patient to report darkening of the urine, a yellow appearance to the skin or whites of the eyes, and an increased tendency to bruise or bleed. Ask the patient about all other drugs in use.	This is an expected and harmless side effect of the drug and will clear some time after the patient stops taking the drug. This drug reduces the effectiveness of oral contraceptives, increasing the risk for an unplanned pregnancy. The drug can cause liver damage. This effect is potentiated by alcohol. These manifestations may indicate liver toxicity or failure. This drug interacts with many drugs.
Pyrazinamide (PZA) 1000-2000 mg orally daily or 3000-6000 mg orally twice each week	Is not inactivated by the acidic environment of macrophages and can effectively kill organisms residing within them.	Ask whether the patient has ever had gout. Teach the patient to drink at least 8 ounces of water when taking this tablet and to increase fluid intake. Teach the patient to wear protective clothing, a hat, and sunscreen when going outdoors in the sunlight. Remind the patient to avoid drinking alcoholic beverages while on this drug. Teach the patient to report darkening of the urine, a yellow appearance to the skin or whites of the eyes, and an increased tendency to bruise or bleed.	This drug increases uric acid formation and will make gout worse. More fluids help prevent uric acid from precipitating and causing gout or kidney problems. The drug causes photosensitivity and greatly increases the risk for sunburn. The drug can cause liver damage. This effect is potentiated by alcohol. These manifestations may indicate liver toxicity or failure.
Ethambutol (EMB) 750-1500 mg orally daily or 2500-5000 mg orally twice each week	Inhibits bacterial RNA synthesis, thus suppressing bacterial growth. It is slow-acting and is bacteriostatic rather than bactericidal. Thus it must be used in combination with other anti-TB drugs.	Remind the patient to avoid drinking alcoholic beverages while on this drug. Teach the patient to report any changes in vision, such as reduced color vision, blurred vision, or reduced visual fields, immediately to his or her health care provider. Ask whether the patient has ever had gout. Teach the patient to drink at least 8 ounces of water when taking this tablet and to increase fluid intake.	The drug induces severe nausea and vomiting when alcohol is ingested. The drug can cause optic neuritis, especially at high doses, and can lead to blindness. When the problem is discovered early, the eye problems are usually reversed when the drug is stopped. This drug increases uric acid formation and will make gout worse. More fluids help prevent uric acid from precipitating and causing gout or kidney problems.

RNA, Ribonucleic acid.

a combination of drugs to which the organism is sensitive. Therapy continues until the disease is under control. The use of multiple-drug regimens destroys organisms as quickly as possible and reduces the emergence of drug-resistant organisms. First-line therapy uses isoniazid (INH) and rifampin (Rifadin) throughout the therapy; pyrazinamide is added for the first 2 months (Chart 31-5). This protocol shortens the therapy from 6 to 12 months to 6 months. Ethambutol (Myambutol) is the recommended fourth drug in first-line therapy. These drugs are now available in two-drug or three-drug combinations. One example is Rifater, which combines isoniazid, pyrazinamide, and rifampin. Variations of the first-line drugs along with other drug types are used when the patient does not tolerate the standard first-line therapy. Nursing interventions focus on patient teaching for drug therapy adherence and INFECTION control.

Strict adherence to the prescribed drug regimen is crucial for suppressing the disease. Thus your major role is teaching the patient about drug therapy and stressing the importance of taking each drug regularly, exactly as prescribed, for as long as it is prescribed. Provide accurate information in multiple formats, such as pamphlets, videos, and drug-schedule worksheets. To determine whether the patient understands how to take the drugs, ask him or her to describe the treatment regimen, side effects, and when to call the health care agency and physician.

! NURSING SAFETY PRIORITY (QSEN)
Drug Alert

The first-line drugs used as therapy for tuberculosis all can damage the liver. Warn the patient to not drink any alcoholic beverages for the entire duration of TB therapy. (Duration of therapy is usually 6 months but can be as long as 2 years for multidrug-resistant [MDR] TB.)

The TB drugs may cause the patient to have nausea. Teach him or her to prevent nausea by taking the daily dose at bedtime. Antiemetics may also prevent this problem. Instruct him or her to eat a well-balanced diet that includes foods that are rich in iron, protein, and vitamins C and B. Collaborate with the registered dietitian for specialized needs.

The patient with TB has reduced physical stamina and also has concerns about the disease prognosis. Offer a positive outlook for the patient who adheres to the drug regimen. Tell him or her that fatigue will diminish as the treatment progresses. *With current resistant strains of TB, however, emphasize that not taking the drugs as prescribed could lead to an infection that is drug resistant.*

Some *multidrug-resistant TB* (MDR TB) strains are emerging as extensively drug-resistant (XDR TB). MDR TB is an INFECTION that resists INH and rifampin. XDR TB is resistant not only to the first-line anti-tuberculosis drugs but also to the second-line antibiotics, including the fluoroquinolones and at least one of the aminoglycosides. In 2011, there were over 690,000 cases of MDR TB worldwide with 9% being XDR TB. The most common cause of MDR TB and XDR TB is mismanagement of drug therapy, either from inappropriate selection or use of antibiotics (WHO, 2013). Patients with acquired immune deficiency syndrome (AIDS) also often have MDR TB (CDC, 2013a). Drug therapy for MDR TB and XDR TB is more limited than standard first-line therapy and requires higher doses for longer periods. A new drug combination of bedaquiline, pyrazinamide, and moxifloxacin (Sirturo) was approved in 2012 to treat multidrug-resistant TB. Another drug, delaminid (OPC-67683), is in clinical trials (Gler et al., 2012).

! NURSING SAFETY PRIORITY (QSEN)
Action Alert

Warn patients with extensively drug-resistant TB that absolute adherence to therapy is critical for survival and cure of the disease. These patients should receive directly observed therapy (DOT).

When teaching the patient and family with either MDR TB or XDR TB, stress that it is the organism, not the patient, that is drug resistant. So a person who acquires the INFECTION and develops TB from a person who is infected with a resistant strain of bacillus will also have drug-resistant disease. Thus teaching infection control strategies is a priority and should be constantly reinforced.

? NCLEX EXAMINATION CHALLENGE
Health Promotion and Maintenance

A client has been admitted to the hospital with suspected TB. What drugs should the nurse plan to teach the client about before discharge? **Select all that apply.**
A. Rifampin (Rifadin); contact lenses can become stained orange
B. Isoniazid (INH); report yellowing of the skin or darkened urine
C. Pyrazinamide (PZA); maintain a fluid restriction of 1200 mL/day
D. Ethambutol (Myambutol); report any changes in vision
E. Amoxicillin (Amoxil); take this drug with food or milk

Other care issues for the patient with TB include teaching about INFECTION prevention and what to expect about disease monitoring and participating in activities. TB is often treated outside the acute care setting, with the patient convalescing in the home setting. Airborne Precautions are not necessary in this setting because family members have already been exposed; however, all members of the household need to undergo TB testing. Teach the patient to cover the mouth and nose with a tissue when coughing or sneezing, to place used tissues in plastic bags, and to wear a mask when in contact with crowds until the drugs suppress infection.

Tell the patient that sputum specimens are needed usually every 2 to 4 weeks once drug therapy is initiated. When the results of three consecutive sputum cultures are negative, the patient is no longer infectious and may return to former employment. Remind him or her to avoid exposure to any inhalation irritants because these can cause further lung damage.

The hospitalized patient with active TB is placed on Airborne Precautions (see Chapter 23) in a well-ventilated room that has at least six exchanges of fresh air per minute. All health care workers must use a personal respirator when caring for the patient. When hand and clothing contamination is a risk, use Standard Precautions with appropriate contact protection (i.e., gowns and gloves). In accordance with The Joint Commission's NPSGs, perform handwashing before and after patient care. Precautions are discontinued when the patient is no longer infectious.

Community-Based Care

Home Care Management. Most patients with TB are managed outside the hospital; however, patients may be diagnosed with TB while in the hospital for another problem. Discharge may be delayed if the living situation is high risk or if nonadherence is likely. Collaborate with the case manager or social service worker in the hospital or the community health nursing agency to ensure that the patient is discharged to the appropriate environment with continued supervision.

Self-Management Education. Teach the patient to follow the drug regimen exactly as prescribed and always to have a supply on hand. Teach about side effects and ways of reducing them to promote adherence. Remind him or her that the disease is usually no longer contagious after drugs have been taken for 2 to 3 consecutive weeks and clinical improvement is seen; however, *he or she must continue with the prescribed drugs for 6 months or longer as prescribed.* **Directly observed therapy (DOT),** in which a health care professional watches the patient swallow the drugs, may be indicated in some situations. This practice leads to more treatment successes, fewer relapses, and less drug resistance.

The patient who has weight loss and severe lethargy should gradually resume usual activities. Proper nutrition is needed to prevent INFECTION recurrence.

To help with concerns about the contagious aspect of the INFECTION, provide the patient with information about TB. A key to preventing transmission is identifying those in close contact with the infected person so that they can be tested and treated if needed. Identified contacts are assessed with a TB test and possibly a chest x-ray to determine infection status. Multi-drug therapy may be indicated as a preventive strategy for heavily exposed individuals or for those who have other health problems that reduce the immune response.

Health Care Resources. Teach the patient to receive follow-up care by a health care provider for at least 1 year during and after active treatment. The American Lung Association (ALA) can provide free information to the patient about the disease and its treatment. In addition, Alcoholics Anonymous (AA) and other health care resources for patients with alcoholism are available if needed. Assist the patient who uses illicit drugs to locate a drug treatment program. In accordance with The Joint Commission's NPSGs, urge smokers to quit, and assist them in finding an appropriate smoking-cessation program (see Chapter 27).

LUNG ABSCESS

A lung abscess is a localized area of subacute INFECTION and necrosis, which is usually related to pyogenic bacteria, and occurs most often in the lung parenchyma. Patients with an abscess often have a history of pneumonia, aspiration of stomach contents, or obstruction as a result of a tumor or foreign body. Other causes of aspiration leading to lung abscesses include any condition that alters the ability to swallow, such as alcoholic blackouts, seizure disorders, neurologic deficits, and swallowing disorders. Bronchial obstruction may cause a necrotizing process in the lung that eventually becomes an abscess (Kamanger, 2013).

Multiple abscesses and cavities form in patients with tuberculosis (TB) or fungal INFECTIONS of the lung. Immunosuppressed patients, such as those receiving cancer chemotherapy or those with AIDS, are at high risk for fungal infections.

Ask the patient about any recent history of influenza, pneumonia, febrile illness, cough, and foul-smelling sputum production. Ask about the sputum color and odor and about any **pleuritic chest pain** (a stabbing pain upon taking a deep breath). Often the patient is febrile, pale, fatigued, and cachectic. Auscultation may reveal decreased breath sounds and dullness on percussion in the involved area. Bronchial breath sounds and crackles may be heard over the site of the lesion. A chest x-ray, sputum sample, and CBC are needed for diagnosis. TB testing should be considered for patients at risk for or with this problem (Zwanger, 2013).

Problems and interventions for the patient with pneumonia also apply to the patient with a lung abscess. Management involves a long course of antibiotics that target organisms acquired by aspiration (Zwanger, 2013).

PULMONARY EMPYEMA

Pulmonary empyema is a collection of pus in the pleural space most commonly caused by pulmonary INFECTION, lung abscess, or infected pleural effusion (Zwanger, 2013). Infections in other body areas also can spread to the lungs by flow of infected lymph into the pleural space. Chest surgery or trauma can introduce bacteria directly into the pleural space, leading to empyema. Blood from trauma may collect in the pleural space, promoting INFECTION.

History findings include febrile illness, pneumonia, chest pain, dyspnea, cough, and trauma. Document the character of the sputum. Chest wall motion may be reduced. If a pleural effusion is present, fremitus may be reduced or absent, percussion is flat, and breath sounds are decreased. Abnormal breath sounds, including bronchial breath sounds, egophony, and whispered pectoriloquy, also may be present. Often the patient has a fever, chills, night sweats, and weight loss.

A chest x-ray or CT scan and a sample of the pleural fluid (obtained via thoracentesis) are needed for diagnosis. Empyema fluid is thick, opaque, exudative, and foul smelling. The fluid is analyzed for color, red blood cell (RBC) count, white blood cell (WBC) count, glucose and protein levels, lactate dehydrogenase (LDH), and pH. Gram stains, acid-fast stains, culture and sensitivity, and cytology studies are also performed.

Therapy involves emptying the empyema cavity, re-expanding the lung, and controlling the INFECTION. Appropriate antibiotics are prescribed. A chest tube(s) to closed-chest drainage is used to promote lung expansion and drainage. The tube is removed when the lung is fully expanded and the infection is under control. Chest surgery may be needed for thick pus or excessive pleural thickening. Nursing interventions are similar to those for patients with a pleural effusion, pneumothorax, or infection. Chapters 30 and 32 discuss these interventions in more detail.

INHALATION ANTHRAX

❖ *PATHOPHYSIOLOGY*

Inhalation anthrax (respiratory anthrax) is a bacterial INFECTION caused by the gram-positive organism *Bacillus anthracis*, which lives as a spore in soil where grass-eating animals live and graze. Most cases of anthrax are on the skin (cutaneous). Inhalation anthrax accounts for only about 5% of cases, and GI anthrax accounts for about 1% of cases of the disease. When infection occurs through the lungs, the disease is nearly 100% fatal without treatment (Cunha, 2014). Inhalation anthrax is a rare natural occurrence in North America and is not spread by person-to-person contact. It is an occupational hazard of veterinarians, farmers, taxidermists, and others who come into frequent contact with animal wool, hides, bone meal, and skin (Cunha, 2014).

> **⚠ NURSING SAFETY PRIORITY** (QSEN)
> *Action Alert*
>
> Because inhalation anthrax is so rare, any occurrence in a person who does not have an occupational risk is considered an intentional act of bioterrorism. Report the presence of manifestations consistent with inhalation anthrax to hospital authorities immediately.

This organism first forms a spore—an encapsulated organism that is inactive. When many spores are inhaled deeply into the lungs, macrophages engulf them. Once inside the macrophage, the organism leaves its capsule and replicates. The active bacteria produce several toxins that are released into the infected

CHART 31-6   Key Features

Inhalation Anthrax

Prodromal Stage (Early)	Fulminant Stage (Late)
• Fever	• Sudden onset of breathlessness
• Fatigue	• Dyspnea
• Mild chest pain	• Diaphoresis
• Dry cough	• Stridor on inhalation and
• No manifestations of upper	exhalation
respiratory infection	• Hypoxia
• Mediastinal "widening" on	• High fever
chest x-ray	• Mediastinitis
	• Pleural effusion
	• Hypotension
	• Septic shock

CHART 31-7   Common Examples of Drug Therapy

Prophylaxis and Treatment of Inhalation Anthrax

PROPHYLAXIS	TREATMENT
Ciprofloxacin (Cipro) 500 mg orally twice daily	Ciprofloxacin (Cipro IV) 400 mg IV every 12 hr
Or	*Or*
Doxycycline (Vibramycin) 100 mg orally twice daily	Doxycycline (Doxy 100) 100 mg IV every 12 hr
Or *(if organism is proven susceptible to penicillin)*	**Plus** *one or two of the following secondary agents (parenteral form (IV); dosage based on patient's weight and age):*
Amoxicillin (Amoxil, Trimox) 500 mg orally every 8 hr or 875 mg orally twice daily	Rifampin (RIF) Clindamycin (Cleocin) Vancomycin (Vancocin, Vancoled)
Prophylaxis must continue for 60 days (or longer if exposure was heavy).	**Treatment with IV drugs continues for at least 7 days. When the response is good and the patient improves, IV drugs are changed to oral agents and are continued for at least 60 days.**

tissues and the blood that make the INFECTION worse. Massive edema occurs along with hemorrhage and destruction of lung cells. Infected macrophages carry the organisms to the lymph nodes, and the organism spreads rapidly, causing bacteremia, sepsis, and meningitis. Lethal toxins produced by the bacteria are the most common cause of death (Cunha, 2014).

❖ **PATIENT-CENTERED COLLABORATIVE CARE**

Inhalation anthrax is a two-stage illness—prodromal and fulminant. Manifestations may not begin until as long as 8 weeks after exposure to the organism (Chart 31-6).

The prodromal stage is early and difficult to distinguish from influenza or pneumonia. Manifestations include low-grade fever, fatigue, mild chest pain, and a dry, harsh cough. *A special feature of inhalation anthrax is that it is **not** accompanied by upper respiratory manifestations of sore throat or rhinitis.* Usually the patient starts to feel better and manifestations improve in 2 to 4 days.

If the patient begins appropriate antibiotic therapy at this stage, the likelihood of survival is high. Diagnostic indicators are positive Gram stain of the serum and a mediastinal "widening" on chest x-ray as the local lymph nodes greatly enlarge. After several days, blood cultures may be positive for the organism and the genetic material of the bacteria may be detected through the amplification process of the polymerase chain reaction (PCR). Positive results for these definitive diagnostic tests may not be evident until the disease has progressed to the fulminant stage.

The fulminant stage begins after the patient feels a little better. Usually there is a sudden onset of severe illness, including respiratory distress, hematemesis (bloody vomit), dyspnea, diaphoresis, stridor, chest pain, and cyanosis. The patient has a high fever. Hemorrhagic mediastinitis and pleural effusions develop. The patient may be admitted with a decreased level of consciousness or frank shock. As the disease spreads through the blood, causing septic shock and hemorrhagic meningitis, death often occurs within 24 to 36 hours even if antibiotics are started in this stage (Cunha, 2014).

The naturally occurring organism is sensitive to common antibiotics; however, organisms grown for bioterrorism may have been altered to be resistant to these antibiotics. Therefore the antibiotics used for suspected or diagnosed inhalation anthrax include combination therapy (Chart 31-7). The same drugs are used for prophylaxis when people have been exposed to inhalation anthrax but do not yet have manifestations. A vaccine is available, but distribution is limited.

Teach patients with any type of lower respiratory INFECTION to be especially vigilant for changes after they think they are getting well. They need to seek medical attention immediately upon having a setback that starts with breathlessness.

PERTUSSIS

Pertussis is a respiratory INFECTION caused by the bacterium *Bordetella pertussis.* It is highly contagious and spreads easily from person to person via respiratory droplets. Once considered a childhood disease, a resurgence is occurring in adults, perhaps due to waning vaccination effectiveness (Bocka, 2014; CDC, 2012). In 2010, there were 27,550 new cases in the United States (CDC, 2012).

The disease occurs in three distinct phases. During the first *(catarrhal)* phase, the patient has manifestations resembling the common cold, including a mild cough. After 1 to 2 weeks, the *paroxysmal* stage begins and the patient has severe coughing "fits" lasting several minutes, during which the coughing spasms are accompanied by turning red and/or vomiting. The patient is frequently exhausted by the coughing. The distinct "whooping" sound common in children at the end of a cough may not be present in adults. This stage can last up to 10 weeks. The recovery *(convalescent)* stage can last for months. During the course of the disease, there is a bloody, purulent, mucinous exudate in the small airways that can lead to atelectasis and pneumonia (Bocka, 2014; Schweon, 2011).

The diagnosis of pertussis can be made clinically, but sputum cultures (obtained by deep suctioning) and PCR laboratory testing are available to aid the diagnosis. Blood cultures will be negative. The CDC recommends testing for anyone who has a cough lasting longer than 3 weeks (Bocka, 2014).

COCCIDIOIDOMYCOSIS

Coccidioidomycosis is a fungal INFECTION caused by the *Coccidioides* organism that is common in the desert southwest regions of the United States, Mexico, and Central and South

America. It is also known as "valley fever," and the incidence is on the rise. The organism is present in the soil as inactive and non-reproducing microfilaments. When the soil is disturbed by excavation or dust storms, the microfilaments become airborne. As the microfilaments are inhaled, they change into the reproductively active spore form of the organism, which can lead to development of an actual pulmonary infection within 1 to 4 weeks after exposure (Buhrow, 2013).

Manifestations of the infection resemble other respiratory viral or bacterial infections with fever, cough, headache, muscle aches, chest pain, and night sweats. The presence of bone and joint pain indicates more severe infection. Often the disorder is misdiagnosed and mistreated as influenza or pneumonia. Neither antibacterial drugs nor antiviral drugs are effective in managing this infection. The disease can become widespread and cause manifestations of hemoptysis, meningitis, and involvement of the skin, adrenal glands, liver, and spleen. It also can become chronic and debilitating with low-grade fever, weight loss, fatigue, chronic cough, and chest pain.

Depending on the health of the infected person and the number of spores present in the respiratory tract, the resulting infection can be mild, moderate, severe, or widely disseminated. Most younger healthy people recover from the infection without treatment. For moderate infection, oral therapy with antifungal agents from the azole class (e.g., fluconazole [Diflucan], ketoconazole [Nizoral], voriconazole [Vfend]) is needed. For those with severe disease or women who are pregnant, IV amphotericin B may be needed. Because the infection is not spread from person to person, Isolation Precautions are not required.

In endemic areas, people working in the soil, such as farm workers or construction workers, are at highest risk for the infection. Older adults and anyone who has reduced immune competence, as well as pregnant women, also are at increased risk for developing more severe disease. Because the areas that naturally harbor this organism are often winter vacation destinations, always ask anyone with respiratory infection manifestations whether they have visited endemic regions so that the possibility of coccidioidomycosis is considered.

NURSING CONCEPTS AND CLINICAL JUDGMENT REVIEW

What might you NOTICE if the patient is experiencing inadequate GAS EXCHANGE and oxygenation as a result of a respiratory INFECTION?

- Respirations rapid and shallow
- Decreased oxygen saturation by pulse oximetry
- Tachycardia
- Skin cyanosis or pallor (in lighter-skinned patients)
- Cyanosis or pallor of the lips and oral mucous membranes (in patients of any skin color)
- Patient appears to work hard to breathe
- Patient is restless, anxious, or confused

What should you INTERPRET and how should you RESPOND to a patient experiencing inadequate GAS EXCHANGE and oxygenation as a result of a respiratory INFECTION?

Perform and interpret physical assessment, including:
- Taking vital signs
- Monitoring oxygen saturation by pulse oximetry
- Auscultating all lung fields
- Checking the accuracy of pulse oximetry readings
- Assessing cognition
- Assessing for the presence and characteristics of sputum production
- Assessing the patient's ability to cough and clear the airway

Interpret laboratory values:
- Elevated white blood cell count
- Arterial blood gas values: pH lower than 7.35, HCO_3^- at or below 24 mEq/L, $Paco_2$ at or below 45 mm Hg; Pao_2 below 90 mm Hg; serum lactate levels above 8 mg/dL

Respond by:
- Administering oxygen
- Assisting the patient to an upright position, with arms resting on a table or armrests
- Prioritizing and pacing activities to prevent fatigue
- Administering prescribed IV, oral, or inhaled drugs
- Ensuring respiratory therapy treatments are administered
- Re-assessing respiratory status after respiratory therapy treatment
- Ensuring a fluid intake of at least 2 liters per day (unless contraindicated)

On what should you REFLECT?
- Observe patient for evidence of improved gas exchange and oxygenation (see Chapter 27).
- Think about what patient teaching focus could help reduce the occurrence of a respiratory infection in the future.

GET READY FOR THE NCLEX® EXAMINATION!

KEY POINTS

Review these Key Points for each NCLEX Examination Client Needs Category.

Safe and Effective Care Environment
- Limit transmission of respiratory INFECTION spread by washing hands after blowing the nose or using a tissue. Safety QSEN

- Receive a yearly influenza vaccination because you are more likely to care for infected people and because you could spread influenza to people who are immunocompromised. Safety QSEN
- Use Airborne Precautions and Isolation Precautions for any patient who has TB manifestations until proven otherwise. Safety QSEN

- If possible, place the patient with a respiratory INFECTION in a private room. **Safety** QSEN
- Keep the door to the room of any patient with a respiratory INFECTION closed until the cause of the infection is identified. **Safety** QSEN

Health Promotion and Maintenance
- Teach everyone the "etiquette" of sneezing or coughing into the upper sleeve rather than the hand when a tissue is not available. **Evidence-Based Practice** QSEN
- Urge all adults older than 50 years, anyone who has a chronic respiratory problem, anyone who is immunocompromised, and anyone who lives with a person who is older or immunocompromised or has a chronic respiratory disease to receive the pneumonia vaccine and yearly influenza vaccinations. **Evidence-Based Practice** QSEN
- Urge patients to complete the anti-infective drug therapy course for any respiratory INFECTION. **Patient-Centered Care** QSEN
- Urge all people to quit smoking or using tobacco in any form. **Patient-Centered Care** QSEN
- Teach people living with patients who have TB to ensure good ventilation of the home with open windows whenever possible.
- Educate the family and the patient with tuberculosis who lives at home about the side effects of anti-tuberculosis (TB) therapy and when to notify the health care provider. **Patient-Centered Care** QSEN
- Teach all people to be prepared for an emergency or disaster by having sufficient food, water, and prescribed drugs for at least 2 weeks (see Chapter 10). **Patient-Centered Care** QSEN
- Teach all people to follow community INFECTION containment procedures if there is a possible outbreak of any pandemic influenza virus. **Patient-Centered Care** QSEN

Psychosocial Integrity
- Assess older patients with acute confusion for pneumonia (cough and fever may not be present).
- Assure the family of an older adult patient with pneumonia who is confused that the new-onset confusion is temporary. **Patient-Centered Care** QSEN

- Teach people who may be afraid of contracting inhalation anthrax that this disease is not transmitted by person-to-person contact. **Patient-Centered Care** QSEN
- Inform patients who have a positive TB test that far more people are infected with the bacillus than have active TB disease. Assess the likelihood of adherence to the drug regimen for patients with TB. **Patient-Centered Care** QSEN
- Identify patients who may require a directly observed therapy (DOT) program in which they must be directly observed by a health care professional while swallowing the drug. **Safety** QSEN

Physiological Integrity
- Assess the respiratory status of anyone suspected of having a respiratory INFECTION by taking vital signs, noting color of nail beds and mucous membranes, measuring oxygen saturation, determining ease of ventilation, determining cognition, and auscultating lung fields. **Evidence-Based Practice** QSEN
- Administer humidified oxygen therapy to patients with inadequate GAS EXCHANGE and hypoxemia. **Evidence-Based Practice** QSEN
- Assess the skin under and around a facemask or nasal cannula for evidence of skin breakdown at least every 8 hours. **Patient-Centered Care** QSEN
- Ask any patient with a respiratory INFECTION if he or she is from a foreign country or has recently visited a foreign country. Ask patients from other countries whether they have had BCG as a vaccination against TB. For patients who have had BCG, the PPD skin test is a less reliable indicator of TB. **Safety** QSEN
- Assess the patient receiving first-line drug therapy for TB for any manifestation of liver impairment (dark urine, clay-colored stools, anorexia, jaundiced sclera or hard palate). **Patient-Centered Care** QSEN
- Teach women taking rifampin or rifapentine as drug therapy for TB that these drugs reduce the effectiveness of oral contraceptives and that an additional form of birth control should be used while on this therapy. **Patient-Centered Care** QSEN

CHAPTER 32

Care of Critically Ill Patients with Respiratory Problems

Meg Blair

PRIORITY CONCEPTS

- GAS EXCHANGE
- PERFUSION
- CLOTTING

LEARNING OUTCOMES

Safe and Effective Care Environment

1. Protect the critically ill patient with respiratory problems from injury, infection, and bleeding.
2. Ensure safe management of endotracheal tubes, tracheostomy tubes, and mechanical ventilators.

Health Promotion and Maintenance

3. Teach people at risk for pulmonary embolism techniques to reduce the risk.
4. Teach patients and family members how to avoid injury during therapy to reduce CLOTTING.

Psychosocial Integrity

5. Reduce the psychological impact for the patient and family experiencing a serious respiratory problem.

Physiological Integrity

6. Assess the respiratory status of any patient who develops sudden-onset respiratory difficulty or acute confusion.
7. Use laboratory data and clinical manifestations to evaluate the adequacy of GAS EXCHANGE with oxygenation and ventilatory interventions.
8. Prioritize nursing care for the patient experiencing a serious or critical respiratory disorder or event.
9. Work with other members of the health care team to coordinate care for the patient being mechanically ventilated.

Any respiratory problem can interfere with GAS EXCHANGE, oxygenation, and tissue PERFUSION, progressing to an emergency and death, even with prompt treatment. These problems may overwhelm the adaptive responses of the cardiac and blood oxygen delivery systems (Fig. 32-1). *Thus prompt recognition and interventions are needed to prevent serious complications and death.*

An acute injury or problem that results in severe respiratory impairment can occur at any age. Older adults, however, are more at risk for developing critical respiratory problems. The patient who is short of breath is also anxious and fearful. Be prepared to manage both the physical and emotional needs of the patient during any respiratory emergency.

PULMONARY EMBOLISM

❖ PATHOPHYSIOLOGY

A pulmonary embolism (PE) is a collection of particulate matter (solids, liquids, or air) that enters venous circulation and lodges in the pulmonary vessels. Large emboli obstruct pulmonary blood flow, leading to reduced GAS EXCHANGE, reduced oxygenation, pulmonary tissue hypoxia, decreased PERFUSION, and potential death. Any substance can cause an embolism, but a blood clot is the most common (McCance et al., 2014). PE is common and may account for as many as 100,000 deaths each year in the United States (Smithburger et al., 2013). It may be the most common preventable death in hospitalized patients but is often misdiagnosed, and patients at risk may not be provided the appropriate preventive measures (Duff et al., 2013; Hussey, 2013).

Most often, a PE occurs when inappropriate blood CLOTTING forms a venous thromboembolism (VTE) (also known as a *deep vein thrombosis* [DVT]) in a vein in the legs or the pelvis and a clot breaks off and travels through the vena cava into the right side of the heart. The clot then lodges in the pulmonary artery or within one or more of its branches. Platelets collect on the embolus, triggering the release of substances that cause blood vessel constriction. Widespread pulmonary vessel constriction and pulmonary hypertension impair GAS EXCHANGE and tissue PERFUSION. Deoxygenated blood moves into arterial circulation, causing hypoxemia (low arterial blood oxygen level), although some patients with PE do *not* have hypoxemia.

NORMAL BALANCE OF TISSUE OXYGEN NEEDS
WITH OXYGEN INTAKE AND OXYGEN DELIVERY

FIG. 32-1 Rapid-onset acute respiratory problems overwhelm the ability of the cardiac oxygen delivery system to adapt and restore balance. The red blood cell (RBC) oxygen delivery system cannot begin to adapt to the acute respiratory problem.

Major risk factors for VTE leading to PE are:
- Prolonged immobility
- Central venous catheters
- Surgery
- Obesity
- Advancing age
- Conditions that increase blood CLOTTING
- History of thromboembolism

Smoking, pregnancy, estrogen therapy, heart failure, stroke, cancer (particularly lung or prostate), and trauma increase the risk for VTE and PE (Hussey, 2013).

Fat, oil, air, tumor cells, amniotic fluid and fetal debris, foreign objects (e.g., broken IV catheters), injected particles, and infected clots can enter a vein and cause PE. Fat emboli from fracture of a long bone and oil emboli from diagnostic procedures do not impede lung blood flow; instead, they injure blood vessels and cause acute respiratory distress syndrome (ARDS) (Powers & Talbot, 2011). Septic clots often arise from a pelvic abscess, an infected IV catheter, and injections of illegal drugs. The effects of sepsis are more serious than the venous blockage.

Health Promotion and Maintenance

Although pulmonary embolism (PE) can occur in healthy people without warning, it occurs more often in some situations. Thus prevention of conditions that lead to PE is a major nursing concern. Preventive actions for PE are those that also prevent venous stasis and VTE. Best nursing practices for PE prevention are outlined in Chart 32-1. Also see Chapter 14 for more information about core measures during the surgical experience for VTE prevention.

Lifestyle changes can help reduce the risk for PE. Tobacco use narrows blood vessels and increases the risk for clot formation. Hormone-based contraceptives also increase blood

---

CHART 32-1 **Best Practice for Patient Safety & Quality Care** QSEN

Prevention of Pulmonary Embolism

- Start passive and active range-of-motion exercises for the extremities of immobilized and postoperative patients.
- Ambulate patients soon after surgery.
- Use antiembolism and pneumatic compression stockings and devices after surgery.
- Evaluate patient for criteria indicating the need for anticoagulant therapy.
- Avoid the use of tight garters, girdles, and constricting clothing.
- Prevent pressure under the popliteal space (e.g., do not place a pillow under the knee, use alternating pressure mattress).
- Perform a comprehensive assessment of peripheral circulation.
- Elevate the affected limb 20 degrees or more above the level of the heart to improve venous return, as appropriate.
- Change patient position every 2 hours, or ambulate as tolerated.
- Prevent injury to the vessel lumen by preventing local pressure, trauma, infection, or sepsis.
- Refrain from massaging leg muscles.
- Instruct patient not to cross legs.
- Administer prescribed prophylactic low-dose anticoagulant and anti-platelet drugs.
- Teach the patient to avoid activities that result in the Valsalva maneuver (e.g., breath-holding, bearing down for bowel movements, coughing).
- Administer prescribed drugs, such as stool softeners, that will prevent episodes of the Valsalva maneuver.
- Teach the patient and family about precautions.
- Encourage smoking cessation.

CLOTTING. Urge patients to stop smoking cigarettes, especially women who use hormone-based contraceptives. Reducing weight and becoming more physically active can reduce risk for PE. Teach patients who are traveling for long periods to drink plenty of water, change positions often, avoid crossing their legs, and get up from the sitting position at least 5 minutes out of every hour to prevent stasis and clot formation.

For patients known to be at risk for PE, small doses of heparin or low–molecular-weight heparin (enoxaparin [Lovenox]), an indirect thrombin inhibitor, may be prescribed every 8 to 12 hours. Oral direct thrombin inhibitors may be used instead of heparin for VTE prevention in patients who have non-valvular atrial fibrillation (Golembiewski, 2011).

❖ PATIENT-CENTERED COLLABORATIVE CARE

◆ Assessment

Physical manifestations range from vague, non-specific discomforts to hemodynamic collapse and death. *It is important to remember that many patients with PE do not have the "classic" manifestations.* This variability in manifestations often leads to PEs being overlooked (Hussey, 2013; Smithburger et al., 2013).

Physical Assessment/Clinical Manifestations. Respiratory manifestations are outlined in Chart 32-2 and are mostly related to decreased GAS EXCHANGE. Assess the patient for difficulty breathing (dyspnea) and pleuritic chest pain (sharp, stabbing-type pain on inspiration). Other manifestations vary depending on the size and the type of embolism. Breath sounds may be normal or include crackles, wheezes, or a pleural friction rub. A dry or productive cough may be present; hemoptysis (bloody sputum) may result from pulmonary infarction.

CHART 32-2 Key Features
Pulmonary Embolism

Classic Manifestations	Signs
• Dyspnea, sudden onset	• Tachypnea
• Sharp, stabbing chest pain	• Crackles
• Apprehension, restlessness	• Pleural friction rub
• Feeling of impending doom	• Tachycardia
• Cough	• S_3 or S_4 heart sound
• Hemoptysis	• Diaphoresis
	• Fever, low-grade
	• Petechiae over chest and axillae
	• Decreased arterial oxygen saturation (SaO_2)

Cardiac manifestations related to decreased tissue PERFUSION include tachycardia, distended neck veins, syncope (fainting or loss of consciousness), cyanosis, and hypotension. Systemic hypotension results from acute pulmonary hypertension and reduced forward blood flow. Abnormal heart sounds, such as an S_3 or S_4, may occur. Electrocardiogram (ECG) changes are nonspecific and transient. T-wave and ST-segment changes may occur as can left-axis or right-axis deviations. Right ventricular dysfunction and failure are extreme manifestations. The patient may have cardiac arrest or frank shock.

! NURSING SAFETY PRIORITY (QSEN)
Critical Rescue

Any patient who has shortness of breath, chest pain, and or/hypotension without an obvious cause should be assessed for PE and the Rapid Response Team notified. If PE is strongly suspected, prompt categorization and management are started before diagnostic studies have been completed (McLenon, 2012; Ouellette, 2014).

Psychosocial Assessment. Manifestations of PE often occur abruptly, and the patient is anxious. Hypoxemia may stimulate a sense of impending doom and cause increased restlessness. The life-threatening nature of PE and admission to an ICU increase the patient's anxiety and fear.

Laboratory Assessment. The hyperventilation triggered by hypoxia and pain first leads to respiratory alkalosis, indicated by low partial pressure of arterial carbon dioxide ($Paco_2$) on arterial blood gas (ABG) analysis. The Pao_2-Fio_2 (fraction of inspired oxygen) ratio falls as a result of "shunting" of blood from the right side of the heart to the left without picking up oxygen from the lungs. Shunting causes the $Paco_2$ level to rise, resulting in respiratory acidosis (McCance et al., 2014). Later, metabolic acidosis results from buildup of lactic acid due to tissue hypoxia. (See Chapter 12 for a more detailed discussion of acidosis.)

Even if ABG studies and pulse oximetry show hypoxemia, these results alone are not sufficient for the diagnosis of PE (McCance et al., 2014). A patient with a small embolus may not be hypoxemic, and PE is not the only cause of hypoxemia.

Other laboratory studies performed when PE is suspected include a general metabolic panel, troponin, brain natriuretic peptide (BNP), and a D-dimer. The D-dimer, a fibrin split product, rises with fibrinolysis. When the value is normal or low, it can rule out a PE. However, even if the value is high, other diagnostic testing is needed to determine whether a PE has occurred (Pagana & Pagana, 2014; Smithburger et al., 2013).

⚛ GENETIC/GENOMIC CONSIDERATIONS
Patient-Centered Care (QSEN)

Factor V Leiden is an inherited thrombophilia (abnormal tendency to develop blood clots) in which the gene coding for blood clotting factor V (the *F5* gene) has a mutation that changes the nature of the factor V produced. With this genetic alteration, factor V functions normally but is not degraded as quickly as it should be. Thus clotting activity continues longer than usual, increasing the chance for developing abnormal blood clots (Lee, 2014). People can inherit either one or both abnormal gene alleles. The risk for developing clots is 8 times greater in those who inherit only one abnormal allele. The risk for developing DVT, PE, or thrombotic strokes increases greatly for people who inherit both abnormal gene alleles (one from each parent), especially if the person also smokes or uses hormone-based contraceptives. This disorder is also known as *activated protein C resistance*. Be aware that testing for factor V Leiden is recommended for people who have developed a VTE without a precipitating event and for those who have a first-degree relative with the disorder (Online Mendelian Inheritance in Man [OMIM], 2013).

Imaging Assessment. Pulmonary angiography is the "gold standard" diagnostic test but is not available in all settings. Computed tomography pulmonary angiography (CT-PA) or helical CT may also be used, which has the added advantage of diagnosing other pulmonary abnormalities causing the patient's manifestations. Ventilation-perfusion ($\dot{V}/\dot{Q}$) scans are not as widely used anymore but may be considered in certain circumstances (e.g., allergy to contrast dye). A chest x-ray may diagnose other conditions that mimic acute PE. Doppler ultrasound may be used to document the presence of VTE and to support a diagnosis of PE (Drumright et al., 2013; Kessenich & Erigo-Backman, 2012).

◆ Analysis

The priority NANDA-I nursing diagnoses and collaborative problems for patients with PE include:

1. Hypoxemia related to mismatch of lung perfusion and alveolar gas exchange with oxygenation
2. Hypotension related to inadequate circulation to the left ventricle
3. Potential for inadequate CLOTTING and bleeding related to anticoagulation or fibrinolytic therapy
4. Anxiety related to hypoxemia and life-threatening illness (NANDA-I)

◆ Planning and Implementation

Managing Hypoxemia. When a patient has a sudden onset of dyspnea and chest pain, immediately notify the Rapid Response Team. Reassure the patient, and elevate the head of the bed. Prepare for oxygen therapy and blood gas analysis while continuing to monitor and assess for other changes.

Planning: Expected Outcomes. The patient with PE is expected to have adequate tissue PERFUSION in all major organs. Indicators of adequate PERFUSION are that the patient has:

• ABGs within normal limits
• Pulse oximetry above 95%
• Cognitive status unimpaired compared with baseline
• Absence of pallor and cyanosis

Interventions. Nonsurgical management of PE is most common. In some cases, invasive procedures also may be needed. Best nursing care practices for the patient with PE are listed in Chart 32-3. Rapid categorization of PE severity and prompt management are required (Table 32-1).

Nonsurgical Management. Management activities for PE focus on increasing GAS EXCHANGE and oxygenation, improving lung PERFUSION, reducing risk for further clot formation, and preventing complications. Priority nursing interventions include implementing oxygen therapy, administering anticoagulation or fibrinolytic therapy to improve tissue perfusion, monitoring the patient's responses to the interventions, and providing psychosocial support.

Oxygen therapy is critical for the patient with PE. The severely hypoxemic patient may need mechanical ventilation and close monitoring with ABG studies. In less severe cases, oxygen may be applied by nasal cannula or mask. Use pulse oximetry to monitor oxygen saturation and hypoxemia.

Monitor the patient continually for any changes in status. Check vital signs, lung sounds, and cardiac and respiratory status at least every 1 to 2 hours. Document increasing dyspnea, dysrhythmias, distended neck veins, and pedal or sacral edema. Assess for crackles and other abnormal lung sounds along with cyanosis of the lips, conjunctiva, oral mucosa, and nail beds.

Drug therapy begins immediately with anticoagulants to prevent embolus enlargement and to prevent more CLOTTING. Unfractionated heparin, low–molecular-weight heparin (enoxaparin [Lovenox]), or fondaparinux (Arixtra) is usually used unless the PE is massive or occurs with hemodynamic instability. Review the patient's partial thromboplastin time (PTT)—also called *activated partial thromboplastin time* (aPTT)—before therapy is started and thereafter according to facility policy. Therapeutic PTT values usually range between 1.5 and 2.5 times the control value for this health problem. Factor anti-Xa levels may be used instead of PTT or aPTT (Riley, 2013).

Fibrinolytic drugs, such as alteplase (Activase, tPA), are used for treatment of PE when specific criteria are met such as shock, hemodynamic collapse, or instability. Fibrinolytic drugs are used to break up the existing clot. (See Chapter 38 for a discussion of fibrinolytic therapy.)

Both heparin and fibrinolytic drugs are *high alert drugs*. These drugs have a high risk to cause harm if given at too high a dose, too low a dose, or to the wrong patient.

CHART 32-3 Best Practice for Patient Safety & Quality Care (QSEN)

Care of the Patient with a Pulmonary Embolism

- Apply oxygen by nasal cannula or mask.
- Reassure patient that the correct measures are being taken.
- Place patient in high-Fowler's position.
- Apply telemetry monitoring equipment.
- Obtain an adequate venous access.
- Assess oxygenation continuously with pulse oximetry.
- Assess respiratory status at least every 30 minutes by:
  - Listening to lung sounds.
  - Measuring the rate, rhythm, and ease of respirations.
  - Checking skin color and capillary refill.
  - Checking position of trachea.
- Assess cardiac status by:
  - Comparing blood pressures in right and left arms.
  - Checking pulse for quality.
  - Checking cardiac monitor for dysrhythmias.
  - Checking for distention of neck veins.
- Ensure prescribed chest imaging and laboratory tests are obtained immediately (may include complete blood count with differential, platelet count, prothrombin time, partial thromboplastin time, D-dimer level, arterial blood gases).
- Examine the thorax for presence of petechiae.
- Administer prescribed anticoagulants.
- Assess for bleeding.
- Handle patient gently.
- Institute Bleeding Precautions.

! NURSING SAFETY PRIORITY (QSEN)
Drug Alert

Heparin comes in a variety of concentrations in vials that have differing amounts, which contributes to possible medication errors. In accordance with The Joint Commission's National Patient Safety Goals (NPSGs), check the prescribed dose carefully and ensure the correct concentration is being used to prevent overdosing or underdosing.

TABLE 32-1 Pulmonary Embolism (PE) Severity and Management Options

CATEGORY	POSSIBLE MANIFESTATIONS	MANAGEMENT OPTIONS
Massive PE Mortality may be as high as 65%	Severe hypotension (SBP <90 mm Hg for at least 15 minutes) Cardiac arrest/cardiopulmonary collapse Severe bradycardia Shock Severe dyspnea/respiratory distress	CPR Inotropic and/or vasopressor support; fluids Fibrinolytic therapy Tissue plasminogen activator (tPA) Alteplase (Activase) Unfractionated heparin initial treatment
Submassive PE	Normotension RV dysfunction on echocardiography RV dilation on echocardiography or CT Right bundle branch block ST elevation or depression T-wave inversion Elevated BNP or troponin	Treatment is controversial; some agents not approved for this group Must weigh benefits of thrombolytic therapy against risk for bleeding Thrombolytics may be preferred if patient appears to be decompensating or if there is RV dysfunction (hypokinesis) or elevation in BNP or troponin LMWH preferred agent Fondaparinux (Arixtra) Unfractionated heparin
Low-risk PE Mortality ranges from 1% to 8%	Normotension No RV dysfunction No elevation in BNP or troponin	Thrombolytics not warranted due to risk for bleeding LMWH Rivaroxaban (Xarelto)

Adapted from Jaff, M.R., McMurtry, M.S., & Archer, S.L. (2011). The use of fibrinolytics in patients with acute pulmonary embolism. *Circulation, 123,* 1788-1830.
BNP, Brain natriuretic peptide; *CPR,* cardiopulmonary resuscitation; *CT,* computed tomography; *LMWH,* low–molecular-weight heparin; *RV,* right ventricle; *SBP,* systolic blood pressure.

Heparin therapy usually continues for 5 to 10 days. Most patients are started on an oral anticoagulant, such as warfarin (Coumadin, Jantoven, Warfilone ♦), on the third day of heparin use. Therapy with both heparin and warfarin continues until the international normalized ratio (INR) reaches 2.0 to 3.0. Monitor the platelet count and INR during this time. A low–molecular-weight heparin (e.g., dalteparin [Fragmin],

enoxaparin [Lovenox]) or a direct thrombin inhibitor (rivaroxaban [Xarelto]) is often used instead of warfarin. Oral anticoagulant use continues for 3 to 6 weeks, but some patients may take it indefinitely. Charts 32-4 and 32-5 list common drugs used and the laboratory tests to monitor in a patient with PE. These drugs and the associated nursing care are discussed in Chapters 36, 38, and 39.

CHART 32-4 Common Examples of Drug Therapy

Pulmonary Embolism

DRUG AND USUAL DOSAGE	PURPOSE	NURSING INTERVENTIONS	RATIONALES
Heparin sodium (Hepalean ♦) 5000-10,000 units as a bolus by IV push initially; then dose adjustment is based on PTT, often at 1300 units/hr on continuous infusion or by intermittent infusion **NOTE:** Some institutions use a weight-based algorithm.	To begin anticoagulation to minimize growth of existing clots and to prevent the development of additional clots	Monitor PTT (or factor anti-Xa) and know expected therapeutic PTT range for each patient. Report PTT (or factor anti-Xa) results. Monitor patient for bleeding or bruising. Adjust infusion based on PTT (or factor anti-Xa) results and institutional protocol. Do not use with salicylates. Monitor platelets daily for thrombocytopenia. Have the antidote *protamine sulfate* available. Avoid puncturing the skin, and apply pressure to venipuncture and IM injection sites. Avoid use of firm toothbrushes, razors, and rectal manipulation.	Ongoing assessment helps detect side effects and prevent complications. Reporting and monitoring enable early management of a prolonged PTT and excessive bleeding. To maintain anticoagulation within consistent therapeutic levels. An increased anticoagulation effect can occur with salicylates. Heparin-induced thrombocytopenia (HIT), a type of adverse reaction, can occur. Being prepared for an emergency helps prevent further complications. Pressure at puncture sites helps promote clotting. Safety measures help prevent bleeding.
Enoxaparin (Lovenox) usually 1 mg/kg subcutaneously every 12 hr	To allow for hospital discharge before complete switch to oral anticoagulants	Monitor platelet count. Have the antidote *protamine sulfate* available. Safety precautions are the same as for heparin.	Heparin-induced thrombocytopenia (HIT), a type of adverse reaction, can occur. This drug is the only antidote for enoxaparin. Safety precautions are the same as for heparin.
Warfarin sodium (Coumadin, Jantoven, Warfilone sodium ♦) 10-15 mg orally once daily for 3 days initially; then dose adjustment is based on INR, usually 5-10 mg orally daily Now available as a parenteral drug for use in hospitalized patients. Dosage is the same as with the oral form of the drug.	To allow for long-term anticoagulation in at-risk patients to prevent the development of future clots	Monitor INR, and know expected therapeutic INR range for each patient. Report INR results. Monitor the patient for bleeding or bruising. Monitor for fever and skin rash. Consult the pharmacist about potential drug interactions, and teach the patient to avoid interacting drugs. Have the antidote *vitamin K (phytonadione)* available. Avoid puncturing the skin, and apply pressure to venipuncture and IM injection sites. Avoid use of firm toothbrushes, razors, and rectal manipulation. Teach the patient which foods are high in vitamin K (e.g., leafy dark green vegetables, herbs, spring onions, Brussels sprouts, broccoli, cabbage, asparagus).	Ongoing assessment helps detect side effects and prevent complications. Reporting enables early management of a prolonged INR. Adverse drug reaction can occur. There are many drug interactions with warfarin. Being prepared for an emergency helps prevent further complications. Pressure at puncture sites helps promote clotting. Safety measures help prevent bleeding. Food sources of vitamin K will alter INR.
Alteplase (tissue plasminogen activator, recombinant; tPA; Activase) 100 mg IV infusion over 2 hr	To promote lysis of large pulmonary emboli in those patients who are hemodynamically unstable	Assess for internal and external bleeding. Reconstitute with sterile water without preservative immediately before use. Administer with caution to patients who have been receiving aspirin, dipyridamole, heparin, or other anticoagulants.	Bleeding is the most common adverse effect. Recommended preparation ensures drug stability. Other drugs with anticoagulation effects increase the risk for bleeding.

INR, International normalized ratio; *PTT,* partial thromboplastin time.

CHART 32-5 Laboratory Profile

Blood Tests Used to Monitor Anticoagulation Therapy

TEST	NORMAL RANGE	SIGNIFICANCE OF ABNORMAL FINDINGS
Partial thromboplastin time (PTT, aPTT [APTT])	Normal values for each local laboratory may vary. When activator reagents are used by the laboratory, the normal clotting time is shortened. Common normal ranges are 20-30 sec in some laboratories and 30-40 sec in others. Therapeutic range for PE is 1.5-2.5 times the normal value (e.g., if normal is 20-30 sec, then therapeutic range is 40-75 sec).	*Subtherapeutic times* may signify that the patient is not receiving enough heparin to prevent extension of the blood clot. An increase in the dosage or rate of infusion is usually indicated. *Therapeutic times* mean that the clotting time is increased from normal but this increase is indicated in the case of PE. *Prolonged times* in patients with PE (i.e., >75 sec) indicate that the patient is at risk for serious spontaneous bleeding. Heparin is usually held or decreased until the PTT drops back into the therapeutic range.
Prothrombin time (pro time, PT)	Common normal range is 11-12.5 sec. Therapeutic range for anticoagulant therapy in PE is 1.5-2.0 times the normal or control value in seconds. Control values can vary day to day because reagents used may vary.	*Subtherapeutic values* may signify that the patient is not receiving enough warfarin. An increase in the dosage is usually indicated. *Therapeutic values* mean that the pro time is increased from normal but this increase is indicated in the case of PE. *Prolonged values* in the treatment of PE indicate that the patient is at risk for bleeding. The warfarin dose is usually decreased or held, the patient is instructed to eat foods high in vitamin K, or an injection of vitamin K may be given.
International Normalized Ratio (INR)	The common normal range is 0.8-1.1. The therapeutic range for PE is 2.5-3.0, or 3.0-4.5 for recurrent PE.	*Subtherapeutic values* may signify that the patient is not receiving enough warfarin. An increase in the dosage is usually indicated. *Therapeutic values* mean that the INR is increased from normal but this increase is indicated in the case of PE. *Prolonged values* (higher than 4.5) in the treatment of PE indicate that the patient is at risk for bleeding. The warfarin dose is usually decreased or held, the patient is instructed to eat foods high in vitamin K, or an injection of vitamin K may be given.

aPTT or *APTT,* Activated partial thromboplastin time; *INR,* international normalized ratio; *PE,* pulmonary embolism.

GENETIC/GENOMIC CONSIDERATIONS

Patient-Centered Care QSEN

Many agencies perform genetic tests before starting warfarin therapy to check for variation in two specific genes. One gene, *VKORC1,* produces an enzyme that alters vitamin K so it can help activate the vitamin K–dependent clotting factors. Warfarin interferes with the activity of this enzyme. Patients who have a variation in the enzyme are resistant to the effects of warfarin, and much higher doses are needed to achieve coagulation. On the other hand, the gene *CYP2C19* produces an enzyme that metabolizes warfarin and prepares it for elimination. Patients who have a variation in this gene do not metabolize warfarin well, so higher blood levels remain and more severe side effects are possible. The dosage of warfarin needs to be much lower in patients with this gene variation. When a patient's response to warfarin therapy is either greater than expected or much less than expected, consider the possibility of a gene mutation.

NCLEX EXAMINATION CHALLENGE

Safe and Effective Care Environment

While assessing a client who has been receiving heparin intravenously for the past 3 days, the nurse notes the IV pump is set at twice the required setting. What orders does the nurse anticipate from the prescriber? **Select all that apply.**
A. Activated partial thromboplastin time
B. International normalized ratio
C. Prothrombin time
D. Vitamin K
E. Protamine sulfate

Surgical Management. Two surgical procedures for the management of PE are embolectomy and inferior vena cava filtration.

Embolectomy is the surgical or percutaneous removal of the embolus. It may be performed when fibrinolytic therapy cannot be used for a patient who has massive or multiple large pulmonary emboli with shock or bleeding complications. Special thrombectomy catheters that mechanically break up clots, such as the AngioJet, allow effective reduction of clots with or without the use of thrombolytic drugs (Drumright et al., 2013).

Inferior vena cava filtration with placement of a vena cava filter prevents further emboli from reaching the lungs in patients

Anticoagulation and fibrinolytic therapy can lead to excessive bleeding. *The antidote for heparin is protamine sulfate; the antidote for warfarin is vitamin K$_1$, which is available as an injectable drug, phytonadione (AquaMEPHYTON, Mephyton). Antidotes for fibrinolytic therapy include clotting factors, fresh frozen plasma, and aminocaproic acid (Amicar).* Keep antidotes to anticoagulant drugs and fibrinolytic drugs on the unit for patients undergoing these therapies.

with ongoing risk for PE. Some filters can be removed when the risk for clot formation decreases, or they can be left in place permanently. Patients for whom filter placement is considered less risky than drug therapy include those with recurrent or major bleeding while receiving anticoagulants, those with septic PE, and those undergoing pulmonary embolectomy (Drumright et al., 2013). Placement of a vena cava filter is detailed in Chapter 36.

Managing Hypotension

Planning: Expected Outcomes. The patient with PE is expected to have adequate circulation and tissue PERFUSION. Indicators of adequate circulation are:

- Maintenance of pulse rate and blood pressure within the normal ranges
- Maintenance of a urine output of at least 30 mL/hr
- Absence of cyanosis

Interventions. In addition to the interventions used for hypoxemia, IV fluid therapy and drug therapy are used to increase cardiac output and maintain blood pressure.

IV fluid therapy involves giving crystalloid solutions to restore plasma volume and prevent shock (see Chapter 37). Continuously monitor the ECG and pulmonary artery and central venous/right atrial pressures of the patient receiving IV fluids because increased fluids can worsen pulmonary hypertension and lead to right-sided heart failure. Also monitor indicators of fluid adequacy including urine output, skin turgor, and moisture of mucous membranes.

Drug therapy with vasopressors is used when hypotension persists despite fluid resuscitation. Commonly used agents include norepinephrine (Levophed), epinephrine (adrenalin), or dopamine (Intropin). Agents that increase myocardial contractility (**positive inotropic agents**), including milrinone (Primacor) and dobutamine (Dobutrex), may be considered. Vasodilators, such as nitroprusside (Nipride, Nitropress), may be used to decrease pulmonary artery pressure if it is impeding cardiac contractility. Assess the patient's cardiac status hourly during therapy with any of these drugs.

Minimizing Bleeding

Planning: Expected Outcomes. The patient with PE is expected to have appropriate CLOTTING and remain free from bleeding. Indicators include that the patient:

- Does not have bruising or petechiae
- Maintains hematocrit, hemoglobin, and platelet count within the normal range

Interventions. Drug therapy that disrupts clots or prevents their formation impairs the patient's ability to start and continue the blood-CLOTTING cascade when injured, increasing the risk for bleeding. Priority nursing actions are ensuring appropriate antidotes are present on the nursing unit, protecting the patient from situations that could lead to bleeding, ensuring correct drug therapy, assessing laboratory values, and monitoring the amount of bleeding that occurs.

Assess for evidence of bleeding (e.g., oozing, bruises that cluster, petechiae, or purpura) at least every 2 hours. Examine all stools, urine, drainage, and vomitus for gross blood, and test for occult blood. Measure any blood loss as accurately as possible. Measure the patient's abdominal girth every 8 hours (increasing girth can indicate internal bleeding). Best practices to prevent bleeding are listed in Chart 32-6.

Monitor laboratory values daily. Review the complete blood count (CBC) results to determine the risk for impaired CLOTTING and whether actual blood loss has occurred. If the patient

---

CHART 32-6 Best Practice for Patient Safety & Quality Care QSEN

Prevention of Injury for the Patient Receiving Anticoagulant, Fibrinolytic, or Antiplatelet Therapy

- Handle the patient gently.
- Use and teach UAP to use a lift sheet when moving and positioning the patient in bed.
- Avoid IM injections and venipunctures.
- When injections or venipunctures are necessary, use the smallest-gauge needle for the task.
- Apply firm pressure to the needle stick site for 10 minutes or until the site no longer oozes blood.
- Apply ice to areas of trauma.
- Test all urine, vomitus, and stool for occult blood.
- Assess IV sites at least every 4 hours for bleeding.
- Instruct alert patients to notify nursing personnel immediately if any trauma occurs and if bleeding or bruising is noticed.
- Avoid trauma to rectal tissues:
  - Do not administer enemas.
  - If suppositories are prescribed, lubricate liberally and administer with caution.
- Instruct the patient and UAP to use an electric shaver rather than a razor.
- When providing mouth care or supervising others in providing mouth care:
  - Use a soft-bristled toothbrush or tooth sponges.
  - Do not use floss.
  - Check to make certain that dentures fit and do not rub.
- Instruct the patient not to blow the nose forcefully or insert objects into the nose.
- Ensure the patient wears shoes with firm soles whenever he or she is ambulating.
- Ensure that antidotes to anticoagulation therapy are on the unit.

UAP, Unlicensed assistive personnel.

---

has severe blood loss, packed red blood cells may be prescribed (see Transfusion Therapy in Chapter 40). Monitor the platelet count. A decreasing count may indicate ongoing CLOTTING or heparin-induced thrombocytopenia (HIT) caused by the formation of anti-heparin antibodies.

Minimizing Anxiety

Planning: Expected Outcomes. The patient with PE is expected to have anxiety reduced to an acceptable level. Indicators include that he or she consistently demonstrates these behaviors:

- States that anxiety is reduced
- Has no distress, irritability, or facial tension
- Uses coping strategies effectively

Interventions. The patient with PE is anxious and fearful and often has pain. Interventions for reducing anxiety in those with PE include oxygen therapy (see Interventions discussion on pp. 605-606 in the Managing Hypoxemia section), communication, and drug therapy.

Communication is critical in allaying anxiety. Acknowledge the anxiety and the patient's perception of a life-threatening situation. Stay with him or her, and speak calmly and clearly, providing assurances that appropriate measures are being taken. Explain the rationale and share information when giving drugs, changing position, taking vital signs, or assessing the patient.

Drug therapy with an antianxiety drug may be prescribed if the patient's anxiety interferes with diagnostic testing, management, or adequate rest. Unless he or she is mechanically ventilated, sedating agents are avoided to reduce the risk for hypoventilation. Pharmacologic therapy is used for pain management. Care is taken to avoid suppressing the respiratory response.

❓ CLINICAL JUDGMENT CHALLENGE

Patient-Centered Care; Safety; Evidence-Based Practice QSEN

The patient is a 70-year-old retiree who had a hip replacement 2 days ago. His hip pain kept him from participating in his usual exercise program for the past 6 months. He is a former two-pack a day smoker. At home he decreased his fluid intake because ambulating to the bathroom was so painful. He resisted getting out of bed with physical therapy yesterday. When you assess him this morning, he reports nausea, some chest pain, mild shortness of breath, and anxiety.

1. What should be your first actions? Provide a rationale for your choice(s).
2. Which of his manifestations are associated with PE, and what risk factors does he have for a PE?
3. What are the common manifestations of PE?
4. The patient is requesting something for his anxiety. Is antianxiety drug therapy appropriate at this time? Why or why not? How else might you be able to reduce his anxiety?
5. What other actions should you take?

Community-Based Care

The patient with a PE is discharged when hypoxemia and hemodynamic instability are resolved and adequate anticoagulation has been achieved. Anticoagulation therapy usually continues after discharge.

Home Care Management. Some patients are discharged to home with minimal risk for recurrence and no permanent physiologic changes. Others have heart or lung damage that requires home and lifestyle modification.

Patients with extensive lung damage may have activity intolerance from reduced GAS EXCHANGE and become fatigued easily. The living arrangements may need to be modified so that patients can spend most of the time on one floor and avoid climbing stairs. Depending on the degree of impairment, patients may require varying amounts of assistance with ADLs.

Self-Management Education. The patient with a PE may continue anticoagulation therapy for weeks, months, or years after discharge, depending on the risks for PE, and have impaired CLOTTING. Teach him or her and the family about Bleeding Precautions, activities to reduce the risk for venous thromboembolism (VTE) and recurrence of PE, complications, and the need for follow-up care (Chart 32-7).

Health Care Resources. Patients using anticoagulation therapy with warfarin are usually seen in a clinic or health care provider's office frequently for blood tests. Those who are homebound may have a visit from a home care nurse to perform these tests. Newer anticoagulation agents (dabigatran [Pradaxa] and enoxaparin [Lovenox]) do not require laboratory monitoring. Patients with severe dyspnea may need home oxygen therapy. Respiratory therapy treatments can be performed in the home. The nurse or case manager coordinates arrangements for oxygen and other respiratory therapy equipment to be available if needed at home. See Chart 32-8 for a focused assessment guide.

CHART 32-7 Patient and Family Education: Preparing for Self-Management

Preventing Injury and Bleeding

During the time you are taking anticoagulants:
- Use an electric shaver.
- Use a soft-bristled toothbrush, and do not floss.
- Do not have dental work performed without consulting your health care provider.
- Do not take aspirin or any aspirin-containing products. Read the label to be sure that the product does not contain aspirin or salicylates.
- Do not participate in contact sports or any activity likely to result in your being bumped, scratched, or scraped.
- If you are bumped, apply ice to the site for at least 1 hour.
- Avoid hard foods that would scrape the inside of your mouth.
- Eat warm, cool, or cold foods to avoid burning your mouth.
- Check your skin and mouth daily for bruises, swelling, or areas with small, reddish purple marks that may indicate bleeding.
- Notify your health care provider if you:
  - Are injured and persistent bleeding results
  - Have excessive menstrual bleeding
  - See blood in your urine or bowel movement
- Avoid anal intercourse.
- Take a stool softener to prevent straining during a bowel movement.
- Do not use enemas or rectal suppositories.
- Do not wear clothing or shoes that are tight or that rub.
- Avoid blowing your nose forcefully or placing objects in your nose. If you must blow your nose, do so gently without blocking either nasal passage.
- Avoid playing musical instruments that raise the pressure inside your head, such as brass wind instruments and woodwinds or reed instruments.
- Keep all appointments for laboratory tests.

◆ Evaluation: Outcomes

Evaluate the care of the patient with PE on the basis of the identified priority patient problems. The expected outcomes are that he or she:
- Attains and maintains adequate GAS EXCHANGE and oxygenation
- Does not experience hypovolemia and shock
- Remains free from bleeding episodes
- States the level of anxiety is reduced
- Uses effective coping strategies

Specific indicators for these outcomes are listed for each patient problem under the Planning and Implementation section (see earlier).

ACUTE RESPIRATORY FAILURE

❖ PATHOPHYSIOLOGY

A near match in the lungs between air movement or ventilation ($\dot{V}$) and blood flow or PERFUSION ($\dot{Q}$) is needed for adequate pulmonary GAS EXCHANGE. When either ventilation or perfusion is mismatched with the other in a lung or lung area, gas exchange is reduced and respiratory failure can result.

Acute respiratory failure (ARF) can be *ventilatory failure, oxygenation (GAS EXCHANGE) failure,* or a *combination of both ventilatory and oxygenation failure* and is classified by abnormal blood gas values. The critical values are:
- Partial pressure of arterial oxygen (Pao_2) less than 60 mm Hg (hypoxemic/oxygenation failure)

CHART 32-8 Home Care Assessment

The Patient After Pulmonary Embolism

Assess respiratory status:
- Observe rate and depth of ventilation.
- Auscultate lungs.
- Examine nail beds and mucous membranes for evidence of cyanosis.
- Take a pulse oximetry reading.
- Ask the patient if chest pain or shortness of breath is experienced in any position.
- Ask the patient about the presence of sputum and its color and character.

Assess cardiovascular status:
- Take vital signs, including apical pulse, pulse pressure; assess for presence or absence of orthostatic hypotension and quality and rhythm of peripheral pulses.
- Note presence or absence of peripheral edema.
- Examine hand vein filling in the dependent position.
- Examine neck vein filling in the recumbent and sitting positions.

Assess lower extremities for deep vein thrombosis:
- Examine lower legs and compare with each other for:
  - General edema
  - Calf swelling
  - Surface temperature
  - Presence of red streaks or cordlike, palpable structure
  - Measure calf circumference:

Assess for evidence of bleeding:
- Examine the mouth and gums for oozing or frank bleeding.
- Examine all skin areas, especially old puncture sites and wounds, for bleeding, bruising, or petechiae.
- If the patient voids during the visit, test the urine for occult blood.

Assess cognition and mental status:
- Check level of consciousness.
- Check orientation to time, place, and person.
- Can the patient accurately read a seven-word sentence containing no words with more than three syllables?

Assess the patient's understanding of illness and adherence to treatment:
- Manifestations to report to health care provider
- Drug therapy plan (correct timing and dose)
- Bleeding Precautions
- Prevention of venous thromboembolism

TABLE 32-2 Common Causes of Ventilatory Failure

EXTRAPULMONARY CAUSES	INTRAPULMONARY CAUSES

• Neuromuscular disorders:
  • Myasthenia gravis
  • Guillain-Barré syndrome
  • Poliomyelitis
• Spinal cord injuries affecting nerves to intercostal muscles
• Central nervous system dysfunction:
  • Stroke
  • Increased intracranial pressure
  • Meningitis
• Chemical depression:
  • Opioid analgesics, sedatives, anesthetics
• Kyphoscoliosis
• Massive obesity
• Sleep apnea
• External obstruction/constriction
	• Airway disease:
	  • Chronic obstructive pulmonary disease (COPD), asthma
	• Ventilation-perfusion ($\dot{V}/\dot{Q}$) mismatch:
	  • Pulmonary embolism
	  • Pneumothorax
	  • Acute respiratory distress syndrome (ARDS)
	  • Amyloidosis
	  • Pulmonary edema
	  • Interstitial fibrosis

the respiratory muscles, especially the diaphragm. The problem is defined by a $Paco_2$ level above 45 mm Hg plus acidemia (pH < 7.35) in patients who have otherwise healthy lungs.

Many disorders can result in ventilatory failure. Causes are either **extrapulmonary** (involving nonpulmonary tissues but affecting respiratory function) or **intrapulmonary** (disorders of the respiratory tract). Table 32-2 lists causes of ventilatory failure.

Oxygenation (Gas Exchange) Failure. In oxygenation (GAS EXCHANGE) failure, chest pressure changes are normal and air moves in and out without difficulty but does not oxygenate the pulmonary blood sufficiently. It occurs in the type of $\dot{V}/\dot{Q}$ mismatch in which air movement and oxygen intake (ventilation) are normal but lung blood flow (PERFUSION) is decreased.

Many lung disorders can cause oxygenation failure. Problems include impaired diffusion of oxygen at the alveolar level, right-to-left shunting of blood in the pulmonary vessels, $\dot{V}/\dot{Q}$ mismatch, breathing air with a low oxygen level, and abnormal hemoglobin that fails to bind oxygen. In one type of $\dot{V}/\dot{Q}$ mismatch, areas of the lungs still have PERFUSION but GAS EXCHANGE does not occur, which leads to hypoxemia. An extreme example of $\dot{V}/\dot{Q}$ mismatch is when systemic venous blood (oxygen-poor) passes through the lungs without being oxygenated and is "shunted" to the left side of the heart and into the systemic arterial system. Normally, less than 5% of cardiac output contains venous blood that has bypassed oxygenation. With poor oxygenation in the lungs or a shunt that allows venous blood to bypass the lungs, even more arterial blood is not oxygenated and applying 100% oxygen does not correct the problem. A classic cause of such a $\dot{V}/\dot{Q}$ mismatch is acute respiratory distress syndrome (ARDS). Table 32-3 lists specific causes of oxygenation failure.

Combined Ventilatory and Oxygenation Failure. Combined ventilatory and oxygenation failure involves **hypoventilation** (poor respiratory movements). Impaired GAS EXCHANGE at the alveolar-capillary membrane results in poor diffusion of oxygen into arterial blood and carbon dioxide retention. The condition may or may not include poor lung perfusion. When lung PERFUSION is not adequate, $\dot{V}/\dot{Q}$ mismatch occurs and

- OR partial pressure of arterial carbon dioxide ($Paco_2$) more than 45 mm Hg occurring with acidemia (pH <7.35) (hypercapnic/ventilatory failure)
- AND arterial oxygen saturation (Sao_2) less than 90% in both cases

Whatever the underlying problem, the patient in acute respiratory failure is always **hypoxemic** (has low arterial blood oxygen levels) (Bekken, 2011; McLean, 2012).

Ventilatory Failure. Ventilatory failure is a problem in oxygen intake (air movement or ventilation) and blood flow (PERFUSION) that causes a ventilation-perfusion ($\dot{V}/\dot{Q}$) mismatch in which blood flow (perfusion) is normal but air movement (ventilation) is inadequate. It occurs when the chest pressure does not change enough to permit air movement into and out of the lungs. As a result, too little oxygen reaches the alveoli and carbon dioxide is retained. Perfusion is wasted in this area of no air movement from either inadequate oxygen intake or excessive carbon dioxide retention leading to poor GAS EXCHANGE and hypoxemia (McLean, 2012).

Ventilatory failure usually results from any of these problems: a physical problem of the lungs or chest wall; a defect in the respiratory control center in the brain; or poor function of

---

TABLE 32-3 **Common Causes of Oxygenation Failure**

- Low atmospheric oxygen concentration:
  - High altitudes, closed spaces, smoke inhalation, carbon monoxide poisoning
- Pneumonia
- Congestive heart failure with pulmonary edema
- Pulmonary embolism (PE)
- Acute respiratory distress syndrome (ARDS)
- Interstitial pneumonitis-fibrosis
- Abnormal hemoglobin
- Hypovolemic shock
- Hypoventilation
- Complications of nitroprusside therapy:
  - Thiocyanate toxicity, methemoglobinemia

---

both ventilation and perfusion are inadequate. This type of respiratory failure leads to a more profound hypoxemia than either ventilatory failure or oxygenation failure alone.

A combination of ventilatory failure and oxygenation (GAS EXCHANGE) failure occurs in patients who have abnormal lungs, such as those who have any form of chronic bronchitis, have emphysema, have cystic fibrosis, or are having an asthma attack. The bronchioles and alveoli are diseased (causing oxygenation failure), and the work of breathing increases until the respiratory muscles cannot function effectively (causing ventilatory failure) leading to acute respiratory failure (ARF). ARF can also occur in patients who have cardiac failure along with respiratory failure and is made worse by the fact that the cardiac system cannot adapt to the hypoxia by increasing the cardiac output.

❖ PATIENT-CENTERED COLLABORATIVE CARE

◆ Assessment

The manifestations of ARF are related to the systemic effects of hypoxia, hypercapnia, and acidosis (Bekken, 2011). Assess for **dyspnea** (perceived difficulty breathing)—the hallmark of respiratory failure. Evaluate dyspnea on the basis of how breathless the patient becomes while performing common tasks. Depending on the nature of the underlying problem, the patient might not be aware of changes in the work of breathing.

Dyspnea is more intense when it develops rapidly. Slowly progressive respiratory failure may first be noticed as dyspnea on exertion (DOE) or when lying down. The patient may have **orthopnea**, finding it easier to breathe in an upright position (Bull, 2014). With chronic respiratory problems, a minor increase in dyspnea may represent severe GAS EXCHANGE problems.

Assess for a change in the patient's respiratory rate or pattern and changes in lung sounds. Pulse oximetry (Spo2) may show decreased oxygen saturation, but end-tidal CO2 (ETCO2 or PETCO2) monitoring may be more valuable for monitoring the patient with ARF (Carlisle, 2014). His or her pulse oximetry may show adequate oxygen saturation but because of increased ETCO2 the patient may be close to respiratory failure. Arterial blood gas (ABG) studies are reviewed to most accurately identify the degree of hypoxia and hypercarbia.

Other manifestations of hypoxic respiratory failure include restlessness, irritability or agitation, confusion, and tachycardia. Manifestations of hypercapnic failure include decreased level of consciousness (LOC), headache, drowsiness, lethargy, and possible seizures. The effects of acidosis may lead to decreased

LOC, drowsiness, confusion, hypotension, bradycardia, and weak peripheral pulses.

◆ Interventions

Oxygen therapy is appropriate for any patient with acute hypoxemia. It is used in acute respiratory failure to keep the arterial oxygen (Pao2) level above 60 mm Hg while treating the cause of the respiratory failure. Oxygen therapy is discussed in detail in Chapter 28. If oxygen therapy does not maintain acceptable Pao2 levels, mechanical ventilation (invasive or noninvasive) may be needed.

Drugs given systemically or by metered dose inhaler (MDI) may be prescribed to dilate the bronchioles and decrease inflammation to promote GAS EXCHANGE. Corticosteroids may be used, but their benefit has not been conclusively demonstrated. Analgesics are needed if the patient has pain. If the patient requires mechanical ventilation, he or she may need neuromuscular blockade drugs for optimal ventilator effect. Other management strategies depend on the underlying condition(s) that predisposed the patient to ARF development.

Help the patient find a position of comfort that allows easier breathing—usually a more upright position. To decrease the anxiety occurring with dyspnea, assist him or her to use relaxation, diversion, and guided imagery. Start energy-conserving measures, such as minimal self-care and no unnecessary procedures. Encourage deep breathing and other breathing exercises.

ACUTE RESPIRATORY DISTRESS SYNDROME

❖ PATHOPHYSIOLOGY

Acute respiratory distress syndrome (ARDS) is acute respiratory failure with these features:
- Hypoxemia that persists even when 100% oxygen is given (**refractory hypoxemia**, a cardinal feature)
- Decreased pulmonary compliance
- Dyspnea
- Noncardiac-associated bilateral pulmonary edema
- Dense pulmonary infiltrates on x-ray (ground-glass appearance)

Often ARDS occurs after an *acute lung injury (ALI)* in people who have no pulmonary disease as a result of other conditions such as sepsis, burns, pancreatitis, trauma, and transfusion. The mortality rate is about 60% depending on the underlying cause (Carroll et al., 2013). Other terms for ARDS include *adult respiratory distress syndrome* and *shock lung.*

Despite different causes of ALI in ARDS, the trigger is a systemic inflammatory response. As a result, ARDS manifestations are similar regardless of the cause. The main site of injury in the lung is the alveolar-capillary membrane, which normally is permeable only to small molecules. It can be injured during sepsis, pulmonary embolism, shock, aspiration, or inhalation injury. When injured, this membrane becomes more permeable to large molecules, which allows debris, proteins, and fluid into the alveoli. Lung tissue normally remains relatively dry, but in patients with ARDS, lung fluid increases and contains more proteins.

Other changes occur in the alveoli and respiratory bronchioles. Normally, the type II pneumocytes produce surfactant, a substance that increases lung **compliance** (elasticity) and prevents alveolar collapse. Surfactant activity is reduced in ARDS because type II pneumocytes are damaged and because the surfactant is diluted by excess lung fluids. As a result, the alveoli become unstable and tend to collapse unless they are filled with fluid. These fluid-filled and collapsed alveoli cannot participate in GAS EXCHANGE. As a result, edema forms around terminal airways, which are compressed and closed and can be destroyed. Lung volume and compliance are further reduced. As fluid continues to leak in more lung areas, fluid, protein, and blood cells collect in the alveoli and in the spaces between the alveoli. Lymph channels are compressed, and more fluid collects. Poorly inflated alveoli receive blood but cannot oxygenate it, increasing the shunt. Hypoxemia and ventilation-perfusion $\dot{V}/\dot{Q}$ mismatch result.

Transfusion-related acute lung injury (TRALI) is the sudden onset (within 6 hours of a transfusion) of hypoxemic lung disease along with infiltrates on x-ray without cardiac problems. TRALI is associated with the activation of the inflammatory response due to a recent transfusion of plasma-containing blood products such as packed red blood cells (PRBCs), platelets, and fresh frozen plasma (Benson, 2012). Other lung complications of transfusion include transfusion-associated circulatory overload (TACO) and transfusion-related immuno-modulation (TRIM) (Benson, 2012).

Etiology and Genetic Risk. ALI leading to ARDS has many causes (Table 32-4). Some causes result in direct injury to lung tissue; other causes do not directly involve the lungs. As a result of sepsis, pancreatitis, trauma, and other conditions, inflammatory mediators spread to the lungs causing damage (Carroll et al., 2013; McCance et al., 2014).

ARDS also can occur from direct lung injury. Aspiration of acidic gastric contents, pneumonia, drowning, and inhaling toxic fumes are examples of conditions causing direct lung injury. With such events, surfactant production is impaired and the remaining surfactant is diluted. This situation leads to atelectasis, decreased lung compliance, and shunting (movement of blood in the lungs without GAS EXCHANGE and oxygenation) (Carroll et al., 2013; Dechert et al., 2012).

🧬 GENETIC/GENOMIC CONSIDERATIONS

Patient-Centered Care QSEN

An increased genetic risk is suspected in the development and progression of ARDS. Variations in the genes responsible for surfactant production appear to increase the predisposition to developing ARDS as does variation in the genes responsible for cytokine production during inflammatory events associated with sepsis (Dechert et al., 2012). Ask about the patient's previous responses to infection or injury. If the patient has consistently had greater-than-expected inflammatory responses, he or she may be at increased risk for ARDS after ALI and should be monitored for manifestations of the disorder.

Incidence and Prevalence. The actual incidence of ARDS is unknown because it is part of other health problems and is not systematically reported as a separate disorder. According to the ARDS Foundation, about 150,000 cases of ARDS occur yearly in North America (ARDS Foundation, 2013) although many health care professionals believe this estimate to be low.

Health Promotion and Maintenance

The nursing priority in the prevention of ARDS is early recognition of patients at high risk for the syndrome. Because patients who aspirate gastric contents are at great risk, closely assess and monitor those receiving tube feedings (because the tube keeps the gastric sphincter open) and those with problems that impair

TABLE 32-4	Common Causes of Acute Lung Injury

- Shock
- Trauma
- Serious nervous system injury
- Pancreatitis
- Fat and amniotic fluid emboli
- Pulmonary infections
- Sepsis
- Inhalation of toxic gases (smoke, oxygen)
- Pulmonary aspiration (especially of stomach contents)
- Drug ingestion (e.g., heroin, opioids, aspirin)
- Hemolytic disorders
- Multiple blood transfusions
- Cardiopulmonary bypass
- Submersion in water with water aspiration (especially in fresh water)

swallowing and gag reflexes. As required by The Joint Commission's NPSGs to prevent ARDS, follow meticulous infection control guidelines, including handwashing, invasive catheter and wound care, and Contact Precautions. Teach unlicensed assistive personnel (UAP) the importance of always adhering to infection control guidelines. Carefully observe patients who are being treated for any health problem associated with ARDS.

❖ PATIENT-CENTERED COLLABORATIVE CARE

◆ Assessment

Physical Assessment/Clinical Manifestations. Assess the breathing of any patient at increased risk for ARDS. Determine whether increased work of breathing is present, as indicated by hyperpnea, noisy respiration, cyanosis, pallor, and retraction **intercostally** (between the ribs) or **substernally** (below the ribs). Document sweating, respiratory effort, and any change in mental status. *Abnormal lung sounds are **not** heard on auscultation because the edema occurs first in the interstitial spaces and not in the airways.* Assess vital signs at least hourly for hypotension, tachycardia, and dysrhythmias.

Diagnostic Assessment. The diagnosis of ARDS is established by a lowered partial pressure of arterial oxygen (Pao_2) value (decreased GAS EXCHANGE and oxygenation), determined by arterial blood gas (ABG) measurements. Because a widening alveolar oxygen gradient (increased fraction of inspired oxygen [Fio_2] that does not lead to increased Pao_2 levels) develops with increased shunting of blood, the patient has a progressive need for higher levels of oxygen. He or she develops refractory hypoxemia and often needs intubation and mechanical ventilation. Sputum cultures obtained by bronchoscopy and by transtracheal aspiration are used to determine if a lung infection also is present.

The chest x-ray may show diffuse haziness or a "whited-out" (ground-glass) appearance of the lung. An ECG rules out cardiac problems and usually shows no specific changes. Hemodynamic monitoring with a pulmonary artery catheter helps diagnose ARDS. In ARDS, the pulmonary capillary wedge pressure (PCWP) is low to normal, whereas in cardiac-induced pulmonary edema, the PCWP is above 18 mm Hg. Chapter 38 explains hemodynamic monitoring in detail.

◆ Interventions

The patient with ARDS often needs intubation and mechanical ventilation with positive end-expiratory pressure (PEEP) or continuous positive airway pressure (CPAP). Best practice involves using "open lung" and lung protective ventilation strategies. Low tidal volumes (6 mL/kg of body weight) have been shown to prevent lung injury. PEEP is started at 5 cm H_2O and increased to keep oxygen saturation adequate. PEEP levels may need to be high. Pressure-controlled ventilation is preferred over volume-controlled ventilation to promote the nonfunctional alveoli to participate in GAS EXCHANGE.

Airway pressure-release ventilation (APRV) and high-frequency oscillatory ventilation are alternative modes of mechanical ventilation that improve GAS EXCHANGE with oxygenation and ventilation in patients with moderate to severe ARDS (Bortolotto & Makic, 2012). Sedation and paralysis may be needed for adequate ventilation and to reduce tissue oxygen needs. Because one of the side effects of PEEP is tension pneumothorax, assess lung sounds hourly and suction as often as needed to maintain a patent airway.

Positioning may be important in promoting GAS EXCHANGE, but the exact position is controversial. Some patients do better in the prone position, especially if it is started early in the disease course. Prone positioning may be achieved using a mechanical turning device, although the turning equipment is awkward and care in the prone position is more difficult. Automated kinetic beds are available to assist with turning. Manually turning the patient every 2 hours has been shown to improve PERFUSION; however, this intervention often is not performed as frequently as needed. Early progressive mobility also has demonstrated benefit in reducing ventilator needs, days on the ventilator, and mortality (Morris et al., 2011; Wright & Flynn, 2011).

For severe ARDS, extracorporeal membrane oxygenation (ECMO) using heart-lung bypass equipment has been a successful life support technique when the patient does not improve with more traditional management. However, the proper timing of ECMO and standardization of this therapy for best outcomes have not been established (Williams, 2013).

Drug and Fluid Therapy. Antibiotics are used to treat infections when organisms are identified. Other drugs are used to manage any underlying cause. Currently, no treatments reverse the pathologic changes in the lungs, although many interventions are under investigation. These include agents that modify the inflammatory responses and reduce oxidative stress, such as vitamins C and E, *N*-acetylcysteine, and nitric oxide, as well as surfactant replacement (Carroll et al., 2013).

Research shows that patients with ARDS who receive conservative fluid therapy have improved lung function and a shorter duration of mechanical ventilation and ICU length of stay compared with those who receive more liberal fluid therapy. Conservative fluid therapy involves infusing smaller amounts of IV fluid and the use of diuretics to maintain fluid balance, whereas liberal fluid therapy often results in an increasingly positive fluid balance and more edema (Ferri, 2013).

Nutrition Therapy. The patient with ARDS is at risk for malnutrition, which further reduces respiratory muscle function and the immune response. Consultation with a dietitian is needed, and enteral nutrition (tube feeding) or parenteral nutrition is started as soon as possible.

Case Management. Case management of the patient with ARDS focuses on the phases of ARDS rather than on day-to-day care. The course of ARDS and its management are divided into three phases:

- *Exudative phase.* This phase includes early changes of dyspnea and tachypnea resulting from the alveoli becoming fluid-filled and from pulmonary shunting and atelectasis. Early interventions focus on supporting the patient and providing oxygen.
- *Fibroproliferative phase.* Increased lung damage leads to pulmonary hypertension and fibrosis. The body attempts to repair the damage, and increasing lung involvement reduces GAS EXCHANGE and oxygenation. Multiple organ dysfunction syndrome (MODS) can occur. Interventions focus on delivering adequate oxygen, preventing complications, and supporting the lungs.
- *Resolution phase.* Usually occurring after 14 days, resolution of the injury can occur; if not, the patient either dies or has chronic disease. Fibrosis may or may not occur. Research indicates that patients surviving ARDS often have neuropsychological deficits and poor quality-of-life scores (Dechert et al., 2012; Mathay & Zemans, 2011).

? CLINICAL JUDGMENT CHALLENGE

Patient-Centered Care; Teamwork and Collaboration **QSEN**

A 50-year-old patient is admitted to the medical-surgical floor from the emergency department with severe abdominal pain thought to be from acute pancreatitis. He has a history of drinking at least a case of beer a day. He also smokes and appears cachectic. His old chart indicates a history of COPD, but he does not take drugs for this. He does have a new productive cough. At change of shift, the nurse finds the patient dyspneic and slightly confused. Lung sounds have wheezes, and he is mildly febrile. Pulse is 120 beats/min, respirations are 32 breaths/min, and blood pressure is 118/64 mm Hg (baseline). Oximetry shows an SpO_2 of 91%.

1. What risk factors for ARDS does this patient have?
2. Explain the relationship between the lung sounds and the oximetry reading.
3. What diagnostic testing should you be prepared to obtain?

Two hours after applying oxygen at 3 liters/nasal cannula, the patient's SpO_2 is now 89%.

4. What additional measures do you anticipate for this patient?

THE PATIENT REQUIRING INTUBATION AND VENTILATION

❖ PATHOPHYSIOLOGY

With mechanical ventilation, the patient who has severe problems of GAS EXCHANGE may be supported until the underlying problem improves or resolves. Usually mechanical ventilation is a temporary life-support technique. The need for this support may be lifelong for those with severe restrictive lung disease or chronic progressive neuromuscular disease that reduces ventilation.

Mechanical ventilation is most often used for patients with hypoxemia and progressive alveolar hypoventilation with respiratory acidosis. The hypoxemia is usually due to pulmonary shunting of blood when other methods of oxygen delivery do not provide a sufficiently high fraction of inspired oxygen (FiO_2). Mechanical ventilation may be used for patients who need ventilatory support after surgery, those who expend too much energy with breathing and barely maintain adequate GAS EXCHANGE, or those who have general anesthesia or heavy sedation.

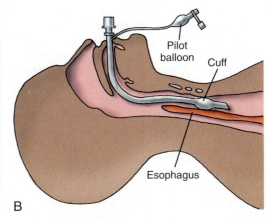

FIG. 32-2 **A,** Endotracheal tubes. **B,** Correct placement of an oral endotracheal tube.

❖ PATIENT-CENTERED COLLABORATIVE CARE

Assess the patient to be intubated in the same way as for other breathing problems. Once mechanical ventilation has been started, assess the respiratory system on an ongoing basis. Monitor and assess for problems related to the artificial airway or ventilator.

Endotracheal Intubation

The patient who needs mechanical ventilation must have an artificial airway. The most common type of airway for a short-term basis is the endotracheal (ET) tube. To reduce tracheal and vocal cord damage, a tracheostomy is considered if an artificial airway is needed for longer than 10 to 14 days (see Chapter 28). The expectations of intubation are to maintain a patent airway, provide a means to remove secretions, and provide ventilation and oxygen.

Endotracheal Tube. An ET tube is a long polyvinyl chloride tube that is passed through the mouth or nose and into the trachea (Fig. 32-2). When properly positioned, the tip of the ET tube rests about 2 cm above the carina (the point at which the trachea divides into the right and left mainstem bronchi). Oral intubation is a fast and easy way to establish an airway and is often performed as an emergency procedure. The nasal route is used for oral surgeries and when oral intubation is not possible but should be avoided with midface trauma or possible basilar skull fracture. This route is not used if the patient has a blood CLOTTING problem. An anesthesiologist, nurse anesthetist, or respiratory therapist usually performs the intubation.

The shaft of the tube has a radiopaque line running the length of the tube. This line shows on x-ray and is used to determine correct tube placement. Short horizontal lines (depth markings) are used to place the tube correctly at the naris or mouth (at the incisor tooth) and to identify how far the tube has been inserted.

The cuff at the distal end of the tube is inflated after placement and creates a seal between the trachea and the cuff. The seal ensures delivery of a set tidal volume when mechanical ventilation is used. The cuff is inflated using a minimal-leak technique: when the cuff is inflated to an adequate sealing volume, a minimal amount of air can pass around the cuff to the vocal cords, nose, or mouth. The patient cannot talk when the cuff is inflated.

The pilot balloon with a one-way valve permits air to be inserted into the cuff and prevents air from escaping. This balloon is a guide for determining whether air is present in the cuff, but it does not show how much or how little air is present.

The adaptor connects the ET tube to ventilator tubing or an oxygen delivery system. The endotracheal tube size is listed on the shaft of the tube. Adult tube sizes range from 7 to 9 mm. Tube size selected is based on the size of the patient.

Preparing for Intubation. Know the proper procedure for summoning intubation personnel in the facility to the bedside in an emergency situation. Explain the procedure to the patient as clearly as possible. *Basic life support measures, such as obtaining a patent airway and delivering 100% oxygen by a manual resuscitation bag with a facemask, are crucial to survival until help arrives.*

> **! NURSING SAFETY PRIORITY** (QSEN)
>
> **Critical Rescue**
>
> For the patient requiring emergency intubation and ventilation, bring the code (or "crash") cart, airway equipment box, and suction equipment (often already on the code cart) to the bedside. Maintain a patent airway through positioning (head-tilt, chin-lift) and the insertion of an oral or nasopharyngeal airway until the patient is intubated. Delivering manual breaths with a bag-valve-mask may also be required.

During intubation, the nurse coordinates the rescue response and continuously monitors the patient for changes in vital signs, signs of hypoxia or hypoxemia, dysrhythmias, and aspiration. Ensure that each intubation attempt lasts no longer than 30 seconds, preferably less than 15 seconds. After 30 seconds, provide oxygen by means of a mask and manual resuscitation bag to prevent hypoxia and cardiac arrest. Suction as necessary (Morton & Fontaine, 2013; Urden et al., 2012).

Verifying Tube Placement. Immediately after an ET tube is inserted, placement should be verified. The most accurate ways to verify placement are by checking end-tidal carbon dioxide levels and by chest x-ray. Assess for breath sounds bilaterally, sounds over the gastric area, symmetric chest movement, and air emerging from the ET tube. If breath sounds and chest wall movement are absent on the left side, the tube may be in the right mainstem bronchus. The person intubating the patient should be able to reposition the tube without repeating the entire intubation procedure.

If the tube is in the stomach, the abdomen may be distended and must be decompressed with a nasogastric (NG) tube after the ET tube is replaced. Monitor chest wall movement and breath sounds until tube placement is verified by chest x-ray.

Stabilizing the Tube. The nurse, respiratory therapist, or anesthesia provider stabilizes the ET tube at the mouth or nose. The tube is marked at the level where it touches the incisor tooth or naris. Two people working together use a head halter technique to secure the tube. An oral airway also may be inserted or a commercial bite block placed to keep the patient from biting an oral endotracheal tube. One person stabilizes the tube at the correct position and prevents head movement while a second person applies the tube holding device. Commercial tube holders are preferred over securing the tube with tape. After the procedure is completed, verify and document the presence of bilateral and equal breath sounds and the level of the tube.

Nursing Care. The priority nursing action when caring for an intubated patient is maintaining a patent airway. Assess tube placement, cuff leak, breath sounds, indications of adequate GAS EXCHANGE and oxygenation, and chest wall movement regularly.

! NURSING SAFETY PRIORITY (QSEN)

Critical Rescue

If an intubated patient shows manifestations of decreased oxygenation, check for DOPE: <u>d</u>isplaced tube, <u>o</u>bstructed tube (most often with secretions), <u>p</u>neumothorax, and <u>e</u>quipment problems (Dennison et al., 2011).

Prevent the patient from pulling or tugging on the tube to avoid tube dislodgment, and check the pilot balloon to ensure that the cuff is inflated. Suctioning, coughing, and speaking can cause dislodgment. Neck flexion, neck extension, and rotation of the head also can cause the tube to move. Tongue movement also can change the tube's position. When other measures fail, obtain a prescription for soft wrist restraints and apply these for the patient who is pulling on the tube. *Restraints are used as a last resort to prevent accidental extubation.* Adequate sedation (chemical restraint) may be needed to decrease agitation or prevent extubation. Obtain permission for restraints from the patient or family. More information on airway management is found in Chapter 28.

Complications of an ET or nasotracheal tube can occur during placement, while in place, during extubation, or after extubation (either early or late). Common complications include tube obstruction, dislodgment, pneumothorax, tracheal tears, bleeding, and infection. Trauma and other problems can occur to the face; eye; nasal and paranasal areas; oral, pharyngeal, bronchial, tracheal, and pulmonary areas; esophageal and gastric areas; and cardiovascular, musculoskeletal, and neurologic systems.

? NCLEX EXAMINATION CHALLENGE

Safe and Effective Care Environment

The nurse caring for a client who is intubated and receiving mechanical ventilation notes that her oxygen saturation is 89%, her heart rate is 120 beats/min, and she is increasingly agitated and restless. On auscultation, the nurse finds that the lung sounds are diminished on one side. Which action does the nurse perform first?

A. Notify the provider, and prepare for re-intubation or repositioning the tube.
B. Document the findings, and request sedation from the provider.
C. Call respiratory therapy to obtain a set of arterial blood gases.
D. Reposition the tube, and call radiology for a stat chest x-ray.

Mechanical Ventilation

Mechanical ventilation to support and maintain GAS EXCHANGE is used in many settings, not just in critical care units. The nurse plays a pivotal role in the coordination of care and the prevention of problems. Chart 32-9 lists best practices for patient care during mechanical ventilation.

The purposes of mechanical ventilation are to improve GAS EXCHANGE and to decrease the work needed for effective breathing. It is used to support the patient until lung function is adequate or until the acute episode has passed. *A ventilator does not cure diseased lungs; it provides ventilation until the patient can resume the process of breathing on his or her own.* Remember *why* the patient is using the ventilator so that management efforts also focus on correcting the causes of the respiratory failure. If normal GAS EXCHANGE with oxygenation, ventilation, and respiratory muscle strength is achieved, mechanical ventilation can be discontinued.

Types of Ventilators. Many types of ventilators are available. The ventilator selected depends on the severity of the breathing problem and the length of time ventilator support is needed. Most ventilators are positive-pressure ventilators. During inspiration, pressure is generated that pushes air into the lungs and expands the chest. Usually an endotracheal (ET) tube or tracheostomy is needed. Positive-pressure ventilators are classified by the mechanism that ends inspiration and starts expiration. Inspiration is cycled in three major ways: pressure-cycled, time-cycled, or volume-cycled.

Pressure-cycled ventilators push air into the lungs until a preset airway pressure is reached. Tidal volumes and inspiratory time vary. These ventilators are used for short periods, such as just after surgery and for respiratory therapy. Bi-level positive airway pressure (Bi-PAP) ventilators are a newer form of pressure-cycled ventilator in which the ventilator provides a preset inspiratory pressure and an expiratory pressure similar to positive end-expiratory pressure (PEEP).

Time-cycled ventilators push air into the lungs until a preset time has elapsed. Tidal volume and pressure vary, depending on the needs of the patient and the type of ventilator.

Volume-cycled ventilators push air into the lungs until a preset volume is delivered. A constant tidal volume is delivered regardless of the pressure needed to deliver the tidal volume. A set pressure limit, however, prevents excessive pressure from being exerted on the lungs. The advantage of this type of ventilator is that a constant tidal volume is delivered regardless of changes in lung or chest wall compliance or in airway resistance.

Microprocessor ventilators are computer-managed positive-pressure ventilators. A computer is built into the ventilator to allow ongoing monitoring of ventilatory functions, alarms, and patient conditions. It often has components of volume-, time-, and pressure-cycled ventilators. This type of ventilator is more responsive to patients who have severe lung disease and those who need prolonged weaning trials. Examples include the Draeger Evita XL (Fig. 32-3) and Puritan-Bennett 840.

Modes of Ventilation. The mode of ventilation is the way in which the patient receives breaths from the ventilator. The most common modes are assist-control ventilation, synchronized intermittent mandatory ventilation, and bi-level positive airway pressure ventilation.

Assist-control (AC) ventilation is the mode used most often as a resting mode. The ventilator takes over the work of breathing for the patient. The tidal volume and ventilatory rate are

Care of the Patient Receiving Mechanical Ventilation

- Assess the patient's respiratory status at least every 4 hours for the first 24 hours and then as needed:
  - Take vital signs at least every 4 hours.
  - Assess the patient's color (especially lips and nail beds).
  - Observe the patient's chest for bilateral expansion.
  - Assess the placement of the nasotracheal or endotracheal tube.
  - Obtain pulse oximetry reading.
  - Evaluate ABGs as available.
  - Maintain head of the bed more than 30 degrees when patient is supine to prevent aspiration and ventilator-associated pneumonia.
- Document pertinent observations in the patient's medical record.
- Check at least every 8 hours to be sure the ventilator setting is as prescribed.
- Check to be sure alarms are set (especially low-pressure and low-exhaled volume).
- If the patient is on PEEP, observe the peak airway pressure dial to determine the proper level of PEEP.
- Check the exhaled volume digital display to be sure the patient is receiving the prescribed tidal volume.
- Empty ventilator tubings when moisture collects. *Never empty fluid in the tubing back into the cascade.*
- Ensure humidity by keeping delivered air temperature maintained at body temperature.
- Be sure the tracheostomy cuff (or endotracheal cuff) is adequately inflated to ensure tidal volume.
- Auscultate the lungs for crackles, wheezes, equal breath sounds, and decreased or absent breath sounds.
- Check the patient's need for tracheal, oral, or nasal suctioning every 2 hours, and suction as needed.
- Assess the patient's mouth around the ET tube for pressure ulcers.
- Perform mouth care every 2 hours.
- Change tracheostomy tube holder or tape or endotracheal tube holder or tape as needed:
  - Carefully move the oral endotracheal tube to the opposite side of the mouth once daily to prevent ulcers.
  - Provide tracheostomy care every 8 hours.
- Assess ventilated patients for GI distress (diarrhea, constipation, tarry stools).
- Maintain accurate intake and output records to monitor fluid balance.
- Turn the patient at least every 2 hours, and get the patient out of bed as prescribed to promote pulmonary hygiene and prevent complications of immobility.
- Schedule treatments and nursing care at intervals for rest.
- Monitor the patient's progress on current ventilator settings, and make appropriate changes, as indicated.
- Monitor the patient for the effectiveness of mechanical ventilation in terms of his or her physiologic and psychological status.
- Monitor for adverse effects of mechanical ventilation: infection, barotrauma, reduced cardiac output.
- Position the patient to facilitate ventilation-perfusion ($\dot{V}/\dot{Q}$) matching ["good lung down"], as appropriate.
- Monitor the effects of ventilator changes on oxygenation and the patient's subjective response.
- Monitor readiness to wean.
- Explain all procedures and treatments; provide access to a call light; visit the patient frequently.
- Provide a method of communication. Request consultation with a speech-language pathologist for assistance, if necessary.
- Initiate relaxation techniques, as appropriate.
- Administer muscle-paralyzing agents, sedatives, and narcotic analgesics, as prescribed.
- Include the patient and family whenever possible (especially during suctioning and tracheostomy care).

ABGs, Arterial blood gases; *ET,* endotrachel; *PEEP,* positive end-expiratory pressure.

FIG. 32-3 Display signals, alarms, and control panel of a typical volume-cycled ventilator.

preset. If the patient does not trigger spontaneous breaths, a ventilatory pattern is established by the ventilator. It is programmed to respond to the patient's inspiratory effort if he or she begins a breath. In this case, the ventilator delivers the preset tidal volume while allowing the patient to control the rate of breathing.

A disadvantage of the AC mode is that the ventilator continues to deliver a preset tidal volume even when the patient's spontaneous breathing rate increases. This can cause hyperventilation and respiratory alkalosis. Investigate and correct causes of hyperventilation, such as pain, anxiety, or acid-base imbalances.

Synchronized intermittent mandatory ventilation (SIMV) is similar to AC ventilation in that tidal volume and ventilatory rate are preset. If the patient does not breathe, a ventilatory pattern is established by the ventilator. Unlike the AC mode, SIMV allows spontaneous breathing at the patient's own rate and tidal volume between the ventilator breaths. It can be used as a main ventilatory mode or as a weaning mode. When used for weaning, the number of mechanical breaths (SIMV breaths) is gradually decreased (e.g., from 12 to 2) as the patient resumes spontaneous breathing. The mandatory ventilator breaths are delivered when the patient is ready to inspire. This action coordinates breathing between the ventilator and the patient.

Bi-level positive airway pressure (BiPAP) provides noninvasive pressure support ventilation by nasal mask or facemask. It is most often used for patients with sleep apnea but also may be used for patients with respiratory muscle fatigue or impending respiratory failure to avoid more invasive ventilation methods.

Other modes of ventilation, such as pressure support and continuous flow (flow-by), are part of most microprocessor ventilators. Both types decrease the work of breathing and are used for weaning patients from mechanical ventilation. Other modes are maximum mandatory ventilation (MMV), inverse inspiration-expiration (I/E) ratio, permissive hypercarbia, airway pressure–release ventilation (APRV), proportional assist ventilation, and high-frequency oscillation. Most modes use special ventilators, tubing, or airways.

Ventilator Controls and Settings. The volume-cycled ventilator is the most widely used type in the acute care setting. Regardless of the type of volume-cycled ventilator used, the controls and types of settings are universal (see Fig. 32-3). The physician prescribes the ventilator settings, and usually the ventilator is readied or set up by the respiratory therapy department. The nurse assists in connecting the patient to the ventilator and monitors the ventilator settings in conjunction with respiratory therapy.

Tidal volume (V_T) is the volume of air the patient receives with each breath, as measured on either inspiration or expiration. The average prescribed V_T ranges between 7 and 10 mL/kg of body weight. Adding a zero to a patient's weight in kilograms gives an estimate of tidal volume.

Rate, or breaths/min, is the number of ventilator breaths delivered per minute. The rate is usually set between 10 and 14 breaths/min.

Fraction of inspired oxygen (Fio_2) is the oxygen level delivered to the patient. The prescribed Fio_2 is based on the ABG values and the patient's condition. The range is 21% to 100% oxygen.

The oxygen delivered to the patient is warmed to body temperature (98.6° F [37° C]) and humidified to 100%. This is needed because upper air passages of the respiratory tree, which normally warm and humidify air, are bypassed. Humidifying and warming prevent mucosal damage.

Peak airway (inspiratory) pressure (PIP) is the pressure used by the ventilator to deliver a set tidal volume at a given lung compliance. The PIP value appears on the display of the ventilator. It is the highest pressure reached during inspiration. Monitoring trends in PIP that reflect changes in resistance of the lungs and resistance in the ventilator. An increased PIP reading means increased airway resistance in the patient or in the ventilator tubing (bronchospasm or pinched tubing), increased secretions, pulmonary edema, or decreased pulmonary compliance (the lungs or chest wall is "stiffer" and harder to inflate). An upper pressure limit is set to prevent barotrauma. When the limit is reached, the high-pressure alarm sounds and the remaining volume is not given.

Continuous positive airway pressure (CPAP) applies positive airway pressure throughout the entire respiratory cycle for spontaneously breathing patients. Sedating drugs are given lightly or not at all when the patient is receiving CPAP so that respiratory effort is not suppressed. CPAP keeps the alveoli open during inspiration and prevents alveolar collapse during expiration. This process increases functional residual capacity (FRC) and improves GAS EXCHANGE and oxygenation.

CPAP is commonly used to help in the weaning process. During CPAP, no ventilator breaths are delivered. The ventilator just delivers oxygen and provides monitoring and an alarm system. The respiratory pattern is determined by the patient's efforts. Normal levels of CPAP are 5 to 15 cm H_2O to promote adequate GAS EXCHANGE and oxygenation. If no pressure is set, the patient receives no positive pressure. The patient is then using the ventilator as a T-piece with alarms. Modifications of CPAP include nasal CPAP and BiPAP, which are used on a temporary basis for select problems.

Positive end-expiratory pressure (PEEP) is positive pressure exerted during expiration. PEEP improves oxygenation by enhancing GAS EXCHANGE and preventing atelectasis. It is used to treat persistent hypoxemia that does not improve with an acceptable oxygen delivery level. It may be added when the arterial oxygen pressure (Pao_2) remains low with an Fio_2 of 50% to 70% or greater.

The need for PEEP indicates a severe GAS EXCHANGE problem. *It is important to lower the Fio_2 delivered whenever possible because prolonged use of a high Fio_2 can damage lungs from the toxic effects of oxygen.* PEEP prevents alveoli from collapsing because the lungs are kept partially inflated so that alveolar-capillary gas exchange is promoted throughout the ventilatory cycle. The effect should be an increase in arterial blood oxygenation so that the Fio_2 can be decreased.

PEEP is "dialed in" on the control panel. The amount of PEEP is usually 5 to 15 cm H_2O (although higher PEEP can be used) and is monitored on the peak airway pressure dial, the same dial used to read the PIP. When PEEP is added, the dial does not return to zero at the end of exhalation; rather, it returns to a baseline that is increased from zero by the amount of PEEP applied.

Flow rate is how fast each breath is delivered and is usually set at 40 L/min. *If a patient is agitated or restless, has a widely fluctuating inspiratory pressure reading, or has other signs of air hunger, the flow may be set too low. Increasing the flow should be tried before using chemical restraints.*

Other settings may be used, depending on the type of ventilator and mode of ventilation. Examples include inspiratory and expiratory cycle, waveform, expiratory resistance, and plateau.

Nursing Management. The use of mechanical ventilation involves a collaborative and complex decision-making process for the patient and family and the health care team. Address the physical and psychological concerns of the patient and family because the mechanical ventilator often causes them anxiety. Explain the purpose of the ventilator, and acknowledge the patient's and family's feelings. Encourage the patient and family to express their concerns. Act as the coach to help and support them through this experience. Patients undergoing mechanical ventilation in ICUs often experience delirium, or "ICU psychosis." These patients need frequent, repeated explanations and reassurance.

When caring for a ventilated patient, be concerned with the patient first and the ventilator second. If the ventilator alarm sounds, examine the patient for breathing, color, and oxygen saturation before assessing the ventilator. It is vital to understand why mechanical ventilation is needed. Some problems requiring ventilation, such as excessive secretions, sepsis, and trauma, require different interventions to successfully wean from the ventilator. The patient's chronic health problems, especially chronic obstructive pulmonary disease (COPD), left-sided heart failure, anemia, and malnutrition, may slow weaning from mechanical ventilation and require close monitoring and intervention.

> **! NURSING SAFETY PRIORITY** (QSEN)
> *Action Alert*
>
> The nursing priorities in caring for the patient during mechanical ventilation are monitoring and evaluating patient responses, managing the ventilator system safely, and preventing complications.

Monitoring the Patient's Response. Monitor, evaluate, and document the patient's response to the ventilator. Assess vital signs and listen to breath sounds every 30 to 60 minutes at first.

Monitor respiratory parameters (e.g., capnography, pulse oximetry), and check ABG values (Carlisle, 2014). Monitoring provides information to guide the patient's activities, such as weaning, physical or occupational therapy, and self-care. Pace activities to ensure effective ventilation with adequate GAS EXCHANGE and oxygenation. Interpret ABG values to evaluate the effectiveness of ventilation and determine whether ventilator settings need to be changed (Lian, 2013).

Assess the breathing pattern in relation to the ventilatory cycle to determine whether the patient is tolerating or fighting the ventilator. Patient asynchrony with mechanical ventilation has many causes and reduces the effectiveness of GAS EXCHANGE (Mellott et al., 2014). Assess and record breath sounds, including bilateral equal breath sounds to ensure proper endotracheal (ET) tube placement. Determine the need for suctioning by observing secretions for type, color, and amount. Assess the area around the ET tube or tracheostomy site at least every 4 hours for color, tenderness, skin irritation, and drainage, and document the findings.

The nurse spends the most time with the patient and is most likely to be the first person to recognize changes in vital signs or ABG values, fatigue, or distress. Promptly coordinate with the physician and respiratory therapist to implement the appropriate interventions.

> ## ! NURSING SAFETY PRIORITY (QSEN)
> ### Critical Rescue
>
> If the patient develops respiratory distress during mechanical ventilation, immediately remove the ventilator and provide ventilation with a bag-valve-mask device. This action allows quick determination of whether the problem is with the ventilator or with the patient.

Serve as a resource for the psychological needs of the patient and family. Anxiety can reduce tolerance for mechanical ventilation. Skilled and sensitive nursing care promotes emotional well-being and synchrony with the ventilator. The patient cannot speak, and communication can be frustrating and anxiety-producing. The patient and family may panic because they believe that the voice has been lost. Reassure them that the ET tube prevents speech only temporarily.

Plan methods of communication to meet the patient's needs, such as a picture board, pen and paper, alphabet board, electronic tablet computer, or programmable speech-generating device (Grossbach et al., 2011). Finding a successful means for communication is important because the patient often feels isolated by the inability to speak. (See Chart 29-2 in Chapter 29.) Anticipate his or her needs, and provide easy access to frequently used belongings. Visits from family, friends, and pets and keeping a call light within reach are some ways of giving patients a sense of control over the environment. Urge them to participate in self-care.

Managing the Ventilator System. Ventilator settings are prescribed by the health care provider in conjunction with the respiratory therapist. Settings include tidal volume, respiratory rate, fraction of inspired oxygen (FiO_2), and mode of ventilation (assist-control [AC] ventilation, synchronized intermittent mandatory ventilation [SIMV], and adjunctive modes, such as positive end-expiratory pressure [PEEP], pressure support, or continuous flow).

Perform and document ventilator checks according to the standards of the unit or facility. Respond promptly to alarms. During a ventilator check, compare the prescribed ventilator settings with the actual settings. Check the level of water in the humidifier and the temperature of the humidifying system to ensure that they are not too high. Temperature extremes damage the airway mucosa. Remove any condensation in the ventilator tubing by draining water into drainage collection receptacles, and empty them every shift.

> ## ! NURSING SAFETY PRIORITY (QSEN)
> ### Action Alert
>
> To prevent bacterial contamination, do not allow moisture and water in the ventilator tubing to enter the humidifier.

Mechanical ventilators have alarm systems that warn of a problem with either the patient or the ventilator. *As required by The Joint Commission's NPSGs, alarm systems must be activated and functional at all times. If the cause of the alarm cannot be determined, ventilate the patient manually with a resuscitation bag until the problem is corrected by another health care professional.* The major alarms on a ventilator indicate either a high pressure or a low exhaled volume. Table 32-5 lists interventions for causes of ventilator alarms.

Assess and care for the ET or tracheostomy tube. Maintain a patent airway by suctioning when any of these conditions are present:

- Secretions
- Increased peak airway (inspiratory) pressure (PIP)
- Rhonchi
- Decreased breath sounds

Proper care of the ET or tracheostomy tube also ensures a patent airway. Assess tube position at least every 2 hours, especially when the airway is attached to heavy ventilator tubing that may pull on the tube. Position the ventilator tubing so that the patient can move without pulling on the ET or tracheostomy tube, possibly dislodging it. To detect changes in tube position, mark it where the tube touches the patient's teeth or nose. Give oral care per facility policy. Standardized oral care has been shown to reduce ventilator-associated pneumonia (VAP), specifically using chlorhexidine oral rinses twice daily (Kiyoshi-Teo et al., 2014; Morton & Fontaine, 2013; Urden et al., 2012).

Special attention is needed for the patient being transported while receiving mechanical ventilation. Monitor SpO_2 during transport to assess adequacy of ventilation. Assess lung sounds each time the patient is moved, transferred, or turned.

> ## ? NCLEX EXAMINATION CHALLENGE
> ### Safe and Effective Care Environment
>
> A student nurse is working with a client in the ICU who is intubated and being mechanically ventilated. What action by the student causes the registered nurse to intervene?
> A. Repositioning the client every 2 hours
> B. Providing oral care with chlorhexidine rinse
> C. Checking tube placement at the client's incisor
> D. Turning off ventilator alarms while working in the room

TABLE 32-5   Nursing Interventions for Various Causes of Ventilator Alarms

CAUSE	NURSING INTERVENTIONS
High-Pressure Alarm (sounds when peak inspiratory pressure reaches the set alarm limit [usually set 10-20 mm Hg above the patient's baseline PIP])	
An increased amount of secretions or a mucus plug is in the airways.	Suction as needed.
The patient coughs, gags, or bites on the oral ET tube.	Insert oral airway to prevent biting on the ET tube.
The patient is anxious or fights the ventilator.	Provide emotional support to decrease anxiety. Increase the flow rate. Explain all procedures to the patient. Provide sedation or paralyzing agent per the health care provider's prescription.
Airway size decreases related to wheezing or bronchospasm.	Auscultate breath sounds. Collaborate with respiratory therapy to provide prescribed bronchodilators.
Pneumothorax occurs.	Alert the health care provider or Rapid Response Team about a new onset of decreased breath sounds or unequal chest excursion, which may be due to pneumothorax. Auscultate breath sounds.
The artificial airway is displaced; the ET tube may have slipped into the right mainstem bronchus.	Assess the chest for unequal breath sounds and chest excursion. Obtain a chest x-ray as ordered to evaluate the position of the ET tube. After the proper position is verified, secure the tube in place.
Obstruction in tubing occurs because the patient is lying on the tubing or there is water or a kink in the tubing.	Assess the system, beginning with the artificial airway and moving toward the ventilator.
There is increased PIP associated with deliverance of a sigh.	Empty water from the ventilator tubing, and remove any kinks. Coordinate with respiratory therapist or physician to adjust the pressure alarm.
Decreased compliance of the lungs is noted; a trend of gradually increasing PIP is noted over several hours or a day.	Evaluate the reasons for the decreased compliance of the lungs. Increased PIP occurs in ARDS, pneumonia, or any worsening of pulmonary disease.
Low Exhaled Volume (or Low-Pressure) Alarm (sounds when there is a disconnection or leak in the ventilator circuit or a leak in the patient's artificial airway cuff)	
A leak in the ventilator circuit prevents breath from being delivered.	Assess all connections and all ventilator tubing for disconnection.
The patient stops spontaneous breathing in the SIMV or CPAP mode or on pressure support ventilation.	Evaluate the patient's tolerance of the mode.
A cuff leak occurs in the ET or tracheostomy tube.	Evaluate the patient for a cuff leak. A cuff leak is suspected when the patient can talk (air escapes from the mouth) or when the pilot balloon on the artificial airway is flat (see Tracheostomy Tubes section in Chapter 28).

ARDS, Acute respiratory distress syndrome; *CPAP,* continuous positive airway pressure; *ET,* endotracheal; *PIP,* peak inspiratory pressure; *SIMV,* synchronized intermittent mandatory ventilation.

Preventing Complications. Most problems are caused by the positive pressure from the ventilator. Nearly every body system is affected.

Cardiac problems from mechanical ventilation include hypotension and fluid retention. Hypotension is caused by positive pressure that increases chest pressure and inhibits blood return to the heart. The decreased blood return reduces cardiac output, causing hypotension, especially in patients who are dehydrated or need high PIP for ventilation. Teach the patient to avoid a **Valsalva maneuver** (bearing down while holding the breath).

Fluid is retained because of decreased cardiac output. The kidneys receive less blood flow, which stimulates the renin-angiotensin-aldosterone system to retain fluid. Humidified air in the ventilator system contributes to fluid retention. Monitor the patient's fluid intake and output, weight, hydration status, and manifestations of hypovolemia.

Lung problems from mechanical ventilation include:
- **Barotrauma** (damage to the lungs by positive pressure)
- **Volutrauma** (damage to the lung by excess volume delivered to one lung over the other)

- **Atelectrauma** (shear injury to alveoli from opening and closing)
- **Biotrauma** (inflammatory response–mediated damage to alveoli)
- **Ventilator-associated lung injury/Ventilator-induced lung injury (VALI/VILI)** (damage from prolonged ventilation causing loss of surfactant, increased inflammation, fluid leakage, and noncardiac pulmonary edema)
- Acid-base imbalance

Barotrauma includes pneumothorax, subcutaneous emphysema, and pneumomediastinum. Patients at highest risk for barotrauma have chronic airflow limitation (CAL), have blebs or bullae, are on PEEP, have dynamic hyperinflation, or require high pressures to ventilate the lungs (because of "stiff" lungs, as seen in acute respiratory distress syndrome [ARDS]). Ventilator-induced lung injury can be prevented by using low tidal volumes combined with moderate levels of PEEP, especially in patients with acute lung injury (ALI) or ARDS (Bortolotto & Makic, 2012). Blood gas problems can be corrected by ventilator changes and adjustment of fluid and electrolyte imbalances.

GI and nutrition problems result from the stress of mechanical ventilation. Stress ulcers occur in many patients receiving mechanical ventilation. These ulcers complicate the nutrition status and, because the mucosa are not intact, increase the risk for systemic infection. Antacids, sucralfate (Carafate, Sulcrate ✦), and histamine blockers such as ranitidine (Zantac) or proton-pump inhibitors such as esomeprazole (Nexium) may be prescribed as soon as the patient is intubated. Because many other acute or life-threatening events occur at the same time, nutrition is often neglected. Malnutrition is an extreme problem for these patients and is a cause of failing to wean from the ventilator. In malnutrition, the respiratory muscles lose mass and strength. The diaphragm, the major muscle of inspiration, is affected early. When it and other respiratory muscles are weak, ineffective breathing results, fatigue occurs, and the patient cannot be weaned.

Balanced nutrition, whether by diet, enteral feedings, or parenteral feeding, is essential during ventilation and should be started within 48 hours of intubation (Morton & Fontaine, 2013). Also, nutrition for the patient with chronic obstructive pulmonary disease (COPD) requires a reduction of dietary carbohydrates. During metabolism, carbohydrates are broken down to glucose, which then produces energy, carbon dioxide, and water. Excessive carbohydrate loads increase carbon dioxide production, which the patient with COPD may be unable to exhale. Hypercarbic respiratory failure results. Nutrition formulas with a higher fat content (e.g., Pulmocare, Nutri-Vent, Intralipid) are calorie sources to combat this problem.

Electrolyte replacement is also important because electrolytes influence muscle function. Monitor potassium, calcium, magnesium, and phosphate levels, and replace them as prescribed.

Infections are a threat for the patient using a ventilator, especially ventilator-associated pneumonia (VAP). The ET or tracheostomy tube bypasses the body's filtering process and provides a direct access for bacteria to enter the lower respiratory system. The artificial airway is colonized with bacteria within 48 hours, which promotes pneumonia development and increases morbidity. Aspiration of colonized fluid from the mouth or the stomach can be a source of infection. *Infection prevention through strict adherence to infection control, especially handwashing during suctioning and care of the tracheostomy or ET tube, is essential (Kiyoshi-Teo et al., 2014).*

To prevent VAP, implement "ventilator bundle" order sets, which typically include these actions (Morton & Fontaine, 2013; Munro & Ruggiero, 2014; Urden et al., 2012):
- Keeping the head of the bed elevated at least 30 degrees
- Performing oral care per agency policy (usually brushing teeth every 8 hours and antimicrobial rinse [chlorhexidine] every 2 hours)
- Ulcer prophylaxis
- Preventing aspiration
- Pulmonary hygiene including chest physiotherapy, postural drainage, and turning and positioning

Using the ventilator bundle has greatly reduced the overall incidence of VAP. Vigilant oral care is a key component of the VAP prevention strategy although there is considerable variation in actual practice for timing, products used, and specific application methods (Booker et al., 2013; Hiller et al., 2013; Kiyoshi-Teo et al., 2014). (See the Evidence-Based Practice box.) Additional information on pneumonia can be found in Chapter 31.

EVIDENCE-BASED PRACTICE QSEN

What is the Best Method and Timing of Oral Hygiene to Prevent Ventilator-Associated Pneumonia?

Hiller, B., Wilson, C., Chamberlain, D., & King, L. (2013). Preventing ventilator-associated pneumonia through oral care, product selection, and application method. *AACN Advanced Critical Care, 24*(1), 38-58.

Ventilator-associated pneumonia (VAP) is a common, costly, and preventable complication of patients receiving mechanical ventilation. During the past decade, implementation of a "ventilator bundle" care approach focusing on prevention of aspiration and prevention of oral bacterial translocation to the lower respiratory tract has been instrumental in reducing the incidence of VAP. At first, more effort was placed on preventing aspiration; however, many studies showed that improved oral care contributed significantly to VAP reduction.

The literature abounds with different methods of oral care and products used. Some methods include toothbrushing, whereas others used sponge swabs. The most commonly used product was chlorhexidine rinse, although the concentration of this solution varied. Some studies also saw a reduction in VAP using sodium chloride solutions combined with mouth swabbing or tooth brushing. Frequency of oral care ranged from twice daily to every 2 hours. Although more vigilant oral care is key to VAP prevention, a clear best practice protocol for frequency, method of care application, and specific product use has yet to be identified. In addition, the qualifications of the person performing the oral assessment and the actual oral care vary among the studies.

Level of Evidence: 1

The results are based on a systematic review and meta-analysis of previous studies related to the outcomes of implementing oral hygiene protocols to help prevent VAP among patients receiving mechanical ventilation. Results of this analysis do indicate that education for nurses and unlicensed assistive personnel (UAP) about oral care needs for the patient receiving mechanical ventilation is needed for optimal outcomes, although no particular practice methods or products emerged as superior in reducing the incidence of VAP.

Commentary: Implications for Practice and Research

For best practice, a protocol must be both effective at preventing VAP and not harmful to the patient. Thus it must demonstrate clear positive outcomes and a lack of harmful outcomes. In addition, the protocol must be viewed as valuable by the people who are supposed to be implementing it. The previous studies analyzed showed that many nurses and UAP did not understand the link between poor oral hygiene and VAP. Thus nursing education needs to stress to students and practicing nurses that good oral hygiene is not just an optional comfort measure but is actually a critical health promotion strategy. In addition, more research is needed into which solutions and solution concentrations provide adequate control of oral flora without causing harm. Chlorhexidine is a drug, and its use requires a health care provider's prescription. In some states, UAP would not be permitted to apply this topical solution in oral care. Thus studies are needed to determine the optimum frequency of chlorhexidine oral hygiene provided by nurses coupled with UAP-implemented sessions of oral hygiene using nonprescription solutions as part of the overall protocol.

Muscle deconditioning and weakness can occur because of immobility. Getting the patient out of bed and having him or her ambulate with help and perform exercises not only improves muscle strength but also boosts morale, enhances GAS EXCHANGE, and promotes oxygen delivery to all muscles. Early progressive mobility decreases ventilator days and ICU stays (Morris et al.,

2011). Early passive exercise may also be beneficial (Amidei & Sole, 2013).

Ventilator dependence is the inability to wean off the ventilator and can have both a physiologic basis and psychological basis. The longer a patient uses a ventilator, the more difficult the weaning process is because the respiratory muscles fatigue and cannot assume breathing. The health care team uses every method of weaning before a patient is declared "unweanable."

Collaborate with the physician, social worker or psychologist, and a member of the clergy to discuss with the patient and family the patient's quality of life, goals, and values. As a result of this discussion, arrange for home ventilation, nursing home placement, or withdrawal of life support (in terminal cases). Special units and facilities can maximize the rehabilitation and weaning of ventilator-dependent patients.

Weaning. Weaning is the process of going from ventilatory dependence to spontaneous breathing. The process is prolonged by complications. Many problems can be avoided with good nursing care. For example, turning and positioning the patient not only promote comfort and prevent skin breakdown but also improve GAS EXCHANGE and prevent pneumonia and atelectasis. Table 32-6 lists various weaning techniques.

CONSIDERATIONS FOR OLDER ADULTS
Patient-Centered Care QSEN

The older patient, especially one who has smoked or who has a chronic lung problem such as COPD, is at risk for ventilator dependence and failure to wean. Age-related changes, such as chest wall stiffness, reduced ventilatory muscle strength, and decreased lung elasticity, reduce the likelihood of weaning. The usual manifestations of ventilatory failure—hypoxemia and hypercarbia—may be less obvious in the older adult. Use other clinical measures of gas exchange and oxygenation, such as a change in mental status, to determine breathing effectiveness.

Extubation. Extubation is the removal of the endotracheal (ET) tube. The tube is removed when the need for intubation has been resolved. Before removal, explain the procedure. Set up the prescribed oxygen delivery system at the bedside, and bring in the equipment for emergency reintubation. Hyperoxygenate the patient, and thoroughly suction both the ET tube and the oral cavity. Then rapidly deflate the cuff of the ET tube and remove the tube at peak inspiration. Immediately instruct the patient to cough. It is normal for large amounts of oral secretions to collect. Give oxygen by facemask or nasal cannula. The fraction of inspired oxygen (FiO_2) is usually prescribed at 10% higher than the level used while the ET tube was in place.

Monitor vital signs after extubation every 5 minutes at first, and assess the ventilatory pattern for manifestations of respiratory distress. It is common for patients to be hoarse and have a sore throat for a few days after extubation. Teach the patient to sit in a semi-Fowler's position, take deep breaths every half-hour, use an incentive spirometer every 2 hours, and limit speaking. These measures help improve GAS EXCHANGE, decrease laryngeal edema, and reduce vocal cord irritation. Observe closely for respiratory fatigue and airway obstruction.

Early manifestations of obstruction are mild dyspnea, coughing, and the inability to expectorate secretions. Stridor is a high-pitched, crowing noise during inspiration caused by laryngospasm or edema around the glottis. It is a late manifestation

of a narrowed airway and requires prompt attention. Racemic epinephrine, a topical aerosol vasoconstrictor, is given, and reintubation may be needed.

TABLE 32-6 Weaning Methods

Synchronous Intermittent Mandatory Ventilation
- The patient breathes between the machine's preset breaths/min rate.
- The machine is initially set on an SIMV rate of 12, meaning the patient receives a minimum of 12 breaths/min by the ventilator.
- The patient's respiratory rate will be a combination of ventilator breaths and spontaneous breaths.
- As the weaning process ensues, the health care provider prescribes gradual decreases in the SIMV rate, usually at a decrease of 1 to 2 breaths/min.

T-Piece Technique
- The patient is taken off the ventilator for short periods (initially 5 to 10 minutes) and allowed to breathe spontaneously.
- The ventilator is replaced with a T-piece (see Chapter 28) or CPAP, which delivers humidified oxygen.
- The prescribed FiO_2 may be higher for the patient on the T-piece than on the ventilator.
- Weaning progresses as the patient can tolerate progressively longer periods off the ventilator.
- Nighttime weaning is not usually attempted until the patient can maintain spontaneous respirations most of the day.

Pressure Support Ventilation
- PSV allows the patient's respiratory effort to be augmented by a predetermined pressure assist from the ventilator.
- As the weaning process ensues, the amount of pressure applied to inspiration is gradually decreased.
- Another method of weaning with PSV is to maintain the pressure but gradually decrease the ventilator's preset breaths/min rate.

CPAP, Continuous positive airway pressure; *FiO₂,* fraction of inspired oxygen; *PSV,* pressure support ventilation; *SIMV,* synchronized intermittent mandatory ventilation.

! NURSING SAFETY PRIORITY QSEN
Critical Rescue

When stridor or other manifestations of obstruction occur after extubation, immediately call the Rapid Response Team before the airway becomes completely obstructed.

CHEST TRAUMA

Chest injuries are responsible for about 25% of traumatic deaths in the United States each year and are a contributing factor in about 50% of deaths related to trauma (Mancini, 2012a). Many of the injured die before arriving at the hospital. A few types of chest injury require thoracotomy. Most can be treated with basic resuscitation, intubation, or chest tube placement. *The first emergency approach to all chest injuries is ABC (airway, breathing, circulation), a rapid assessment and treatment of life-threatening conditions.* See Chapter 8 for more information on care of the trauma patient.

Pulmonary Contusion

Pulmonary contusion, a potentially lethal injury, is a common chest injury and occurs most often by rapid deceleration during car crashes. After a contusion, respiratory failure can develop immediately or over time. Hemorrhage and edema occur in and between the alveoli, reducing both lung movement and the area available for GAS EXCHANGE. The patient becomes hypoxemic and dyspneic.

Patients may be asymptomatic at first and can later develop various degrees of respiratory failure. These patients often have decreased breath sounds or crackles and wheezes over the affected area. Other manifestations include bruising over the injury, dry cough, tachycardia, tachypnea, and dullness to percussion. At first, the chest x-ray may show no abnormalities. A hazy opacity in the lobes or parenchyma may develop over several days. If there is no disruption of the parenchyma, bruise resorption often occurs without treatment (Dennison et al., 2011; Mancini, 2012a).

Management includes maintenance of ventilation and oxygenation. Provide oxygen, give IV fluids as prescribed, and place the patient in a moderate-Fowler's position. When side-lying, the "good lung down" position may be helpful. The patient in obvious respiratory distress may need mechanical ventilation with positive end-expiratory pressure (PEEP) to inflate the lungs.

A vicious cycle occurs in which more muscle effort is needed for ventilating a lung with a contusion and the patient becomes progressively hypoxemic. This situation causes him or her to tire easily, have reduced GAS EXCHANGE, and become more fatigued and hypoxemic. This condition often leads to acute respiratory distress syndrome (ARDS).

Rib Fracture

Rib fractures are a common injury to the chest wall, often resulting from direct blunt trauma to the chest. The force applied to the ribs fractures them and drives the bone ends into the chest. Thus there is a risk for deep chest injury, such as pulmonary contusion, pneumothorax, and hemothorax.

The patient has pain on movement and splints the chest defensively. Splinting reduces breathing depth and clearance of secretions. If the patient has pre-existing lung disease, the risk for atelectasis and pneumonia increases. Those with injuries to the first or second ribs, flail chest, seven or more fractured ribs, or expired volumes of less than 15 mL/kg often have a deep chest injury and a poor prognosis.

Management of uncomplicated rib fractures is simple because the fractured ribs reunite spontaneously. The chest is usually not splinted by tape or other materials. The main focus is to decrease pain so that adequate ventilation is maintained. An intercostal nerve block may be used if pain is severe. Analgesics that cause respiratory depression are avoided.

Flail Chest

Flail chest is the result of fractures of at least two neighboring ribs in two or more places causing **paradoxical chest wall movement** (inward movement of the thorax during inspiration, with outward movement during expiration) (Fig. 32-4). It usually involves one side of the chest and results from blunt chest trauma—often high-speed car crashes. Because the force required to produce a flail chest is great, it is important to assess for other possible underlying injuries (Bjerke, 2012; Poirier & Vacca, 2013).

Flail chest can also occur from bilateral separations of the ribs from their cartilage connections to each other anteriorly, without an actual rib fracture. This condition can occur as a complication of cardiopulmonary resuscitation. Other injuries to the lung tissue under the flail segment may be present. GAS

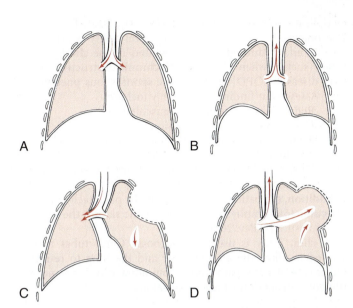

FIG. 32-4 Flail chest. Normal respiration: **A,** Inspiration; **B,** Expiration. Paradoxic motion: **C,** Inspiration—area of the lung underlying unstable chest wall sucks in on inspiration; **D,** Expiration—unstable area balloons out. Note movement of mediastinum toward opposite lung during inspiration.

EXCHANGE, coughing, and clearance of secretions are impaired. Splinting further reduces the patient's ability to exert the extra effort to breathe and may contribute later to failure to wean.

Assess the patient with a flail chest for paradoxical chest movement, dyspnea, cyanosis, tachycardia, and hypotension. The patient is often anxious, short of breath, and in pain. Work of breathing is increased from the paradoxical movement of the involved segment of the chest wall (Bjerke, 2012).

Interventions include humidified oxygen, pain management, promotion of lung expansion through deep breathing and positioning, and secretion clearance by coughing and tracheal suction.

The patient with a flail chest may be managed with vigilant respiratory care. Mechanical ventilation is needed if respiratory failure or shock occurs. Monitor ABG values and vital capacity closely. With severe hypoxemia and hypercarbia, the patient is intubated and mechanically ventilated with PEEP. With lung contusion or an underlying pulmonary disease, the risk for respiratory failure increases. Usually flail chest is stabilized by positive-pressure ventilation. Surgical stabilization is used only in extreme cases of flail chest (Messing et al., 2014).

Monitor the patient's vital signs and fluid and electrolyte balance closely so that hypovolemia or shock can be managed immediately. If he or she has a lung contusion, provide oxygen as needed and give IV fluids as prescribed. Assess for and relieve pain with prescribed analgesic drugs by IV, epidural, or nerve block route. Give psychosocial support to the anxious patient by explaining all procedures, talking slowly, and allowing time for expression of feelings and concerns.

Pneumothorax

Any chest injury that allows air to enter the pleural space results in a rise in chest pressure and a reduction in vital capacity. Severity depends on the amount of lung collapse produced. Pneumothorax is often caused by blunt chest trauma and may occur with some degree of hemothorax. It can also occur as a complication of medical procedures (Day, 2011; Ruiz, 2011). The pneumothorax can be *open* (pleural cavity is exposed to outside air, as through an open wound in the chest wall) or *closed* (such as when a patient with chronic obstructive pulmonary disease [COPD] experiences a spontaneous pneumothorax). Assessment findings commonly include:

- Reduced breath sounds on auscultation
- Hyperresonance on percussion
- Prominence of the involved side of the chest, which moves poorly with respirations
- Deviation of the trachea *away* from the side of injury (tension pneumothorax)

In addition, the patient may have pleuritic pain, tachypnea, and subcutaneous emphysema (air under the skin in the subcutaneous tissues (Daley, 2014).

A chest x-ray is used for diagnosis. Chest tubes may be needed to allow the air to escape and the lung to re-inflate. Other care includes pain control, pulmonary hygiene, and continued assessment for respiratory failure.

Tension Pneumothorax

Tension pneumothorax, a rapidly developing and life-threatening complication of blunt chest trauma, results from an air leak in the lung or chest wall. Air forced into the chest cavity causes complete collapse of the affected lung. Air that enters the pleural space during inspiration does not exit during expiration. As a result, air collects under pressure, compressing blood vessels and limiting blood return. This process leads to decreased filling of the heart and reduced cardiac output. *If not promptly detected and treated, tension pneumothorax is quickly fatal.* Causes include blunt chest trauma, mechanical ventilation with positive end-expiratory pressure (PEEP), closed–chest drainage (chest tubes), and insertion of central venous access catheters.

Assessment findings with tension pneumothorax include:

- Asymmetry of the thorax
- Tracheal movement *away* from midline toward the *unaffected* side
- Extreme respiratory distress
- Absence of breath sounds on one side
- Distended neck veins
- Cyanosis
- Hypertympanic sound on percussion over the affected side
- Hemodynamic instability

Pneumothorax is detectable on a chest x-ray but also can be diagnosed by the patient's manifestations. ABG assays show hypoxia and respiratory alkalosis.

Initial management is an immediate needle thoracostomy, with a large-bore needle inserted by the health care provider into the second intercostal space in the midclavicular line of the affected side. Then a chest tube is placed into the fourth intercostal space and the other end is attached to a water seal drainage system until the lung re-inflates. Chest tubes are discussed in detail in Chapter 30.

Nursing care also involves pain control and pulmonary hygiene.

Hemothorax

Hemothorax is a common problem occurring after blunt chest trauma or penetrating injuries. A *simple* hemothorax is a blood loss of less than 1000 mL into the chest cavity; a *massive* hemothorax is a blood loss of more than 1000 mL (Mancini, 2012b).

Bleeding is caused by injury to the lung tissue, such as lung contusions or lacerations, that can occur with rib and sternal fractures. Massive internal chest bleeding in blunt chest trauma may stem from the heart, the great vessels, or the intercostal arteries.

Assessment findings vary with the size of the hemothorax. If the hemothorax is small, the patient may not have manifestations. With a large hemothorax, the patient may have respiratory distress with breath sounds reduced on auscultation. Percussion on the involved side produces a dull sound. Blood in the pleural space is visible on a chest x-ray and is confirmed by thoracentesis.

Interventions focus on removing the blood in the pleural space to normalize breathing and to prevent infection. Chest tubes are inserted to empty the pleural space; multiple chest tubes may be needed. Closely monitor the chest tube drainage. Serial chest x-rays are used to determine treatment effectiveness. Aggressive pain management and pulmonary hygiene are also part of care.

An open thoracotomy is needed when there is initial blood loss of 1000 mL from the chest or persistent bleeding at the rate of 150 to 200 mL/hr over 3 to 4 hours (Mancini, 2012b). Monitor the vital signs, blood loss, and intake and output. Assess the patient's response to the chest tubes, and infuse IV fluids and blood as prescribed. The blood lost through chest drainage can be infused back into the patient after processing if needed.

Tracheobronchial Trauma

Most tears of the tracheobronchial tree result from severe blunt trauma or rapid deceleration and often involve the mainstem bronchi. These injuries are rare, and patients often die before reaching the hospital. Injuries to the trachea usually occur at the junction of the trachea and cricoid cartilage, often by striking the neck against the dashboard or steering wheel during a car crash. Patients with tracheal lacerations develop massive air leaks, which cause air to enter the mediastinum and lead to extensive subcutaneous emphysema. Upper airway obstruction may occur, causing severe respiratory distress and stridor.

Airway management is the priority. If possible, an ET tube is placed distal to the injury. Cricothyroidotomy or tracheotomy below the level of injury may be required. A patient with a torn mainstem bronchus may develop a tension pneumothorax rapidly when intubated and ventilated with positive pressure (Dennison et al., 2011; Mancini, 2012a).

Assess for hypoxemia by ABG assays. Apply oxygen as needed. Depending on the degree of injury, the patient may need mechanical ventilation or surgical repair. Assess vital signs every 15 minutes because hypotension and shock are likely. Assess for subcutaneous emphysema and listen to the lungs every 1 to 2 hours. Decreased breath sounds or wheezing may indicate further obstruction, atelectasis, or pneumothorax. Care of the patient with a tracheostomy is discussed in Chapter 28.

NURSING CONCEPTS AND CLINICAL JUDGMENT REVIEW

What might you NOTICE if the patient is experiencing inadequate GAS EXCHANGE and tissue PERFUSION as a result of a critical respiratory problem?

- Respirations rapid and shallow
- Change in cognition, acute confusion (especially in older adults)
- Decreased oxygen saturation by pulse oximetry
- Cyanosis or pallor of the lips and oral mucous membranes
- Tachycardia
- Patient appears to strain to catch breath
- Patient is restless or anxious

What should you INTERPRET and how should you RESPOND to a patient experiencing inadequate GAS EXCHANGE and tissue PERFUSION as a result of a critical respiratory problem?

Perform and interpret physical assessment, including:
- Taking vital signs
- Auscultating all lung fields
- Monitoring oxygen saturation by pulse oximetry
- Checking the accuracy of pulse oximetry readings
- Checking most recent laboratory values for ABG levels
- Assessing chest symmetry
- Assessing accessory muscle use
- Assessing cognition
- Assessing for the presence of hemoptysis
- Assessing the patient's ability to cough and clear the airway
- Asking the patient if he or she has chest pain

- Checking for the presence of petechiae, especially over the chest

Respond by:
- Applying oxygen and assessing the patient's responses
- Keeping the patient's head elevated to about 30 degrees (unless the potential for cervical spine trauma exists)
- Suctioning (oral, pharyngeal, endotracheal, tracheostomy), if needed
- Notifying the physician or Rapid Response Team
- Staying with the patient
- Calling for the emergency cart to be brought to the patient's bedside
- Reassuring the patient that appropriate interventions are being instituted
- Preparing for intubation
- Using a manual resuscitation bag if the patient's Spo_2 falls below 60% while receiving oxygen by mask
- Starting an IV

On what should you REFLECT?
- Observe patient for evidence of restored GAS EXCHANGE and oxygenation (see Chapter 27).
- Think about what may have precipitated this episode and what steps could be taken to either prevent a similar episode or identify it earlier.
- Think about what additional resources might improve the nursing response to this situation.

GET READY FOR THE NCLEX® EXAMINATION!

KEY POINTS

Review these Key Points for each NCLEX Examination Client Needs Category.

Safe and Effective Care Environment
- Use aseptic technique when caring for a patient requiring pulmonary suctioning. **Safety** QSEN
- Identify patients in your setting who are at risk for developing a pulmonary embolism. **Safety** QSEN
- Use Bleeding Precautions for patients receiving anticlotting therapy (see Chart 32-6). **Safety** QSEN
- Keep antidotes available when patients are receiving heparin (antidote is protamine) or warfarin (antidote is phytonadione). **Safety** QSEN
- Inspect the mouth and perform oral care every 2 hours for anyone who has an endotracheal tube or is being mechanically ventilated. **Safety** QSEN
- Check and document ventilator settings hourly. **Safety** QSEN
- Ensure that alarm systems on mechanical ventilators are activated and functional at all times. **Safety** QSEN
- Ensure that bag-valve-mask device and suction equipment are at the bedside at all times. **Safety** QSEN
- Evaluate the need for chemical restraint or soft wrist restraints.

Health Promotion and Maintenance
- Teach patients ways to promote venous return and avoid venous thromboembolism (VTE), especially when traveling long distances (see Chart 32-1). **Patient-Centered Care** QSEN
- Teach patients ways to prevent injury when taking drugs that reduce CLOTTING (see Chart 32-7). **Patient-Centered Care** QSEN

Psychosocial Integrity
- Allow the patient and family members the opportunity to express feelings and concerns about a change in breathing status or the possibility of intubation and mechanical ventilation. **Patient-Centered Care** QSEN
- Use alternate ways to communicate with a patient who is intubated or being mechanically ventilated. **Patient-Centered Care** QSEN
- Reassure intubated patients that speech loss is temporary. **Patient-Centered Care** QSEN
- Remember that patients who are receiving mechanical ventilation and are being chemically paralyzed usually can hear and can feel pain. **Patient-Centered Care** QSEN
- Provide appropriate pain management. **Patient-Centered Care** QSEN

Physiological Integrity

- Use Aspiration Precautions for any patient with an altered level of consciousness, poor gag reflex, or neurologic impairment or who has an endotracheal tube. **Evidence-Based Practice** QSEN
- Check the patient with ARDS hourly for oxygen saturation, vital sign changes, or any indication of increased work of breathing such as cyanosis, pallor, and retractions. **Patient-Centered Care** QSEN
- Assess all patients with blunt chest trauma for tracheal position and bilateral breath sounds. **Patient-Centered Care** QSEN
- Notify the physician immediately for any patient who develops sudden-onset respiratory difficulty. **Safety** QSEN
- Check oxygen saturation by pulse oximetry for any patient who has trouble breathing or who develops acute confusion. **Patient-Centered Care** QSEN
- Evaluate ABG values to assess the severity of hypoxia and the patient's response to therapy. **Patient-Centered Care** QSEN

- Apply oxygen to anyone who is hypoxemic. **Evidence-Based Practice** QSEN
- Ensure that oxygen therapy delivered to the patient is humidified. **Evidence-Based Practice** QSEN
- Assess lung sounds bilaterally each hour for patients who are receiving PEEP. **Patient-Centered Care** QSEN
- Check all ventilator settings against the prescription at least once per shift. **Safety** QSEN
- Administer drugs for pain to patients who have rib fractures, and encourage deep breaths. **Patient-Centered Care** QSEN
- Evaluate nutrition status, and collaborate with the dietitian to meet the patient's nutrition needs. **Teamwork and Collaboration** QSEN
- If a patient experiences respiratory distress during mechanical ventilation, remove him or her from the ventilator and provide ventilation by bag-valve-mask device. **Safety** QSEN

CHAPTER 33

Assessment of the Cardiovascular System

Donna Ignatavicius

 http://evolve.elsevier.com/Iggy/

PRIORITY CONCEPTS

- PERFUSION
- FLUID AND ELECTROLYTE BALANCE

LEARNING OUTCOMES

Safe and Effective Care Environment
1. Prioritize care for patients having invasive cardiac diagnostic tests.

Health Promotion and Maintenance
2. Identify patients at risk for cardiovascular (CV) problems.
3. Differentiate modifiable and nonmodifiable risk factors for CV disease.
4. Teach patients about evidence-based ways to decrease their risk for CV health problems.
5. Explain nursing implications related to CV changes that affect PERFUSION in older adults.

Psychosocial Integrity
6. Describe common psychological responses to CV disease.

Physiological Integrity
7. Review the anatomy and physiology of the CV system.
8. Describe the unique characteristics of heart disease in women.
9. Perform focused physical assessment for patients with CV problems.
10. Interpret laboratory test findings for patients with suspected or actual CV disease.

As the name implies, the cardiovascular (CV) system is made up of the heart and blood vessels (both arteries and veins). It is responsible for supplying oxygen to body organs and other tissues (PERFUSION). The heart muscle, called the myocardium, must receive sufficient oxygen to pump blood to other parts of the body. The arteries must be patent so that the pumped blood can reach the rest of the body. *Oxygen in the blood* is needed for cells to live and function properly. When diseases or other problems of the CV systems occur, oxygenation and PERFUSION decrease, often resulting in life-threatening events or a risk for these events.

The CV system works with the respiratory and hematologic systems to meet the human need for oxygenation and tissue PERFUSION (see Fig. 1 of the *Concept Overview*). Any problem in these systems requires the CV system to work harder to meet oxygenation and tissue perfusion needs.

Cardiovascular disease (CVD) continues to be the number-one cause of death in the United States. An average of one death in the United States occurs every 40 seconds from CVD (Go

et al., 2013). The disease kills more people than the next four causes of death combined, including cancer, chronic lower respiratory diseases, accidents, and diabetes. *Of particular concern is that CVD is the leading cause of death for women.* In addition, the American Heart Association (AHA) estimates that more than one in three adults is living with some form of the disease. About 20% of people who experience a myocardial infarction will die within 1 year from the initial cardiac event (Go et al., 2013).

ANATOMY AND PHYSIOLOGY REVIEW

Heart

Structure
The human heart is a fist-sized, muscular organ located in the mediastinum between the lungs (Fig. 33-1). Each beat of the heart pumps about 60 mL of blood, or 5 L/min. During strenuous physical activity, it can double the amount of blood pumped

FIG. 33-1 Surface anatomy of the heart.

to meet the body's increased oxygenation needs. The heart is protected by a covering called the *pericardium*. A muscular wall (septum) separates the heart into two halves: right and left. Each half has an atrium and a ventricle (Fig. 33-2).

The *right atrium (RA)* receives *deoxygenated* venous blood, which is returned from the body through the superior and inferior venae cavae. It also receives blood from the heart muscle through the coronary sinus. Most of this venous return flows passively from the RA, through the opened tricuspid valve, and to the right ventricle during ventricular diastole, or filling. The remaining venous return is actively propelled by the RA into the right ventricle during atrial systole, or contraction.

The *right ventricle (RV)* is a muscular pump located behind the sternum. It generates enough pressure to close the tricuspid valve, open the pulmonic valve, and propel blood into the pulmonary artery and the lungs.

After blood is *reoxygenated* in the lungs, it flows freely from the four pulmonary veins into the left atrium. Blood then flows through an opened mitral valve into the left ventricle during ventricular diastole. When the left ventricle is almost full, the *left atrium (LA)* contracts, pumping the remaining blood volume into the left ventricle. With systolic contraction, the *left ventricle (LV)* generates enough pressure to close the mitral valve and open the aortic valve. Blood is propelled into the aorta and into the systemic arterial circulation. Blood flow through the heart is shown in Fig. 33-2.

Blood moves from the aorta throughout the systemic circulation to the various tissues of the body. The pressure of blood in the aorta of a young adult averages about 100 to 120 mm Hg, whereas the pressure of blood in the RA averages about 0 to 5 mm Hg. These differences in pressure produce a pressure gradient, with blood flowing from an area of higher pressure to an area of lower pressure. The heart and vascular structures are responsible for maintaining these pressures.

The four *cardiac valves* are responsible for maintaining the forward flow of blood through the chambers of the heart (see

Fig. 33-2). These valves open and close when pressure and volume change within the heart's chambers. The cardiac valves are classified into two types: atrioventricular (AV) valves and semilunar valves.

The *AV valves* separate the atria from the ventricles. The *tricuspid valve* separates the RA from the RV. The *mitral (bicuspid) valve* separates the LA from the LV. During ventricular diastole, these valves act as funnels and help move the flow of blood from the atria to the ventricles. During systole, the valves close to prevent the backflow (**valvular regurgitation**) of blood into the atria.

The *semilunar valves* are the pulmonic valve and the aortic valve, which prevent blood from flowing back into the ventricles during diastole. The *pulmonic valve* separates the right ventricle from the pulmonary artery. The *aortic valve* separates the left ventricle from the aorta.

The heart muscle receives blood to meet its metabolic needs through the coronary arterial system (Fig. 33-3). The coronary arteries originate from an area on the aorta just beyond the aortic valve. All of the coronary arteries feeding the left heart originate from the left main coronary artery (LMCA). The right coronary artery (RCA) branches from the aorta to perfuse the right heart and inferior wall of the left heart.

Coronary artery blood flow to the myocardium occurs primarily during diastole, when coronary vascular resistance is minimized. *To maintain adequate blood flow through the coronary arteries,* **mean arterial pressure (MAP)** *must be at least 60 mm Hg. A MAP of between 60 and 70 mm Hg is necessary to maintain perfusion of major body organs, such as the kidneys and brain.*

The *left main artery* divides into two branches: the left anterior descending (LAD) branch and the left circumflex (LCX) branch. The LAD branch descends toward the anterior wall and the apex of the left ventricle. It supplies blood to portions of the left ventricle, ventricular septum, chordae tendineae, papillary muscle, and, to a lesser extent, the right ventricle.

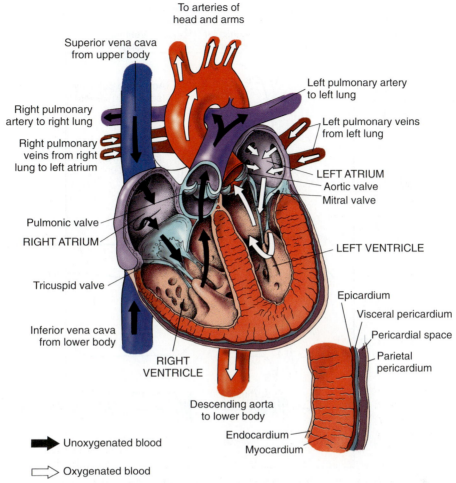

FIG. 33-2 Blood flow through the heart.

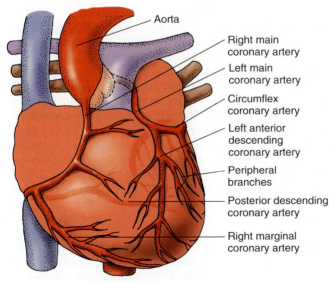

FIG. 33-3 Coronary arterial system.

The LCX branch descends toward the lateral wall of the left ventricle and apex. It supplies blood to the left atrium, the lateral and posterior surfaces of the left ventricle, and sometimes portions of the interventricular septum. In about half of people, the LCX branch supplies the sinoatrial (SA) node. In a very small number of people, it supplies the AV node. Peripheral

branches arise from the LAD and LCX branches and form an abundant network of vessels throughout the entire myocardium.

The *right coronary artery (RCA)* originates from the right sinus of Valsalva, encircles the heart, and descends toward the apex of the right ventricle. The RCA supplies the RA, RV, and inferior portion of the LV. In about half of people, the RCA supplies the SA node, and in almost everyone, it supplies the AV node.

Function

The *electrophysiologic properties* of heart muscle are responsible for regulating heart rate (HR) and rhythm. Cardiac muscle cells possess the characteristics of automaticity, excitability, conductivity, contractility, and refractoriness. Chapter 34 describes these properties and cardiac conduction in detail.

Sequence of Events During the Cardiac Cycle. The phases of the cardiac cycle are generally described in relation to changes in pressure and volume in the left ventricle during filling (diastole) and ventricular contraction (systole) (Fig. 33-4). **Diastole,** normally about two thirds of the cardiac cycle, consists of relaxation and filling of the atria and ventricles. **Systole** consists of the contraction and emptying of the atria and ventricles.

Myocardial contraction results from the release of large numbers of calcium ions from the sarcoplasmic reticulum and from the blood. These ions diffuse into the myofibril sarcomere (the basic contractile unit of the myocardial cell). Calcium ions

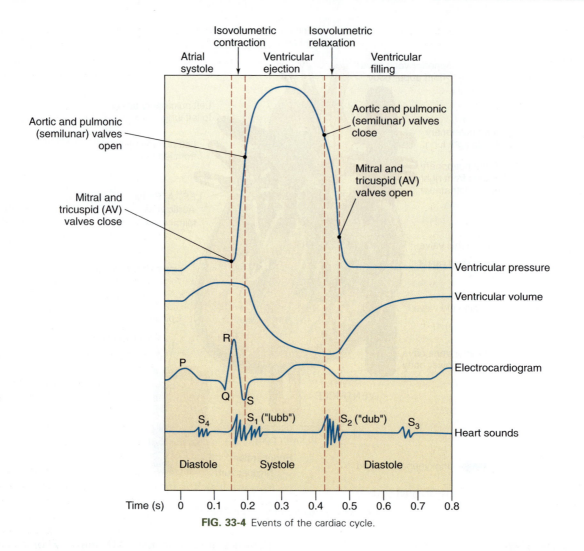

FIG. 33-4 Events of the cardiac cycle.

promote the interaction of actin and myosin protein filaments, causing these filaments to link and overlap. Cross-bridges, or linkages, are formed as the protein filaments slide over or overlap each other. These cross-bridges act as force-generating sites. The sliding of these protein filaments shortens the sarcomeres, producing myocardial contraction.

Cardiac muscle relaxes when calcium ions are pumped back into the sarcoplasmic reticulum, causing a decrease in the number of calcium ions around the myofibrils. This reduced number of ions causes the protein filaments to disengage, the sarcomere to lengthen, and the muscle to relax.

Mechanical Properties of the Heart. The electrical and mechanical properties of cardiac muscle determine the function of the cardiovascular system. The healthy heart can adapt to various pathophysiologic conditions (e.g., stress, infections, hemorrhage) to maintain PERFUSION to the various body tissues. Blood flow from the heart into the systemic arterial circulation is measured clinically as **cardiac output (CO)**, the amount of blood pumped from the left ventricle each minute. *CO depends on the relationship between heart rate (HR) and stroke volume (SV);* it is the product of these two variables:

Cardiac output = Heart rate × Stroke volume

In adults, the CO ranges from 4 to 7 L/min. Because CO requirements vary according to body size, the cardiac index is calculated to adjust for differences in body size. The **cardiac**

index can be determined by dividing the CO by the body surface area. The normal range is 2.7 to 3.2 L/min/m² of body surface area.

Heart rate (HR) refers to the number of times the ventricles contract each minute. The normal resting HR for an adult is between 60 and 100 beats/min. Increases in rate increase myocardial oxygen demand. The HR is extrinsically controlled by the autonomic nervous system (ANS), which adjusts rapidly when necessary to regulate cardiac output. *The parasympathetic (vagus nerve) system slows the HR, whereas sympathetic stimulation increases the heart rate.* An increase in circulating catecholamines (e.g., epinephrine and norepinephrine) usually causes an increase in HR and contractility. Many cardiovascular drugs, particularly beta blockers, block this sympathetic (fight or flight) pattern by decreasing the HR.

Stroke volume (SV) is the amount of blood ejected by the left ventricle during each contraction. Several variables influence SV and, ultimately, CO. These variables include HR, preload, afterload, and contractility.

Preload refers to the degree of myocardial fiber stretch at the end of diastole and just before contraction. The stretch imposed on the muscle fibers results from the volume contained within the ventricle at the end of diastole. *Preload is determined by the amount of blood returning to the heart from both the venous system (right heart) and the pulmonary system (left heart) (left ventricular end-diastolic [LVED] volume).*

An increase in ventricular volume increases muscle-fiber length and tension, thereby enhancing contraction and improving stroke volume. This statement is derived from Starling's law of the heart: The more the heart is filled during diastole (within limits), the more forcefully it contracts. Excessive filling of the ventricles results in excessive LVED volume and pressure, however, and may result in decreased cardiac output.

Another factor affecting stroke volume, **afterload,** is the pressure or resistance that the ventricles must overcome to eject blood through the semilunar valves and into the peripheral blood vessels. The amount of resistance is directly related to arterial blood pressure and the diameter of the blood vessels.

Impedance, the peripheral component of afterload, is the pressure that the heart must overcome to open the aortic valve. The amount of impedance depends on aortic compliance and total systemic vascular resistance, a combination of blood viscosity (thickness) and arteriolar constriction. A decrease in stroke volume can result from an increase in afterload without the benefit of compensatory mechanisms, thus leading to a decrease in cardiac output.

Myocardial contractility affects stroke volume and CO and is the force of cardiac contraction independent of preload. Contractility is increased by factors such as sympathetic stimulation, calcium release, and positive inotropic drugs. It is decreased by factors such as hypoxia and acidemia.

Vascular System

The vascular system serves several purposes:
- Provides a route for blood to travel from the heart to nourish the various tissues of the body
- Carries cellular wastes to the excretory organs
- Allows lymphatic flow to drain tissue fluid back into the circulation
- Returns blood to the heart for recirculation

The vascular system is divided into the arterial system and the venous system. In the arterial system, blood moves from the larger arteries to a network of smaller blood vessels, called *arterioles*, which meet the capillary bed. In the venous system, blood travels from the capillaries to the venules and to the larger system of veins, eventually returning in the vena cava to the heart for recirculation.

Arterial System

The primary function of the arterial system is to deliver oxygen and nutrients to various tissues in the body. Nutrients are carried through arteries to arterioles, then branch into smaller terminal arterioles, and finally join with capillaries and venules to form a capillary network. Within this network, nutrients are exchanged across capillary membranes by three primary processes: osmosis, filtration, and diffusion. (See Chapter 11 for detailed discussions of these processes.)

The arterial system delivers blood to various tissues for oxygen and nourishment. At the tissue level, nutrients, chemicals, and body defense substances are distributed and exchanged for cellular waste products, depending on the needs of the particular tissue. The arteries transport the cellular wastes to the excretory organs (e.g., kidneys and lungs) to be reprocessed or removed. These vessels also contribute to temperature regulation in the tissues. Blood can be either directed toward the skin to promote heat loss or diverted away from the skin to conserve heat.

Blood pressure (BP) *is the force of blood exerted against the vessel walls.* Pressure in the larger arterial blood vessels is greater (about 80 to 100 mm Hg) and decreases as blood flow reaches the capillaries (about 25 mm Hg). By the time blood enters the right atrium, the BP is about 0 to 5 mm Hg. Volume, ventricular contraction, and vascular tone are necessary to maintain blood pressure.

BP is determined primarily by the quantity of blood flow or cardiac output (CO), as well as by the resistance in the arterioles:

Blood pressure = Cardiac output × Peripheral vascular resistance

Any factor that increases CO or total peripheral vascular resistance increases the BP. In general, BP is maintained at a relatively constant level. Therefore an increase or decrease in total peripheral vascular resistance is associated with a decrease or an increase in CO, respectively. Three mechanisms mediate and regulate BP:
- The autonomic nervous system (ANS), which excites or inhibits sympathetic nervous system activity in response to impulses from chemoreceptors and baroreceptors
- The kidneys, which sense a change in blood flow and activate the renin-angiotensin-aldosterone mechanism
- The endocrine system, which releases various hormones (e.g., catecholamine, kinins, serotonin, histamine) to stimulate the sympathetic nervous system at the tissue level

Systolic BP is the amount of pressure/force generated by the left ventricle to distribute blood into the aorta with each contraction of the heart. It is a measure of how effectively the heart pumps and is an indicator of vascular tone. **Diastolic BP** is the amount of pressure/force against the arterial walls during the relaxation phase of the heart.

BP is regulated by balancing the sympathetic and parasympathetic nervous systems of the autonomic nervous system. Changes in autonomic activity are responses to messages sent by the sensory receptors in the various tissues of the body. These receptors, including the baroreceptors, chemoreceptors, and stretch receptors, respond differently to the biochemical and physiologic changes of the body.

Baroreceptors in the arch of the aorta and at the origin of the internal carotid arteries are stimulated when the arterial walls are stretched by an increased BP. Impulses from these baroreceptors inhibit the vasomotor center, which is located in the pons and the medulla. Inhibition of this center results in a drop in BP.

Several 1- to 2-mm collections of tissue have been identified in the carotid arteries and along the aortic arch known as **peripheral chemoreceptors.** These receptors are sensitive primarily to hypoxemia (a decrease in the partial pressure of arterial oxygen [Pao_2]). When stimulated, these chemoreceptors send impulses along the vagus nerves to activate a vasoconstrictor response and raise BP.

The central chemoreceptors in the respiratory center of the brain are also stimulated by **hypercapnia** (an increase in partial pressure of arterial carbon dioxide [$Paco_2$]) and acidosis. The direct effect of carbon dioxide on the central nervous system (CNS), however, is 10 times stronger than the effect of hypoxia on the peripheral chemoreceptors.

Stretch receptors in the vena cavae and the right atrium are sensitive to pressure or volume changes. When a patient is hypovolemic, stretch receptors in the blood vessels sense a reduced volume or pressure and send fewer impulses to the CNS. This reaction stimulates the sympathetic nervous system to increase the heart rate (HR) and constrict the peripheral blood vessels.

The *kidneys* also help regulate cardiovascular activity. When renal blood flow or pressure decreases, the kidneys retain sodium and water. BP tends to rise because of fluid retention and activation of the renin-angiotensin-aldosterone mechanism (see Fig. 11-6 in Chapter 11). This mechanism results in vasoconstriction and sodium retention (and thus fluid retention). Vascular volume is also regulated by the release of antidiuretic hormone (vasopressin) from the posterior pituitary gland (see Chapter 11).

Other factors can also influence the activity of the cardiovascular system. Emotional behaviors (e.g., excitement, pain, anger) stimulate the sympathetic nervous system to increase blood pressure (BP) and heart rate (HR). Increased physical activity such as exercise also increases BP and HR during the activity. Body temperature can affect the metabolic needs of the tissues, thereby influencing the delivery of blood. In hypothermia, tissues require fewer nutrients and blood pressure falls. In hyperthermia, the metabolic requirement of the tissues is greater and BP and pulse rate rise.

Venous System

The primary function of the venous system is to complete the circulation of blood by returning blood from the capillaries to the right side of the heart. It is composed of a series of veins that are located next to the arterial system. A second superficial venous circulation runs parallel to the subcutaneous tissue of the extremity. These two venous systems are connected by communicating veins that provide a means for blood to travel from the superficial veins to the deep veins. Blood flow is directed toward the deep venous circulation.

Veins have the ability to accommodate large shifts in volume with minimal changes in venous pressure. This flexibility allows the venous system to accommodate the administration of IV fluids and blood transfusions, as well as to maintain pressure during blood loss and dehydration. Veins in the superficial and deep venous systems (except the smallest and the largest veins) have valves that direct blood flow back to the heart and prevent backflow. Skeletal muscles in the extremities provide a force that helps push the venous blood forward. The superior vena cava and inferior vena cava are valveless and large enough to allow blood flow to return easily to the heart.

Gravity exerts an increase in **hydrostatic pressure** in the capillaries when the patient is in an upright position, delaying venous return. Hydrostatic pressure is decreased in dependent areas such as the legs when the patient is lying down, and thus there is less hindrance of venous return to the heart.

Cardiovascular Changes Associated with Aging

A number of physiologic changes in the cardiovascular system occur with advancing age (Chart 33-1). Many of these changes result in a loss of cardiac reserve. Thus these changes are usually not evident when the older adult is resting. They become apparent only when the person is physically or emotionally stressed and the heart cannot meet the increased metabolic demands of the body.

ASSESSMENT METHODS

Patient History

The focus of the patient history is on obtaining information about risk factors and symptoms of cardiovascular disease. Assess *nonmodifiable* (uncontrollable) risk factors including the

patient's age, gender, ethnic origin, and family history of cardiovascular disease. Ask about any chronic disease or illness that the patient may have. The incidence of conditions such as coronary artery disease (CAD) and valvular disease increases with age. The incidence of CAD also varies with the patient's gender. Men have a higher risk for CAD than women of all ages except in the oldest age-group of 80 years and older (Go et al., 2013).

GENDER HEALTH CONSIDERATIONS
Patient-Centered Care **QSEN**

Postmenopausal women are 2 to 3 times more likely than premenopausal women to have CAD. The incidence for the disease in women is about 10 years later than in men and 20 years later for myocardial infarction (MI) and death to occur. After an acute MI, women tend to have a higher mortality rate and suffer more complications when compared with men (Go et al., 2013).

Women with waist and abdominal obesity (greater waist-hip ratio) are more likely to experience cardiovascular disease (CVD) than are women with excess fat in their buttocks, hips, and thighs.

Heart disease is the leading cause of diabetes-related death for both men and women. Adults with diabetes have heart disease death rates 2 to 4 times higher than those without diabetes. The risk for stroke is also 2 to 4 times higher among people with diabetes. The number of premature deaths (younger than 65 years) from heart disease is greatest among American Indians and Alaska Natives and lowest among Asians (Go et al., 2013).

Modifiable (controllable) risk factors should also be assessed. *Modifiable* risk factors are personal lifestyle habits, including cigarette use, physical inactivity, obesity, and psychological variables. Ask the patient about each of these common risk factors.

Cigarette smoking is a major risk factor for CVD, specifically coronary artery disease (CAD) and peripheral vascular disease (PVD). Three compounds in cigarette smoke have been implicated in the development of CAD: tar, nicotine, and carbon monoxide. The smoking history should include the number of cigarettes smoked daily, the duration of the smoking habit, and the age of the patient when smoking started. Record the smoking history in **pack-years**, which is the number of packs per day multiplied by the number of years the patient has smoked.

Ask about the patient's desire to quit, past attempts to quit, and the methods used. Determine nicotine dependence by asking questions such as:

- How soon after you wake up in the morning do you smoke?
- Do you wake up in the middle of your sleep time to smoke?
- Do you find it difficult not to smoke in places where smoking is prohibited?
- Do you smoke when you are ill?

Three to four years after a patient has stopped smoking, his or her CVD risk appears to be similar to that of a person who has never smoked. Be sure to ask those who do not currently smoke whether they have ever smoked and when they quit. Passive smoke significantly reduces blood flow in healthy young adults' coronary arteries, and the risk for dying increases among those who are exposed to secondhand smoke (American Heart Association [AHA], 2013).

A *sedentary lifestyle* is also a major risk factor for heart disease. Regular physical activity promotes cardiovascular

CHART 33-1 Nursing Focus on the Older Adult

Changes in the Cardiovascular System Related to Aging

CHANGE	NURSING INTERVENTIONS	RATIONALES
Cardiac Valves Calcification and mucoid degeneration occur, especially in mitral and aortic valves.	Assess heart rate and rhythm and heart sounds for murmurs. Question patients about dyspnea.	Murmurs may be detected before other symptoms. Valvular abnormalities may result in rhythm changes.
Conduction System Pacemaker cells decrease in number. Fibrous tissue and fat in the sinoatrial node increase. Few muscle fibers remain in the atrial myocardium and bundle of His. Conduction time increases.	Assess the electrocardiogram (ECG) and heart rhythm for dysrhythmias or a heart rate less than 60 beats/min.	The sinoatrial (SA) node may lose its inherent rhythm. Atrial dysrhythmias occur in many older adults; 80% of older adults experience premature ventricular contractions (PVCs).
Left Ventricle The size of the left ventricle increases. The left ventricle becomes stiff and less distensible. Fibrotic changes in the left ventricle decrease the speed of early diastolic filling by about 50%.	Assess the ECG for a widening QRS complex and a longer QT interval. Assess the heart rate at rest and with activity. Assess for activity intolerance.	Ventricular changes result in decreased stroke volume, ejection fraction, and cardiac output during exercise; the heart is less able to meet increased oxygen demands. Maximum heart rate with exercise is decreased. The heart is less able to meet increased oxygen demands.
Aorta and Other Large Arteries The aorta and other large arteries thicken and become stiffer and less distensible. Systolic blood pressure increases to compensate for the stiff arteries. Systemic vascular resistance increases as a result of less distensible arteries; therefore the left ventricle pumps against greater resistance, contributing to left ventricular hypertrophy.	Assess blood pressure. Note increases in systolic, diastolic, and pulse pressures. Assess for activity intolerance and shortness of breath. Assess the peripheral pulses.	Hypertension may occur and must be treated to avoid target organ damage.
Baroreceptors Baroreceptors become less sensitive.	Assess the patient's blood pressure with the patient lying and then sitting or standing. Assess for dizziness when the patient changes from a lying to a sitting or standing position. Teach the patient to change positions slowly.	Orthostatic (postural) and postprandial changes occur because of ineffective baroreceptors. Changes may include blood pressure decreases of 10 mm Hg or more, dizziness, and fainting.

fitness and produces beneficial changes in blood pressure and levels of blood lipids and clotting factors. Unfortunately, few people in the United States follow the recommended exercise guidelines: 30 minutes daily of light to moderate exercise, which is equivalent to a 30-minute brisk walk. According to the AHA (2013), fewer than two thirds of people in the United States engage in this much exercise 5 times a week and fewer engage in more vigorous physical activity to promote cardiopulmonary fitness. Encourage increased physical exercise as part of a life-style change to reduce the risk for CAD. Ask patients about the type of exercise they perform, how long a period they have participated in the exercise, and the frequency and intensity of the exercise.

About two thirds of American adults are overweight when defined as a body mass index (BMI) of 25 to 30. Obesity, defined as a BMI greater than 30, is particularly a problem for African-American women, Mexican Americans, and native Hawaiians, but the exact cause of this cultural difference is unknown (AHA, 2013). Obesity is also associated with hypertension, hyperlipidemia, and diabetes; all are known contributors to CVD.

The American Heart Association provides guidelines to combat obesity and improve cardiac health, including ingesting more nutrient-rich foods that have vitamins, minerals, fiber, and other nutrients but are low in calories. To get the necessary nutrients, teach patients to choose foods like vegetables, fruits, unrefined whole-grain products, and fat-free dairy products most often. Also teach patients to not eat more calories than they can burn every day (AHA, 2013).

A variety of *psychological factors* make people more vulnerable to the development of heart disease. Those who are highly competitive, overly concerned about meeting deadlines, and often hostile or angry are at higher risk for heart disease. Psychological stress, anger, depression, and hostility are all closely associated with risk for developing heart disease.

You might ask the patient "How do you respond when you have to wait for an appointment?" Chronic anger and hostility appear to be closely associated with CVD. The constant arousal of the sympathetic nervous system as a result of anger may influence blood pressure, serum fatty acids and lipids, and clotting mechanisms. Observe the patient, and assess his or her response to stressful situations.

Review the patient's medical history, noting any major illnesses such as diabetes mellitus, renal disease, anemia, high BP, stroke, bleeding disorders, connective tissue diseases, chronic pulmonary diseases, heart disease, and thrombophlebitis. These conditions can influence the patient's cardiovascular status.

Ask about previous treatment for CVD, identify previous diagnostic procedures (e.g., electrocardiography [ECG], cardiac catheterization), and request information about any medical or invasive treatment of CVD. Ask specifically about recurrent tonsillitis, streptococcal infections, and rheumatic fever, because these conditions may lead to valvular abnormalities of the heart. In addition, inquire about any known congenital heart defects. Many patients with congenital heart problems live into adulthood because of improved treatment and surgeries.

Ask patients about their drug history, beginning with any current or recent use of prescription or over-the-counter (OTC) medications or herbal/natural products. Inquire about known sensitivities to any drug and the nature of the reaction (e.g., nausea, rash). Patients should be asked whether they have recently used cocaine or any IV "street" drugs, because these substances are often associated with heart disease.

GENDER HEALTH CONSIDERATIONS
Patient-Centered Care QSEN

Ask young women whether they are taking oral contraceptives or an estrogen replacement. The incidence of myocardial infarction (MI) and stroke in women older than 35 years who take oral contraceptives is increased if they smoke, have diabetes, or have hypertension. Ask menopausal women and transgender women if they are on hormone therapy, because these drugs can also cause an increased incidence of MIs and strokes.

The *social history* includes information about the patient's living situation, including having a domestic partner, other household members, environment, and occupation. Identification of support systems is especially important in exploring the possibility that the patient might have difficulty paying for medications or treatment. People who are from a low socioeconomic (SE) group have a greater chance of having MIs than those from a higher SE status (Wright et al., 2009).

Ask about occupation, including the type of work performed and the requirements of the specific job. For instance, does the job involve physical exertion such as lifting heavy objects? Is the job emotionally stressful? What does a day's work entail? Does the patient's job require him or her to be outside in extreme weather conditions?

Nutrition History

A nutrition history includes the patient's recall of food and fluid intake during a 24-hour period, self-imposed or medically prescribed dietary restrictions or supplementations, and the amount and type of alcohol consumption. If needed, the dietitian may review the type of foods selected by the patient for the amount of sodium, sugar, cholesterol, fiber, and fat. Cultural beliefs and economic status can influence the choice of food items and therefore are seriously considered. Family members or significant others who are responsible for shopping and cooking should be included in this screening.

NCLEX EXAMINATION CHALLENGE
Health Promotion and Maintenance

The nurse is providing education to help reduce cardiovascular risks for a women's book club. Which statement made by a participant indicates a need for further teaching?
A. "We are more likely to die from cardiovascular disease than men."
B. "We need to walk or do other exercise every day for 30 minutes."
C. "We need to stay away from people who smoke."
D. "We should take hormones for menopause to decrease the risk for heart attack."

Family History and Genetic Risk

Review the family history, and obtain information about the age, health status, and cause of death of immediate family members. A positive family history for CAD in a first-degree relative (parent, sibling, or child) is a major risk factor. It is *more* important than other factors such as hypertension, obesity, diabetes, or sudden cardiac death.

GENETIC/GENOMIC CONSIDERATIONS
Patient-Centered Care QSEN

Cardiovascular disease has many contributory factors, including a genetic tendency. A significant association between familial cardiac history and cardiovascular disease is consistently demonstrated in the evidence of multiple large-scale prospective epidemiology studies (Go, et al., 2013). Although several genes have been reported to be associated with heart disease, stroke, and hypertension, the impact of each individual gene is not fully understood. Numerous genetic association studies are underway to determine more specific genetic variants that may underlie the family history (Go, et al., 2013). Additional discussions about genetic factors related to specific CV diseases are found in other chapters in this unit.

Current Health Problems

Ask the patient to describe his or her health concerns. Expand on the description of these concerns by obtaining information about their onset, duration, sequence, frequency, location, quality, intensity, associated symptoms, and precipitating, aggravating, and relieving factors. Major symptoms usually identified by patients with CVD include chest pain or discomfort, dyspnea, fatigue, palpitations, weight gain, syncope, and extremity pain.

Pain or discomfort, considered a traditional symptom of heart disease, can result from ischemic heart disease, pericarditis, and aortic dissection. Chest pain can also be due to noncardiac conditions such as pleurisy, pulmonary embolus, hiatal hernia, gastroesophageal reflux disease, neuromuscular abnormalities, and anxiety.

NURSING SAFETY PRIORITY QSEN
Action Alert

Thoroughly evaluate the nature and characteristics of the chest pain. Because pain resulting from myocardial ischemia is life threatening and can lead to serious complications, its cause should be considered ischemic (reduced or obstructed blood flow to the myocardium) until proven otherwise. When assessing for symptoms, ask the patient if he or she has "discomfort," "heaviness," "pressure," and "indigestion."

GENDER HEALTH CONSIDERATIONS
Patient-Centered Care QSEN

Some patients, especially women, do not experience pain in the chest but, instead, feel discomfort or indigestion. Women often present with a "triad" of symptoms. In addition to indigestion or feeling of abdominal fullness, chronic fatigue despite adequate rest and feelings of an "inability to catch my breath" (dyspnea) are also common in heart disease. The patient may also describe the sensation as aching, choking, strangling, tingling, squeezing, constricting, or viselike. Others with severe neuropathy may experience few or no traditional symptoms except shortness of breath, despite major ischemia.

Ask the patient to identify when the symptoms were first noticed (onset):
- Did the symptoms begin suddenly or develop gradually (manner of onset)?
- How long did the symptoms last (duration)?

If he or she has repeated painful episodes, assess how often the symptoms occur (frequency). If pain is present, ask whether it is different from any other episodes of pain. Ask the patient to describe what activities he or she was doing when it first occurred, such as sleeping, arguing, or running (precipitating factors). If possible, the patient should point to the area where the chest pain occurred (location) and describe if and how the pain radiated (spread).

In addition, ask how the pain feels and whether it is sharp, dull, or crushing (quality of pain). To understand the severity of the pain, ask the patient to grade it from 0 to 10, with 10 indicating severe pain (intensity). He or she may also report other signs and symptoms that occur at the same time (associated symptoms), such as dyspnea, diaphoresis (excessive sweating), nausea, and vomiting. Other factors that need to be addressed are those that may have made the chest pain worse (aggravating factors) or less intense (relieving factors). Chest pain can arise from a variety of sources (Table 33-1). By obtaining the appropriate information, you can help identify the source of the chest discomfort.

Dyspnea (difficult or labored breathing) can occur as a result of both cardiac and pulmonary disease. It is experienced by the patient as uncomfortable breathing or shortness of breath. When obtaining the history, ask what factors precipitate and relieve dyspnea, what level of activity produces dyspnea, and what the patient's body position was when dyspnea occurred.

Dyspnea that is associated with activity, such as climbing stairs, is referred to as **dyspnea on exertion (DOE)**. *This is usually an early symptom of heart failure and may be the only symptom experienced by women.*

The patient with advanced heart disease may experience **orthopnea** (dyspnea that appears when he or she lies flat). Several pillows may be needed to elevate the head and chest, or a recliner to prevent breathlessness may be used. *The severity of orthopnea is measured by the number of pillows or the amount of head elevation needed to provide restful sleep.* This symptom is usually relieved within a matter of minutes by sitting up or standing.

Paroxysmal nocturnal dyspnea (PND) develops after the patient has been lying down for several hours. In this position, blood from the lower extremities is redistributed to the venous system, which increases venous return to the heart. A diseased heart cannot compensate for the increased volume and is ineffective in pumping the additional fluid into the circulatory system. Pulmonary congestion results. The patient awakens abruptly, often with a feeling of suffocation and panic. He or she sits upright and dangles the legs over the side of the bed to relieve the dyspnea. This sensation may last for 20 minutes.

Fatigue may be described as a feeling of tiredness or weariness resulting from activity. The patient may report that an activity takes longer to complete or that he or she tires easily after activity. Although fatigue in itself is not diagnostic of heart disease, many people with heart failure are limited by leg fatigue during exercise. Fatigue that occurs after mild activity and exertion usually indicates inadequate cardiac output (due to low stroke volume) and anaerobic metabolism in skeletal muscle. *It can also accompany other symptoms or may be an early indication of heart disease in women.*

Ask about the time of day the patient experiences fatigue and the activities that he or she can perform. Fatigue resulting from decreased cardiac output is often worse in the evening. Ask whether the patient can perform the same activities as he or she could perform a year ago or the same activities as others of the same age. Often he or she limits activities in response to fatigue and, unless questioned, is unaware how much less active he or she has become.

A feeling of fluttering or unpleasant feeling in the chest caused by an irregular heartbeat is referred to as **palpitations**. They may result from a change in heart rate or rhythm or from an increase in the force of heart contractions. Rhythm disturbances that may cause palpitations include paroxysmal supraventricular tachycardia, premature contractions, and sinus tachycardia. Those that occur during or after strenuous physical activity, such as running and swimming, may indicate overexertion or possibly heart disease. Noncardiac factors that may precipitate palpitations include anxiety, stress, fatigue, insomnia, hyperthyroidism, and the ingestion of caffeine, nicotine, or alcohol. Ask the patient about specific factors that cause his or her palpitations.

A sudden weight increase of 2.2 pounds (1 kg) can result from excess FLUID (1 L) in the interstitial spaces. *The best indicator of fluid balance is weight.* Excess FLUID accumulation is commonly known as **edema**. It is possible for weight gains of up to 10 to 15 pounds (4.5 to 6.8 kg, or 4 to 7 L of fluid) to occur before edema is apparent. Ask whether the patient has noticed a tightness of shoes, indentations from socks, or tightness of rings.

Syncope refers to a brief loss of consciousness. The most common cause is decreased perfusion to the brain. Any condition that suddenly reduces cardiac output, resulting in decreased cerebral blood flow, can lead to a syncopal episode. Conditions such as cardiac rhythm disturbances, especially ventricular dysrhythmias, and valvular disorders, such as aortic stenosis, may trigger this symptom. **Near-syncope** refers to dizziness with an inability to remain in an upright position. Explore the circumstances that lead to dizziness or syncope.

CONSIDERATIONS FOR OLDER ADULTS
Patient-Centered Care QSEN

Syncope in the aging person may result from hypersensitivity of the carotid sinus bodies in the carotid arteries. Pressure applied to these arteries while turning the head, shrugging the shoulders, or performing a Valsalva maneuver (bearing down during defecation) may stimulate a vagal response. A decrease in blood pressure and heart rate can result, which can produce syncope. This type of syncopal episode may also result from postural (orthostatic) or postprandial (after eating) hypotension.

TABLE 33-1	Assessment of Chest Discomfort: How Various Types of Chest Pain Differ		
ONSET	QUALITY AND SEVERITY	LOCATION AND RADIATION	DURATION AND RELIEVING FACTORS
Angina			
Sudden, usually in response to exertion, emotion, or extremes in temperature	Squeezing, viselike pain	Usually the left side of chest without radiation Substernal; may spread across the chest and the back and/or down the arms	Usually lasts less than 15 min; relieved with rest, nitrate administration, or oxygen therapy
Myocardial Infarction			
Sudden, without precipitating factors, often in early morning	Intense stabbing, viselike pain or pressure, severe	Substernal; may spread throughout the anterior chest and to the arms, jaw, back, or neck	Continuous or no chest discomfort; relieved with morphine, cardiac drugs, and oxygen therapy
Pericarditis			
Sudden	Sharp, stabbing, moderate to severe	Substernal; usually spreads to the left side or the back	Intermittent; relieved with sitting upright, analgesia, or administration of anti-inflammatory agents
Pleuropulmonary			
Variable	Moderate ache, worse on inspiration	Lung fields	Continuous until the underlying condition is treated or the patient has rested
Esophageal-Gastric			
Variable	Squeezing, heartburn, variable severity	Substernal; may spread to the shoulders or the abdomen	Variable; may be relieved with antacid administration, food intake, or taking a sitting position
Anxiety			
Variable, may be in response to stress or fatigue	Dull ache to sharp stabbing; may be associated with numbness in fingers	Not well located and usually does not radiate to other parts of the body as pain	Usually lasts a few minutes

Extremity pain may be caused by two conditions: ischemia from atherosclerosis and venous insufficiency of the peripheral blood vessels. Patients who report a moderate to severe cramping sensation in their legs or buttocks associated with an activity such as walking have intermittent claudication related to decreased arterial tissue PERFUSION. *Claudication pain is usually relieved by resting or lowering the affected extremity to decrease tissue demands or to enhance arterial blood flow.* Leg pain that results from prolonged standing or sitting is related to venous insufficiency from either incompetent valves or venous obstruction. This pain may be relieved by elevating the extremity.

Functional History

After the history of the patient's cardiovascular status is obtained, he or she may be classified according to the New York Heart Association Functional Classification (Table 33-2) or other system. The four classifications (I, II, III, and IV) depend on the degree to which ordinary physical activities (routine ADLs) are affected by heart disease. The Killip Classification provides a more objective description of the hemodynamics of heart failure and is described in Chapter 38.

Physical Assessment

A thorough physical assessment is the foundation for the nursing database and the patient's priority problems. Any changes noted during the course of illness can be compared with this initial database. Evaluate the patient's vital signs on admission to the hospital or during the initial visit to the clinic or primary care provider's office.

TABLE 33-2	New York Heart Association Functional Classification of Cardiovascular Disability

Class I
- Patients with cardiac disease but without resulting limitations of physical activity
- Ordinary physical activity does not cause undue fatigue, palpitation, dyspnea, or anginal pain

Class II
- Patients with cardiac disease resulting in slight limitation of physical activity
- They are comfortable at rest
- Ordinary physical activity results in fatigue, palpitation, dyspnea, or anginal pain

Class III
- Patients with cardiac disease resulting in marked limitation of physical activity
- They are comfortable at rest
- Less than ordinary physical activity causes fatigue, palpitation, dyspnea, or anginal pain

Class IV
- Patients with cardiac disease resulting in inability to carry on any physical activity without discomfort
- Symptoms of cardiac insufficiency or of the anginal syndrome may be present, even at rest
- If any physical activity is undertaken, discomfort is increased

Excerpted from The New York Heart Association. (1964). *Diseases of the heart and blood vessels: Nomenclature and criteria for diagnosis* (6th ed.). Boston: Little, Brown.

General Appearance

Physical assessment begins with the patient's general appearance. Assess general build and appearance, skin color, distress level, level of consciousness, shortness of breath, position, and verbal responses.

Patients can have left- or right-sided heart failure, or both. They can also be diagnosed with systolic and/or diastolic heart failure. *As a result, poor cardiac output and decreased cerebral* PERFUSION *may cause confusion, memory loss, and slowed verbal responses, especially in older adults.* Patients with chronic heart failure may also appear malnourished, thin, and cachectic. Late signs of severe right-sided heart failure are ascites, jaundice, and anasarca (generalized edema) as a result of prolonged congestion of the liver. Heart failure may also cause fluid retention and may be manifested by obvious generalized dependent edema. Chapter 35 differentiates right and left failure and systolic from diastolic heart failure in detail.

Skin

Skin assessment includes color and temperature. The best areas in which to assess circulation include the nail beds, mucous membranes, and conjunctival mucosa, because small blood vessels are located near the surface of the skin in those areas.

If there is normal blood flow or adequate perfusion to a given area in *light-colored skin*, it appears pink, perhaps rosy, and is warm. *Decreased* PERFUSION *is manifested as cool, pale, and moist skin. Pallor is characteristic of anemia and can be seen in areas such as the nail beds, palms, and conjunctival mucous membranes in any patient.*

A bluish or darkened discoloration of the skin and mucous membranes in *light-skinned* people is referred to as cyanosis. This condition results from an increased amount of deoxygenated hemoglobin. It is not an early sign of decreased perfusion but occurs later with other symptoms. *Dark-skinned patients may experience cyanosis as a graying of the same tissues.*

Central cyanosis involves decreased oxygenation of the arterial blood in the lungs and appears as a bluish tinge of the conjunctivae and the mucous membranes of the mouth and tongue. Central cyanosis may indicate impaired lung function or a right-to-left shunt found in congenital heart conditions. Because of impaired circulation, there is marked desaturation of hemoglobin in the peripheral tissues, which produces a bluish or darkened discoloration of the nail beds, earlobes, lips, and toes.

Peripheral cyanosis occurs when blood flow to the peripheral vessels is decreased by peripheral vasoconstriction. Constriction results from a low cardiac output or an increased extraction of oxygen from the peripheral tissues. Peripheral cyanosis localized in an extremity is usually a result of arterial or venous insufficiency. Rubor (dusky redness) that replaces pallor in a dependent foot suggests arterial insufficiency.

Skin *temperature* can be assessed for symmetry by touching different areas of the body with the dorsal (back) surface of the hand or fingers. Decreased blood flow results in decreased skin temperature. It is lowered in several clinical conditions, including heart failure, peripheral vascular disease, and shock.

Extremities

Assess the patient's hands, arms, feet, and legs for skin changes, vascular changes, clubbing, and edema. Skin mobility and turgor are affected by fluid status. Dehydration and aging reduce skin turgor, and edema decreases skin elasticity. Vascular changes in an affected extremity may include paresthesia, muscle fatigue and discomfort, numbness, pain, coolness, and loss of hair distribution from a reduced blood supply.

Clubbing of the fingers and toes is caused by *chronic* oxygen deprivation in body tissues. It is common in patients with advanced chronic pulmonary disease, congenital heart defects, and cor pulmonale (right-sided heart failure). The angle of the normal nail bed is 160 degrees. With clubbing, the nail straightens out to an angle of 180 degrees and the base of the nail becomes spongy. Fig. 30-12 in Chapter 30 shows late clubbing.

Peripheral edema (FLUID accumulation in the legs and feet) is a common finding in patients with cardiovascular problems. The location of edema helps determine its potential cause. Bilateral edema of the legs may be seen in those with heart failure or chronic venous insufficiency. Abdominal and leg edema can be seen in patients with heart disease and cirrhosis of the liver. Localized edema in one extremity may be the result of venous obstruction (thrombosis) or lymphatic blockage of the extremity (lymphedema). Edema may also be noted in dependent areas, such as the sacrum, when a patient is confined to bed. In other patients, edema results from third spacing when plasma proteins decrease. Dependent foot and ankle edema is also a common side effect of certain antihypertensive drugs, such as amlodipine (Norvasc).

Document the location of edema as precisely as possible (e.g., midtibial or sacral) and the number of centimeters from an anatomic landmark. The extent of edema can be assessed as mild, moderate, or severe (or 1+, 2+, 3+, or 4+). However, these values are not precise and are very unreliable. Determine whether the edema is pitting (the skin can be indented) (Fig. 33-5) or nonpitting.

The finger is typically used for pulse oximetry as a noninvasive method for assessing oxygenation and PERFUSION of many medical-surgical nursing patients. Correct placement of the pulse oximetry sensor is essential for accurate readings. Oxygen saturation levels of above 90% are considered normal, depending on the patient's age. Detailed information about this assessment method can be found in Chapter 27.

Blood Pressure

Arterial blood pressure is measured *indirectly* by sphygmomanometry. This technique of measurement is described in detail in nursing skills textbooks.

The 8th National High Blood Pressure Education Program Joint National Committee (JNC) on Prevention, Detection, Evaluation, and Treatment of High Blood Pressure (2013)

FIG. 33-5 Peripheral pitting edema.

defines hypertension as a systolic pressure of 140 mm Hg or higher or a diastolic pressure of 90 mm Hg or higher, or taking drugs to control blood pressure. Specific treatment goals were outlined for patients based on age and co-morbidities. Chapter 36 describes hypertension in detail.

A BP less than 90/60 mm Hg (hypotension) may not be adequate for providing enough oxygen and sufficient nutrition to body cells. In certain circumstances, such as shock, the Korotkoff sounds are less audible or are absent. In these cases, palpate the BP, use an ultrasonic device (Doppler device), or obtain a direct measurement by arterial catheter in the critical care setting. When BP is palpated, only the systolic pressure can be determined. Patients may report dizziness or light-headedness when they move from a flat, supine position to a sitting or a standing position at the edge of the bed. Normally these symptoms are transient and pass quickly; pronounced symptoms may be due to postural hypotension. *Postural (orthostatic) hypotension occurs when the BP is not adequately maintained while moving from a lying to a sitting or standing position. It is defined as a decrease of more than 20 mm Hg of the systolic pressure or more than 10 mm Hg of the diastolic pressure, as well as a 10% to 20% increase in heart rate.* The causes of postural hypotension include cardiovascular drugs, blood volume decrease, prolonged bedrest, age-related changes, or disorders of the ANS.

To detect orthostatic changes in BP, first measure the BP when the patient is supine. After remaining supine for at least 3 minutes, the patient changes position to sitting or standing. Normally systolic pressure drops slightly or remains unchanged as the patient rises, whereas diastolic pressure rises slightly. After the position change, wait for at least 1 minute before auscultating BP and counting the radial pulse. The cuff should remain in the proper position on the patient's arm. Observe and record any signs or symptoms of dizziness. If the patient cannot tolerate the position change, return him or her to the previous position of comfort.

Paradoxical blood pressure is an exaggerated decrease in systolic pressure by more than 10 mm Hg during the inspiratory phase of the respiratory cycle (normal is 3 to 10 mm Hg). Certain clinical conditions that potentially alter the filling pressures in the right and left ventricles may produce a paradoxical BP. Such conditions include pericardial tamponade, constrictive pericarditis, and pulmonary hypertension. During inspiration, the filling pressures normally decrease slightly. However, decreased fluid volume in the ventricles resulting from these pathologic conditions produces a marked reduction in cardiac output. The difference between the systolic and diastolic values is referred to as pulse pressure. This value can be used as an indirect measure of cardiac output. Narrowed pulse pressure is rarely normal and results from increased peripheral vascular resistance or decreased stroke volume in patients with heart failure, hypovolemia, or shock. It can also be seen in those with mitral stenosis or regurgitation. An increased pulse pressure may occur in patients with slow heart rates, aortic regurgitation, atherosclerosis, hypertension, and aging.

The ankle-brachial index (ABI) can be used to assess the vascular status of the lower extremities. A BP cuff is applied to the lower extremity just above the malleolus. The systolic pressure is measured by Doppler ultrasound at both the dorsalis pedis and posterior tibial pulses. The higher of these two pressures is then divided by the higher of the two brachial pulses to obtain the ABI.

Normal values for the ABI are 1.00 or higher because BP in the legs is usually higher than BP in the arms. ABI values less than 0.80 usually indicate moderate vascular disease, whereas values less than 0.50 indicate severe vascular compromise. Although used primarily to help identify peripheral vascular disease, the ABI may be effective as a risk factor in predicting other CV disease in women, especially coronary artery disease (Pearson, 2010).

A toe brachial pressure index (TBPI) may be performed instead of or in addition to the ABI to determine arterial perfusion in the feet and toes. TBPI is the toe systolic pressure divided by the brachial (arm) systolic pressure.

Venous and Arterial Pulses

Observe the *venous pulsations* in the neck to assess the adequacy of blood volume and central venous pressure (CVP). Specially educated or critical care nurses can assess jugular venous pressure (JVP) to estimate the filling volume and pressure on the right side of the heart. An increase in JVP causes jugular venous distention (JVD).

Normally the JVP is 3 to 10 cm H_2O. Increases are usually caused by right ventricular failure. Other causes include tricuspid regurgitation or stenosis, pulmonary hypertension, cardiac tamponade, constrictive pericarditis, hypervolemia, and superior vena cava obstruction.

Assessment of *arterial pulses* provides information about vascular integrity and circulation. For patients with suspected or actual vascular disease, all major peripheral pulses should be assessed for presence or absence, amplitude, contour, rhythm, rate, and equality. Palpate the peripheral arteries in a head-to-toe approach with a side-to-side comparison (Fig. 33-6).

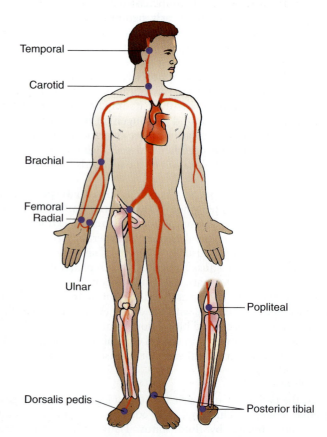

FIG. 33-6 Pulse points for assessment of arterial pulses.

A *hypokinetic* pulse is a weak pulse indicative of a narrow pulse pressure. It is seen in patients with hypovolemia, aortic stenosis, and decreased cardiac output. A *hyperkinetic* pulse is a large, "bounding" pulse caused by an increased ejection of blood. It occurs in patients with a high cardiac output (with exercise, sepsis, or thyrotoxicosis) and in those with increased sympathetic system activity (with pain, fever, or anxiety).

Auscultation of the major arteries (e.g., carotid and aorta) is necessary to assess for bruits. **Bruits** are swishing sounds that may occur from turbulent blood flow in narrowed or atherosclerotic arteries. Assess for the absence or presence of bruits by placing the bell of the stethoscope on the neck over the carotid artery while the patient holds his or her breath. Normally there are no sounds if the artery has uninterrupted blood flow. A bruit may develop when the internal diameter of the vessel is narrowed by 50% or more, but this does not indicate the severity of disease in the arteries. Once the vessel is blocked 90% or greater, the bruit often cannot be heard.

Precordium

Assessment of the precordium (the area over the heart) involves inspection, palpation, percussion, and auscultation. *In most settings, the medical-surgical nurse seldom performs precordial palpation and percussion. Critical care nurses and advanced practice nurses are qualified to perform the complete assessment.* Therefore only inspection and auscultation are described here. Begin by placing the patient in a supine position, with the head of the bed slightly elevated for comfort. Some patients may require elevation of the head of the bed to 45 degrees for ease and comfort in breathing.

Inspection. A cardiac examination is usually performed in a systematic order, beginning with inspection. Inspect the chest from the side, at a right angle, and downward over areas of the precordium where vibrations are visible. Cardiac motion is of low amplitude, and sometimes the inward movements are more easily detected by the naked eye.

Examine the entire precordium (Fig. 33-7), and note any prominent pulses. Movement over the aortic, pulmonic, and tricuspid areas is abnormal. Pulses in the mitral area (the apex of the heart) are considered normal and are referred to as the **apical impulse,** or the **point of maximal impulse (PMI).** The PMI should be located at the left fifth intercostal space (ICS) in the midclavicular line. If it appears in more than one ICS and has shifted lateral to the midclavicular line, the patient may have left ventricular hypertrophy.

Auscultation. Auscultation evaluates heart rate and rhythm, cardiac cycle (systole and diastole), and valvular function. The technique of auscultation requires a good-quality stethoscope and extensive clinical practice. Identifying specific abnormal heart sounds is most important in critical care and telemetry.

Listen to heart sounds in a systematic order. Examination usually begins at the aortic area and progresses slowly to the apex of the heart. The diaphragm of the stethoscope is pressed tightly against the chest to listen for high-frequency sounds and is useful in listening to the first and second heart sounds and high-frequency murmurs. Repeat the progression from the base to the apex of the heart using the bell of the stethoscope, which is held lightly against the chest. The bell can screen out high-frequency sounds and is useful in listening for low-frequency gallops (diastolic filling sounds) and murmurs.

Normal Heart Sounds. The **first heart sound (S1)** is created by the closure of the mitral and tricuspid valves (atrioventricular valves) (see Fig. 33-4). When auscultated, S_1 is softer and longer; it is of a low pitch and is best heard at the lower left sternal border or the apex of the heart. It may be identified by palpating the carotid pulse while listening. S_1 marks the beginning of ventricular systole and occurs right after the QRS complex on the ECG.

S_1 can be accentuated or intensified in conditions such as exercise, hyperthyroidism, and mitral stenosis. A decrease in sound intensity occurs in patients with mitral regurgitation and heart failure. If you have difficulty hearing heart sounds, have the patient lean forward or roll to his or her left side.

The *second heart sound (S_2)* is caused mainly by the closing of the aortic and pulmonic valves (semilunar valves) (see Fig. 33-4). S_2 is characteristically shorter. It is higher pitched and is heard best at the base of the heart at the end of ventricular systole.

The splitting of heart sounds is often difficult to differentiate from diastolic filling sounds (gallops). A splitting of S_1 (closure of the mitral valve followed by closure of the tricuspid valve) occurs physiologically because left ventricular contraction

The **aortic area** is a valvular outflow tract located in the second intercostal space just right of the sternum.

The **epigastric area** is located over the lower right sternal border.

The **tricuspid area** is a valvular outflow tract located in the fifth intercostal space at the lower left of the sternal border.

The **pulmonic area** is a valvular outflow tract located in the second intercostal space just left of the sternum.

The **right ventricular area** is located over the lower half of the sternum and the left parasternal area.

The **mitral area** is a valvular outflow tract located in the fifth intercostal space at the apex of the heart.

FIG. 33-7 Areas for myocardial inspection and auscultation.

occurs slightly before right ventricular contraction. Closure of the mitral valve is louder than closure of the tricuspid valve, however, so splitting is often not heard. Normal splitting of S_2 occurs because of the longer systolic phase of the right ventricle. Splitting of S_1 and S_2 can be accentuated by inspiration (due to increased venous return), and it narrows during expiration.

Abnormal Heart Sounds. Abnormal splitting of S_2 is referred to as **paradoxical splitting** and has a wider split heard on expiration. Paradoxical splitting of S_2 is heard in patients with severe myocardial depression that causes early closure of the pulmonic valve or a delay in aortic valve closure. Such conditions include myocardial infarction (MI), left bundle-branch block, aortic stenosis, aortic regurgitation, and right ventricular pacing.

Gallops and murmurs are common abnormal heart sounds that may occur with heart disease, but they can occur in some healthy people. Diastolic filling sounds (S_3 and S_4) are produced when blood enters a noncompliant chamber during rapid ventricular filling. The third heart sound (S_3) is produced during the rapid passive filling phase of ventricular diastole when blood flows from the atrium to a noncompliant ventricle. The sound arises from vibrations of the valves and supporting structures. The fourth heart sound (S_4) occurs as blood enters the ventricles during the active filling phase at the end of ventricular diastole.

S_3 is called a **ventricular gallop,** and S_4 is referred to as **atrial gallop**. These sounds can be caused by decreased compliance of either or both ventricles. Left ventricular diastolic filling sounds are best heard with the patient on his or her left side. The bell of the stethoscope is placed at the apex and at the left lower sternal border during expiration.

An S_3 heart sound is most likely to be a normal finding in those younger than 35 years. An S_3 gallop in patients older than 35 years is considered abnormal and represents a decrease in left ventricular compliance. It can be detected as an early sign of heart failure or as a ventricular septal defect.

An atrial gallop (S_4) may be heard in patients with hypertension, anemia, ventricular hypertrophy, MI, aortic or pulmonic stenosis, and pulmonary emboli. *It may be heard also with advancing age because of a stiffened ventricle.*

Murmurs reflect turbulent blood flow through normal or abnormal valves. They are classified according to their timing in the cardiac cycle: *systolic* murmurs (e.g., aortic stenosis and mitral regurgitation) occur between S_1 and S_2, whereas *diastolic* murmurs (e.g., mitral stenosis and aortic regurgitation) occur between S_2 and S_1. Murmurs can occur during presystole, midsystole, or late systole or diastole or can last throughout both phases of the cardiac cycle. They are also graded by the primary care provider according to their intensity, depending on their level of loudness (Table 33-3).

Although you are not expected to grade murmurs as a medical-surgical nurse, describe their location based on where they are best heard. Some murmurs transmit or radiate from their loudest point to other areas, including the neck, the back, and the axilla. The configuration is described as *crescendo* (increases in intensity) or *decrescendo* (decreases in intensity). The quality of murmurs can be further characterized as harsh, blowing, whistling, rumbling, or squeaking. They are also described by pitch—usually *high* or *low*.

A **pericardial friction rub** originates from the pericardial sac and occurs with the movements of the heart during the cardiac cycle. Rubs are usually transient and are a sign of inflammation, infection, or infiltration. They may be heard in patients with pericarditis resulting from MI, cardiac tamponade, or post-thoracotomy.

Psychosocial Assessment

To most people, the heart is a symbol of their ability to exist, survive, and love. A patient with a heart-related illness, whether acute or chronic, usually perceives it as a major life crisis. The patient and family confront not only the possibility of death but also fears about pain, disability, lack of self-esteem, physical dependence, and changes in family dynamics. Assess the meaning of the illness to the patient and family by asking "What do you understand about what happened to you (or the patient)?" and "What does that mean to you?" When they perceive the stressor as overwhelming, formerly adequate support systems may no longer be effective. In these circumstances, the patient and family members attempt to cope to regain a sense or feeling of control.

Coping behaviors vary among patients and their families. Those who feel helpless to meet the demands of the situation may exhibit behaviors such as disorganization, fear, and anxiety. Ask them "Have you ever encountered such a situation before?" "How did you manage that situation?" and "To whom can you turn for help?" The answers to these questions often reassure the patient and family that they have encountered difficult situations in the past and have the ability and resources to cope with them.

A common and normal response is denial, which is a defense mechanism that enables the patient to cope with threatening circumstances. He or she may deny the current cardiovascular condition, may state that it was present but is now absent, or may be excessively cheerful. Denial becomes maladaptive when the patient is noncompliant or does not adhere to the interdisciplinary plan of care.

Family members and significant others may be more anxious than the patient. Often they recall all events of the illness, are unprotected by denial, and are afraid of recurrence. Disagreements may occur between the patient and family members over adherence to appropriate follow-up care.

Diagnostic Assessment
Laboratory Assessment

Assessment of the patient with cardiovascular dysfunction includes examination of the blood for abnormalities. The examination is performed to help establish a diagnosis, detect concurrent disease, assess risk factors, and monitor response to treatment. Normal values for serum cardiac enzymes and serum lipids are listed in Chart 33-2.

Serum Markers of Myocardial Damage. Events leading to cellular injury cause a release of enzymes from intracellular

TABLE 33-3	**Grading of Heart Murmurs**
Grade I	Very faint
Grade II	Faint but recognizable
Grade III	Loud but moderate in intensity
Grade IV	Loud and accompanied by a palpable thrill
Grade V	Very loud, accompanied by a palpable thrill, and audible with the stethoscope partially off the patient's chest
Grade VI	Extremely loud, may be heard with the stethoscope slightly above the patient's chest, accompanied by a palpable thrill

CLINICAL JUDGMENT CHALLENGE

Safety; Teamwork and Collaboration QSEN

A middle-aged man is admitted to the cardiac unit after reports of a severe headache and flushing of the face. He is diagnosed with severe hypertension. The patient is alert and oriented; BP = 192/104 and HR = 88. You are the RN assigned to his care. There is an unlicensed nursing technician working with you.

1. What assessment data will you perform upon his arrival to the unit? Why?
2. The cardiologist prescribes IV fluids, hourly blood pressure checks, blood pressure medication, and oxygen at 2 liters per nasal cannula. What part of the patient's care will you delegate to the unlicensed nursing technician? What information will you communicate upon delegation?
3. What interventions will you implement to ensure this patient's safety?
4. The patient's wife is very concerned about her husband returning to work as owner of a roofing company. What education will you provide the patient and his wife at this time? With what health care team members will you collaborate to ensure positive patient outcomes?

CHART 33-2 Laboratory Profile

Cardiovascular Assessment

NORMAL RANGE	SIGNIFICANCE OF ABNORMAL FINDINGS
Serum Cardiac Enzymes	

Creatine kinase (CK)
  Females: 30-135 units/L
  Males: 55-170 units/L
Values higher after exercise
	Elevations indicate possible brain, myocardial, and skeletal muscle necrosis or injury.

CK-MB (CK$_2$) 0% of total CK	Elevations occur with myocardial injury or after percutaneous transluminal angioplasty and intracoronary streptokinase infusion.
Serum Lipids	
Total lipids 400-1000 mg/dL	Elevation indicates increased risk for coronary artery disease (CAD).
Cholesterol Less than 200 mg/dL	Elevation indicates increased risk for CAD.

Triglycerides
  Females: 35-135 mg/dL
  Males: 40-160 mg/dL
	Elevation indicates increased risk for CAD.

Plasma high-density lipoproteins (HDLs)
  Females: >55 mg/dL
  Males: >45 mg/dL
  Older adults: range increases with age
	Elevations protect against CAD.

Plasma low-density lipoproteins (LDLs) <130 mg/dL	Elevation indicates increased risk for CAD.
HDL:LDL ratio 3:1	Elevated ratios may protect against CAD.
VLDL 7-32 ng/dL	Elevated level indicates risk for CAD.
C-reactive protein (CRP) <1.0 mg/dL	Elevation may indicate tissue infarction or damage.
Serum Markers	
Troponins Cardiac troponin T <0.10 ng/mL Cardiac troponin I <0.03 ng/mL	Elevations indicate myocardial injury or infarction.
Myoglobin <90 mcg/L	Elevation indicates myocardial infarction.

VLDL, Very-low-density lipoproteins.

storage, and circulating levels of these enzymes are dramatically elevated. Acute myocardial infarction (MI), also known as **acute coronary syndrome,** can be confirmed by abnormally high levels of certain proteins or isoenzymes. These serum studies are commonly referred to as **cardiac markers** and include troponin, creatine kinase–MB, and myoglobin.

Troponin is a myocardial muscle protein released into the bloodstream with injury to myocardial muscle. Troponins T and I are not found in healthy patients, so any rise in values indicates cardiac necrosis or acute MI. Specific markers of myocardial injury, troponins T and I, have a wide diagnostic time frame, making them useful for patients who present several hours after the onset of chest pain. Even low levels of troponin T are treated aggressively because of increased risk for death from cardiovascular disease (CVD). Obtaining cardiac markers at the bedside in the emergency department can be done as "point of care" (POC) testing for patients experiencing or at risk for acute MI, with results available within 15 to 20 minutes. These markers are evaluated in addition to clinical signs and symptoms and ECG changes when identifying at-risk patients.

Creatine kinase (CK) is an enzyme specific to cells of the brain, myocardium, and skeletal muscle. The appearance of CK in the blood indicates tissue necrosis or injury, with levels following a predictable rise and fall during a specified period. Cardiac specificity must be determined by measuring isoenzyme activity. There are three isoenzymes of CK: CK-MM is the predominant isoenzyme of skeletal muscle; CK-MB is found in myocardial muscle; and CK-BB occurs in the brain. CK-MB activity is most specific for MI and shows a predictable rise and fall during 3 days; a peak level occurs about 24 hours after the onset of chest pain.

Treatment modalities for early intervention after acute MI and acute ischemia require more rapid diagnosis of MI. An assay using monoclonal anti–CK-MB antibodies (stat CK) can detect myocardial necrosis accurately 3 hours after emergency department admission when examined with an ECG. Two subforms of CK-MB (CK-MB$_1$ and CK-MB$_2$) have also been identified. Abnormal elevations of these CK subforms may occur as early as 2 hours after MI. They remain elevated for up to 12 hours after MI and appear to be very sensitive and specific early diagnostic markers of MI.

Another early marker of an MI is myoglobin. **Myoglobin,** a low–molecular-weight heme protein found in cardiac and skeletal muscle, is the earliest marker detected—as early as 2 hours after an MI with rapid decline after 7 hours. Because myoglobin is not cardiac specific and is found in skeletal and cardiac muscle, its clinical usefulness is more limited than troponin.

Serum Lipids. Elevated lipid levels are considered a risk factor for coronary artery disease (CAD). **Cholesterol, triglycerides,** and the protein components of **high-density lipoproteins (HDLs)** and **low-density lipoproteins (LDLs)** are evaluated to assess the risk for CAD. The desired ranges for lipids are (Pagana & Pagana, 2014):

- Total cholesterol less than 200 mg/dL
- Triglycerides between 40 and 160 mg/dL for men and between 35 and 135 mg/dL for women
- HDL more than 45 mg/dL for men; more than 55 mg/dL for women ("good" cholesterol)
- LDL less than 130 mg/dL

Each of the lipoproteins contains varying proportions of cholesterol, triglyceride, protein, and phospholipid. HDL contains mainly protein and 20% cholesterol, whereas LDL is mainly cholesterol. Elevated LDL levels are positively correlated with CAD, whereas elevated HDL levels are negatively correlated and appear to be protective for heart disease. LDL pattern size is of significant importance in determining risk for CVD. LDL pattern A is associated with non–insulin resistance; normal glucose, insulin, and HDL levels; and a normal blood pressure. LDL pattern B is associated with insulin resistance; increased glucose, insulin, and triglyceride levels; and hypertension.

A fasting blood sample for the measurement of serum cholesterol levels is preferable to a nonfasting sample. If triglycerides are to be evaluated with cholesterol, the health care provider requests the specimen after a 12-hour fast

Lipoprotein-a, or Lp(a), is a modified form of LDL, the most common familial lipoprotein disorder in patients with premature coronary artery disease. Lp(a) is atherogenic (increases atherosclerotic plaques) and prothrombotic (increases clots). Therefore the desired outcome is a value less than 30 mg/dL. The patient should be fasting and avoid smoking before the test (Pagana & Pagana, 2014).

Other Laboratory Tests. **Homocysteine** is an amino acid that is produced when proteins break down. A certain amount of homocysteine is present in the blood, but elevated values may be an independent risk factor for the development of CVD. Although the relationship between homocysteine and CVD remains controversial, elevated levels of homocysteine may increase the risk for disease as much as smoking and hyperlipemia, especially in women. High-risk patients who have a personal or family history of premature heart disease should be screened. A level less than 14 mmol/dL is considered optimal, but this level increases as one ages (Pagana & Pagana, 2014).

Inflammation is a common and critical component to the development of atherothrombosis. **Highly sensitive C-reactive protein (hsCRP)** has been the most studied marker of inflammation. Any inflammatory process can produce CRP in the blood. Elevations are seen also with hypertension, infection, and smoking. A level less than 1 mg/dL is considered low risk; a level over 3 mg/dL places the patient at high risk for heart disease. The CRP is very helpful in determining treatment outcomes in patients at risk for coronary disease and in managing statin therapy after an acute myocardial infarction. The most useful time to measure CRP appears to be for risk assessment in middle-aged or older persons.

Microalbuminuria, or small amounts of protein in the urine, has been shown to be a clear marker of widespread endothelial dysfunction in cardiovascular disease (along with elevated CRP). It should be screened annually in all patients with hypertension, metabolic syndrome, or diabetes mellitus. Microalbuminuria has also been used as a marker for renal disease, particularly in patients with hypertension and diabetes.

Blood coagulation studies evaluate the ability of the blood to clot. They are important in patients with a greater tendency to form thrombi (e.g., those with atrial fibrillation, prosthetic valves, or infective endocarditis). These tests are also essential for monitoring patients receiving anticoagulant therapy (e.g., during cardiac surgery, during treatment of an established thrombus).

Prothrombin time (PT) and *international normalized ratio (INR)* are used when initiating and maintaining therapy with oral anticoagulants, such as sodium warfarin (Coumadin, Warfilone ✦). They measure the activity of prothrombin, fibrinogen, and factors V, VII, and X. INR is the most reliable way to monitor anticoagulant status in warfarin therapy. The therapeutic ranges vary significantly based on the reason for the anticoagulation and the patient's history. The normal INR is 1.

Partial thromboplastin time (PTT) is assessed in patients who are receiving heparin (Hepalean ✦). It measures deficiencies in all coagulation factors except VII and XIII.

Arterial blood gas (ABG) determinations are often obtained in patients with CVD. Determination of tissue oxygenation, carbon dioxide removal, and acid-base status is essential to appropriate treatment. (See Chapter 12 for a complete discussion of ABGs.)

FLUID AND ELECTROLYTE BALANCE is essential for normal cardiovascular performance. Cardiac manifestations often occur when there is an imbalance in either fluids or electrolytes in the body. For example, the cardiac effects of hypokalemia (low serum potassium level) include increased electrical instability, ventricular dysrhythmias, and an increased risk for digitalis toxicity. The effects of hyperkalemia on the myocardium include slowed ventricular conduction, peaked T waves on the ECG, and contraction followed by asystole (cardiac standstill).

Cardiac manifestations of hypocalcemia are ventricular dysrhythmias, a prolonged QT interval, and cardiac arrest. Hypercalcemia shortens the QT interval and causes AV block, digitalis hypersensitivity, and cardiac arrest. Serum sodium values reflect fluid balance and may be decreased, indicating a fluid excess in patients with heart failure (dilutional hyponatremia).

Because magnesium regulates some aspects of myocardial electrical activity, hypomagnesemia has been implicated in some forms of ventricular dysrhythmias known as *torsades de pointes.* Hypomagnesemia prolongs the QT interval, causing this specific type of ventricular tachycardia. Chapter 11 describes these electrolytes in more detail.

The *erythrocyte (red blood cell [RBC]) count* is usually decreased in rheumatic fever and infective endocarditis. It is increased in heart diseases as needed to compensate for decreased available oxygen.

Decreased *hematocrit and hemoglobin* levels (e.g., caused by hemorrhage or hemolysis from prosthetic valves) indicate anemia and can lead to angina or aggravate heart failure. Vascular volume depletion with hemoconcentration (e.g., hypovolemic shock and excessive diuresis) results in an elevated hematocrit.

The *leukocyte (white blood cell [WBC]) count* is typically elevated after an MI and in various infectious and inflammatory diseases of the heart (e.g., infective endocarditis and pericarditis). An increased WBC has been implicated as a strong independent risk factor for stroke and heart disease, particularly in postmenopausal women (Go et al., 2013).

Other Diagnostic Assessment

Posteroanterior (PA) and left lateral *x-ray* views of the chest are routinely obtained to determine the size, silhouette, and

TABLE 33-4 Indications For Cardiac Catheterization
• To confirm suspected heart disorders, including congenital abnormalities, coronary artery disease, myocardial disease, valvular disease, and valvular dysfunction
• To determine the location and extent of the disease process
• To assess:
• Stable, severe angina unresponsive to medical management
• Unstable angina pectoris
• Uncontrolled heart failure, ventricular dysrhythmias, or cardiogenic shock associated with acute myocardial infarction, papillary muscle dysfunction, ventricular aneurysm, or septal perforation
• To determine best therapeutic option (percutaneous transluminal coronary angioplasty, stents, coronary artery bypass graft, valvulotomy versus valve replacement)
• To evaluate effects of medical or invasive treatment on cardiovascular function, percutaneous transluminal coronary angioplasty, or coronary artery bypass graft patency

TABLE 33-5 Complications of Cardiac Catheterization
Right-Sided Heart Catheterization
• Thrombophlebitis
• Pulmonary embolism
• Vagal response
Left-Sided Heart Catheterization and Coronary Arteriography
• Myocardial infarction
• Stroke
• Arterial bleeding or thromboembolism
• Dysrhythmias
Right-Sided or Left-Sided Heart Catheterization*
• Cardiac tamponade
• Hypovolemia
• Pulmonary edema
• Hematoma or blood loss at insertion site
• Reaction to contrast medium

*In addition to those cited for each procedure.

position of the heart. In acutely ill patients, a simple anteroposterior (AP) view may be obtained at the bedside. Cardiac enlargement, pulmonary congestion, cardiac calcifications, and placement of central venous catheters, endotracheal tubes, and hemodynamic monitoring devices are assessed by x-ray.

Angiography of the arterial vessels, or **arteriography**, is an invasive diagnostic procedure that involves fluoroscopy and the use of contrast media. This procedure is performed when an arterial obstruction, narrowing, or aneurysm is suspected. The interventional radiologist performs selective arteriography to evaluate specific areas of the arterial system. For example, a coronary arteriography, which is performed during left-sided cardiac catheterization, assesses arterial circulation within the heart. It can also be performed on arteries in the extremities, mesentery, and cerebrum. Angiography is discussed under the appropriate associated diseases elsewhere in this text.

Cardiac Catheterization. The most definitive but most invasive test in the diagnosis of heart disease is cardiac catheterization. **Cardiac catheterization** may include studies of the right or left side of the heart and the coronary arteries. Some of the most common indications for cardiac catheterization are listed in Table 33-4.

Patient Preparation. Assess the patient's physical and psychosocial readiness and knowledge level about the procedure because many patients have anxiety and fear about cardiac catheterization. Review the purpose of the procedure, inform the patient about the length of the procedure, state who will be present, and describe the appearance of the catheterization laboratory. Tell the patient about the sensations he or she may experience during the procedure, such as palpitations (as the catheter is passed up to the left ventricle), a feeling of heat or a hot flash (as the medium is injected into either side of the heart), and a desire to cough (as the medium is injected into the right side of the heart). Written, electronic, or illustrated materials or DVDs may be used to assist in understanding.

The risks of cardiac catheterization are usually explained by the cardiologist. The risks vary with the procedures to be performed and the patient's physical status (Table 33-5). Although not common, several serious complications may follow coronary arteriography, such as:
• Myocardial infarction (MI)
• Stroke
• Arterial bleeding
• Thromboembolism
• Lethal dysrhythmias
• Arterial dissection
• Death

The cardiologist or interventional radiologist obtains a written informed consent from the patient or responsible party before the procedure.

The patient is admitted to the hospital on the day of the catheterization procedure. He or she may be admitted earlier if there is renal dysfunction. Fluids may be given 12 to 24 hours before the procedure for renal protection. Contrast-induced renal dysfunction can result from vasoconstriction and the direct toxic effect of the contrast agent on the renal tubules. Hydration and the administration of acetylcysteine pre- and post-study help eliminate or minimize contrast-induced renal toxicity.

Standard preoperative tests are performed, which usually include a chest x-ray, complete blood count, coagulation studies, and 12-lead ECG. The patient receives nothing by mouth after midnight or has only a liquid breakfast if the catheterization is scheduled for the afternoon. The catheterization site is antiseptically prepared with hairs clipped according to agency policy.

Before the procedure, take the patient's vital signs, auscultate the heart and the lungs, and assess the peripheral pulses. Question him or her about any history of allergy to iodine-based contrast agents. An antihistamine or steroid may be given to a patient with a positive history or to prevent a reaction. Be sure that the signed informed consent is completed, as required by The Joint Commission's National Patient Safety Goals (NPSGs). A mild sedative is usually administered before the procedure. If the patient normally takes a digitalis preparation or diuretic, it is usually withheld before the catheterization. Analysis of electrolytes, blood urea nitrogen (BUN), creatinine, coagulation profile, and complete blood count (CBC) is essential before and after the procedure, and abnormalities are discussed with the health care provider.

Procedure. The patient is taken to the cardiac catheterization laboratory (sometimes referred to as the "cath lab"), placed in the supine position on the x-ray table, and securely strapped to the table. The physician injects a local anesthetic at the insertion site. During the procedure, the patient is instructed to report any chest pain, pressure, or other symptoms to the staff.

The *right side of the heart* is catheterized first and may be the only side examined. The cardiologist inserts a catheter through the femoral vein to the inferior vena cava or through the basilic vein to the superior vena cava. The catheter is advanced through either the inferior or the superior vena cava and, guided by fluoroscopy, is advanced through the right atrium, through the right ventricle, and, at times, into the pulmonary artery. Intracardiac pressures (right atrial, right ventricular, pulmonary artery, and pulmonary artery wedge pressures) and blood samples are obtained. A contrast medium is usually injected to detect any cardiac shunts or regurgitation from the pulmonic or tricuspid valves.

In a *left-sided heart catheterization*, the cardiologist advances the catheter against the blood flow from the femoral, brachial, or radial artery up the aorta, across the aortic valve, and into the left ventricle (Fig. 33-8). Alternatively, the catheter may be passed from the right side of the heart through the atrial septum, using a special needle to puncture the septum. Intracardiac pressures and blood samples are obtained. The pressures of the left atrium, left ventricle, and aorta, as well as mitral and aortic valve status, are evaluated. The cardiologist injects contrast dye into the ventricle; digital subtraction angiography evaluates left ventricular motion. Calculations are made regarding end-systolic volume, end-diastolic volume, stroke volume, and ejection fraction.

The technique for *coronary arteriography* is the same as for left-sided heart catheterization. The catheter is advanced into the aortic arch and positioned selectively in the right or left coronary artery. Injection of a contrast medium permits viewing the coronary arteries. By assessing the flow of the medium through the coronary arteries, information about the site and severity of coronary lesions is obtained.

An alternative to injecting a medium into the coronary arteries is **intravascular ultrasonography (IVUS)**, which introduces a flexible catheter with a miniature transducer at the distal tip to view the coronary arteries. The transducer emits sound waves, which reflect off the plaque and the arterial wall to create an image of the blood vessel. IVUS is more reliable than angiography in indicating plaque distribution and composition, arterial dissection, and degree of stenosis of the occluded artery.

Follow-up Care. The patient recovers in a specialty area equipped with monitored beds. After cardiac catheterization, restrict the patient to bedrest and keep the insertion site extremity straight. A soft knee brace can be applied to prevent bending of the affected extremity. Some cardiologists allow the head of the bed to be elevated up to 30 degrees during the period of bedrest, whereas other cardiologists prefer that the patient remain supine. Current practice is for patients to remain in bed for 2 to 6 hours depending on the type of vascular closure device used. Various types of vascular closure devices are used to eliminate the need for manual compression after the catheterization. Examples include arteriotomy sutures and collagen plugs to seal the insertion site.

Monitor the patient's vital signs every 15 minutes for 1 hour, then every 30 minutes for 2 hours or until vital signs are stable, and then every 4 hours or according to hospital policy. Assess the insertion site for bloody drainage or hematoma formation. Complications with vascular closure devices are not common but can be very serious. Assess peripheral pulses in the affected extremity, as well as skin temperature and color, with every vital sign check. Observe for complications of cardiac catheterization (see Table 33-5).

> **! NURSING SAFETY PRIORITY** (QSEN)
>
> ### Critical Rescue
>
> If the patient experiences symptoms of cardiac ischemia such as chest pain, dysrhythmias, bleeding, hematoma formation, or a dramatic change in peripheral pulses in the affected extremity, contact the Rapid Response Team or physician immediately to provide prompt intervention! Neurologic changes indicating a possible stroke, such as visual disturbances, slurred speech, swallowing difficulties, and extremity weakness, should also be reported immediately.

Because the contrast medium acts as an osmotic diuretic, monitor urine output and ensure that the patient receives sufficient oral and IV fluids for adequate excretion of the medium. Pain medication for insertion site or back discomfort may be given as prescribed.

Review home instructions and risk factor modification with the patient before discharge. Remind the patient to:

- Limit activity for several days, including avoiding lifting and exercise.
- Leave the dressing in place for at least the first day at home.
- Observe the insertion site over the next few weeks for increased swelling, redness, warmth, and pain. Bruising or a small hematoma is expected.

Electrocardiography. The electrocardiogram (ECG) is a routine part of every cardiovascular evaluation and is one of the most valuable diagnostic tests. Various forms are available: resting ECG, continuous ambulatory ECG (Holter monitoring), exercise ECG (stress test), signal-averaged ECG, and 30-day

FIG. 33-8 Left-sided cardiac catheterization.

Aortic arch

Left atrium

Left ventricle

Catheter

Catheter entering femoral artery

FIG. 33-9 Patient using a treadmill for a stress test.

event monitoring. The resting ECG provides information about cardiac dysrhythmias, myocardial ischemia, the site and extent of MI, cardiac hypertrophy, electrolyte imbalances, and the effectiveness of cardiac drugs. The normal ECG pattern and a detailed discussion of the interpretation of abnormal patterns are discussed in Chapter 34.

Electrophysiologic Studies. An **electrophysiologic study (EPS)** is an invasive procedure during which programmed electrical stimulation of the heart is used to cause and evaluate lethal dysrhythmias and conduction abnormalities. Patients who have survived cardiac arrest, have recurrent tachydysrhythmias, or experience unexplained syncopal episodes may be referred for EPS. Induction of the dysrhythmia during EPS helps find an accurate diagnosis and aids in effective treatment. These procedures have risks similar to those for cardiac catheterization and are performed in a special catheterization laboratory, where conditions are strictly controlled and immediate treatment is available for any adverse effects.

Exercise Electrocardiography (Stress Test). The **exercise electrocardiography** test (also known as **exercise tolerance**, or **stress test**) assesses cardiovascular response to an increased workload. The stress test helps determine the functional capacity of the heart and screens for asymptomatic coronary artery disease. Dysrhythmias that develop during exercise may be identified, and the effectiveness of antidysrhythmic drugs can be evaluated.

Patient Preparation. Because risks are associated with exercising, the patient must be adequately informed about the purpose of the test, the procedure, and the risks involved. Written consent must be obtained. Anxiety and fear are common before stress testing. Therefore assure the patient that the procedure is performed in a controlled environment in which prompt nursing and medical attention are available.

Instruct the patient to get plenty of rest the night before the procedure. He or she may have a light meal 2 hours before the test but should avoid smoking or drinking alcohol or caffeine-containing beverages on the day of the test. The cardiologist decides whether the patient should stop taking any cardiac medications. Usually cardiovascular drugs such as beta blockers or calcium channel blockers are withheld on the day of the test to allow the heart rate to increase during the stress portion of the test. Patients are advised to wear comfortable, loose clothing and rubber-soled, supportive shoes. Remind them to tell the physician if symptoms such as chest pain, dizziness, shortness of breath, and an irregular heartbeat are experienced during the test.

Before the stress test, a resting 12-lead ECG, cardiovascular history, and physical examination are performed to check for any ECG abnormalities or medical factors that might interfere with the test. Check to see that all emergency supplies such as

cardiac drugs, a defibrillator, and other necessary resuscitation equipment are available in the room in which the stress test is performed. It is important to be proficient in the use of resuscitation equipment when assisting the physician because chest pain, dysrhythmias, and other ECG changes may occur.

Procedure. The technician places electrodes on the patient's chest and attaches them to a multilead monitoring system. Note baseline blood pressure (BP), heart rate (HR), and respiratory rate. The two major modes of exercise available for stress testing are pedaling a bicycle ergometer and walking on a treadmill. A bicycle ergometer has a wheel operated by pedals that can be adjusted to increase the resistance to pedaling. The treadmill is a motorized device with an adjustable conveyor belt. It can reach speeds of 1 to 10 miles/hr and can also be adjusted from a flat position to a 22-degree incline.

After the patient is shown how to use the bicycle or to walk on the treadmill, he or she begins to exercise. During the test, the BP and ECG are closely monitored as the resistance to cycling or the speed and incline of the treadmill are increased (Fig. 33-9). The patient exercises until one of these findings occurs:

- A predetermined HR is reached and maintained.
- Signs and symptoms such as chest pain, fatigue, extreme dyspnea, vertigo, hypotension, and ventricular dysrhythmias appear.
- Significant ST-segment depression or T-wave inversion occurs.
- The 20-minute protocol is completed.

Follow-up Care. After the test, the nurse or other qualified health care team member monitors the ECG and BP until the patient has completely recovered. After recovery, he or she can return home if the test was performed on an ambulatory basis. Advise him or her to avoid a hot shower for 1 to 2 hours after the test because this may cause hypotension. If he or she does not recover but continues to have pain or ventricular dysrhythmias or appears medically unstable, admission to a telemetry unit for observation is needed.

For patients who cannot exercise because of conditions such as peripheral vascular disease or arthritis, pharmacologic stress testing with agents such as dobutamine (Dobutrex) may be indicated. The nursing considerations are similar to those for the patient who has undergone an exercise ECG.

Echocardiography. As a noninvasive, risk-free test, echocardiography is easily performed at the bedside or on an ambulatory care basis. **Echocardiography** uses ultrasound waves to assess cardiac structure and mobility, particularly of the valves. It helps assess and diagnose cardiomyopathy, valvular disorders, pericardial effusion, left ventricular function, ventricular aneurysms, and cardiac tumors.

There is no special *preparation* for echocardiography. Inform the patient that the test is painless and takes 30 to 60 minutes to complete. The patient is instructed to lie quietly during the test and on his or her left side with the head elevated 15 to 20 degrees.

During an echocardiogram, a small transducer lubricated with gel to facilitate movement and conduction is placed on the patient's chest at the level of the third or fourth intercostal space near the left sternal border. The transducer transmits high-frequency sound waves and receives them as they are reflected from different structures. These echoes are usually videotaped simultaneously with the echocardiogram and can be recorded on graph paper for a permanent record.

After the images are taped, cardiac measurements that require several images can be obtained. Routine measurements include chamber size, ejection fraction, and flow gradient across the valves. There is no specific *follow-up care* for a patient who has undergone an echocardiogram.

A slightly more aggressive form of echocardiogram is a **pharmacologic stress echocardiogram** using either dobutamine or dipyridamole. This test is usually used when patients cannot tolerate exercise. Dobutamine (Dobutrex) increases the heart's contractility; dipyridamole (Persantine, Apo-Dipyridamole ✦) is a coronary artery dilator. Patients are required to be NPO status for 3 to 6 hours before the test except for sips of water with medications. The technician ensures that IV access is present before the procedure and monitors BP and pulse continuously throughout the procedure. After the procedure, vital signs are monitored until BP returns to baseline and the pulse rate slows to less than 100 beats/min.

Transesophageal Echocardiography. Echocardiograms may also be performed transesophageally (through the esophagus). **Transesophageal echocardiography (TEE)** examines cardiac structure and function with an ultrasound transducer placed immediately behind the heart in the esophagus or stomach. The transducer provides especially detailed views of posterior cardiac structures such as the left atrium, mitral valve, and aortic arch. Preparation and follow-up are similar to that for an upper GI endoscopic examination (see Chapter 52).

Myocardial Nuclear Perfusion Imaging. The use of radionuclide techniques in cardiovascular assessment is called **myocardial nuclear perfusion imaging (MNPI)**. Cardiovascular abnormalities can be viewed, recorded, and evaluated using radioactive tracer substances. These studies are useful for detecting myocardial infarction (MI) and decreased myocardial blood flow and for evaluating left ventricular ejection. Conducting myocardial nuclear imaging tests, in conjunction with exercise or the administration of vasodilating agents, allows clearer identification of how the heart responds to stress.

Inform the patient that these tests are noninvasive. Because the amount of radioisotope is small, radiation exposure risks are minimal. If a dilating agent is to be used, advise the patient to avoid cigarettes and caffeinated food or drinks for 4 hours before administration of the vasodilator.

Common tests in nuclear cardiology include technetium (^{99m}Tc) pyrophosphate scanning, thallium imaging, and multigated cardiac blood pool imaging. Each test requires the injection of different types of radioactive isotopes into the antecubital vein. After the cells and tissues have time to take up the radioactive substances, usually 10 minutes to 2 hours, nuclear imaging can detect the difference between healthy and unhealthy tissue.

During the *technetium scan*, radioisotopes (^{99m}Tc pyrophosphate) accumulate in damaged myocardial tissue, which appears as a "hot spot" during the scan. This test helps detect the location and size of acute myocardial infarctions.

Alternatively, during the *thallium imaging scan*, necrotic or ischemic tissue does not absorb the radioisotope (thallium-201) and appears as "cold spots" on the scan. Thallium imaging is used to assess myocardial scarring and perfusion, to detect the location and extent of an acute or chronic myocardial infarction, to evaluate graft patency after coronary bypass surgery, and to evaluate antianginal therapy, thrombolytic therapy, or balloon angioplasty.

Thallium imaging may be performed during an exercise test or with the patient at rest. Thallium imaging performed during an exercise test may demonstrate perfusion deficits not apparent at rest. First, the stress test procedure is performed. After the patient reaches maximum activity level, a small dose of thallium-201 is injected IV. The patient continues to exercise for about 1 to 2 minutes, after which the scanning is performed. Nuclear cardiologists often compare the resting and stress images to differentiate between fixed and reversible defects in the myocardium.

If a patient cannot exercise on a bike or treadmill, dipyridamole (Persantine, Apo-Dipyridamole ✦) or dobutamine hydrochloride (Dobutrex) is administered to simulate the effects of exercise. Tell the patient that these vasodilators may cause flushing, headache, dyspnea, and chest tightness for a few moments after injection.

Cardiac blood pool imaging is a noninvasive test for evaluating cardiac motion and calculating ejection fraction. It uses a computer to synchronize the patient's ECG with pictures taken by a special camera. The technician attaches the patient to an ECG and injects a small amount of ^{99m}Tc IV. The radioisotope is not taken up by tissue but remains "tagged" to red blood cells in the circulation. The camera may take pictures of the radioactive material as it makes its first pass through the heart.

During **multigated blood pool scanning**, the computer breaks the time between R waves on the ECG into fractions of a second, called "gates." The camera records blood flow through the heart during each of these gates. By analyzing the information from multiple gates, the computer can evaluate the ventricular wall motion and calculate ejection fraction (percentage of the left ventricular volume that is ejected with each contraction) and ejection velocity. Areas of decreased, absent, or paradoxical movement of the left ventricle may also be identified.

Positron emission tomography (PET) scans are used to compare cardiac perfusion and metabolic function and differentiate normal from diseased myocardium. The technician administers the first radioisotope (nitrogen-13-ammonia) and then begins a 20-minute scan to detect myocardial perfusion. Next, the technician administers a second radioisotope (fluoro-18-deoxyglucose). After a pause, a second scan is performed to detect the metabolically active myocardium, which is using glucose.

The two scans are compared. In a normal heart, performance and metabolic function will match. In an ischemic heart, there will be a mismatch—a reduction in perfusion and increased glucose uptake by the ischemic myocardium. The scanning procedure takes 2 to 3 hours, and the patient may be asked to use a treadmill or exercise bicycle in conjunction with the scan.

Depending on which test is performed, the patient may report fatigue or discomfort at the antecubital injection site. If a stress test was paired with the study, he or she will need follow-up care for the stress test.

Magnetic Resonance Imaging. Magnetic resonance imaging (MRI) is a noninvasive diagnostic option. An image of the heart or great vessels is produced through the interaction of magnetic fields, radio waves, and atomic nuclei showing hydrogen density. Simply put, the radio waves "bounce off" the body tissue being examined. Because each tissue has its own density, the computer image clearly differentiates between various types of tissues. MRI permits determination of cardiac wall thickness, chamber dilation, valve and ventricular function, and blood movement in the great vessels. Improved MRI techniques allow coronary artery blood flow to be mapped with nearly the accuracy of a cardiac catheterization.

Before an MRI, ensure that the patient has removed all metallic objects, including watches, jewelry, clothing with metal fasteners, and hair clips. Patients with pacemakers or implanted defibrillators may not be able to have an MRI because the magnetic fields can deactivate them. However, some newer MRI machines have eliminated this complication. A few patients experience claustrophobia during the 15 to 60 minutes required to complete the scan.

NURSING CONCEPTS AND CLINICAL JUDGMENT REVIEW

What might you NOTICE in a patient with adequate oxygenation and PERFUSION related to the cardiovascular system?

Physical assessment:
- Vital signs within normal limits or baseline
- No abnormal heart sounds
- Strong and equal peripheral pulses
- Even and unlabored respirations
- Regular heartbeat
- No pallor, cyanosis, or clubbing

- No syncope, fatigue, or chest pain
- No edema
- Can perform ADLs without dyspnea

Diagnostic assessment:
- No serum markers of myocardial damage
- Serum lipids within normal ranges
- Normal C-reactive protein and homocysteine
- Normal electrocardiogram (ECG)

GET READY FOR THE NCLEX® EXAMINATION!

KEY POINTS

Review these Key Points for each NCLEX Examination Client Needs Category.

Safe and Effective Care Environment
- Assess patients for allergy to iodine-based contrast media before having invasive diagnostic tests requiring an iodine-based contrast agent. **Safety** **QSEN**
- After invasive cardiovascular diagnostic testing, such as angiography and cardiac catheterization, monitor the insertion site for bleeding and hematoma formation. **Safety** **QSEN**
- Assess vital signs carefully in patients having invasive cardiovascular testing; report and document any new dysrhythmias after testing. **Informatics** **QSEN**

Health Promotion and Maintenance
- Identify patients at risk for cardiovascular disease, especially those with hyperlipidemia, hypertension, excess weight, physical inactivity, smoking, psychological stress, a positive family history, and diabetes. **Evidence-Based Practice** **QSEN**
- Teach patients how to reduce the risk for heart disease through modifiable factors such as exercise, diet modification, smoking cessation, and medications, as needed. **Patient-Centered Care** **QSEN**
- Inform patients that genetics and other nonmodifiable risk factors, such as family history and gender, contribute to the development of CAD.

- Assess the older adult for cardiovascular changes associated with aging as described in Chart 33-1.

Psychosocial Integrity
- Discuss with the patient any feelings or concerns he or she might have about the stress of cardiac illness, diagnostic testing, or other issues, and use therapeutic measures to decrease anxiety. **Patient-Centered Care** **QSEN**
- Recognize that denial is a common and normal response to help patients cope with threatening circumstances.
- Be aware that coping behaviors of those who have cardiovascular problems vary from patient to patient. **Patient-Centered Care** **QSEN**
- Allow the patient to express feelings about an actual or perceived loss of health or social status related to cardiovascular disease.

Physiological Integrity
- Be aware of the importance of recalling the anatomy and physiology of the cardiovascular (CV) system to best understand how to care for patients with CV health problems.
- Assess the patient's report of pain to differentiate the pain of angina and myocardial infarction (MI) from other noncardiac causes; *discomfort, indigestion, squeezing, heaviness,* and *viselike* are common terms used to describe chest pain of cardiac origin.

- Recall that syncope is a transient loss of consciousness and is common in older adults.
- Be aware that women often present with different indicators of heart disease when compared with men; examples include dyspnea, chest discomfort, indigestion, and fatigue.

Evidence-Based Practice QSEN

- Use jugular venous pressure to assess the filling volume and pressure on the right side of the heart.
- Assess for bruits, which are swishing sounds that develop in narrowed arteries.

- Auscultate the heart for normal first and second sounds, as well as for abnormalities such as an S_3, S_4, murmur, or gallop.
- Monitor serum markers of myocardial damage and other cardiac-related laboratory tests as listed in Chart 33-2.
- Prepare patients having a cardiac catheterization for expectations of the procedure and postprocedure care.
- Assess patients having cardiac catheterizations for potential complications as listed in Table 33-5. **Safety** QSEN

CHAPTER 34

Care of Patients with Dysrhythmias

Laura Dechant

 http://evolve.elsevier.com/Iggy/

PRIORITY CONCEPTS

- PERFUSION

LEARNING OUTCOMES

Safe and Effective Care Environment

1. Provide a safe environment for patients and staff when using a cardiac defibrillator.

Health Promotion and Maintenance

2. Teach patients and their families about drug therapy used for common dysrhythmias.
3. Educate patients and families about procedures and other interventions for common dysrhythmias.

Physiological Integrity

4. Identify typical physical assessment findings associated with common dysrhythmias.
5. Explain how to perform an electrocardiogram (ECG) test.

6. Analyze an ECG rhythm strip to identify normal sinus rhythm and common or life-threatening dysrhythmias.
7. Plan collaborative care for patients experiencing common dysrhythmias.
8. Explain the purpose and types of pacing used as interventions for patients with dysrhythmias to promote PERFUSION.
9. Explain the need to perform evidence-based emergency care procedures, such as cardiopulmonary resuscitation (CPR) and automated external defibrillation.
10. Teach patients with a pacemaker or implantable cardioverter/defibrillator about self-management when in the community.

Cardiac dysrhythmias are abnormal rhythms of the heart's electrical system that can affect its ability to effectively pump *oxygenated* blood throughout the body. Some dysrhythmias are life threatening, and others are not. They are the result of disturbances of cardiac electrical impulse formation, conduction, or both. When the heart does not work effectively as a pump, PERFUSION to vital organs and peripheral tissues can be impaired, resulting in organ dysfunction or failure.

Many health problems, especially coronary artery disease (CAD), electrolyte imbalances, impaired oxygenation, and drug toxicity (both legal and illicit drugs), can cause abnormal heart rhythms. Dysrhythmias can occur in people of any age but occur most often in older adults. To provide collaborative patient-centered care using best practices, a *basic* understanding of cardiac electrophysiology, the conduction system of the heart, and the principles of electrocardiography is needed as a medical-surgical nurse. Specialty nurses and advanced practice nurses have a more in-depth knowledge as they manage patients with these cardiac problems in critical care and ambulatory care settings.

REVIEW OF CARDIAC CONDUCTION SYSTEM

The cardiac conduction system consists of specialized myocardial cells (Fig. 34-1). The electrophysiologic properties of those cells regulate heart rate and rhythm and possess unique properties: automaticity, excitability, conductivity, and contractility.

Automaticity (pacing function) is the ability of cardiac cells to generate an electrical impulse spontaneously and repetitively. Normally, only primary pacemaker cells (sinoatrial [SA] node) can generate an electrical impulse. Under certain conditions, such as myocardial ischemia (decreased blood flow), electrolyte imbalance, hypoxia, drug toxicity, and infarction (cell death), any cardiac cell may produce electrical impulses independently and create dysrhythmias. Disturbances in automaticity may involve either an increase or a decrease in pacing function.

Excitability is the ability of non-pacemaker heart cells to respond to an electrical impulse that begins in pacemaker cells and to depolarize. **Depolarization** occurs when the normally negatively charged cells within the heart muscle develop a positive charge.

Conductivity is the ability to send an electrical stimulus from cell membrane to cell membrane. As a result, excitable cells depolarize in rapid succession from cell to cell until all cells have depolarized. *The wave of depolarization causes the deflections of the electrocardiogram (ECG) waveforms that are recognized as the P wave and the QRS complex.* Disturbances in conduction result when conduction is too rapid or too slow, when the pathway is totally blocked, or when the electrical impulse travels an abnormal pathway.

FIG. 34-1 The cardiac conduction system.

Contractility is the ability of atrial and ventricular muscle cells to shorten their fiber length in response to electrical stimulation, causing sufficient pressure to push blood forward through the heart. In other words, *contractility is the mechanical activity of the heart.*

Specialized cells of the myocardium are responsible for cardiac conduction. They consist of the sinoatrial node, atrioventricular junctional area, and bundle branch system.

Conduction begins with the **sinoatrial (SA) node** (also called the *sinus node*), located close to the surface of the right atrium near its junction with the superior vena cava. *The SA node is the heart's primary pacemaker.* It can spontaneously and rhythmically generate electrical impulses at a rate of 60 to 100 beats per minute and therefore has the greatest degree of automaticity.

The SA node is richly supplied by the sympathetic and parasympathetic nervous systems, which increase and decrease the rate of discharge of the sinus node, respectively. This process results in changes in the heart rate.

Impulses from the sinus node move directly through atrial muscle and lead to atrial depolarization, which is *reflected in a P wave on the ECG.* Atrial muscle contraction should follow. Within the atrial muscle are slow and fast conduction pathways leading to the atrioventricular (AV) node.

The **atrioventricular (AV) junctional** area consists of a transitional cell zone, the AV node itself, and the bundle of His. The AV node lies just beneath the right atrial endocardium, between the tricuspid valve and the ostium of the coronary sinus. Here T-cells (transitional cells) cause impulses to slow down or to be delayed in the AV node before proceeding to the ventricles. This delay is *reflected in the PR segment on the ECG.* This slow conduction provides a short delay, allowing the atria to contract and the ventricles to fill. The contraction is known as "atrial kick" and contributes additional blood volume for a greater cardiac output. The AV node is also controlled by both the sympathetic and the parasympathetic nervous systems. The bundle of His connects with the distal portion of the AV node and continues through the interventricular septum.

The *bundle of His* extends as a right bundle branch down the right side of the interventricular septum to the apex of the right ventricle. On the left side, it extends as a left bundle branch, which further divides.

At the ends of both the right and the left bundle branch systems are the Purkinje fibers. These fibers are an interweaving network located on the endocardial surface of both ventricles, from apex to base. The fibers then partially penetrate into the myocardium. **Purkinje cells** make up the bundle of His, bundle branches, and terminal Purkinje fibers. These cells are responsible for the rapid conduction of electrical impulses throughout the ventricles, leading to ventricular depolarization and the subsequent ventricular muscle contraction. A few nodal cells in the ventricles also occasionally demonstrate automaticity, giving rise to ventricular beats or rhythms.

ELECTROCARDIOGRAPHY

The **electrocardiogram (ECG)** provides a graphic representation, or picture, of cardiac electrical activity. The cardiac electrical currents are transmitted to the body surface. Electrodes, consisting of a conductive gel on an adhesive pad, are placed on specific sites on the body and attached to cables connected to an ECG machine or to a monitor. The cardiac electrical current is transmitted via the electrodes and through the lead wires to the machine or monitor, which displays the cardiac electrical activity.

A **lead** provides one view of the heart's electrical activity. Multiple leads, or views, can be obtained. Electrode placement is the same for male and female patients.

Lead systems are made up of a positive pole and a negative pole. An imaginary line joining these two poles is called the **lead axis**. The direction of electrical current flow in the heart is the **cardiac axis**. The relationship between the cardiac axis and the lead axis is responsible for the deflections seen on the ECG pattern:

- The baseline is the **isoelectric** line. It occurs when there is no current flow in the heart after complete depolarization and also after complete repolarization. Positive deflections occur above this line, and negative deflections occur below it. Deflections represent depolarization and repolarization of cells.

- If the direction of electrical current flow in the heart (cardiac axis) is toward the positive pole, a **positive deflection** (above the baseline) is viewed (Fig. 34-2, *A*).
- If the direction of electrical current flow in the heart (cardiac axis) is moving away from the positive pole toward the negative pole, a **negative deflection** (below the baseline) is viewed (Fig. 34-2, *B*).
- If the cardiac axis is moving neither toward nor away from the positive pole, a biphasic complex (both above and below baseline) will result (Fig. 34-2, *C*).

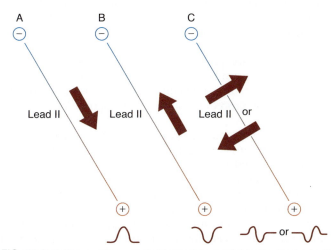

FIG. 34-2 A, The cardiac axis *(bold arrow)* is parallel to the lead axis *(the line between the negative and the positive electrodes)*, going toward the positive electrode; a positive deflection is inscribed. **B,** The cardiac axis is parallel to the lead axis, going toward the negative electrode; a negative deflection is inscribed. **C,** The cardiac axis is perpendicular to the lead axis, going neither toward the positive electrode nor toward the negative electrode; a biphasic deflection is inscribed.

Lead Systems

The standard 12-lead ECG consists of 12 leads (or views) of the heart's electrical activity. Six of the leads are called *limb leads* because the electrodes are placed on the four extremities in the frontal plane. The remaining six leads are called *chest (precordial) leads* because the electrodes are placed on the chest in the horizontal plane.

Standard bipolar *limb leads* consist of three leads (I, II, and III) that each measures the electrical activity between two points and a fourth lead (right leg) that acts as a ground electrode. Of the three measuring leads, the right arm is always negative, the left leg is always positive, and the left arm can be either positive or negative.

Other lead systems include the 18-lead ECG, which adds six leads placed on the horizontal plane on the right side of the chest to view the right side of the heart. This is sometimes referred to as a "right-sided ECG." The extra leads are sometimes placed on the back. The latest evidence indicates an 80-lead ECG, which looks at the heart from 80 views instead of only 12 and gives a 360-degree view of the heart. Evaluation of this 80-lead ECG revealed an increase in diagnosing myocardial infarctions (MIs), particularly in the posterior wall and right ventricular region, which was missed in the 12-lead ECG (Franks & Lawson, 2012). This device consists of a vest which contains 58 anterior leads, 12 lateral leads, and 10 posterior leads. One limitation is that vests are available in only four sizes and therefore may not be appropriate for some patients.

Unipolar limb leads consist of a positive electrode only. The unipolar limb leads are aVR, aVL, and aVF, with *a* meaning augmented. *V* is a designation for a unipolar lead. The third letter denotes the positive electrode placement: *R* for right arm, *L* for left arm, and *F* for foot (left leg). The positive electrode is at one end of the lead axis. The other end is the center of the electrical field, at about the center of the heart (Table 34-1).

There are six unipolar (or V) *chest leads*, determined by the placement of the chest electrode. The four limb electrodes are placed on the extremities, as designated on each electrode (right arm, left arm, right leg, and left leg). The fifth (chest) electrode

LEAD	NEGATIVE ELECTRODE	POSITIVE ELECTRODE	GROUND ELECTRODE
I	Right arm or under the right clavicle	Left arm or under the left clavicle	Right leg or lowest rib, left midclavicular line
II	Right arm or under the right clavicle	Left leg or lowest rib, left midclavicular line	Right leg or under the left clavicle
III	Left arm or under the left clavicle	Left leg or lowest rib, left midclavicular line	Right leg or under the right clavicle
aVR	Average potential of left arm (or under the left clavicle) and left leg (or lowest rib, left midclavicular line)	Right arm or under the right clavicle	Right leg or lowest rib, right midclavicular line
aVL	Average potential of right arm (or under the right clavicle) and left leg (or lowest rib, left midclavicular line)	Left arm or under the left clavicle	Same as for aVR
aVF	Average potential of right arm (or under the right clavicle) and left arm (or under the left clavicle)	Left leg or lowest rib, left midclavicular line	Same as for aVR
V$_1$	Average potential of right arm, left arm, and left leg	Fourth intercostal space (ICS), right sternal border	Same as for aVR
V$_2$	Same as for V$_1$	Fourth ICS, left sternal border	Same as for aVR
V$_3$	Same as for V$_1$	Midway between V$_2$ and V$_4$	Same as for aVR
V$_4$	Same as for V$_1$	Fifth ICS, left midclavicular line	Same as for aVR
V$_5$	Same as for V$_1$	Horizontal to V$_4$, left anterior axillary line	Same as for aVR
V$_6$	Same as for V$_1$	Horizontal to V$_4$, left midaxillary line	Same as for aVR

TABLE 34-1 Electrode Placement for 12 Leads

on a monitor system is the positive, or exploring, electrode and is placed in one of six designated positions to obtain the desired chest lead. With a 12-lead ECG, four leads are placed on the limbs and six are placed on the chest, eliminating the need to move any electrodes about the chest.

Positioning of the electrodes is crucial in obtaining an accurate ECG. Comparisons of ECGs taken at different times will be valid only when electrode placement is accurate and identical at each test. Positioning is particularly important when working with patients with chest deformities or large breasts. Patients may be asked to move the breasts to ensure proper electrode placement.

While obtaining a 12-lead ECG, remind the patient to be as still as possible in a semi-reclined position, breathing normally. Any repetitive movement will cause artifact and could lead to inaccurate interpretation of the ECG.

Nurses are sometimes responsible for obtaining 12-lead ECGs, but more commonly, technicians are trained to perform this skill. Remind the technician to notify the nurse or physician of any suspected abnormality. A nurse may direct a technician to take a 12-lead ECG on a patient experiencing chest pain to observe for diagnostic changes, but it is ultimately the health care provider's responsibility to definitively interpret the ECG.

Continuous Electrocardiographic Monitoring

For continuous ECG monitoring, the electrodes are not placed on the limbs because movement of the extremities causes "noise," or motion artifact, on the ECG signal. Place the electrodes on the trunk, a more stable area, to minimize such artifacts and to obtain a clearer signal. If the monitoring system provides five electrode cables, place the electrodes as follows:

- Right arm electrode just below the right clavicle
- Left arm electrode just below the left clavicle
- Right leg electrode on the lowest palpable rib, on the right midclavicular line
- Left leg electrode on the lowest palpable rib, on the left midclavicular line
- Fifth electrode placed to obtain one of the six chest leads

With this placement, the monitor lead select control may be changed to provide lead I, II, III, aVR, aVL, or aVF or one chest lead. The monitor automatically alters the polarity of the electrodes to provide the lead selected.

The clarity of continuous ECG monitor recordings is affected by skin preparation and electrode quality. To ensure the best signal transmission and to decrease skin impedance, clean the skin and clip hairs if needed. Make sure the area for electrode placement is dry. The gel on each electrode must be moist and fresh. Attach the electrode to the lead cable and then to the contact site. The contact site should be free of any lotion, tincture, or other substance that increases skin impedance. Electrodes cannot be placed on irritated skin or over scar tissue. The application of electrodes may be done by unlicensed assistive personnel (UAP), but the nurse determines which lead to select and checks for correct electrode placement. Assess the quality of the ECG rhythm transmission to the monitoring system.

The ECG cables can be attached directly to a wall-mounted monitor (a hard-wired system) if the patient's activity is restricted to bedrest and sitting in a chair, as in a critical care unit. For an ambulatory patient, the ECG cable is attached to a battery-operated transmitter (a **telemetry** system) held in a pouch. The ECG is transmitted to a remote monitor via antennae located in strategic places, usually in the ceiling. Telemetry

allows freedom of movement within a certain area without losing transmission of the ECG.

Most acute care facilities have monitor technicians (monitor "techs") who are educated in ECG rhythm interpretation and are responsible for:

- Watching a bank of monitors on a unit
- Printing ECG rhythm strips routinely and as needed
- Interpreting rhythms
- Reporting the patient's rhythm and significant changes to the nurse

The technical support is particularly helpful on a telemetry unit that does not have monitors at the bedside. The nurse is responsible for accurate patient assessment and management.

Some units have full-disclosure monitors, which continuously store ECG rhythms in memory up to a certain amount of time. This system allows nurses and health care providers to access and print rhythm strips for more thorough patient assessment. Routine strips, as well as any changes in rhythm, are printed and documented in the patient's record.

The health care provider is responsible for determining when monitoring can be suspended, such as during showering. He or she also determines whether monitoring is needed during off-unit testing procedures and for transportation to other facilities.

Prehospital personnel, such as paramedics and emergency medical technicians (EMTs) with advanced training, frequently monitor ECG rhythms at the scene and on the way to a health care facility. They function under medical direction and protocols but may also be communicating with a nurse in the emergency department.

The ECG strip is printed on graph paper (Fig. 34-3), with each small block measuring 1 mm in height and width. ECG recorders and monitors are standardized at a speed of 25 mm/sec. Time is measured on the horizontal axis. At this speed, each small block represents 0.04 second. Five small blocks make up one large block, defined by darker bold lines and representing 0.20 second. Five large blocks represent 1 second, and 30 large blocks represent 6 seconds. Vertical lines in the top margin of the graph paper are usually 15 large blocks apart, representing 3-second segments (Fig. 34-4).

Electrocardiographic Complexes, Segments, and Intervals

Complexes that make up a normal ECG consist of a P wave, a QRS complex, a T wave, and possibly a U wave. Segments include the PR segment, the ST segment, and the TP segment. Intervals include the PR interval, the QRS duration, and the QT interval (Fig. 34-5).

The **P wave** is a deflection representing atrial depolarization. The shape of the P wave may be a positive, negative, or biphasic (both positive and negative) deflection, depending on the lead selected. When the electrical impulse is consistently generated from the sinoatrial (SA) node, the P waves have a consistent shape in a given lead. If an impulse is then generated from a different (ectopic) focus, such as atrial tissue, the shape of the P wave changes in that lead, indicating that an ectopic focus has fired.

The **PR segment** is the isoelectric line from the end of the P wave to the beginning of the QRS complex, when the electrical impulse is traveling through the atrioventricular (AV) node, where it is delayed. It then travels through the ventricular conduction system to the Purkinje fibers.

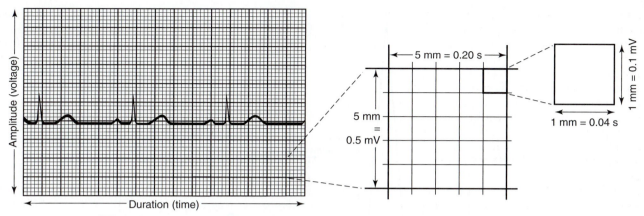

FIG. 34-3 Electrocardiographic waveforms are measured in amplitude (voltage) and duration (time).

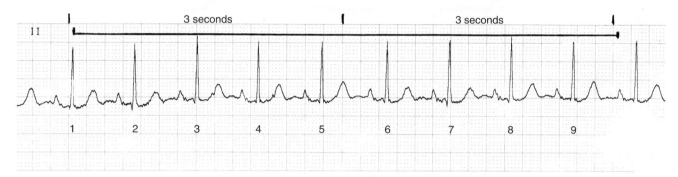

FIG. 34-4 Each segment between the dark lines *(above the monitor strip)* represents 3 seconds when the monitor is set at a speed of 25 mm per second. To estimate the ventricular rate, count the QRS complexes in a 6-second strip and then multiply that number by 10 to estimate the rate for 1 minute. In this example, there are 9 QRS complexes in 6 seconds. Therefore the heart rate can be estimated to be 90 beats per minute.

The **PR interval** is measured from the beginning of the P wave to the end of the PR segment. It represents the time required for atrial depolarization as well as the impulse delay in the AV node and the travel time to the Purkinje fibers. It normally measures from 0.12 to 0.20 second (five small blocks).

The **QRS complex** represents ventricular depolarization. The shape of the QRS complex depends on the lead selected. The Q wave is the first negative deflection and is not present in all leads. When present, it is small and represents initial ventricular septal depolarization. When the Q wave is abnormally present in a lead, it represents myocardial necrosis (cell death). The R wave is the first positive deflection. It may be small, large, or absent, depending on the lead. The S wave is a negative deflection following the R wave and is not present in all leads.

The **QRS duration** represents the time required for depolarization of both ventricles. It is measured from the beginning of the QRS complex to the J point (the junction where the QRS complex ends and the ST segment begins). It normally measures from 0.04 to 0.12 second (up to three small blocks).

The **ST segment** is normally an isoelectric line and represents early ventricular repolarization. It occurs from the J point to the beginning of the T wave. Its length varies with changes in the heart rate, the administration of medications, and electrolyte disturbances.

The **T wave** follows the ST segment and represents ventricular repolarization. It is usually positive, rounded, and slightly asymmetric. T waves may become tall and peaked, inverted (negative), or flat as a result of myocardial ischemia, potassium or calcium imbalances, medications, or autonomic nervous system effects.

The *TP segment* begins at the end of the T wave and ends at the beginning of the P wave. It is the true isoelectric interval in the ECG.

The **U wave,** when present, follows the T wave and may result from slow repolarization of ventricular Purkinje fibers. It is of the same polarity as the T wave, although generally it is smaller. It is not normally seen in all leads and is more common in lead V_3. An abnormal U wave may suggest an electrolyte abnormality (particularly hypokalemia) or other disturbance. Correct identification is important so that it is not mistaken for a P wave. If in doubt, notify the health care provider and request that a potassium level be obtained.

The **QT interval** represents the total time required for ventricular depolarization and repolarization. The QT interval is measured from the beginning of the Q wave to the end of the T wave. This interval varies with the patient's age and gender and changes with the heart rate, lengthening with slower heart rates and shortening with faster rates. It may be prolonged by certain medications, electrolyte disturbances, or subarachnoid hemorrhage. A prolonged QT interval may lead to a unique type of ventricular tachycardia called *torsades de pointes.*

Artifact is interference seen on the monitor or rhythm strip, which may look like a wandering or fuzzy baseline. It can be caused by patient movement, loose or defective electrodes,

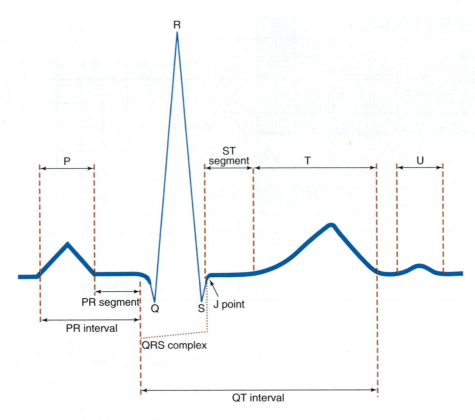

P wave:	Represents atrial depolarization.
PR segment:	Represents the time required for the impulse to travel through the AV node, where it is delayed, and through the bundle of His, bundle branches, and Purkinje fiber network, just before ventricular depolarization.
PR interval:	Represents the time required for atrial depolarization as well as impulse travel through the conduction system and Purkinje fiber network, inclusive of the P wave and PR segment. It is measured from the beginning of the P wave to the end of the PR segment.
QRS complex:	Represents ventricular depolarization and is measured from the beginning of the Q (or R) wave to the end of the S wave.
J point:	Represents the junction where the QRS complex ends and the ST segment begins.
ST segment:	Represents early ventricular repolarization.
T wave:	Represents ventricular repolarization.
U wave:	Represents late ventricular repolarization.
QT interval:	Represents the total time required for ventricular depolarization and repolarization and is measured from the beginning of the QRS complex to the end of the T wave.

FIG. 34-5 The components of a normal electrocardiogram.

improper grounding, or faulty ECG equipment, such as broken wires or cables. Some artifact can mimic lethal dysrhythmias like ventricular tachycardia (with tooth brushing) or ventricular fibrillation (with tapping on the electrode). *Assess the patient to differentiate artifact from actual lethal rhythms! Do not rely only on the ECG monitor.*

Determination of Heart Rate

The heart rate can be estimated by counting the number of QRS complexes in 6 seconds and multiplying that number by 10 to calculate the rate for a full minute. This is called the *6-second strip method* and is a quick method to determine the mean or average heart rate. This method is the least accurate; however, it is the method of choice for irregular rhythms.

For accuracy, the *big block method* is used if the QRS complexes are regular or evenly spaced. Count the number of big blocks between the same point in any two successive QRS complexes (usually R wave to R wave) and divide into 300. There are 300 big blocks in 1 minute. It is easiest to use a QRS that falls on a dark line. If little blocks are left over when counting big blocks, count each little block as 0.2, add this to the number of big blocks, and then divide that total into 300 (Fig. 34-6).

Count the number of large blocks in an interval and divide into 300 (the number of large blocks in 1 minute). For example, three large blocks equals a heart rate of 100 beats per minute (300 ÷ 3 = 100).

Another method (called the *memory method*) relies on memorizing this sequence: 300, 150, 100, 75, 60, 50, 43, 37, 33, 30. This is the big block method with the math already done. Find a QRS complex that falls on the dark line representing 0.2 second or a big block, and count backwards to the next QRS complex. Each dark line is a memorized number. This is the method most widely used in hospitals for calculating heart rates for regular rhythms.

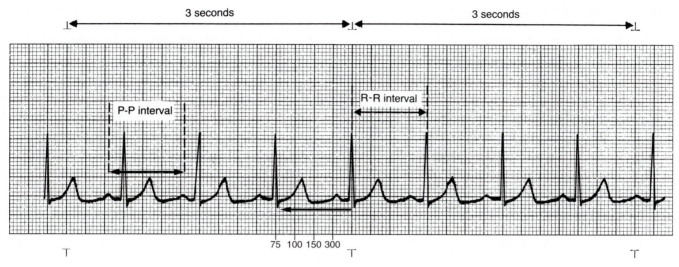

FIG. 34-6 In this example, the heart rate using the big block method is 300 ÷ 4 big blocks (between QRS complexes), or 75 beats per minute. The memory method is also demonstrated with a heart rate of 75 beats per minute.

Commercially prepared ECG rate rulers are based on these calculations and may be used for regular rhythms. Current monitoring systems will display a continuous heart rate and print the heart rate on the ECG strip. *Use caution and confirm that the rate is correct by assessing the patient's heart rate directly.* Many factors can incorrectly alter the rate displayed by the monitor.

Electrocardiographic Rhythm Analysis

Analysis of an ECG rhythm strip requires a systematic approach using an eight-step method facilitated by use of a measurement tool called an **ECG caliper** (Palmer, 2011):

1. ***Determine the heart rate.*** If the atrial and ventricular rhythms are regular, use any of the methods previously described to calculate the heart rate. If the rhythms are irregular, use the 6-second strip method for accuracy. Normal heart rates fall between 60 and 100 beats/min. A rate less than 60 beats/min is called **bradycardia**. A rate greater than 100 beats/min is called **tachycardia**.
2. ***Determine the heart rhythm.*** Assess for atrial and/or ventricular regularity. Heart rhythms can be either regular or irregular. Irregular rhythms can be regularly irregular, occasionally irregular, or irregularly irregular. Check the regularity of the atrial rhythm by assessing the PP intervals, placing one caliper point on a P wave and placing the other point on the precise spot on the next P wave. Then move the caliper from P wave to P wave along the entire strip ("walking out" the P waves) to determine the regularity of the rhythm. P waves of a different shape (ectopic waves), if present, create an irregularity and do not walk out with the other P waves. A slight irregularity in the PP intervals, varying no more than three small blocks, is considered essentially regular if the P waves are all of the same shape. This alteration is caused by changes in intrathoracic pressure during the respiratory cycle.

   Check the regularity of the ventricular rhythm by assessing the RR intervals, placing one caliper point on a portion of the QRS complex (usually the most prominent portion of the deflection) and the other point on the precise spot of the next QRS complex. Move the caliper from QRS complex to QRS complex along the entire strip (walking out the QRS complexes) to determine the regularity of the rhythm. QRS complexes of a different shape (ectopic QRS complexes), if present, create an irregularity and do not walk out with the other QRS complexes. A slight irregularity of no more than three small blocks between intervals is considered essentially regular if the QRS complexes are all of the same shape.

3. ***Analyze the P waves.*** Check that the P-wave shape is consistent throughout the strip, indicating that atrial depolarization is occurring from impulses originating from one focus, normally the SA node. Determine whether there is one P wave occurring before each QRS complex, establishing that a relationship exists between the P wave and the QRS complex. This relationship indicates that an impulse from one focus is responsible for both atrial and ventricular depolarization. The nurse may observe more than one P wave shape, more P waves than QRS complexes, absent P waves, or P waves coming after the QRS, each indicating that a dysrhythmia exists. Ask these five questions when analyzing P waves:
   - Are P waves present?
   - Are the P waves occurring regularly?
   - Is there one P wave for each QRS complex?
   - Are the P waves smooth, rounded, and upright in appearance, or are they inverted?
   - Do all the P waves look similar?
4. ***Measure the PR interval.*** Place one caliper point at the beginning of the P wave and the other point at the end of the PR segment. The PR interval normally measures between 0.12 and 0.20 second. The measurement should be constant throughout the strip. The PR interval cannot be determined if there are no P waves or if P waves occur after the QRS complex. Ask these three questions about the PR interval:
   - Are PR intervals greater than 0.20 second?
   - Are PR intervals less than 0.12 second?
   - Are PR intervals constant across the ECG strip?
5. ***Measure the QRS duration.*** Place one caliper point at the beginning of the QRS complex and the other at the

J point, where the QRS complex ends and the ST segment begins. The QRS duration normally measures between 0.04 and 0.10 second. The measurement should be constant throughout the entire strip. Check that the QRS complexes are consistent throughout the strip. When the QRS is narrow (0.10 second or less), this indicates that the impulse was not formed in the ventricles and is referred to as supraventricular or above the ventricles. When the QRS complex is wide (greater than 0.10 second), this indicates that the impulse is either of ventricular origin or of supraventricular origin with aberrant conduction, meaning deviating from the normal course or pattern. More than one QRS complex pattern or occasionally missing QRS complexes may be observed, indicating a dysrhythmia.

Ask these questions to evaluate QRS intervals:
- Are QRS intervals less than or greater than 0.12 second?
- Are the QRS complexes similar in appearance across the ECG paper?

6. ***Examine the ST segment.*** The normal ST segment begins at the isoelectric line. ST elevation or depression is significant if displacement is 1 mm (one small box) or more above or below the line and is seen in two or more leads. ST elevation may indicate problems such as myocardial infarction, pericarditis, and hyperkalemia. ST depression is associated with hypokalemia, myocardial infarction, or ventricular hypertrophy.

7. ***Assess the T wave.*** Note the shape and height of the T wave for peaking or inversion. Abnormal T waves may indicate problems such as myocardial infarction and ventricular hypertrophy.

8. ***Measure the QT interval.*** A normal QT interval should be equal to or less than one-half the distance of the R-to-R interval.

Using steps 1 through 8, you can interpret the cardiac rhythm and differentiate normal and abnormal cardiac rhythms (dysrhythmias).

OVERVIEW OF NORMAL CARDIAC RHYTHMS

Normal sinus rhythm (NSR) is the rhythm originating from the sinoatrial (SA) node (dominant pacemaker) that meets these ECG criteria (Fig. 34-7):

- *Rate:* Atrial and ventricular rates of 60 to 100 beats/min
- *Rhythm:* Atrial and ventricular rhythms regular
- *P waves:* Present, consistent configuration, one P wave before each QRS complex
- *PR interval:* 0.12 to 0.20 second and constant
- *QRS duration:* 0.04 to 0.10 second and constant

Sinus arrhythmia is a variant of NSR. It results from changes in intrathoracic pressure during breathing. In this context, the term *arrhythmia* does not mean an absence of rhythm, as the term suggests. Instead, the heart rate increases slightly during inspiration and decreases slightly during exhalation. This irregular rhythm is frequently observed in healthy adults.

Sinus arrhythmia has all the characteristics of NSR except for its irregularity. The PP and RR intervals vary, with the difference between the shortest and the longest intervals being greater than 0.12 second (three small blocks):

- *Rate:* Atrial and ventricular rates between 60 and 100 beats/min
- *Rhythm:* Atrial and ventricular rhythms irregular, with the shortest PP or RR interval varying at least 0.12 second from the longest PP or RR interval
- *P waves:* One P wave before each QRS complex; consistent configuration
- *PR interval:* Normal, constant
- *QRS duration:* Normal, constant

Sinus arrhythmias occasionally are due to nonrespiratory causes, such as digitalis or morphine. These drugs enhance vagal tone and cause decreased heart rate and irregularity unrelated to the respiratory cycle.

COMMON DYSRHYTHMIAS

Any disorder of the heartbeat is called a **dysrhythmia**. Historically, the term *arrhythmia* has been used in the literature. Although the terms are often used interchangeably, *dysrhythmia* is more accurate. Although many dysrhythmias have no clinical manifestations, many others have serious consequences if not treated.

❖ *PATHOPHYSIOLOGY*

Dysrhythmias are classified in several ways. As broad categories, they include premature complexes, bradydysrhythmias (bradycardias), and tachydysrhythmias (tachycardias). **Premature complexes** are early rhythm complexes. They occur when a

FIG. 34-7 Normal sinus rhythm. Both atrial and ventricular rhythms are essentially regular (a slight variation in rhythm is normal). Atrial and ventricular rates are both 87 beats per minute. There is one P wave before each QRS complex, and all the P waves are of a consistent morphology, or shape. The PR interval measures 0.18 second and is constant; the QRS complex measures 0.06 second and is constant.

cardiac cell or cell group, other than the sinoatrial (SA) node, becomes irritable and fires an impulse before the next sinus impulse is produced. The abnormal focus is called an *ectopic focus* and may be generated by atrial, junctional, or ventricular tissue. After the premature complex, there is a pause before the next normal complex, creating an irregularity in the rhythm. The patient with premature complexes may be unaware of them or may feel **palpitations** or a "skipping" of the heartbeat. If premature complexes, especially those that are ventricular, become more frequent, the patient may experience symptoms of decreased cardiac output.

Premature complexes may occur *repetitively in a rhythmic fashion:*

- **Bigeminy** exists when normal complexes and premature complexes occur alternately in a repetitive two-beat pattern, with a pause occurring after each premature complex so that complexes occur in pairs.
- **Trigeminy** is a repeated three-beat pattern, usually occurring as two sequential normal complexes followed by a premature complex and a pause, with the same pattern repeating itself in triplets.
- **Quadrigeminy** is a repeated four-beat pattern, usually occurring as three sequential normal complexes followed by a premature complex and a pause, with the same pattern repeating itself in a four-beat pattern.

Bradydysrhythmias occur when the heart rate is less than 60 beats per minute. These rhythms can also be significant because:

- Myocardial oxygen demand is reduced from the slow heart rate, which can be beneficial.
- Coronary perfusion time may be adequate because of a prolonged diastole, which is desirable.
- Coronary perfusion pressure may decrease if the heart rate is too slow to provide adequate cardiac output and blood pressure; this is a serious consequence.

Therefore the patient may tolerate the bradydysrhythmia well if the blood pressure is adequate. If the blood pressure is not adequate, symptomatic bradydysrhythmias may lead to myocardial ischemia or infarction, dysrhythmias, hypotension, and heart failure.

Tachydysrhythmias are heart rates greater than 100 beats per minute. They are a major concern in the adult patient with coronary artery disease (CAD). Coronary artery blood flow occurs mostly during diastole when the aortic valve is closed and is determined by diastolic time and blood pressure in the root of the aorta. Tachydysrhythmias are serious because they:

- Shorten the diastolic time and therefore the coronary perfusion time (the amount of time available for blood to flow through the coronary arteries to the myocardium).
- Initially increase cardiac output and blood pressure. However, a continued rise in heart rate decreases the ventricular filling time because of a shortened diastole, decreasing the stroke volume. Consequently, cardiac output and blood pressure will begin to decrease, reducing aortic pressure and therefore coronary PERFUSION pressure.
- Increase the work of the heart, increasing myocardial oxygen demand.

The patient with a tachydysrhythmia may have:

- Palpitations
- Chest discomfort (pressure or pain from myocardial ischemia or infarction)

CHART 34-1 Key Features

Sustained Tachydysrhythmias and Bradydysrhythmias

- Chest discomfort, pressure, or pain, which may radiate to the jaw, the back, or the arm
- Restlessness, anxiety, nervousness, confusion
- Dizziness, syncope
- Palpitations (in tachydysrhythmias)
- Change in pulse strength, rate, and rhythm
- Pulse deficit
- Shortness of breath, dyspnea
- Tachypnea
- Pulmonary crackles
- Orthopnea
- S_3 or S_4 heart sounds
- Jugular venous distention
- Weakness, fatigue
- Pale, cool, skin; diaphoresis
- Nausea, vomiting
- Decreased urine output
- Delayed capillary refill
- Hypotension

- Restlessness and anxiety
- Pale, cool skin
- Syncope ("blackout") from hypotension

Tachydysrhythmias may also lead to heart failure. Presenting symptoms of heart failure may include dyspnea, lung crackles, distended neck veins, fatigue, and weakness (see Chapter 35). Chart 34-1 summarizes key features of sustained bradydysrhythmias and tachydysrhythmias.

Etiology

Dysrhythmias occur for many reasons, including myocardial infarction (MI), electrolyte imbalances (especially potassium and magnesium), hypoxia, drug toxicity, and hypovolemia (decreased blood volume). People who use cocaine and illicit inhalants are particularly at risk for potentially fatal dysrhythmias. Stress, fear, anxiety, and caffeine can cause an increased heart rate (tachycardia or premature ventricular contractions). Nicotine and alcohol excess can lead to abnormal heart rates such as atrial fibrillation. Specific etiologies are described for each common dysrhythmia discussed in this chapter.

❖ PATIENT-CENTERED COLLABORATIVE CARE

Dysrhythmias may also be classified by their site of origin in the heart. These include common sinus, atrial, and ventricular dysrhythmias. Although there are many specific dysrhythmias that can occur, general assessment and interventions for patient care may be similar (Chart 34-2). Assess the patient's apical and radial pulses for a full minute for any irregularity, which may occur with premature beats or atrial fibrillation. If the apical pulse differs from the radial pulse rate, a **pulse deficit** exists and indicates that the heart is not pumping adequately to achieve optimal PERFUSION to the body.

Dysrhythmias are often managed with antidysrhythmic drug therapy. Specific drugs and other treatments are discussed for common dysrhythmias starting on p. 667.

Drug Classifications

When dysrhythmias are sustained and/or life threatening, drug therapy from one or more classes of antidysrhythmic agents is

Care of the Patient with Dysrhythmias

- Assess vital signs at least every 4 hours and as needed.
- Monitor patient for cardiac dysrhythmias.
- Evaluate and document the patient's response to dysrhythmias.
- Encourage the patient to notify the nurse when chest pain occurs.
- Assess chest pain (e.g., location, intensity, duration, radiation, and precipitating and alleviating factors).
- Assess peripheral circulation (e.g., palpate for presence of peripheral pulses, edema, capillary refill, color, and temperature of extremity).
- Provide antidysrhythmic therapy according to unit policy (e.g., antidysrhythmic medication, cardioversion, or defibrillation), as appropriate.
- Monitor and document patient's response to antidysrhythmic medications or interventions.
- Monitor appropriate laboratory values (e.g., cardiac enzymes, electrolyte levels).
- Monitor the patient's activity tolerance and schedule exercise/rest periods to avoid fatigue.
- Observe for respiratory difficulty (e.g., shortness of breath, rapid breathing, labored respirations).
- Promote stress reduction.
- Offer spiritual support to the patient and/or family (e.g., contact clergy), as appropriate.

often used (Chart 34-3). The Vaughn-Williams classification is commonly used to categorize drugs according to their effects on the action potential of cardiac cells (classes I though IV). Other drugs also have antidysrhythmic effects but do not fit the Vaughn-Williams classification.

Class I antidysrhythmics are membrane-stabilizing agents used to decrease automaticity. The three subclassifications in this group include type IA drugs, which moderately slow conduction and prolong repolarization, prolonging the QT interval. These drugs are used to treat or to prevent supraventricular and ventricular premature beats and tachydysrhythmias, but they are not as commonly used as other drugs. An example is procainamide hydrochloride (Pronestyl). Type IB drugs shorten repolarization. These drugs are used to treat or prevent ventricular premature beats, ventricular tachycardia (VT), and ventricular fibrillation (VF). Examples include lidocaine and mexiletine hydrochloride (Mexitil). Type IC drugs markedly slow conduction and widen the QRS complex. These agents are used primarily to treat or to prevent recurrent, life-threatening ventricular premature beats, VT, and VF. Examples include flecainide acetate (Tambocor) and propafenone hydrochloride (Rythmol).

Class II antidysrhythmics control dysrhythmias associated with excessive beta-adrenergic stimulation by competing for

Common Dysrhythmias

DRUG	USUAL DOSAGE	NURSING INTERVENTIONS	RATIONALES
Class I Drugs			
Type IA			
Disopyramide phosphate (Norpace)	100-200 mg orally every 6 hr	Monitor BP.	Hypotension is a common side effect.
Used for AF, WPW syndrome, PSVT, PVCs, VT		Watch for shortness of breath and weight gain.	Disopyramide can cause heart failure in a patient with CAD.
		Monitor for widening QRS complex, prolonged QT or PR interval, or heart block.	Toxic side effects necessitate stopping disopyramide administration.
Type IB			
Lidocaine (Xylocaine) Used for PVCs, VT, VF	1-1.5 mg/kg IV bolus, then 0.5-0.75 mg/kg IV boluses every 5-10 min to a loading dose of 3 mg/kg, followed by 2-4 mg/min infusion For VF or pulseless VT: 1-1.5 mg/kg IV bolus every 3-5 min to a loading dose of 3 mg/kg, followed by 1-4 mg/min infusion	Watch for confusion, paresthesias, slurring of speech, drowsiness, or seizure activity.	CNS adverse effects predominate; they may require a decrease in dosage or discontinuation of the infusion.
Mexiletine hydrochloride (Mexitil)	200-300 mg orally every 8 hr with food	Monitor BP and heart rate.	Hypotension and bradycardia may occur.
Used for PVCs, VT, VF	125-250 mg IV bolus over 5-10 min 0.5-1.5 mg/min infusion	Assess for tremors, blurred vision, dizziness, ataxia, or confusion.	CNS adverse reactions predominate.
Tocainide hydrochloride (Tonocard)	400 mg orally every 8 hr initially Increase to 800 mg orally every 8 hr if needed Maximum of 2.4 g daily Take with food	Watch for tremors.	Tremors indicate that the maximum dose is being approached.
Used for PVCs, VT, VF		Monitor heart rate and BP.	Bradycardia and hypotension may occur.
		Teach patient to report shortness of breath, wheezing, chest pain, or cough, as well as dyspnea and distended neck veins or swelling of the extremities.	Pulmonary fibrosis is a serious side effect, which necessitates discontinuation of the drug; the drug may also cause CHF.

CHART 34-3   Common Examples of Drug Therapy—cont'd

Common Dysrhythmias

DRUG	USUAL DOSAGE	NURSING INTERVENTIONS	RATIONALES
Type IC			
Flecainide acetate (Tambocor) Used for AF, PSVT, life-threatening ventricular dysrhythmias	100 mg orally twice daily Maximum dose of 400 mg daily	Monitor for an increase in frequency and severity of dysrhythmias. Monitor heart rate and BP. Monitor for CHF, dizziness, visual disturbances, paresthesias, and tremors.	Flecainide can induce dysrhythmias. Bradycardia and hypotension may occur. Side effects may require a decrease in dosage or discontinuation of the drug.
Propafenone hydrochloride (Rythmol) Used for PAF, WPW syndrome, life-threatening ventricular dysrhythmias	150-300 mg orally every 8 hr	Monitor for an increase in dysrhythmias. Monitor heart rate and BP. Monitor for CNS effects, dizziness, anxiety, ataxia, insomnia, confusion, and seizures, as well as CHF and GI distress.	Propafenone can induce dysrhythmias. Bradycardia and hypotension may occur. Side effects may require a decrease in dosage or discontinuation of the drug.
Class II Drugs			
Propranolol hydrochloride (Inderal, Apo-Propranolol ✦) Used for AF, atrial flutter, PSVT, PVCs	10-80 mg orally four times daily before meals 0.1 mg/kg slow IV bolus divided into 3 equal doses given at intervals of 2-3 min at rate of 1 mg/min	Monitor heart rate and BP. Assess for shortness of breath or wheezing. Assess for insomnia, fatigue, and dizziness.	Bradycardia and decreased BP are expected effects. Beta$_2$-blocking effects on the lungs can cause bronchospasm. Side effects may require decrease in dosage or discontinuation of the drug.
Acebutolol hydrochloride (Sectral) Used for AF, atrial flutter, PSVT, PVCs	600-1200 mg orally daily	Monitor heart rate and BP. Assess for shortness of breath or wheezing. Assess for insomnia, fatigue, and dizziness.	Bradycardia and decreased BP are expected effects. Beta$_2$-blocking effects on the lungs can cause bronchospasm. Side effects may require a decrease in dosage or discontinuation of the drug.
Esmolol hydrochloride (Brevibloc) Used for AF, atrial flutter, PSVT, PVCs	Initially, 500 mcg/kg/min over 1 min, then 50 mcg/kg/min for 4 min IV Titrate up if necessary	Monitor heart rate and BP. Assess for shortness of breath or wheezing. Assess for insomnia, fatigue, and seizures.	Bradycardia and decreased BP are expected effects. Beta$_2$-blocking effects on the lungs can cause bronchospasm. Side effects may require a decrease in dosage or discontinuation of the drug.
Sotalol hydrochloride (Betapace) Used for AF, PAF, PSVT, life-threatening ventricular dysrhythmias	Initial dose of 80 mg orally twice daily Dosage may be increased every 2-3 days, if necessary, to 240-320 mg daily in 2-3 divided doses	Assess ECG rhythm for torsades de pointes and other serious new ventricular dysrhythmias. Assess for fatigue, bradycardia, dyspnea, CHF, chest pain, hypotension, dizziness, hypoglycemia, nausea, and vomiting. Sotalol should not be administered to patients with hypokalemia or hypomagnesemia before correction of these imbalances. Sotalol is contraindicated in patients with bronchial asthma, sinus bradycardia, or second- and third-degree AV block (unless a functioning pacemaker is present), prolonged QT syndrome, cardiogenic shock, or CHF.	Sotalol may have proarrhythmic effects. Adverse reactions may warrant drug discontinuation. Hypokalemia or hypomagnesemia may prolong the QT interval and cause torsades de pointes. Sotalol has beta-blocking (class II) effects and class III effects.

Continued

CHART 34-3 **Common Examples of Drug Therapy—cont'd**

Common Dysrhythmias

DRUG	USUAL DOSAGE	NURSING INTERVENTIONS	RATIONALES
Class III Drugs			
Amiodarone hydrochloride (Cordarone) Used for AF, PAF, PSVT, life-threatening ventricular dysrhythmias	800-1600 mg orally daily in divided doses for 1-3 wk, then 600-800 mg daily for 1 mo, then 200-600 mg daily (average of 400 mg daily) Rapid loading dose: 150 mg IV over first 10 min (15 mg/min); slow loading dose: 360 mg IV over next 6 hr (1 mg/min); maintenance infusion: 540 mg IV over next 18 hr (0.5 mg/min), then 720 mg/24 hr (0.5 mg/min) For pulseless VT/Vfib: 300 mg IV/IO push; may repeat 150 mg IV/IO if necessary	Use volumetric infusion pump and polyvinyl chloride tubing with in-line filter, and infuse via central line. Rapid-loading IV dose must not be administered faster than 10 min. Must stay with patient and monitor heart rate and BP. Continually monitor ECG rhythm during IV infusion; measure QT and QTc. Assess the patient's knowledge of the treatment regimen and side effects. Monitor heart rate, BP, and cardiac rhythm when initiating therapy. Teach patients to report any muscle weakness, tremors, or difficulty with ambulation. Teach patients to report shortness of breath, cough, pleuritic pain, or fever. Teach patients to report any visual disturbances and to wear sunglasses outdoors in the daytime if they have photophobia. Teach patients to use barrier sunscreens. Teach patients to report any signs of thyroid problems or hepatotoxicity.	Drug is irritating to peripheral vasculature; drug is more stable in glass bottle. Hypotension may occur. It should be treated by slowing the infusion or using other standard therapy. Cordarone should not be discontinued unless necessary. Bradycardia and AV block may occur and are treated by slowing the infusion rate and providing pacemaker therapy, if necessary. May cause a worsening of ventricular dysrhythmias. Drug has major side effects, which make noncompliance a problem; patients may take the drug for 1½-3 mo before full clinical effects are apparent. Bradycardia, hypotension, and worsening dysrhythmia can occur. Muscle-related side effects usually develop during the first week of treatment. Pulmonary side effects may indicate drug-induced pulmonary toxicity. Corneal pigmentation occurs in most patients but generally does not interfere with vision; if it does, the dosage is decreased. Photosensitivity reactions may occur. Thyroid problems or hepatotoxicity may occur, necessitating a decrease in dosage or discontinuation of the drug.
Dronedarone (Multaq) Used for AF, atrial flutter	400 mg twice daily with meals	Monitor heart rate, BP, and cardiac rhythm when initiating therapy. Monitor BUN, creatinine, and liver function panel. Teach patients to take with a meal. Do not take with grapefruit juice. Teach patients to notify the doctor if signs of worsening heart failure such as weight gain, dependent edema, or increasing shortness of breath. Teach patients that if a dose is missed, take at next regularly scheduled dose. Do not double dose. Advise patients to report all medications to doctor (prescription, OTC, and herbal products, especially St. John's wort).	Bradycardia and worsening dysrhythmia can occur. May cause worsening renal function. Drug is contraindicated for patients with severe hepatic impairment. Better absorbed with food. Grapefruit juice alters drug effectiveness. Drug is contraindicated for patients with heart failure. May have serious drug interaction and cause potentially fatal dysrhythmias.

Common Dysrhythmias

DRUG	USUAL DOSAGE	NURSING INTERVENTIONS	RATIONALES
Ibutilide fumarate (Corvert) Used for AF, atrial flutter	1 mg IV over 10 min for patients >60 kg; 0.01 mg/kg over 10 min for patients <60 kg May repeat dose 10 min after completion of first infusion if necessary	Stop infusion as soon as dysrhythmia is terminated, or in event of sustained or nonsustained VT, or marked prolongation of QT or QTc. Observe patients with continuous ECG monitoring and measure QT or QTc for at least 4 hr after infusion or until QTc has returned to baseline. Patients with atrial fibrillation of >2-3 days' duration must be adequately anticoagulated for at least 2 wk. Hypokalemia and hypomagnesemia must be corrected before Corvert infusion.	Drug may cause potentially fatal dysrhythmias. Acute ventricular dysrhythmias must be promptly identified and treated. Patient may develop heart blocks. Atrial fibrillation is associated with formation of thrombi in atrial chambers. This is important to reduce potential for proarrhythmic effects.
Dofetilide (Tikosyn) Used for AF, atrial flutter	125-500 mcg orally twice daily	Teach patients to change positions slowly. Inform patients that dosages will be adjusted, depending on their creatinine clearance level. Monitor patients on telemetry for several days; observe for and report bradycardia and hypotension.	Orthostatic hypotension is a common side effect of the drug. The patient must have adequate creatinine clearance to prevent drug toxicity. Bradycardia and hypotension are common side effects.
Class IV Drugs Verapamil hydrochloride (Calan, Isoptin ✦) Used for AF, atrial flutter, PSVT	2.5-5 mg IV over 1-2 min for narrow-complex SVT or PSVT; after 15-30 min may give 5-10 mg IV over 1-2 min, if necessary, and repeat to a maximum of 20 mg 80-120 mg orally every 6-8 hr	Monitor heart rate and BP. Teach patients to remain recumbent for at least 1 hr after IV administration. Teach patients to change positions slowly when receiving oral therapy. Teach patients to report dyspnea, orthopnea, distended neck veins, or swelling of the extremities.	Bradycardia and hypotension are common side effects. Hypotension may occur; may be reversed with calcium chloride (CaCl₂), 0.5-1 g slow IV. Dizziness and orthostatic hypotension often occur until tolerance develops. Heart failure may occur, necessitating a decrease in dosage or discontinuation of the drug.
Diltiazem hydrochloride (Cardizem) Used for AF, atrial flutter, PSVT	0.25 mg/kg IV over 2 min After 15 min, give 0.35 mg/kg IV over 2 min 5-15 mg/hr IV infusion	Monitor heart rate and BP. Teach patients to remain recumbent for at least 1 hr after IV administration. Teach patients to report dyspnea, orthopnea, distended neck veins, or swelling of the extremities.	Bradycardia and hypotension are common side effects. Hypotension may occur. Heart failure may occur, necessitating a decrease in dosage or discontinuation of the drug.
Other Drugs Digoxin (Lanoxin, Novo-Digoxin ✦) Used for CHF, AF, atrial flutter, PSVT	Rapid digitalization: 0.5-1 mg orally or IV initially; 0.125-0.5 mg orally every 6 hr or IV until a total of 1-1.5 mg is reached Maintenance: 0.125-0.25 mg orally or IV daily or every other day (may be less for older adults)	Assess apical heart rate for 1 min before each dose. Assess for sudden increase in heart rate and change of rhythm from regular to irregular, or irregular to regular. Teach patients to report anorexia, nausea, vomiting, diarrhea, paresthesias, confusion, or visual disturbances. Monitor serum potassium levels. Monitor serum creatinine levels.	Decreased heart rate is an expected response, but bradycardia may indicate toxicity. Changes in heart rate or rhythm may indicate toxicity. Side effect can indicate toxicity. Hypokalemia increases the risk for toxicity and ventricular dysrhythmias. Impaired renal function can cause toxicity; the dosage is altered if this occurs.

Continued

CHART 34-3 **Common Examples of Drug Therapy—cont'd**

Common Dysrhythmias

DRUG	USUAL DOSAGE	NURSING INTERVENTIONS	RATIONALES
Atropine sulfate Used for bradycardia	0.5 mg IV bolus may be repeated every 3-5 min, if necessary, to a maximum of 0.04 mg/kg (total 3 mg)	Monitor heart rate and rhythm after administration. Assess for chest pain after administration. Assess for urinary retention and dry mouth after administration. Avoid using in patients with acute angle-closure glaucoma.	Increased heart rate is expected. Increased heart rate may cause ischemia in patients with CAD. Atropine is an anticholinergic agent. Atropine increases intraocular pressure.
Adenosine (Adenocard) Used for PSVT, WPW syndrome	6 mg rapid IV over 1-3 sec followed by 20-mL saline flush; repeat in 1-2 min at 12 mg IV over 1-3 sec with 20-mL flush	Monitor heart rate and rhythm after administration. Assess patients for facial flushing, shortness of breath, dyspnea, and chest pain. Assess patients for recurrence of PSVT or ventricular ectopy.	A short period of asystole is common after administration; bradycardia and hypotension may occur. These side effects commonly occur. Recurrence of PSVT is common; PVCs may occur.
Magnesium sulfate Used for torsades de pointes	1-2 g diluted in 100 mL of D₅W administered IV over 1-2 min for VF or VT 1-2 g in 50-100 mL of D₅W for 5-60 min for loading dose; 0.5-1 g/hr over 24 hr for supplementation	Assess ECG rhythm for conversion to sinus rhythm. Assess patients for facial flushing, hypotension, and respiratory and CNS depression.	Hypomagnesemia may precipitate refractory VF. Magnesium sulfate causes vasodilation and respiratory and CNS depression.

AF, Atrial fibrillation; *AV,* atrioventricular; *BP,* blood pressure; *BUN,* blood urea nitrogen; *CAD,* coronary artery disease; *CHF,* congestive heart failure; *CNS,* central nervous system; *D₅W,* 5% dextrose in water; *ECG,* electrocardiogram; *EMD,* electromechanical dissociation; *IO,* intraosseous; *OTC,* over-the-counter; *PAF,* paroxysmal atrial fibrillation/flutter; *PSVT,* paroxysmal supraventricular tachycardia; *PVC,* premature ventricular complex; *SVT,* supraventricular tachycardia; *V fib,* ventricular fibrillation; *VF,* ventricular fibrillation; *VT,* ventricular tachycardia; *WPW syndrome,* Wolff-Parkinson-White syndrome.

receptor sites and thereby decreasing heart rate and conduction velocity. Beta-adrenergic blocking agents, such as propranolol (Inderal) and esmolol hydrochloride (Brevibloc), are class II drugs. They are used to treat or to prevent supraventricular and ventricular premature beats and tachydysrhythmias. Sotalol hydrochloride (Betapace, Sotacor ✦) is an antidysrhythmic agent with both non-cardioselective beta-adrenergic blocking effects (class II) and action potential duration prolongation properties (class III). It is an oral agent that may be used for the treatment of documented ventricular dysrhythmias, such as VT, that are life threatening.

Class III antidysrhythmics lengthen the absolute refractory period and prolong repolarization and the action potential duration of ischemic cells. Class III drugs include amiodarone (Cordarone) and ibutilide (Corvert) and are used to treat or prevent ventricular premature beats, VT, and VF.

Class IV antidysrhythmics slow the flow of calcium into the cell during depolarization, thereby depressing the automaticity of the sinoatrial (SA) and atrioventricular (AV) nodes, decreasing the heart rate, and prolonging the AV nodal refractory period and conduction. Calcium channel blockers, such as verapamil hydrochloride (Calan, Isoptin ✦) and diltiazem hydrochloride (Cardizem), are class IV drugs. They are used to treat supraventricular tachycardia (SVT) and atrial fibrillation (AF) to slow the ventricular response.

Other drugs, such as digoxin, atropine, adenosine, and magnesium sulfate, may be used to treat dysrhythmias. Digoxin (Lanoxin, Novo-Digoxin ✦) increases vagal tone, slowing AV nodal conduction. It is useful in treating chronic AF by controlling the rate of ventricular response. However, digoxin does not convert AF to sinus rhythm. Atropine is a parasympatholytic or vagolytic agent used to treat vagally induced symptomatic

bradydysrhythmias. Adenosine is an endogenous nucleoside that slows AV nodal conduction to interrupt re-entry pathways. Magnesium sulfate is an electrolyte administered to treat refractory VT or VF because these patients may be hypomagnesemic, with increased ventricular irritability. The drug is also used for a life-threatening VT called **torsades de pointes** that can result from certain antidysrhythmics, such as amiodarone.

Sinus Dysrhythmias

The sinoatrial (SA) node in the right atrium is the pacemaker in all sinus dysrhythmias. Innervation from sympathetic and parasympathetic nerves is normally in balance to ensure a normal sinus rhythm (NSR). An imbalance increases or decreases the rate of SA node discharge either as a normal response to activity or physiologic changes or as a pathologic response to disease. Sinus tachycardia and sinus bradycardia are the two most common types of sinus dysrhythmias.

Sinus Tachycardia. Sympathetic nervous system stimulation or vagal (parasympathetic) inhibition results in an increased rate of SA node discharge, which increases the heart rate. When the rate of SA node discharge is more than 100 beats per minute, the rhythm is called **sinus tachycardia** (Fig. 34-8, *A*). From age 10 years to adulthood, the heart rate normally does not exceed 100 beats per minute except in response to activity and then usually does not exceed 160 beats per minute. Rarely does the heart rate reach 180 beats per minute.

Sinus tachycardia initially increases cardiac output and blood pressure. However, continued increases in heart rate decrease coronary PERFUSION time, diastolic filling time, and coronary perfusion pressure while increasing myocardial oxygen demand.

Increased sympathetic stimulation is a normal response to physical activity but may also be caused by anxiety, pain, stress,

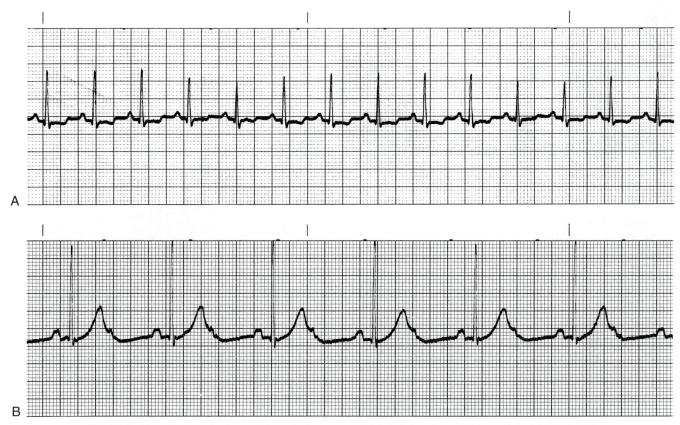

FIG. 34-8 Sinus rhythms. **A,** Sinus tachycardia (heart rate, 115 beats per minute; PR interval, 0.12 second; QRS complex, 0.08 second). **B,** Sinus bradycardia (heart rate, 52 beats per minute; PR interval, 0.18 second; QRS complex, 0.08 second).

fever, anemia, hypoxemia, and hyperthyroidism. Drugs such as epinephrine, atropine, caffeine, alcohol, nicotine, cocaine, aminophylline, and thyroid medications may also increase the heart rate. In some cases, sinus tachycardia is a compensatory response to decreased cardiac output or blood pressure, as occurs in dehydration, hypovolemic shock, myocardial infarction (MI), infection, and heart failure. Assess patients for clinical manifestations of hypovolemia and dehydration, including increased pulse rate, decreased urinary output, decreased blood pressure, and dry skin and mucous membranes.

The patient may be asymptomatic except for an increased pulse rate. However, if the rhythm is not well tolerated, he or she may have symptoms.

The desired outcome is to decrease the heart rate to normal levels by treating the underlying cause. Remind the patient to remain on bedrest if the tachycardia is causing hypotension or

weakness. Teach the patient to avoid substances that increase cardiac rate, including caffeine, alcohol, and nicotine. Help patients develop stress management strategies, or refer the patient to a mental health professional.

> ### ? NCLEX EXAMINATION CHALLENGE
>
> ### *Physiological Integrity*
>
> A client who had open abdominal surgery 4 hours ago reports feeling weak and dizzy. The client's current blood pressure has decreased to 98/50, and pulse rate is 108. What is the nurse's best action at this time?
> A. Document the vital signs, and continue to monitor the client.
> B. Remind the client to stay in bed if feeling weak and dizzy.
> C. Call the health care provider immediately.
> D. Increase the client's IV rate to restore fluid volume.

Sinus Bradycardia. Excessive vagal (parasympathetic) stimulation to the heart causes a decreased rate of sinus node discharge. It may result from carotid sinus massage, vomiting, suctioning, Valsalva maneuvers (e.g., bearing down for a bowel movement or gagging), ocular pressure, or pain. Increased parasympathetic stimuli may also result from hypoxia, inferior wall MI, and the administration of drugs such as beta-adrenergic blocking agents, calcium channel blockers, and digitalis. Bradycardia may also be caused by Lyme disease and hypothyroidism.

The stimuli slow the heart rate and decrease the speed of conduction through the heart. When the sinus node discharge rate is less than 60 beats per minute, the rhythm is called **sinus bradycardia** (Fig. 34-8, *B*). Sinus bradycardia increases coronary PERFUSION time, but it may decrease coronary perfusion pressure. However, myocardial oxygen demand is *decreased*. Well-conditioned athletes who are bradycardic have a hypereffective heart in which the strong heart muscle provides an adequate stroke volume and a low heart rate to achieve a normal cardiac output.

Assessment. The patient with sinus bradycardia may be asymptomatic except for the decreased pulse rate. In many cases, the cause of sinus bradycardia is unknown. Assess the medication administration record (MAR) to determine if the patient is receiving medications that slow the conduction through the SA or AV node. Assess the patient for:

- Syncope ("blackouts" or fainting)
- Dizziness and weakness
- Confusion
- Hypotension
- Diaphoresis (excessive sweating)
- Shortness of breath
- Chest pain

Interventions. If the patient has any of these symptoms and the underlying cause cannot be determined, the treatment is to administer drug therapy with atropine 0.5 mg IV, increase intravascular volume via IV fluids, and apply oxygen. Drugs suspected of causing the bradycardia are discontinued. If the heart rate does not increase sufficiently, prepare for transcutaneous or transvenous pacing to increase the heart rate. If treatment of the underlying cause does not restore normal sinus rhythm, the patient will require permanent pacemaker implantation.

Temporary Pacing. Temporary pacing is a nonsurgical intervention that provides a timed electrical stimulus to the heart when either the impulse initiation or the conduction system of the heart is defective. The electrical stimulus then spreads throughout the heart to depolarize the cells, which should be followed by contraction and cardiac output. Electrical stimuli may be delivered to the right atrium or right ventricle (single-chamber pacemakers) or to both (dual-chamber pacemakers).

Temporary pacing is used for patients with symptomatic, atropine-refractory bradydysrhythmias or for patients with asystole (discussed on p. 671 in this chapter). The two basic types of *temporary* pacing are transcutaneous and transvenous pacing. *Transcutaneous pacing* is accomplished through the application of two large external electrodes. The electrodes are attached to an external pulse generator. The generator emits electrical pulses, which are transmitted through the electrodes and then transcutaneously to stimulate ventricular depolarization when the patient's heart rate is slower than the rate set on the pacemaker. A transvenous system consists of an external battery-operated pulse generator and pacing electrodes, or lead wires. These wires attach to the generator on one end and are threaded to the right atrium via the subclavian or femoral vein (Fig. 34-9). Electrical pulses, or stimuli, are emitted from the negative terminal of the generator, flow through a lead wire, and stimulate the cardiac cells to depolarize. The current seeks ground by returning through the other lead wire to the positive terminal of the generator, thus completing a circuit. The intensity of electrical current is set by selecting the appropriate current output, measured in milliamperes.

The two major modes of pacing are synchronous (demand) pacing and asynchronous (fixed-rate) pacing. Temporary pacing is *usually* done in the synchronous (demand) pacing mode. The

FIG. 34-9 Placement of pacemaker in chest and heart leads.

pacemaker's sensitivity is set to sense the patient's own beats. When the patient's heart rate is above the rate set on the pulse generator, the pacemaker does not fire (inhibits itself). When the patient's heart rate is less than the generator setting, the pacemaker provides electrical impulses (paces).

Transcutaneous pacing is used as an *emergency* measure to provide demand ventricular pacing in a profoundly bradycardic or asystolic patient until invasive pacing can be used or the patient's heart rate returns to normal. It may be used prophylactically when performing procedures or transporting patients at risk for bradydysrhythmias. However, it is used only as a temporary measure to maintain heart rate and PERFUSION until a more permanent method of pacing is used.

When a pacing stimulus is delivered to the heart, a spike (or pacemaker artifact) is seen on the monitor or ECG strip. The spike should be followed by evidence of depolarization (i.e., a P wave, indicating atrial depolarization, or a QRS complex, indicating ventricular depolarization). This pattern is referred to as *capture*, indicating that the pacemaker has successfully depolarized, or captured, the chamber.

Permanent Pacemaker. Pacemaker insertion is performed to treat conduction disorders that are not temporary, including complete heart block. These pacemakers are usually powered by a lithium battery and have an average life span of 10 years. After the battery power is depleted, the generator must be replaced by a procedure done with the patient under local anesthesia. Some pacemakers are nuclear-powered and have a life span of 20 years or longer. Other pacemakers can be recharged externally. Combination pacemaker/defibrillator devices are also available.

A biventricular pacemaker may be utilized to coordinate contractions between the right and left ventricles. In addition to pacing used in the right side of the heart, an additional lead is placed in the left lateral wall of the left ventricle through the coronary sinus. This procedure allows synchronized depolarization of the ventricles and is used in patients with moderate to severe heart failure to improve functional ability.

The electrophysiologist implants the pulse generator in a surgically made subcutaneous pocket at the shoulder in the

FIG. 34-10 Permanent pacemaker, programmer, and rhythm strip.

right or left subclavicular area, which may create a visible bulge. The leads are introduced transvenously via the cephalic or the subclavian vein to the endocardium on the right side of the heart. After the procedure, monitor the ECG rhythm to check that the pacemaker is working correctly. Assess the implantation site for bleeding, swelling, redness, tenderness, and infection. The dressing over the site should remain clean and dry. The patient should be afebrile and have stable vital signs. The physician prescribes initial activity restrictions, which are then gradually changed. Complications of permanent pacemakers are similar to those of temporary invasive pacing.

Pacemaker checks are done on an ambulatory care basis at regular intervals. Reprogramming may be needed if pacemaker problems develop. The pulse generator is interrogated using an electronic device to determine the pacemaker settings and battery life (Fig. 34-10). In addition, most pacemaker manufacturers offer wireless home transmitter devices. Data are then sent via landline telephone to a database, which is then accessed by the device clinic or health care provider. Stress the need to keep follow-up appointments for more detailed pacemaker checks and reprogramming, if necessary, as well as for assessment.

Atrial Dysrhythmias

In patients with atrial dysrhythmias, the focus of impulse generation shifts away from the sinus node to the atrial tissues. The shift changes the axis (direction) of atrial depolarization, resulting in a P-wave shape that differs from normal P waves. The most common atrial dysrhythmias are:

- Premature atrial complexes
- Supraventricular tachycardia
- Atrial fibrillation

Premature Atrial Complexes. A **premature atrial complex (contraction) (PAC)** occurs when atrial tissue becomes irritable. This ectopic focus fires an impulse before the next sinus impulse is due. The premature P wave may not always be clearly visible because it can be hidden in the preceding T wave. Examine the T wave closely for any change in shape, and compare with other T waves. A PAC is usually followed by a pause.

The causes of atrial irritability include:

- Stress
- Fatigue
- Anxiety
- Inflammation
- Infection
- Caffeine, nicotine, or alcohol
- Drugs such as epinephrine, sympathomimetics, amphetamines, digitalis, or anesthetic agents

PACs may also result from myocardial ischemia, hypermetabolic states, electrolyte imbalance, or atrial stretch. Atrial stretch can result from congestive heart failure, valvular disease, and pulmonary hypertension with cor pulmonale.

The patient usually has no symptoms except for possible heart palpitations. No intervention is needed except to treat causes such as heart failure. If PACs occur frequently, they may lead to more serious atrial tachydysrhythmias and therefore may need treatment. Administration of prescribed antidysrhythmic drugs may be necessary (see Chart 34-3). Teach the patient measures to manage stress and substances to avoid, such as caffeine and alcohol, that are known to increase atrial irritability.

Supraventricular Tachycardia. **Supraventricular tachycardia (SVT)** involves the rapid stimulation of atrial tissue at a rate of 100 to 280 beats per minute in adults. During SVT, P waves may not be visible, especially if there is a 1:1 conduction with rapid rates, because the P waves are embedded in the preceding T wave. *SVT may occur in healthy young people, especially women.*

SVT is usually due to a re-entry mechanism in which one impulse circulates repeatedly throughout the atrial pathway, re-stimulating the atrial tissue at a rapid rate. The term **paroxysmal supraventricular tachycardia (PSVT)** is used when the rhythm is intermittent. It is initiated suddenly by a premature complex such as a PAC and terminated suddenly with or without intervention.

Assessment. The clinical manifestations depend on the duration of the SVT and the rate of the ventricular response. In patients with a *sustained* rapid ventricular response, assess for palpitations, chest pain, weakness, fatigue, shortness of breath, nervousness, anxiety, hypotension, and syncope. Cardiovascular deterioration may occur if the rate does not sustain adequate blood pressure. In that case, SVT can result in angina, heart failure, and cardiogenic shock. With a *nonsustained* or slower ventricular response, the patient may be asymptomatic except for occasional palpitations.

Interventions. If SVT occurs in a healthy person and stops on its own, no intervention may be needed other than eliminating identified causes. If it continues, the patient should be studied in the electrophysiology study (EPS) laboratory. The preferred treatment for recurrent SVT is radiofrequency catheter ablation, described later in this chapter on p. 668. In sustained SVT with a rapid ventricular response, the desired outcomes of treatment are to decrease the ventricular response, convert the dysrhythmia to a sinus rhythm, and treat the cause.

Vagal maneuvers induce vagal stimulation of the cardiac conduction system, specifically the SA and AV nodes. Although not as common today, vagal maneuvers may be attempted to treat supraventricular tachydysrhythmias and include carotid sinus massage and Valsalva maneuvers. The results of these interventions, however, are often temporary and may cause "rebound" tachycardia or severe bradycardia. Further therapy must be initiated.

In *carotid sinus massage*, the physician massages over one carotid artery for a few seconds, observing for a change in cardiac rhythm. This intervention causes vagal stimulation, slowing SA and AV nodal conduction. Prepare the patient for the procedure. Instruct him or her to turn the head slightly away from the side to be massaged, and observe the cardiac monitor for a change in rhythm. An ECG rhythm strip is recorded before, during, and after the procedure. After the procedure, assess vital signs and the level of consciousness. Complications include bradydysrhythmias, asystole, ventricular fibrillation (VF), and cerebral damage. Because of these risks, carotid massage is not commonly performed. *A defibrillator and resuscitative equipment must be immediately available during the procedure.*

To stimulate a *vagal reflex*, the health care provider instructs the patient to bear down as if straining to have a bowel movement. Assess the patient's heart rate, heart rhythm, and blood pressure. Observe the cardiac monitor; and record an ECG rhythm strip before, during, and after the procedure to determine the effect of therapy.

Drug therapy is prescribed for some patients to convert SVT to a normal sinus rhythm (NSR). Adenosine (Adenocard) is used to terminate the acute episode and given rapidly (over several seconds) followed by a normal saline bolus.

! NURSING SAFETY PRIORITY (QSEN)
Drug Alert

Side effects of adenosine include significant bradycardia with pauses, nausea, and vomiting. When administering adenosine, be sure to have emergency equipment readily available!

AV nodal blocking agents, such as beta and calcium channel blockers, are also given to treat SVT. Chart 34-3 lists medications that may be used for SVT.

If symptoms of poor PERFUSION are severe and persistent, the patient may require synchronized cardioversion to immediately terminate the SVT. For long-term treatment, patients are referred to an electrophysiologist for radiofrequency catheter ablation. Synchronized cardioversion and catheter ablation are discussed in detail on p. 668 of this chapter.

Atrial Fibrillation. **Atrial fibrillation (AF)** is the most common dysrhythmia seen in clinical practice. It can impair quality of life, cause considerable morbidity and mortality, and impose a large economic burden on health care systems (Dagres & Anastasiou-Nana, 2010).

AF is associated with atrial fibrosis and loss of muscle mass. A mutation in the *lamin AC* (LMAC) gene has been linked to atrial fibrosis and dilation (Hardin & Steele, 2008). These structural changes are common in heart diseases such as hypertension, heart failure, and coronary artery disease. As AF progresses, cardiac output decreases by as much as 20 to 30 percent.

Currently, about 2.3 million people in the United States are diagnosed with AF; it is estimated that more than 12 million people will have AF by the year 2050 (Tedrow et al., 2010). The incidence of AF increases with age; AF causes serious problems in older people, leading to stroke and/or heart failure. Risk factors include hypertension (HTN), previous ischemic stroke, transient ischemic attack (TIA) or other thromboembolic event,

EVIDENCE-BASED PRACTICE (QSEN)
Is There a Relationship Between Obesity and Atrial Fibrillation?

Tedrow, U.B., Conen, D., Ridker, P.M., Cook, N.R., Koplan, B.A., Manson, J.E., et al. (2010). The long- and short-term impact of elevated body mass index on the risk of new atrial fibrillation: The WHS (Women's Health Study). *Journal of the American College of Cardiology, 55*(21), 2319-2327.

There has been an increase in atrial fibrillation (AF) in recent years that is not explained by aging alone. Modifiable risk factors must be identified. Recent evidence estimates that 32.2% of adults are obese (body mass index [BMI] >30) and 6.9% of women are extremely obese (BMI >40). This study used data from the Women's Health Study (WHS) and included 34,309 women who were followed for about 12.9 years. Participants reported their weight on questionnaires at 24-, 36-, 60-, 72-, and 108-month intervals. During this time, 834 AF events were confirmed. BMI was linearly associated with AF risk, and being overweight and/or obese was associated with short-term increases in AF risk. Participants who became obese had a 41% risk for developing AF. Study limitations include the heterogeneous population with self-reported height/weight and lack of electrocardiograph (ECG) screening. The researchers concluded that weight-control strategies may reduce AF incidence.

Level of Evidence: 1
The evidence was obtained from a randomized trial of a very large longitudinal national study using multiple methods of data collection.

Commentary: Implications for Practice and Research
Obesity is a major health concern in the United States. Cases of AF are increasing. Both affect the economy of health care because of complications and hospital admissions. Nurses need to recognize AF risk factors and provide proactive education to patients at risk for obesity, cardiovascular disease, and atrial fibrillation. Further research is needed to replicate the study on different populations, to determine the economic impact on health care, and to determine if weight loss reduces the incidence of AF.

---

coronary heart disease, diabetes mellitus, heart failure, and mitral valve disease.

In addition to advanced age, obesity, Caucasian race, and excessive alcohol have been identified as risk factors for AF (see the Evidence-Based Practice box). About half of obese adults may develop AF (Chilukuri et al., 2010). Caucasians are more at risk for AF than African Americans and other ethnic groups, perhaps because of the larger left atrial diameter in Caucasians (Marcus et al., 2010). AF that is temporary and reversible is associated with excessive alcohol consumption (sometimes called "*holiday heart syndrome*").

Assessment. In patients with AF, multiple rapid impulses from many atrial foci depolarize the atria in a totally disorganized manner at a rate of 350 to 600 times per minute; ventricular response is usually 120 to 200 beats per minute. The result is a chaotic rhythm with no clear P waves, no atrial contractions, loss of atrial kick, and an irregular ventricular response (Fig. 34-11). The atria merely quiver in fibrillation (commonly called "A fib"). Often the ventricles beat with a rapid rate in response to the numerous atrial impulses. The rapid and irregular ventricular rate decreases ventricular filling and reduces cardiac output, further impairing the heart's PERFUSION ability.

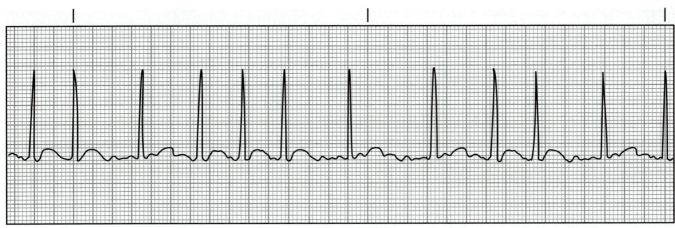

FIG. 34-11 Atrial fibrillation. Note wavy baseline with atrial electrical activity and irregular ventricular rhythm.

! NURSING SAFETY PRIORITY (QSEN)
Action Alert

The loss of coordinated atrial contractions in AF can lead to pooling of blood resulting in thrombus formation. *The patient is at high risk for pulmonary embolism!* Thrombi may form within the right atrium and then move through the right ventricle to the lungs. In addition, the patient is at risk for systemic emboli, particularly an embolic stroke, which may cause severe neurologic impairment or death. Patients with AF who have valvular disease are particularly at risk for venous thromboembolism (VTE). Monitor patients carefully for these complications discussed elsewhere in this text.

Interventions. Interventions for AF depend on the severity of the problem and the patient's response. Drug therapy is often effective for treating AF.

Drug Therapy. Traditional interventions for AF include anti-dysrhythmic drugs to slow the ventricular conduction or to convert the AF to normal sinus rhythm (NSR). Examples of these drugs are calcium channel blockers like diltiazem (Cardizem) or, for more difficult-to-control AF, amiodarone (Cordarone). Dronedarone (Multaq) is a new drug similar to amiodarone, yet better tolerated by patients, for maintenance of sinus rhythm after cardioversion (Cheng, 2010). However, dronedarone should not be used in patients with a history or current congestive heart failure because it can cause an exacerbation of cardiac symptoms.

Beta blockers, such as metoprolol (Toprol, Dutoprol) and esmolol (Brevibloc), may also be used to slow ventricular response. Digoxin (Lanoxin, Novo-Digoxin♣) is given for patients with heart failure and AF. These drugs are described in Chart 34-3. Carefully monitor the pulse rate of patients taking these drugs.

Health care providers use the **CHADS₂ scoring system** (Congestive heart failure, Hypertension, Age ≥75, Diabetes mellitus, Stroke) to determine if the patient with atrial fibrillation needs preventive anticoagulant therapy (Table 34-2). If the patient scores a 0 or 1 on the scale, aspirin is utilized as the anticoagulant of choice. Patients with a score of 2 or more are considered high risk for clot development and are placed on anticoagulants, such as heparin, enoxaparin (Lovenox), and warfarin (Coumadin). Because of the unpredictable drug response and many food-drug interactions, laboratory test

---

TABLE 34-2 CHADS₂ Scoring System for Risk of Stroke in Patients Who Have Atrial Fibrillation

RISK FACTOR	PRESENT	SCORE
History of **c**ongestive heart failure	Yes	1
	No	0
History of **h**ypertension	Yes	1
	No	0
Age ≥75 years	Yes	1
	No	0
History of **d**iabetes	Yes	1
	No	0
History of **s**troke or TIA	Yes	2
	No	0

Score of 0: Low risk—recommended 325 mg of aspirin
Score of 1: Moderate risk—recommended aspirin or warfarin
Score of 2: High risk—warfarin with INR goal of 2.0-3.0 or other anticoagulant (see Chart 34-3)

Source: Gage, B.F., Waterman, A.D., Shannon, W., Boechler, M., Rich, M.W., & Radford, M.J. (2001). Validation of clinical classification schemes for predicting stroke: Results from the National Registry of Atrial Fibrillation. *Journal of the American Medical Association, 285*(22), 2864-2870; MDCalc.com. (2013). *CHADS₂ score for atrial fibrillation stroke risk.* Retrieved July 2014, from www.mdcalc.com/chads2-score-for-atrial-fibrillation-stroke-risk/; QxMD.com.(2013). *HADS₂.* Retrieved July 2014, from www.qxmd.com/calculate-online/cardiology/chads2-stroke-risk-in-atrial-fibrillation. *INR,* International normalized ratio; *TIA,* transient ischemic attack.

---

monitoring (e.g., international normalized ratio [INR]) is required when a patient is taking warfarin. Teach patients the importance of avoiding high vitamin K foods and avoiding herbs, such as ginger, ginseng, goldenseal, *Ginkgo biloba,* and St. John's wort, which could interfere with the drug's action. Chapter 36 describes care of patients receiving anticoagulant therapy in detail on p. 731.

Because of the problems associated with warfarin, alternative anticoagulant agents such as dabigatran (Pradaxa), rivaroxaban (Xarelto), or apixaban (Eliquis) may be given on a long-term basis to prevent strokes associated with nonvalvular AF (Chart 34-4). Because these drugs achieve a steady state, there is no need for laboratory test monitoring. However, if the patient does experience severe bleeding, reversal agents are not available and prothrombin time (PT) and INR are not accurate predictors of bleeding time. These drugs should be used cautiously in patients older than 75 years because of their risk for falls (Sellers & Newby, 2011).

CHART 34-4 **Common Examples of Drug Therapy**

Nonvalvular Atrial Fibrillation

DRUG	USUAL DOSAGE	NURSING INTERVENTIONS	RATIONALES	REVERSAL AGENT
Rivaroxaban (Xarelto) (factor Xa inhibitor)	20 mg orally daily with evening meal 15 mg orally daily if CrCl <15-50 mL	Monitor for signs and symptoms of bleeding. Teach patient the importance of taking as directed.	Abrupt discontinuation may put patient at high risk for stroke.	None
Dabigatran (Pradaxa) (thrombin inhibitor)	150 mg orally twice daily	Monitor for signs and symptoms of bleeding. Teach patient the importance of taking as directed.	Abrupt discontinuation may put patient at high risk for stroke.	None Hemodialysis may remove dabigatran—limited data available.
Apixaban (Eliquis) (factor Xa inhibitor)	5 mg orally twice daily 2.5 mg orally twice daily used in patients with at least 2 of these characteristics: age ≥80 years, body weight ≤60 kg, or serum creatinine ≥1.5mg/dL	Monitor for signs and symptoms of bleeding. Teach patient the importance of taking as directed.	Abrupt discontinuation may put patient at high risk for stroke.	None

CrCl, Creatinine clearance.

⚠ NURSING SAFETY PRIORITY (QSEN)

Drug Alert

Teach patients taking any type of anticoagulant drug to report bruising, bleeding nose or gums, and other signs of bleeding to their health care provider immediately. Also remind them to take aspirin with food to prevent GI distress.

❓ NCLEX EXAMINATION CHALLENGE

Physiological Integrity

The health care provider prescribes warfarin (Coumadin) for a client with atrial fibrillation. Which foods will the nurse teach the client taking this drug to avoid? **Select all that apply.**
A. Spinach
B. Corn
C. Tomatoes
D. Brussels sprouts
E. Potatoes

Cardioversion. **Cardioversion** is a *synchronized* countershock that may be performed (1) in emergencies for unstable ventricular or supraventricular tachydysrhythmias or (2) electively for stable tachydysrhythmias that are resistant to medical therapies. If the patient has been taking digoxin, the drug is withheld for up to 48 hours before an elective cardioversion. Digoxin increases ventricular irritability and puts the patient at risk for VF after the countershock. For elective cardioversion for atrial fibrillation, the patient must take anticoagulants for 4 to 6 weeks before the procedure to prevent clots from moving from the heart to the brain or lungs. If unsure of onset of AF, a transesophageal echocardiogram (TEE) may be performed to assess for clot formation in the left atrium.

The shock depolarizes a large amount of myocardium during the cardiac depolarization. It is intended to stop the re-entry circuit and allow the sinus node to regain control of the heart. Emergency equipment must be available during the procedure. The physician, advanced practice nurse, or other qualified nurse explains the procedure to the patient and family. Assist the patient in signing a consent form unless the procedure is an emergency for a life-threatening dysrhythmia. Because he or she

is usually conscious, a short-acting anesthetic agent is administered for sedation.

One electrode is placed to the left of the precordium, and the other is placed on the right next to the sternum and below the clavicle. The defibrillator should be set in the synchronized mode. This avoids discharging the shock during the T wave, which may increase ventricular irritability, causing ventricular fibrillation (VF). Charge the defibrillator to the energy level requested, usually starting at a low rate of 120 to 200 joules for biphasic machines.

⚠ NURSING SAFETY PRIORITY (QSEN)

Critical Rescue

For safety before cardioversion, turn oxygen off and away from patient; fire could result. Shout "CLEAR" before shock delivery for electrical safety!

After cardioversion, assess the patient's response and heart rhythm. Therapy is repeated, if necessary, until the desired result is obtained or alternative therapies are considered. If the patient's condition deteriorates into VF after cardioversion, check to see that the synchronizer is turned off so that immediate defibrillation can be administered.

Nursing care after cardioversion includes:
- Maintaining a patent airway
- Administering oxygen
- Assessing vital signs and the level of consciousness
- Administering antidysrhythmic drug therapy, as prescribed
- Monitoring for dysrhythmias
- Assessing for chest burns from electrodes
- Providing emotional support
- Documenting the results of cardioversion

Radiofrequency Catheter Ablation. **Radiofrequency catheter ablation** is an invasive procedure that may be used to destroy an irritable focus causing a supraventricular or ventricular tachydysrhythmia. The patient must first undergo electrophysiologic studies and mapping procedures to locate the focus. Then radiofrequency waves are delivered to abolish the irritable focus. When ablation is performed in the AV nodal or His bundle area, damage may also occur to the normal conduction system, causing heart blocks and requiring implantation of a permanent pacemaker. In AF, pulmonary vein isolation and ablation creates scar tissue that blocks impulses and disconnects the pathway of the abnormal rhythm. Patients with AF with a rapid ventricular rate not responsive to drug therapy may have AV nodal ablation performed to totally disconnect the conduction from the atria to the ventricles, which requires implantation of a permanent pacemaker

Other Nonsurgical Management. *Bi-ventricular pacing* may be another alternative for patients with heart failure and conduction disorders. Bi-atrial pacing, anti-tachycardia pacing, and implantable atrial defibrillators are other methods used to suppress or resolve AF.

Patients in AF with heart failure (discussed in Chapter 35) may benefit from the *surgical* maze procedure, an open-chest surgical technique often performed with coronary artery bypass grafting (CABG). Before this procedure, electrophysiologic mapping studies are done to confirm the diagnosis of AF. The surgeon places a maze of sutures in strategic places in the atrial myocardium, pulmonary artery, and possibly the superior vena cava to prevent electrical circuits from developing and continuing AF. Sinus impulses can then depolarize the atria before reaching the AV node and preserve the atrial kick. Postoperative care is similar to that after other open-heart surgical procedures (see Chapter 38).

The *catheter* maze procedure is done by inserting a catheter through a leg vein into the atria and dragging a heated ablating catheter along the atria to create lines (scars) of conduction block. Patients having this minimally invasive form of the procedure have fewer complications, less pain, and a quicker recovery than those with the open, surgical maze procedure.

? NCLEX EXAMINATION CHALLENGE
Physiological Integrity

A client is prescribed to take rivaroxaban (Xarelto) 20 mg orally every day. What is the nurse's priority when teaching the client about this drug?
A. "Be sure to keep laboratory appointments to check your clotting times."
B. "Take the medication every morning before breakfast."
C. "Report any signs of bleeding to your health care provider."
D. "Have vitamin K available in case you need it."

Ventricular Dysrhythmias

Ventricular dysrhythmias are potentially more life threatening than atrial dysrhythmias because the left ventricle pumps oxygenated blood throughout the body to perfuse vital organs and other tissues. The most common or life-threatening ventricular dysrhythmias include:
- Premature ventricular complexes
- Ventricular tachycardia
- Ventricular fibrillation
- Ventricular asystole

Premature Ventricular Complexes. **Premature ventricular complexes (PVCs)**, also called *premature ventricular contractions*, result from increased irritability of ventricular cells and are seen as early ventricular complexes followed by a pause. When multiple PVCs are present, the QRS complexes may be unifocal or uniform, meaning that they are of the same shape (Fig. 34-12, *A*), or multifocal or multiform, meaning that they are of different shapes (Fig. 34-12, *B*). PVCs frequently occur in repetitive rhythms, such as bigeminy (two), trigeminy (three),

FIG. 34-12 Premature ventricular contractions. **A,** Normal sinus rhythm with unifocal premature ventricular complexes (PVCs). **B,** Normal sinus rhythm with multifocal PVCs (one negative and the other positive).

and quadrigeminy (four). Two sequential PVCs are a pair, or couplet. Three or more successive PVCs are usually called **non-sustained ventricular tachycardia (NSVT)**.

Premature ventricular contractions are common, and their frequency increases with age. They may be insignificant or may occur with problems such as myocardial infarction, chronic heart failure, chronic obstructive pulmonary disease (COPD), and anemia. PVCs may also be present in patients with hypokalemia or hypomagnesemia. Sympathomimetic agents, anesthesia drugs, stress, nicotine, caffeine, alcohol, infection, or surgery can also cause PVCs, especially in older adults. Postmenopausal women often find that caffeine causes palpitations and PVCs.

Assessment. The patient may be asymptomatic or experience palpitations or chest discomfort caused by increased stroke volume of the normal beat after the pause. Peripheral pulses may be diminished or absent with the PVCs themselves because the decreased stroke volume of the premature beats may *decrease peripheral* PERFUSION.

> ### ⚠ NURSING SAFETY PRIORITY ◲QSEN◳
> #### *Action Alert*
>
> Because other dysrhythmias can cause widened QRS complexes, assess whether the premature complexes perfuse to the extremities. Palpate the carotid, brachial, or femoral arteries while observing the monitor for widened complexes or auscultating apical heart sounds. With acute MI, PVCs may be considered as a warning, possibly triggering life-threatening ventricular tachycardia (VT) or ventricular fibrillation (VF).

Interventions. If there is no underlying heart disease, PVCs are not usually treated other than by eliminating or managing any contributing cause (e.g., caffeine, stress). Potassium or magnesium is given for replacement therapy if hypokalemia or hypomagnesemia is the cause. People with more than 5000 PVCs in a 24-hour period are usually placed on beta-adrenergic blocking agents (beta blockers) (see Chart 34-3).

Ventricular Tachycardia. **Ventricular tachycardia (VT)**, sometimes referred to as "V tach," occurs with repetitive firing of an irritable ventricular ectopic focus, usually at a rate of 140 to 180 beats/min or more (Fig. 34-13). VT may result from increased automaticity or a re-entry mechanism. It may be intermittent (nonsustained VT) or sustained, lasting longer than 15 to 30 seconds. The sinus node may continue to discharge independently, depolarizing the atria but not the ventricles, although P waves are seldom seen in sustained VT.

Ventricular tachycardia may occur in patients with ischemic heart disease, MI, cardiomyopathy, hypokalemia, hypomagnesemia, valvular heart disease, heart failure, drug toxicity (e.g., steroids), or hypotension. Patients who use cocaine or illicit inhalants are at a high risk for VT. *In patients who go into cardiac arrest, VT is commonly the initial rhythm before deterioration into ventricular fibrillation (VF) as the terminal rhythm!*

Clinical manifestations of sustained VT partially depend on the ventricular rate. Slower rates are better tolerated.

> ### ⚠ NURSING SAFETY PRIORITY ◲QSEN◳
> #### *Critical Rescue*
>
> In some patients, VT causes cardiac arrest. Assess the patient's airway, breathing, circulation, level of consciousness, and oxygenation level. For the *stable* patient with sustained VT, administer oxygen and confirm the rhythm via a 12-lead ECG. Amiodarone (Cordarone), lidocaine, or magnesium sulfate may be given.

Current Advanced Cardiac Life Support (ACLS) guidelines state that elective cardioversion is highly recommended for stable VT. The physician may prescribe an oral antidysrhythmic agent, such as mexiletine (Mexitil) or sotalol (Betapace, Sotacor♣), to prevent further occurrences. Patients who persist with episodes of stable VT may require radiofrequency catheter ablation (see p. 668 of this chapter). *Unstable* VT without a pulse is treated the same way as ventricular fibrillation as described below.

Ventricular Fibrillation. **Ventricular fibrillation (VF)**, sometimes called "V fib," is the result of electrical chaos in the ventricles and is *life threatening*! Impulses from many irritable foci fire in a totally disorganized manner so that ventricular contraction cannot occur. There are no recognizable ECG deflections (Fig. 34-14, *A*). The ventricles merely quiver, consuming a tremendous amount of oxygen. *There is no cardiac output or pulse and therefore no cerebral, myocardial, or systemic perfusion. This rhythm is rapidly fatal if not successfully ended within 3 to 5 minutes.*

VF may be the first manifestation of coronary artery disease (CAD). Patients with myocardial infarction (MI) are at great risk for VF. It may also occur in those with hypokalemia, hypomagnesemia, hemorrhage, drug therapy, rapid supraventricular

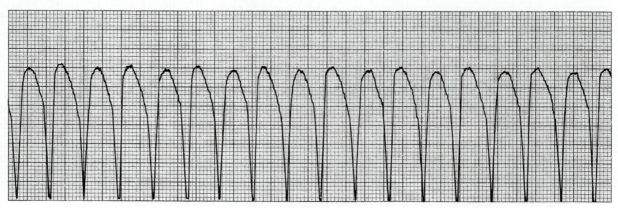

FIG. 34-13 Sustained ventricular tachycardia at a rate of 166 beats per minute.

tachycardia (SVT), or shock. Surgery or trauma may also cause VF.

Emergency Care: Ventricular Fibrillation. When VF begins, the patient becomes faint, immediately loses consciousness, and becomes pulseless and apneic (no breathing). There is no blood pressure, and heart sounds are absent. Respiratory and metabolic acidosis develop. Seizures may occur. Within minutes, the pupils become fixed and dilated and the skin becomes cold and mottled. *Death results without prompt intervention.*

The desired outcomes of collaborative care are to resolve VF promptly and convert it to an organized rhythm. *Therefore the priority is to defibrillate the patient immediately according to ACLS protocol.* If a defibrillator is not readily available, high quality CPR must be initiated and continued until the defibrillator arrives. An automated external defibrillator (AED) is frequently used because it is simple for both medical and lay personnel. Defibrillation is discussed on p. 672.

Ventricular Asystole. **Ventricular asystole**, sometimes called *ventricular standstill*, is the complete absence of any ventricular rhythm (Fig. 34-14, *B*). There are no electrical impulses in the ventricles and therefore *no* ventricular depolarization, no QRS complex, no contraction, no cardiac output, and no PERFUSION to the rest of the body.

Assessment. The patient in ventricular asystole has no pulse, respirations, or blood pressure. *The patient is in full cardiac arrest.* The sinoatrial (SA) node, in some cases, may continue to fire and depolarize the atria, with only P waves seen on the ECG. The sinus impulses, however, do not conduct to the ventricles, and QRS complexes remain absent. In most cases, the entire conduction system is electrically silent, with no P waves seen on the ECG.

Ventricular asystole usually results from myocardial hypoxia, which may be a consequence of advanced heart failure. It may also be caused by severe hyperkalemia and acidosis. If P waves are seen, asystole is likely because of severe ventricular conduction blocks.

Interventions. *When cardiac arrest occurs, cardiac output stops.* The underlying rhythm is usually ventricular tachycardia (VT), ventricular fibrillation (VF), or asystole. Without cardiac output, the patient is pulseless and becomes unconscious because of inadequate cerebral PERFUSION and oxygenation. Shortly after cardiac arrest, respiratory arrest occurs. Therefore cardiopulmonary resuscitation is essential to prevent brain damage and death.

Cardiopulmonary Resuscitation and Defibrillation. Cardiopulmonary resuscitation (CPR), also known as **Basic Cardiac Life Support (BCLS)**, must be initiated immediately when asystole occurs. When finding an unresponsive patient, confirm unresponsiveness and call 911 (in community or long-term care setting) or the emergency response team (in the hospital). Gather the AED or defibrillator *before initiating CPR*. Guidelines for CPR have changed from an ABC (airway-breathing-compressions) approach to the initial priorities of CAB (compressions-airway-breathing) (American Heart Association [AHA], 2010).

- Check for a carotid pulse for 5 to 10 seconds
- *If carotid pulse is absent*, start chest **c**ompressions of at least 100 compressions per minute and a compression depth of at least 2 inches. Push hard and fast!

FIG. 34-14 Ventricular dysrhythmias. **A,** Coarse ventricular fibrillation. **B,** Ventricular asystole with one idioventricular complex.

- Maintain a patent **a**irway.
- Ventilate (**b**reathing) with a mouth-to-mask device. Give rescue breaths at a rate of 10 to 12 breaths/min. If an advanced airway is in place, one breath should be given every 6 to 8 seconds (8 to 10 breaths/min).
- Ventilation to compression ratio should be maintained at 30 compressions to 2 breaths if advanced airway is not in place

Be sure to use Standard Precautions when administering CPR. Be aware that complications of CPR include:

- Rib fractures
- Fracture of the sternum
- Costochondral separation
- Lacerations of the liver and spleen
- Pneumothorax
- Hemothorax
- Cardiac tamponade
- Lung contusions
- Fat emboli

As soon as help arrives, place a board under the patient who is not on a firm surface. To make room for the resuscitation team and the crash cart, ask that the area be cleared of movable items and unnecessary personnel. When the AED or defibrillator arrives, *do not stop chest compressions while the defibrillator is being set up.* If trained to use the AED or defibrillator, apply hands-off defibrillator pads to the patient's chest and turn on the monitor. If the patient is in VF or pulseless VT, the immediate priority is to defibrillate! **Defibrillation**, an *asynchronous countershock,* depolarizes a critical mass of myocardium simultaneously to stop the re-entry circuit, allowing the sinus node to regain control of the heart. After defibrillation, CPR is resumed. CPR must continue at all times except during defibrillation.

! NURSING SAFETY PRIORITY (QSEN)

Critical Rescue

Early defibrillation is critical in resolving pulseless ventricular tachycardia (VT) or ventricular fibrillation (VF). It must not be delayed for any reason after the equipment and skilled personnel are present. The earlier defibrillation is performed, the greater the chance of survival! *Do not defibrillate ventricular asystole.*

Before defibrillation, loudly and clearly command all personnel to clear contact with the patient and the bed and check to see they are clear before the shock is delivered. Deliver shock and immediately resume CPR for 5 cycles or about 2 minutes. Reassess the rhythm every 2 minutes and if indicated. Charge the defibrillator to deliver an additional shock at the same energy level previously used. During the 2-minute intervals while high-quality CPR is being delivered, the Advanced Cardiac Life Support (ACLS) team administers medications and performs interventions to try and restore an organized cardiac rhythm. *Discussion of ACLS protocol is beyond the scope of this text.*

After the ACLS team initiates interventions, the role of the medical-surgical nurse is to provide information about the patient. Specific nursing responsibilities include providing a brief summary of the patient's medical condition and the events that occurred up until the time of cardiac arrest. Report the patient's initial cardiac rhythm. Remain in the room to answer questions, document the event, and assist with compressions. If family is present, provide emotional support and explanation of events in the room.

An emerging clinical practice is allowing or encouraging family presence at resuscitation attempts. This can be a positive experience for family members and significant others because it promotes closure after the death of a loved one. Although there may be staff resistance and some limits to family presence, overall it is a beneficial practice that should be considered in all resuscitation attempts.

When spontaneous circulation resumes, the patient is transported to the intensive care unit. Be ready to give hand-off report to the ICU nurse using SBAR communication or other agency system, and assist with patient transport

---

? CLINICAL JUDGMENT CHALLENGE

Teamwork and Collaboration; Evidence-Based Practice; Safety (QSEN)

A 72-year-old woman is transported to the ED with a diagnosis of chest pain to rule out myocardial infarction (MI). During the initial assessment, the nurse notes the cardiac rhythm changes from sinus tachycardia to ventricular tachycardia (VT) with a pulse. Her vital signs are: blood pressure, 84/40 mm Hg; pulse, 154/min; and respirations, 30/min.

1. What is the initial treatment for this patient at this time?
2. What drugs should you anticipate administering to this patient? Why are they indicated?
3. What evidence-based precautions must be taken to promote safety for both the patient and the ACLS team?
4. If this rhythm deteriorates to ventricular fibrillation or VT without a pulse, what steps should you take? Why?

Automated External Defibrillation. The American Heart Association promotes the use of automated external defibrillators (AEDs) for use by laypersons and health care professionals responding to cardiac arrest emergencies (Fig. 34-15). These devices are found in many public places such as malls, airports, and commercial jets. The patient in cardiac arrest must be on a firm, dry surface. The rescuer places two large adhesive-patch electrodes on the patient's chest in the same positions as for defibrillator electrodes. The rescuer stops CPR and commands anyone present to move away, ensuring that no one is touching the patient. This measure eliminates motion artifact when the machine analyzes the rhythm. The rescuer presses the "analyze" button on the machine. After rhythm analysis, which may take up to 30 seconds, the machine either advises that a shock is necessary or advises that a shock is not indicated. *Shocks are recommended for VF or pulseless VT only.*

If a shock is indicated, issue a command to clear all contact with the patient and press the charge button. Once the AED is

FIG. 34-15 Automated external defibrillator.

charged, press the shock button and the shock will be delivered. The shock is delivered through the patches, so it is hands-off defibrillation, which is safer for the rescuer. The rescuer then resumes CPR until the AED instructs to "stop CPR" to analyze the rhythm. If the rhythm is VF or VT and another shock is indicated, the AED will instruct the rescuer to charge and deliver another shock. Newer AEDs perform rhythm analysis and defibrillation without the need for a rescuer to press a button to analyze or to shock the victim. It is essential that Advanced Cardiac Life Support (ACLS) be provided as soon as possible. Use of AEDs allows for earlier defibrillation. Therefore there is a greater chance of successful rhythm conversion and patient survival.

Implantable Cardioverter/Defibrillator. The implantable cardioverter/defibrillator (ICD) is indicated for patients who have experienced one or more episodes of spontaneous sustained ventricular tachycardia (VT) or ventricular fibrillation (VF) not caused by an MI. Collaborate with the physician and the electrophysiology nurse to prepare the patient for this procedure. A psychological profile is done to determine whether the patient can cope with the discomfort and fear associated with internal defibrillation from the ICD. Many patients report anxiety, depression, and decreased quality of life, which improves for the majority of patients after 12 months (Hallas et al., 2010).

The leads of the device are introduced through the skin, and the generator is implanted in the left pectoral area, similar to a permanent pacemaker insertion procedure. This procedure is performed in the electrophysiology laboratory. If the patient experiences a VT or VF episode after ICD placement and the ICD therapies are not successful, the qualified nurse or health care provider promptly externally defibrillates and initiates high-quality CPR.

The generator may be activated or deactivated by the physician placing a magnet over the implantation site for a few moments. The patient requires close monitoring in the postoperative period for dysrhythmias and complications such as bleeding and cardiac tamponade. The nurse must know whether the ICD is activated or deactivated. Care of the patient is similar to that after implantation of a permanent pacemaker, discussed on p. 664 of this chapter.

Some patients use a lightweight, automated wearable cardioverter/defibrillator (WCD). This external vest-like device is worn 24 hours a day except when the patient showers or bathes. A family member must be present to call 911 and initiate CPR if the patient experiences pulseless VT or VF while in the shower. One popular brand is the Zoll Lifecore LifeVest, which is programmed to monitor for VT and VF. If the patient is conscious while experiencing VT, he or she can press a button to prevent a shock. This precaution is an advantage over implantable devices because ICDs are programmed to always deliver a shock when VT or VF occurs.

NCLEX EXAMINATION CHALLENGE

Safe and Effective Care Environment

A client in the telemetry unit is on a cardiac monitor. The monitor technician notices there are no ECG complexes and the alarm sounds. What is the first action by the nurse?
A. Begin CPR immediately.
B. Call the emergency response team.
C. Press the record button to get an ECG strip.
D. Assess the client and check lead placement.

Community-Based Care

For many patients, dysrhythmias are a disorder resulting from chronic cardiac and pulmonary diseases. Patients may be cared for in a variety of settings, including the acute care hospital, subacute unit, traditional nursing home, or their own home. They are admitted to the hospital when they experience life-threatening or potentially life-threatening dysrhythmias, often associated with an acute disorder.

Home Care Management. Patients discharged from the hospital may have considerable needs, often more related to their underlying chronic diseases than to their dysrhythmias. A case manager or care coordinator can assess the need for health care resources and coordinate access to services.

The focus of the home care nurse's interventions is assessment and health teaching. Patients and families often fear recurrence of a life-threatening dysrhythmia. Patients with an ICD may dread or fear the activation of the device. The community-based nurse provides the patient and family members with an opportunity to verbalize their concerns and fears. Provide emotional support as well as information about support groups and referrals in the community. Assess the patient for possible side effects of antidysrhythmic agents or complications from a pacemaker or ICD.

Self-Management Education. Teach the patient who has had a dysrhythmia caused by an acute problem, such as electrolyte imbalance or MI, about prevention, early recognition, and management of that disorder. Instruct the patient and family about lifestyle modifications designed to prevent, decrease, or control the occurrence of dysrhythmias, as outlined in Chart 34-5. This

---

CHART 34-5   Patient and Family Education: Preparing for Self-Management

How to Prevent or Decrease Dysrhythmias

For Patients at Risk for Vasovagal Attacks Causing Bradydysrhythmias
• Avoid doing things that stimulate the vagus nerve, such as raising your arms above your head, applying pressure over your carotid artery, applying pressure on your eyes, bearing down or straining during a bowel movement, and stimulating a gag reflex when brushing your teeth or putting objects in your mouth.

For Patients with Premature Beats and Ectopic Rhythms
• Take the medications that have been prescribed for you, and report any adverse effects to your physician.
• Stop smoking, avoid caffeinated beverages and energy drinks as much as possible, and drink alcohol only in moderation.
• Learn ways to manage stress and avoid getting too tired.

For Patients with Ischemic Heart Disease
• If you have an angina attack, treat it promptly with rest and nitroglycerin administration as prescribed by your physician. This decreases your chances of experiencing a dysrhythmia.
• If chest pain is not relieved after taking the amount of nitroglycerin that has been prescribed for you, seek medical attention promptly. Also, seek prompt medical attention if the pain becomes more severe or you experience other symptoms, such as sweating, nausea, weakness, and palpitations.

For Patients at Risk for Potassium Imbalance
• Know the symptoms of decreased potassium levels, such as muscle weakness and cardiac irregularity.
• Eat foods high in potassium, such as tomatoes, beans, prunes, avocados, bananas, strawberries, and lettuce.
• Take the potassium supplements that have been prescribed for you.

teaching may be provided in the acute care setting, primary care provider's office, health care clinic, or home setting.

CONSIDERATIONS FOR OLDER ADULTS
Patient-Centered Care QSEN

Older adults are at increased risk for dysrhythmias because of normal physiologic changes in their cardiac conduction system. The sinoatrial node has fewer pacemaker cells. There is a loss of fibers in the bundle branch system. Therefore older adults are at risk for sinus node dysfunction and may require pacemaker therapy. The most common dysrhythmias are premature atrial contractions, premature ventricular contractions, and atrial fibrillation. Dysrhythmias tend to be more serious in older patients because of underlying heart disease, causing cardiac decompensation. Consequently, blood flow to organs that may already be decreased because of the aging process may be further compromised, leading to multisystem organ dysfunction. Chart 34-6 highlights special considerations for older adults receiving antidysrhythmic therapy.

Patients and their families must have a thorough understanding of the prescribed *drug therapy*, including antidysrhythmic agents. Pharmacies provide written instructions with filled prescriptions. Teach patients and families the generic and trade names of their drugs, as well as the drugs' purposes, using basic terms that are easily understood. Clear instructions regarding dosage schedules and common side effects are important (see Chart 34-3). Emphasize the importance of reporting these side effects and any dizziness, nausea, vomiting, chest discomfort, or shortness of breath to the primary care provider.

Teach all patients and their family members how to take a pulse and blood pressure. Some patients may want to use technology to calculate and record their pulse rate. Several applications (apps) for handheld mobile devices (such as the iPhone) are available, but their accuracy varies. "Instant Health Rate" and "Quick Heart Rate" are examples of apps used to calculate pulse rate.

Remind patients to report any signs of a change in heart rhythm, such as a significant decrease in pulse rate, a rate more than 100 beats/min, or increased rhythm irregularity. Smart Blood Pressure (SmartBP) is a blood pressure and pulse management system that records, tracks, and analyzes data to share via an iPhone or iPad. The patient can send these readings to their health care provider as needed to maintain frequent vital sign monitoring.

Give written and verbal information to patients who have a *permanent pacemaker* about the type and settings of their pacemaker. Teach the patient to report any pulse rate lower than that set on the pacemaker. Review the proper care of the pacemaker insertion site and the importance of reporting any fever or any redness, swelling, or drainage at the pacemaker insertion site. If the surgical incision is near either shoulder, teach and demonstrate range-of-motion exercises to perform to prevent shoulder stiffness.

CHART 34-6   Nursing Focus on the Older Adult
Dysrhythmias

Special nursing considerations for the older patient with dysrhythmias are:
- Evaluate the patient with dysrhythmias immediately for the presence of a life-threatening dysrhythmia or hemodynamic deterioration.
- Assess the patient with a dysrhythmia for angina, hypotension, heart failure, and decreased cerebral and renal perfusion.
- Consider these causes of dysrhythmias when taking the patient's history: hypoxia, drug toxicity, electrolyte imbalances, heart failure, and myocardial ischemia or infarction.
- Assess the patient's level of education, hearing, learning style, and ability to understand and recall instructions to determine the best approaches for teaching.
- Assess the patient's ability to read written instructions.
- Teach the patient the generic and trade names of prescribed antidysrhythmic drugs, as well as their purposes, dosage, side effects, and special instructions for their use.
- Provide clear written instructions in basic language and easy-to-read print.
- Provide a written drug dosage schedule for the patient, considering all the drugs the patient is taking and possible drug interactions.
- Assess the patient for possible side effects or adverse reactions to drugs considering age and health status.
- Teach the patient to take his or her pulse and to report significant changes in heart rate or rhythm to the health care provider.
- Inform the patient of available resources for blood pressure and pulse checks, such as blood pressure clinics, home health agencies, and cardiac rehabilitation programs.
- Instruct the patient on the importance of keeping follow-up appointments with the health care provider and reporting symptoms promptly.
- Include the patient's family members or significant other in all teaching whenever possible.
- Teach the patient to avoid drinking caffeinated beverages, to stop smoking, to drink alcohol only in moderation, and to follow his or her prescribed diet.

! NURSING SAFETY PRIORITY QSEN
Action Alert

Teach patients who have permanent pacemakers to:
- Keep handheld cellular phones at least 6 inches away from the generator, with the handset on the ear opposite the side of the generator.
- Avoid sources of strong electromagnetic fields, such as magnets and telecommunications transmitters. These may cause interference and could change the pacemaker settings, causing a malfunction. Magnetic resonance imaging (MRI) is usually contraindicated, depending on the machine's technology.
- Carry a pacemaker identification card provided by the manufacturer and wear a medical alert bracelet at all times.

Chart 34-7 outlines the major points for patient and family teaching after the insertion of a permanent pacemaker.

Patients with an *implantable cardioverter/defibrillator (ICD)* usually continue to receive antidysrhythmic drugs after discharge from the hospital. Provide health teaching about the purposes of drug therapy, dosage schedules, special instructions, and side effects that need to be reported. If patients experience an internal defibrillator shock, remind them to sit or lie down immediately and notify the primary care provider. Some patients describe the experience of a shock as a quick thud or kick in the chest, whereas others relate severe discomfort similar to that of external defibrillation. Usually the shock is not as severe because the heart is situated between the defibrillation pads, thus requiring less electrical current to convert the dysrhythmia. Inform family members that they may feel an electrical shock if they are touching the patient during delivery of the shock but that it is not harmful. Provide information about how to access the emergency medical services (EMS) system in the community. Recommend resources for the family to learn how to perform CPR.

Remind patients with an ICD to avoid sources of strong electromagnetic fields, such as large electrical generators and radio and television transmitters. Tell the patient that these items may inhibit tachydysrhythmia detection and therapy or may cause pacing or shocks. MRI should not be used for patients with ICDs unless the patient has an MRI-conditional ICD. Handheld cellular phones must be at least 6 inches away from the generator, with the handset held to the ear opposite the side of the ICD. If the pulse generator emits a beeping sound or provides some other indicator, the patient must move away from the area as quickly as possible to prevent deactivation of the device. Teach the patient with an ICD to carry an ICD identification card and wear a medical alert bracelet. Chart 34-8 highlights the important points for health teaching.

CHART 34-7 Patient and Family Education: Preparing for Self-Management

Permanent Pacemakers

- Follow the instructions for pacemaker site skin care that have been specifically prepared for you. Report any fever or redness, swelling, or drainage from the incision site to your physician.
- Do not manipulate the pacemaker generator site.
- Keep your pacemaker identification card in your wallet, and wear a medical alert bracelet.
- Take your pulse for 1 full minute at the same time each day, and record the rate in your pacemaker diary. Take your pulse any time you feel symptoms of a possible pacemaker failure, and report your heart rate and symptoms to your physician.
- Know the rate at which your pacemaker is set and the basic functioning of your pacemaker. Know what rate changes to report to your physician.
- Do not apply pressure over your generator. Avoid tight clothing or belts.
- You may take baths or showers without concern for your pacemaker.
- Inform all health care providers that you have a pacemaker. Certain tests they may wish to perform (e.g., magnetic resonance imaging) could affect or damage your pacemaker.
- Know the indications of battery failure for your pacemaker as you were instructed, and report these findings to your health care provider if they occur.
- Do not operate electrical appliances directly over your pacemaker site because this may cause your pacemaker to malfunction.
- Do not lean over electrical or gasoline engines or motors. Be sure that electrical appliances or motors are properly grounded.
- Avoid all transmitter towers for radio, television, and radar. Radio, television, other home appliances, and antennas do not pose a hazard.
- Be aware that antitheft devices in stores may cause temporary pacemaker malfunction. If symptoms develop, move away from the device.
- Inform airport personnel of your pacemaker before passing through a metal detector, and show them your pacemaker identification card. The metal in your pacemaker will trigger the alarm in the metal detector device.
- Stay away from any arc welding equipment.
- Be aware that it is safe to operate a microwave oven unless it does not have proper shielding (old microwave ovens) or is defective.
- Report any of these symptoms to your physician if you experience them: difficulty breathing, dizziness, fainting, chest pain, weight gain, and prolonged hiccupping. If you have any of these symptoms, check your pulse rate and call your health care provider.
- If you feel symptoms when near any device, move 5 to 10 feet away from it and then check your pulse. Your pulse rate should return to normal.
- Keep all of your health care provider and pacemaker clinic appointments.
- Take all medications prescribed for you as instructed.
- Follow your prescribed diet.
- Follow instructions on restrictions on physical activity, such as no sudden, jerky movement, for 8 weeks to allow the pacemaker to settle in place.

CHART 34-8 Patient and Family Education: Preparing for Self-Management

Implantable Cardioverter/Defibrillator

- Follow the instructions for implantable cardioverter/defibrillator (ICD) site skin care that have been specifically prepared for you.
- Report to your health care provider any fever or redness, swelling, soreness, or drainage from your incision site.
- Do not wear tight clothing or belts that could cause irritation over the ICD generator.
- Do not manipulate your generator site
- Avoid activities that involve rough contact with the ICD implantation site.
- Keep your ICD identification card in your wallet, and consider wearing a medical alert bracelet.
- Know the basic functioning of your ICD device and its rate cutoff, as well as the number of consecutive shocks it can deliver.
- Avoid magnets directly over your ICD because they can inactivate the device. If beeping tones are coming from the ICD, move away from the electromagnetic field immediately (within 30 seconds) before the inactivation sequence is completed, and notify your health care provider.
- Inform all health care providers caring for you that you have an ICD implanted, because certain diagnostic tests and procedures must be avoided to prevent ICD malfunction. These include diathermy, electrocautery, and nuclear magnetic resonance tests.
- Avoid other sources of electromagnetic interference, such as devices emitting microwaves (not microwave ovens); transformers; radio, television, and radar transmitters; large electrical generators; metal detectors, including handheld security devices at airports; antitheft devices; arc welding equipment; and sources of 60-cycle (Hz) interference. Also avoid leaning directly over the alternator of a running motor of a car or boat.
- Report to your health care provider symptoms such as fainting, nausea, weakness, blackout, and rapid pulse rates.
- Take all medications prescribed for you as instructed.
- Follow instructions on restrictions on physical activity, such as not swimming, driving motor vehicles, or operating dangerous equipment.
- Follow your prescribed diet.
- Keep all health care provider and ICD clinic appointments.
- Sit or lie down immediately if you feel dizzy or faint to avoid falling if the ICD discharges.
- Post emergency telephone numbers.
- Know how to contact the local emergency medical services (EMS) systems in your community. Inform them in advance that you have an ICD so that they can be prepared if they need to respond to an emergency call for you.
- Encourage family members to learn how to perform CPR. Family members should know that if they are touching you when the device discharges, they may feel a slight shock but that this is not harmful to them.
- Follow instructions on what to do if the ICD successfully discharges, after which you feel well. This may include maintaining a diary of the date, the time, activity preceding the shock, symptoms, the number of shocks delivered, and how you feel after the shock. The physician may wish to be notified each time the device discharges.
- Avoid strenuous activities that may cause your heart rate to meet or exceed the rate cutoff of your ICD because this causes the device to discharge inappropriately.
- Notify your health care provider for information regarding access to health care if you are leaving town or are relocating.

Health Care Resources. The cardiac rehabilitation nurse typically provides written and oral information about dysrhythmias, antidysrhythmic drugs, pacemakers, and ICDs, as well as information about cardiac exercise programs, educational programs, and support groups. The office or ambulatory care nurse may also provide information about resources. Teach the patient how to contact the local chapter of the American Heart Association (www.americanheart.org) or the provincial chapter of the Heart and Stroke Foundation in Canada (www.heartandstroke.ca) for information about dysrhythmias, pacemakers, and CPR training.

Manufacturers of pacemakers and ICDs provide helpful booklets and CDs to give patients and their families a better understanding of these therapies. Teach patients how to use telephonic systems for transmission of their rhythms to the ambulatory care setting or health care provider's office. Stress the importance of keeping scheduled appointments for visits with the cardiologist and pacemaker or ICD clinic. Instruct patients to contact the local ambulance or paramedic services and emergency facilities to let them know that they have these devices implanted. Encourage the patient and family to attend pacemaker or ICD support groups.

NURSING CONCEPTS AND CLINICAL JUDGMENT REVIEW

What might you NOTICE if the patient is experiencing inadequate oxygenation and tissue PERFUSION as a result of dysrhythmias?
- Report of chest discomfort or pain
- Report of dizziness or syncope
- Shortness of breath
- Weakness and fatigue
- Decreased urine output
- Pale, cool skin
- Diaphoresis
- Anxiety or restlessness

What should you INTERPRET and how should you RESPOND to a patient experiencing inadequate oxygenation and PERFUSION as a result of dysrhythmias?

Perform and interpret physical assessment, including:
- Taking vital signs (may have hypotension and weak pulse)
- Checking for pulse deficit
- Asking if patient has palpitations
- Checking capillary refill (decreased)
- Listening to lung and heart sounds
- Assessing cognition
- Taking an ECG
- Checking oxygen saturation

Respond by:
- Applying oxygen
- Keeping the head of the bed elevated unless patient is very hypotensive
- Maintaining or starting an IV line
- Notifying the health care provider or Rapid Response Team
- Giving drug therapy as prescribed
- Initiating CPR for asystole
- Defibrillating the patient in VF
- Assisting with other procedures as needed, for example, defibrillation

On what should you REFLECT?
- Evaluate patient's response to drug therapy.
- Observe for evidence of increased oxygenation and perfusion.
- Think about what else you could have done to assist the patient with this problem.

GET READY FOR THE NCLEX® EXAMINATION!

KEY POINTS

Review these Key Points for each NCLEX Examination Client Needs Category.

Safe and Effective Care Environment
- Be very careful to protect patients and staff to prevent electrical injury when assisting with invasive pacemakers, cardioversion, and defibrillation. **Safety** **QSEN**
- For safety during cardioversion, turn oxygen off and away from the patient to prevent a fire. Shout "CLEAR" before shock delivery for electrical safety. **Safety** **QSEN**
- Teach patients who have permanent pacemakers to keep cell phones at least 6 inches away from the generator, avoid electromagnetic fields such as telecommunication transmitters, wear a medical alert bracelet at all times, and carry a pacemaker identification card. **Safety** **QSEN**

Health Promotion and Maintenance
- Teach patients with dysrhythmias the correct drug, dose, route, time, and side effects of prescribed drugs, and teach them to notify their primary care provider if adverse effects occur (see Chart 34-3).
- Teach patients taking anticoagulant therapy to report any signs of bruising or unusual bleeding immediately to their health care provider.
- Teach family members where to learn cardiopulmonary resuscitation (CPR) to decrease their anxiety while living with a patient with dysrhythmias or ICD/pacemaker. **Patient-Centered Care** **QSEN**
- Teach patients the importance of adhering to their prescribed cardiac regimen, such as checking their pulse to ascertain pacemaker function.

Physiological Integrity

- Assess patients with dysrhythmias for a decrease in cardiac output resulting in inadequate oxygenation and perfusion to vital organs (see Chart 34-2); typical assessment findings include shortness of breath, dizziness or syncope, weakness and fatigue, and irregular pulse.
- Monitor patients with dysrhythmias, including conducting a physical assessment and health history, as well as interpreting ECG rhythm strips. Report significant changes to the health care provider.
- Interpret common dysrhythmias, especially bradycardia, tachycardia, atrial fibrillation (AF) and ventricular fibrillation (VF), premature ventricular contractions (PVCs), and asystole, using the steps of ECG analysis.
- Use special considerations when caring for older adults with dysrhythmias, as described in Chart 34-6. **Patient-Centered Care** QSEN

- Recognize that noninvasive pacing is an emergency measure to provide demand ventricular pacing in patients with profound bradycardia or asystole. Teach patients to expect possible discomfort.
- Identify and intervene in life-threatening situations by providing cardiopulmonary resuscitation, electrical therapy, or drug administration. **Evidence-Based Practice** QSEN
- Be aware that automated external defibrillators (AEDs) are used by medical and lay personnel as an essential intervention for VF.
- Do not perform CPR while the patient is being defibrillated. **Safety** QSEN
- Educate patients who have permanent pacemakers or ICDs about self-management (see Charts 34-7 and 34-8).

35 | CHAPTER

Care of Patients with Cardiac Problems

Laura M. Dechant

http://evolve.elsevier.com/Iggy/

This chapter focuses on heart failure and its common causes in the adult population; coronary artery disease is discussed in Chapter 38. Heart failure is the most common reason for hospital stays in patients older than 65 years in the United States. When the heart is diseased, it cannot effectively pump an adequate amount of arterial blood to the rest of the body. Arterial blood carries *oxygen* and nutrients to vital organs, such as the kidneys and brain, and to peripheral tissues. When these organs and other body tissues are not adequately *perfused*, they may not function properly.

HEART FAILURE

Heart failure, sometimes referred to as *pump failure*, is a general term for the inability of the heart to work effectively as a pump. It results from a number of acute and chronic cardiovascular problems that are discussed later in this chapter and elsewhere in the cardiovascular unit.

❖ PATHOPHYSIOLOGY

Heart failure (HF) is a common *chronic* health problem, with acute episodes often causing hospitalization. Acute coronary disease and other structural or functional problems of the heart can lead to *acute* heart failure. Both acute and chronic HF can be life threatening if they are not adequately treated or if the patient does not respond to treatment.

Types of Heart Failure

The major types of heart failure are:
- Left-sided heart failure
- Right-sided heart failure
- High-output failure

Because the two ventricles of the heart represent two separate pumping systems, it is possible for one to fail by itself for a short period. *Most heart failure begins with failure of the left ventricle and progresses to failure of both ventricles.* Typical causes of **left-sided heart (ventricular) failure** include hypertension, coronary artery disease, and valvular disease involving the mitral or aortic valve. Decreased tissue PERFUSION from poor cardiac output and pulmonary congestion from increased pressure in the pulmonary vessels indicate left ventricular failure (LVF).

Left-sided heart failure was formerly referred to as **congestive heart failure (CHF)**; however, not all cases of LVF involve fluid accumulation. In the clinical setting, though, the term *CHF* is still commonly used. Left-sided failure may be acute or chronic and mild to severe. It can be further divided into two subtypes: systolic heart failure and diastolic heart failure.

Systolic heart failure (systolic ventricular dysfunction) results when the heart cannot contract forcefully enough during systole to eject adequate amounts of blood into the circulation. Preload increases with decreased contractility, and afterload increases as a result of increased peripheral resistance (e.g., hypertension) (McCance et al., 2014). The **ejection fraction** (the percentage of blood ejected from the heart during systole) drops from a normal of 50% to 70% to below 40% with ventricular dilation. As it decreases, tissue perfusion diminishes and blood accumulates in the pulmonary vessels. Manifestations of systolic dysfunction may include symptoms of inadequate tissue PERFUSION or pulmonary and systemic congestion. Systolic heart failure is often called "forward failure" because cardiac output is decreased and fluid backs up into the pulmonary system. Because these patients are at high risk for sudden cardiac death, patients with an ejection fraction of less than 30% are considered candidates for an implantable cardioverter/defibrillator (ICD; also known as an *internal cardioverter/defibrillator*) (see Chapter 34).

In contrast, **diastolic heart failure** (heart failure with preserved left ventricular function) occurs when the left ventricle cannot relax adequately during diastole. Inadequate relaxation or "stiffening" prevents the ventricle from filling with sufficient blood to ensure an adequate cardiac output. Although ejection fraction is more than 40%, the ventricle becomes less compliant over time because more pressure is needed to move the same amount of volume as compared with a healthy heart. Diastolic failure represents about 20% to 40% of all heart failure, primarily in older adults and in women who have chronic hypertension and undetected coronary artery disease. Clinical

manifestations and management of diastolic failure are similar to those of systolic dysfunction (McCance et al., 2014).

Right-sided heart (ventricular) failure may be caused by left ventricular failure, right ventricular myocardial infarction (MI), or pulmonary hypertension. In this type of heart failure (HF), the right ventricle cannot empty completely. Increased volume and pressure develop in the venous system, and peripheral edema results.

High-output heart failure can occur when cardiac output remains normal or above normal, unlike left- and right-sided heart failure, which are typically low-output states. High-output failure is caused by increased metabolic needs or hyperkinetic conditions, such as septicemia, high fever, anemia, and hyperthyroidism. This type of heart failure is not as common as other types.

Classification and Staging of Heart Failure

The American College of Cardiology (ACC) and American Heart Association (AHA) have developed evidence-based guidelines for staging and managing heart failure as a chronic, progressive disease. These guidelines do not replace the New York Heart Association (NYHA) functional classification system, which is used to describe symptoms a patient may exhibit (see Table 33-2 in Chapter 33).

The ACC/AHA staging system when compared with the NYHA system categorizes patients as:
- A. Patients at high risk for developing heart failure (class I NYHA)
- B. Patients with cardiac structural abnormalities or remodeling who have not developed HF symptoms (class I NYHA)
- C. Patients with current or prior symptoms of heart failure (class II or III NYHA)
- D. Patients with refractory end-stage heart failure (class IV NYHA)

Another method for staging HF is the Killip classification system, which is based on the heart's hemodynamic ability. Table 38-3 in Chapter 38 outlines this system.

Compensatory Mechanisms

When cardiac output is insufficient to meet the demands of the body, compensatory mechanisms work to improve cardiac output (Fig. 35-1). Although these mechanisms may initially increase cardiac output, they eventually have a damaging effect on pump function. Major compensatory mechanisms include:
- Sympathetic nervous system stimulation
- Renin-angiotensin system (RAS) activation (also called renin-angiotensin-aldosterone [RAAS] activation)
- Other chemical responses
- Myocardial hypertrophy

In heart failure (HF), *stimulation of the sympathetic nervous system* (i.e., increasing catecholamines) as a result of tissue hypoxia represents the most immediate compensatory mechanism. Stimulation of the adrenergic receptors causes an increase in heart rate (beta adrenergic) and blood pressure from vasoconstriction (alpha adrenergic).

Because cardiac output (CO) is the product of heart rate (HR) and stroke volume (SV), an increase in HR results in an immediate *increase in cardiac output.* The HR is limited, though, in its ability to compensate for decreased CO. If it becomes too rapid, diastolic filling time is limited and CO may start to

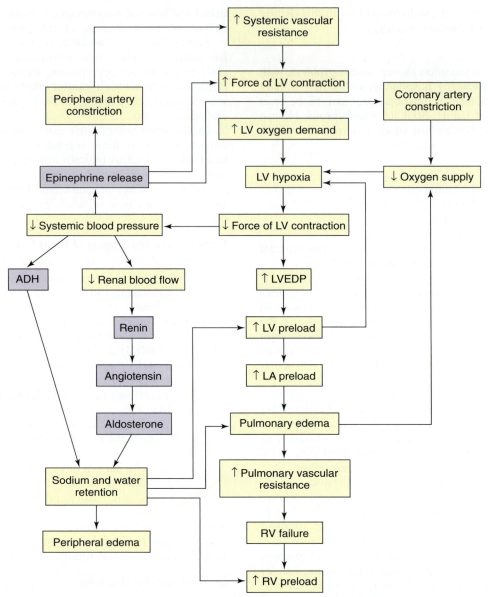

FIG. 35-1 Left-sided heart failure from elevated systemic vascular resistance. Left heart failure leads to right heart failure. Systemic vascular resistance and preload are exacerbated by renal and adrenal mechanisms. *ADH,* Antidiuretic hormone; *LA,* left atrial; *LV,* left ventricular; *LVEDP,* left ventricular end-diastolic pressure; *RV,* right ventricular.

decline. An increase in HR also significantly increases oxygen demand by the myocardium. If the heart is poorly perfused because of arteriosclerosis, HF may worsen.

Stroke volume (SV) is also *improved* by sympathetic stimulation. Sympathetic stimulation increases venous return to the heart, which further stretches the myocardial fibers causing dilation. According to Starling's law, increased myocardial stretch results in more forceful contraction. More forceful contractions increase SV and CO. After a critical point is reached within the cardiac muscle, further volume and stretch reduce the force of contraction and cardiac output.

Sympathetic stimulation also results in *arterial vasoconstriction.* Vasoconstriction has the benefit of maintaining blood pressure and improving tissue perfusion in low-output states. However, constriction of the arteries increases **afterload,** the resistance against which the heart must pump. Afterload is the major determinant of myocardial oxygen requirements. As it

increases, the left ventricle requires more energy to eject its contents and SV may decline.

Reduced blood flow to the kidneys, a common occurrence in low-output states, results in *activation of the renin-angiotensin system (RAS).* Vasoconstriction becomes more pronounced in response to angiotensin II, and aldosterone secretion causes sodium and water retention. Preload and afterload increase. Angiotensin II contributes to *ventricular remodeling* resulting in progressive myocyte (myocardial cell) contractile dysfunction over time (McCance et al., 2014).

In addition to the sympathetic nervous system and RAS responses, other mechanisms are activated when a patient experiences heart failure (HF). Most of these actions contribute to worsening of the condition.

For example, in those who have had an MI, heart muscle cell injury causes an *immune response.* Pro-inflammatory cytokines, such as tumor necrosis factor (TNF) and interleukins (IL-1 and

IL-6), are released, especially with left-sided HF. These substances contribute to ventricular remodeling.

Natriuretic peptides are neurohormones that work to promote vasodilation and diuresis through sodium loss in the renal tubules. The **B-type natriuretic peptide (BNP)** is produced and released by the ventricles when the patient has fluid overload as a result of HF. It increases with age and has a greater concentration in women (Jessup et al., 2009). People who are obese have lower BNP levels compared with those who are not (Clerico et al., 2012).

Low cardiac output (CO) causes decreased cerebral perfusion. As a result, the posterior pituitary gland secretes *vasopressin* (antidiuretic hormone [ADH]). The hormone causes vasoconstriction and fluid retention, which worsen HF.

Endothelin is secreted by endothelial cells when they are stretched. As the myocardial fibers are stretched in patients with HF, this potent vasoconstrictor is released, which increases peripheral resistance and hypertension. HF worsens as a result of these actions.

Myocardial hypertrophy (enlargement of the myocardium), with or without chamber dilation, is another compensatory mechanism. The walls of the heart thicken to provide more muscle mass, which results in more forceful contractions, further increasing cardiac output. Cardiac muscle, however, may hypertrophy more rapidly than collateral circulation can provide adequate blood supply to the muscle. Often a hypertrophied heart is slightly oxygen deprived.

All the compensatory mechanisms contribute to an increase in the consumption of myocardial oxygen. When the demand for oxygen increases and the myocardial reserve has been exhausted, clinical manifestations of HF develop.

Etiology

Heart failure (HF) is caused by systemic hypertension in most cases. Some patients experiencing myocardial infarction (MI, "heart attack") also develop HF. The next most common cause is structural heart changes, such as valvular dysfunction, particularly pulmonic or aortic stenosis, which leads to pressure or volume overload on the heart. Common direct causes and risk factors for HF are listed in Table 35-1.

CONSIDERATIONS FOR OLDER ADULTS

Patient-Centered Care QSEN

Heart failure is a common problem among older adults. The use of certain drugs can contribute to the development or exacerbation of the problem in this population. For example, long-term use of NSAIDs for arthritis and other chronic pain can cause fluid and sodium retention. NSAIDs may cause peripheral vasoconstriction and increase the toxicity of diuretics and angiotensin-converting enzyme inhibitors (ACEIs). Thiazolidinediones (TZDs) (e.g., pioglitazone [Actos]) used for diabetics also cause fluid and sodium retention. Rosiglitazone (Avandia), another TZD drug, has recently been found to cause acute myocardial infarction (AMI) in patients with type 2 diabetes. These drugs should be used with caution and restrictions in the older adult population.

Right-sided HF in the absence of left-sided HF is usually the result of pulmonary problems such as chronic obstructive pulmonary disease (COPD) or pulmonary hypertension. Acute respiratory distress syndrome (ARDS) may also cause right-sided HF. These problems are discussed elsewhere in this text.

TABLE 35-1   Common Causes and Risk Factors For Heart Failure

- Hypertension
- Coronary artery disease
- Cardiomyopathy
- Substance abuse (alcohol and illicit/prescribed drugs)
- Valvular disease
- Congenital defects
- Cardiac infections and inflammations
- Dysrhythmias
- Diabetes mellitus
- Smoking/tobacco use
- Family history
- Obesity
- Severe lung disease
- Sleep apnea
- Hyperkinetic conditions (e.g., hyperthyroidism)

TABLE 35-2   Meeting *Healthy People 2020* Objectives

Cardiac Disease

To reduce hospitalizations of older adults with heart failure as the principal diagnosis.

- For patients hospitalized for heart failure, collaborate with the case manager for discharge planning, including adequate support in the community.
- Provide a continuing plan of care for patients and their families or other caregivers when the patient is discharged from the hospital.
- If the patient is discharged to home, call to check that he or she has no impending signs and symptoms of heart failure (the case manager may make calls).
- Teach the patient and family or other caregiver about when to call the health care provider for health changes so the patient can be treated at home.
- Ensure that the interdisciplinary team provides the patient with follow-up care in the home or nursing home.

Incidence and Prevalence

Over five million people in the United States have HF, causing about 875,000 hospitalizations each year. HF is the most common reason for hospital admission for people older than 65 years. African Americans are affected more often than Euro-Americans, probably because they have more risk factors that can lead to HF (Go et al., 2013). The disease is a major cause of disability and death after MI, often due to nonadherence to the treatment plan and recommended lifestyle changes.

CONSIDERATIONS FOR OLDER ADULTS

Patient-Centered Care QSEN

Heart failure has been referred to as a U.S. epidemic, although it is a major problem worldwide. One of the U.S. *Healthy People 2020* objectives is to reduce the number of hospitalizations of older adults with HF as the principal diagnosis. Patient and family education can help meet this objective (Table 35-2). As the "baby boomer" population reaches 65 years of age, the numbers of hospital stays and deaths from HF are likely to increase dramatically.

❖ PATIENT-CENTERED COLLABORATIVE CARE

◆ Assessment

History. When obtaining a history, keep in mind the many conditions that can lead to HF. Carefully question the patient about his or her medical history, including hypertension, angina (cardiac pain), MI, rheumatic heart disease, valvular disorders, endocarditis, and pericarditis. Ask about the patient's perception of his or her activity tolerance, breathing pattern, sleeping pattern, urinary pattern, and fluid volume status, as well as his or her knowledge about HF.

Left-Sided Heart Failure. With left ventricular systolic dysfunction, cardiac output (CO) is diminished, leading to impaired tissue perfusion, anaerobic metabolism, and unusual fatigue. Assess activity tolerance by asking whether the patient can perform normal ADLs or climb flights of stairs without *fatigue* or dyspnea. Many patients with heart failure (HF) experience weakness or fatigue with activity or have a feeling of heaviness in their arms or legs. Ask about their ability to perform simultaneous arm and leg work (e.g., walking while carrying a bag of groceries). Such activity may place an unacceptable demand on the failing heart. Ask the patient to identify his or her most strenuous activity in the past week. Many people unconsciously limit their activities in response to fatigue or dyspnea and may not realize how limited they have become.

PERFUSION to the myocardium is often impaired as a result of left ventricular failure, especially with cardiac hypertrophy. The patient may report *chest discomfort* or may describe palpitations, skipped beats, or a fast heartbeat.

As the amount of blood ejected from the left ventricle diminishes, hydrostatic pressure builds in the pulmonary venous system and results in fluid-filled alveoli and pulmonary congestion, which results in a *cough*. The patient in early HF describes the cough as irritating, nocturnal (at night), and usually nonproductive. *As HF becomes very severe, he or she may begin expectorating frothy, pink-tinged sputum—a sign of life-threatening pulmonary edema.*

Dyspnea also results from increasing pulmonary venous pressure and pulmonary congestion. Carefully question about the presence of dyspnea and when and how it developed. The patient may refer to dyspnea as "trouble in catching my breath," "breathlessness," or "difficulty in breathing."

As **exertional dyspnea** develops (also called *dyspnea upon* or *on exertion [DUE/DOE]*), the patient often stops previously tolerated levels of activity because of shortness of breath. Dyspnea at rest in the recumbent (lying flat) position is known as **orthopnea**. Ask how many pillows are used to sleep or whether the patient sleeps in an upright position in a bed, recliner, or other type of chair.

Patients who describe sudden awakening with a feeling of breathlessness 2 to 5 hours after falling asleep have **paroxysmal nocturnal dyspnea (PND)**. Sitting upright, dangling the feet, or walking usually relieves this condition.

Right-Sided Heart Failure. Signs of systemic congestion occur as the right ventricle fails, fluid is retained, and pressure builds in the venous system. Edema develops in the lower legs and may progress to the thighs and abdominal wall. Patients may notice that their shoes fit more tightly, or their shoes or socks may leave indentations on their swollen feet. They may have removed their rings because of swelling in their fingers and hands. Ask about weight gain. An adult may retain 4 to 7 liters of fluid (10 to 15 lb [4.5 to 6.8 kg]) before pitting edema occurs.

Reports of *nausea and anorexia* may be a direct consequence of liver engorgement (congestion) resulting from fluid retention. In *advanced* heart failure (HF), *ascites* and an increased abdominal girth may develop from severe liver congestion. Another common finding related to fluid retention is *diuresis at rest*. At rest, fluid in the peripheral tissue is mobilized and excreted and the patient describes frequent awakening at night to urinate.

CHART 35-1   Key Features

Left-Sided Heart Failure

DECREASED CARDIAC OUTPUT	PULMONARY CONGESTION
• Fatigue	• Hacking cough, worse at night
• Weakness	• Dyspnea/breathlessness
• Oliguria during the day (nocturia at night)	• Crackles or wheezes in lungs
• Angina	• Frothy, pink-tinged sputum
• Confusion, restlessness	• Tachypnea
• Dizziness	• S_3/S_4 summation gallop
• Tachycardia, palpitations	
• Pallor	
• Weak peripheral pulses	
• Cool extremities	

CHART 35-2   Key Features

Right-Sided Heart Failure

Systemic Congestion

• Jugular (neck vein) distention	• Swollen hands and fingers
• Enlarged liver and spleen	• Polyuria at night
• Anorexia and nausea	• Weight gain
• Dependent edema (legs and sacrum)	• Increased blood pressure (from excess volume) or decreased blood pressure (from failure)
• Distended abdomen	

Obtain a careful nutritional history, questioning about the use of salt and the types of food consumed. Ask about daily fluid intake. Patients with HF may experience increased thirst and drink excessive fluid (4000 to 5000 mL/day) because of sodium retention.

Physical Assessment/Clinical Manifestations. Manifestations of HF depend on the type of failure, the ventricle involved, and the underlying cause. Impaired tissue perfusion, pulmonary congestion, and edema are associated with *left* ventricular failure (Chart 35-1). Conversely, systemic venous congestion and peripheral edema are associated with *right* ventricular failure (Chart 35-2).

Left-Sided Heart Failure. Left ventricular failure is associated with decreased cardiac output and elevated pulmonary venous pressure. It may appear clinically as:

- Weakness
- Fatigue
- Dizziness
- Acute confusion
- Pulmonary congestion
- Breathlessness
- Oliguria (scant urine output)

Decreased blood flow to the major body organs can cause dysfunction, especially renal failure. Nocturia may occur when the patient is at rest.

The pulse may be tachycardic, or it may alternate in strength (**pulsus alternans**). Take the apical pulse for a full minute, noting any irregularity in heart rhythm. *An irregular heart rhythm resulting from premature atrial contractions (PACs), premature ventricular contractions (PVCs), or atrial fibrillation (AF) is common in HF* (see Chapter 34). The sudden development of an irregular rhythm may further compromise CO. Carefully monitor the patient's respiratory rate, rhythm, and character, as well as oxygen saturation. The respiratory rate typically exceeds 20 breaths/min.

Assess whether the patient is oriented to person, place, and time. A short mental status examination may be used if there are concerns about orientation. Objective data are important because in daily conversation many people are skillful at covering up memory losses. Older adults are frequently disoriented or confused when the heart fails due to brain hypoxia (decreased oxygen).

Increased heart size is common with a displacement of the apical impulse to the left. A third heart sound, **S₃ gallop,** is an early diastolic filling sound indicating an increase in left ventricular pressure. This sound is often the first sign of HF. A fourth heart sound (S₄) also can occur; it is not a sign of failure but is a reflection of decreased ventricular compliance.

Auscultate for crackles and wheezes of the lungs. Late inspiratory crackles and fine profuse crackles that repeat themselves from breath to breath and do not diminish with coughing indicate HF. *Crackles are produced by intra-alveolar fluid and are often noted first in the bases of the lungs and spread upward as the condition worsens.* Wheezes indicate a narrowing of the bronchial lumen caused by engorged pulmonary vessels. Identify the precise location of crackles and wheezes and whether the wheezes are heard on inspiration, expiration, or both.

Right-Sided Heart Failure. Right ventricular failure is associated with increased systemic venous pressures and congestion. On inspection, assess the neck veins for distention and measure abdominal girth. Hepatomegaly (liver engorgement), hepatojugular reflux, and ascites may also be assessed. Abdominal fluid can reach volumes of more than 10 liters.

Assess for dependent edema. In ambulatory patients, edema commonly presents in the ankles and legs. When patients are restricted to bedrest, the sacrum is dependent and fluid accumulates there.

❗ NURSING SAFETY PRIORITY (QSEN)
Action Alert

Edema is an extremely unreliable sign of HF. Be sure that accurate daily weights are taken every morning to document fluid retention. *Weight is the most reliable indicator of fluid gain and loss!*

❓ NCLEX EXAMINATION CHALLENGE
Physiological Integrity

A client is diagnosed with left-sided heart failure. Which assessment findings will the nurse expect the client to have? **Select all that apply.**
A. Peripheral edema
B. Crackles in both lungs
C. Breathlessness
D. Ascites
E. Tachypnea

Psychosocial Assessment. Chronic heart failure (HF) is typically a slow, debilitating disease. Anxiety and frustration are common. Symptoms such as dyspnea increase the patient's anxiety level.

Patients with HF, especially those with advanced disease, are at high risk for depression. It is not certain whether the

functional impairments contribute to the depression or depression affects functional ability. Older hospitalized patients may be depressed, particularly those who have been re-admitted for an acute episode of HF. Lifestyle changes and quality-of-life issues can also cause depression many months after the initial diagnosis of HF.

Assess patients and their families for anxiety and depression. Ask them about their usual methods of coping, as well as any history of depression. If anxiety or depression is present, notify the health care provider for further assessment. Social workers, certified clinical chaplains, or psychologists may administer specific assessment tools to determine the extent of the problem. Some patients need drug therapy and nonpharmacologic modalities, such as cognitive behavior therapy, biofeedback, or relaxation training.

Hope is a major indicator of well-being for patients with HF. Those who are hopeful tend to feel better and are more socially involved. Ask patients about their daily activities and how often they interact with the significant people in their life to help determine patient and family coping strategies.

Laboratory Assessment. Electrolyte imbalance may occur from complications of HF or as side effects of drug therapy, especially diuretic therapy. Regular evaluations of a patient's *serum electrolytes,* including sodium, potassium, magnesium, calcium, and chloride, are essential. Any impairment of renal function resulting from inadequate perfusion causes elevated blood urea nitrogen and serum creatinine and decreased creatinine clearance levels. *Hemoglobin* and *hematocrit* tests should be performed to identify HF resulting from anemia. If the patient has fluid volume excess, the hematocrit levels may be low as a result of hemodilution.

B-type natriuretic peptide (BNP) is used for diagnosing HF (in particular, diastolic HF) in patients with acute dyspnea. As discussed earlier, it is part of the body's response to decreased cardiac output from either left or right ventricular dysfunction. An increase in BNP, in conjunction with history and physical, best differentiates between the dyspnea of HF and that associated with lung dysfunction (Fard et al., 2012). However, patients with renal disease may also have elevated BNP levels (Chen et al., 2010). In the ambulatory care arena, BNP is trended over time to guide ambulatory care treatment of heart failure (DeBeradinis & Januzzi, 2012); as therapy is optimized, levels decrease. If levels increase, alternate causes such as ischemia are looked at prior to intensifying treatment.

Urinalysis may reveal proteinuria and high specific gravity. *Microalbuminuria* is an early indicator of decreased compliance of the heart and occurs before the BNP rises. It serves as an "early warning detector" that lets the health care provider know that the heart is experiencing early signs of decreased compliance, long before symptoms occur.

CONSIDERATIONS FOR OLDER ADULTS
Patient-Centered Care (QSEN)

Thyroxine (T₄) and thyroid-stimulating hormone (TSH) levels should be assessed in patients who are older than 65 years, have atrial fibrillation, or have evidence of thyroid disease. Heart failure (HF) may be caused or aggravated by hypothyroidism or hyperthyroidism.

Arterial blood gas (ABG) values often reveal hypoxemia (low blood oxygen level) because oxygen does not diffuse easily through fluid-filled alveoli. Respiratory alkalosis may occur because of hyperventilation; respiratory acidosis may occur because of carbon dioxide retention. Metabolic acidosis may indicate an accumulation of lactic acid.

Imaging Assessment. *Chest x-rays* can be helpful in diagnosing left ventricular failure. Typically the heart is enlarged (cardiomegaly), representing hypertrophy or dilation. Pleural effusions develop less often and generally reflect biventricular failure. *Echocardiography is considered the best tool in diagnosing heart failure.* Cardiac valvular changes, pericardial effusion, chamber enlargement, and ventricular hypertrophy can be diagnosed using this noninvasive technique. The test can also be used to determine ejection fraction.

Radionuclide studies (thallium imaging or technetium pyrophosphate scanning) can also indicate the presence and cause of HF. Multigated acquisition (MUGA) scans, also called multigated blood pool scans, provide information about left ventricular ejection fraction and velocity, which are typically low in patients with HF. These tests are discussed in Chapter 33.

Other Diagnostic Assessment. An *electrocardiogram* (ECG) is also performed. It may show ventricular hypertrophy, dysrhythmias, and any degree of myocardial ischemia, injury, or infarction. However, it is *not* helpful in determining the presence or extent of HF.

Invasive hemodynamic monitoring allows the direct assessment of cardiac function and volume status in acutely ill patients. Although medical-surgical nurses do not manage these systems on general hospital units, they should be familiar with the interpretation of some of the major hemodynamic pressures as they relate to patient assessment. These measurements can confirm the diagnosis and guide the management of HF. For example, right atrial pressure is either normal or elevated in left ventricular failure and elevated in right ventricular failure. Pulmonary artery pressure (PAP) and pulmonary artery wedge pressure (PAWP) are elevated in left-sided HF because volumes and pressures are increased in the left ventricle. Hemodynamic monitoring is described in detail in Chapter 38.

◆ *Analysis*

The priority NANDA-I nursing diagnoses and collaborative problems for patients with heart failure (HF) include:

1. Impaired Gas Exchange related to ventilation/perfusion imbalance (NANDA-I)
2. Decreased Cardiac Output related to altered contractility, preload, and afterload (NANDA-I)
3. Fatigue related to hypoxemia (NANDA-I)
4. Potential for pulmonary edema related to left-sided HF

◆ *Planning and Implementation*

The patient-centered collaborative care that patients with HF need depends on their disease stage and severity of signs and symptoms. Be sure to individualize care based on the patient's values and preferences, your clinical expertise, and best current evidence.

Improving Gas Exchange

Planning: Expected Outcomes. The expected outcome is that the patient will have an optimal spontaneous breathing pattern that increases GAS EXCHANGE and oxygenation and maintains a serum carbon dioxide level that is within normal limits.

Interventions. The purpose of collaborative care is to help promote GAS EXCHANGE and oxygenation. *Ventilation assistance* may be needed because the oxygen content of the blood is often

---

TABLE 35-3 **Commonly Used Drug Classifications for Patients with Systolic Heart Failure**
Angiotensin-converting enzyme (ACE) inhibitors or angiotensin-receptor blockers (ARBs)
Diuretics:
• High-ceiling
• Potassium-sparing
Human B-type natriuretic peptides
Nitrates
Inotropics:
• Beta-adrenergic agonists
• Phosphodiesterase inhibitors
• Calcium sensitizers
• Digoxin (Lanoxin)
Beta-adrenergic blockers

---

decreased in patients who have pulmonary congestion. Monitor or have assistive personnel monitor the patient's respiratory rate, rhythm, and quality every 1 to 4 hours. Auscultate breath sounds every 4 to 8 hours.

! NURSING SAFETY PRIORITY (QSEN)

Action Alert

Provide the necessary amount of supplemental oxygen within a range prescribed by the health care provider *to maintain oxygen saturation at 90% or greater*. If the patient has dyspnea, place him or her in a high-Fowler's position with pillows under each arm to maximize chest expansion and improve oxygenation. Repositioning and performing coughing and deep-breathing exercises every 2 hours help improve oxygenation and prevent atelectasis. Collaborate with the respiratory therapist, if available, to plan the most effective methods for assisting with ventilation.

Improving Cardiac Output

Planning: Expected Outcomes. The expected outcome is that the patient will have increased cardiac output by improving stroke volume (SV) (determined by preload, afterload, and contractility) and heart rate (HR).

Interventions. Collaborative care begins with nonsurgical interventions, but the patient may need surgery if these are not successful in meeting optimal outcomes.

Nonsurgical Management. Nonsurgical management relies primarily on a variety of drugs (Table 35-3). If drug therapy is ineffective, other nonsurgical options are available. Drugs to improve stroke volume include those that reduce afterload, reduce preload, and improve cardiac muscle contractility. A major role of the nurse is to give medications as prescribed, monitor for their therapeutic and adverse effects, and teach the patient and family about drug therapy. A variety of classes of drugs that reduce afterload and preload are used to manage heart failure (see Table 35-3).

Drugs That Reduce Afterload. By relaxing the arterioles, arterial vasodilators can reduce the resistance to left ventricular ejection (afterload) and improve CO. These drugs do not cause excessive vasodilation but reverse some of the inappropriate or excessive vasoconstriction common in HF.

Angiotensin-Converting Enzyme Inhibitors (ACEIs) and Angiotensin-Receptor Blockers (ARBs). Patients with even mild heart failure (HF) resulting from left ventricular dysfunction are given a trial of ACE inhibitors or ARBs. Both ACE inhibitors (e.g., enalapril [Vasotec] and fosinopril [Monopril]) and ARBs (e.g., valsartan [Diovan], irbesartan [Avapro], and losartan [Cozaar]) improve function and quality of life for patients with HF. ACE inhibitors are the first-line drug of choice, but some health care providers prefer to start the patient on an ARB because ACE inhibitors can cause a nagging, dry cough. For patients with *acute* HF, the health care provider may prescribe an IV-push ACE inhibitor such as Vasotec IV.

The ACE inhibitors and ARBs suppress the renin-angiotensin system (RAS), which is activated in response to decreased renal blood flow. ACE inhibitors prevent conversion of angiotensin I to angiotensin II, resulting in arterial dilation and increased stroke volume. ARBs block the effect of angiotensin II receptors and thus decrease arterial resistance and arterial dilation. In addition, these drugs block aldosterone, which prevents sodium and water retention, thus decreasing fluid overload. *Both ACEIs and ARBs work more effectively for Euro-Americans than for African-American populations.* Volume-depleted patients should receive a low starting dose, or the fluid volume should be restored before beginning the prescribed drug. Monitor for hyperkalemia, a potential adverse drug effect in patients who have renal dysfunction.

> ### ! NURSING SAFETY PRIORITY (QSEN)
> #### Drug Alert
>
> ACEIs and ARBs are started slowly and cautiously. The first dose may be associated with a rapid drop in blood pressure (BP). Patients at risk for hypotension usually have an initial systolic BP less than 100 mm Hg, are older than 75 years, have a serum sodium level less than 135 mEq/L, or are volume depleted. Monitor BP every hour for several hours after the initial dose and each time the dose is increased. Immediately report to the health care provider and document a systolic blood pressure of less than 90 mm Hg (or designated protocol level). If this problem occurs, place the patient flat and elevate legs to increase cerebral perfusion and promote venous return.

Assess for orthostatic hypotension, acute confusion, poor peripheral perfusion, and reduced urine output in patients with low systolic blood pressure. Monitor serum potassium and creatinine levels to determine renal dysfunction. Additional nursing implications for selected ACE inhibitor/ARB drugs are described in Chapter 38 on p. 766 in the Drug Therapy section.

Human B-type Natriuretic Peptides. Human B-type natriuretic peptides (hBNPs) such as nesiritide (Natrecor) are often used to treat *acute* HF. Endogenous BNP is released in response to decreased CO and causes *natriuresis,* or loss of sodium in the renal tubules, as well as vasodilation. Natrecor lowers pulmonary capillary wedge pressure (PCWP) and improves renal glomerular filtration. It is given as an IV bolus over 60 seconds followed with a continuous infusion for up to 48 hours.

> ### ! NURSING SAFETY PRIORITY (QSEN)
> #### Drug Alert
>
> When giving Natrecor, monitor BP and pulse carefully because significant decreases in BP may occur. Although the patient's systolic BP may be between 90 and 100 mm Hg, he or she is usually asymptomatic. *Give Natrecor through a separate infusion line because it is incompatible with heparin and most other parenteral medications.* Expect an increase in the serum BNP after drug administration.

Interventions That Reduce Preload. Ventricular fibers contract less forcefully when they are overstretched, such as in a failing heart. Interventions aimed at reducing preload attempt to decrease volume and pressure in the left ventricle, increasing ventricular muscle stretch and contraction. Preload reduction is appropriate for HF accompanied by congestion with total body sodium and water overload.

Nutrition Therapy. In HF, nutrition therapy is aimed at reducing sodium and water retention to decrease the workload of the heart. The primary care provider may restrict sodium intake in an attempt to decrease fluid retention. Many patients need to omit table salt (no added salt) from their diet, thus reducing sodium intake to about 3 g daily.

If salt intake must be reduced further, the patient may need to eliminate all salt in cooking and high-sodium foods (e.g., ham, bacon, pickles), thus reducing sodium intake to 2 g daily. If needed, collaborate with the dietitian to help the patient select foods that meet such a restricted therapeutic diet.

Few patients are placed on severe fluid restrictions. However, patients with excessive aldosterone secretion may experience thirst and drink 3 to 5 liters of fluid each day. As a result, their fluid intake may be limited to a more normal 2 liters daily. *Supervise unlicensed assistive personnel (UAP) to ensure that they limit the prescribed intake and accurately record intake and output.*

Weigh the patient daily, or delegate this activity to UAP and supervise that it is done. Keep in mind that *1 kg of weight gain or loss equals 1 liter of retained or lost fluid.* The same scale should be used every morning before breakfast for the most accurate assessment of weight. Monitor for an expected *decrease* in weight because excess fluid is excreted from the body.

Drug Therapy. Common drugs prescribed to reduce preload are diuretics and venous vasodilators. *Morphine sulfate* is also given for patients in *acute* heart failure to reduce anxiety, decrease preload and afterload, slow respirations, and reduce the pain associated with a myocardial infarction (MI).

The health care provider adds *diuretics* to the regimen when diet and fluid restrictions have not been effective in managing the symptoms of HF. Diuretics are the first-line drug of choice in older adults with HF and fluid overload. These drugs enhance the renal excretion of sodium and water by reducing circulating blood volume, decreasing preload, and reducing systemic and pulmonary congestion.

The type and dosage of diuretic prescribed depend on the severity of HF and renal function. High-ceiling (loop) diuretics, such as furosemide (Lasix, Furoside ✦, Novosemide ✦), torsemide (Demadex), and bumetanide (Bumex), are most effective for treating fluid volume overload.

> ### CONSIDERATIONS FOR OLDER ADULTS
> #### Patient-Centered Care (QSEN)
>
> Loop diuretics continue to work even after excess fluid is removed. As a result, some patients, especially older adults, can become dehydrated. Observe for manifestations of dehydration in the older adult, especially acute confusion, decreased urinary output, and dizziness. Provide evidence-based interventions to reduce the risk for falls, as discussed in Chapter 2.

For those patients with *acute* HF, Lasix or Bumex can be administered by IV push (IVP). Lasix can be given in doses of 20 to 40 mg IVP and increased by 20 mg every 2 hours until the desired diuresis is obtained. The usual IVP initial dose for Bumex is 1 to 2 mg once or twice daily, but it is more often given in a continuous infusion of 10 mg over 24 hours.

The practitioner may initially use a thiazide diuretic, such as hydrochlorothiazide (HCTZ) (HydroDIURIL, Urozide ✦) and metolazone (Zaroxolyn), for *older adults* with *mild* volume overload. Zaroxolyn is a long-acting agent and is therefore often given every second, third, or fourth day, depending on patient need and tolerance.

Unlike loop diuretics, the action of thiazides is self-limiting (i.e., diuresis decreases after edema fluid is lost). Therefore the dehydration that may occur with loop diuretics is not common with these drugs. Patients also prefer thiazides because of the gradual onset of diuresis.

As HF progresses, many patients develop diuretic resistance with refractory edema. The health care provider may choose to manage this problem by prescribing both types of diuretics. Other strategies include IV continuous infusion of furosemide or bumetanide or rotating loop diuretics.

Monitor for and prevent potassium deficiency (hypokalemia) from diuretic therapy. The primary signs of hypokalemia are nonspecific neurologic and muscular symptoms, such as generalized weakness, depressed reflexes, and irregular heart rate. A potassium supplement may be prescribed for some patients. Other practitioners prescribe a potassium-sparing diuretic, such as spironolactone (Aldactone), for patients at risk for dysrhythmias from hypokalemia. Although not as effective as other diuretics, Aldactone helps retain potassium and thus decrease the risk for ventricular dysrhythmias and is usually used in stage III/IV heart failure. Monitor for hyperkalemia and renal failure if Aldactone inhibitors are utilized, and anticipate stopping the medication if potassium or creatinine levels rise.

Patients being managed with ACE inhibitors or ARBs and diuretics at the same time may not experience hypokalemia. However, if their kidneys are not functioning well, they may develop hyperkalemia (elevated serum potassium level). Review the patient's serum creatinine level. *If the creatinine is greater than 1.8 mg/dL, notify the health care provider before administering supplemental potassium.*

The health care provider may prescribe *venous vasodilators* (e.g., nitrates) for the patient with HF who has persistent dyspnea. Significant constriction of venous and arterial blood vessels occurs to compensate for reduced CO. Constriction reduces the volume of fluid that the vascular bed can hold and increases preload. Venous vasodilators may benefit by:

- Returning venous vasculature to a more normal capacity
- Decreasing the volume of blood returning to the heart
- Improving left ventricular function

Nitrates may be administered IV, orally, or topically. IV nitrates are used most often for *acute* HF. These drugs cause primarily venous vasodilation but also a significant amount of arteriolar vasodilation. Monitor the patient's blood pressure when starting nitrate therapy or increasing the dosage. Patients may initially report headache, but assure them that they will develop a tolerance to this effect and that the headache will cease or diminish. Acetaminophen (Tylenol, Exdol ✦) can be given to help relieve discomfort.

Unfortunately, tolerance to the vasodilating effects develops when nitrates are given around-the-clock. To prevent this tolerance, the health care provider may prescribe at least one 12-hour nitrate-free period out of every 24 hours (usually overnight).

Nitrates such as isosorbide (Imdur, ISMO) are prescribed to provide nitrate-free periods and reduce the problem of tolerance. Chapter 38 discusses nitrates in more detail.

Drugs That Enhance Contractility. Contractility of the heart can also be enhanced with drug therapy. Positive inotropic drugs are most commonly used, but vasodilators and beta-adrenergic blockers may also be administered. For *chronic* HF, low-dose beta blockers are most commonly used. Digoxin (Lanoxin) may be prescribed to improve symptoms, thereby decreasing dyspnea and improving functional activity. This older and long-used drug is not expensive. In some settings, nesiritide (Natrecor) may be administered for end-stage HF, although this drug is very expensive (see discussion of Natrecor for acute HF on p. 685).

Digoxin. Although not as commonly used today, digoxin (Lanoxin, Novodigoxin ✦), a cardiac glycoside, has been demonstrated to provide symptomatic benefits for patients in *chronic* heart failure (HF) with sinus rhythm and atrial fibrillation. Digoxin (sometimes called "dig") therapy reduces exacerbations of HF and hospitalizations when added to a regimen of ACE inhibitors or ARBs, beta blockers, and diuretics. However, it may increase mortality due to drug toxicity, especially in older adults.

The potential benefits of digoxin include:

- Increased contractility
- Reduced heart rate (HR)
- Slowing of conduction through the atrioventricular node
- Inhibition of sympathetic activity while enhancing parasympathetic activity

Digoxin is erratically absorbed from the GI tract. Many drugs, especially antacids, interfere with its absorption. It is eliminated primarily by renal excretion. Older patients should be maintained on lower doses of the drug than younger patients.

Other Inotropic Drugs. Patients experiencing *acute* heart failure are candidates for IV drugs that increase contractility. For example, *beta-adrenergic agonists,* such as dobutamine (Dobutrex), are used for short-term treatment of *acute* episodes of HF. Dobutamine improves cardiac contractility and thus cardiac output and myocardial-systemic perfusion.

A more potent drug used for *acute* HF, milrinone (Primacor), functions as a vasodilator/inotropic medication with phosphodiesterase activity. Also known as a *phosphodiesterase inhibitor,* this drug increases cyclic adenosine monophosphate (cAMP), which enhances the entry of calcium into myocardial cells to increase contractile function. Like the beta-adrenergic agonists, Primacor is given IV.

Levosimendan (Simdax) is a calcium-sensitizing medication and a positive inotropic drug. It appears to bind to troponin C in the heart muscle and therefore increases the contraction of the heart. Simdax is used most often in patients who have had

! NURSING SAFETY PRIORITY (QSEN)

Drug Alert

Increased cardiac automaticity occurs with toxic digoxin levels or in the presence of hypokalemia, resulting in ectopic beats (e.g., premature ventricular contractions [PVCs]). Changes in potassium level, especially a decrease, cause patients to be more sensitive to the drug and cause toxicity.

The clinical manifestations of **digoxin toxicity** are often vague and nonspecific and include anorexia, fatigue, blurred vision, and changes in mental status, especially in older adults. Toxicity may cause nearly any dysrhythmia, but PVCs are most commonly noted. Assess for early signs of toxicity such as bradycardia and loss of the P wave on the ECG. Carefully monitor the apical pulse rate and heart rhythm of patients receiving digoxin.

The health care provider determines the desirable heart rate (HR) to achieve. Some health care providers prefer a rate between 50 and 60 beats per minute. Report the development of either an irregular rhythm in a patient with a previously regular rhythm or a regular rhythm in a patient with a previously irregular one. Monitor serum digoxin and potassium levels (hypokalemia potentiates digoxin toxicity) to identify toxicity. Older adults are more likely than other patients to become toxic because of decreased renal excretion.

Any drug that increases the workload of the failing heart also increases its oxygen requirement. Be alert for the possibility that the patient may experience angina (chest pain) in response to digoxin.

? NCLEX EXAMINATION CHALLENGE

Physiological Integrity

An older adult taking digoxin and hydrochlorothiazide (HCTZ) for chronic heart failure is admitted to the emergency department (ED) with an apical pulse of 48. A family member states that the client has reported blurred vision and loss of appetite for 2 weeks. What is the nurse's first action?

A. Call the ED physician immediately.
B. Draw a serum digoxin level.
C. Assess for signs of hypokalemia.
D. Establish the client's airway.

or are at high risk for myocardial infarction. Chapter 38 discusses inotropic drugs in more detail.

Beta-Adrenergic Blockers. Beta-adrenergic blockers (commonly referred to as "beta blockers") improve the condition of some patients in HF. Prolonged exposure to increased levels of sympathetic stimulation and catecholamines worsens cardiac function. Beta-adrenergic blockade reverses this effect, improving morbidity, mortality, and quality of life for patients in HF.

Beta blockers must be started slowly for HF. *Patients in acute HF should not be started on these drugs.* Carvedilol (Coreg), metoprolol succinate (Toprol XL), and bisoprolol (Zebeta) are approved for treatment of *chronic* HF. ***Do not confuse metoprolol tartrate with metoprolol succinate.*** Current guidelines only recommend the sustained-release formulation of metoprolol for chronic HF treatment. The first dose is extremely low. Monitor the patient either in the hospital or in the health care provider's office to assess for bradycardia or hypotension after the first dose is given.

Instruct the patient to weigh daily and to report any signs of worsening HF immediately. The health care provider gradually increases the drug dose if HF worsens. The patient is evaluated at least weekly for changes in BP, pulse, activity tolerance, and orthopnea. A modest drop in BP is acceptable if he or she

remains asymptomatic and can stand without experiencing dizziness or a further drop in BP. The resting heart rate (HR) should remain between 55 and 60 and increase slightly with exercise. Activity tolerance improves, and less orthopnea is experienced. Most patients with mild and moderate HF demonstrate improved ejection fraction, decreased hospital admissions, and improvement in symptoms when beta blockers are added to their treatment regimens. The benefits of this therapy are seen over a long period rather than immediately.

For patients with *diastolic* HF, drug therapy has not been as effective. Calcium channel blockers, ACE inhibitors, and beta blockers have been used with various degrees of success.

Other Nonsurgical Options. In addition to drug therapy, other nonsurgical options, both noninvasive and invasive, may be used and include:

- Continuous positive airway pressure (CPAP)
- Cardiac resynchronization therapy (CRT)
- Investigative gene therapy

Continuous positive airway pressure (CPAP) is a respiratory treatment that improves obstructive sleep apnea in patients with HF. It also improves cardiac output (CO) and ejection fraction (EF) by decreasing afterload and preload, blood pressure (BP), and dysrhythmias. Sleep apnea is directly correlated with coronary artery disease as a result of diminished oxygen supply to the heart during apneic episodes. This respiratory problem is discussed in detail in Chapter 29.

Cardiac resynchronization therapy (CRT), also called *biventricular pacing*, uses a permanent pacemaker alone or is combined with an implantable cardioverter/defibrillator. Electrical stimulation causes more synchronous ventricular contractions to improve EF, CO, and mean arterial pressure. This modality is indicated for patients with class III or IV HF and an EF of less than 35%. CRT improves the patient's ability to perform ADLs. Chapter 34 discusses pacing in more detail.

Gene therapy may be indicated for patients in end-stage HF who are not candidates for heart transplantation. This therapy replaces damaged genes with normal or modified genes by a series of injections of growth factor into the left ventricle. Although still investigative, this therapy may result in improved exercise tolerance and regrowth of cardiac cells.

Surgical Management. Heart transplantation is still the ultimate choice for end-stage HF (see discussion on p. 702). Several surgical procedures are available to improve CO in patients who are *not* candidates for a transplant or are awaiting transplant.

Ventricular Assist Devices. Patients with debilitating end-stage heart failure are often sent home on drug therapy and referred to hospice. However, ventricular assist devices (VADs) can dramatically improve the lives of many patients. In this procedure, a mechanical pump is implanted to work with the patient's own heart (Fig. 35-2). Both left and right VADs are available, depending on the type of heart failure the patient has. Those with end-stage kidney disease, severe chronic lung disease, clotting disorders, and infections that do not respond to antibiotics are not candidates for this surgery. Postoperative complications include bleeding, infective endocarditis, ventricular dysrhythmias, and stroke. Nursing care is similar to that described for cardiac surgery in Chapter 38.

Ventricular assist devices can be used short-term while awaiting heart transplantation (a "bridge-to-transplant" procedure) or long-term (destination therapy). Most patients survive with a VAD until a transplant is available. The evidence shows

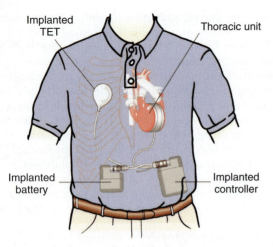

FIG. 35-2 The AbioCor Implantable Replacement Heart has four main parts that are placed inside the body. *TET,* Transtelephonic electrocardiographic transmission device.

Labels on figure: Implanted TET; Thoracic unit; Implanted battery; Implanted controller

that patients who have long-term devices live longer and have an improved quality of life (Rogers et al., 2010).

Other Surgical Therapies. Heart failure causes ventricular remodeling, or dilation, which worsens as the disease progresses. Several new therapies are used to reshape the left ventricle in patients with HF. Perioperative care is similar to that for the patient having a coronary artery bypass graft (CABG) (see Chapter 38). The most common ventricular reconstructive procedures include:

- Partial left ventriculectomy (PLV)
- Endoventricular circular patch cardioplasty
- Acorn cardiac support device
- Myosplint

Also known as *heart reduction surgery,* PLV (sometimes referred to as the *Batista procedure*) involves removing a triangle-shaped section of the weakened heart in the left lateral ventricle to reduce the ventricle's diameter and decrease wall tension. In *endoventricular circular patch cardioplasty,* the surgeon removes portions of the cardiac septum and left ventricular wall and grafts a circular patch (synthetic or autologous) into the opening. This procedure provides a more normal shape to the left ventricle to improve the heart's ejection fraction (EF) and cardiac output (CO).

The Acorn cardiac support device is a polyester mesh jacket that is placed over the ventricles to provide support and to avoid overstretching the myocardial muscle. The material for the jacket has been used for other procedures, such as vascular grafts. The jacket appears to reduce hypertrophy of the heart muscle and assists with improvement of the EF.

The Myosplint has recently been approved for use in the United States. Electrical stimulation of several tension pads (splints) on the outside of the ventricle changes it to a more normal shape to improve function.

Decreasing Fatigue

Planning: Expected Outcomes. The expected outcome is that the patient will have decreased fatigue and will gain energy as heart failure improves.

Interventions. The patient in severe heart failure initially requires physical and emotional rest for *energy management.* On the first day of hospitalization, he or she may sit up in a chair for meals and perform basic leg exercises while out of bed. Organize nursing care to allow periods of rest. Collaborate with

the interdisciplinary team to observe and document the patient's physiologic response to activity.

As the patient's condition improves, the physical therapist (PT) starts ambulation, usually on hospital day 2. The PT or nurse checks the BP, pulse, and oxygen saturation before and after the activity. A BP change of more than 20 mm Hg or a pulse increase of more than 20 beats per minute may indicate that the activity is too stressful. Other indications of activity intolerance include dyspnea, fatigue, and chest pain. Ask a patient having any of these symptoms to rate how hard he or she has been working on a scale of 1 to 20, with 20 being the maximum perceived exertion. If the patient rates the exertion more than 12, remind him or her to slow down. If activity is tolerated, the PT steadily increases the activity level until the patient is ambulating 200 to 400 feet several times per day.

If the patient is able, the PT (or assistive nursing or PT personnel) might time him or her for 6 minutes while walking at a comfortable pace. The distance the patient can walk can be used to determine his or her functional level and activity plan.

Preventing or Managing Pulmonary Edema

Planning: Expected Outcomes. The most desirable outcome is that the patient will not develop pulmonary edema as a result of heart failure (HF). However, if the patient progresses to pulmonary edema, the expected outcome is that he or she will recover from this complication without other problems.

Interventions. Monitor for manifestations of acute pulmonary edema, a life-threatening event that can result from severe HF (with fluid overload), acute myocardial infarction (MI), mitral valve disease, and possibly dysrhythmias. In pulmonary edema, the left ventricle fails to eject sufficient blood and pressure increases in the lungs as a result. The increased pressure causes fluid to leak across the pulmonary capillaries and into the lung airways and tissues.

! NURSING SAFETY PRIORITY (QSEN)

Critical Rescue

Assess for and report early manifestations, such as crackles in the lung bases, dyspnea at rest, disorientation, and confusion, especially in older patients. Document the precise location of the crackles because the level of the fluid progresses from the bases to higher levels in the lungs when the condition worsens. The patient in acute pulmonary edema is also typically extremely anxious, tachycardic, and struggling for air. As pulmonary edema becomes more severe, he or she may have a moist cough productive of frothy, blood-tinged sputum and his or her skin may be cold, clammy, or cyanotic. Chart 35-3 lists the major clinical manifestations of this complication.

CHART 35-3   Key Features

Pulmonary Edema

- Crackles
- Dyspnea at rest
- Disorientation or acute confusion (especially in older adults as early symptom)
- Tachycardia
- Hypertension or hypotension
- Reduced urinary output
- Cough with frothy, pink-tinged sputum
- Premature ventricular contractions and other dysrhythmias
- Anxiety
- Restlessness
- Lethargy

The patient diagnosed with pulmonary edema is admitted to the acute care hospital, often in a critical care unit. Reassure the patient and family that his or her distress will decrease with proper management.

! NURSING SAFETY PRIORITY (QSEN)

Critical Rescue

If the patient is not hypotensive, place him or her in a sitting (high-Fowler's) position with his or her legs down to decrease venous return to the heart. The *priority nursing action* is to administer high-flow oxygen therapy at 5 to 6 L/min by facemask or at 10 to 15 L/min by non-rebreather mask with reservoir (which may deliver up to 100% oxygen) to promote GAS EXCHANGE and PERFUSION. Apply a pulse oximeter, and titrate the oxygen flow to keep the patient's oxygen saturation above 90%. If supplemental oxygen does not resolve the patient's respiratory distress, collaborate with the respiratory therapist, physician, advanced practice nurse, or physician assistant for more aggressive therapy, such as continuous positive airway pressure (CPAP) or bi-level positive airway pressure (BiPAP) ventilation. Intubation and mechanical ventilation may be needed for some patients.

If the patient's systolic blood pressure is above 100, give sublingual nitroglycerin (NTG) to decrease afterload and preload every 5 minutes for three doses while establishing IV access for additional drug therapy. The health care provider prescribes rapid-acting diuretics, such as Lasix or Bumex. Give Lasix IV push (IVP) over 1 to 2 minutes, usually at a starting dose of 20 to 40 mg for diuretic-naive patients, and another 40 mg if needed in 30 minutes. Patients already on oral diuretic therapy should be given an amount that is the same or doubled in milligrams as initial IV diuretic therapy. Administer each increment of 40 mg of Lasix over 1 to 2 minutes to avoid oto-toxicity. Bumex may be administered 1 to 2 mg IVP or as a continuous infusion to provide consistent fluid removal over 24 hours. Monitor vital signs frequently, at least every 30 to 60 minutes.

If the patient's blood pressure is adequate, IV morphine sulfate may be prescribed, 1 to 2 mg at a time, to reduce venous return (preload), decrease anxiety, and reduce the work of breathing. Monitor respiratory rate and BP closely. Other drugs, such as IV NTG and drugs to treat HF, may be administered. Monitor the patient's vital signs closely (especially BP) while these drugs are being given.

In severe cases of fluid overload and renal dysfunction or diuretic resistance, ultrafiltration may be used. The benefits of ultrafiltration include:
- Decrease in cardiac filling pressures
- Decrease in pulmonary arterial pressure
- Increase in cardiac index
- Reduction in norepinephrine, rennin, and aldosterone

Ultrafiltration can remove up to 500 mL/hr and uses a blood flow rate of 10 to 40 mL/hr. Peripheral lines are used for IV access. See Chapter 68 for discussion of this procedure and nursing implications.

Community-Based Care

Patients who are not adequately prepared for discharge or do not have adequate community support and follow-up for self-management are at high risk for repeated hospital admissions for heart failure. Collaborate with the case manager or care coordinator to assess the patient's needs for health care resources.

? CLINICAL JUDGMENT CHALLENGE

Safety; Patient-Centered Care; Evidence-Based Practice; Informatics (QSEN)

A 71-year-old man is admitted to the telemetry unit with right-sided heart failure, type 2 diabetes mellitus, hypertension, and COPD. He is married but has no children. During your assessment, you observe that his color is pale, he is dyspneic, and he reports new onset of chest discomfort. Even though he has oxygen via nasal cannula at 2 L/min., you note that he seems a little confused and is oriented only to person. His oxygen saturation has decreased from 95% to 88%.
1. What lung sounds do you expect to hear and why?
2. What evidence-based actions will you plan to implement at this time based on your observations? What is the source of the evidence?
3. The patient's physician prescribes an initial dose of furosemide (Lasix) 40 mg IVP. What assessments will you perform to determine if the drug was effective?
4. What will you tell the patient's wife about his condition at this time? Should the patient's wife be present during his emergency treatment? Why or why not?
5. After two doses of Lasix, the patient's condition improves. What data will you document in the electronic medical record (EMR)?

The Heart Failure Core Measure Set must be determined for hospitals accredited by The Joint Commission. These measures include that the patient with heart failure has:
- Discharge instructions (including information on diet, activity, medications, weight monitor, and plan for worsening symptoms)
- Evaluation of left ventricular systolic function
- An ACEI or ARB for left ventricular systolic dysfunction
- Adult smoking-cessation advice/counseling (if appropriate)

An inability to obtain help in activities such as food shopping and obtaining medications is a major contributor to hospital readmission. If home support is available, the patient may be discharged home in the care of a family member or other caregiver. Home care nurses may direct the care and assess for adherence to the discharge plan; home health aides may provide assistance with ADLs for a short time. If the patient has multiple health problems or has been severely compromised by heart disease, he or she may require admission to a skilled unit for either transitional or long-term care.

Home Care Management. The focus of the home care nurse's interventions is assessment and health teaching, which are reimbursable by Medicare and other third-party payers. Chart 35-4 lists the major areas of home health assessment.

Patients with chronic HF need to make many adjustments in their lifestyles. They must adhere to the collaborative plan of care that includes dietary restrictions, activity, prescriptions, and drug therapy. They need careful, concise explanations of the self-management plan. The community-based nurse in any setting encourages the patient to verbalize fears and concerns about his or her illness and assists in exploring coping skills. Patient participation in self-management can help alleviate and control symptoms.

Self-Management Education. Health teaching is essential for promoting self-management (also called *self-care*). Many patients are re-admitted to hospitals because they do not maintain their prescribed treatment plan, including lifestyle changes. Because of the need for extensive discharge instructions, most

CHART 35-4 Home Care Assessment

The Patient with Heart Failure

Assess for signs of heart failure, including:
- Changes in vital signs (heart rate >100 beats/min at rest, new atrial fibrillation, blood pressure <90 or >150 systolic)
- Indications of poor tissue perfusion:
  - Fatigue
  - Angina
  - Activity intolerance
  - Changes in mental status
  - Pallor or cyanosis
  - Cool extremities
- Indications of congestion:
  - Presence of cough or dyspnea
  - Weight gain
  - Jugular venous distention and peripheral edema

Assess functional ability, including:
- Performance of ADLs
- Mobility and ambulation (review frequency and duration of walking, development of symptoms, and pulse rate)
- Cognitive ability

Assess nutritional status, including:
- Food and fluid intake
- Intake of sodium-rich foods
- Alcohol consumption
- Skin turgor

Assess home environment, including:
- Safety hazards, especially related to oxygen therapy
- Structural barriers affecting functional ability
- Social support (family, home health services)

Assess the patient's adherence and understanding of illness and its treatment, including:
- Signs and symptoms to report to health care provider
- Dosages, effects, and side or toxic effects of medications
- When to report for laboratory and health care provider visits
- Ability to accurately weigh self on scale
- Presence of advance directive
- Use of home oxygen, if appropriate

Assess patient and caregiver coping skills

TABLE 35-4 Heart Failure Self-Management Health Teaching (MAWDS)

Medications:
- Take medications as prescribed, and do not run out.
- Know the purpose and side effects of each drug.
- Avoid NSAIDs to prevent sodium and fluid retention.

Activity:
- Stay as active as possible, but don't overdo it.
- Know your limits.
- Be able to carry on a conversation while exercising.

Weight:
- Weigh each day at the same time on the same scale to monitor for fluid retention.

Diet:
- Limit daily sodium intake to 2 to 3 grams as prescribed.
- Limit daily fluid intake to 2 liters.

Symptoms:
- Note any new or worsening symptoms, and notify the health care provider immediately.

EVIDENCE-BASED PRACTICE QSEN

What is the Most Effective Education Method to Provide Heart Failure Education to Heart Failure Patients?

Boyde, M., Turner, C., Thompson, D., & Stewart, S. (2011). Educational interventions for patients with heart failure: A systematic review of randomized controlled trials. *Journal of Cardiovascular Nursing, 26*(4), E27-E35.

The purpose of this meta-analysis research was to determine the most effective educational interventions provided by nurses to improve outcomes of the heart failure population. Randomized control trials from CINAHL, MEDLINE, PsycINFO, EMBASE, and Cochrane between the years 1998 and 2008 were identified. A total of 1515 abstracts were reviewed by two independent reviewers, and a total of 19 met inclusion criteria. To be included, studies needed to have evaluation of a specific education intervention or learning activity. Interventions studied included one-on-one didactic education, video, interactive CDs, TV programs, and mailings. Although it is acknowledged that patients have different learning styles, only four studies provided learning needs assessment. The ultimate goal was not only to improve the knowledge base but also to change patient behavior and improve outcomes. Of the 19 studies, 8 evaluated self-care in which 7 showed significant improvements in self-care after intervention. Re-admission rates were evaluated in 13 studies; 4 showed decreased rates of admission, and 3 showed decreased death rates. Various outcomes were measured, and 15 studies were able to demonstrate statistically significant changes in outcomes related to the education initiative.

Level of Evidence: 1
The researchers used a systematic review of randomized controlled trials.

Commentary: Implications for Practice and Research
Gaining knowledge does not equate to a change in behavior and, therefore, improved outcomes. To impart knowledge, a learning needs assessment must be performed before tailoring an education program for the patient. It is not enough to measure the amount of knowledge transmitted; changes in behavior and outcomes need to be the endpoint of studies related to nursing education.

hospitals are using teaching packets with videos, CDs, and easy-to-read information about the importance of adhering to specific self-management strategies at home. One standardized and commonly used self-management plan called *MAWDS* is outlined in Table 35-4. Medication reconciliation is also important to be sure that similar drugs are not being prescribed and that patients meet the Core Measure requirements for HF. It is important to perform a learning needs assessment and tailor education to the patient's particular need to see changes in behavior and improved outcomes (see the Evidence-Based Practice box).

Ambulatory care clinics for heart failure patients are also becoming increasingly common. Their purpose is to offer assessments, drug therapy, and health teaching. Some nurses specialize in caring for patients with health failure.

Activity Schedule. Encourage patients with heart failure to stay as active as possible and to develop a regular exercise regimen (e.g., home walking program). However, teach the patient not to overdo it. Medicare and third-party payers typically do not reimburse for cardiac rehabilitation for HF. Paying for a cardiac rehabilitation program out of pocket is expensive.

Remind patients with persistent crackles and uncontrolled edema to begin exercise after their condition stabilizes. When exercise is indicated, teach the patient to begin walking 200 to 400 feet per day. At home the patient should try to walk at least 3 times a week and should slowly increase the amount of time walked over several months. If chest pain or severe dyspnea occurs while exercising or the patient has fatigue the next day, he or she is probably advancing the activity too quickly and

---

CHART 35-5 Patient and Family Education: Preparing for Self-Management

Beta Blocker/Digoxin Therapy

- Establish same time of day to take this medication every day.
- Continue taking this medication unless your health care provider tells you to stop.
- Do not take digoxin at the same time as antacids or cathartics (laxatives).
- Take your pulse rate before taking each dose of digoxin. Notify your health care provider of a change in pulse rate (60 to 100 beats/min is typically normal, depending on your baseline pulse rate) or rhythm, as well as increasing fatigue, muscle weakness, confusion, or loss of appetite (signs of digoxin toxicity).
- If you forget to take a dose, it may be delayed a few hours. However, if you do not remember it until the next day, you should take only your usual daily dose.
- Report for scheduled laboratory tests (e.g., potassium and digoxin levels).
- If potassium supplements are prescribed, continue the dose until told to stop by your health care provider.

---

should slow down. Encourage him or her to keep a diary that documents the time and duration of each exercise session, as well as HR and any symptoms that occur with exercise.

Indications of Worsening or Recurrent Heart Failure. Many patients who are re-admitted to hospitals for treatment of HF fail to seek medical attention promptly when symptoms recur.

⚠ NURSING SAFETY PRIORITY (QSEN)

Action Alert

Per the HF Core Measure for discharge instructions, teach the patient and caregiver to immediately report to the health care provider the occurrence of *any* of these symptoms, which could indicate worsening or recurrent heart failure:
- Rapid weight gain (3 lb in a week or 1 to 2 lb overnight)
- Decrease in exercise tolerance lasting 2 to 3 days
- Cold symptoms (cough) lasting more than 3 to 5 days
- Excessive awakening at night to urinate
- Development of dyspnea or angina at rest or worsening angina
- Increased swelling in the feet, ankles, or hands

Drug Therapy. Provide oral, written, and video instructions about the drug regimen. Teach the caregiver and patient how to count a pulse rate, especially if the patient is on digoxin or beta blockers. Chart 35-5 lists instructions for the patient taking either of these drugs at home.

Advise the patient taking diuretics to take them in the morning to avoid waking during the night for voiding. After determining whether he or she has a weight scale and can use it, emphasize the importance of weighing each morning at the same time. Daily weights indicate whether the patient is losing or retaining fluid. Some patients are taught to use a sliding scale to adjust their daily diuretic dose depending on their daily weight, similar to the way a diabetic patient adjusts an insulin dose based on the capillary glucose level.

Teach patients taking ACEIs or ARBs to move slowly when changing positions, especially from a lying to a sitting position. Remind them to report dizziness, light-headedness, and cough to the health care provider.

Serum potassium level and renal function are monitored at least every few months for patients taking diuretics and ACE inhibitors or ARBs. Diuretics, especially loop diuretics such as Lasix and Bumex, deplete potassium and often cause hypokalemia. Conversely, ACE inhibitors, ARBs, or potassium-sparing diuretics may result in potassium retention. If serum potassium levels drop below 4.0 mEq/L, the health care provider may prescribe potassium supplements or add a potassium-sparing diuretic such as spironolactone (Aldactone) or eplerenone (Inspra). Provide information about potassium-rich foods to include in the diet for patients at risk for hypokalemia (see Chapter 11).

Nutrition Therapy. Remind patients with chronic HF to restrict their dietary sodium. In collaboration with the home care nurse or dietitian, provide written instructions on low- or restricted-sodium diets. A 3-g sodium diet is recommended for *mild to moderate* disease. Remind the patient to avoid salty foods and table salt. Patients usually find this diet acceptable and fairly easy to follow.

A 2-g sodium diet may be needed for patients with *severe* HF. They should not add salt during or after meal preparation, avoid milk and milk products, use few canned or prepared foods, and read food labels to determine sodium content. This diet is not easily tolerated for many patients, and the cost of low-sodium foods can be a financial burden.

Commercial salt substitutes typically contain potassium. Teach patients that their renal status and serum potassium level must be evaluated while using these products. Suggest that patients try lemon, spices, and herbs to enhance the flavor of low-salt foods.

Advance Directives. About 50% of deaths from HF are sudden—many without any warning or worsening of symptoms. Assess whether the patient has written advance directives. If not, provide information about them during his or her hospital stay. Because most of these deaths occur at home, it is important for the health care provider or home care nurse to discuss advance directives with the patient and family. The family should be prepared to act in agreement with the patient's wishes in the event of cardiac arrest. If resuscitation is desired, be sure that the family knows how to activate the emergency medical system (EMS) and how to provide cardiopulmonary resuscitation (CPR) until an ambulance arrives. If CPR is not desired, the patient, family, and nurse plan how the family will respond. For some patients with end-stage disease, hospice care is an option. Chapter 7 discusses hospice and end-of-life care in detail.

Health Care Resources. A home care nurse, ambulatory care clinic, or nurse-led follow-up program may be needed to assess the patient's adherence to drug and nutrition therapy and to monitor for worsening or recurrent HF. Many large hospitals use follow-up telephone calls or teleconferencing/videoconferencing devices to monitor patients at home. Teleconferencing can also assess the patient's heart and lung sounds. These follow-up processes have been very successful in decreasing repeated hospital stays for chronic HF patients.

In addition to home care support, other resources are available for patient education and family support. The American Heart Association is an excellent community resource for print and electronic pamphlets, books, newsletters, and videotapes or DVDs related to HF and heart disease. The organization also provides referrals to various local support groups for patients and their caregivers.

CHART 35-6 Key Features

Valvular Heart Disease

MITRAL STENOSIS	MITRAL REGURGITATION	MITRAL VALVE PROLAPSE	AORTIC STENOSIS	AORTIC REGURGITATION
Fatigue	Fatigue	Atypical chest pain	Dyspnea on exertion	Palpitations
Dyspnea on exertion	Dyspnea on exertion	Dizziness, syncope	Angina	Dyspnea
Orthopnea	Orthopnea	Palpitations	Syncope on exertion	Orthopnea
Paroxysmal nocturnal dyspnea	Palpitations	Atrial tachycardia	Fatigue	Paroxysmal nocturnal dyspnea
Hemoptysis	Atrial fibrillation	Ventricular tachycardia	Orthopnea	Fatigue
Hepatomegaly	Neck vein distention	Systolic click	Paroxysmal nocturnal dyspnea	Angina
Neck vein distention	Pitting edema		Harsh, systolic crescendo-decrescendo murmur	Sinus tachycardia
Pitting edema	High-pitched holosystolic murmur			Blowing, decrescendo diastolic murmur
Atrial fibrillation				
Rumbling, apical diastolic murmur				

For equipment needs

For equipment needs (e.g., home oxygen therapy, hospital bed), medical supply companies provide setup and maintenance services. Chapter 30 provides a detailed description of home oxygen therapy.

⚡ CLINICAL JUDGMENT CHALLENGE

Quality Improvement; Informatics [QSEN]

At a recent staff meeting, the medical-surgical nurse manager reports that the rate of repeated hospitalizations for patients with chronic heart failure has increased 50% in the past 3 months. As a staff nurse, you agree to be part of the unit quality improvement (QI) team to examine the cause(s) of the increase and make evidence-based recommendations for improving the outcomes for this patient population. Specific patient data and summaries are available for the team to review as needed.

1. Where will your team begin with this process during the first meeting of the team?
2. Formulate a PICOT clinical question using the format described in Chapter 5.
3. What Internet sites will your team use to determine best practices for decreasing repeated hospital stays and why?
4. How will your team interpret and use the evidence that you obtain? (See Chapter 5 for assistance.)
5. After your team assembles and analyzes the evidence to determine best practices, what will be done with the information?
6. How will you know if the plan of action to improve care was effective?

◆ Evaluation: Outcomes

Evaluate the care of the patient with HF on the basis of the identified patient problems. The expected outcomes include that the patient will:

- Have adequate pulmonary tissue PERFUSION
- Have increased cardiac pump effectiveness
- Take actions to manage energy
- Be free of pulmonary edema

VALVULAR HEART DISEASE

❖ PATHOPHYSIOLOGY

Acquired valvular dysfunctions include mitral stenosis, mitral regurgitation, mitral valve prolapse, aortic stenosis, and aortic regurgitation (Chart 35-6). The tricuspid valve is not affected often and may occur following endocarditis in IV drug abusers.

Mitral Stenosis

Mitral stenosis usually results from rheumatic carditis, which can cause valve thickening by fibrosis and calcification. Rheumatic fever is the most common cause of the problem. In more developed nations, congenital anomalies affect the majority of patients with mitral stenosis (Ray, 2010).

In mitral stenosis, the valve leaflets fuse and become stiff and the chordae tendineae contract and shorten. The valve opening narrows, preventing normal blood flow from the left atrium to the left ventricle. As a result of these changes, left atrial pressure rises, the left atrium dilates, pulmonary artery pressures increase, and the right ventricle hypertrophies.

Pulmonary congestion and right-sided heart failure occur first. Later, when the left ventricle receives insufficient blood volume, preload is decreased and cardiac output (CO) falls.

People with mild mitral stenosis are usually asymptomatic. As the valvular orifice narrows and pressure in the lungs increases, the patient experiences dyspnea on exertion, orthopnea, paroxysmal nocturnal dyspnea (sudden dyspnea at night), palpitations, and dry cough. Hemoptysis (coughing up blood) and pulmonary edema occur as pulmonary hypertension and congestion progress. Right-sided HF can cause hepatomegaly (enlarged liver), neck vein distention, and pitting dependent edema late in the disorder.

On palpation, the pulse may be normal, rapid, or irregularly irregular (as in atrial fibrillation). Because the development of atrial fibrillation indicates that the patient may decompensate, the physician should be notified immediately of the development of an irregularly irregular rhythm. A rumbling, apical diastolic murmur is noted on auscultation.

Mitral Regurgitation (Insufficiency)

The fibrotic and calcific changes occurring in **mitral regurgitation** (insufficiency) prevent the mitral valve from closing completely during *systole*. Incomplete closure of the valve allows the backflow of blood into the left atrium when the left ventricle contracts (Ray, 2010). During *diastole*, regurgitant output again flows from the left atrium to the left ventricle along with the normal blood flow. The increased volume must be ejected during the next systole. To compensate for the increased volume and pressure, the left atrium and ventricle dilate and hypertrophy.

The primary causes of mitral regurgitation are "degenerative" due to aging and infective endocarditis (Ray, 2010). Other causes include papillary muscle dysfunction or rupture resulting from ischemic heart disease or congenital anomalies. Rheumatic heart disease is the number-one cause in developing nations. When it results from rheumatic heart disease, it usually coexists with some degree of mitral stenosis; it affects women more often than men.

Mitral regurgitation usually progresses slowly; patients may remain symptom-free for decades. Symptoms begin to occur when the left ventricle fails in response to chronic blood volume overload. They include fatigue and chronic weakness as a result of reduced cardiac output (CO). Dyspnea on exertion and orthopnea develop later. A significant number of patients report anxiety, atypical chest pains, and palpitations. Assessment may reveal normal BP, atrial fibrillation, or changes in respirations characteristic of left ventricular failure.

When right-sided HF develops, the neck veins become distended, the liver enlarges (hepatomegaly), and pitting edema develops. A high-pitched systolic murmur at the apex, with radiation to the left axilla, is heard on auscultation. Severe regurgitation often exhibits a third heart sound (S$_3$).

Mitral Valve Prolapse

Mitral valve prolapse (MVP) occurs because the valvular leaflets enlarge and prolapse into the left atrium during systole. This abnormality is usually benign but may progress to pronounced mitral regurgitation in some patients.

The etiology of MVP is variable and has been associated with conditions such as Marfan syndrome and other congenital cardiac defects. MVP also has a familial tendency. Usually, however, no other cardiac abnormality is found.

Most patients with MVP are asymptomatic. However, some may report chest pain, palpitations, or exercise intolerance. Chest pain is usually atypical with patients describing a sharp pain localized to the left side of the chest. Dizziness, **syncope** ("blackouts"), and palpitations may be associated with atrial or ventricular dysrhythmias.

A normal heart rate and BP are usually found on physical examination. A midsystolic click and a late systolic murmur may be heard at the apex of the heart. The intensity of the murmur is not related to the severity of the prolapse.

Aortic Stenosis

Aortic stenosis is the most common cardiac valve dysfunction in the United States and is often considered a disease of "wear and tear." In **aortic stenosis**, the aortic valve orifice narrows and obstructs left ventricular outflow during systole. This increased resistance to ejection or afterload results in ventricular hypertrophy. As stenosis worsens, cardiac output becomes fixed and cannot increase to meet the demands of the body during exertion. Symptoms then develop. Eventually the left ventricle fails, blood backs up in the left atrium, and the pulmonary system becomes congested. Right-sided HF can occur late in the disease. *When the surface area of the valve becomes 1 cm or less, surgery is indicated on an urgent basis!*

Congenital bicuspid or unicuspid aortic valves are the primary causes for aortic stenosis in many patients. Rheumatic aortic stenosis occurs with rheumatic disease of the mitral valve and develops in young and middle-aged adults. Atherosclerosis and degenerative calcification of the aortic valve are the major causative factors in older adults. *Aortic stenosis has become the most common valvular disorder in all countries with aging populations.*

The classic symptoms of aortic stenosis result from fixed cardiac output: dyspnea, angina, and syncope occurring on exertion. When cardiac output falls in the late stages of the disease, the patient experiences marked fatigue, debilitation, and peripheral cyanosis. A narrow pulse pressure is noted when the BP is measured. A diamond-shaped, systolic crescendo-decrescendo murmur is usually noted on auscultation.

Aortic Regurgitation (Insufficiency)

In patients with **aortic regurgitation**, the aortic valve leaflets do not close properly during diastole and the *annulus* (the valve ring that attaches to the leaflets) may be dilated, loose, or deformed. This allows flow of blood from the aorta back into the left ventricle during diastole. The left ventricle, in compensation, dilates to accommodate the greater blood volume and eventually hypertrophies.

Aortic insufficiency usually results from nonrheumatic conditions such as infective endocarditis, congenital anatomic aortic valvular abnormalities, hypertension, and Marfan syndrome (a rare, generalized, systemic disease of connective tissue).

Patients with aortic regurgitation remain asymptomatic for many years because of the compensatory mechanisms of the left ventricle. As the disease progresses and left ventricular failure occurs, the major symptoms are exertional dyspnea, orthopnea, and paroxysmal nocturnal dyspnea. Palpitations may be noted with severe disease, especially when the patient lies on the left side. Nocturnal angina with diaphoresis often occurs.

On palpation, the nurse notes a "bounding" arterial pulse. The pulse pressure is usually widened, with an elevated systolic pressure and diminished diastolic pressure. The classic auscultatory finding is a high-pitched, blowing, decrescendo diastolic murmur.

❖ PATIENT-CENTERED COLLABORATIVE CARE

◆ Assessment

A patient with valvular disease may suddenly become ill or slowly develop symptoms over many years. Collect information about the patient's family health history, including valvular or other forms of heart disease to which he or she may be genetically predisposed. Question about attacks of rheumatic fever and infective endocarditis, the specific dates when these occurred, and the use of antibiotics to prevent recurrence of these diseases. Also question the patient about a history of IV drug abuse, a common cause of infective endocarditis. Discuss the patient's fatigue level and tolerated activity level, the presence of angina or dyspnea, and the occurrence of palpitations, if present.

As part of the physical assessment, obtain vital signs, inspect for signs of edema, palpate and auscultate the heart and lungs, and palpate the peripheral pulses. Assessment findings are summarized in Chart 35-6.

Echocardiography is the noninvasive diagnostic procedure of choice to visualize the structure and movement of the heart. The more invasive transesophageal echocardiography (TEE) or transthoracic echocardiography (TTE) is also performed to assess most valve problems. Exercise tolerance testing (ETT) and stress echocardiography are sometimes done to evaluate symptomatic response and assess functional capacity. With either mitral or aortic stenosis, cardiac catheterization may be indicated to assess the severity of the stenosis and its other effects on the heart.

In patients with mitral stenosis, the chest x-ray shows left atrial enlargement, prominent pulmonary arteries, and an enlarged right ventricle. In those with mitral regurgitation (insufficiency), the chest x-ray reveals an increased cardiac shadow, indicating left ventricular and left atrial enlargement.

In the later stages of aortic stenosis, the chest x-ray may show left ventricular enlargement and pulmonary congestion. Left atrial and left ventricular dilation appear on the chest x-ray of patients with aortic regurgitation (insufficiency). If HF is present, pulmonary venous congestion is also evident.

The health care provider also requests an ECG to assess abnormalities such as left ventricular hypertrophy, as seen with mitral regurgitation and aortic regurgitation, or right ventricular hypertrophy, as seen in severe mitral stenosis. Atrial fibrillation is a common finding in both mitral stenosis and mitral regurgitation and may develop in aortic stenosis because of left atrial dilation.

◆ **Interventions**

Management of valvular heart disease depends on which valve is affected and the degree of valve impairment. Some patients can be managed with yearly monitoring and drug therapy, whereas others require invasive procedures or heart surgery.

Nonsurgical Management. Nonsurgical management focuses on drug therapy and rest. During the course of valvular disease, left ventricular failure with pulmonary or systemic congestion may develop.

Drug Therapy. Diuretics, beta blockers, digoxin, and oxygen are often administered to improve the symptoms of heart failure. Nitrates are administered cautiously to patients with aortic stenosis because of the potential for syncope associated with a reduction in left ventricular volume (preload). Vasodilators such as calcium channel blockers may be used to reduce the regurgitant flow for patients with aortic or mitral stenosis.

> ⚠ **NURSING SAFETY PRIORITY** (QSEN)
>
> **Drug Alert**
>
> Teach patients with valve disease the importance of prophylactic antibiotic therapy before any invasive dental or respiratory procedure. Prophylactic antibiotics are *not* recommended prior to gastrointestinal procedures such as upper GI endoscopy, colonoscopy, or procedures requiring genitourinary instrumentation.

A major concern in valvular heart disease is maintaining cardiac output if atrial fibrillation develops. With mitral valvular disease, left ventricular filling is especially dependent on atrial contraction. When atrial fibrillation develops, there is no longer a single coordinated atrial contraction. Cardiac output can decrease, and HF may occur. Ineffective atrial contraction may also lead to the stasis of blood and thrombi in the left atrium. Monitor the patient for the development of an irregular rhythm, and notify the primary care provider if it develops. (See Chapter 34 for a detailed explanation of atrial fibrillation.)

The primary care provider usually starts drug therapy first to control the heart rate and maintain cardiac output (<100 for heart rate is considered a controlled ventricular response). After those outcomes are met, drugs are used in an attempt to restore normal sinus rhythm (NSR). In some cases, the provider elects to convert a patient from atrial fibrillation to sinus rhythm using IV diltiazem (Cardizem, Apo-Diltiaz ✦) or amiodarone (Cordarone, Pacerone). Monitor the patient on a unit where both cardiac rhythm and BP can be closely watched. Synchronized countershock (cardioversion) may be attempted if atrial fibrillation is rapid, the patient's condition worsens, and the rhythm is unresponsive to medical treatment (see Chapter 34).

If the patient remains in atrial fibrillation, low-dose amiodarone (Cordarone) is often prescribed to slow ventricular rate. Procainamide hydrochloride (Pronestyl hydrochloride, Procanbid) may be added to the regimen. A beta-blocking agent (e.g., metoprolol) may also be considered to slow the ventricular response.

For valvular heart disease and chronic atrial fibrillation, anticoagulation with sodium warfarin (Coumadin, Warfilone ✦) is usually a part of the plan of care to prevent thrombus formation. Thrombi (clots) may form in the atria or on defective valve segments, resulting in systemic emboli. If a portion breaks off and travels to the brain, one or more strokes may occur. Assess the patient's baseline neurologic status, and monitor for changes. A transesophageal echocardiography (TEE) is often done before synchronized cardioversion to ensure that thrombi are not present that could embolize when this therapy is administered. The newer direct thrombin inhibitors *rivaroxaban* (Xarelto) and *dabigatran* (Pradaxa) are *not recommended* to anticoagulate patients with atrial fibrillation related to valvular disease.

Rest is often an important part of treatment. Activity may be limited because cardiac output (CO) cannot meet increased metabolic demands and angina or HF can result. A balance of rest and exercise is needed to prevent skeletal muscle atrophy and fatigue.

Noninvasive Heart Valve Reparative Procedures. Reparative procedures are becoming more popular because of continuing problems with thrombi, endocarditis, and left ventricular dysfunction after valve replacement. Reparative procedures do not result in a normal valve, but they usually "turn back the clock," resulting in a more functional valve and an improvement in cardiac output. Turbulent blood flow through the valve may persist, and degeneration of the repaired valve is possible.

Balloon valvuloplasty, an invasive nonsurgical procedure, is possible for stenotic mitral and aortic valves; however, careful selection of patients is needed. It may be the initial treatment of choice for people with noncalcified, mobile mitral valves. Patients selected for *aortic* valvuloplasty are usually older and are at high risk for surgical complications or have refused operative treatment. The benefits of this procedure for aortic stenosis tend to be short lived, rarely lasting longer than 6 months.

When performing *mitral* valvuloplasty, the physician passes a balloon catheter from the femoral vein, through the atrial

A   B   C   D

FIG. 35-3 Transcatheter aortic valve replacement (TAVR) procedure.

septum, and to the mitral valve. The balloon is inflated to enlarge the mitral orifice. For *aortic* valvuloplasty, the physician inserts the catheter through the femoral artery and advances it to the aortic valve, where it is inflated to enlarge the orifice. The procedure usually offers immediate relief of symptoms because the balloon has dilated the orifice and improved leaflet mobility. The results are comparable with those of surgical commissurotomy for appropriately selected patients.

Minimally invasive techniques have expanded. For patients who are not surgical candidates, *transcatheter aortic valve replacement (TAVR)* is an alternative option for treatment of aortic stenosis (Fig. 35-3). A bioprosthetic valve is placed percutaneously via either the transfemoral or transapical route under general anesthesia in a hybrid operating room (a combination of a catheterization laboratory and cardiovascular operating room). After initial balloon aortic valvuloplasty, the new valve, which is wrapped around a balloon on a large catheter, is inserted via the femoral artery. The patient is transvenously paced at a rate of about 200 beats per minute to mimic ventricular standstill. The balloon is then inflated and the valve deployed. In the transapical approach, a small incision is made at the apex of the heart. The catheter is then threaded through the incision and the left ventricle to gain access to the aortic valve. As in the transvenous approach, the balloon and catheter is deployed during rapid transvenous pacing. This procedure is performed by a health care team consisting of interventional cardiologists and cardiovascular surgeons. The team must be prepared to convert to an open or traditional aortic valve replacement (AVR) if necessary. Care of the patient is similar to the care of the patient undergoing CABG (see Chapter 38); however, this patient population only needs anticoagulation with aspirin and clopidogrel postprocedure.

The pulmonary valve can also be replaced percutaneously by a device from Medtronic using a similar procedure to the TAVR. The Mitraclip, approved for use in Europe and under investigation for use in the United States, is used to repair the mitral valve in patients with mitral regurgitation. Under general anesthesia, access is gained percutaneously via the femoral vein, and the catheter and Mitraclip is advanced in the left atria and then the left ventricle. The Mitraclip is then retracted and deployed to hold the leaflets of the valve together. Care is similar to the care of the patient undergoing CABG (see Chapter 38).

> **⚠ NURSING SAFETY PRIORITY** (QSEN)
>
> **Action Alert**
>
> After valvuloplasty, observe the patient closely for bleeding from the catheter insertion site and institute post-angiogram precautions. Bleeding is likely because of the large size of the catheter. Assess for signs of a regurgitant valve by closely monitoring heart sounds, CO, and heart rhythm. Because vegetations (thrombi) may have been dislodged from the valve, observe for any indication of systemic emboli (see the Infective Endocarditis section, p. 697).

Surgical Management. Surgeries for patients with valvular heart disease include invasive reparative procedures and replacement. These procedures are performed after symptoms of left ventricular failure have developed but before irreversible dysfunction occurs. Surgical therapy is the *only* definitive treatment of *aortic stenosis* and is recommended when angina, syncope, or dyspnea on exertion develops.

Invasive Heart Valve Reparative Procedures. *Direct (open) commissurotomy* is accomplished with cardiopulmonary bypass during open heart surgery. The surgeon visualizes the valve, removes thrombi from the atria, incises the fused commissures (leaflets), and débrides calcium from the leaflets, widening the orifice.

Mitral valve annuloplasty (reconstruction) is the reparative procedure of choice for most patients with acquired mitral insufficiency. To make the annulus (the valve ring that attaches to and supports the leaflets) smaller, the surgeon may suture the leaflets to an annuloplasty ring or take tucks in the patient's annulus. Leaflet repair is often performed at the same time. Elongated leaflets may be shortened, and shortened leaflets may be repaired by lengthening the chordae that bind them in place. Perforated leaflets may be patched with synthetic grafts.

Annuloplasty and leaflet repair result in an annulus of the appropriate size and in leaflets that can close completely. Thus regurgitation is eliminated or markedly reduced.

Heart Valve Replacement Procedures. The development of a wide variety of *prosthetic* (synthetic) and *biologic* (tissue) valves has improved the surgical therapy and prognosis of valvular heart disease. Each type has advantages and disadvantages. An aortic valve can be replaced only with a prosthetic valve for symptomatic adults with aortic stenosis and aortic

FIG. 35-4 Examples of biologic (tissue) heart valves. **A,** Freestyle, a stentless pig valve with no frame. **B,** Hancock II, a stented pig valve. **C,** Carpentier-Edwards pericardial bioprosthesis.

insufficiency. A biologic valve cannot be used because of the high pressure within the aorta.

Biologic valve replacements may be **xenograft** (from other species), such as a porcine valve (from a pig) (Fig. 35-4) or a bovine valve (from a cow). Because tissue valves are associated with little risk for clot formation, long-term anticoagulation is *not* indicated. Xenografts are not as durable as prosthetic valves and usually must be replaced every 7 to 10 years. The durability of the graft is related to the age of the recipient. Calcium in the blood, which is present in larger quantities in younger patients, breaks down the valves. The older the patient, the longer the xenograft will last. Valves donated from human cadavers and **pulmonary autographs** (relocation of the patient's own pulmonary valve to the aortic position [Ross procedure]) are also being used for valve replacement.

Patients having a valve replacement have open heart surgery similar to the procedure for a coronary artery bypass graft (CABG) (see Chapter 38). Ideally, surgery is an elective and planned procedure. Inform the patient and family about the management of postoperative pain, incision care, and strategies to prevent respiratory complications (see Chapters 14 and 16). Teach patients receiving oral anticoagulants to stop taking them before surgery, usually at least 72 hours before the procedure. Patients also need to have a preoperative dental examination. If dental caries or periodontal disease is present, these problems must be resolved before valve replacement.

Postoperative nursing interventions for patients with valve replacement are similar to those for a CABG (see Chapter 38).

> ### ⚠ NURSING SAFETY PRIORITY (QSEN)
> #### *Critical Rescue*
> Patients with mitral stenosis often have pulmonary hypertension and stiff lungs. Therefore monitor respiratory status closely during weaning from the ventilator. Be especially alert for bleeding in those with aortic valve replacements because of a higher risk for postoperative hemorrhage. If heart rate or blood pressure decreases, call the Rapid Response Team or other health care provider immediately!

Patients with valve replacements are also more likely to have significant reductions in cardiac output (CO) after surgery, especially those with aortic stenosis or left ventricular failure from mitral valve disease. Carefully monitor CO, and assess for indications of heart failure. Report any manifestations of HF to the surgeon immediately, and prepare for collaborative

management (see earlier discussion on heart failure in this chapter).

Community-Based Care

The patient with valvular heart disease may be discharged home on medical therapy or postoperatively after valve repair or replacement. Because fatigue is a common problem, ensure that the home environment can provide rest while moving the patient toward increased activity levels. Some older adults with aortic stenosis live in long-term care settings.

Home Care Management. A home care nurse may be needed to help the patient adhere to drug therapy and activity schedules and to detect any problems, particularly with anticoagulant therapy. Patients who have undergone surgery may require a nurse for assistance with incision care. A home care aide may assist with ADLs if the patient lives alone or is older.

Self-Management Education. The teaching plan for the patient with valvular heart disease includes:

- The disease process and the possibility of heart failure
- Drug therapy, including diuretics, vasodilators, beta blockers, calcium channel blockers, antibiotics, and anticoagulants
- The prophylactic use of antibiotics
- A plan of activity and rest to conserve energy

Because patients with defective or repaired valves are at risk for infective endocarditis, teach them to adhere to the precautions described for endocarditis. *Remind them to inform all health care providers of the valvular heart disease history. Tell providers that they require antibiotic administration before all invasive procedures and tests.* Health teaching for the patient is summarized in Chart 35-7.

Patients who have had valve replacements with prosthetic valves require lifetime prophylactic anticoagulation therapy to prevent thrombus formation. Teach patients taking anticoagulants how to manage their drug therapy successfully, including nutritional considerations (if taking warfarin) and the prevention of bleeding. For example, the patient should be taught to avoid foods high in vitamin K, especially dark green leafy vegetables, and to use an electric razor to avoid skin cuts. In addition, teach him or her to report any bleeding or excessive bruising to the health care provider.

For patients who have surgery, reinforce how to care for the sternal incision and instruct them to watch for and report any fever, drainage, or redness at the site. Most patients can usually return to normal activity after 6 weeks but should avoid heavy

---

physical activity involving their upper extremities for 3 to 6 months to allow the incision to heal. Those who have had valvular surgery should also avoid invasive dental procedures for 6 months because of the potential for endocarditis. Those with prosthetic valves need to avoid any procedure using magnetic resonance unless the newest technology is available. Remind patients to obtain a medical alert bracelet, card, or necklace to indicate they have a valve replacement and are taking anticoagulants.

Patients with valvular heart disease may have complicated medication schedules that can potentially lead to inadequate self-management. Provide clear, concise instructions about drug therapy, and discuss the risks associated with nonadherence. Patients with a failed valve or those who do not follow the treatment plan are at high risk for heart failure. Teach them to report any changes in cardiovascular status, such as dyspnea, syncope, dizziness, edema, and palpitations.

The psychological response to valve surgery is similar to that after coronary artery bypass surgery. Patients may experience an altered self-image as a result of the required lifestyle changes or the visible medial sternotomy incision. In addition, those with prosthetic valves may need to adjust to a soft but audible clicking sound of the prosthetic valve. Encourage patients to verbalize their feelings about the prosthetic heart valve. Patients may display a variety of emotions postoperatively, especially after hospital discharge.

Health Care Resources. The American Heart Association's *Mended Hearts, Inc.* (www.mendedhearts.org) is a community resource that provides information about valvular heart disease. A wallet-size card can be obtained to identify the patient as needing prophylactic antibiotics. An identification bracelet or necklace that states the name of the drugs the patient is taking should also be worn.

INFLAMMATIONS AND INFECTIONS

INFECTIVE ENDOCARDITIS

❖ PATHOPHYSIOLOGY

Infective endocarditis (previously called *bacterial endocarditis*) is a microbial INFECTION (e.g., viruses, bacteria, fungi) of the endocardium. The most common infective organism is *Streptococcus viridans* or *Staphylococcus aureus*.

Infective endocarditis occurs primarily in patients who abuse IV drugs, have had valve replacements, have experienced systemic INFECTION, or have structural cardiac defects. With a cardiac defect, blood may flow rapidly from a high-pressure area to a low-pressure zone, eroding a section of endocardium. Platelets and fibrin adhere to the denuded endocardium, forming a vegetative lesion. During bacteremia, bacteria become trapped in the low-pressure "sinkhole" and are deposited in the vegetation. Additional platelets and fibrin are deposited, which causes the vegetative lesion to grow. The endocardium and valve are destroyed. Valvular insufficiency may result when the lesion interferes with normal alignment of the valve. If vegetations become so large that blood flow through the valve is obstructed, the valve appears stenotic and then is very likely to *embolize* (i.e., cause emboli to be released into the systemic circulation) (McCance et al., 2010).

Possible ports of entry for infecting organisms include:
- The oral cavity (especially if dental procedures have been performed)
- Skin rashes, lesions, or abscesses
- Infections (cutaneous, genitourinary, GI, systemic)
- Surgery or invasive procedures, including IV line placement

❖ PATIENT-CENTERED COLLABORATIVE CARE

◆ Assessment

Because the mortality rate remains high, early detection of infective endocarditis is essential. Unfortunately, many patients (especially older adults) are misdiagnosed. Clinical manifestations typically occur within 2 weeks of a bacteremia (Chart 35-8).

Most patients have recurrent fevers from 99° to 103° F (37.2° to 39.4° C). As a result of physiologic changes associated with aging, however, older adults may be afebrile. The severity of symptoms may depend on the virulence of the infecting organism.

Physical Assessment/Clinical Manifestations. Assess the patient's *cardiovascular status.* Almost all patients with infective endocarditis develop murmurs. Carefully auscultate the precordium, noting and documenting any new murmurs (usually regurgitant in nature) or any changes in the intensity or quality of an old murmur. An S_3 or S_4 heart sound also may be heard.

Heart failure is the most common complication of infective endocarditis. Assess for right-sided HF (as evidenced by peripheral edema, weight gain, and anorexia) and left-sided HF (as evidenced by fatigue, shortness of breath, and crackles on auscultation of breath sounds). See discussion of HF earlier in this chapter.

Arterial embolization is a major complication in up to half of patients with infective endocarditis. Fragments of vegetation (clots) break loose and travel randomly through the circulation. When the left side of the heart is involved, vegetation fragments are carried to the spleen, kidneys, GI tract, brain, and extremities. When the right side of the heart is involved, emboli enter the pulmonary circulation.

Splenic infarction with sudden abdominal PAIN and radiation to the left shoulder can also occur. When performing an *abdominal assessment,* note rebound tenderness on palpation. The classic pain described with renal infarction is flank pain that radiates to the groin and is accompanied by hematuria (red blood cells in the urine) or pyuria (white blood cells in the urine). Mesenteric emboli cause diffuse abdominal pain, often after eating, and abdominal distention.

About a third of patients have *neurologic changes;* others have signs and symptoms of pulmonary problems. Emboli to the central nervous system cause either transient ischemic attacks (TIAs) or a stroke. Confusion, reduced concentration, and aphasia or dysphagia may occur. Pleuritic chest pain, dyspnea, and cough are symptoms of pulmonary infarction related to embolization.

Petechiae (pinpoint red spots) occur in many patients with endocarditis. Examine the mucous membranes, the palate, the conjunctivae, and the skin above the clavicles for small, red, flat lesions. Assess the distal third of the nail bed for **splinter hemorrhages,** which appear as black longitudinal lines or small red streaks.

Diagnostic Assessment. The most reliable criteria for diagnosing endocarditis include positive blood cultures, a new regurgitant murmur, and evidence of endocardial involvement by echocardiography.

A positive *blood culture* is a prime diagnostic test. Both aerobic and anaerobic specimens are obtained for culture. Some slow-growing organisms may take 3 weeks and require a specialized medium to isolate. Low hemoglobin and hematocrit levels may also be present.

Echocardiography has improved the ability to diagnose infective endocarditis accurately. Transesophageal echocardiography (TEE) allows visualization of cardiac structures that are difficult to see with transthoracic echocardiography (TTE) (see Chapter 33).

◆ **Interventions**

Care of the patient with endocarditis usually includes antimicrobials, rest balanced with activity, and supportive therapy for HF. If these interventions are successful, surgery is usually not required.

Nonsurgical Management. The major component of treatment for endocarditis is drug therapy. Other interventions help prevent the life-threatening complications of the disease.

Antimicrobials are the main treatment, with the choice of drug depending on the specific organism involved. Because vegetations surround and protect the offending microorganism, an appropriate drug must be given in a sufficiently high dose to ensure its destruction. Antimicrobials are usually given IV, with the course of treatment lasting 4 to 6 weeks. For most bacterial cases, the ideal antibiotic is one of the penicillins or cephalosporins.

Patients may be hospitalized for several days to institute IV therapy and then are discharged for continued IV therapy at home. After hospitalization, most patients who respond to therapy may continue it at home when they become afebrile, have negative blood cultures, and have no signs of HF or embolization.

Anticoagulants do not prevent embolization from vegetations. Because they may result in bleeding, these drugs are avoided unless they are required to prevent thrombus formation (clotting) on a prosthetic valve.

The patient's activities are balanced with *adequate rest.* Consistently use appropriate aseptic technique to protect the patient from contact with potentially infective organisms. Continue to assess for signs of HF (e.g., rapid pulse, fatigue, cough, dyspnea) throughout the antimicrobial regimen, and report significant changes.

Surgical Management. The cardiac surgeon may be consulted if antibiotic therapy is ineffective in sterilizing a valve, if refractory HF develops secondary to a defective valve, if large valvular vegetations are present, or if multiple embolic events occur. Current surgical interventions for infective endocarditis include:

- Removing the infected valve (either biologic or prosthetic)
- Repairing or removing congenital shunts
- Repairing injured valves and chordae tendineae
- Draining abscesses in the heart

Preoperative and postoperative care of patients having surgery involving the valves is similar to that described earlier for valve replacement (pp. 695-696).

Community-Based Care

Community-based care for patients with infective endocarditis is essential to resolve the problem, prevent relapse, and avoid complications. Patients and families need to be willing and have the knowledge, physical ability, and resources to administer IV antibiotics at home. Collaborate with the home care nurse to complete health teaching started in the hospital and to monitor patient adherence and health status as directed by The Joint Commission's National Patient Safety Goals.

In collaboration with the case manager, the home care nurse and pharmacist arrange for appropriate supplies to be available to the patient at home. Supplies include the prepared antibiotic, IV pump with tubing, alcohol wipes, IV access device, normal saline solution, and a saline flush solution drawn up in syringes. A saline lock, peripherally inserted central catheter (PICC) line, or central catheter is positioned at a venous site that is easily accessible to the patient or a family member.

Teach the patient and family how to administer the antibiotic and care for the infusion site while maintaining aseptic technique. The patient or family member should demonstrate this technique before the patient is discharged from the hospital. Emphasize the importance of maintaining a blood level of the antibiotic by administering the antibiotics as scheduled. After stabilization at home, the case manager or other nurse contacts the patient every week to determine whether he or she is adhering to the antibiotic therapy and whether any problems have been encountered.

Encourage proper oral hygiene. Advise patients to use a soft toothbrush, to brush their teeth at least twice per day, and to rinse the mouth with water after brushing. They should not use irrigation devices or floss the teeth because bacteremia may result. Teach them to clean any open skin areas well and apply an antibiotic ointment.

> ### ❗ NURSING SAFETY PRIORITY (QSEN)
> #### Action Alert
>
> Patients must remind health care providers (including their dentists) of their endocarditis. Guidelines for antibiotic prophylaxis have been revised and are recommended only if the patient with a prosthetic valve, a history of infective endocarditis, or an unrepaired cyanotic congenital heart disease undergoes invasive dental, oral, or upper respiratory procedure.
>
> Instruct patients to note any indications of recurring endocarditis such as fever. Remind them to monitor and record their temperature daily for up to 6 weeks. Teach them to report fever, chills, malaise, weight loss, increased fatigue, sudden weight gain, or dyspnea to their primary care provider.

❖ PERICARDITIS
❖ PATHOPHYSIOLOGY

Acute pericarditis is an inflammation or alteration of the pericardium (the membranous sac that encloses the heart). The problem may be fibrous, serous, hemorrhagic, purulent, or neoplastic. Acute pericarditis is most commonly associated with:

- Infective organisms (bacteria, viruses, or fungi) (usually respiratory)
- Post–myocardial infarction (MI) syndrome (Dressler's syndrome)
- Post-pericardiotomy syndrome
- Acute exacerbations of systemic connective tissue disease

Chronic constrictive pericarditis occurs when chronic pericardial inflammation causes a fibrous thickening of the pericardium. It is caused by tuberculosis, radiation therapy, trauma, renal failure, or metastatic cancer. In chronic constrictive pericarditis, the pericardium becomes rigid, preventing adequate filling of the ventricles and eventually resulting in cardiac failure.

❖ PATIENT-CENTERED COLLABORATIVE CARE
◆ Assessment

Assessment findings for patients with *acute pericarditis* include substernal precordial PAIN that radiates to the left side of the neck, the shoulder, or the back. PAIN is classically grating and oppressive and is aggravated by breathing (mainly on inspiration), coughing, and swallowing. The PAIN is worse when the patient is in the supine position and may be relieved by sitting up and leaning forward. Ask specific questions to evaluate chest discomfort to differentiate it from the pain associated with an acute MI (see Chapter 38).

A pericardial friction rub may be heard with the diaphragm of the stethoscope positioned at the left lower sternal border. This scratchy, high-pitched sound is produced when the inflamed, roughened pericardial layers create friction as their surfaces rub together.

Patients with acute pericarditis may have an elevated white blood cell count and usually have a fever. Therefore blood culture and sensitivity may be analyzed in the laboratory. The ECG usually shows ST-T spiking in almost all leads simultaneously, and aVR with ST depression with the onset of inflammation, which returns to baseline with treatment. Atrial fibrillation is also common. Echocardiograms may be used to determine a pericardial effusion.

Patients with *chronic constrictive pericarditis* have signs of right-sided HF, elevated systemic venous pressure with jugular distention, hepatic engorgement, and dependent edema. Exertional fatigue and dyspnea are common complications. Thickening of the pericardium is seen on echocardiography or a computed tomography (CT) scan.

◆ Interventions

The focus of collaborative management is to relieve pain and treat the cause of pericarditis before severe complications occur.

Pain Management. The health care provider usually prescribes NSAIDs for PAIN associated with pericarditis. Patients who do not obtain pain relief and who do not have bacterial pericarditis may receive corticosteroid therapy. Assist the patient to assume positions of comfort—usually sitting upright and leaning slightly forward. If the pain is not relieved within 24 to 48 hours, notify the health care provider. Colchicine 1 to 2 mg orally on Day 1 followed by 0.5 to 1 mg orally daily for 6 months has been shown to prevent pericarditis reoccurrence.

The various causes of pericarditis require specific therapies. For example, bacterial pericarditis (acute) usually requires antibiotics and pericardial drainage. The usual clinical course of acute pericarditis is short term (2 to 6 weeks), but episodes may recur. Chronic pericarditis caused by malignant disease may be treated with radiation or chemotherapy, whereas uremic pericarditis is treated by hemodialysis. The definitive treatment for chronic constrictive pericarditis is surgical excision of the pericardium (**pericardiectomy**).

Monitor all patients for **pericardial effusion**, which occurs when the space between the parietal and visceral layers of the pericardium fills with fluid. This complication puts the patient at risk for **cardiac tamponade**, or excessive fluid within the pericardial cavity.

Emergency Care: Acute Cardiac Tamponade. Acute cardiac tamponade may occur when small volumes (20 to 50 mL) of fluid accumulate rapidly in the pericardium and cause a sudden decrease in cardiac output (CO). If the fluid accumulates slowly, the pericardium may stretch to accommodate several hundred milliliters of fluid. Report any suspicion of this complication to the physician immediately. Findings of cardiac tamponade include:

- Jugular venous distention
- **Paradoxical pulse**, also known as *pulsus paradoxus* (systolic blood pressure 10 mm Hg or more higher on expiration than on inspiration) (Chart 35-9)
- Increased heart rate, dyspnea, and fatigue
- Muffled heart sounds
- Hypotension

Care of the Patient with Pericarditis

- Assess the nature of the patient's chest discomfort. (Pericardial pain is typically substernal. It is worse on inspiration and decreases when the patient leans forward.)
- Auscultate for a pericardial friction rub.
- Assist the patient to a position of comfort.
- Provide anti-inflammatory agents as prescribed.
- Explain that anti-inflammatory agents usually decrease the pain within 48 hours.
- Avoid the administration of aspirin and anticoagulants because these may increase the possibility of tamponade.
- Auscultate the blood pressure carefully to detect paradoxical blood pressure (pulsus paradoxus), a sign of tamponade:
  - Palpate the blood pressure, and inflate the cuff above the systolic pressure.
  - Deflate the cuff gradually, and note when sounds are first audible on expiration.
  - Identify when sounds are also audible on inspiration.
  - Subtract the inspiratory pressure from the expiratory pressure to determine the amount of pulsus paradoxus (>10 mm Hg is an indication of tamponade).
- Inspect for other indications of tamponade, including jugular venous distention with clear lungs, muffled heart sounds, and decreased cardiac output.
- Notify the physician if tamponade is suspected.

Cardiac tamponade is an emergency! The physician may initially manage the decreased cardiac output (CO) with increased fluid volume administration while awaiting an echocardiogram or x-ray to confirm the diagnosis. Unfortunately, these tests are not always helpful because the fluid volume around the heart may be too small to visualize. Hemodynamic monitoring in a specialized critical care unit usually demonstrates compression of the heart, with all pressures (right atrial, pulmonary artery, and wedge) being similar and elevated (plateau pressures).

The physician may elect to perform a **pericardiocentesis** to remove fluid and relieve the pressure on the heart. Under echocardiographic or fluoroscopic and hemodynamic monitoring, the cardiologist inserts an 8-inch (20.3-cm), 16- or 18-gauge pericardial needle into the pericardial space. When the needle is properly positioned, a catheter is inserted and all available pericardial fluid is withdrawn. A pericardial drain may be temporarily placed. Monitor the pulmonary artery, wedge, and right atrial pressures during the procedure. The pressures should return to normal as the fluid compressing the heart is removed, and the clinical manifestations of tamponade should resolve. In situations in which the cause of the tamponade is unknown, pericardial fluid specimens may be sent to the laboratory for culture and sensitivity tests and cytology.

! NURSING SAFETY PRIORITY QSEN

Action Alert

After the pericardiocentesis, closely monitor the patient for the recurrence of tamponade. Pericardiocentesis alone often does not resolve acute tamponade. Be prepared to provide adequate fluid volumes to increase CO and to prepare the patient for emergency sternotomy if tamponade recurs.

If the patient has a recurrence of tamponade or recurrent effusions or adhesions from chronic pericarditis, a portion or all of the pericardium may need to be removed to allow adequate ventricular filling and contraction. The surgeon may create a pericardial window, which involves removing a portion of the pericardium to permit excessive pericardial fluid to drain into the pleural space. In more severe cases, removal of the toughened encasing pericardium (pericardiectomy) may be necessary.

RHEUMATIC CARDITIS

❖ PATHOPHYSIOLOGY

Rheumatic carditis, also called *rheumatic endocarditis,* is a sensitivity response that develops after an upper respiratory tract infection with group A beta-hemolytic *Streptococci.* It occurs in almost half of patients with rheumatic fever. The precise mechanism by which the infection causes inflammatory lesions in the heart is not established; however, inflammation is evident in all layers of the heart. The inflammation results in impaired contractile function of the myocardium, thickening of the pericardium, and valvular damage.

Rheumatic carditis is characterized by the formation of Aschoff bodies (small nodules in the myocardium that are replaced by scar tissue). A diffuse cellular infiltrate also develops and may be responsible for the resulting heart failure (HF). The pericardium becomes thickened and covered with exudate, and a serosanguineous pleural effusion may develop. The most serious damage occurs to the endocardium, with inflammation of the valve leaflets developing. Hemorrhagic and fibrous lesions form along the inflamed surfaces of the valves, resulting in stenosis or regurgitation of the mitral and aortic valves (McCance et al., 2010).

❖ PATIENT-CENTERED COLLABORATIVE CARE

Rheumatic carditis is one of the major indicators of rheumatic fever. The common manifestations are:
- Tachycardia
- **Cardiomegaly** (enlarged heart)
- Development of a new murmur or a change in an existing murmur
- Pericardial friction rub
- Precordial pain
- Electrocardiogram (ECG) changes (prolonged PR interval)
- Indications of heart failure (HF)
- Evidence of an existing streptococcal infection

Primary prevention is extremely important. Teach all patients to remind their health care providers to provide appropriate antibiotic therapy if they develop the indications of streptococcal pharyngitis:
- Moderate to high fever
- Abrupt onset of a sore throat
- Reddened throat with exudate
- Enlarged and tender lymph nodes

Penicillin is the antibiotic of choice for treatment. Erythromycin (Eryc, Erythromid ✦) is the alternative for penicillin-sensitive patients.

Once a diagnosis of rheumatic fever is made, antibiotic therapy is started immediately. Teach the patient to continue the antibiotic administration for the full 10 days to prevent re-infection. Suggest ways to manage fever, such as maintaining hydration and taking antipyretics. Encourage the patient to get adequate rest.

Explain to the patient and family that a recurrence of rheumatic carditis is most likely the result of reinfection by *Streptococcus*. Antibiotic prophylaxis is necessary for the rest of the patient's life to prevent infective endocarditis (see Infective Endocarditis, p. 697).

CARDIOMYOPATHY

❖ *PATHOPHYSIOLOGY*

Cardiomyopathy is a subacute or chronic disease of cardiac muscle, and the cause may be unknown. Cardiomyopathies are classified into four categories on the basis of abnormalities in structure and function: dilated cardiomyopathy, hypertrophic cardiomyopathy, restrictive cardiomyopathy, and arrhythmogenic right ventricular cardiomyopathy (Table 35-5). Mortality at 1 year is 20% and 70% to 80% at year 8 for patients who develop heart failure (Go et al., 2013).

Dilated cardiomyopathy (DCM) is the structural abnormality most commonly seen. DCM involves extensive damage to the myofibrils and interference with myocardial metabolism.

Ventricular wall thickness is normal, but both ventricles are dilated (left ventricle is usually worse) and systolic function is impaired. Causes may include alcohol abuse, chemotherapy, infection, inflammation, and poor nutrition. Decreased CO from inadequate pumping of the heart causes the patient to experience dyspnea on exertion (DOE), decreased exercise capacity, fatigue, and palpitations.

The cardinal features of hypertrophic cardiomyopathy (HCM) are asymmetric ventricular hypertrophy and disarray of the myocardial fibers. Left ventricular hypertrophy leads to a stiff left ventricle, which results in diastolic filling abnormalities. Obstruction in the left ventricular outflow tract is seen in most patients with HCM. In about half of patients, HCM is transmitted as a single-gene autosomal dominant trait (McCance et al., 2010). Some patients die without any symptoms, whereas others have dyspnea on exertion (DOE), syncope, dizziness, and palpitations. Many athletes who die suddenly probably had hypertrophic cardiomyopathy.

Restrictive cardiomyopathy, the rarest of the cardiomyopathies, is characterized by stiff ventricles that restrict filling during diastole. Symptoms are similar to left or right heart failure (HF) or both. The disease can be primary or caused by endocardial or myocardial disease such as sarcoidosis

TABLE 35-5 Pathophysiology, Signs and Symptoms, and Treatment of Common Cardiomyopathies

| DILATED CARDIOMYOPATHY | HYPERTROPHIC CARDIOMYOPATHY | |
	NONOBSTRUCTED	OBSTRUCTED
Pathophysiology		
Fibrosis of myocardium and endocardium Dilated chambers Mural wall thrombi prevalent	Hypertrophy of all walls Hypertrophied septum Relatively small chamber size	Same as for nonobstructed except for obstruction of left ventricular outflow tract associated with the hypertrophied septum and mitral valve incompetence
Signs and Symptoms		
Fatigue and weakness Heart failure (left side) Dysrhythmias or heart block Systemic or pulmonary emboli S_3 and S_4 gallops Moderate to severe cardiomegaly	Dyspnea Angina Fatigue, syncope, palpitations Mild cardiomegaly S_4 gallop Ventricular dysrhythmias Sudden death common Heart failure	Same as for nonobstructed except with mitral regurgitation murmur Atrial fibrillation
Treatment		
Symptomatic treatment of heart failure Vasodilators Control of dysrhythmias Surgery: heart transplant	For both: Symptomatic treatment Beta blockers Conversion of atrial fibrillation Surgery: ventriculomyotomy or muscle resection with mitral valve replacement Nitrates and other vasodilators *contraindicated* with the obstructed form	

or amyloidosis. The prognosis for this type of cardiomyopathy is poor.

Arrhythmogenic right ventricular cardiomyopathy (dysplasia) results from replacement of myocardial tissue with fibrous and fatty tissue. Although the name implies right ventricle disease, about a third of patients also have left ventricle (LV) involvement. This disease has a familial association and most often affects young adults. Some patients have symptoms, and others do not.

❖ PATIENT-CENTERED COLLABORATIVE CARE

◆ Assessment

Findings in cardiomyopathy depend on the structural and functional abnormalities. For example, left ventricular or biventricular failure is characteristic of *dilated* cardiomyopathy (DCM). Some patients with DCM are asymptomatic for months to years and have left and/or right ventricular dilation confirmed on x-ray examination or echocardiography. Others experience sudden, pronounced symptoms of left ventricular failure, such as progressive dyspnea on exertion, orthopnea, palpitations, and activity intolerance. Right-sided HF develops late in the disease and is associated with a poor prognosis. Atrial fibrillation occurs in some patients and is associated with embolism.

The clinical picture of *hypertrophic* cardiomyopathy (HCM) results from the hypertrophied septum causing a reduced stroke volume (SV) and cardiac output (CO). Most patients are asymptomatic until late adolescence or early adulthood. The primary symptoms of HCM are exertional dyspnea, angina, and syncope. The chest pain is atypical in that it usually occurs at rest, is prolonged, has no relation to exertion, and is not relieved by the administration of nitrates. A high incidence of ventricular dysrhythmias is associated with HCM. Sudden death occurs and may be the first manifestation of the disease.

Echocardiography, radionuclide imaging, and angiocardiography during cardiac catheterization are performed to diagnose and differentiate cardiomyopathies.

◆ Interventions

The treatment of choice for the patient with cardiomyopathy varies with the type of cardiomyopathy and may include both medical and surgical interventions.

Nonsurgical Management. The care of patients with dilated or restrictive cardiomyopathy is initially the same as for HF. Drug therapy includes the use of diuretics, vasodilating agents, and cardiac glycosides to increase cardiac output (CO). Because patients are at risk for sudden death, teach them to report any palpitations, dizziness, or fainting, which might indicate a dysrhythmia. Antidysrhythmic drugs or implantable cardiac defibrillators may be used to control life-threatening dysrhythmias. To block inappropriate sympathetic stimulation and tachycardia, beta blockers (e.g., metoprolol) are used. If cardiomyopathy has developed in response to a toxin (such as alcohol), further exposure to that toxin must be avoided.

Management of obstructive HCM includes administering negative inotropic agents such as beta-adrenergic blocking agents (carvedilol) and calcium antagonists (diltiazem). These drugs decrease the outflow obstruction that accompanies exercise. They also decrease heart rate (HR), resulting in less angina, dyspnea, and syncope. Vasodilators, diuretics, nitrates, and cardiac glycosides are contraindicated in patients with obstructive HCM because vasodilating and positive inotropic effects may worsen the obstruction (Sherrid & Arabadjian, 2012). Strenuous exercise is also prohibited because it can increase the risk for sudden death.

Surgical Management

Myomectomy and Ablation. The type of surgery performed depends on the type of cardiomyopathy. The most commonly used surgical treatment for obstructive HCM involves excising a portion of the hypertrophied ventricular septum to create a wider outflow tract (**ventriculomyomectomy**; also called *ventricular septal myectomy*). This procedure results in long-term improvement in activity tolerance for most patients.

Percutaneous alcohol septal ablation is another option for patients with HCM. Absolute alcohol is injected into a target septal branch of the left anterior descending coronary artery to produce a small septal infarction.

The patient with arrhythmogenic right ventricular cardiomyopathy who does not respond to drug therapy may have a radiofrequency catheter ablation or placement of an implantable defibrillator (see Chapter 34 for discussion of these procedures).

Heart Transplantation. Heart transplantation (surgical replacement with a donor heart) is the treatment of choice for patients with severe DCM and may be considered for patients with restrictive cardiomyopathy. The procedure may be done also for end-stage heart disease due to coronary artery disease, valvular disease, or congenital heart disease.

Preoperative Care. Criteria for candidate selection for heart transplantation include:

- Life expectancy less than 1 year
- Age generally less than 65 years
- New York Heart Association (NYHA) class III or IV
- Normal or only slightly increased pulmonary vascular resistance
- Absence of active infection
- Stable psychosocial status
- No evidence of current drug or alcohol abuse

Once the candidate is eligible and a heart is available, provide preoperative care as described in Chapter 14.

Operative Procedures. The surgeon transplants a heart from a donor with a comparable body weight and ABO compatibility into a recipient less than 6 hours after procurement. In the most common procedure (**bicaval technique**), the intact right atrium of the donor heart is preserved by anastomoses at the patient's (recipient's) superior and inferior venae cavae. In the more traditional **orthotopic** technique, cuffs of the patient's right and left atria are attached to the donor's atria. Anastomoses are made between the recipient and donor atria, aorta, and pulmonary arteries (Fig. 35-5). Because the remaining remnant of the recipient's atria contains the sinoatrial (SA) node, two unrelated P waves are visible on the ECG.

Postoperative Care. The postoperative care of the heart transplant recipient is similar to that for conventional cardiac surgery (see Chapter 38). However, the nurse must be especially observant to identify occult bleeding into the pericardial sac with the potential for tamponade (see earlier discussion of this complication on p. 699). The patient's pericardium has usually stretched considerably to accommodate the diseased, hypertrophied heart, predisposing him or her to have concealed postoperative bleeding.

The transplanted heart is denervated (disconnected from the body's autonomic nervous system) and is unresponsive to vagal

1. After the recipient is placed on cardiopulmonary bypass, the heart is removed.

2. The posterior walls of the recipient's left and right atria are left intact.

3. The left atrium of the donor heart is anastomosed to the recipient's residual posterior atrial walls, and the other atrial walls, the atrial septum, and the great vessels are joined.

POSTOPERATIVE RESULT

FIG. 35-5 One technique for heart transplantation.

stimulation. In the early postoperative phase, isoproterenol (Isuprel) may be titrated to support the HR and maintain cardiac output. Atropine, digoxin, and carotid sinus pressure are not used because they do not have their usual effects on the new heart. Denervation of the heart may cause pronounced orthostatic hypotension in the immediate postoperative phase. Caution the patient to change position slowly to help prevent this complication. Some patients also require a permanent pacemaker that is rate responsive to his or her activity level. The purpose is to increase CO and improve activity tolerance.

To suppress natural defense mechanisms (especially T- and B-cell function) and prevent transplant rejection, patients require a combination of immunosuppressants for the rest of their lives. Chapter 17 describes transplant rejection and prevention in detail.

> ⚠ **NURSING SAFETY PRIORITY** (QSEN)
>
> **Critical Rescue**
>
> After surgery, perform comprehensive cardiovascular and respiratory assessments frequently according to agency or heart transplant surgical protocol. Chart 35-10 lists the signs and symptoms of rejection that are specific to heart transplant. Report any of these manifestations to the surgeon immediately! To detect rejection, the surgeon performs right endomyocardial biopsies at regularly scheduled intervals and whenever symptoms occur.

Be very careful about handwashing and aseptic technique because patients are immunosuppressed from drug therapy. *Infection is the major cause of death* and usually develops in the immediate post-transplant period or during treatment for acute rejection.

About 50% of patients survive 10 years after transplantation (Eisen, 2014). Many of the surviving patients have a form of

---

> **CHART 35-10   Best Practice for Patient Safety & Quality Care** (QSEN)
>
> ### Assessing for Clinical Manifestations of Heart Transplant Rejection
>
> - Shortness of breath
> - Fatigue
> - Fluid gain (edema, increased weight)
> - Abdominal bloating
> - New bradycardia
> - Hypotension
> - Atrial fibrillation or flutter
> - Decreased activity tolerance
> - Decreased ejection fraction (late sign)

coronary artery disease (CAD) called **coronary artery vasculopathy (CAV)**, which presents as diffuse plaque in the arteries of the donor heart. The cause is thought to involve a combination of immunologic and non-immunologic processes that result in vascular endothelial injury and an inflammatory response (Eisen, 2014). Because the heart is denervated, patients do not usually experience angina. Regularly scheduled exercise tolerance tests and angiography are required to identify CAV. Only a small percentage of patients with CAV benefit from revascularization procedures like balloon angioplasty or coronary artery bypass surgery. Stents are beginning to show some promise in managing these patients. Retransplantation may be done in select patients.

To delay the development of CAV, encourage patients to follow lifestyle changes similar to those with primary CAD (see Chapter 38). The physician may prescribe a calcium channel blocker such as diltiazem (Cardizem) to prevent coronary spasm and closure. Stress the importance of strict adherence to nutritional modifications and drug regimens. Teach the patient the importance of participating in a regular exercise program.

Collaborate with the physical therapist to plan the most appropriate exercise plan for the patient.

Discharge planning involves a collaborative, interdisciplinary approach. Patients require extensive health teaching for self-management and community resources for support.

Counseling and support groups can help patients cope with their fear of organ rejection. Drug therapy adherence is crucial to prevent this problem. Continuing community-based care for patients with a heart transplant is similar to that for heart failure as discussed on p. 689.

NURSING CONCEPTS AND CLINICAL JUDGMENT REVIEW

What might you NOTICE if a patient is experiencing inadequate GAS EXCHANGE and tissue PERFUSION as a result of heart failure?
- Report of shortness of breath, especially on exertion
- Report of dizziness
- Report of weight gain within days
- Syncope
- Dyspnea on exertion
- Report of palpitations
- Report of fatigue and weakness
- Disorientation or acute confusion (especially in older adults)
- Peripheral or abdominal ascites

What should you INTERPRET and how should you RESPOND to a patient experiencing inadequate GAS EXCHANGE and tissue PERFUSION as a result of heart failure?

Perform and interpret physical assessment, including:
- Taking vital signs
- Monitoring oxygen saturation by pulse oximetry
- Performing a complete cardiovascular assessment
- Performing a complete respiratory assessment (listen for crackles or wheezes)
- Weighing patient

- Assessing cognition
- Assessing for pain or other symptoms

Respond by:
- Seeing health care provider immediately or calling 911 if patient is not in hospital setting …OR
- Notifying physician or Rapid Response Team in hospital setting
- Raising the head of the bed to a sitting position
- Giving oxygen
- Maintaining or starting IV line
- Administering furosemide IV push (IVP) as prescribed
- Monitoring intake and output
- Giving ACE inhibitors or ARBs as prescribed IV or orally

On what should you REFLECT?
- Observe patient for increased urinary output.
- Monitor for decreased respiratory distress.
- Continue to monitor for improvement.
- Think about the possible cause(s) of the patient's heart failure.
- Think about your response to the patient.
- Develop a teaching plan for the patient to help prevent worsening or recurrent acute episodes of heart failure.

GET READY FOR THE NCLEX® EXAMINATION!

KEY POINTS

Review these Key Points for each NCLEX Examination Client Needs Category.

Safe and Effective Care Environment
- Provide information about continuing care for patients with heart failure (HF) after discharge to the community.
- Assess whether patients with end-stage HF have advance directives. If not, provide information about them.
- Collaborate with members of the health care team when developing and implementing a plan of care for patients with heart failure. **Teamwork and Collaboration** QSEN
- Teach patients about community support groups and resources such as the American Heart Association.

Health Promotion and Maintenance
- Provide teaching about self-management at home for patients with HF (see Table 35-4).
- Monitor older adults who are taking digoxin for manifestations of toxicity. Monitor potassium levels to check for hypokalemia (see Chart 35-5). **Safety** QSEN
- Teach patients taking ACE inhibitors or ARBs to change positions slowly to avoid orthostatic hypotension, especially older adults. **Safety** QSEN

- Teach the patient with valvular dysfunction, cardiac infection, or cardiomyopathy the necessity of taking preventive antibiotic therapy before any invasive procedure. **Evidence-Based Practice** QSEN

Psychosocial Integrity
- Assess the patient for depression resulting from altered self-concept and anxiety.
- Assess the patient's coping skills. **Patient-Centered Care** QSEN

Physiological Integrity
- Assess the patient for manifestations of right- and left-sided HF (see Charts 35-1 and 35-2).
- Weigh daily and record intake and output of patients with HF.
- Assess for early signs and symptoms of pulmonary edema (e.g., crackles in the lung bases, dyspnea at rest, disorientation, confusion), especially in older adults. **Safety** QSEN
- Assess for symptoms of worsening HF: rapid weight gain (3 lb in a week), a decrease in exercise tolerance lasting 2 to 3 days, cold symptoms (cough) lasting more than 3 to 5 days,

nocturia, development of dyspnea or angina at rest, or unstable angina. **Safety** [QSEN]

- Monitor the HF patient on beta blockers carefully for hypotension and bradycardia. **Safety** [QSEN]
- Monitor the pulse of patients taking digoxin before administration, and report to the health care provider a pulse that is not within the desired parameters.
- Monitor for manifestations of pulmonary edema as listed in Chart 35-3.
- Place the patient in a sitting position and provide oxygen therapy at a high flow rate (unless otherwise contraindicated) if pulmonary edema is suspected. **Evidence-Based Practice** [QSEN]
- Recognize that home care nurses perform and document focused physical assessments for cardiac patients as delineated in Chart 35-4. **Informatics** [QSEN]

- Monitor the patient with valvular dysfunction for atrial fibrillation, which may lead to hemostasis and mural thrombi. Monitor for an irregularly irregular cardiac rhythm, and administer warfarin as indicated.
- Document neurovascular status frequently because emboli from valvular disease may cause strokes. **Informatics** [QSEN]
- Differentiate major types of cardiomyopathy as described in Table 35-5.
- Observe for symptoms of heart transplant rejection as listed in Chart 35-10.
- Provide care for patients with pericarditis as outlined in Chart 35-9.

Care of Patients with Vascular Problems

Donna D. Ignatavicius

http://evolve.elsevier.com/Iggy/

PRIORITY CONCEPTS

- Perfusion
- Clotting
- Pain
- Inflammation

LEARNING OUTCOMES

Safe and Effective Care Environment

1. Collaborate with interdisciplinary health care team members when providing care for patients with PERFUSION and CLOTTING problems.
2. Prioritize care for patients with hypertension.

Health Promotion and Maintenance

3. Identify risk factors for vascular problems.
4. Teach patients about lifestyle modifications to prevent vascular problems.

Physiological Integrity

5. Explain the INFLAMMATION process that is associated with the development of arteriosclerosis and atherosclerosis.
6. Interpret essential laboratory data related to risk for atherosclerosis.
7. Discuss the role of nutrition therapy in the management of patients with arteriosclerosis.

8. Describe the differences between essential and secondary hypertension.
9. Develop an evidence-based plan of care for a patient with essential hypertension.
10. Document a teaching plan for patients receiving drug therapy for hypertension.
11. Compare common assessment findings present in patients with peripheral arterial and peripheral venous disease.
12. Identify when venous thromboembolism (VTE) and complications of VTE occur.
13. Plan evidence-based nursing interventions to help prevent VTE.
14. Explain the nurse's role in monitoring patients who are receiving anticoagulants.
15. Compare assessment findings associated with Raynaud's phenomenon and Buerger's disease.

The *peripheral* vascular system is essential for transporting blood to and from distal tissues in the extremities. When peripheral blood vessels are diseased or damaged, especially in the legs, arterial blood flow is impaired, preventing distal areas like the feet from having adequate PERFUSION. The result can be ischemia and necrosis (cell death). Venous disease causes blood to back up into the distal areas and can lead to edema and thromboses (clots) that can become emboli, a life-threatening complication.

ARTERIOSCLEROSIS AND ATHEROSCLEROSIS

❖ PATHOPHYSIOLOGY

Arteriosclerosis is a thickening, or hardening, of the arterial wall that is often associated with aging. **Atherosclerosis**, a type of arteriosclerosis, involves the formation of plaque within the arterial wall and is the leading risk factor for cardiovascular disease. Usually the disease affects the larger arteries, such as

coronary artery beds; aorta; carotid and vertebral arteries; renal, iliac, and femoral arteries; or any combination of these.

The exact pathophysiology of atherosclerosis is not known, but the condition is thought to occur from blood vessel damage that causes INFLAMMATION (see the discussion of inflammation in Chapter 17) (Fig. 36-1). After the vessel becomes inflamed, a fatty streak appears on the intimal surface (inner lining) of the artery. Through the process of cellular proliferation, collagen migrates over the fatty streak, forming a fibrous plaque. The fibrous plaque is often elevated and protrudes into the vessel lumen, partially or completely obstructing blood flow through the artery. Plaques are either stable or unstable. Unstable plaques are prone to rupture and are often clinically silent until they rupture (McCance et al., 2014).

In the final stage, the fibrous plaques become calcified, hemorrhagic, ulcerated, or thrombosed and affect all layers of the vessel. The rate of progression of the process may be influenced by genetic factors; certain chronic diseases (e.g., diabetes

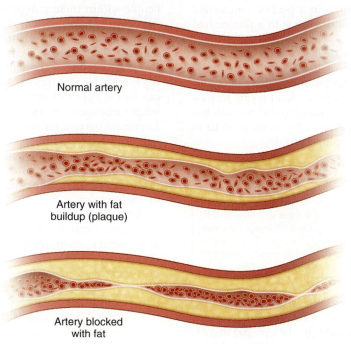

Normal artery

Artery with fat
buildup (plaque)

Artery blocked
with fat

FIG. 36-1 Pathophysiology of atherosclerosis.

mellitus); and lifestyle habits, including smoking, eating habits, and level of exercise.

When *stable* plaque ruptures, thrombosis (blood clot) and constriction obstruct the vessel lumen, causing inadequate perfusion and oxygenation to distal tissues. *Unstable* plaque rupture causes more severe damage. After the rupture occurs, the exposed underlying tissue causes platelet adhesion and rapid thrombus formation. The thrombus may suddenly block a blood vessel, resulting in ischemia and infarction (e.g., myocardial infarction) (McCance et al., 2014).

Endothelial (intimal) injury of the major arteries of the body can be caused by many factors. Elevated levels of **lipids** (fats) like low-density lipoprotein cholesterol (LDL-C) and decreased levels of high-density lipoprotein cholesterol (HDL-C) can cause chemical injuries to the vessel wall. (Chapter 33 discusses lipids in detail.) Chemical injury can also be caused by elevated levels of toxins in the bloodstream, which may occur with renal failure or by carbon monoxide circulating in the bloodstream from cigarette smoking. The vessel wall can be weakened by the natural process of aging or by diseases such as hypertension.

Genetic predisposition and diabetes have a major effect on the development of atherosclerosis. Some patients have familial **hyperlipidemia**, an elevation of serum lipid levels. In these people, the liver makes excessive cholesterol and other fats. However, some people with hereditary atherosclerosis have a normal blood cholesterol level. The reason for the development and progression of plaque in these patients is not understood (McCance et al., 2014).

Adult patients of any age with severe diabetes mellitus frequently have premature and severe atherosclerosis from microvascular damage. The premature atherosclerosis occurs because diabetes promotes an increase in LDL-C and triglycerides (lipids) in plasma. In addition, arterial damage may result from the effect of hyperglycemia.

Other factors are indirectly related to atherosclerosis development. A list of risk factors is found in Table 36-1.

TABLE 36-1	Risk Factors for Atherosclerosis
• Low HDL-C	• Sedentary lifestyle
• High LDL-C	• Smoking
• Increased triglycerides	• Stress
• Genetic predisposition	• African-American or Hispanic
• Diabetes mellitus	ethnicity
• Obesity	• Older adult

HDL-C, High-density lipoprotein cholesterol; *LDL-C,* low-density lipoprotein cholesterol.

It is not known exactly how many people have atherosclerosis, but small plaques are almost always present in the arteries of young adults. The incidence can be better quantified by assessing the number of cardiovascular diseases (CVDs) that result from atherosclerosis. An estimated 81 million U.S. adults have one or more types of CVD (Go et al., 2013). About half of those with CVD are older than 60 years, and many more are middle-aged. The number of people affected by atherosclerosis is likely to increase as the population ages.

❖ PATIENT-CENTERED COLLABORATIVE CARE

◆ Assessment

Physical Assessment/Clinical Manifestations. The assessment of a patient with atherosclerosis includes a complete cardiovascular assessment because associated heart disease is often present. Because of the high incidence of hypertension in patients with atherosclerosis, assess the blood pressure in both arms.

Palpate pulses at all of the major sites on the body, and note any differences. *Palpate each carotid artery separately to prevent blocking blood flow to the brain!* Also feel for temperature differences in the lower extremities, and check capillary filling. Prolonged capillary filling (>3 seconds in young to middle-aged adults; >5 seconds in older adults) generally indicates poor circulation, *although this indicator is not the most reliable indicator of* PERFUSION. An extremity in a person with severe atherosclerotic disease may be cool or cold with a diminished or absent pulse.

Many patients with vascular disease have a bruit in the larger arteries, which can be heard with a stethoscope or Doppler probe. A **bruit** is a turbulent, swishing sound, which can be soft or loud in pitch. It is heard as a result of blood trying to pass through a narrowed artery. A bruit is considered abnormal, but it does not indicate the severity of disease. Bruits often occur in the carotid, aortic, femoral, and popliteal arteries.

> ### ! NURSING SAFETY PRIORITY (QSEN)
> #### Critical Rescue
>
> A decrease in intensity or a complete loss of a pulse in a patient with atherosclerosis may indicate an arterial occlusion (blockage) in the area supplied by the artery. Immediately report pulselessness to the health care provider and document for emergency management (described later in this chapter under Acute Peripheral Arterial Occlusion).

Laboratory Assessment. Patients with atherosclerosis often have elevated lipids, including cholesterol and triglycerides. Total serum *cholesterol* levels should be below 200 mg/dL. Elevated cholesterol levels are confirmed by HDL and LDL measurements. Increased low-density lipoprotein cholesterol (LDL-C) ("bad" cholesterol) levels indicate that a person is at an increased risk for atherosclerosis. Low high-density lipoprotein cholesterol (HDL-C) ("good" cholesterol) levels also indicate an increased risk. In general, a desirable LDL-C level is one below 130 mg/dL for healthy people and below 70 mg/dL for those diagnosed with CVD or who are diabetic. A desirable HDL-C level is 45 mg/dL or above for men and 55 mg/dL for women (Pagana & Pagana, 2014). These values differ based on age and comorbidities.

Triglyceride level may also be elevated with atherosclerosis and is an emerging lipid risk factor by the classic Adult Treatment Panel Report No. 3 (ATP III) released by the National Heart, Lung, and Blood Institute (National Cholesterol Education Program, 2002). A level of 160 mg/dL or above indicates **hypertriglyceridemia** in men. Women should have a level below 135 mg/dL (Pagana & Pagana, 2014). Elevated triglycerides are considered a marker for other lipoproteins. They also suggest metabolic syndrome, which increases the risk for coronary heart disease (see Table 38-1 and discussion in Chapter 38).

◆ Interventions

Atherosclerosis progresses for years before clinical manifestations occur. Adults who are at risk for the disease can often be identified through cholesterol screening and history. Because of the high incidence in the United States, low-risk people 20 years of age and older are advised to have their total serum cholesterol level evaluated at least once every 5 years. More frequent measurements are suggested for people with multiple risk factors and those older than 40 years.

People with multiple risk factors are grouped into high-risk patient categories termed "coronary heart disease equivalents." These groups include:

- Patients with diabetes but without signs of vascular disease
- Patients with a Framingham Heart Study 10-year absolute risk score of over 20% for coronary heart disease events
- Patients identified with multiple metabolic risk factors

People within these groups are at the same risk level as those who already have vascular disease.

Interventions for patients with atherosclerosis or those at high risk for the disease focus on lifestyle changes. Teach patients about the need to make daily changes by avoiding or minimizing modifiable risk factors. *Modifiable risk factors* are those that can be changed or controlled by the patient, such as smoking, weight management, and exercise. Nutrition is one of the most important parts of the risk-reduction plan. Chapter 38 describes how to manage modifiable risk factors in detail in the Health Promotion and Maintenance section, p. 759. If lipoprotein levels do not improve after lifestyle changes, the health care provider may prescribe drug therapy to lower cholesterol and/or triglycerides.

Nutrition Therapy. The American College of Cardiology and American Heart Association (ACC/AHA) recently published new dietary recommendations for lowering LDL-C levels (Eckel et al., 2014). These recommendations were based on the best current evidence from randomized controlled trials and include:

- Consume a dietary pattern that emphasizes intake of vegetables, fruits, and whole grains.
- Consume low-fat dairy products, poultry, fish, legumes, nontropical (e.g., canola) vegetable oils, and nuts.
- Limit intake of sweets, sugar-sweetened beverages, and red meats.
- Aim for a dietary pattern that includes 5% to 6% of calories from saturated fat.
- Reduce percent of calories from *trans* fat.

These guidelines are similar to the Dietary Approaches to Stop Hypertension (DASH), which also recommend daily sodium, potassium, and fiber amounts (National Heart, Lung, and Blood Institute, 2012). In collaboration with the dietitian as needed, teach the patient about the types of fat content in food. Meats and eggs contain mostly saturated fats and are high in cholesterol. Instruct patients about increasing dietary fiber to 30 g each day, which is consistent with DASH guidelines.

Physical Activity. The ACC/AHA also recommends that adults engage in aerobic physical activity 3 or 4 times a week to reduce LDL-C levels. Each session should last for 40 minutes on average and involve moderate-to-vigorous physical activity (Eckel et al., 2014).

Drug Therapy. For patients with elevated total and LDL-C levels that do not respond adequately to dietary intervention, the health care provider prescribes a cholesterol-lowering agent. Drug choice and dosing depend on the serum cholesterol level, the degree to which the level needs to be decreased, and the patient's age (Stone et al., 2014). Because most of these drugs can produce major side effects, they are generally given only when nonpharmacologic management has been unsuccessful.

A class of drugs known as *3-hydroxy-3-methylglutaryl coenzyme A (HMG-CoA) reductase inhibitors (statins)* successfully reduces total cholesterol in most patients when used for an extended period. Examples include lovastatin (Mevacor), simvastatin (Zocor), and pitavastatin (Livalo), which lower both LDL-C and triglyceride levels (Table 36-2).

The American College of Cardiology/American Heart Association recently published new recommendations for treatment of high cholesterol to reduce atherosclerotic cardiovascular disease (ASCVD) in adults (Stone et al., 2014). These evidence-based recommendations are highlighted in Table 36-3.

TABLE 36-2 Commonly Used Drugs for Lowering LDL-C Levels

HMG-CoA Reductase Inhibitors (Statins)	Combination Drugs
• Lovastatin (Mevacor) • Atorvastatin (Lipitor) • Simvastatin (Zocor) • Fluvastatin (Lescol) • Rosuvastatin (Crestor) • Pravastatin (Pravachol) • Pitavastatin (Livalo)	• Ezetimibe and simvastatin (Vytorin) • Amlodipine and atorvastatin (Caduet) • Niacin and lovastatin (Advicor)

HMG-CoA, 3-hydroxy-3-methylglutaryl coenzyme A.

! NURSING SAFETY PRIORITY (QSEN)

Drug Alert

Statins reduce cholesterol synthesis in the liver and increase clearance of LDL-C from the blood. Therefore they are contraindicated in patients with active liver disease or during pregnancy because they can cause muscle myopathies and marked decreases in liver function. Statins also have the potential for interactions with other drugs, such as warfarin, cyclosporine, and selected antibiotics. Statins are discontinued if the patient has muscle cramping or elevated liver enzyme levels. Some patients also report abdominal bloating, flatulence, diarrhea, and/or constipation as side effects of these drugs. Remind patients to have laboratory testing follow-up as prescribed by their health care provider (Lilley et al., 2014).

Teach patients taking statin drugs, especially those taking atorvastatin, lovastatin, and simvastatin, to *avoid grapefruit and grapefruit juice in their diet.* Grapefruit contains a group of chemicals called *furanocoumarins* that bind to and inactivate the enzyme *CYP3A4.* This enzyme is important for metabolism of many drugs, including statins. If it is inactivated, too much of the statin drug can remain in the patient's bloodstream, causing possible kidney failure, heart failure, GI bleeding, or even death (Bailey et al., 2013).

A different type of lipid-lowering agent, ezetimibe (Zetia), may be used in place of or in combination with statin-type drugs. This drug inhibits the absorption of cholesterol through the small intestine. Vytorin is a combination drug containing ezetimibe and simvastatin. This drug works two ways—by reducing the absorption of cholesterol and by decreasing the amount of cholesterol synthesis in the liver. Other statin combinations have been developed to improve lipid levels, such as Advicor—a combination of niacin and lovastatin. Aspirin and pravastatin are combined as Pravigard. Amlodipine (Norvasc) and atorvastatin are combined as Caduet to decrease blood pressure while decreasing triglycerides (TGs), increasing HDL, and lowering LDL. Combining drugs may improve adherence for the patient who is often taking multiple drugs.

Complementary and Alternative Therapies. Nicotinic acid or niacin (Niaspan), a B vitamin, may lower LDL-C and very-low-density lipoprotein (VLDL) cholesterol levels and increase HDL-C levels in some patients, although the evidence supporting its use is lacking. It is used as a single agent or in combination with an acid-binding resin drug or a statin. Low doses are recommended because many patients experience flushing and a very warm feeling all over. Higher doses can result in an elevation of hepatic enzymes.

Lovaza (omega-3 ethyl esters) is approved by the Food and Drug Administration (FDA) as an adjunct to diet to reduce TGs that are greater than 500 mg/dL. This drug also decreases plaque growth and INFLAMMATION and reduces clot formation.

TABLE 36-3 Selected 2013 ACC/AHA Recommendations for the Treatment of Serum Cholesterol to Reduce Atherosclerotic Cardiovascular Disease Risk in Adults

Primary Prevention
- All people with LDL-C equal to or greater than 190 mg/dL should be evaluated for secondary causes of hyperlipidemia and treated with statin therapy.
- Adults with diabetes mellitus who are 40 to 75 years of age should be treated with high-intensity statin therapy.
- Adults 40 to 75 years of age with LDL-C of 70 to 189 mg/dL without clinical signs of ASCVD or diabetes should be treated with moderate- to high-intensity statin therapy.

Secondary Prevention
- High-intensity statin therapy should be initiated or continued as first-line treatment in adults 75 years of age or younger who have clinical manifestations of ASCVD, unless contraindicated.
- In people older than 75 years, the potential for ASCVD risk-reduction benefits, adverse drug effects, and drug-drug interactions should be evaluated.

Data from Stone, N.J., Robinson, J., Lichtenstein, A.H., Merz, N.B., Blum, C.B., Eckel, R.H., et al. (2014). 2013 ACC/AHA guidelines on the treatment of blood cholesterol to reduce atherosclerotic cardiovascular risk in adults: A report of the American College of Cardiology/American Heart Association Task Force on Practice Guidelines. *Circulation, 129*(25 Suppl 2), S1-S45.
ASCVD, Atherosclerotic cardiovascular disease; *LDL-C,* low-density lipoprotein cholesterol.

? NCLEX EXAMINATION CHALLENGE

Health Promotion and Maintenance

A client diagnosed with atherosclerosis has been prescribed lovastatin (Mevacor). Which statement by the client indicates a need for further teaching?
A. "I won't need to change my diet because now I'm taking a pill."
B. "I'll follow up with my nurse practitioner on a regular basis."
C. "I need to quit smoking as soon as I possibly can."
D. "I shouldn't drink grapefruit juice while on this drug."

HYPERTENSION

Hypertension, or high blood pressure (BP), is the most common health problem seen in primary care settings and can cause stroke, myocardial infarction (heart attack), kidney failure, and death if not treated early and effectively. The Eighth Joint National Committee (JNC 8) on Prevention, Detection, Evaluation, and Treatment of High Blood Pressure recently published its *2014 Evidence-Based Guidelines for the Management of High Blood Pressure in Adults* based on the results of randomized controlled trials, the gold standard for establishing recommendations for best clinical practice (James et al., 2014). These new guidelines replace the JNC 7 recommendations and hypertension classifications.

According to JNC 8, in the general population ages 60 years and older, the desired BP is below 150/90. For people younger than 60 years, the desired BP is below 140/90. Patients whose blood pressures are above these desired goals should be treated with drug therapy (James et al., 2014). Adult patients with specific risk factors for developing hypertension should be treated at any age, as described later under Drug Therapy.

❖ PATHOPHYSIOLOGY

To best understand the pathophysiology of hypertension, a review of normal blood pressure and how it is normally maintained is essential.

Mechanisms That Influence Blood Pressure. The systemic arterial blood pressure is a product of cardiac output (CO) and total peripheral vascular resistance (PVR). Cardiac output is determined by the stroke volume (SV) multiplied by heart rate (HR) (CO = SV × HR). Control of peripheral vascular resistance (i.e., vessel constriction or dilation) is maintained by the autonomic nervous system and circulating hormones, such as norepinephrine and epinephrine. Consequently, any factor that increases peripheral vascular resistance, heart rate, or stroke volume increases the systemic arterial pressure. Conversely, any factor that decreases peripheral vascular resistance, heart rate, or stroke volume decreases the systemic arterial pressure and can cause decreased PERFUSION to body tissues.

Stabilizing mechanisms exist in the body to exert an overall regulation of systemic arterial pressure and to prevent circulatory collapse. Four control systems play a major role in maintaining blood pressure:
- The arterial baroreceptor system
- Regulation of body fluid volume
- The renin-angiotensin-aldosterone system
- Vascular autoregulation

Arterial baroreceptors are found primarily in the carotid sinus, aorta, and wall of the left ventricle. They monitor the level of arterial pressure and counteract a rise in arterial pressure through vagally mediated cardiac slowing and vasodilation with decreased sympathetic tone. Therefore reflex control of circulation elevates the systemic arterial pressure when it falls and lowers it when it rises. Why baroreceptor control fails in hypertension is not clear (McCance et al., 2014).

Changes *in fluid volume* also affect the systemic arterial pressure. For example, if there is an excess of sodium and/or water in a person's body, the blood pressure rises through complex physiologic mechanisms that change the venous return to the heart, producing a rise in cardiac output. If the kidneys are functioning adequately, a rise in systemic arterial pressure produces diuresis (excessive voiding) and a fall in pressure. Pathologic conditions change the pressure threshold at which the kidneys excrete sodium and water, thereby altering the systemic arterial pressure.

The *renin-angiotensin-aldosterone* system also regulates blood pressure (see discussion in Chapter 11). The kidney produces renin, an enzyme that acts on angiotensinogen (a plasma protein substrate) to split off angiotensin I, which is converted by an enzyme in the lung to form angiotensin II. Angiotensin II has strong vasoconstrictor action on blood vessels and is the controlling mechanism for aldosterone release. Aldosterone then works on the collecting tubules in the kidneys to reabsorb sodium. Sodium retention inhibits fluid loss, thus increasing blood volume and subsequent blood pressure.

Inappropriate secretion of renin may cause increased peripheral vascular resistance in patients with hypertension. When the blood pressure is high, renin levels should decrease because the increased renal arteriolar pressure usually inhibits renin secretion. However, for most people with essential hypertension, renin levels remain normal.

The process of *vascular autoregulation,* which keeps perfusion of tissues in the body relatively constant, appears to be important in causing hypertension. However, the exact mechanism of how this system works is poorly understood.

Classifications of Hypertension. Hypertension can be essential (primary) or secondary. **Essential hypertension** is the most common type and is not caused by an existing health problem. However, a number of risk factors can increase a person's likelihood of becoming hypertensive. Continuous BP elevation in patients with essential hypertension results in damage to vital organs by causing medial hyperplasia (thickening) of the arterioles. As the blood vessels thicken and PERFUSION decreases, body organs are damaged. These changes can result in myocardial infarctions, strokes, peripheral vascular disease (PVD), or kidney failure.

Specific disease states and drugs can increase a person's susceptibility to hypertension. A person with this type of elevation in blood pressure has **secondary hypertension.**

Malignant hypertension is a severe type of elevated blood pressure that rapidly progresses. A person with this health problem usually has symptoms such as morning headaches, blurred vision, and dyspnea and/or symptoms of uremia (accumulation in the blood of substances ordinarily eliminated in the urine). Patients are often in their 30s, 40s, or 50s with their systolic blood pressure greater than 200 mm Hg. The diastolic blood pressure is greater than 150 mm Hg or greater than 130 mm Hg when there are pre-existing complications. Unless intervention occurs promptly, a patient with malignant hypertension may experience kidney failure, left ventricular heart failure, or stroke.

Etiology and Genetic Risk. *Essential* hypertension can develop when a patient has any one or more of the risk factors listed in Table 36-4.

Kidney disease is one of the most common causes of *secondary* hypertension. Hypertension can develop when there is any sudden damage to the kidneys. Renovascular hypertension is associated with narrowing of one or more of the main arteries carrying blood directly to the kidneys, known as *renal artery stenosis (RAS).* Many patients have been able to reduce the use of their antihypertensive drugs when the narrowed arteries are dilated through angioplasty with stent placement.

Dysfunction of the adrenal medulla or the adrenal cortex can also cause secondary hypertension. *Adrenal-mediated hypertension* is due to primary excesses of aldosterone, cortisol, and catecholamines. In *primary aldosteronism,* excessive aldosterone causes hypertension and hypokalemia (low potassium levels). It usually arises from benign adenomas of the adrenal cortex.

TABLE 36-4	**Etiology of Hypertension**
Essential (Primary)	**Secondary**
• Family history of hypertension	• Kidney disease
• African-American ethnicity	• Primary aldosteronism
• Hyperlipidemia	• Pheochromocytoma
• Smoking	• Cushing's disease
• Older than 60 years or postmenopausal	• Coarctation of the aorta
• Excessive sodium and caffeine intake	• Brain tumors
• Overweight/obesity	• Encephalitis
• Physical inactivity	• Pregnancy
• Excessive alcohol intake	• Drugs:
• Low potassium, calcium, or magnesium intake	• Estrogen (e.g., oral contraceptives)
• Excessive and continuous stress	• Glucocorticoids
	• Mineralocorticoids
	• Sympathomimetics

Pheochromocytomas are tumors that originate most commonly in the adrenal medulla and result in excessive secretion of catecholamines, resulting in life-threatening high blood pressure. In *Cushing's syndrome,* excessive glucocorticoids are excreted from the adrenal cortex. The most common cause of Cushing's syndrome is either adrenocortical hyperplasia or adrenocortical adenoma (tumor).

Drugs that can cause secondary hypertension include estrogen, glucocorticoids, mineralocorticoids, sympathomimetics, cyclosporine, and erythropoietin. The use of estrogen-containing oral contraceptives is likely the most common cause of secondary hypertension in women. Drugs that cause hypertension are discontinued to reverse this problem.

Incidence and Prevalence. Hypertension is a worldwide epidemic. In the United States, one in every three adults has high blood pressure or is being treated for hypertension (Go et al., 2013). The disease can shorten life expectancy.

GENDER HEALTH CONSIDERATIONS
Patient-Centered Care QSEN

A higher percentage of men than women have hypertension until age 45 years. From 45 to 54 years, women have a slightly higher percentage of hypertension than men. After age 54 years, women have a much higher percentage of the disease (Go et al., 2013). The causes for these differences are not known.

CULTURAL CONSIDERATIONS
Patient-Centered Care QSEN

The prevalence of hypertension in African Americans in the United States is among the highest in the world and is constantly increasing. When compared with Euro-Americans, they develop high BP earlier in life, making them much more likely to die from strokes, heart disease, and kidney disease (Go et al., 2013). The exact reasons for these differences are not known, but genetics and environmental factors may play a role. Efforts to raise awareness of hypertension through education within African-American communities, including the importance of receiving treatment and controlling blood pressure, have been somewhat successful. Geographic differences still exist (Go et al., 2013).

Health Promotion and Maintenance

Control of hypertension has resulted in major decreases in cardiovascular morbidity and mortality. The U.S. *Healthy People 2020* campaign includes a number of objectives related to hypertension to decrease cardiovascular mortality (Table 36-5).

The *2013 ACA/AHA Guidelines on Lifestyle Management to Reduce Cardiovascular Risk* outlines evidence-based dietary and exercise practices to help lower blood pressure (Eckel et al., 2014). These guidelines are similar to the Dietary Approaches to Stop Hypertension (DASH) and include:

- Consume a dietary pattern that emphasizes intake of vegetables, fruits, and whole grains.
- Consume low-fat dairy products, poultry, fish, legumes, nontropical vegetable oils, and nuts.
- Limit intake of sweets, sugar-sweetened beverages, and red meats.
- Lower sodium intake to no more than 2400 mg per day; a limit of 1500 mg of sodium per day is preferred.
- Engage in aerobic physical activity 3 or 4 times a week. Each session should last for 40 minutes on average and involve moderate-to-vigorous physical activity.

TABLE 36-5 **Meeting** *Healthy People 2020* **Objectives**

Heart Disease and Stroke

Selected objectives retained from *Healthy People 2010:*
- Increase the proportion of adults with high blood pressure who are taking action to help control their blood pressure.
- Increase the proportion of adults who have had their blood pressure measured within the preceding 2 years and can state whether their blood pressure was normal or high.

Selected objectives retained but modified from *Healthy People 2010:*
- Reduce the proportion of persons in the population with hypertension.
- Increase the proportion of adults with prehypertension who meet the recommended guidelines for:
  a. Body mass index (BMI)
  b. Saturated fat consumption
  c. Sodium intake
  d. Physical activity
  e. Moderate alcohol consumption
- Increase the proportion of adults with hypertension who meet the [above] recommended guidelines.

New objectives for *Healthy People 2020:*
- Increase the proportion of adults with hypertension who are taking the recommended medications to decrease their blood pressure.

Data from www.healthypeople.gov/2020.

In addition to following specific dietary and physical activity guidelines, teach patients ways to decrease other modifiable risk factors for hypertension, such as smoking and excessive alcohol intake. Risk factor prevention and lifestyle changes are discussed in more detail in Chapter 38.

❖ PATIENT-CENTERED COLLABORATIVE CARE
◆ Assessment

History. During history taking, review the patient's risk factors for hypertension. Collect data on the patient's age; ethnic origin or race; family history of hypertension; average dietary intake of calories, sodium- and potassium-containing foods, and alcohol; and exercise habits. Also assess any past or present history of kidney or cardiovascular disease and current use of drug therapy or illicit drugs.

Physical Assessment/Clinical Manifestations. When a diagnosis of hypertension is made, most people have no symptoms. However, some patients experience headaches, facial flushing (redness), dizziness, or fainting as a result of the elevated blood pressure. Obtain blood pressure readings in both arms. Two or more readings may be taken at each visit (Fig. 36-2). Some patients have high blood pressure due to anxiety associated with visiting a health care provider. Be sure to take an accurate blood pressure by using an appropriate-size cuff. Anderson et al. (2010) found that forearm blood pressure measurements are as accurate as upper arm blood pressures, especially in patients who are obese.

To detect postural (orthostatic) changes, take readings with the patient in the supine (lying) or sitting position and at least 2 minutes later when standing. Orthostatic hypotension is a decrease in blood pressure (20 mm Hg systolic and/or 10 mm Hg diastolic) when the patient changes position from lying to sitting.

Funduscopic examination of the eyes to observe vascular changes in the retina is done by a skilled health care practitioner.

FIG. **36-2** Blood pressure screening during history and physical examination.

The appearance of the retina can be a reliable index of the severity and prognosis of hypertension.

Physical assessment is helpful in diagnosing several conditions that produce secondary hypertension. The presence of abdominal bruits is typical of patients with renal artery stenosis. Tachycardia, sweating, and pallor may suggest a pheochromocytoma (adrenal medulla tumor). Coarctation of the aorta is evidenced by elevation of blood pressure in the arms, with normal or low blood pressure in the lower extremities. Femoral pulses are also delayed or absent.

Psychosocial Assessment. Assess for psychosocial stressors that can worsen hypertension and affect the patient's ability to adhere to treatment. Evaluate job-related, economic, and other life stressors, as well as the patient's response to these stressors. Some patients may have difficulty coping with the lifestyle changes needed to control hypertension. Be sure to assess past coping strategies.

Diagnostic Assessment. Although no laboratory tests are diagnostic of essential hypertension, several laboratory tests can assess possible causes of secondary hypertension. Kidney disease can be diagnosed by the presence of protein and red blood cells in the urine, elevated levels of blood urea nitrogen (BUN), and elevated serum creatinine levels. The creatinine clearance test directly indicates the glomerular filtration ability of the kidneys. The normal value is 107 to 139 mL/min for men and 87 to 107 mL/min for women (Pagana & Pagana, 2014). Decreased levels indicate acute or chronic kidney disease.

Urinary test results are positive for the presence of catecholamines in patients with a pheochromocytoma (tumor of the adrenal medulla). An elevation in levels of serum corticoids and 17-ketosteroids in the urine is diagnostic of Cushing's disease.

No specific x-ray studies can diagnose hypertension. Routine chest radiography may help recognize cardiomegaly (heart enlargement).

An electrocardiogram (ECG) determines the degree of cardiac involvement. Left atrial and ventricular hypertrophy is the first ECG sign of heart disease resulting from hypertension. Left ventricular remodeling can be detected on the 12-lead ECG (see Chapter 38 for discussion of remodeling).

◆ ***Analysis***

The priority collaborative problems for patients with hypertension include:

1. Need for health teaching related to the plan of care for hypertension management
2. Risk for nonadherence related to side effects of drug therapy and necessary changes in lifestyle

◆ ***Planning and Implementation***

Health Teaching

Planning: Expected Outcomes. The patient with hypertension is expected to verbalize his or her individualized plan of care for hypertension (see the Concept Map on Hypertension).

Interventions. Lifestyle changes are considered the foundation of hypertension control. If these changes are unsuccessful, the primary care provider considers the use of antihypertensive drugs. There is no surgical treatment for essential hypertension. However, surgery may be indicated for certain causes of secondary hypertension, such as kidney disease, coarctation of the aorta, and pheochromocytoma.

Lifestyle Changes. In collaboration with the health care team, teach the patient to (Baldwin, 2011):

• Restrict sodium intake in the diet per the ACA/AHA guidelines
• Reduce weight, if overweight or obese
• Use alcohol sparingly (no more than 1 drink a day for women and 2 drinks a day for men [1 drink = 12 oz. beer, 5 oz. wine, or 1.5 oz. liquor such as vodka or gin.])
• Exercise 3 or 4 days a week for 40 minutes each day per the ACA/AHA guidelines
• Use relaxation techniques to decrease stress
• Avoid tobacco and caffeine

Strategies to help patients make these changes are discussed in Chapter 38.

Complementary and Alternative Therapies. Garlic and coenzyme Q_{10} have been used for a number of health problems, but evidence to support their use to prevent hypertension is controversial. Evidence by consensus and case reports does support garlic's cholesterol-lowering ability and its ability to decrease blood pressure in patients with hypertension (National Center for Complementary and Alternative Medicine, 2013). Teach patients to check with their health care provider before starting garlic or any herbal therapy because of possible side effects and interactions with other herbs, foods, or drugs. Garlic can damage the liver and cause bleeding in some patients, especially if they have invasive procedures such as surgery.

Some patients have also had success with biofeedback, meditation, and acupuncture as part of their overall management plan. These methods may be most useful as adjuncts for patients who experience continuous and severe stress.

Drug Therapy. Drug therapy is individualized for each patient, with consideration given to culture, age, other existing illness, severity of blood pressure elevation, and cost of drugs and follow-up. Once-a-day drug therapy is best, especially for the older adult, because the more doses required each day, the higher the risk that a patient will not follow the treatment regimen. However, many patients with hypertension need two or more drugs to adequately control blood pressure.

In the largest hypertensive trial done to date, Antihypertensive and Lipid-Lowering Treatment to Prevent Heart Attack Trial (ALLHAT), the use of diuretics has been practically

CONCEPT MAP

HYPERTENSION

PAIN · PERFUSION · CLOTTING

Concept Map by Deanne A. Blach, MSN, RN

INTERVENTIONS

1. Data Collection
- Assess risk factors: age, ethnicity, family history, diet history, alcohol consumption, drug use, history of renal or CV disease. *Reviews modifiable and nonmodifiable risk factors that decrease PERFUSION and provides a foundation for teaching lifestyle changes.*

2. Physical Assessment
- Assess BP in both arms with accurately sized BP cuff. *Determines orthostatic changes; increased incidence of hypertension in patients with atherosclerosis.*
- Palpate all pulses and note differences; palpate each carotid artery separately. *Assesses for heart blocking PERFUSION to the brain.*
- Check temperature differences in lower extremities; check capillary filling. *Assesses heart disease that is often present in patients with DM.*

3. Lifestyle Modifications
- Teach the patient to restrict sodium, identify potassium-rich foods, control weight, consume alcohol sparingly, increase exercise, use relaxation techniques, and avoid tobacco and caffeine. *Educates about decreasing modifiable risk factors to control hypertension and stresses the importance of lifestyle choices.*
- Identify ways to encourage drug adherence. *Encourages the patient without physical symptoms, economic restraints, or forgetfulness, the importance of taking medications as prescribed to prevent decreased PERFUSION*

4. Psychosocial Assessment
- Evaluate economic and other life stressors as well as patient's response to stressors. Assess past coping strategies. *Determines the patient's coping ability and gauges probability of treatment compliance; stressors can worsen hypertension and affect the patient's ability to follow treatment*

5. Interpretation of Lab Values
- Review and intervene with abnormal lab values: total cholesterol, HDL-C, LDL-C, triglycerides, blood sugar. *Monitors lipid levels; patients with DM can have increased lipid levels leading to early severe atherosclerosis, arterial damage, and CAD.*

6. Drug Therapy
- Administer antihypertensive and antihyperlipoproteinemic drugs as prescribed. *Controls hypertension and lipid levels; medications are instituted if lifestyle changes prove unsuccessful.*
- Monitor for signs of orthostatic hypotension. *Promotes safety in the older patient who is at greatest risk for postural hypotension because of perfusion changes associated with aging.*

7. Nursing Safety Priority: Drug Alert!
Monitor K+ levels and assess for irregular pulse and muscle weakness, which may indicate decreased K+. Patients taking potassium-depleting diuretics should eat foods high in K+; supplements may be needed. *Helps prevent electrolyte imbalance which can cause cardiac dysrhythmias.*

8. Complementary and Alternative Therapies
- Help the patient explore complementary and alternative therapies. *Gives the patient alternatives to replace or supplement conventional therapies. Garlic and Q₁₀ may prevent/treat hypertension and have short-term lipid-lowering abilities; biofeedback, meditation, and acupuncture may help with continuous and severe stress.*

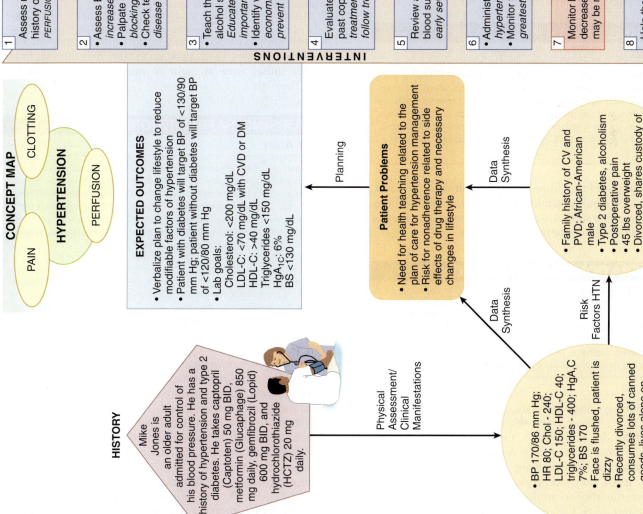

HISTORY
Mike Jones is an older adult admitted for control of his blood pressure. He has a history of hypertension and type 2 diabetes. He takes captopril (Capoten) 50 mg BID, metformin (Glucaphage) 850 mg daily, gemfibrozil (Lopid) 600 mg BID, and hydrochlorothiazide (HCTZ) 20 mg daily.

Physical Assessment/Clinical Manifestations
- BP 170/86 mm Hg; HR 80; Chol - 240; LDL-C 150; HDL-C 40; triglycerides - 400; HgA₁C 7%; BS 170
- Face is flushed, patient is dizzy
- Recently divorced, consumes lots of canned goods, lives alone on fixed income

Data Synthesis
- Family history of CV and PVD; African-American male
- Type 2 diabetes, alcoholism
- Postoperative pain
- 45 lbs overweight
- Divorced, shares custody of 2 teenagers with ex-wife

Risk Factors HTN

Patient Problems
- Need for health teaching related to the plan of care for hypertension management
- Risk for nonadherence related to side effects of drug therapy and necessary changes in lifestyle

Planning

EXPECTED OUTCOMES
- Verbalize plan to change lifestyle to reduce modifiable factors of hypertension
- Patient with diabetes will target BP of <130/90 mm Hg; patient without diabetes will target BP of <120/80 mm Hg
- Lab goals:
  Cholesterol: <200 mg/dL
  LDL-C: <70 mg/dL with CVD or DM
  HDL-C: >40 mg/dL
  Triglycerides <150 mg/dL
  HgA₁c: 6%
  BS <130 mg/dL

unmatched in preventing the cardiovascular complications of hypertension. The *2014 Evidence-Based Guidelines for the Management of High Blood Pressure in Adults* presented by JNC 8 recommends the use of one or more of these four classes of drugs: thiazide-type diuretics, calcium channel blockers (CCBs), angiotensin-converting enzyme inhibitors (ACEIs), and angiotensin II receptor blockers (ARBs). Patients who do not respond to these first-line drugs may be placed on an aldosterone receptor antagonist (blocker), beta-adrenergic blocker, or renin inhibitor. Examples of commonly used drug classes for hypertension are listed in Chart 36-1. JNC 8 recommendations for pharmacologic management are summarized in Table 36-6.

Diuretics. Diuretics are the first type of drugs for managing hypertension. Three basic types of diuretics are used to decrease blood volume and lower blood pressure in order of how commonly they are typically prescribed:

- Thiazide (low-ceiling) diuretics, such as hydrochlorothiazide (HydroDIURIL, Microzide, Oretic, Urozide ✽), inhibit sodium, chloride, and water reabsorption in the distal tubules while promoting potassium, bicarbonate, and magnesium excretion. However, they decrease calcium excretion, which helps prevent kidney stones and bone loss. Because of the low cost and high effectiveness of thiazide-type diuretics, they are usually the drugs of choice for patients with uncomplicated hypertension. These drugs can be prescribed as a single agent or in combination with other classes of drugs.

! NURSING SAFETY PRIORITY (QSEN)
Drug Alert

Teach men that they may experience decreased libido (desire for sex) and decreased sexual performance when taking thiazides. Thiazides should be used with caution in patients with diabetes mellitus because they can interfere with serum glucose control. Caution is also indicated for patients with gout or a history of significant hyponatremia (decreased serum sodium level) because these problems can worsen when thiazides are taken.

- Loop (high-ceiling) diuretics, such as furosemide (Lasix, Furoside ✽) and torsemide (Demadex), inhibit sodium, chloride, and water reabsorption in the ascending loop of Henle and promote potassium excretion.

CONSIDERATIONS FOR OLDER ADULTS
Patient-Centered Care (QSEN)

Loop diuretics are not used commonly for older adults because they can cause dehydration and orthostatic hypotension. These complications increase the patient's risk for falls. Teach families to monitor for and report patient dizziness, falls, or confusion to the health care provider as soon as possible and discontinue the medication.

- Potassium-sparing diuretics, such as spironolactone (Aldactone, Novospiroton ✽), triamterene (Dyrenium), and amiloride (Midamor), act on the distal renal tubule to inhibit reabsorption of sodium ions in exchange for potassium, thereby *retaining* potassium in the body. When used, they are typically in combination with another diuretic or antihypertensive drug to *conserve* potassium.

TABLE 36-6   Selected 2014 Evidence-Based Recommendations for the Management of High Blood Pressure in Adults (JNC 8)

- In the general population ages 60 years and older, start drug therapy to lower blood pressure at systolic blood pressure (SBP) equal to or greater than 150 mm Hg or diastolic blood pressure (DBP) equal to or greater than 90 mm Hg. The goal is to decrease blood pressure (BP) to below 150/90.
- In the general population younger than 60 years, start drug therapy to lower blood pressure at SBP equal to or greater than 140 mm Hg or DBP equal to or greater than 90 mm Hg. The goal is to decrease blood pressure to below 140/90.
- In people ages 18 years and older with chronic kidney disease (CKD), start drug therapy to lower BP to less than 140/90.
- In the general *nonblack* population, including those with diabetes mellitus, initial drug therapy should include a thiazide-type diuretic, calcium channel blocker (CCB), angiotensin-converting enzyme inhibitor (ACEI), or angiotensin receptor blocker (ARB).
- In the general *black* population, including those with diabetes mellitus, initial drug therapy should include a thiazide-type diuretic or CCB.
- If the goal BP is not reached within a month of treatment, increase drug dosage or add a second drug from one of the recommended classes.

Data from James, P.A., Oparil, S., Carter, B.L., Cushman, W.C., Dennison-Himmelfarb, C., Handler, J., et al. (2014). 2014 evidence-based guidelines for the management of high blood pressure in adults: Report from the panel members appointed to the Eighth National Committee (JNC 8). *Journal of the American Medical Association, 311*(5), 507-520. Retrieved December 2013, from http://jama.jamanetwork.com/article.aspx?articleid=1791497.

Frequent voiding caused by any type of diuretic may interfere with daily activities. Teach patients to take their diuretic in the morning rather than at night to prevent nocturia (voiding during the night).

! NURSING SAFETY PRIORITY (QSEN)
Drug Alert

The most frequent side effect associated with *thiazide and loop diuretics* is hypokalemia (low potassium level). Monitor serum potassium levels, and assess for irregular pulse, dysrhythmias, and muscle weakness, which may indicate hypokalemia. Teach patients taking potassium-depleting diuretics to eat foods high in potassium, such as bananas, potatoes, and orange juice. Most people also need a potassium supplement to maintain adequate serum potassium levels.

Assess for hyperkalemia (high potassium level) for patients taking potassium-sparing diuretics, such as spironolactone. Like hypokalemia, an increased potassium level can also cause weakness, irregular pulse, and cardiac dysrhythmias. In some cases, patients may have painful muscle spasms (cramping) in their legs. These electrolyte imbalances are described in detail in Chapter 11.

Other Antihypertensive Drugs. Calcium channel blockers, such as verapamil hydrochloride (Calan, Nu-Verap ✽) and amlodipine (Norvasc), lower blood pressure by interfering with the transmembrane flux of calcium ions. This results in vasodilation, which *decreases* blood pressure. These drugs also block SA and AV node conduction, resulting in a decreased heart rate. Calcium channel blockers are most effective in older adults and African Americans (Go et al., 2013).

Some calcium channel blockers (CCBs), especially felodipine (Plendil, Renedil ✽) and nifedipine (Adalat, Apo-Nifed ✽), react with grapefruit and grapefruit juice. Grapefruit contains

CHART 36-1   Common Examples of Drug Therapy

Hypertension Management

DRUG/USUAL DOSAGE	PURPOSE/ACTION	NURSING INTERVENTIONS	RATIONALES
Diuretics			
Hydrochlorothiazide (HCTZ) (Microzide, Oretic, Urozide ✦) 25-100 mg orally daily	Low-ceiling diuretic that inhibits Na^+, Cl^-, and water reabsorption in the distal tubules of the kidney.	Teach patient to eat foods high in K^+ and have follow-up laboratory tests to monitor electrolyte levels. Teach older adults to rise slowly from chair or bed. Use with caution for patients with diabetes. Use with caution for patients with gout.	Drug causes K^+ and Mg^{2+} excretion. Drug causes diuresis, which can cause orthostatic hypotension. Drug can affect glucose control. Drug can cause uric acid retention.
Furosemide (Lasix, Furoside ✦) 40-600 mg orally daily	High-ceiling diuretic that inhibits Na^+, Cl^-, and water reabsorption in the kidney's loop of Henle.	Report to the health care provider weakness or dizziness or new-onset confusion. Same as for HCTZ, except safer to give to patients with diabetes and gout.	Drug can cause hypovolemia, dehydration, and hypokalemia. Same as for HCTZ.
Spironolactone (Aldactone, Novo-Spiroton ✦) 50-400 mg orally daily	Acts on distal tubules of kidneys to inhibit reabsorption of Na^+ in exchange for K^+.	Teach patients to *decrease* intake of foods high in potassium and have follow-up laboratory tests for electrolyte levels. Teach patients to report weakness and irregular pulse to health care provider.	Drug causes K^+ retention in the body. These symptoms may indicate hyperkalemia.
Calcium Channel Blockers			
Verapamil (Calan, Nu-Verap ✦) Up to 480 mg orally in 3 divided doses; *Extended-release* form (ER) also available as 240-480 mg orally daily	Interferes with flux of calcium ions to cause vasodilation, which lowers blood pressure (BP).	Monitor pulse and blood pressure before taking each day; do not take without contacting health care provider if pulse is less than 60 or systolic BP is below 100 mm Hg. Teach patients and their families that patients should avoid grapefruit juice and grapefruits when taking calcium channel blockers.	Drug slows SA and AV conduction in the heart, thus decreases heart rate; vasodilation causes decreased blood pressure. Grapefruit and its juice can enhance the action of the drug causing organ dysfunction or death.
Amlodipine (Norvasc) 5-10 mg orally daily	Same as above for verapamil.	Same as above for verapamil, but safe to drink grapefruit juice.	Same as above for verapamil, but safe to drink grapefruit juice.
Angiotensin-Converting Enzyme (ACE) Inhibitors			
Lisinopril (Prinivil, Zestril) 10-80 mg orally daily	Blocks action of ACE in converting angiotensin I to angiotensin II (vasoconstrictor).	Report nagging cough to health care provider. Monitor blood pressure carefully, especially orthostatic checks; remind patients to move slowly from sitting to standing to prevent dizziness and possible falls. Do not give drug without checking with health care provider if systolic blood pressure is below 100.	Cough is a common and annoying side effect, and drug should be discontinued if it occurs. Drug prevents vasoconstriction by angiotensin II, resulting in vasodilation and decreased blood pressure.
Enalapril (Vasotec) 10-40 mg orally daily or in divided doses; also available in IV form	Same as above for lisinopril.	Monitor blood pressure as described above for lisinopril.	Same as above for lisinopril.
Angiotensin II Receptor Blockers (ARBs)			
Valsartan (Diovan) 80-320 mg orally daily	Blocks binding of angiotensin II to receptor sites in vascular smooth muscle and adrenal glands.	Teach patients to avoid foods high in potassium. Monitor blood pressures to ensure that hypotension does not occur. Do not take drug without checking with a health care provider if systolic BP is below 100.	ARBs can cause hyperkalemia, especially when combined with other antihypertensive drugs. Vasodilation causes decreased blood pressure.
Losartan (Cozaar) 25-100 mg orally daily or in divided doses twice a day	Same as above for valsartan.	Same as above for valsartan.	Same as above for valsartan.

Continued

CHART 36-1   Common Examples of Drug Therapy—cont'd

Hypertension Management

DRUG/USUAL DOSAGE	PURPOSE/ACTION	NURSING INTERVENTIONS	RATIONALES
Aldosterone Receptor Antagonists			
Eplerenone (Inspra) 25-50 mg orally daily	Blocks aldosterone binding at receptor sites in kidney, heart, blood vessels, and brain to inhibit sodium reabsorption by the kidneys.	Teach patients to follow up with laboratory tests as scheduled; decrease intake of high-potassium foods. Avoid taking the drug with grapefruit, grapefruit juice, and St. John's wort.	Drug can cause increases in K^+ and triglycerides and a decreased Na^+. Grapefruit, grapefruit juice, and St. John's wort increase the risk for adverse drug events (including death) when taking eplerenone due to enhancing the drug's action.
		Avoid taking the drug with itraconazole (Sporanox) and ketoconazole (Nizoral). Check with the pharmacist about interactions with other drugs or herbs that the patient is taking.	These drugs interact with eplerenone. Drug interacts with many other drugs and herbs and is either not prescribed or drug dosage is adjusted.
Beta-Adrenergic Blockers			
Metoprolol (Toprol, Toprol XL, Lopressor, Betaloc ♦) 100-400 mg orally daily or in divided doses (one dose daily for XL form)	Cardioselective drugs block beta$_1$ receptors in the heart and peripheral blood vessels.	Monitor carefully for orthostatic hypotension; teach patients to rise slowly from the sitting position to prevent dizziness; do not take drug without contacting the health care provider if systolic BP is below 100. Monitor pulse rate every day; do not take drug without contacting the health care provider if pulse is below 60.	Orthostatic hypotension is a common adverse effect of the drug and can contribute to falls and confusion, especially in older adults. The beta$_1$-blocking action of the drug decreases the rate, contractility, and output of the heart.
		Teach the patient that the drug can cause fatigue, depression, and sexual dysfunction; report any of these problems to the health care provider. Use the drug with caution in patients who are diabetic.	The drug has many side and adverse effects because of its potent action. Because of the sympathetic blocking action of the drug, glucose production may be affected.
Atenolol (Tenormin, Apo-Atenol ♦) 50-100 mg orally daily	Same as above for metoprolol.	Same as above for metoprolol.	Same as above for metoprolol.
Renin Inhibitors			
Aliskiren (Tekturna) 150-300 mg orally daily	Inhibits renin production, which prevents conversion of angiotensinogen to angiotensin I; decreased vasoconstriction, peripheral resistance, and cardiac output result.	Teach patients that side effects (cough and diarrhea) are not common; in a few cases, respiratory distress has occurred.	Drug is relatively safe with few side effects.

AV, Atrioventricular; **SA,** sinoatrial.

a group of chemicals called *furanocoumarins* that bind to and inactivate the enzyme *CYP3A4.* This enzyme is important for metabolism of many drugs, including some CCBs. If it is inactivated, too much of the CCB drug can remain in the patient's bloodstream causing possible kidney failure, heart failure, GI bleeding, or even death (Bailey et al., 2013).

A newer CCB, clevidipine butyrate (Cleviprex), is available only in IV form and must be administered using an infusion pump. This drug is indicated when oral therapy is not possible and is most often used for hypertensive urgency or severe hypertension. The most common side effects are headache and nausea. Monitor the patient's blood pressure frequently to

check for hypotension. A dosage increase of 1 to 2 mg/hr generally produces an additional 2– to 4–mm Hg decrease in systolic blood pressure (Lilley et al., 2014).

Angiotensin-converting enzyme inhibitors (ACE inhibitors or ACEIs), known as the *"pril"* drugs, are also used as single or combination agents in the treatment of hypertension. These drugs block the action of the angiotensin-converting enzyme as it attempts to convert angiotensin I to angiotensin II, one of the most powerful vasoconstrictors in the body. This action also decreases sodium and water retention and lowers peripheral vascular resistance, both of which lower blood pressure. ACE inhibitors include captopril (Capoten), lisinopril (Prinivil,

Zestril), and enalapril (Vasotec). *The most common side effect of this group of drugs is a nagging, dry cough.* Teach patients to report this problem to their health care provider as soon as possible. If a cough develops, the drug is discontinued.

> ### ⚠ NURSING SAFETY PRIORITY (QSEN)
> **Drug Alert**
>
> Instruct the patient receiving an ACE inhibitor for the first time to get out of bed slowly to avoid the severe hypotensive effect that can occur with initial use. Orthostatic hypotension may occur with subsequent doses, but it is usually less severe. If dizziness continues or there is a significant decrease in the systolic blood pressure (more than a change of 20 mm Hg), notify the health care provider or teach the patient to notify his or her provider. *The older patient is at the greatest risk for postural hypotension because of the cardiovascular changes associated with aging.*

Angiotensin II receptor antagonists, also called *angiotensin II receptor blockers (ARBs)* or the *-sartan drugs,* make up a group of drugs that selectively block the binding of angiotensin II to receptor sites in the vascular smooth muscle and adrenal tissues by competing directly with angiotensin II but not inhibiting ACE. Examples of drugs in this group are candesartan (Atacand), valsartan (Diovan), losartan (Cozaar), and azilsartan (Edarbi). ARBs can be used alone or in combination with other antihypertensive drugs. These drugs are excellent options for patients who report a nagging cough associated with ACE inhibitors. In addition, these drugs do not require initial adjustment of the dose for older adults or for any patient with renal impairment. Like the ACEs, the ARBs are not as effective in African Americans unless these drugs are taken with diuretics or another category such as a beta blocker or calcium channel blocker (Go et al., 2013).

Aldosterone receptor antagonists block the hypertensive effect of the mineralocorticoid hormone *aldosterone.* Aldosterone increases sodium reabsorption by the kidney and is a significant contributor to hypertension, cardiac and vascular remodeling, and heart failure. Eplerenone (Inspra) lowers blood pressure by blocking aldosterone binding at the mineralocorticoid receptor sites in the kidney, heart, blood vessels, and brain. Generally well tolerated, eplerenone has dose-related adverse effects of hypertriglyceridemia, hyponatremia, and hyperkalemia. Teach patients taking eplerenone to avoid grapefruit or grapefruit juice in their diet to prevent severe complications, including death. Using ACE inhibitors or ARBs at the same time increases the risk for hyperkalemia. Therefore monitor potassium levels carefully, initially every 2 weeks for the first few months and then monthly thereafter.

> ### ⚠ NURSING SAFETY PRIORITY (QSEN)
> **Drug Alert**
>
> When taking eplerenone, itraconazole (Sporanox) and ketoconazole (Nizoral) should not be taken. Drug interactions are common. Patients taking erythromycin, fluconazole (Diflucan), saquinavir (Fortovase), and verapamil (Calan) can take eplerenone but with a reduction in dosage by half to 25 mg daily. Teach patients that grapefruit juice and the popular herb *St. John's wort* can also increase the chance of adverse effects. Similar to all antihypertensives, remind patients not to get up quickly, drive, or climb stairs until they adjust to the effects of the drug.

Beta-adrenergic blockers, identified by the ending -olol, are categorized as cardioselective (working only on the cardiovascular system) and non-cardioselective. Cardioselective beta blockers, affecting only beta$_1$ receptors, may be prescribed to lower blood pressure by blocking beta receptors in the heart and peripheral vessels. By blocking these receptors, the drugs decrease heart rate and myocardial contractility. Teach patients about common side effects of beta blockers, including fatigue, weakness, depression, and sexual dysfunction. The potential for side effects depends on the "selective" blocking effects of the drug. Atenolol (Tenormin, Apo-Atenol ✦), bisoprolol (Zebeta), and metoprolol (Lopressor, Toprol, Toprol-XL, Betaloc ✦) are cardioselective beta blockers given for hypertension.

Patients with diabetes who take beta blockers may not have the usual manifestations of hypoglycemia because the sympathetic nervous system is blocked. The body's responses to hypoglycemia such as gluconeogenesis may also be inhibited by certain beta blockers.

Beta blockers are often the drug of choice for hypertensive patients with ischemic heart disease (IHD) because the heart is the most common target of end-organ damage with hypertension. If this drug is not tolerated, a long-acting calcium channel blocker can be used. In patients with unstable angina or myocardial infarction (MI), beta blockers or calcium channel blockers should be used initially in combination with ACE inhibitors or ARBs, with addition of other drugs if needed to control the blood pressure (see Chapter 38).

Renin inhibitors are effective for mild to moderate hypertension. Aliskiren (Tekturna) is an example and can be used alone or with a thiazide diuretic. Renin is an enzyme produced in the kidneys that causes vasoconstriction, increases peripheral resistance, and increases cardiac output. The result is an increase in blood pressure. Renin inhibitors prevent renin from producing this action. Side effects are minimal and not common, although respiratory distress may occur.

> ### ❓ NCLEX EXAMINATION CHALLENGE
> **Physiological Integrity**
>
> A client is prescribed enalapril (Vasotec) for control of hypertension. What health teaching will the nurse provide before the client begins therapy?
> A. "You may develop a higher pulse rate."
> B. "You may notice some swelling in your feet."
> C. "You may develop a nagging cough."
> D. "Your diet should include foods high in sodium."

Promoting Adherence to the Plan of Care

Planning: Expected Outcomes. The patient with hypertension is expected to adhere to the plan of care, including making necessary lifestyle changes.

Interventions. Patients who require medications to control essential hypertension usually need to take them for the rest of their lives. Some patients stop taking them because they have no symptoms and have troublesome side effects.

In the hospital setting, collaborate with the pharmacist, as needed, to discuss the outcomes of therapy with the patient, including potential side effects. Assist the patient in tailoring the therapeutic regimen to his or her lifestyle and daily schedule.

Patients who do not adhere to antihypertensive treatment are at a high risk for target organ damage and **hypertensive**

Emergency Care of Patients with Hypertensive Urgency or Crisis

Assess
- Severe headache
- Extremely high blood pressure (BP)
- Dizziness
- Blurred vision
- Shortness of breath
- Epistaxis (nosebleed)
- Severe anxiety

Intervene
- Place patient in a semi-Fowler's position.
- Administer oxygen.
- Start IV of 0.9% normal saline (NS) solution slowly to prevent fluid overload (which would increase blood pressure).
- Administer IV beta blocker or nicardipine (Cardene IV) or other infusion drug as prescribed; when stable, switch to oral antihypertensive drug.
- Monitor BP every 5 to 15 minutes until the diastolic pressure is below 90 and not less than 75; then monitor BP every 30 minutes to ensure that BP is not lowered too quickly.
- Observe for neurologic or cardiovascular complications, such as seizures; numbness, weakness, or tingling of extremities; dysrhythmias; or chest pain (possible indicators of target organ damage).

crisis, a severe elevation in blood pressure (greater than 180/120), which can cause organ damage in the kidneys or heart (target organs) (Chart 36-2). Patients in hypertensive crisis are admitted to critical care units, where they receive IV antihypertensive therapy such as nitroprusside (Nipride), nicardipine (Cardene IV), fenoldopam (Corlopam), or labetalol (Normodyne). These drugs act quickly as vasodilators to decrease blood pressure (BP) by no more that 25% within 2 to 6 hours. Provide oxygen to the patient, and monitor oxygen saturation levels. When the patient's blood pressure stabilizes, oral antihypertensive drugs are given (Day, 2011).

Community-Based Care

Home Care Management. Hypertension is a chronic illness. Allow patients to verbalize feelings about the disease and its treatment. Emphasize that their involvement in the collaborative plan of care can lead to control of the disease and can prevent complications.

Some patients do not adhere to their drug therapy regimen at home because they have no symptoms or they simply forget to take their drugs. Others may think they are not sick enough to need medication. Some patients may assume that once their blood pressure returns to normal levels, they no longer need treatment. They may also stop taking their drugs because of side effects or cost. Develop a plan with the patient and family, and identify ways to encourage adherence to the plan of care.

Self-Management Education. Health teaching is essential to help patients become successful in managing their blood pressure. Provide oral and written information about the indications, dosage, times for administration, side effects, and drug interactions for antihypertensives. Stress that medication must be taken as prescribed; when all of it has been consumed, the prescription must be renewed on a continual basis. Suddenly stopping drugs such as beta blockers can result in angina (chest pain),

myocardial infarction (MI), or rebound hypertension. Urge patients to report unpleasant side effects such as excessive fatigue, cough, or sexual dysfunction. In many instances, an alternative drug can be prescribed to minimize certain side effects.

Teach the patient to obtain an ambulatory blood pressure monitoring (ABPM) device for use at home so that the pressure can be checked. Evaluate the patient's and family's ability to use this device. If weight reduction is a desired outcome, suggest having a scale in the home for weight monitoring. For patients who do not want to self-monitor, are not able to self-monitor, or have "white-coat" syndrome when they go to their health care provider (causing elevated BP), continuous ABPM may be used. The monitor is worn for 24 hours or longer while patients perform their normal daily activities. Blood pressure is automatically taken every 15 to 30 minutes and recorded for review later. The advantage of this technique is that the health care provider can view the changes in BP readings throughout the 24-hour period to get a picture of a true BP value. Research strongly supports 24-hour ambulatory blood pressure monitoring as a first-line procedure to determine the need for antihypertensive therapy (Verdecchia et al., 2009).

Instruct the patient about sodium restriction, weight maintenance or reduction, alcohol restriction, stress management, and exercise. If necessary, also explain about the need to stop using tobacco, especially smoking.

Health Care Resources. A home care nurse may be needed for follow-up to monitor the blood pressure. Evaluate the patient's or family's ability to obtain accurate BP measurements, and assess adherence with treatment. The American Heart Association (www.aha.org), the Red Cross, or a local pharmacy may be used for free blood pressure checks if patients cannot buy equipment to monitor their blood pressure. Health fairs are also available in most locations.

◆ Evaluation: Outcomes

Evaluate the care of the patient with hypertension on the basis of the identified patient problems. The expected outcomes are that the patient will:
- Verbalize understanding of the plan of care, including drug therapy and any necessary lifestyle changes
- Report adverse drug effects, such as coughing, dizziness, or sexual dysfunction, to the health care provider immediately
- Consistently adhere to the plan of care, including regular follow-up health care provider visits

PERIPHERAL ARTERIAL DISEASE

Peripheral vascular disease (PVD) includes disorders that change the natural flow of blood through the arteries and veins of the peripheral circulation, causing decreased PERFUSION to body tissues. It affects the legs much more frequently than the arms. Generally, a diagnosis of PVD implies arterial disease (peripheral arterial disease [PAD]) rather than venous involvement. Some patients have both arterial and venous disease. The cost of the disease is very high and is expected to increase as baby boomers age and obesity in the United States continues to be a major health problem.

❖ PATHOPHYSIOLOGY

PAD is a result of systemic atherosclerosis. It is a chronic condition in which partial or total arterial occlusion (blockage)

💡 CLINICAL JUDGMENT CHALLENGE

Patient-Centered Care; Teamwork and Collaboration; Evidence-Based Practice QSEN

A nursing home administrator reports having severe headache and facial flushing for the past 3 weeks. He does not smoke but is overweight. Both of his parents have hypertension and cardiac disease. One of his nurses takes his blood pressure, which is 210/116. He states that he will see his primary care provider as soon as possible. At the physician's office, his heart rate is 88 beats/min, blood pressure is 190/110, and respiratory rate is 24 breaths/min.

1. What additional information will you need from his past and current family and personal history?
2. What physical assessment data will you collect as the office nurse?
3. What type of drug therapy may be prescribed for this patient? What are your nursing responsibilities when giving these drugs?
4. What health teaching will you provide for the patient? What evidence do you have to support your answer?
5. What members of the health care team may be involved in this patient's care?
6. What community resources are available to assist this patient to self-manage his hypertension?

decreases PERFUSION to the extremities. The tissues below the narrowed or obstructed arteries cannot live without an adequate *oxygen* and nutrient supply. PAD in the legs is sometimes referred to as *lower extremity arterial disease (LEAD)*.

Obstructions are classified as inflow or outflow, according to the arteries involved and their relationship to the inguinal ligament (Fig. 36-3). *Inflow* obstructions involve the distal end of the aorta and the common, internal, and external iliac arteries. They are located above the inguinal ligament. *Outflow* obstructions involve the femoral, popliteal, and tibial arteries and are below the superficial femoral artery (SFA). Gradual inflow occlusions may not cause significant tissue damage. Gradual outflow occlusions typically do.

Atherosclerosis is the most common cause of chronic arterial obstruction; therefore the risk factors for atherosclerosis apply to PAD as well. Common risk factors include hypertension, hyperlipidemia, diabetes mellitus, cigarette smoking, obesity, high cholesterol and lipid levels, and familial predisposition. Advancing age also increases the risk for disease related to atherosclerosis. Patients with PAD have an increased risk for developing chronic angina, MI, or stroke and are much more likely to die within 10 years compared with those who do not have the disease (Go et al., 2013).

About 10 to 12 million people in the United States have PAD, most of them older than 65 years. African Americans are affected more often than any other group, most likely because they have many risk factors such as diabetes and hypertension (Go et al., 2013).

❖ PATIENT-CENTERED COLLABORATIVE CARE

◆ Assessment

The clinical course of chronic PAD can be divided into four stages (Chart 36-3). Patients do not experience symptoms in the early stages of disease. Most patients are not diagnosed until they develop leg pain.

Physical Assessment/Clinical Manifestations. Most patients initially seek medical attention for a classic leg pain known as

- Aorta
- Common iliac artery
- External iliac artery
- Inguinal ligament
- Internal iliac (hypogastric) artery
- Common femoral artery
- Deep femoral (profunda femoris) artery
- Superficial femoral artery
- Popliteal artery
- Peroneal artery
- Anterior tibial artery
- Posterior tibial artery
- Dorsalis pedis artery

FIG. 36-3 Common locations of inflow and outflow lesions.

CHART 36-3   Key Features

Chronic Peripheral Arterial Disease

Stage I: Asymptomatic
- No claudication is present.
- Bruit or aneurysm may be present.
- Pedal pulses are decreased or absent.

Stage II: Claudication
- Muscle pain, cramping, or burning occurs with exercise and is relieved with rest.
- Symptoms are reproducible with exercise.

Stage III: Rest Pain
- Pain while resting commonly awakens the patient at night.
- Pain is described as numbness, burning, toothache-type pain.
- Pain usually occurs in the distal portion of the extremity (toes, arch, forefoot, or heel), rarely in the calf or the ankle.
- Pain is relieved by placing the extremity in a dependent position.

Stage IV: Necrosis/Gangrene
- Ulcers and blackened tissue occur on the toes, the forefoot, and the heel.
- Distinctive gangrenous odor is present.

intermittent claudication (a term derived from a word meaning "to limp"). Usually they can walk only a certain distance before a cramping, burning muscle discomfort or PAIN forces them to stop. The pain stops after rest. When patients resume walking, they can walk the same distance before it returns. Thus the pain is considered reproducible. As the disease progresses, they can walk only shorter and shorter distances before pain recurs. Ultimately, it may occur even while at rest.

Rest pain, which may begin while the disease is still in the stage of intermittent claudication, is a numbness or burning sensation, often described as feeling like a toothache that is severe enough to awaken patients at night. It is usually located in the toes, the foot arches, the forefeet, the heels, and, rarely, in the calves or ankles. Patients can sometimes get PAIN relief by keeping the limb in a dependent position (below the heart). Those with rest pain often have advanced disease that may result in limb loss.

Patients with **inflow disease** have discomfort in the lower back, buttocks, or thighs. Patients with *mild* inflow disease have discomfort after walking about two blocks. This discomfort is not severe but causes them to stop walking. It is relieved with rest. Patients with *moderate* inflow disease experience pain in these areas after walking about one or two blocks. The discomfort is described as being more like PAIN, but it eases with rest most of the time. *Severe* inflow disease causes severe pain after walking less than one block. These patients usually have rest pain.

Patients with **outflow disease** describe burning or cramping in the calves, ankles, feet, and toes. Instep or foot discomfort indicates an obstruction below the popliteal artery. Those with *mild* outflow disease experience discomfort after walking about five blocks. This discomfort is relieved by rest. Patients with *moderate* outflow disease have pain after walking about two blocks. Intermittent rest pain may be present. Those with *severe* outflow disease usually cannot walk more than one-half block and usually experience rest PAIN. They may hang their feet off the bed at night for comfort and report more frequent rest pain than do those with inflow disease.

Specific findings for PAD depend on the severity of the disease. Observe for loss of hair on the lower calf, ankle, and foot; dry, scaly, dusky, pale, or mottled skin; and thickened toenails. With severe arterial disease, the extremity is cold and gray-blue (cyanotic) or darkened. Pallor may occur when the extremity is elevated. Dependent **rubor** (redness) may occur when the extremity is lowered (Fig. 36-4). Muscle atrophy can result from prolonged chronic arterial disease.

🌐 CULTURAL CONSIDERATIONS

Patient-Centered Care QSEN

Only severe cyanosis is evident in the skin of dark-skinned patients. To detect cyanosis, assess the skin and nail beds for a dull, lifeless color. The soles of the feet and the toenails are less pigmented and allow detection of cyanosis or duskiness in the lower extremities.

Palpate all pulses in both legs. The most sensitive and specific indicator of arterial function is the quality of the posterior tibial pulse, because the pedal pulse is not palpable in a small percentage of people. The strength of each pulse should be compared bilaterally.

Note early signs of ulcer formation or complete ulcer formation, a complication of PAD. Arterial and venous stasis ulcers differ from diabetic ulcers (Chart 36-4). Initially, **arterial ulcers** are painful and develop on the toes (often the great toe), between the toes, or on the upper aspect of the foot. With prolonged occlusion, the toes can become gangrenous. Typically, the ulcer is small and round with a "punched out" appearance and well-defined borders. Skin lesions are discussed in further detail in Chapter 25.

FIG. 36-4 Dependent rubor in the left leg of a patient with peripheral arterial disease.

Imaging Assessment. *Magnetic resonance angiography (MRA)* is commonly used to assess blood flow in the peripheral arteries. A contrast medium such as gadolinium is used to help visualize blood flow through peripheral arteries. This test is often the only one used to diagnose PAD, although a computed tomography angiography (CTA) may also be performed.

Other Diagnostic Assessment. Using a Doppler probe, *segmental systolic blood pressure measurements* of the lower extremities at the thigh, calf, and ankle are an inexpensive, noninvasive method of assessing PAD. Normally, blood pressure readings in the thigh and calf are higher than those in the upper extremities. With the presence of arterial disease, these pressures are lower than the brachial pressure.

With *inflow* disease, pressures taken at the thigh level indicate the severity of disease. Mild inflow disease may cause a difference of only 10 to 30 mm Hg in pressure on the affected side compared with the brachial pressure. Severe inflow disease can cause a pressure difference of more than 40 to 50 mm Hg. The ankle pressure is normally equal to or more than the brachial pressure.

To evaluate *outflow* disease, compare ankle pressure with the brachial pressure, which provides a ratio known as the **ankle-brachial index (ABI)**. The value can be derived by dividing the ankle blood pressure by the brachial blood pressure. *An ABI of less than 0.90 in either leg is diagnostic of PAD. Patients with diabetes are known to have a falsely elevated ABI.*

Doppler-derived maximal systolic acceleration is a newer technique that has demonstrated successful evaluations of peripheral arterial disease in patients with diabetes (Van Tongeren et al., 2010).

Exercise tolerance testing (by chemical stress test or treadmill) may give valuable information about claudication (muscle

CHART 36-4 Key Features

Lower Extremity Ulcers

FEATURE	ARTERIAL ULCERS	VENOUS ULCERS	DIABETIC ULCERS
History	Patient reports claudication after walking about 1-2 blocks Rest pain usually present Pain at ulcer site Two or three risk factors present	Chronic nonhealing ulcer No claudication or rest pain Moderate ulcer discomfort Patient reports of ankle or leg swelling	Diabetes Peripheral neuropathy No reports of claudication
Ulcer location and appearance	End of the toes Between the toes Deep Ulcer bed pale, with even edges Little granulation tissue	Ankle area Brown pigmentation Ulcer bed pink Usually superficial, with uneven edges Granulation tissue present	Plantar area of foot Metatarsal heads Pressure points on feet Deep Pale, with even edges Little granulation tissue
Other assessment findings	Cool or cold foot Decreased or absent pulses Atrophy of skin Hair loss Pallor with elevation Dependent rubor Possible gangrene When acute, neurologic deficits noted	Ankle discoloration and edema Full veins when leg slightly dependent No neurologic deficit Pulses present May have scarring from previous ulcers	Pulses usually present Cool or warm foot Painless
Treatment	Treat underlying cause (surgical, revascularization) Prevent trauma and infection Patient education, stressing foot care	Long-term wound care (Unna boot, damp-to-dry dressings) Elevate extremity Patient education Prevent infection	Rule out major arterial disease Control diabetes Patient education regarding foot care Prevent infection

Photograph of arterial ulcer from Bonow, R.O., Mann, D.L., Zipes, D.P., & Libby, P. (2011). *Braunwald's heart disease: A textbook of cardiovascular medicine* (9th ed.). Philadelphia: Saunders. Photograph of venous ulcer from Bryant, R., & Nix, D. (2012). *Acute and chronic wounds: Current management concepts* (4th ed.). Philadelphia: Saunders. Photograph of diabetic ulcer from Bryant, R., & Nix, D. (2007). *Acute and chronic wounds: Current management concepts* (3rd ed.). Philadelphia: Saunders.

pain) without rest PAIN. The technician obtains resting pulse volume recordings and asks the patient to walk on a treadmill until the symptoms are reproduced. At the time of symptom onset or after about 5 minutes, the technician obtains another pulse volume recording. Normally, there may be an increased waveform with minimal, if any, drop in the ankle pressure. In patients with arterial disease, the waveforms are decreased (dampened) and there is a decrease in the ankle pressure of 40 to 60 mm Hg for 20 to 30 seconds in the affected limb. If the return to normal pressure is delayed (longer than 10 minutes), the results suggest abnormal arterial flow in the affected limb.

Plethysmography can also be performed to evaluate arterial flow in the lower extremities. The measurement provides graphs or tracings of arterial flow in the limb. If an occlusion is present, the waveforms are decreased to flattened, depending on the degree of occlusion.

◆ *Interventions*

Collaborative management of PAD may include nonsurgical interventions and/or surgery. The patient must first be assessed to determine if the altered tissue PERFUSION is due to arterial disease, venous disease, or both.

Nonsurgical Management. Exercise, positioning, promoting vasodilation, drug therapy, and invasive nonsurgical procedures are used to increase *arterial* flow to the affected leg(s).

Using Exercise and Positioning. *Exercise* may improve arterial blood flow to the affected leg through buildup of the collateral circulation. Collateral circulation provides blood to the affected area through smaller vessels that develop and compensate for the occluded vessels. Exercise is individualized for each patient, but people with severe rest pain, venous ulcers, or gangrene should not participate. Others with PAD can benefit from exercise that is started gradually and slowly increased. Instruct the patient to walk until the point of claudication, stop and rest, and then walk a little farther. Eventually, he or she can walk longer distances as collateral circulation develops. Collaborate with the health care provider and physical therapist in determining an appropriate exercise program. Exercise rehabilitation has been used to relieve symptoms but requires a motivated patient. Supervised sessions are generally not reimbursed by health care insurance.

Positioning to promote circulation has been somewhat controversial. Some patients have swelling in their extremities. Teach them to avoid raising their legs above the heart level because extreme elevation slows arterial blood flow to the feet. In severe cases, patients with PAD and swelling may sleep with the affected leg hanging from the bed or sit upright in a chair for comfort.

> ## ! NURSING SAFETY PRIORITY (QSEN)
> ### Action Alert
>
> Instruct all patients with the disease to avoid crossing their legs and avoid wearing restrictive clothing (e.g., garters to hold up nylon stockings, particularly common among older women), which interfere with blood flow. Teach them the importance of inspecting their feet daily for color or other changes.

Promoting Vasodilation. Vasodilation can be achieved by providing warmth to the affected extremity and preventing long periods of exposure to cold. Encourage the patient to maintain a warm environment at home and to wear socks or insulated shoes at all times. *Caution him or her to never apply direct heat to the limb such as with the use of heating pads or extremely hot water. Sensitivity is decreased in the affected limb. Burns may result.*

Encourage patients to prevent exposure of the affected limb to the cold because cold temperatures cause vasoconstriction (decreasing of the diameter of the blood vessels) and therefore decrease arterial PERFUSION. Patients should also drink adequate fluids to prevent increased blood viscosity.

Emotional stress, caffeine, and nicotine also can cause vasoconstriction. *Emphasize that complete abstinence from smoking or chewing tobacco is essential to prevent vasoconstriction.* The vasoconstrictive effects of each cigarette may last up to 1 hour after the cigarette is smoked.

> ## ? NCLEX EXAMINATION CHALLENGE
> ### Physiological Integrity
>
> The nurse is caring for a client with lower extremity peripheral arterial disease. Which statement made by the client regarding self-management requires further health teaching?
> A. "I need to quit smoking as soon as I can."
> B. "I will elevate my legs above the level of my heart."
> C. "I will use a heating pad to promote circulation."
> D. "I will avoid crossing my legs at all times."

Drug Therapy. For patients with chronic PAD, prescribed drugs include hemorheologic and antiplatelet agents. Pentoxifylline (Trental) is a hemorheologic agent that increases the flexibility of red blood cells. It decreases blood viscosity by inhibiting platelet aggregation and decreasing fibrinogen and thus increases blood flow in the extremities. Many patients report limited improvement in their daily lives after taking pentoxifylline. However, those with extremely limited endurance for walking have reported improvement to the point that they can perform some activities (e.g., walk to the mailbox or dining room) that were previously impossible.

Antiplatelet agents, such as aspirin (acetylsalicylic acid, Ancasal ✦) and clopidogrel (Plavix), are commonly used. Aspirin 325 or 81 mg daily may be recommended for patients with chronic PAD. However, clopidogrel is better than aspirin for reducing the risk for myocardial infarction (MI), ischemic stroke,

and vascular death. Patients with PAD and no contraindications to antiplatelet therapy should receive either aspirin or clopidogrel. Some patients receive both drugs (dual antiplatelet therapy).

Remind patients not to eat grapefruit or drink grapefruit juice while on clopidogrel. Grapefruit contains a group of chemicals called *furanocoumarins* that bind to and inactivate the enzyme *CYP3A4*. This enzyme is important for metabolism of many drugs, including clopidogrel. If it is inactivated, too much of the drug can remain in the patient's bloodstream causing possible kidney failure, heart failure, GI bleeding, or even death (Bailey et al., 2013).

Patients who experience disabling intermittent claudication may also benefit from phosphodiesterase inhibitors such as cilostazol (Pletal). This drug can also increase HDL-C levels. Teach patients taking the drug that it may cause headaches and GI disturbances, especially flatulence (gas) and diarrhea.

Controlling hypertension can improve tissue PERFUSION by maintaining pressures that are adequate to perfuse the periphery but not constrict the vessels. Teach about the effect of blood pressure on the circulation, and instruct in methods of control. For example, patients taking beta blockers may have drug-related claudication or a worsening of symptoms. The health care provider closely monitors those who are receiving beta blockers. If the patient has high serum lipids, lipid-lowering drugs such as statins are used (see earlier discussion of statins under Drug Therapy for Atherosclerosis, p. 712).

Invasive Nonsurgical Procedures. A nonsurgical but invasive approach for improving arterial flow is the use of **percutaneous vascular intervention,** also called **percutaneous transluminal coronary angioplasty (PTCA).** This procedure requires an arterial puncture in the patient's groin. One or more arteries are dilated with a balloon catheter advanced through a cannula, which is inserted into or above an occluded or stenosed artery. When the procedure is successful, it opens the vessel and improves arterial blood flow. Patients who are candidates for percutaneous procedures such as PTA must have occlusions or stenoses that are accessible to the catheter. Reocclusion may occur, and the procedure may be repeated. Some patients are occlusion-free for up to 3 to 5 years, whereas others may experience reocclusion within a year.

During percutaneous vascular intervention, intravascular stents (wire meshlike devices) are usually inserted to ensure adequate blood flow in a stenosed vessel. Candidates for stents are patients with stenosis of the common or external iliac arteries. Stents are also available to effectively treat superficial femoral artery disease. Patients have these procedures in same-day surgery or ambulatory care centers.

Another arterial technique to improve blood flow to ischemic legs in people with PAD is mechanical rotational abrasive **atherectomy.** The Rotablator device is designed to scrape plaque from inside the artery while minimizing damage to the vessel surface.

> ## ! NURSING SAFETY PRIORITY (QSEN)
> ### Critical Rescue
>
> The priority for nursing care following a PTA or atherectomy is to observe for bleeding at the arterial puncture site, which is sealed with a special collagen plug. Monitor for manifestations of impending hypovolemic shock, including a decrease in blood pressure, increased pulse rate, and decreased urinary output. Perform frequent checks of the distal pulses in both legs to ensure adequate PERFUSION and oxygenation.

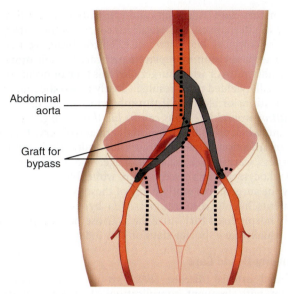

FIG. 36-5 In aortoiliac and aortofemoral bypass surgery, a midline incision into the abdominal cavity is required, with an additional incision in each groin.

Most patients receive anticoagulant or antiplatelet therapy, such as heparin or clopidogrel (Plavix), before and/or during the procedure. An antiplatelet drug may also be prescribed for 1 to 3 months or longer after the procedure to prevent arterial clotting.

Surgical Management. Patients with severe rest pain or claudication that interferes with the ability to work or threatens loss of a limb become surgical candidates. **Arterial revascularization** is the surgical procedure most commonly used to increase arterial blood flow in an affected limb.

Surgical procedures are classified as *inflow* or *outflow*. Inflow procedures involve bypassing arterial occlusions above the superficial femoral arteries (SFAs). Outflow procedures involve surgical bypassing of arterial occlusions at or below the SFAs. For those who have both inflow and outflow problems, the inflow procedure (for larger arteries) is done before the outflow repair.

Inflow procedures include aortoiliac, aortofemoral, and axillofemoral bypasses. Outflow procedures include femoropopliteal and femorotibial bypasses. Inflow procedures are more successful, with less chance of reocclusion or postoperative ischemia. Outflow procedures are less successful in relieving ischemic pain and are associated with a higher incidence of reocclusion.

Graft materials for bypasses are selected on an individual basis. For outflow procedures, the preferred graft material is the patient's own **(autogenous)** saphenous vein. However, some patients experience coronary artery disease and may need this vein for coronary artery bypass. When the saphenous vein is not usable, the cephalic or basilic arm veins may be used. Grafts made of synthetic materials have also been used when autogenous veins were not available.

Preoperative Care. Preparing the patient for surgery is similar to procedures described for general or epidural anesthesia (see Chapter 14). Documentation of vital signs and peripheral pulses provides a baseline of information for comparison during the postoperative phase. Depending on the surgical procedure, the patient may have one or more IV lines, urinary catheter, central venous catheter, and/or arterial line. To prevent

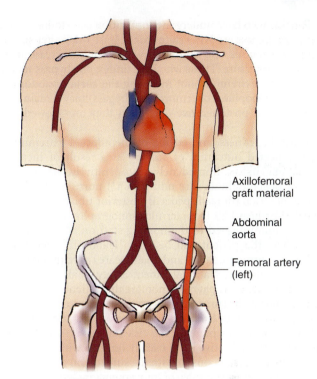

FIG. 36-6 An axillofemoral bypass graft

postoperative infection, antibiotic therapy is typically given before the procedure.

Operative Procedures. The anesthesia provider places the patient under general, epidural, or spinal anesthesia. Epidural or spinal induction is preferred for older adults to decrease the risk for cardiopulmonary complications in this age-group. If arterial bypass is to be accomplished by autogenous grafts, the surgeon removes the veins through an incision. The blocked artery is then exposed through an incision, and the replacement vein or synthetic graft material is sutured above and below the occlusion to increase blood flow around the occlusion.

For conventional open *aortoiliac* and *aortofemoral* bypass (AFB) surgery, the surgeon makes a midline incision into the abdominal cavity to expose the abdominal aorta, with additional incisions in each groin (Fig. 36-5). Graft material is tunneled from the aorta to the groin incisions, where it is sutured in place.

In an open *axillofemoral* bypass (Fig. 36-6), the surgeon makes an incision beneath the clavicle and tunnels graft material subcutaneously with a catheter from the chest to the iliac crest, into a groin incision, where it is sutured in place. Neither the thoracic nor the abdominal cavity is entered. For that reason, the axillofemoral bypass is used for high-risk patients who cannot tolerate a procedure requiring abdominal surgery.

Minimally invasive surgical techniques are beginning to be performed by vascular surgeons in large urban medical centers using robotic-assisted laparoscopic procedures. These newer surgical techniques require extensive training and do not shorten surgical time.

Postoperative Care. Thorough and ongoing nursing assessment for postoperative arterial revascularization patients is crucial to detect complications. Deep breathing every 1 to 2 hours and using an incentive spirometer are essential to prevent respiratory complications.

Patients who have undergone conventional aortoiliac or aortofemoral bypass are NPO status for at least 1 day after surgery to prevent nausea and vomiting, which could increase intra-abdominal pressure. Those who have undergone bypass surgery of the lower extremities not involving the aorta or abdominal wall (femoropopliteal or femorotibial bypass) may remain NPO until the first postoperative day, when they are allowed clear liquids.

Warmth, redness, and edema of the affected extremity are often expected outcomes of surgery as a result of increased arterial PERFUSION. Immediately postoperatively, the operating suite or postanesthesia care unit (PACU) nurse marks the site where the distal (dorsalis pedis or posterior tibial) pulse is best palpated or heard by Doppler ultrasonography. This information is communicated to the nursing staff on the critical care unit where the patient will be sent. "Hand-off" reporting is essential to promote safety and quality care (as required by The Joint Commission's National Patient Safety Goals).

To promote graft patency, monitor the patient's blood pressure and notify the surgeon if the pressure increases or decreases beyond the patient's baseline. Hypotension may indicate hypovolemia, which can increase the risk for CLOTTING. Range of motion of the operative leg is usually limited, with no bending of the hip and knee. Consult with the surgeon on a case-by-case basis regarding limitations of movement, including turning. Patients having open procedures may be restricted to bedrest for 24 hours or longer after surgery to prevent disruption of the suture lines. Patients having minimally invasive surgical (MIS) procedures may be ambulatory and eat within the day of surgery. Pain and surgical complications tend to occur less often in patients who have MIS procedures.

⚠ NURSING SAFETY PRIORITY (QSEN)

Critical Rescue

Graft occlusion (blockage) is a postoperative emergency that can occur within the first 24 hours after arterial revascularization. Monitor the patient for and report severe continuous and aching pain, which may be the first indicator of postoperative graft occlusion and ischemia. Many people experience a throbbing PAIN caused by the increased blood flow to the extremity. Because this sensation is different from ischemic pain, be sure to assess the type of pain that is experienced. Pain from occlusion may be masked by patient-controlled analgesia (PCA). Some patients have ischemic pain that is not relieved by PCA.

Monitor the patency of the graft by checking the extremity every 15 minutes for the first hour and then hourly for changes in color, temperature, and pulse intensity. Compare the operative leg with the unaffected one. *If the operative leg feels cold; becomes pale, ashen, or cyanotic; or has a decreased or absent pulse, contact the surgeon immediately!*

Emergency **thrombectomy** (removal of the clot), which the surgeon may perform at the bedside, is the most common treatment for acute graft occlusion. Thrombectomy is associated with excellent results in prosthetic grafts. Results of thrombectomy in autogenous vein grafts are not as successful and often necessitate graft revision and even replacement.

Local intra-arterial thrombolytic (clot-dissolving) therapy with an agent such as tissue plasminogen activator (t-PA) or an infusion of a platelet inhibitor such as abciximab (ReoPro) may be used for acute graft occlusions. This therapy is provided in select settings in which health care providers are experts in its use. Other antiplatelet drugs such as the glycoprotein IIb/IIIa

inhibitors *tirofiban (Aggrastat)* and *eptifibatide (Integrilin)* may be used as alternatives. The physician considers these therapies when the surgical alternative (e.g., thrombectomy with or without graft revision or replacement) carries high morbidity or mortality rates or when surgery for this type of occlusion has traditionally yielded poor results. Closely assess the patient for manifestations of bleeding if thrombolytics are used.

Graft or wound infections can be life threatening. Use sterile technique when providing incisional care, and observe for symptoms of infection. Assess the area for induration, erythema, tenderness, warmth, edema, or drainage. Also monitor for fever and leukocytosis (increased serum white blood cell count). Notify the surgeon promptly if any of these symptoms occur.

Patients having conventional open bypass procedures are usually hospitalized for 5 to 7 days. Those having MIS procedures usually have shorter stays of 2 or 3 days.

Community-Based Care

Peripheral arterial disease (PAD) is a chronic, long-term problem with frequent complications. Patients may benefit from a case manager who can follow them across the continuum of care. The desired outcome is that the patient can be maintained in the home.

Management at home often requires an interdisciplinary team approach, including several home care visits. Chart 36-5 outlines the assessment highlights for home care patients with peripheral vascular disease (PVD).

Instruct patients on methods to promote vasodilation. Teach them to avoid raising their legs above the level of the heart unless venous stasis is also present. Provide written and oral instructions on foot care and methods to prevent injury and ulcer development (Chart 36-6).

Patients who have had surgery require additional instruction on incision care (see Chapter 16). Encourage all patients to avoid smoking and to limit dietary fat intake to 5% to 6% of the total daily calories (Eckel et al., 2014). Remind them to drink adequate fluids to prevent dehydration.

Patients with chronic arterial obstruction may fear recurrent occlusion or further narrowing of the artery. They often fear that they might lose a limb or become debilitated in other ways.

CHART 36-5　Home Care Assessment

The Patient with Peripheral Vascular Disease

Assess tissue perfusion to affected extremity(ies), including:
- Distal circulation, sensation, and motion
- Presence of pain, pallor, paresthesias, pulselessness, paralysis, poikilothermy (coolness)
- Ankle-brachial index

Assess adherence to therapeutic regimen, including:
- Following foot care instructions
- Quitting smoking
- Maintaining dietary restrictions
- Participating in exercise regimen
- Avoiding exposure to cold and constrictive clothing

Assess ability to manage wound care and prevent further injury, including:
- Use of compression stockings or compression pumps as directed
- Use of various dressing materials
- Signs and symptoms to report to nurse

Assess coping ability of patient and family members.

Assess home environment, including:
- Safety hazards, especially related to falls

Indeed, chronic PAD may worsen, especially in those with diabetes mellitus. Reassure them that participation in prescribed exercise, nutrition therapy, and drug therapy, along with cessation of smoking, can limit further formation of atherosclerotic plaques.

Patients with arterial compromise may need assistance with ADLs if activity is limited by PAIN. They may need to limit or avoid stair climbing, depending on the severity of disease. Patients who have undergone surgery or need to limit activity usually need temporary help with daily activities by the family or other caregiver.

Patients who must limit activity because of PAD may benefit from the assistance of a home care aide. Those who have undergone surgery may require a home care nurse to assist with incision care. In collaboration with the case manager, arrange for home care resources before discharge.

ACUTE PERIPHERAL ARTERIAL OCCLUSION

❖ PATHOPHYSIOLOGY

Although chronic peripheral arterial disease (PAD) progresses slowly, the onset of acute arterial occlusions is sudden and dramatic. An embolus (piece of clot that travels and lodges in a new area) is the most common cause of peripheral occlusions, although a local thrombus may be the cause. Occlusion may affect the upper extremities, but it is more common in the lower extremities. Emboli originating from the heart are the most common cause of acute arterial occlusions. Most patients with an embolic occlusion have had an acute myocardial infarction (MI) and/or atrial fibrillation within the previous weeks.

❖ PATIENT-CENTERED COLLABORATIVE CARE

Patients with an acute arterial occlusion describe severe pain below the level of the occlusion that occurs even at rest. The affected extremity is cool or cold, pulseless, and mottled. Small areas on the toes may be blackened or gangrenous due to lack of PERFUSION. *Those with acute arterial insufficiency often present with the "six P's" of ischemia:*

- Pain
- Pallor
- Pulselessness
- Paresthesia
- Paralysis
- Poikilothermy (coolness)

The health care provider must initiate treatment promptly to avoid permanent damage or loss of an extremity. Anticoagulant therapy with unfractionated heparin (UFH, Hepalean ✦) is usually the first intervention to prevent further clot formation. A bolus of up to 10,000 units may be prescribed. The patient may undergo angiography.

A surgical *thrombectomy* or *embolectomy* with local anesthesia may be performed to remove the occlusion. The physician makes a small incision, which is followed by an arteriotomy (a surgical opening into an artery). A catheter is inserted into the artery to retrieve the embolus. It may be necessary to close the artery with a synthetic or autologous (patient's own blood vessel) patch graft.

⚠ NURSING SAFETY PRIORITY (QSEN)

Critical Rescue

After an arterial thrombectomy, observe the affected extremity for improvement in color, temperature, and pulse every hour for the first 24 hours or according to the postoperative surgical protocol. Monitor patients for manifestations of new thrombi or emboli, especially pulmonary emboli (PE). Chest pain, dyspnea, and acute confusion (older adults) typically occur in patients with PE. Notify the health care provider or Rapid Response Team immediately if these symptoms occur.

PAIN should significantly diminish after the surgical procedure, although mild incisional pain remains. Watch closely for complications caused by reperfusing the artery after thrombectomy or embolectomy, which include spasms and swelling of the skeletal muscles. Swelling of the skeletal muscles can result in compartment syndrome.

Compartment syndrome occurs when tissue pressure within a confined body space becomes elevated and restricts blood flow. The resulting ischemia can lead to tissue damage and eventually tissue death. Assess the motor and sensory function of the affected extremity. Monitor for increasing pain, swelling, and tenseness. Report any of these symptoms to the health care provider immediately. Fasciotomy (surgical opening into the tissues) may be necessary to prevent further injury and save the limb.

The use of *systemic thrombolytic therapy* for acute arterial occlusions has been disappointing because bleeding complications often outweigh the benefits obtained. Catheter-directed intra-arterial thrombolytic therapy with *fibrinolytics,* such as alteplase (Activase) or t-PA, has emerged as an alternative to surgical treatment in selected settings. A catheter is placed percutaneously (through the skin) into the artery with or without ultrasound guidance by the vascular surgeon or interventional radiologist. The tip of the catheter is embedded in the clot to directly deliver the thrombolytic infusion for 24 to 36 hours until the clot dissolves.

During infusion, monitor the patient for complications such as bleeding and hemorrhagic stroke. Maintain a normal blood pressure for the patient by monitoring fluids to prevent a potential stroke. As the clot dissolves, the patient typically experiences severe pain that requires patient-controlled analgesia (PCA).

ANEURYSMS OF CENTRAL ARTERIES

❖ PATHOPHYSIOLOGY

An **aneurysm** is a permanent localized dilation of an artery, which enlarges the artery to at least 2 times its normal diameter. It may be described as *fusiform* (a diffuse dilation affecting the entire circumference of the artery) or *saccular* (an outpouching affecting only a distinct portion of the artery). Aneurysms may also be described as *true* or *false.* In true aneurysms, the arterial wall is weakened by congenital or acquired problems. False aneurysms occur as a result of vessel injury or trauma to all three layers of the arterial wall. *Dissecting aneurysms* differ from aneurysms in that they are formed when blood accumulates in the wall of an artery.

Aneurysms tend to occur at specific anatomic sites (Fig. 36-7), most commonly in the abdominal aorta. They often occur at a point where the artery is not supported by skeletal muscles or on the lines of curves or flexion in the arterial tree. This chapter discussed aneurysms of the central arteries. Brain aneurysms are discussed in Chapter 45.

An aneurysm forms when the middle layer (media) of the artery is weakened, producing a stretching effect in the inner layer (intima) and outer layers of the artery. As the artery widens, tension in the wall increases and further widening occurs, thus enlarging the aneurysm and increasing the risk for arterial rupture. Elevated blood pressure can also increase the rate of aneurysmal enlargement and risk for early rupture. When *dissecting* aneurysms occur, the aneurysm enlarges, blood is lost, and blood flow to organs is diminished.

Abdominal aortic aneurysms (AAAs) account for most aneurysms, are commonly asymptomatic, and frequently rupture. Most of these are located between the renal arteries and the aortic bifurcation (dividing area).

Thoracic aortic aneurysms (TAAs) are not quite as common and are frequently misdiagnosed. They are typically discovered when advanced imaging is used to assess other conditions. TAAs commonly develop between the origin of the left subclavian artery and the diaphragm. They are located in the descending, ascending, and transverse sections of the aorta. They can also occur in the aortic arch and are very difficult to manage surgically.

Aneurysms can cause symptoms by exerting pressure on surrounding structures or by rupturing. *Rupture is the most frequent complication and is life threatening because abrupt and massive hemorrhagic shock results.* Thrombi within the wall of an aneurysm can also be the source of emboli in distal arteries below the aneurysm.

Atherosclerosis is the most common cause of aneurysms, with hypertension, hyperlipidemia, and cigarette smoking being contributing factors. Age, gender, and family history also play a

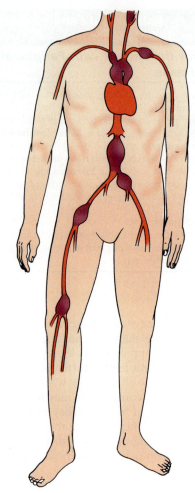

FIG. 36-7 Common anatomic sites of arterial aneurysms.

role (McCance et al., 2014). Syphilis (a sexually transmitted disease), Marfan syndrome (a connective tissue disease), and Ehlers-Danlos syndrome (a rare genetic disorder) are other causes of AAAs. Chronic INFLAMMATION (aortitis) and blunt trauma, usually from motor vehicle crashes, can cause aneurysms in the descending thoracic aorta (Hiratzka et al., 2010).

❖ PATIENT-CENTERED COLLABORATIVE CARE

◆ Assessment

Most patients with abdominal or thoracic aneurysms are asymptomatic when their aneurysms are first discovered by routine examination or during an imaging study performed for another reason. However, a few patients do have symptoms that bring them to their health care provider or the emergency department.

Physical Assessment/Clinical Manifestations. Assess patients with a known or suspected *abdominal aortic aneurysm (AAA)* for abdominal, flank, or back pain. Pain is usually described as steady with a gnawing quality, unaffected by movement, and lasting for hours or days.

A pulsation in the upper abdomen slightly to the left of the midline between the xyphoid process and the umbilicus may be present. A detectable aneurysm is at least 5 cm in diameter. *Auscultate for a bruit over the mass, but avoid palpating the mass because it may be tender and there is risk for rupture!* If expansion and impending rupture of an AAA are suspected, assess for severe PAIN of sudden onset in the back or lower abdomen, which may radiate to the groin, buttocks, or legs.

Patients with a rupturing AAA are critically ill and are at risk for hypovolemic shock due to hemorrhage. Clinical manifestations include hypotension, diaphoresis, decreased level of consciousness, oliguria (scant urine output), loss of pulses distal to the rupture, and dysrhythmias. Retroperitoneal hemorrhage is manifested by hematomas in the flanks (lower back). Rupture into the abdominal cavity causes abdominal distention.

When *a thoracic aortic aneurysm* is suspected, assess for back PAIN and manifestations of compression of the aneurysm on adjacent structures. Signs include shortness of breath, hoarseness, and difficulty swallowing. TAAs are not often detected by physical assessment, but occasionally a mass may be visible above the suprasternal notch. Assess the patient with suspected rupture of a thoracic aneurysm for sudden and excruciating back or chest pain. Hypovolemic shock also occurs with TAA.

Imaging Assessment. Computed tomography (CT) scanning with contrast is the standard tool for assessing the size and location of an abdominal or thoracic aneurysm. *Ultrasonography* is also used.

◆ **Interventions**

The size of the aneurysm and the presence of symptoms determine patient management. The nurse's role is to perform frequent patient assessments, including blood pressure, pulse, and peripheral circulation checks.

Nonsurgical Management. The desired outcome of nonsurgical management is to monitor the growth of the aneurysm and maintain the blood pressure at a normal level to decrease the risk for rupture. Patients with hypertension are treated with antihypertensive drugs to decrease the rate of enlargement and the risk for early rupture.

For those with small or asymptomatic aneurysms, frequent ultrasound or CT scans are necessary to monitor the growth of the aneurysm. Emphasize the importance of following through with scheduled tests to monitor the growth. Also explain the clinical manifestations of aneurysms that need to be promptly reported.

Surgical Management. Surgical management of an aneurysm may be an elective or an emergency procedure. *For patients with a rupturing abdominal aortic or a thoracic aneurysm, emergency surgery is performed.* Patients with smaller aneurysms that are producing symptoms are advised to have elective surgery. Those with smaller aneurysms that are not causing symptoms are treated nonsurgically until symptoms occur or the aneurysm enlarges.

The most common surgical procedure for AAA has traditionally been a resection or repair (**aneurysmectomy**). However, the mortality rate for elective resection is high and markedly increases for emergency surgery. Endovascular stent grafts have improved mortality rates and shortened the hospital stay for select patients who need AAA repair.

The repair of AAAs with **endovascular stent grafts** is the procedure of choice for almost all patients on an elective or emergent basis. Stents (wirelike devices) are inserted percutaneously (through the skin), avoiding abdominal incisions and therefore decreasing the risk for a prolonged postoperative recovery. Postoperative care is similar to care required after an arteriogram (angiogram).

Different designs of endovascular stent grafts are used, depending on the anatomic involvement of the aneurysm. The stent graft is flexible with either Dacron or polytetrafluoroethylene (PTFE) material. It is inserted through a skin incision into the femoral artery by way of a catheter-based system. The catheter is advanced to a level above the aneurysm away from the renal arteries. The graft is released from the catheter, and the stent graft is placed with a series of hooks. This procedure is done in collaboration with the vascular surgeon, interventional radiologist, operating suite team, and, at some centers, vascular medicine physician.

Complications for stent repair include:
- Conversion to open surgical repair
- Bleeding
- Aneurysm rupture
- Peripheral embolization
- Misplacement of the stent graft

The endovascular repair of AAAs has decreased the length of hospital stay for patients requiring repair of abdominal aneurysms. However, the patient needs to be closely monitored, in the hospital and at home, for the development of complications after the procedure. Expert nursing care is required to allow for early identification of problems, and complications require timely surgical intervention. In addition, coordination and collaboration with the health care team are required for discharge planning and follow-up care for patients at home.

Community-Based Care

Most patients are discharged to home after aneurysm repair. However, in the absence of family or other support systems, the postoperative patient may be discharged to a transitional care or long-term care facility for rehabilitation.

If discharged to home, the patient must follow instructions regarding activity level and incisional care. Because stair climbing may be restricted initially, he or she may need a bedside commode if the bathroom is inaccessible. Teach the patient who has undergone surgical repair about activity restrictions, wound care, and pain management. Patients may not perform activities that involve lifting heavy objects (usually more than 15 to 20 pounds [6.8 to 9.1 kg]) for 6 to 12 weeks postoperatively. Advise them to use caution for activities that involve pulling, pushing, or straining. Those who usually engage in vigorous activities should discuss them with their health care provider. Most patients are restricted from driving a car for several weeks after discharge.

For patients who have not undergone surgical aneurysm repair, the teaching plan emphasizes the importance of compliance with the schedule of frequent ultrasound scanning to monitor the size of the aneurysm.

> **! NURSING SAFETY PRIORITY** (QSEN)
> *Action Alert*
>
> Teach patients receiving treatment for hypertension about the importance of continuing to take prescribed drugs. Instruct them about the signs and symptoms that must promptly be reported to the health care provider, which include:
> - Abdominal fullness or pain or back pain
> - Chest or back pain
> - Shortness of breath
> - Difficulty swallowing or hoarseness

In collaboration with the case manager or social worker, assess the availability of transportation to and from appointments for patients needing ultrasound monitoring. Those who have undergone surgery may require the services of a home care nurse for initial assistance with dressing changes. A home care aide may be needed to assist with ADLs, depending on the patient's support system.

ANEURYSMS OF THE PERIPHERAL ARTERIES

Although femoral and popliteal aneurysms are not common, they may be associated with an aneurysm in another location of the arterial tree (see Fig. 36-7). To detect a popliteal aneurysm, assess for a pulsating mass in the popliteal space. To detect a femoral aneurysm, observe a pulsatile mass over the femoral artery. *To prevent its rupture, do not palpate the mass!* Evaluate both extremities because more than one femoral or popliteal aneurysm may be present.

The patient may have symptoms of limb ischemia (decreased PERFUSION), including diminished or absent pulses, cool to cold skin, and pain. PAIN also may be present if an adjacent nerve is compressed. The recommended treatment for either type of aneurysm, regardless of the size, is surgery because of the risk for thromboembolic complications.

To treat a femoral aneurysm, the surgeon removes the aneurysm and restores circulation using a synthetic or an autogenous saphenous vein graft-stent repair. Most surgeons prefer to bypass rather than resect a popliteal aneurysm.

After surgery, monitor for lower limb ischemia. Palpate pulses below the graft to assess graft patency. Often, Doppler ultrasonography is necessary to assess blood flow when pulses are not palpable. *Report sudden development of pain or discoloration of the extremity immediately to the physician because it may indicate graft occlusion.*

AORTIC DISSECTION

❖ *PATHOPHYSIOLOGY*

Aortic dissection was previously referred to as a *dissecting aneurysm.* However, because this condition is more accurately described as a *dissecting hematoma,* the term *aortic dissection* is more commonly used. Aortic dissection is not common but is a life-threatening problem.

Aortic dissection is thought to be caused by a sudden tear in the aortic intima, opening the way for blood to enter the aortic wall. Degeneration of the aortic media may be the primary cause for this condition, with hypertension being an important contributing factor. It is often associated with connective tissue disorders such as Marfan syndrome. It occurs also in middle-aged and older people, peaking in adults in their 50s and 60s. Men are more commonly affected than women (Hiratzka et al., 2010).

The circulation of any major artery arising from the aorta can be impaired in patients with aortic dissection; therefore this condition is highly lethal and represents an emergency situation. Although the ascending aorta and descending thoracic aorta are the most common sites, dissections can also occur in the abdominal aorta and other arteries.

❖ *PATIENT-CENTERED COLLABORATIVE CARE*

◆ *Assessment*

The most common symptom is PAIN. It is described as "sharp," "tearing," "ripping," and "stabbing" and tends to move from its point of origin. Depending on the site of dissection, the patient may feel pain in the anterior chest, back, neck, throat, jaw, or teeth at a level of 10 on a 0-to-10 PAIN intensity scale.

Diaphoresis (excessive sweating), nausea, vomiting, faintness, and apprehension are also common. Blood pressure is usually elevated unless complications such as cardiac tamponade or rupture have occurred. In these cases, the patient becomes rapidly hypotensive. A decrease or absence of peripheral pulses is common, as is aortic regurgitation, which is characterized by a musical murmur best heard along the right sternal border. Neurologic deficits such as an altered level of consciousness, paraparesis, and strokes also can occur.

Chest x-ray, computed tomography (CT), magnetic resonance imaging (MRI), and aortic angiography may be used to confirm the diagnosis. However, MRI scanning is very time-consuming and may not be the test of choice. Transthoracic echocardiography (TTE) or transesophageal echocardiography (TEE) may be performed at the bedside for patients who cannot be moved (Braverman, 2010).

◆ *Interventions*

The expected outcomes for emergency care for a patient with an aortic dissection are elimination of PAIN and reduction of systolic blood pressure to 100 to 120 mm Hg. Make sure that the patient has two large-bore IV catheters to infuse 0.9% sodium chloride and give medication. Insert an indwelling urinary catheter. The physician prescribes IV morphine sulfate to relieve PAIN and an IV beta blocker, such as esmolol (Brevibloc), to lower heart rate and blood pressure (Carlson, 2012). If this regimen is not effective, nicardipine hydrochloride (Cardene) or other antihypertensive may be used.

Subsequent treatment depends on the location of the dissection. Patients receive continued medical treatment for uncomplicated distal dissections and surgical treatment for proximal dissections. For those receiving long-term medical treatment, the systolic blood pressure must be maintained at or below 130 to 140 mm Hg. Beta blockers (e.g., propranolol) and calcium channel antagonists (e.g., amlodipine) are prescribed to assist with blood pressure maintenance once the patient is stabilized.

Patients having surgical intervention for a proximal dissection typically require cardiopulmonary bypass (CPB) (see Chapter 38). The surgeon removes the intimal tear and sutures edges of the dissected aorta. Usually a synthetic graft is used.

OTHER ARTERIAL HEALTH PROBLEMS

Fewer health problems affect peripheral and central arteries. Examples of some of these problems are summarized in Table 36-7.

PERIPHERAL VENOUS DISEASE

To function properly, veins must be patent (open) with competent valves. Vein function also requires the assistance of the surrounding muscle beds to help pump blood toward the heart. If one or more veins are not operating properly, they become distended and clinical manifestations occur.

Three health problems alter the blood flow in veins:
- Thrombus formation (*venous thrombosis*) can lead to pulmonary embolism (PE), a life-threatening complication. Venous thromboembolism (VTE) is the current term that includes both deep vein thrombosis and PE.

TABLE 36-7   Assessment and Interventions for Other Arterial Health Problems

DISEASE/HEALTH PROBLEM	ASSESSMENT	COLLABORATIVE MANAGEMENT	NURSING CARE
Buerger's Disease	Claudication in feet and lower extremities worse at night; causes ischemia and fibrosis of vessels in extremities with increased sensitivity to cold. Ulcerations and gangrene occur on digits. Cause unknown but is associated with smoking.	Vasodilating drugs, such as nifedipine (Procardia); management of ulceration and gangrene; chronic pain management modalities.	Teach patient about smoking cessation, avoid cold by wearing gloves and warm clothes, manage stress, avoid caffeine; teach patient taking nifedipine to avoid grapefruit and grapefruit juice to prevent severe adverse effects, including possible death; teach patients on vasodilators about side effects such as facial flushing, hypotension, headaches.
Raynaud's Phenomenon/ Disease	Painful vasospasms of arteries and arterioles in extremities, especially digits; causes red-white-blue skin color changes on exposure to cold or stress; cause unknown, occurs more in women, and may be autoimmune because it is associated with many rheumatic diseases like systemic lupus erythematosus.	Same as above	Same as above
Subclavian Steal	Occurs in upper extremities as result of subclavian artery occlusion or stenosis causing ischemia in the arm and pain; paresthesias and dizziness are also common; BP difference in arms and presence of subclavian bruit on the affected side.	Surgical interventions for cyanosis or unrelenting pain, such as endarterectomy, bypass, or dilation of subclavian artery.	Monitor patient closely for new signs and symptoms; postoperative, check pulses and observe for ischemic changes, including severe pain or color changes (e.g., cyanosis).
Thoracic Outlet Syndrome	Compression of subclavian artery by rib or muscle that is more common in women and those who have to keep arms moving or above their heads (e.g., golfers, swimmers); also present with trauma; causes neck, arm, and shoulder pain with numbness and possible cyanosis.	Physical therapy for exercise program, avoiding aggravating positions; surgery as last resort for severe pain.	Health teaching about avoiding activities and positions that aggravate pain; monitor for new signs and symptoms; neurovascular assessments; postoperative care if needed.

- Defective valves lead to *venous insufficiency* and *varicose veins*, which are not life threatening but are problematic.
- Skeletal muscles do not contract to help pump blood in the veins. This problem can occur when weight bearing is limited or muscle tone decreases.

VENOUS THROMBOEMBOLISM

❖ PATHOPHYSIOLOGY

Venous thromboembolism (VTE) is one of health care's greatest challenges and includes both thrombus and embolus complications. A thrombus (also called a *thrombosis*) is a blood clot believed to result from an endothelial injury, venous stasis, or hypercoagulability. The thrombosis may be specifically attributable to one element, or it may involve all three elements. It is often associated with an inflammatory process. When a thrombus develops, INFLAMMATION occurs around the clot, thickening the vein wall and consequently possibly leading to embolization (the formation of an embolus). Pulmonary embolism (PE) is the most common type of embolus and is discussed in detail in Chapter 32.

Thrombophlebitis refers to a thrombus that is associated with INFLAMMATION. Phlebothrombosis is a thrombus without inflammation. Thrombophlebitis can occur in superficial veins. However, it most frequently occurs in the deep veins of the lower extremities.

Deep vein thrombophlebitis, commonly referred to as deep vein thrombosis (DVT), is the most common type of thrombophlebitis. Deep vein thrombophlebitis (thrombosis) is more serious than superficial thrombophlebitis because it presents a greater risk for PE. In PE, a dislodged blood clot travels to the pulmonary artery—a medical emergency! DVT develops most often in the legs but can occur also in the upper arms as a result of increased use of central venous devices.

Thrombus formation has been associated with stasis of blood flow, endothelial injury, and/or hypercoagulability, known as Virchow's triad. The precise cause of these events remains unknown; however, a few predisposing factors have been identified.

The highest incidence of clot formation occurs in patients who have undergone hip surgery, total knee replacement, or open prostate surgery. Other conditions that seem to promote thrombus formation are ulcerative colitis, heart failure, cancer, oral contraceptives, and immobility. Complications of immobility occur during prolonged bedrest such as when a patient is confined to bed for an extensive illness. People who sit for long periods (e.g., on an airplane or at a computer) are also at risk. Phlebitis (vein INFLAMMATION) associated with invasive procedures such as IV therapy can also predispose patients to thrombosis.

A systematic literature review by Anthony (2013) found a valid and reliable model for placing patients in high- and low-risk groups for DVT. This model is highly predictive of DVT development. During the nursing assessment, one point is given for each of nine characteristics, which include:

- Active cancer, paralysis, or casting of an extremity
- Bedridden for more than 3 days
- Major surgery with general anesthesia during the previous 3 months
- Localized tenderness along the deep venous system
- Swelling of the entire leg
- Calf swelling of greater than 3 cm larger when compared with the other leg
- Pitting edema in one leg
- Dilated superficial veins in one leg
- Previously documented DVT

A score of 2 or more indicates that a DVT is likely to occur.

Millions of people in the United States are affected by deep vein thrombosis each year, and many die from pulmonary embolism. The largest number of deaths occur in older adults.

Health Promotion and Maintenance

In the *community*, if a person has a history of any type of VTE, these precautions should be taken:

- Avoid oral contraceptives.
- Drink adequate fluids to avoid dehydration.
- Exercise legs during long periods of bedrest or sitting.

The Joint Commission's VTE Core Measure Set requires that hospitals report data on 6 areas related to VTE prophylaxis and management (Table 36-8). If VTE is not prevented or adequately managed, the hospital may not be paid by the third party payer (e.g., Medicare) for the patient's care. In the *inpatient setting*, all patients must be assessed for risk for VTE on admission. For those at moderate to high risk, initiate these interventions to prevent VTE:

- Patient education
- Leg exercises
- Early ambulation
- Adequate hydration
- Graduated compression stockings
- Intermittent pneumatic compression, such as sequential compression devices (SCDs)
- Venous plexus foot pump
- Anticoagulant therapy

❖ PATIENT-CENTERED COLLABORATIVE CARE

◆ Assessment

People with DVT may have symptoms or may be asymptomatic. *The classic signs and symptoms of DVT are calf or groin tenderness and pain and sudden onset of unilateral swelling of the leg.* PAIN in the calf on dorsiflexion of the foot (positive Homans' sign) appears in only a small percentage of patients with DVT, and false-positive findings are common (Anthony, 2013). *Therefore checking a Homans' sign is not advised because it is an unreliable tool!* Examine the area described as painful, comparing this site with the other limb. *Gently* palpate the site, observing for **induration** (hardening) along the blood vessel and for warmth and edema. Redness may also be present (Fig. 36-8).

Although diagnostic tests are available, physical examination findings are often adequate for diagnosis. If a definitive diagnosis is lacking from physical assessment findings alone, diagnostic tests may be performed.

The preferred diagnostic test for DVT is *venous duplex ultrasonography,* a noninvasive ultrasound that assesses the flow of blood through the veins of the arms and legs. *Doppler flow studies* may also be useful in the diagnosis, but they are more sensitive in detecting proximal rather than distal DVT. Normal venous circulation creates audible signals, whereas thrombosed veins produce little or no sound. The accuracy of the scanning depends on the technical skill of the health care professional performing the test. If the test is negative but a DVT is still

TABLE 36-8	Venous Thromboembolism (VTE) Core Measure Set	
CORE MEASURE	**ASSESSMENT OF MEASURE**
VTE-1	**VTE Prophylaxis:** Number of patients who received VTE prophylaxis or have documented why no VTE prophylaxis was given the day of or the day after hospital admission or surgery
VTE-2	**ICU VTE:** Number of patients who received VTE prophylaxis on ICU admission or have documented why no VTE prophylaxis was given the day of admission, transfer, or surgery
VTE-3	**VTE Patients with Anticoagulant Overlap Therapy:** Number of patients diagnosed with confirmed VTE who received overlap of parenteral anticoagulant and warfarin
VTE-4	**VTE Patients Receiving Unfractionated Heparin:** Number of patients receiving heparin with dosages/platelet count monitoring by protocol or nomogram
VTE-5	**VTE Warfarin Therapy Discharge Instructions:** Number of patients who received written instructions that address these four criteria: • Compliance issues • Dietary advice • Follow-up monitoring • Information about potential for adverse drug reactions/interactions
VTE-6	**Hospital-Acquired Potentially Preventable VTE:** Number of patients who developed VTE while hospitalized

Data from www.jointcommission.org/venous_thromboembolism/.
ICU, Intensive care unit.

FIG. 36-8 Deep vein thrombosis (DVT) of lower left leg.

suspected, a venogram may be needed to make an accurate diagnosis.

Impedance plethysmography assesses venous outflow and can detect most DVTs that are located above the popliteal vein. It is not helpful in locating clots in the calf and is less sensitive than Doppler studies.

Magnetic resonance direct thrombus imaging (MRI), another noninvasive test, is useful in finding a DVT in the proximal deep veins and is better than traditional venography in finding DVT in the inferior vena cava or pelvic veins.

A D-dimer test is a global marker of coagulation activation and measures fibrin degradation products produced from fibrinolysis (clot breakdown). The test is used for the diagnosis of DVT when the patient has few clinical signs and stratifies patients into a high-risk category for reoccurrence. Useful as an adjunct to noninvasive testing, a negative D-dimer test can exclude a DVT without an ultrasound.

Physical and diagnostic assessment of patients with pulmonary embolism is described in Chapter 32.

◆ Interventions

The focus of managing thrombophlebitis is to prevent complications such as pulmonary emboli, prevent further thrombus formation, and prevent an increase in size of the thrombus. Patients with deep vein thrombosis (DVT) may be hospitalized for treatment, although this practice is changing as a result of the use of newer drugs.

Nonsurgical Management. DVT is usually treated medically using a combination of rest and drug therapy. Prevention of DVT and other types of venous thromboembolism (VTE) is crucial for patients at risk. Preventive measures are listed on p. 730 in the Health Promotion and Maintenance section.

Rest. Supportive therapy for DVT has typically included bedrest and elevation of the extremity. However, a review and synthesis of the literature showed that outcomes are not different if the patient is allowed to ambulate (Gay et al., 2009). Ambulation did not cause pulmonary embolus, and the DVT did not worsen any more with ambulation than with bedrest. Allowing patients to ambulate may decrease their fear and anxiety about dislodging the clot and life-threatening complications.

Teach the patient to elevate his or her legs when in bed and chair. To help prevent chronic venous insufficiency, instruct patients with active and resolving DVT to wear knee- or thigh-high sequential or graduated compression stockings for an extended period. Be sure to select the correct stocking size for the patient according to the sizing chart provided.

Some health care providers prescribe intermittent or continuous warm, moist soaks to the affected area. *To prevent the thrombus from dislodging and becoming an embolus, do not massage the affected extremity.* Monitor all patients for signs and symptoms of pulmonary embolism (PE), which include shortness of breath, chest pain, and acute confusion (in older adults). Emboli may also travel to the brain or heart, but these complications are not as common as PE. Chapter 32 describes PE manifestations in detail.

Drug Therapy. *Anticoagulants are the drugs of choice for actual DVT and for patients at risk for DVT.* However, these drugs are known to cause medical complications and even death. Therefore The Joint Commission's National Patient Safety Goals (NPSGs) include the need for agencies to reduce the likelihood of patient harm associated with the use of anticoagulant therapy.

The conventional treatment has been IV unfractionated heparin followed by oral anticoagulation with warfarin (Coumadin). However, unfractionated heparin can be problematic because each patient's response to the drug is unpredictable and hospital admission is usually required for laboratory monitoring and dose adjustments. The use of low–molecular-weight heparin (LMWH) has changed the management of both DVT and PE.

Unfractionated Heparin Therapy. Some patients with a confirmed diagnosis of an existing blood clot are started on a regimen of IV unfractionated heparin (UFH, Hepalean ✦) therapy. UFH is an anticoagulant agent that at low doses interacts with antithrombin III to produce selective inhibition of clotting factors IIa (thrombin) and Xa. At higher doses, it inhibits practically all CLOTTING factors. The ultimate result is inhibition of fibrin formation. The health care provider prescribes UFH to prevent the formation of further clots, which often develop in the presence of an existing clot, and to prevent enlargement of the existing clot. Over a long period, the existing clot is slowly absorbed by the body.

Before UFH administration, a baseline prothrombin time (PT), activated partial thromboplastin time (APTT or aPTT), international normalized ratio (INR), complete blood count (CBC) with platelet count, urinalysis, stool for occult blood, and creatinine level are required. Notify the physician if the platelet count is below 100,000 to 120,000/mm^3, depending on agency protocol.

UFH is initially given in a bolus IV dose of about 80 to 100 units/kg of body weight in a prefilled syringe or 5000 units followed by continuous infusion via an infusion pump. The infusion is regulated by a reliable electronic pump that protects against accidental free flow of solution. The physician or clinical pharmacist prescribes concentrations of UFH (in 5% dextrose in water) and the number of units or milliliters per hour needed to maintain a therapeutic aPTT (usually 18-20 units/kg/hr or at least 30,000 units over 24 hours). aPTT is measured at least daily, and results are reported to the health care provider as soon as results are available to allow adjustment of heparin dosage. Therapeutic levels of aPTTs are usually 1½ to 2 times normal control levels.

> **! NURSING SAFETY PRIORITY** (QSEN)
> *Critical Rescue*
>
> Notify the physician if the aPTT value is greater than 70 seconds, or follow hospital protocol for reporting critical laboratory values. Assess patients for signs and symptoms of bleeding, which include hematuria, frank or occult blood in the stool, ecchymosis (bruising), petechiae, an altered level of consciousness, or pain. If bleeding occurs, stop the anticoagulant immediately and call the health care provider or Rapid Response Team!

UFH can also decrease platelet counts. Mild reductions are common and are resolved with continued heparin therapy. Severe platelet reductions, although rare, result from the development of antiplatelet bodies within 6 to 14 days after the beginning of treatment. Platelets aggregate into "white clots" that can cause thrombosis, usually in the form of an acute arterial occlusion. The provider discontinues heparin administration if severe **heparin-induced thrombocytopenia (HIT)** (platelet count <150,000), or "white clot syndrome," occurs. Low–molecular-weight heparin is used more commonly today because of the complications involved with unfractionated heparin.

CHART 36-7 Best Practice for Patient Safety & Quality Care QSEN

The Patient Receiving Anticoagulant Therapy

- Carefully check the dosage of anticoagulant to be administered, even if the pharmacy prepared the drug.
- Monitor the patient for signs and symptoms of bleeding, including hematuria, frank or occult blood in the stool, ecchymosis, petechiae, altered mental status (indicating possible cranial bleeding), or pain (especially abdominal pain, which could indicate abdominal bleeding).
- Monitor vital signs frequently for decreased blood pressure and increased pulse (indicating possible internal bleeding).
- Have antidotes available as needed (e.g., protamine sulfate for heparin; vitamin K for warfarin [Coumadin, Warfilone]).
- Monitor activated partial thromboplastin time (aPTT) for patients receiving unfractionated heparin. Monitor prothrombin time (PT)/international normalized ratio (INR) for patients receiving warfarin or low–molecular-weight heparin (LMWH).
- Apply prolonged pressure over venipuncture sites and injection sites.
- When administering *subcutaneous* heparin, apply pressure over the site and do not massage.
- Teach the patient going home while taking an anticoagulant to:
  - Use only an electric razor
  - Take precautions to avoid injury; for example, do not use tools such as hammers or saws, where accidents commonly occur
  - Report signs and symptoms of bleeding, such as blood in the urine or stool, nosebleeds, ecchymosis, or altered mental status
  - Take the prescribed dosage of drug at the precise time that it was prescribed to be taken
  - Not stop taking the drug abruptly; the physician usually tapers the anticoagulant gradually

Bivalirudin (Angiomax), lepirudin (Refludan), and argatroban injection are *highly selective direct thrombin inhibitors* that may be used as alternatives to heparin or for patients who have had HIT. Like heparin, these drugs increase the risk for bleeding. Monitor hemoglobin, hematocrit, aPTT, platelet count, urinalysis, fecal occult blood test, and blood pressure for indications of this complication. An oral anticoagulant like warfarin (Coumadin) may also be substituted for heparin if necessary.

Ensure that protamine sulfate, the antidote for heparin, is available if needed for excessive bleeding. Chart 36-7 highlights information important to nursing care and patient education associated with anticoagulant therapy.

To *prevent* DVT, unfractionated heparin may be given in low doses subcutaneously for high-risk patients, especially after orthopedic surgery. Commonly used alternatives to unfractionated heparin include:

- Low–molecular-weight heparin (e.g., enoxaparin [Lovenox]) (drug class of choice after orthopedic surgery)
- Selective factor Xa inhibitors (e.g., fondaparinux [Arixtra]; rivaroxaban [Xarelto] used most often for orthopedic surgery)
- Warfarin (Coumadin, Warfilone ♦)

Low–Molecular-Weight Heparin. Subcutaneous low–molecular-weight heparins (LMWHs) such as enoxaparin (Lovenox), dalteparin (Fragmin), and ardeparin (Normiflo) have a consistent action and are preferred for prevention and treatment of DVT. Danaparoid (Orgaran) is also classified as an LMWH but is actually a heparinoid. LMWHs bind less to plasma proteins, blood cells, and vessel walls, resulting in a longer half-life and more predictable response. These drugs inhibit thrombin formation because of reduced factor IIa activity and enhanced inhibition of factor Xa and thrombin.

Some patients taking LMWH may be safely managed at home with visits from a home care nurse. Candidates for home therapy must have stable DVT or PE, low risk for bleeding, adequate renal function, and normal vital signs. They must be willing to learn self-injection or have a family member, friend, or home care nurse administer the subcutaneous injections.

Some health care providers place the patient on a regimen of IV unfractionated heparin (UFH) for several days and then follow up with an LMWH. In this case, the UFH is discontinued at least 30 minutes before the first LMWH injection. The usual dose of enoxaparin is 1 mg/kg of body weight, not to exceed 90 mg, and is repeated every 12 hours. If the patient's creatinine level is greater than 2 mg/dL (indicating renal insufficiency), the health care provider lowers the dose. Dalteparin can be given once daily at 200 units/kg of body weight and does not require dose adjustment for renal insufficiency. The usual dose of ardeparin is 50 units/kg of body weight and is given every 12 hours.

Assess all stools for occult blood. The aPTTs are not checked on an ongoing basis because the doses of LMWH are not adjusted.

Warfarin Therapy. If the patient is receiving continuous UFH, warfarin (Coumadin), an oral anticoagulant, may be *added* at least 5 days later. Patients receiving LMWH are placed on the oral drug after the first dose. This anticoagulant drug overlap is necessary because heparin and warfarin work differently. Warfarin works in the liver to inhibit synthesis of the four vitamin K–dependent clotting factors and takes 3 to 4 days before it can exert therapeutic anticoagulation. The heparin continues to provide therapeutic anticoagulation until this effect is achieved. IV heparin is then discontinued.

According to the National Patient Safety Goals, therapeutic levels of warfarin must be monitored by measuring the international normalized ratio (INR) at frequent intervals. Because prothrombin times are often inconsistent and misleading, the INR was developed. Most laboratories report both results. Most patients receiving warfarin should have an INR between 1.5 and 2.0 to prevent future DVT and to minimize the risk for stroke or hemorrhage (Pagana & Pagana, 2014). For patients with additional cardiovascular problems or pulmonary embolus, the desired INR is higher, up to 3.5 or 4.0. The health care provider specifies the desired INR level to obtain. Be aware of the critical value for INR according to agency policy (ranges between 4.5 and 6.0). Notify the health care provider immediately if your patient's INR is at a critical value.

After obtaining the patient's baseline INR, warfarin therapy should be started with low doses, at least 5 mg, and gradually titrated up according to the INR. Patients usually receive this drug for 3 to 6 months or longer after an episode of DVT if no precipitating factors were discovered, with recurrence, or if there are continuing risk factors.

❗ NURSING SAFETY PRIORITY QSEN

Drug Alert

For patients taking warfarin, assess for any bleeding, such as hematuria or blood in the stool. *Ensure that vitamin K, the antidote for warfarin, is available in case of excessive bleeding* (see Chart 36-7). Report any bleeding to the health care provider, and document in the patient's health record. Teach patients to avoid foods with high concentrations of Vitamin K, especially dark green leafy vegetables. These foods interfere with the action of warfarin.

? NCLEX EXAMINATION CHALLENGE

Physiological Integrity

The nurse is providing care to a client who has started warfarin after being diagnosed with a deep vein thrombosis. What health teaching will the nurse provide to the client related to self-management of warfarin therapy?

A. "You must have your partial thromboplastin time checked every 2 weeks."

B. "Massage the injection site after the warfarin is injected."

C. "Eat plenty of dark green leafy vegetables while taking warfarin."

D. "Report any signs of bleeding to your primary care provider."

CHART 36-8 Patient and Family Education: Preparing for Self-Management

Foods and Drugs That Interfere with Warfarin (Coumadin)

Eat small amounts of foods rich in vitamin K each day, including any of these:	If possible, avoid:
• Broccoli	• Allopurinol
• Cauliflower	• NSAIDs
• Spinach	• Acetaminophen
• Kale	• Vitamin E
• Other green leafy vegetables	• Histamine blockers
• Brussels sprouts	• Cholesterol-reducing drugs
• Cabbage	• Antibiotics
• Liver	• Oral contraceptives
	• Antidepressants
	• Thyroid drugs
	• Antifungal agents
	• Other anticoagulants
	• Corticosteroids
	• Herbs, such as St. John's wort, garlic, ginseng, Ginkgo biloba

---

Thrombolytic Therapy. Thrombolytic therapy using fibrinolytics is not commonly prescribed unless it is the treatment of last resort.

Surgical Management. A deep vein thrombus is rarely removed surgically unless there is a massive occlusion that does not respond to medical treatment and the thrombus is of recent (1 to 2 days) onset. **Thrombectomy** is a common surgical procedure for removing the clot. Preoperative and postoperative care of patients undergoing thrombectomy is similar to the care for those undergoing arterial surgery (see pp. 723-725 in the Peripheral Arterial Disease section).

For patients with recurrent deep vein thrombosis (DVT) or pulmonary emboli that do not respond to medical treatment and for patients who cannot tolerate anticoagulation, **inferior vena cava filtration** may be indicated. The surgeon usually inserts a filter device, or "umbrella," into the femoral vein. The device is meant to trap emboli in the inferior vena cava before they progress to the lungs. Holes in the device allow blood to pass through, thus not significantly interfering with the return of blood to the heart. There are several new filter brands available and designed to allow for removal if and when DVT risks diminish.

Preoperative care is similar to that provided for patients receiving local anesthesia (see Chapter 14). If they have recently been taking anticoagulants, collaborate with the physician about interrupting this therapy in the preoperative period to avoid hemorrhage.

Postoperatively, inspect the groin insertion site for bleeding and signs or symptoms of infection. Other postoperative nursing care is similar to that for any patient undergoing local anesthesia (see Chapter 16).

Community-Based Care

Patients recovering from thrombophlebitis or DVT are ambulatory when they are discharged from the hospital. The primary focus of planning for discharge is to educate the patient and family about anticoagulation therapy.

Teach patients recovering from DVT to stop smoking and avoid the use of oral contraceptives to decrease the risk for recurrence. Alternative forms of birth control may be used. Most patients are discharged on a regimen of warfarin (Coumadin, Warfilone ♣) or low–molecular-weight heparin (LMWH). The VTE Core Measures and the Joint Commission's National Patient Safety Goals require that the patients be given written discharge instructions about anticoagulant therapy that address:

- Drug compliance issues (need to take drug as prescribed)
- Dietary advice (e.g., foods to avoid)
- Follow-up monitoring (e.g., Coumadin clinic, INR testing)
- Information about potential for adverse drug reactions/interactions (e.g., bleeding, bruising)

Instruct patients and their families to avoid potentially traumatic situations, such as participation in contact sports. Provide written and oral information about the signs and symptoms of bleeding (see Chart 36-7). Reinforce the need to report any of these manifestations to the health care provider immediately.

The anticoagulant effect of warfarin may be reversed by omitting one or two doses of the drug or by the administration of vitamin K. In case of injury, teach patients to apply pressure to bleeding wounds and to seek medical assistance immediately. Encourage them to carry an identification card or wear a medical alert bracelet that states that they are taking warfarin or any other anticoagulant.

Instruct patients to tell their dentist and other health care providers before receiving treatment or prescriptions that they are taking warfarin. Prothrombin times are affected by many prescription and over-the-counter drugs such as NSAIDs. Teach patients to avoid high-fat and vitamin K–rich foods, such as cabbage, cauliflower, broccoli, asparagus, turnips, spinach, kale, fish, and liver (Chart 36-8). Remind them to drink adequate fluids to stay well hydrated, avoid alcohol (which can cause dehydration), and avoid sitting for prolonged periods.

If possible, in collaboration with the case manager (CM) or other discharge planner, arrange for the patient to obtain a device to self-monitor INR at home. Some insurance companies do not pay for the INR monitoring device. Clinical studies show that self-monitoring of the INR and self-adjusting of anticoagulation therapy result in better anticoagulation control, improve patient satisfaction, and improve quality of life (Michaels & Regan, 2013). The device used to self-monitor is similar to a glucometer for glucose testing and requires a fingerstick blood sample applied to a test strip or plastic cuvette, which is then inserted into the machine. Self-monitoring can be used either for the testing alone or for self-management, in which the patient uses the test results to adjust drug dosages based on a dosing protocol. If the patient cannot use a monitoring device, teach a family member or other caregiver how to perform the procedure. If the patient lives alone, collaborate with the CM to arrange for follow-up laboratory appointments to have blood drawn at frequent intervals—usually every week until the patient's values are stabilized. Communication with the primary care provider is essential while patients are receiving warfarin.

Patients receiving subcutaneous LMWH injections at home need instruction on self-injection. Teach the appropriate caregiver and family members or friends, if necessary, to administer the injections.

Patients who have experienced DVT may fear recurrence of a thrombus. They may also be concerned about treatment with warfarin and the risk for bleeding. Assure them that the prescribed treatment will help resolve this problem and that ongoing assessment of prothrombin times and INR values decreases the risks for bleeding.

VENOUS INSUFFICIENCY

❖ PATHOPHYSIOLOGY

Venous insufficiency occurs as a result of prolonged venous hypertension that stretches the veins and damages the valves. Valvular damage can lead to a backup of blood and further venous hypertension, resulting in edema and decreased tissue perfusion. With time, this stasis (stoppage) results in venous stasis ulcers, swelling, and cellulitis.

The veins cannot function properly when thrombosis occurs or when valves are not working correctly. Venous hypertension can occur in people who stand or sit in one position for long periods (e.g., teachers, office personnel). Obesity can also cause chronically distended veins, which lead to damaged valves. Thrombus formation can contribute to valve destruction. Chronic venous insufficiency also often occurs in patients who have had thrombophlebitis. In severe cases, venous ulcers develop.

Venous leg ulcers are a major cause of death, PAIN, and health care costs. Most venous ulcer care is delivered in the community setting by home care nurses or through self-management.

❖ PATIENT-CENTERED COLLABORATIVE CARE

◆ Assessment

Venous insufficiency may result in edema of both legs. There may be **stasis dermatitis** or reddish brown discoloration along the ankles, extending up to the calf. In people with long-term venous insufficiency, **stasis ulcers** often form. They can result from the edema or from minor injury to the limb. Ulcers typically occur over the malleolus, more often medially (inner ankle) than laterally (outer ankle). The ulcer usually has irregular borders. In general, these ulcers are chronic and difficult to heal (see Chart 36-4). Many people live with ulcers for years, and recurrence is common. Some may lose one or both legs if ulcers are not controlled.

◆ Interventions

The focus of treating venous insufficiency is to decrease edema and promote venous return from the affected leg. Patients are

not usually hospitalized for venous insufficiency alone unless it is complicated by an ulcer or another disorder is occurring at the same time.

Nonsurgical Management. Treatment of chronic venous insufficiency is nonsurgical unless it is complicated by a venous stasis ulcer that requires surgical débridement. The desired outcomes of managing venous stasis ulcers are to heal the ulcer, prevent infection, and prevent stasis with recurrence of ulcer formation. Collaborate with the wound care nurse or wound, ostomy, and continence nurse (WOCN) to make recommendations for ulcer care. A dietitian can suggest dietary supplements, such as zinc and vitamins A and C, as well as high-protein foods, to promote wound healing.

Patients with chronic venous insufficiency wear graduated compression stockings, which fit from the middle of the foot to just below the knee or to the thigh. Stockings should be worn during the day and evening. Explain the purpose and importance of wearing the compression stockings. Be sure to use the sizing chart that comes with the stockings to select the best fit. Teach patients to not roll them down and to report if they become too tight or uncomfortable.

Teach the patient to elevate his or her legs for at least 20 minutes 4 or 5 times per day. When the patient is in bed, remind him or her to elevate the legs above the level of the heart (Chart 36-9).

Coordinate with the physician about the use of intermittent sequential pneumatic compression or foot plexus pumps for patients with past or present venous stasis ulcers. If an open venous ulcer is present, the device may be applied over a dressing such as an Unna boot. Instruct the patient to apply the pump as directed during the period of healing. Because of the high incidence of venous ulcer recurrence, encourage patients with chronic venous insufficiency whose ulcers have healed to continue compression therapy for life.

CHART 36-9 **Patient and Family Education: Preparing for Self-Management**

Venous Insufficiency

Graduated Compression Stockings (GCSs)
- Wear stockings as prescribed, usually during the day and evening.
- Put the stockings on upon awakening and before getting out of bed.
- When applying the stockings, do not "bunch up" and apply like socks. Instead, place your hand inside the stocking and pull out the heel. Then place the foot of the stocking over your foot and slide the rest of the stocking up. Be sure that rough seams on the stocking are on the outside, not next to your skin.
- Do not push stockings down for comfort, because they may function like a tourniquet and further impair venous return.
- Put on a clean pair of stockings each day. Wash them by hand (not in a washing machine) in a gentle detergent and warm water.
- If the stockings seem to be "stretched out," replace them with a new pair.

Dos and Don'ts
- Elevate your legs for at least 20 minutes 4 or 5 times a day. When in bed, elevate your legs above the level of your heart.
- Avoid prolonged sitting or standing.
- Do not cross your legs. Crossing at the ankles is acceptable for short periods.
- Do not wear tight, restrictive pants. Avoid girdles and garters.

Venous stasis ulcers are slightly more manageable than ulcers resulting from arterial disease. They are chronic in nature, with some patients having the same ulcer for years. Ulcers often heal, only to recur in the same area several years later.

Two types of occlusive dressings are used for venous stasis ulcers: oxygen-permeable dressings and oxygen-impermeable dressings. Because the role of atmospheric oxygen in wound healing is controversial, opinions vary with regard to which type of dressing is preferred. An oxygen-permeable polyethylene film and an oxygen-impermeable hydrocolloid dressing (e.g., DuoDERM) are common. Hydrocolloid dressings are left in place for a minimum of 3 to 5 days for best effect. Use medical aseptic technique when changing dressings. If the wound is infected, use Contact Precautions in addition to Standard Precautions.

Artificial skin products can be used for difficult-to-heal venous leg ulcers. These first-generation products are very expensive but are laying the foundation in the field, with costs anticipated to come down in the future. Except for cultured epithelial autografts, artificial skins are only temporary. Artificial skin serves as a biologic cover to secrete growth factors to promote more growth factor secretion from the patient's own skin to speed the wound healing process.

If the patient is ambulatory, an **Unna boot** may be used. An Unna boot dressing is constructed of gauze that has been moistened with zinc oxide. Apply the boot to the affected limb, from the toes to the knee, after the ulcer has been cleaned with normal saline solution. It is then covered with an elastic wrap and hardens like a cast. This promotes venous return and prevents stasis. The Unna boot also forms a sterile environment for the ulcer. The physician or advanced practice nurse changes the boot about once a week. Instruct the patient to report increased pain, which indicates that the boot may be too tight.

The health care provider may prescribe topical agents, such as Accuzyme, to chemically débride the ulcer, eliminating necrotic tissue and promoting healing. Remind patients that they may temporarily feel a burning sensation when the agent is applied. If an infection or cellulitis develops, systemic antibiotics are necessary.

Surgical Management. Surgery for chronic venous insufficiency is not usually performed because it is not successful. Attempts at transplanting vein valves have had limited success. Surgical débridement of venous ulcers is similar to that performed for arterial ulcers.

NCLEX EXAMINATION CHALLENGE

Health Promotion and Maintenance

The nurse is caring for a client with chronic venous stasis ulcers. Which statement by the client indicates a need for further health teaching?
A. "I'll wear compression stockings at night."
B. "I'll keep my affected leg above my heart."
C. "I'll eat protein and vitamin C foods to help heal the ulcer"
D. "I'll change my dressing every 3 to 5 days as needed."

Community-Based Care

The desired outcome for the patient with chronic venous insufficiency is to be managed in the home. For patients with frequent acute complications and repeated hospital admissions, case management can help meet appropriate clinical and cost outcomes.

Help patients plan for opportunities and facilities that allow for elevation of the lower extremities in and outside the home. In addition, collaborate with the wound specialist to plan care of the ulcers at home.

If the physician prescribes graduated compression stockings, teach patients to apply these stockings before they get out of bed in the morning and to remove them just before going to bed at night (see Chart 36-9). Also advise them that they will probably need to wear these stockings for the rest of their lives.

To improve circulation and aid in weight reduction, collaborate with the physical therapist to prescribe an exercise program on an individual basis. Encourage all patients to maintain an optimal weight and consult with the dietitian to plan a weight-reduction diet.

Patients with venous stasis disease, especially those with venous stasis ulcers, may require long-term emotional support to assist them in meeting long-term needs. They may also need assistance in coping with necessary lifestyle adjustments, such as possible changes in occupation.

Patients with venous stasis ulcers may need the assistance of a home care nurse to perform dressing changes. Those with Unna boots need weekly transportation to their health care provider for dressing changes. Collaborate with the case manager to arrange for a sequential compression device in the home if the health care provider prescribes one.

VARICOSE VEINS

❖ PATHOPHYSIOLOGY

Varicose veins are distended, protruding veins that appear darkened and tortuous. They can occur in anyone, but they are common in adults older than 30 years whose occupations require prolonged standing or heavy physical activity. Varicose veins are frequently seen also in patients with systemic problems (e.g., heart disease), obesity, high estrogen states, and a family history of varicose veins.

Both *superficial* and *deep* veins can become distended. As the vein wall weakens and dilates, venous pressure increases and the valves become incompetent (defective), causing venous reflux (Armstrong, 2013). The incompetent valves enhance the vessel dilation, and the veins become tortuous and distended. The severity of the disease depends on the extent of the distention and reflux. **Telangiectasias** (spider veins) are dilated *intradermal* veins less than 1 to 3 mm in diameter that are visible on the skin surface. Most patients are not bothered by them but may consider them unattractive. Most telangiectasias do not develop into the more severe varicose vein disease.

More advanced disease causes venous distention (bulging), edema, a feeling of fullness in the legs, and pruritus (itching). As a result, signs and symptoms of venous insufficiency may occur, including venous stasis ulcers, brown pigmentation from extravasated red blood cells (also called *skin staining*), and pain.

Varicose veins and reflux are diagnosed by simple ultrasonography or duplex ultrasonography. Informal assessments of venous reflux can be made with the patient lying down to determine the direction of flow within a vein. For the duplex ultrasound procedure, the patient is upright and BP cuffs are placed at the thigh, calf, and ankle. The cuffs are serially inflated and deflated while the scanner tests for reflux. A reflux time greater than 0.5 second in the saphenous vein is considered abnormal (Armstrong, 2013).

❖ PATIENT-CENTERED COLLABORATIVE CARE

The overall purpose of management for patients with varicose veins is to improve and maintain optimal venous return to the heart and prevent disease progression. Conservative measures are the treatment of choice, including the three Es: **e**lastic compression hose, **e**xercise, and **e**levation. Graduated compression stockings (GCSs) rely on graduated external pressure to improve venous return by applying pressure to the muscles. They are available in many grades or strengths, ranging from 8 to 50 mm Hg pressure. Exercise increases venous return by helping the muscles pump blood back to the heart. Teach patients to avoid high-impact exercises such as horseback riding and running. Daily walks and ankle flexion exercises while sitting are common exercises that are helpful in promoting circulation. Elevating the extremities as much as possible allows gravity to work with the valves in promoting venous return and prevent reflux.

Patients who continue to have pain or unsightly veins despite using the three Es may opt for more invasive approaches. Surgical ligation and/or removal of veins ("stripping") were the procedures of choice for many years. Sclerotherapy to occlude the affected vessel is also an option.

However, newer, less-invasive treatments are more common today. They are less painful and have a shorter recovery time. A common procedure is an endovenous ablation, which occludes the varicose vein, most commonly the saphenous vein. Using ultrasound guidance, the clinician advances a catheter into the vein and injects an anesthetic agent around it. Then the vessel is ablated (occluded) while the catheter is slowly removed. The two modalities for ablation are (1) endovenous laser treatment (EVLT) using laser heat and (2) radiofrequency ablation (RFA) using a radiofrequency heating element.

After the procedure, teach the patient the importance of using a GCS or other form of compression (such as elastic compression bandages) for 24 hours a day, except for showers, for at least the first week. Follow-up ultrasonography ensures that the treated vein is closed. The patient is monitored carefully for the first 6 to 8 weeks to determine how healing has progressed. Some patients require continued use of the three Es for many years, depending on the severity of their disease.

Assess the affected limb for vascular status, including any changes in color or temperature of the leg. Monitor for PAIN, edema, and paresthesias that could indicate complications such as DVT or nerve damage. Nerve damage is usually temporary and minimal; it usually resolves within a few months (Armstrong, 2013).

VASCULAR TRAUMA

Many types of trauma can result in vascular injury. Vascular injuries include punctures, lacerations, and transections. Acute blunt or penetrating trauma may result in a false aneurysm or hematoma. Arteriovenous fistulas may be seen after penetrating injuries. The more common causes of penetrating injuries to the blood vessels are gunshot and knife wounds.

Blunt trauma can result from high-speed automobile crashes as a result of the shearing force of rapid deceleration. Vascular trauma can also occur during arterial puncture for arteriographic or hemodynamic studies in which a dissection, hematoma, or occlusive lesion occurs.

The history and physical examination aid in establishing the diagnosis of vascular injury. Ask the patient or family about the mechanism of injury, the site of injury, the amount of blood loss, and symptoms present after the injury. Assess for circulatory, sensory, and motor impairment. Be aware that, despite significant trauma, impairment may not be apparent, especially if deep vessels have been injured. Arteriography can provide essential information about the vascular injury.

Management of vascular injuries is often initiated in a hospital emergency department. Careful patient triage is crucial. The most important principles in the management of vascular trauma are establishing a patent airway, controlling bleeding, and restoring blood flow. Emergency or urgent surgical intervention is needed for ischemia to maximize successful revascularization.

The method of repair varies with the type of vascular injury. Techniques include vein bypass grafting, lateral suture repair, thrombectomy (excision of blood clot), resection with end-to-end anastomosis, and vein patch grafting. Vascular repair can sometimes be done via angiographic access (covered stent sealing an injury or embolizing a branch artery where appropriate).

NURSING CONCEPTS AND CLINICAL JUDGMENT REVIEW

What might you NOTICE if the patient is experiencing inadequate GAS EXCHANGE and tissue PERFUSION as a result of vascular problems?

- Redness and swelling in lower leg (venous)
- Pallor, cyanosis (darkened), mottling, or rubor in lower leg (arterial)
- Report of pain/cramping in lower legs or hands (at rest or during activity)
- Ulcers on ankles, feet, or digits
- Pulsating mass in abdomen (abdominal aortic aneurysm)
- Decreased level of consciousness (LOC), diaphoresis, decreased urine output (rupturing aortic aneurysm)

What should you INTERPRET and how should you RESPOND to a patient experiencing inadequate GAS EXCHANGE and tissue PERFUSION as a result of peripheral vascular disease?

Perform and interpret physical assessment, including:

- Taking vital signs
- Assessing peripheral pulses
- Assessing capillary refill
- Checking for sensation and temperature
- Completing a pain assessment
- Assessing ulcer

Respond by:
- Notifying physician immediately or calling Rapid Response Team if aortic rupture suspected
- Monitoring vital signs
- Giving oxygen if aneurysm rupture suspected
- Starting an IV line if aneurysm rupture suspected
- Documenting abnormal peripheral vascular assessment findings

- Elevating legs if swollen unless arterial blood flow is poor

On what should you REFLECT?
- Think about how you responded.
- Continue to monitor patient for changes in peripheral blood flow, including pulse assessments.
- Observe patient for decreased report of pain.

GET READY FOR THE NCLEX® EXAMINATION!

KEY POINTS

Review these Key Points for each NCLEX Examination Client Needs Category.

Safe and Effective Care Environment
- Plan care for the patient with atherosclerosis and hypertension, in collaboration with the health care team, including the dietitian, pharmacist, and primary health care provider as needed. **Teamwork and Collaboration** QSEN
- To reduce the risk for injury, caution patients about orthostatic hypotension when taking antihypertensive drugs. **Safety** QSEN
- Monitor blood pressure carefully in patients who have hypertension; be aware that they may develop a hypertensive crisis, a life-threatening medical emergency (see Chart 36-2).

Health Promotion and Maintenance
- In collaboration with the dietitian, assist the patient to incorporate healthy eating behaviors to lower cholesterol and saturated fats and increase fresh fruits, vegetables, and fiber in the diet. For overweight patients, assist in a weight-reduction plan. **Teamwork and Collaboration** QSEN
- Teach patients to engage in 40 minutes of moderate-to-vigorous physical activity 3 or 4 times a week to lower blood pressure and LDL-C levels.
- Assess the patient for modifiable and nonmodifiable risk factors for vascular disease, and teach health promotion behaviors to the patient and family. Pay particular attention to the patient with a family history of cardiovascular disease (see Table 36-1). **Patient-Centered Care** QSEN

Physiological Integrity
- Remember that risk factors such as smoking increase the pathophysiologic process of atherosclerosis (see Table 36-1).
- Remember that atherosclerosis occurs when fatty plaques occlude arteries and prevent adequate PERFUSION to vital body tissues.
- Monitor total cholesterol, HDL-C, and LDL-C levels to assess patient risk for atherosclerosis.
- Teach patients taking any of the statins in Table 36-2 to report any adverse effects including muscle cramping to their health care provider. Monitor the patient's liver enzymes carefully.
- Teach patients to decrease saturated and *trans* fats in their diet; instruct them to consume a diet rich in fruits, vegetables, and whole grains; and instruct them to include legumes, poultry, fish, and low-fat dairy products. Remind them to

limit sweets, red meats, and sugar-sweetened beverages. **Evidence-Based Practice** QSEN
- Hypertension is categorized as either essential or secondary; the risk factors and causes for each type are described in Table 36-4. Essential hypertension is called *primary hypertension* and is not caused by another health problem or drug. *Secondary hypertension* is caused by other health problems or drug therapy.
- Closely observe the patient receiving anticoagulants or fibrinolytics for signs of bleeding, and monitor appropriate laboratory values for desired outcome values (see Chart 36-7). **Safety** QSEN
- Monitor for decreased serum potassium levels when patients are taking thiazide or loop diuretics; hypokalemia could cause life-threatening cardiac dysrhythmias (see Chart 36-1). **Safety** QSEN
- Teach patients to move slowly when changing position if taking any of the antihypertensive drugs listed in Chart 36-1. **Safety** QSEN
- Recognize that clinical manifestations of peripheral vascular disease (PVD) depend on whether it affects the arteries or veins. In addition to pallor, rubor, or cyanosis, key features of chronic peripheral arterial disease are listed in Chart 36-3.
- Vasodilating drugs or surgery is used for arterial vascular diseases.
- Deep vein thrombosis (DVT) is the most common type of peripheral vascular problem. When symptoms are present, they include swelling, redness, localized pain, and warmth.
- Be aware that DVT can lead to pulmonary embolism, a life-threatening emergency!
- Teach patients to prevent VTE by leg exercises, early ambulation, adequate hydration, graduated compression stockings (GCSs), sequential compression devices (SCDs), and anticoagulant therapy.
- Monitor aPTT values for patients receiving unfractionated heparin; monitor INR for patients receiving warfarin (Coumadin). **Safety** QSEN
- Assess for venous and arterial ulcers as described in Chart 36-4.
- Teach foot care for patients with PVD as outlined in Chart 36-6.
- Teach patients about precautions for anticoagulant therapy as described in Chart 36-7. Teach about food and drugs that interfere with warfarin (Coumadin) as listed in Chart 36-8. **Evidence-Based Practice** QSEN

- Monitor for indications of aneurysm rupture: diaphoresis, nausea, vomiting, pallor, hypotension, tachycardia, severe pain, and decreased level of consciousness. **Safety** OSEN
- Varicose veins can cause severe pain and reflux requiring the three *E*s: **e**lastic compression hose, **e**xercise, and **e**levation. Endovascular ablation can occlude the affected vessel with minimal pain and the risk for few complications. Postprocedure compression with graduated stockings or other elastic bandages is essential for this procedure to be successful.
- Raynaud's and Buerger's disease affect the digits of the fingers and toes as outlined in Table 36-7.

CHAPTER 37

Care of Patients with Shock

M. Linda Workman

ℯ http://evolve.elsevier.com/Iggy/

PRIORITY CONCEPTS

- PERFUSION
- CLOTTING

- INFLAMMATION
- INFECTION

LEARNING OUTCOMES

Safe and Effective Care Environment

1. Evaluate patient risk for hypovolemic shock or sepsis and septic shock.
2. Apply principles of infection control to prevent INFECTION and sepsis in susceptible patients, especially older adults.

Health Promotion and Maintenance

3. Teach all people how to prevent and recognize hypovolemic shock or sepsis.

Psychosocial Integrity

4. Reduce the psychological impact for the patient and family regarding the assessment and management of hypovolemic or septic shock.

Physiological Integrity

5. Use laboratory data and clinical manifestations of PERFUSION to determine the effectiveness of therapy for hypovolemic shock and sepsis.
6. Prioritize the nursing care for the patient experiencing any stage of hypovolemic shock.
7. Prioritize the nursing care for the patient with sepsis or septic shock, especially when impaired CLOTTING is present.

OVERVIEW

All organs, tissues, and cells need a continuous supply of oxygen to function properly. The lungs first bring oxygen into the body through ventilation and gas exchange, and the cardiovascular system (heart, blood, and blood vessels) delivers oxygen by PERFUSION to all tissues and removes cellular wastes (Fig. 37-1). Shock is widespread abnormal cellular metabolism that occurs when gas exchange with oxygenation and tissue perfusion needs are not met sufficiently to maintain cell function (McCance et al., 2014). It is a condition rather than a disease and is the "whole-body" response that occurs when too little oxygen is delivered to the tissues. All body organs are affected by shock and either work harder to adapt and compensate for reduced gas exchange or perfusion (see Fig. 37-1) or fail to function because of hypoxia. Shock is a "syndrome" because the problems resulting from it occur in a predictable sequence.

Any problem that impairs oxygen PERFUSION to tissues and organs can start the syndrome of shock and lead to a life-threatening emergency. Shock is often a result of cardiovascular problems. Patients in acute care settings are at higher risk, but shock can occur in any setting. For example, older patients in long-term care settings are at risk for sepsis and shock related to urinary tract infections. When the body's adaptive adjustments (compensation) or health care interventions are not effective and shock progresses, severe hypoxia can lead to cell loss, multiple organ dysfunction syndrome (MODS), and death.

Shock is classified by the type of impairment causing it into the categories of hypovolemic shock, cardiogenic shock, distributive shock (which includes septic shock, neurogenic shock, and anaphylactic shock), and obstructive shock. Table 37-1 describes this classification and common causes of shock.

Most manifestations of shock are similar regardless of what starts the process or which tissues are affected first. These manifestations result from physiologic adjustments *(compensatory mechanisms)* that the body makes in the attempt to ensure continued PERFUSION of vital organs. These adjustment actions are triggered by the sympathetic nervous system's stress response activating the endocrine and cardiovascular systems. Manifestations unique to any one type of shock result from specific tissue dysfunction. The common features of shock are listed in Chart 37-1.

Review of Oxygenation and Tissue Perfusion

Oxygenation with gas exchange and PERFUSION depend on how much oxygen from arterial blood perfuses the tissue. Perfusion

Specific Human Need

Organs/Tissues Important
in Meeting the Need

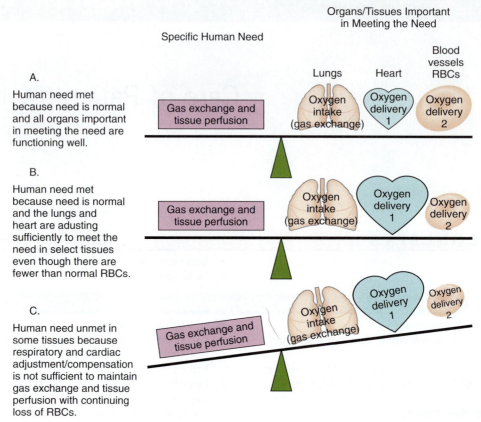

FIG. 37-1 Gas exchange and tissue perfusion affected by hypovolemic shock and adjustment/compensation. *RBCs,* Red blood cells.

is related to mean arterial pressure (MAP). The factors that influence MAP include:

- Total blood volume
- Cardiac output
- Size and integrity of the vascular bed, especially capillaries

Total blood volume and cardiac output are directly related to MAP, so increases in either total blood volume or cardiac output *raise* MAP. Decreases in either total blood volume or cardiac output *lower* MAP.

The size of the vascular bed is inversely (negatively) related to MAP. This means that increases in the size of the vascular bed *lower* MAP and decreases *raise* MAP (Fig. 37-2). The small arteries and veins connected to capillaries can increase in diameter by relaxing the smooth muscle in vessel walls (**dilation**) or decrease in diameter by contracting the muscle (**vasoconstriction**). When blood vessels dilate and total blood volume remains the same, blood pressure decreases and blood flow is slower. When blood vessels constrict and total blood volume remains the same, blood pressure increases and blood flow is faster.

Blood vessels are innervated by the sympathetic nervous system. Some nerves continuously stimulate vascular smooth muscle so that the blood vessels are normally partially constricted, a condition called **sympathetic tone**. Increases in sympathetic stimulation constrict smooth muscle even more, raising MAP. Decreases in sympathetic tone relax smooth muscle, dilating blood vessels and lowering MAP.

PERFUSION (blood flow) to organs varies and adjusts to changes in tissue oxygen needs. The body can selectively increase blood flow to some areas while reducing flow to others. The skin and skeletal muscles can tolerate low levels of oxygen for hours without dying or being damaged. Other organs (e.g., heart, brain, liver, pancreas) do not tolerate **hypoxia** (low levels of tissue oxygenation), and a few minutes without oxygen results in serious damage and cell death.

Types of Shock

Types of shock vary because shock is a manifestation of a pathologic condition rather than a disease state (see Table 37-1). *More than one type of shock can be present at the same time.* For example, trauma caused by a car crash may trigger hemorrhage (leading to hypovolemic shock) and a myocardial infarction (leading to cardiogenic shock).

Hypovolemic shock occurs when too little circulating blood volume decreases MAP, resulting in inadequate total body PERFUSION and oxygenation. Common problems leading to hypovolemic shock are poor CLOTTING with hemorrhage and dehydration. A complete discussion of the pathophysiology and management of hypovolemic shock begins on p. 741.

Cardiogenic shock occurs when the heart muscle is unhealthy and pumping is impaired. Myocardial infarction is the most common cause of direct pump failure. Other causes are listed in Table 37-1. Any type of pump failure decreases cardiac output and MAP. Chapter 38 discusses the pathophysiology and care for the person with shock from myocardial infarction.

Distributive shock occurs when blood volume is not lost from the body but is distributed to the interstitial tissues where it cannot perfuse organs. It can be caused by blood vessel dilation, pooling of blood in venous and capillary beds, and increased capillary leak. All these factors decrease mean arterial

TABLE 37-1 Causes and Types of Shock by Functional Impairment

Hypovolemic Shock
Overall Cause

Total body fluid decreased (in all fluid compartments).

Specific Cause or Risk Factors
- Hemorrhage
  - Trauma
  - GI ulcer
  - Surgery
  - Inadequate clotting
    - Hemophilia
    - Liver disease
    - Cancer therapy
    - Anticoagulation therapy
- Dehydration
  - Vomiting
  - Diarrhea
  - Heavy diaphoresis
  - Diuretic therapy
  - Nasogastric suction
  - Diabetes insipidus

Cardiogenic Shock
Overall Cause

Direct pump failure (fluid volume not affected).

Specific Cause or Risk Factors
- Myocardial infarction
- Cardiac arrest
- Ventricular dysrhythmias
- Cardiac amyloidosis
- Cardiomyopathies
- Myocardial degeneration

Distributive Shock
Overall Cause

Fluid shifted from central vascular space (total body fluid volume normal or increased).

Specific Cause or Risk Factors
- Neural-induced
  - Pain
  - Anesthesia
  - Stress
  - Spinal cord injury
  - Head trauma
- Chemical-induced
  - Anaphylaxis
  - Sepsis
  - Capillary leak
    - Burns
    - Extensive trauma
    - Liver impairment
    - Hypoproteinemia

Obstructive Shock
Overall Cause

Cardiac function decreased by noncardiac factor (indirect pump failure). Total body fluid is not affected although central volume is decreased.

Specific Cause or Risk Factors
- Cardiac tamponade
- Arterial stenosis
- Pulmonary embolus
- Pulmonary hypertension
- Constrictive pericarditis
- Thoracic tumors
- Tension pneumothorax

CHART 37-1 Key Features
Shock

Cardiovascular Manifestations
- Decreased cardiac output
- Increased pulse rate
- Thready pulse
- Decreased blood pressure
- Narrowed pulse pressure
- Postural hypotension
- Low central venous pressure
- Flat neck and hand veins in dependent positions
- Slow capillary refill in nail beds
- Diminished peripheral pulses

Respiratory Manifestations
- Increased respiratory rate
- Shallow depth of respirations
- Increased $PaCO_2$
- Decreased PaO_2
- Cyanosis, especially around lips and nail beds

Gastrointestinal Manifestations
- Decreased motility
- Diminished or absent bowel sounds
- Nausea and vomiting
- Constipation

Neuromuscular Manifestations
Early
- Anxiety
- Restlessness
- Increased thirst

Late
- Decreased central nervous system activity (lethargy to coma)
- Generalized muscle weakness
- Diminished or absent deep tendon reflexes
- Sluggish pupillary response to light

Kidney Manifestations
- Decreased urine output
- Increased specific gravity
- Sugar and acetone present in urine

Integumentary Manifestations
- Cool to cold
- Pale to mottled to cyanotic
- Moist, clammy
- Mouth dry; pastelike coating present

$PaCO_2$, Partial pressure of arterial carbon dioxide; PaO_2, partial pressure of arterial oxygen.

pressure (MAP) and may be started either by nerve changes (*neural-induced*) or by the presence of some chemicals (*chemical-induced*).

Neural-induced distributive shock is a loss of MAP that occurs when sympathetic nerve impulses are decreased and blood vessel smooth muscles relax, causing vasodilation and poor perfusion. Shock results when vasodilation is widespread. Problems leading to loss of sympathetic tone are listed in Table 37-1.

Chemical-induced distributive shock has three common origins: anaphylaxis, sepsis, and capillary leak syndrome. It occurs when certain body chemicals or foreign substances in the blood and vessels start widespread changes in blood vessel walls. The chemicals are usually exogenous (originate outside the body), but this type of shock also can be induced by substances normally found in the body, such as excessive amounts of histamine.

Anaphylaxis is an extreme type I allergic reaction. It begins within seconds to minutes after exposure to a specific allergen in a susceptible person. The result is widespread loss of blood vessel tone, with decreased blood pressure and decreased cardiac output. Table 20-2 (in Chapter 20) lists common allergens that can cause anaphylaxis. Chapter 20 describes the pathophysiology, prevention, and care of the patient with anaphylactic shock.

Sepsis is a widespread infection that triggers whole-body INFLAMMATION. It leads to distributive shock when infectious microorganisms are present in the blood and is most commonly called septic shock. A complete discussion of the pathophysiology, prevention, and care for the patient with sepsis and septic shock begins on p. 748.

Capillary leak syndrome is the response of capillaries to the presence of body chemicals that enlarge capillary pores and allow fluid to shift from the capillaries into the interstitial tissues. Once in the interstitial tissue, these fluids are stagnant and cannot deliver oxygen or remove tissue waste products. Problems causing fluid shifts include severe burns, liver disorders, ascites, peritonitis, large wounds, kidney disease, hypoproteinemia, and trauma.

Obstructive shock is caused by problems that impair the ability of the normal heart to pump effectively. The heart itself remains normal, but conditions outside the heart prevent either adequate filling of the heart or adequate contraction of the healthy heart muscle. The most common cause of obstructive shock is cardiac tamponade (Table 37-1). Care of the person with cardiac tamponade is presented in Chapter 35 (pericarditis) and Chapter 38.

Although the causes and initial manifestations associated with the different types of shock vary, eventually the effects of hypotension and anaerobic cellular metabolism (metabolism without oxygen) result in the common key features of shock listed in Chart 37-1.

FIG. 37-2 Interaction of blood volume and the size of the capillary bed affecting mean arterial pressure (MAP).

HYPOVOLEMIC SHOCK

❖ *PATHOPHYSIOLOGY*

The basic problem of hypovolemic shock is a loss of blood volume from the vascular space, resulting in a decreased mean arterial pressure (MAP) (see Fig. 37-2) and a loss of oxygen-carrying capacity from the loss of circulating red blood cells (RBCs). The reduced MAP slows blood flow, decreasing tissue PERFUSION. The loss of RBCs decreases the ability of the blood to oxygenate the tissue it does reach. These oxygenation and perfusion problems lead to *anaerobic* (without oxygen) cellular metabolism.

The main trigger leading to hypovolemic shock is a sustained decrease in MAP from decreased circulating blood volume. A decrease in MAP of 5 to 10 mm Hg below the patient's normal baseline value is detected by pressure-sensitive nerve receptors *(baroreceptors)* in the aortic arch and carotid sinus. This information is transmitted to brain centers, which stimulate adjustments *(compensatory mechanisms)* to help ensure continued blood flow and oxygen delivery to vital organs while limiting blood flow to less vital areas. The movement of blood into selected areas while bypassing others ("shunting") results in some shock manifestations.

If the events that caused the initial decrease in MAP are halted now, compensatory mechanisms provide adequate oxygenation and PERFUSION without intervention. If events continue and MAP decreases further, some tissues function under anaerobic conditions. This condition increases lactic acid levels and other harmful metabolites (e.g., protein-destroying enzymes, oxygen free radicals) (McCance et al., 2014). These substances cause acid-base imbalances with tissue-damaging

effects and depressed heart muscle activity. These effects are temporary and reversible if the cause of shock is corrected within 1 to 2 hours after onset. When shock conditions continue for longer periods without help, the resulting acid-base imbalance and increased metabolites cause so much cell damage in vital organs that they are unable to perform their critical functions. When this problem, known as multiple organ dysfunction syndrome (MODS), occurs to the extent that vital organs die, recovery from shock is no longer possible (see the section on the Refractory Stage of Shock on p. 742). Table 37-2 summarizes the progression of shock.

Stages of Shock

The syndrome of shock progresses in four stages when the conditions that cause shock remain uncorrected and poor cellular oxygenation continues. These stages are:
1. Initial stage
2. Nonprogressive stage
3. Progressive stage
4. Refractory stage

Initial Stage of Shock. The initial (early) stage of shock is present when the patient's baseline MAP is decreased by less than 10 mm Hg. Compensatory mechanisms are so effective at returning systolic pressure to normal during this stage that oxygen PERFUSION to vital organs is maintained. The cellular change in this stage is increased anaerobic metabolism in some tissues with production of lactic acid, although overall metabolism is still aerobic. The compensation responses of vascular constriction and increased heart rate are effective, and both cardiac output and MAP are maintained within the normal range. Because vital organ function is not disrupted, the

TABLE 37-2 Adaptive Responses and Events During Hypovolemic Shock

Initial Stage
- Decrease in mean arterial pressure (MAP) of 5-10 mm Hg from baseline value
- Increased sympathetic stimulation
  - Mild vasoconstriction
  - Increased heart rate

Nonprogressive Stage
- Decrease in MAP of 10-15 mm Hg from baseline value
- Continued sympathetic stimulation
  - Moderate vasoconstriction
  - Increased heart rate
  - Decreased pulse pressure
- Chemical compensation
  - Renin, aldosterone, and antidiuretic hormone secretion
    Increased vasoconstriction
    Decreased urine output
    Stimulation of the thirst reflex
- Some anaerobic metabolism in nonvital organs
  - Mild acidosis
  - Mild hyperkalemia

Progressive Stage
- Decrease in MAP of >20 mm Hg from baseline value
- Anoxia of nonvital organs
- Hypoxia of vital organs
- Overall metabolism is anaerobic
  - Moderate acidosis
  - Moderate hyperkalemia
  - Tissue ischemia

Refractory Stage
- Severe tissue hypoxia with ischemia and necrosis
- Release of myocardial depressant factor from the pancreas
- Buildup of toxic metabolites
- Multiple organ dysfunction syndrome (MODS)
- Death

manifestations of shock are difficult to detect at this stage. *A heart and respiratory rate increased from the patient's baseline level or a slight* **increase** *in diastolic blood pressure may be the only manifestation of this stage of shock.*

Nonprogressive Stage. The nonprogressive (compensatory) stage of shock occurs when MAP decreases by 10 to 15 mm Hg from baseline. Kidney and hormonal compensatory mechanisms are activated because cardiovascular responses alone are not enough to maintain MAP and supply oxygen to vital organs.

The ongoing decrease in MAP triggers the release of renin, antidiuretic hormone (ADH), aldosterone, epinephrine, and norepinephrine to start kidney compensation. Urine output decreases, sodium reabsorption increases, and widespread blood vessel constriction occurs. ADH increases water reabsorption in the kidney, further reducing urine output, and increases blood vessel constriction in the skin and other less vital tissue areas. Together these actions compensate for shock by maintaining the fluid volume within the central blood vessels.

Tissue hypoxia occurs in nonvital organs (e.g., skin, GI tract) and in the kidney, but it is not great enough to cause permanent damage. Acid-base and electrolyte changes occur in response to the buildup of metabolites. Changes include **acidosis** (low blood pH) and **hyperkalemia** (increased blood potassium level).

Manifestations of this stage include changes resulting from decreased tissue PERFUSION. Subjective changes include thirst and anxiety. Objective changes include restlessness, tachycardia, increased respiratory rate, decreased urine output, falling systolic blood pressure, rising diastolic blood pressure, narrowing pulse pressure, cool extremities, and a 2% to 5% decrease in oxygen saturation. *Comparing these changes with the values and manifestations obtained earlier is critical to identifying this stage of shock.*

If the patient is stable and compensatory mechanisms are supported by medical and nursing interventions, he or she can remain in this stage for hours without having permanent damage. *Stopping the conditions that started shock and providing supportive interventions can prevent the shock from progressing.* The effects of this stage are reversible when nurses recognize the problem and coordinate the health care team to start appropriate interventions.

Progressive Stage of Shock. The progressive stage of shock occurs when there is a sustained decrease in MAP of more than 20 mm Hg from baseline. Compensatory mechanisms are functioning but can no longer deliver sufficient oxygen, even to vital organs. Vital organs develop hypoxia, and less vital organs become **anoxic** (no oxygen) and **ischemic** (cell dysfunction or death from lack of oxygen). As a result of poor PERFUSION and a buildup of metabolites, some tissues die.

Manifestations of the progressive stage of shock include a *worsening* of changes resulting from decreased tissue PERFUSION. The patient may express a sense of "something bad" (impending doom) about to happen. He or she may seem confused, and thirst increases. Objective changes are a rapid, weak pulse; low blood pressure; pallor to cyanosis of oral mucosa and nail beds; cool and moist skin; anuria; and a 5% to 20% decrease in oxygen saturation. Laboratory data at this stage may show a low blood pH, along with rising lactic acid and potassium levels.

! NURSING SAFETY PRIORITY (QSEN)

Critical Rescue

The progressive stage of shock is a life-threatening emergency. Vital organs can tolerate this situation for only a short time before developing multiple organ dysfunction syndrome (MODS) and being damaged permanently. Immediate interventions are needed to reverse the effects of this stage of shock. The patient's life usually can be saved if the conditions causing shock are corrected within 1 hour or less of the onset of the progressive stage. Continuously monitor and compare with earlier findings to assess therapy effectiveness and determine when therapy changes are needed.

Refractory Stage of Shock and Multiple Organ Dysfunction Syndrome. The refractory stage of shock occurs when too much cell death and tissue damage result from too little oxygen reaching the tissues. Vital organs have extensive damage and cannot respond effectively to interventions, and shock continues. So much damage has occurred with release of metabolites and enzymes that damage to vital organs continues despite interventions.

The sequence of cell damage caused by massive release of toxic metabolites and enzymes is termed **multiple organ dysfunction syndrome (MODS)**. Once the damage has started, the sequence becomes a vicious cycle as more dead and dying cells open and release metabolites. These trigger small clots (microthrombi) to form, which block tissue PERFUSION and damage more cells, continuing the devastating cycle. Liver, heart, brain, and kidney function are lost first. The most profound change is damage to the heart muscle.

Manifestations are a rapid loss of consciousness; nonpalpable pulse; cold, dusky extremities; slow, shallow respirations; and unmeasurable oxygen saturation. *Therapy is not effective in saving the patient's life, even if the cause of shock is corrected and MAP temporarily returns to normal.*

Etiology

Hypovolemic shock occurs when too little circulating blood volume causes a MAP decrease that prevents total body PERFUSION and oxygenation. Problems leading to hypovolemic shock are listed in Table 37-1.

Hypovolemic shock from external hemorrhage is common after trauma and surgery. Hypovolemic shock from internal hemorrhage occurs with blunt trauma, GI ulcers, and poor control of surgical bleeding. Hemorrhage leading to hypovolemia also can be caused by any problem that reduces the levels of CLOTTING factors (see Table 37-1). Hypovolemia as a result of dehydration can be caused by any problem that decreases fluid intake or increases fluid loss (see Table 37-1).

Incidence and Prevalence

The exact incidence of hypovolemic shock is not known because it is a response rather than a disease. It is a common complication among hospitalized patients in emergency departments and after surgery or invasive procedures.

Health Promotion and Maintenance

Hypovolemic shock from most causes can be prevented. Teach all people to prevent dehydration by having an adequate fluid intake during exercise and when in hot, dry environments. Urge people to prevent trauma and hemorrhage by using proper safety equipment and seat belts and being aware of hazards in the home or workplace.

Recognizing hypovolemic shock is a major nursing responsibility. Keep in mind that just being a patient in the acute care setting is a risk factor. Also identify patients at risk for dehydration, and assess for early manifestations. This is especially important for those who have reduced cognition or reduced mobility or who are on NPO status.

Assess all patients with invasive procedures or trauma for obvious or occult impaired CLOTTING with bleeding. Compare pulse quality and rate with baseline. Compare urine output with fluid intake. Check vital signs of patients who have persistent thirst. Assess for shock in any patient who develops a change in mental status, an increase in pain, or an increase in anxiety.

Teach patients who have invasive procedures in an ambulatory setting the manifestations of shock. Stress the importance of seeking immediate help for obvious heavy bleeding, persistent thirst, decreased urine output, light-headedness, or a sense of impending doom (a feeling that something bad is happening or going to happen).

❖ PATIENT-CENTERED COLLABORATIVE CARE

The Concept Map on p. 744 addresses assessment and nursing care issues related to hypovolemic shock.

◆ Assessment

History. Ask about risk factors related to hypovolemic shock. If the patient is alert, question him or her directly. If the patient is not alert, collect information from family members. *Age is important because shock from trauma is more common in* young adults and other types of shock are more common in older adults. Ask about recent illness, trauma, procedures, or chronic health problems that may lead to shock (e.g., GI ulcers, general surgery, hemophilia, liver disorders, prolonged vomiting or diarrhea). Ask about the use of drugs such as aspirin, other NSAIDs, and diuretics that may cause changes leading to hypovolemic shock.

Ask about fluid intake and output during the previous 24 hours. *Information about urine output is especially important because urine output is reduced during the first stages of shock, even when fluid intake is normal.*

Assess the patient for factors that can lead to shock. Areas to examine for poor CLOTTING and hemorrhage include the gums, wounds, and sites of dressings, drains, and vascular accesses. Also check *under* the patient for blood. Observe for any swelling or skin discoloration that may indicate an internal hemorrhage.

Physical Assessment/Clinical Manifestations. Most manifestations of hypovolemic shock are caused by the changes resulting from compensatory efforts. Compensatory mechanisms are physiologic responses that try to keep an adequate PERFUSION to vital organs. Shock may be first evident as changes in cardiovascular function. As shock progresses, changes in the renal, respiratory, integumentary, musculoskeletal, and central nervous systems become evident. Ensure that vital sign measurements are accurate, and monitor them for trends indicating shock.

! NURSING SAFETY PRIORITY (QSEN)
Action Alert

Assign a registered nurse rather than a licensed practical nurse/licensed vocational nurse (LPN/LVN) or unlicensed assistive personnel (UAP) to assess the vital signs of a patient who is at risk for or suspected of having hypovolemic shock.

Cardiovascular changes that occur with hypovolemic shock start with decreased mean arterial pressure (MAP) leading to compensatory responses. Assess the central and peripheral pulses for rate and quality. In the initial stage of shock, the pulse rate increases to keep cardiac output and MAP at normal levels, even though the actual stroke volume (amount of blood pumped out from the heart) per beat is decreased. *Increased heart rate is the first manifestation of shock.* Because stroke volume is decreased, the peripheral pulses are difficult to palpate and are blocked with light pressure. As shock progresses, peripheral pulses may be absent.

When assessing the blood pressure (BP), consider the patient's normal baseline blood pressure. Although a blood pressure of 90/50 mm Hg may indicate severe shock in one person, it may be the normal blood pressure for another healthy adult.

! NURSING SAFETY PRIORITY (QSEN)
Action Alert

Because changes in systolic blood pressure are not always present in the initial stage of shock, use changes in pulse rate and quality as the main indicators of shock presence or progression.

CONCEPT MAP

HYPOVOLEMIC SHOCK
- CLOTTING
- PERFUSION
- INFLAMMATION
- INFECTION

EXPECTED OUTCOMES

Maintain normal aerobic cellular metabolism as evidenced by:
- Clear thought processes
- MAP <10 mm Hg from baseline
- BP, HR, RR, ABGs, O_2 saturation return to baseline
- U/O significantly >30 mL/hr
- No development of complications by supportive and drug therapies

Planning

Patient Problems
- Hypoxia related to hypovolemia
- Inadequate PERFUSION related to active fluid volume loss and hypotension
- Anxiety related to potential for death and decreased cerebral PERFUSION
- Acute confusion related to decreased cerebral PERFUSION

Data Synthesis

- Hemorrhage after blunt trauma
- Hemorrhage that reduces levels of clotting factors.

Causes

HISTORY

A 59 year-old involved in a motor vehicle crash comes to the ED in a confused and restless state with HR 120 (weak and thready), RR 24, BP 102/76 mm Hg. No open wounds, abdomen distended, hypoactive bowel sounds.

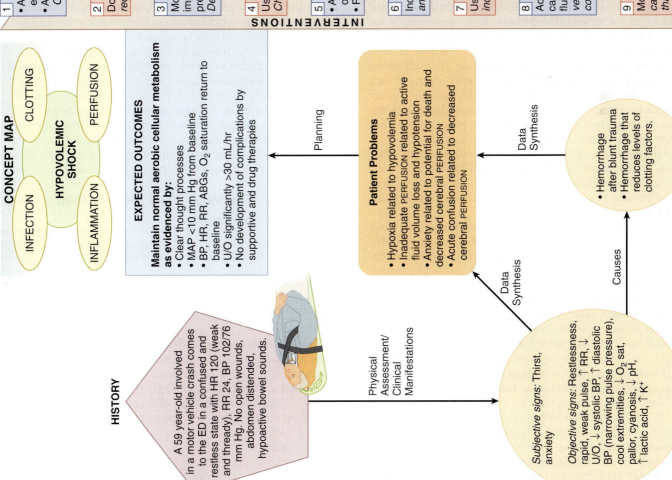

Physical Assessment/Clinical Manifestations

Data Synthesis

Subjective signs: Thirst, anxiety

Objective signs: Restlessness, rapid, weak pulse, ↑RR, ↓ U/O, ↓ systolic BP, ↑ diastolic BP (narrowing pulse pressure), cool extremities, ↓ O_2 sat, pallor, cyanosis, ↓ pH, ↑ lactic acid, ↑ K^+

INTERVENTIONS

1 **Nursing Priority – Ensuring a Patent Airway**
- Administer oxygen; monitor and respond to: ↑ RR, shallow depth; ↓ $PaCO_2$; ↓ PaO_2; cyanosis, especially around lips and nail beds. *Monitors for progression of shock and inadequate PERFUSION.*
- Assess oxygen saturation through pulse oximetry. *Indicates life-threatening emergency when O_2 saturation is below 70%.*

2 **Nursing Safety Priority: Critical Rescue!**
Do not leave the patient. RN (not LPN or UAP) must assess vital signs. *An unstable patient requires the assessment skills of an RN.*

3 **Assessment of Vital Signs in Shock**
Monitor vital signs at least every 15 minutes until shock is controlled and patient's condition improves. Assess pulse (rate, regularity, quality), blood pressure, pulse pressure, central venous pressure, respiratory rate, skin and mucosal color, oxygen saturation, cognition, and urine output. *Determines the patient's condition and the effectiveness of therapy.*

4 **Nursing Safety Priority: Action Alert!**
Use changes in pulse rate and quality as the main indicators of shock presence or progression. *Changes in systolic blood pressure are not always present in the initial stage of shock.*

5 **Minimizing Bleeding**
- Apply direct pressure for overt bleeding. Check *under* the patient for blood. Observe for swelling or skin discoloration. *Discoloration may indicate internal hemorrhage.*
- Prepare the patient for surgical intervention. *Corrects internal bleeding for the patient's survival.*

6 **Fluid Replacement Therapy**
Increase the rate of IV fluid delivery: crystalloids, colloids, and/or blood products. *Restores fluid volume and improves perfusion to vital organs which is the primary intervention for hypovolemic shock.*

7 **Nursing Safety Priority: Action Alert!**
Use only normal saline for infusion with blood or blood products. *Calcium in Ringer's lactate induces clotting of the infusing blood.*

8 **Drug Therapy**
Administer drugs for shock, vasoconstrictors, inotropic agents, and/or drugs that enhance cardiac perfusion when volume loss is severe and the patient does not respond sufficiently to fluid replacement and blood products. *Increases likelihood to recover from shock by increasing venous return, improving cardiac contractility, or improving cardiac PERFUSION by dilating the coronary vessels.*

9 **Nursing Safety Priority: Drug Alert!**
Monitor the patient closely. *Drugs that dilate coronary blood vessels, such as nitroprusside, can cause systemic vasodilation and increase shock if the patient is volume depleted. Drugs that increase heart muscle contraction increase heart oxygen consumption and can cause angina or infarction.*

Concept Map by Deanne A. Blach, MSN, RN

With vasoconstriction, diastolic pressure increases but systolic pressure remains the same. As a result, the difference between the systolic and diastolic pressures *(pulse pressure)* is smaller or "narrower." Monitor blood pressure for changes from baseline levels and for changes from the previous measurement. For accuracy, use the same equipment on the same extremity. Validate an abnormal electronic BP reading with a manual BP reading.

Systolic pressure decreases as shock progresses and cardiac output decreases. A reduced systolic pressure narrows the pulse pressure even further. When shock continues and interventions are not adequate, compensation fails and both systolic and diastolic pressures decrease and blood pressure is difficult to hear. Palpation or a Doppler device may be needed to detect the systolic blood pressure.

Oxygen saturation is assessed through pulse oximetry. Pulse oximetry values between 90% and 95% occur with the nonprogressive stage of shock, and values between 75% and 80% occur with the progressive stage of shock. *Any value below 70% is considered a life-threatening emergency and may signal the refractory stage of shock.*

Respiratory changes with shock are an adaptive response to help maintain oxygenation when tissue PERFUSION is decreased. Assess the rate and depth of respiration. Respiratory rate increases during shock to ensure that oxygen intake is increased so that it can be delivered to critical tissues. When shock progresses to the stage at which lactic acidosis is present, the respiratory depth also increases.

Kidney and urinary changes occur with shock to compensate for decreased MAP by saving body water through decreased filtration and increased water reabsorption. Assess urine for volume, color, specific gravity, and the presence of blood or protein. *Decreased urine output is a sensitive indicator of early shock. Measure urine output at least every hour. In severe shock, urine output may be absent.* Of the four vital organs (heart, brain, liver, and kidney), only the kidney can tolerate hypoxia and anoxia for up to 1 hour without permanent damage. When hypoxia or anoxia persists beyond this time, patients are at risk for acute kidney injury (AKI) and kidney failure.

Skin changes occur because of reduced blood flow in the skin. An early compensatory mechanism is skin blood vessel constriction, which reduces skin PERFUSION. This allows more blood to perfuse the vital organs, which cannot tolerate low oxygen levels.

Assess the skin for temperature, color, and moisture. With shock, it feels cool or cold to the touch and is moist. Color changes appear first in oral mucous membranes and in the skin around the mouth. In dark-skinned patients, pallor or cyanosis is best assessed in the oral mucous membranes. Other color changes are noted first in the skin of the extremities and then in the central trunk area. The skin feels clammy or moist to the touch, not because sweating increases but because the normal fluid lost through the skin does not evaporate well on cool skin. As shock progresses, skin becomes mottled. Lighter-skinned patients have an overall grayish blue color and darker-skinned patients appear darker, without an underlying reddish glow.

Evaluate capillary refill time by pressing on the patient's fingernail until it blanches and then observing how fast the nail bed resumes color when pressure is released. Normally these capillaries resume color as soon as pressure is released. With shock, capillary refill is slow or may be absent. Capillary refill is not a reliable indicator for peripheral blood flow in older patients or those with anemia, diabetes, or peripheral vascular disease.

Central nervous system (CNS) changes with shock first manifest as thirst. Thirst is caused by stimulation of the thirst centers in the brain in response to decreased blood volume.

Assess the patient's level of consciousness (LOC) and orientation. CNS changes with shock are caused by cerebral hypoxia. In the initial and nonprogressive stages, patients may be restless or agitated and may be anxious or have a feeling of impending doom that has no obvious cause. As hypoxia progresses, confusion and lethargy occur. Lethargy progresses to somnolence and loss of consciousness as cerebral hypoxia worsens with shock progression.

Skeletal muscle changes during shock include weakness and pain in response to tissue hypoxia and anaerobic metabolism, which are later manifestations. Weakness is generalized and has no specific pattern. Deep tendon reflexes are decreased or absent.

Assess muscle strength by having the patient squeeze your hand and by trying to keep his or her arms flexed while you attempt to straighten them. Assess deep tendon reflexes by lightly tapping the patellar tendons and Achilles tendons with a reflex hammer and observing the degree of responsive movement.

Psychosocial Assessment. *Changes in mental status and behavior occur early in shock.* Observe the patient closely, and document behavior. Assess mental status by evaluating LOC and noting whether the patient is asleep or awake. If the patient is asleep, attempt to awaken him or her and document how easily he or she is aroused. If the patient is awake, determine whether he or she is oriented to person, place, and time. Avoid asking questions that can be answered with a "yes" or a "no" response. Consider these points during assessment:

- Is it necessary to repeat questions to obtain a response?
- Does the response answer the question asked?
- Does the patient have difficulty making word choices?
- Is the patient irritated or upset by the questions?
- Can the patient concentrate on a question long enough to answer, or is the attention span limited?

Talk with the family to determine whether the patient's behavior and cognition are typical or represent a change.

❓ NCLEX EXAMINATION CHALLENGE
Physiological Integrity

Which manifestations of shock are a result of compensatory mechanisms to maintain circulating blood volume?
A. Edema and weight gain
B. Confusion and lethargy
C. Decreased urine output and thirst
D. Increased pulse and respiratory rates

Laboratory Assessment. Although no single test confirms or rules out shock, changes in laboratory data may support the diagnosis. Chart 37-2 lists laboratory changes occurring with hypovolemic shock. As shock progresses, arterial blood gas values become abnormal. The pH decreases, the partial pressure of arterial oxygen (Pao_2) decreases, and the partial pressure of arterial carbon dioxide ($Paco_2$) increases. Other laboratory changes occur with specific causes of hypovolemic shock.

Hematocrit and hemoglobin levels decrease if shock is caused by poor CLOTTING and hemorrhage. When shock is

CHART 37-2   Laboratory Profile

Hypovolemic Shock

TEST	NORMAL RANGE FOR ADULTS	SIGNIFICANCE OF ABNORMAL FINDINGS
pH (arterial)	7.35-7.45	Decreased: insufficient tissue oxygenation causing anaerobic metabolism and acidosis
PaO_2	80-100 mm Hg	Decreased: anaerobic metabolism
$PaCO_2$	35-45 mm Hg	Increased: anaerobic metabolism
Lactic acid (arterial)	3-7 mg/dL 0.3-0.8 mmol/L	Increased: anaerobic metabolism with buildup of metabolites
Hematocrit	*Females:* 37%-47% *Males:* 42%-52%	Increased: fluid shift, dehydration Decreased: hemorrhage
Hemoglobin	*Females:* 12-16 g/dL *Males:* 14-18 g/dL	Increased: fluid shift, dehydration Decreased: hemorrhage
Potassium	3.5-5.0 mEq/L or mmol/L	Increased: dehydration, acidosis

Pagana, K., & Pagana, T. (2014). *Mosby's manual of diagnostic and laboratory tests* (5th ed.). St. Louis: Mosby.
$PaCO_2$, Partial pressure of arterial carbon dioxide; PaO_2, partial pressure of arterial oxygen.

caused by dehydration or a fluid shift, hematocrit and hemoglobin levels are elevated.

◆ Analysis

The priority NANDA-I nursing diagnoses and collaborative problems for patients with hypovolemic shock include:

- Hypoxia related to hypovolemia
- Inadequate perfusion related to active fluid volume loss and hypotension
- Anxiety related to potential for death and decreased cerebral perfusion (NANDA-I)
- Acute Confusion related to decreased cerebral perfusion (NANDA-I)

❓ CLINICAL JUDGMENT CHALLENGE

Patient-Centered Care; Evidence-Based Practice; Safety QSEN

Your patient is a 40-year-old woman who is returned to your ambulatory care unit after having a cholecystectomy (gall bladder removal) performed as minimally invasive surgery by laparoscopy. After moving her from the stretcher to her bed, you take her vital signs. Her pulse is 118 and thready, blood pressure is 88/72, respiratory rate is 28, and pulse oxymetry is 88%. When you call her name, she opens her eyes but does not answer any questions.
1. What should you do first?
2. What manifestations of shock are present based on the information you currently have?
3. How would you classify this stage of shock? Provide a rationale for your evaluation.
4. What other assessment data should you obtain?
5. Given the type of surgery she has undergone, where would you expect bleeding to occur and what manifestations would indicate possible bleeding?
6. She still has an IV in her left hand infusing dextrose 5% in 0.45% saline. The post-surgical orders indicate that it should be removed when she is stable. Should you remove it now? Why or why not?

CHART 37-3   Best Practice for Patient Safety & Quality Care QSEN

The Patient in Hypovolemic Shock

- Ensure a patent airway.
- Insert an IV catheter, or maintain an established catheter.
- Administer oxygen.
- Elevate the patient's feet, keeping his or her head flat or elevated to no more than a 30-degree angle.
- Examine the patient for overt bleeding.
- If overt bleeding is present, apply direct pressure to the site.
- Administer drugs as prescribed.
- Increase the rate of IV fluid delivery.
- Do not leave the patient.

◆ Interventions

Medical and nursing interventions for patients in hypovolemic shock focus on reversing the shock, restoring fluid volume to the normal range, and preventing complications. Monitoring is critical to determine whether the patient is responding to therapy or whether shock is progressing and a change in intervention is needed. Surgery may be needed to correct the cause of shock. Chart 37-3 lists best practices for patients in hypovolemic shock.

Nonsurgical Management. The purposes of shock management are to maintain tissue oxygenation, increase vascular volume, and support compensatory mechanisms. Oxygen therapy, fluid replacement therapy, and drug therapy are useful.

Oxygen therapy is used at any stage of shock and is delivered by mask, hood, nasal cannula, endotracheal tube, or tracheostomy tube. It is given in liters per minute (L/min) by cannula or percentage concentration with a mask.

IV therapy for fluid resuscitation is a primary intervention for hypovolemic shock. Crystalloids and colloids are often used for volume replacement. Crystalloid solutions contain nonprotein substances (e.g., minerals, salts, sugars). Colloid solutions contain large molecules of proteins or starches (see Chapter 11).

Crystalloid fluids help maintain an adequate fluid and electrolyte balance. Two common solutions are normal saline and Ringer's lactate. Normal saline (0.9% sodium chloride in water) is a replacement solution used to increase plasma volume and can be infused with any blood product. Ringer's lactate contains sodium, chloride, calcium, potassium, and lactate. This isotonic solution expands volume, and the lactate buffers acidosis.

⚠ NURSING SAFETY PRIORITY QSEN

Action Alert

Use only normal saline for infusion with blood or blood products because the calcium in Ringer's lactate induces clotting of the infusing blood.

Protein-containing colloid fluids help restore osmotic pressure and fluid volume. Blood and blood products are used when shock is caused by blood loss. These fluids include whole blood, packed red blood cells, and plasma.

Whole blood and packed red blood cells (PRBCs) increase hematocrit and hemoglobin levels along with fluid volume. PRBCs are given for moderate blood loss because they restore

CHART 37-4 Common Examples of Drug Therapy
Hypovolemic Shock

DRUGS	NURSING INTERVENTIONS	RATIONALES
Vasoconstrictors	**Improve mean arterial pressure by increasing peripheral resistance, increasing venous return, and increasing myocardial contractility.**	
Dopamine (Intropin, Revimine ♣)	Assess patient for chest pain.	Drugs increase myocardial oxygen consumption.
Norepinephrine (Levophed)	Monitor urine output hourly.	Higher doses decrease kidney perfusion and urine output.
Phenylephrine HCl	Assess blood pressure every 15 min.	Hypertension is a manifestation of overdose.
	Assess the patient for headache.	Headache is an early manifestation of drug excess.
	Assess every 30 min for extravasation; check extremities for color and perfusion.	If the drug gets into the tissues, it can cause severe vasoconstriction, tissue ischemia, and tissue necrosis.
	Assess for chest pain.	Drug can cause rapid onset of vasoconstriction in the myocardium and impair cardiac oxygenation.
Inotropic Agents	**Directly stimulate beta adrenergic receptors on the heart muscle, improving contractility**	
Dobutamine (Dobutrex)	Assess for chest pain.	Drugs increase myocardial oxygen consumption and can cause angina or infarction.
Milrinone (Primacor)	Assess blood pressure every 15 min.	Hypertension is a manifestation of overdose.
Agents Enhancing Myocardial Perfusion	**Improve myocardial perfusion by dilating coronary arteries rapidly for a short time.**	
Sodium nitroprusside (Nitropress, Nipride ♣)	Protect drug container from light.	Light degrades drug quickly.
	Assess blood pressure at least every 15 min.	Drug can cause systemic vasodilation and hypotension, especially in older adults.

the red blood cell deficit and improve oxygen-carrying capacity without adding excessive fluid volume. Massive transfusion therapy, defined as 10 units of PRBCs given within the first 6 hours of severe hemorrhage, can improve outcomes and prevent death from acute traumatic coagulopathy (Day et al., 2013). See Chapter 40 for nursing care during transfusion therapy.

Plasma, an acellular blood product containing clotting factors, is given to restore osmotic pressure when hematocrit and hemoglobin levels are normal. Plasma protein fractions (e.g., Plasmanate) and synthetic plasma expanders (e.g., hetastarch [hydroxyethyl starch, Hespan]) increase volume and are used for hypovolemic shock before a cause is identified.

Drug therapy is used in addition to fluid therapy when the volume lost is severe and the patient does not respond sufficiently to fluid replacement and blood products. Drugs for shock increase venous return, improve cardiac contractility, or improve cardiac PERFUSION by dilating the coronary vessels. Chart 37-4 lists common drugs used to treat shock.

> **! NURSING SAFETY PRIORITY** (QSEN)
> **Drug Alert**
>
> Monitor the patient closely because drugs that dilate coronary blood vessels, such as nitroprusside, can cause systemic vasodilation and increase shock if the patient is volume depleted. Drugs that increase heart muscle contraction increase heart oxygen consumption and can cause angina or infarction.

Monitoring vital signs and level of consciousness is a major nursing action to determine the patient's condition and the effectiveness of therapy. Monitor these vital signs:
- Pulse (rate, regularity, and quality)
- Blood pressure
- Pulse pressure
- Central venous pressure (CVP)
- Respiratory rate

- Skin and mucosal color
- Oxygen saturation
- Cognition
- Urine output

Assess these parameters at least every 15 minutes until the shock is controlled and the patient's condition improves. Hemodynamic monitoring in critical care settings includes intra-arterial monitoring, mixed venous oxygen saturation (Svo_2), pulmonary artery monitoring, and pulmonary capillary wedge pressures.

Insertion of a CVP catheter allows pressure to be monitored in the patient's right atrium or superior vena cava while providing venous access. A decrease in CVP from baseline levels reflects hypovolemic shock with reduced venous return to the right atrium.

Intra-arterial catheters allow continuous blood pressure monitoring and are an access for arterial blood sampling. They are inserted into an artery (radial, brachial, femoral, or dorsalis pedis). The catheter is attached to pressure tubing and a transducer, which converts arterial pressure into an electrical signal seen as a waveform on an oscilloscope and as a numeric value.

Surgical Management. Surgical intervention in addition to nonsurgical management may be needed to correct the cause of shock. Such procedures include vascular repair, surgical hemostasis of major wounds, closure of bleeding ulcers, and chemical scarring (chemosclerosis) of varicosities.

Community-Based Care
Hypovolemic shock is a complication of another condition and is resolved before patients are discharged from the acute care setting. Because surgery and many other invasive procedures now occur on an ambulatory care basis, more patients at home are at increased risk for hypovolemic shock. Teach patients and family members the early manifestations of shock (increased thirst, decreased urine output, light-headedness, sense of apprehension) and to seek immediate medical attention if they appear.

SEPSIS AND SEPTIC SHOCK

❖ PATHOPHYSIOLOGY

Sepsis leading to septic shock is a complex type of distributive shock that usually begins as a bacterial or fungal infection and progresses to a critical emergency over a period of days. The progression of sepsis to septic shock is outlined in Fig. 37-3. *As progression occurs, the pathologic problems occur faster and to a greater degree. Thus control of sepsis and prevention of severe sepsis and septic shock are easier to achieve early in the process. Failure to recognize and intervene in early sepsis is a major factor for progression to septic shock and death.*

Infection

When INFECTION is confined to a local area, it should not lead to sepsis and shock. In the person whose immune system and inflammatory responses are effective, the presence of organism invasion first starts a helpful, local response of INFLAMMATION to confine and eliminate the organism and to prevent the infection from becoming worse or widespread.

The white blood cells (WBCs) in the area of invasion secrete cytokines to trigger local inflammation and bring more WBCs to kill the invading organisms. The results of this response constrict the small veins and dilate the arterioles in the area, which increases PERFUSION to locally infected tissues.

Capillary leak occurs, allowing plasma to leak into the tissues. This response causes swelling. The duration of INFLAMMATION depends on the size and severity of the INFECTION, but usually it subsides within a few days, when the infection has been managed by these responses. A benefit of inflammation is that it is limited only to the area of infection and stops as soon as it is no longer needed. The patient does not have fever, tachycardia, decreased oxygen saturation, or reduced urine output.

Sepsis and Systemic Inflammatory Response Syndrome

Sepsis is the presence of infection systemic manifestations (Dellinger et al., 2013). Infectious organisms have entered the bloodstream. As their numbers increase, widespread INFLAMMATION, known as *systemic inflammatory response syndrome (SIRS)*, is triggered as a result of INFECTION escaping local control. With the organisms and their toxins in the bloodstream and entering other body areas, inflammation is an enemy, leading to extensive hormonal, tissue, and vascular changes and oxidative stress that further impair oxygenation and tissue PERFUSION. The WBCs produce many pro-inflammation cytokines, especially interleukin-1 (IL-1), interleukin-6 (IL-6), and tumor necrosis factor-alpha (TNF-A or TNF-α) (Abbas et al., 2012). (See Chapter 17 for a discussion of cytokines.) As a result, there is widespread vasodilation and blood pooling (Schell-Chaple &

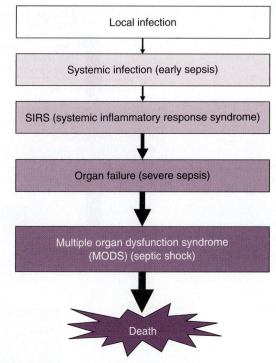

FIG. 37-3 Common progression of events leading to septic shock and multiple organ dysfunction syndrome (MODS).

Lee, 2014). The patient has mild hypotension, a low urine output, and an increased respiratory rate. These responses result in a hypodynamic state with decreased cardiac output. Body temperature varies depending on the duration of the sepsis and on WBC function. Some patients have a low-grade fever and others have a high fever. Still others may have a below-normal body temperature. Fever and hypotension result from SIRS. The reduced urine output and increased respiratory rate are compensatory responses to impaired oxygenation and perfusion. Often the patient has the elevated WBC count expected with a systemic infection.

Inappropriate CLOTTING with microthrombi forming in some organ capillaries causes hypoxia and reduces organ function. This problem is hard to detect, but if sepsis is stopped at this point, the organ damage is completely reversible. The microthrombi increase hypoxic conditions, which then generate more toxic metabolites. These damage more cells and increase the production of pro-inflammatory cytokines, leading to an amplification of SIRS and a vicious repeating cycle of poor oxygenation and PERFUSION (Fig. 37-4). Although these manifestations are subtle, they indicate sepsis and SIRS and will progress unless intervention begins now.

Unfortunately, this early hypodynamic state has a relatively short duration and manifestations are so subtle that the condition is often missed or misdiagnosed. When early sepsis and SIRS are identified and treated aggressively at this stage, the cycle of progression is stopped and the outcome is good. When sepsis and SIRS are not identified and treated at this stage, it progresses to severe sepsis, which is much harder to control. Nurses, as well as all other health care professionals, have a responsibility to identify cues that indicate sepsis before it becomes severe (Kleinpell et al., 2013). Identifying criteria have been established (Table 37-3) and must be used to ensure interventions are instituted at this stage.

FIG. 37-4 Vicious cycle of systemic inflammatory response syndrome (SIRS) and multiple organ dysfunction syndrome (MODS) in septic shock.

TABLE 37-3 Sepsis with Systemic Inflammatory Response Syndrome (SIRS) Criteria

Suspected or identified infection with some of the following:

- Temperature of more than 101°F (38.3°C) or less than 96.8°F (36°C)
- Heart rate of more than 90 beats per minute
- Respiratory rate of more than 20 breaths per minute
- Abnormal WBC count (>12,000/mm³ or <4000/mm³)
- Normal WBC count with >10% bands
- Plasma C-reactive protein >2 standard deviations above normal
- Plasma prolactin >2 standard deviations above normal
- Arterial hypotension (SBP <90 mm Hg; MAP <70 mm Hg)
- Arterial hypoxemia (PaO₂/FiO₂ <300)
- Urine output <0.5 mL/kg/hr for 2 hours despite adequate fluid resuscitation
- Creatinine increase >0.5 mg/dL
- INR >1.5 or aPTT >60
- Absent bowel sounds
- Platelet count <100,000/mm³
- Total bilirubin >4 mg/dL
- Elevated lactic acid (lactate) levels
- Decreased capillary refill or presence of mottling
- Hyperglycemia (plasma glucose >140 mg/dL or 7.7 mmol/L) in absence of diabetes
- Unexplained change in mental status
- Significant edema or positive fluid balance

Adapted from Dellinger, R.P., Levy, M., Rhodes, A., Annane, D., Gerlach, H., Opal, S.M., et al. (2013). Surviving sepsis campaign: International guidelines for management of severe sepsis and septic shock: 2012. *Critical Care Medicine, 41*(2), 580-637.

aPTT, Activated partial thromboplastin time; *FiO₂,* fraction of inspired oxygen; *INR,* international normalized ratio; *MAP,* mean arterial pressure; *PaO₂,* partial pressure of arterial oxygen; *SBP,* systolic blood pressure; *WBC,* white blood cell.

! NURSING SAFETY PRIORITY (QSEN)
Critical Rescue

Notify the health care provider or the Rapid Response Team for any patient who has vital signs or other conditions that meet the sepsis with SIRS criteria.

Severe Sepsis

Severe sepsis is sepsis plus sepsis-induced organ dysfunction or tissue hypoperfusion (Dellinger et al., 2013). It represents the progression of sepsis with an amplified SIRS (see Fig. 37-4). All tissues are involved and are hypoxic to some degree. Some organs are experiencing cell death and dysfunction at this time. Microthrombi formation is widespread with clots forming where they are not needed. This process uses up or consumes much of the available platelets and clotting factors, a condition known as *disseminated intravascular coagulation (DIC).* The amplified SIRS and cytokine release increase capillary leakiness, injure cells, and increase cell metabolism. Damage to endothelial cells reduces anticlotting actions and triggers the formation of even more small clots, increasing DIC. Anaerobic metabolism continues, and cell uptake of oxygen is poor. The continued stress response triggers the continued release of glucose from the liver and causes hyperglycemia. The more severe the response, the higher the blood glucose level (Kleinpell et al., 2013; Schell-Chaple & Lee, 2014).

Despite the severity of this stage and the fact that it may be present for 24 hours or more, it is often missed. One of the reasons it may be missed is that the cardiac function is hyperdynamic in this phase. The pooling of blood and the widespread capillary leak stimulate the heart, and cardiac output is *increased* with a more rapid heart rate and an elevated systolic blood pressure. In addition, the patient's extremities may feel warm and there is little or no cyanosis. Even though the patient may "look" better, the pathologic changes occurring at the tissue level are serious and have caused significant damage. The WBC count at this time may no longer be elevated. The reason for this is that a prolonged sepsis stage may have exceeded the bone marrow's ability to keep producing and releasing new mature neutrophils and other WBCs. The WBC count may be extremely low, especially the segmented neutrophils (segs).

Clinical manifestations of this stage include a lower oxygen saturation, rapid respiratory rate, decreased to absent urine output, and a change in the patient's cognition and affect. Appropriate and aggressive interventions at this stage can still prevent septic shock, although mortality after a patient reaches this stage is much higher than for sepsis and SIRS. *At this point, the down-hill course leading to septic shock is extremely rapid.*

Septic Shock

Septic shock is sepsis-induced hypotension persisting despite adequate fluid resuscitation. It is the stage of sepsis and SIRS when multiple organ dysfunction syndrome (MODS) with organ failure is evident and poor CLOTTING with uncontrolled bleeding occurs (see Fig. 37-4). *Even with appropriate intervention, the death rate among patients in this stage of sepsis is very high* (Dellinger et al., 2013). Severe hypovolemic shock and hypodynamic cardiac function are present as a result of an inability of the blood to clot because the platelets and clotting factors were consumed earlier. Vasodilation and capillary leak continue from vascular endothelial cell disruption, and cardiac contractility is poor from cellular ischemia. The clinical manifestations resemble the late stage of hypovolemic shock.

Etiology

The major cause of sepsis is a bacterial infection that escapes local control, although in immunocompromised patients, fungal infections also cause sepsis. Common organisms causing sepsis include gram-negative bacteria (*Pseudomonas aeruginosa, Escherichia coli,* and *Klebsiella pneumoniae*) and gram-positive bacteria (*Staphylococcus* and *Streptococcus*). Patients especially at risk for sepsis are those who are immunocompromised in any way and those who have central lines. Central lines in place even for short periods create a direct access point for microorganisms and can lead to central line–associated bloodstream infections (CLABSIs) (Dumont & Nesselrodt, 2012; Earhart, 2013). Table 37-4 lists some of the health problems that increase the risk for sepsis and septic shock.

TABLE 37-4 Conditions Predisposing to Sepsis and Septic Shock

• Malnutrition	• Infection with resistant
• Immunosuppression	microorganisms
• Large, open wounds	• Receiving cancer
• Mucous membrane fissures in	chemotherapy
prolonged contact with bloody	• Alcoholism
or drainage-soaked packing	• Diabetes mellitus
• GI ischemia	• Chronic kidney disease
• Exposure to invasive procedures	• Transplantation recipient
• Cancer	• Hepatitis
• Older than 80 years	• HIV/AIDS

AIDS, Acquired immune deficiency syndrome; *HIV,* human immune deficiency virus.

Incidence and Prevalence

Sepsis and septic shock are common events in the United States and throughout the world (Dellinger et al., 2013). Although sepsis management has improved, the incidence is increasing as a result of more drug-resistant organisms and the fact that patients are discharged from the hospital "quicker and sicker" (Lopez-Bushnell et al., 2014). Sepsis takes time to develop, and the patient may be discharged before manifestations are obvious.

Health Promotion and Maintenance

Prevention is the best management strategy for sepsis and septic shock. Evaluate all patients for their risk for sepsis, especially older adults because the death rate from sepsis in people older than 65 years is nearly twice that of younger adults. Table 37-4 lists some of the health problems that increase the risk for septic shock. Use aseptic technique during invasive procedures and when working with nonintact skin and mucous membranes in immunocompromised patients. Remove indwelling urinary catheters and IV access lines as soon as they are no longer needed. Ensure that patients receiving mechanical ventilation are weaned from the ventilator as soon as possible (Kleinpell et al., 2013).

Because sepsis can be a complication of many conditions found in acute care settings, always consider its possibility.

QUALITY IMPROVEMENT QSEN

Improving Nurse Recognition of Sepsis Indicators in the Emergency Department

Kilburn, F., Baily, P., & Price, D. (2013). Sepsis: Recognizing the next event. *Nursing2013, 43*(10), 14-16.

After prevention, the greatest positive factor for surviving sepsis is early recognition of the condition, which leads to implementation of the evidence-based interventions through early goal-directed therapy (EGDT). Recognition of the condition while patients are being seen in the emergency department (ED) can be challenging; however, delay of diagnosis significantly increases the risk for death (Dellenger et al., 2013). One rural Midwestern emergency department found that of the 42 patients admitted through the ED who were diagnosed after admission with sepsis or systemic inflammatory response syndrome (SIRS), 21 had two or more defining criteria while in the ED. Of these 21, only 3 were actually recognized and diagnosed in the ED. The Quality Management department determined that the greatest obstacle to early recognition of SIRS or sepsis was the seven-page assessment document that, although comprehensive, was time-consuming and minimally used by the ED nurses.

The stakeholders in the process developed a shorter, clearer, and more user-friendly SIRS and sepsis protocol consisting of a recognition and treatment order set based on the 2012 sepsis guidelines. In the first 3 months after developing this tool and incorporating it into the triage nurse admission data set, there was a 37% increase in the recognition of patients meeting SIRS and sepsis criteria in the ED.

Commentary: Implications for Practice and Research

Evidence-based practice has demonstrated that early recognition of patients with SIRS or sepsis is the first step in improving survival from this devastating condition. The implementation of a more user-friendly protocol in one ED has improved the step of recognition at one facility. Research measuring the final survival and cost outcomes based on speed of implementing EGDT is needed to determine how well early recognition is turned into early intervention through communication and teamwork.

Early detection of sepsis before progression to septic shock is a major nursing responsibility. The nurse is the health care professional most in contact with the patient and is in a unique position to detect subtle changes in appearance and behavior that can indicate sepsis. Use the assessment techniques described below for changes in vital signs, laboratory findings, appearance, and behavior to identify early any characteristics of sepsis and sepsis progression at least every shift for potentially infected, seriously ill patients (Kleinpell & Schorr, 2014). Using an evidence-based protocol to identify patients in the emergency department who may be in early sepsis on admission can improve the timing of implementing an appropriate sepsis bundle intervention (see the Quality Improvement box).

Early detection can be made by patients and families, as well as by health care personnel. This is especially important for patients discharged to home after invasive procedures or surgery. Teach patients the manifestations of local infection (local redness, pain, swelling, purulent drainage, loss of function) and of early sepsis (fever, urine output less than intake, lightheadedness). Teach them how to use a thermometer and to take the temperature twice a day and whenever they are not feeling well. Urge those with manifestations of early sepsis to immediately contact their health care provider. Teach them that if antibiotics are prescribed, to take these drugs as prescribed and to complete the entire course.

❖ PATIENT-CENTERED COLLABORATIVE CARE

◆ Assessment

Sepsis and septic shock differ from other types of shock in many ways. The entire syndrome may occur over many hours to days, and the manifestations are less obvious. The chance for recovery is good when the patient is recognized as having sepsis with SIRS and appropriate interventions are started within 6 hours. Septic shock, on the other hand, has a rapid downhill course and chances for recovery are relatively poor. Nurses identifying patients in the earlier stages of sepsis can make the greatest difference in survival.

History. Age is important because sepsis develops more easily among older, debilitated patients who are immunosuppressed (Touhy & Jett, 2014). Chart 37-5 lists factors that increase the older adult's risk for shock. Ask about the patient's medical

history including recent illness, trauma, invasive procedures, or chronic conditions that may lead to sepsis. Check which drugs the patient has used in the past week. Some drugs may directly cause changes leading to shock. Also, a drug regimen may indicate a disorder or problem that can contribute to sepsis. These drugs include aspirin, corticosteroids, antibiotics, and cancer therapy drugs.

Physical Assessment/Clinical Manifestations. Manifestations of sepsis and septic shock occur over many hours, and some change during the progression. See Table 37-3 for a listing of specific manifestations and laboratory changes that often occur with sepsis and septic shock.

Cardiovascular changes differ in the different stages of sepsis and septic shock. Cardiac output and blood pressure are low in early sepsis and very low in septic shock. In severe sepsis, cardiac output is higher as are heart rate and blood pressure, although this is an indication of a worsening condition rather than an improvement. Increased cardiac output is reflected by tachycardia, increased stroke volume, a normal systolic blood pressure, and a normal central venous pressure (CVP). Increased cardiac output and vasodilation make the skin color appear normal with pink mucous membranes, and the skin is warm to the touch. This situation is temporary, and eventually the cardiac output is greatly reduced.

With progression, disseminated intravascular coagulation (DIC) occurs as a result of excessive CLOTTING with formation of thousands of small clots in the tiny capillaries of the liver, kidney, brain, spleen, and heart. DIC reduces PERFUSION and oxygenation and decreases oxygen saturation, causing hypoxia and ischemia.

The huge number of small clots uses clotting factors and fibrinogen faster than they can be produced, which eventually leads to poor CLOTTING. This increases the risk for hemorrhage, which occurs in the septic shock stage. Coupled with the continued capillary leak, the bleeding causes hypovolemia and a dramatic decrease in cardiac output, blood pressure, and pulse pressure. The manifestations of this phase are the same as those of the later stages of hypovolemic shock.

Respiratory changes are first caused by compensatory mechanisms that try to maintain oxygenation with a rate increase. As tissue hypoxia becomes more profound and acidosis is present, the depth of respiration also increases. The lungs are susceptible to damage, and the complication of acute respiratory distress syndrome (ARDS) may occur in septic shock. ARDS in septic shock is caused by the continued systemic inflammatory response syndrome (SIRS) increasing the formation of oxygen free radicals, which damage lung cells. *ARDS in a patient with septic shock has a high mortality rate.*

Skin changes differ at different stages of sepsis. In the hyperdynamic stage, the skin is warm and no cyanosis is evident. With progression to septic shock and compromised circulation, the skin is cool and clammy with pallor, mottling, or cyanosis. In DIC, petechiae and ecchymoses can occur anywhere. Blood may ooze from the gums, other mucous membranes, and venipuncture sites, as well as around IV catheters.

A kidney/urinary change of low urine output compared with fluid intake indicates shock. When a patient who has no known kidney or bladder problem suddenly starts having a low urine output, be suspicious of severe sepsis or septic shock. Reduced output is caused by capillary leak, low circulating volume, and hormonal changes. Kidney function decreases, and serum creatinine levels increase.

CHART 37-5   Nursing Focus on the Older Adult

Risk Factors for Shock

Hypovolemic Shock
- Diuretic therapy
- Diminished thirst reflex
- Immobility
- Use of aspirin-containing products
- Use of complementary therapies such as *Ginkgo biloba*
- Anticoagulant therapy

Cardiogenic Shock
- Diabetes mellitus
- Presence of cardiomyopathies

Distributive Shock
- Diminished immune response
- Reduced skin integrity
- Presence of cancer
- Peripheral neuropathy
- Strokes
- Being in a hospital or extended-care facility
- Malnutrition
- Anemia

Obstructive Shock
- Pulmonary hypertension
- Presence of cancer

Psychosocial Assessment. The indicator that patients may be in the beginning of severe sepsis is often a change in affect or behavior. Compare the patient's current behavior, verbal responses, and general affect with those assessed earlier in the day or the day before. They may seem just slightly different in their reactions to greetings, comments, or jokes. They may be less patient than usual or act restless or fidgety. Patients may make statements such as "I feel as if something is wrong, but I don't know what." If behavior is changed from prior assessments, consider the possibility of severe sepsis and shock.

Laboratory Assessment. No single laboratory test confirms the presence of sepsis and septic shock, although the hallmark of sepsis is an increasing serum lactate level, a normal or low total white blood cell (WBC) count, and a decreasing segmented neutrophil level with a rising band neutrophil level (left shift, see Chapter 17). The presence of bacteria in the blood supports the diagnosis of sepsis although this finding may not be present. Obtain specimens of urine, blood, sputum, and any drainage for culture to identify the causative organisms. Blood cultures should be taken before antibiotic therapy is started provided that this action does not delay antibiotic therapy by more than 45 minutes (Dellinger et al., 2013). Other abnormal laboratory findings that occur with septic shock include changes in the white blood cell (WBC) count; the differential leukocyte count may show a left shift. Hematocrit and hemoglobin levels usually do not change until late in septic shock. At that point, the hematocrit and hemoglobin levels, fibrinogen levels, and platelet count are low from disseminated intravascular coagulation (DIC). The serum lactate level is above normal, and the serum bicarbonate levels are lower than normal. Unfortunately, these parameters may take time to change and cannot be relied on as sensitive indicators of the patient's worsening condition.

Another indicator of sepsis and septic shock is a low blood level of activated protein C. Protein C is an enzyme that prevents inappropriate clot formation. It is activated when it binds to healthy vascular endothelial cells. In severe sepsis, the injured endothelial cells cannot activate protein C and thousands of small clots form in the capillaries of vascular organs. Decreasing levels of activated protein C indicate the beginning of severe sepsis even before other manifestations are evident.

Other biologic indicators of severe sepsis and septic shock are changes in plasma D-dimer levels and cytokine (interleukin-6 [IL-6] and interleukin-10 [IL-10]) levels. Plasma D-dimer levels rise during sepsis as the fibrin in clots is broken down. IL-6 is a pro-inflammatory cytokine, and IL-10 is an anti-inflammatory cytokine. In sepsis, IL-6 levels rise and IL-10 levels either remain normal or decrease. These indicators have a lag time, and changes may not be present soon enough to identify sepsis with SIRS before severe sepsis or septic shock develops.

Because the results of blood cultures may not be available until the patient's condition has progressed to severe sepsis or septic shock, other biomarkers for sepsis and SIRS are needed to help identify the condition when it can be managed and cured. Two such markers are increasing lactic acid levels and increasing prolactin levels.

The actual diagnosis of sepsis is difficult to make, yet the best outcome depends on an early diagnosis and the implementation of appropriate aggressive interventions within 6 hours. In general, sepsis is considered to exist when an infection is present along with some of the additional established criteria listed in Table 37-3.

TABLE 37-5 Bundles for Resuscitation and Management of Severe Sepsis

Surviving Sepsis Care Bundle

Within the first 3 hours of suspecting severe sepsis:

1. Measure serum lactate levels.
2. Obtain blood cultures *before* administering antibiotics.
3. Administer broad-spectrum antibiotics.
4. If either hypotension or a serum lactate level greater than 4 mmol/L (36 mg/dL) is present, administer 30 mL/kg crystalloids intravenously.

Within 6 hours of initial manifestations of suspected septic shock:

5. Administer prescribed vasopressors for hypotension that does not respond to initial fluid resuscitation measures to maintain MAP ≥65 mm Hg.
6. If arterial hypotension persists despite fluid volume resuscitation (indicating septic shock) or lactic acid remains ≥4 mmol/L (36 mg/dL), institute these assessments:
   - Measure central venous pressure.
   - Measure central venous oxygen saturation.
7. Re-measure lactic acid (lactate) level if initial value was elevated.

Data from Dellinger, R.P., Levy, M., Rhodes, A., Annane, D., Gerlach, H., Opal, S.M., et al. (2013). Surviving sepsis campaign: International guidelines for management of severe sepsis and septic shock: 2012. *Critical Care Medicine, 41*(2), 580-637; Kleinpell, R., Aitken, L., & Schorr, C. (2013). Implications of the new international sepsis guidelines for nursing care. *American Journal of Critical Care, 22*(3), 212-222.
MAP, Mean arterial pressure.

❓ NCLEX EXAMINATION CHALLENGE

Safe and Effective Care Environment

Which clinical manifestation in a client alerts the nurse to the probability of septic shock instead of hypovolemic shock?

A. Hypotension
B. Pale, clammy skin
C. Decreased urine output
D. Oozing of blood at the IV site

◆ Planning and Implementation

The priority problem for patients with septic shock is potential for multiple organ dysfunction syndrome (MODS).

Planning: Expected Outcomes. With appropriate interventions, the patient with sepsis or septic shock is expected to have normal aerobic cellular metabolism. Indicators include:

- Arterial blood gases (pH, Pao_2, and $Paco_2$) within the normal range
- Maintenance of a urine output of at least 20 mL/hr
- Maintenance of mean arterial blood pressure within 10 mm Hg of baseline
- Absence of multiple organ dysfunction syndrome (MODS)

Interventions. Interventions for sepsis and septic shock focus on identifying the problem as early as possible, correcting the conditions causing it, and preventing complications. The use of a sepsis resuscitation bundle for treatment of sepsis within 6 hours is the standard of practice. A *bundle* is a group of two or more specific interventions that have been shown to be effective when applied together or in sequence. The sepsis management bundle is presented in Table 37-5. Target outcomes of implementing the bundle are obtaining and maintaining a central venous pressure of 8 mm Hg or higher, central venous oxygen saturation of at least 70%, and return of lactic acid levels to normal (Kleinpell et al., 2013).

Oxygen therapy is useful whenever poor tissue PERFUSION and poor oxygenation are present. Oxygen is delivered in the same ways as for hypovolemic shock. However, the patient with septic shock is more likely to be mechanically ventilated. Care of the patient being mechanically ventilated is discussed in detail in Chapter 32.

Drug therapy to enhance cardiac output and restore vascular volume is essentially the same as that used in hypovolemic shock (see Chart 37-4). In addition, drug therapy is needed to combat sepsis, adrenal insufficiency, hyperglycemia, and clotting problems.

Although septic shock can be caused by any organism, the most common agents are gram-negative bacteria. In accordance with the recommendations of The Joint Commission's National Patient Safety Goals (NPSGs), IV antibiotics with known activity against gram-negative bacteria are given before organisms are identified, preferably within 1 hour of a sepsis diagnosis. Multiple drugs with wide activity are prescribed, based on the site of infection and the most common geographic infections, until the actual causative organism is known.

The stress of severe sepsis can cause adrenal insufficiency. Adrenal support may involve providing the patient with low-dose corticosteroids during the treatment period. Drugs used for this purpose are IV hydrocortisone and oral fludrocortisone (Florinef).

Patients with sepsis or septic shock usually have elevated blood glucose levels (>180 mg/dL), which is associated with a poor outcome. Insulin therapy is used to maintain blood glucose levels between 110 mg/dL and 150 mg/dL. Keeping the blood glucose level below 110 mg/dL is associated with increased mortality.

During severe sepsis, patients have microvascular abnormalities and form many small clots. Heparin therapy with fractionated heparin is used to limit inappropriate CLOTTING and to prevent the excessive consumption of clotting factors.

Blood replacement therapy is used when poor CLOTTING with hemorrhage occurs and may include clotting factors, platelets, fresh frozen plasma (FFP), or packed red blood cells. Chapter 40 discusses in detail the care of the patient during blood replacement. The use of platelet transfusion is recommended ahead of other blood products for patients with septic shock to improve CLOTTING (Dellinger et al., 2013).

Community-Based Care

Identified sepsis should be resolved before patients are discharged from the acute care setting. Because more patients are receiving treatment on an ambulatory care basis and are being discharged earlier from acute care settings, more patients at home are at increased risk for sepsis.

Home Care Management. Evaluate the home environment for safety regarding infection hazards. Note the general cleanliness, especially in the kitchen and bathrooms. Chart 37-6 lists focused patient and environmental assessment data to obtain during a home visit.

Self-Management Education. Protecting frail patients from infection and sepsis at home is an important nursing function. Teach about the importance of self-care strategies, such as good hygiene, handwashing, balanced diet, rest and exercise, skin care, and mouth care. If patients or family members do not know how to take a temperature or read a thermometer, teach

---

CHART 37-6 Home Care Assessment

The Patient at Risk for Sepsis

- Assess the patient for any clinical manifestations of infection, including:
  - Temperature, pulse, respiration, and blood pressure
  - Color of skin and mucous membranes
  - The mouth and perianal area for fissures or lesions
  - Any nonintact skin area for the presence of exudates, redness, increased warmth, swelling
  - Any pain, tenderness, or other discomfort anywhere
  - Cough or any other symptoms of a cold or the flu
  - Urine; or ask patient whether urine is dark or cloudy, has an odor, or causes pain or burning during urination
- Assess patient's and caregiver's adherence to and understanding of infection prevention techniques.
- Assess home environment, including:
  - General cleanliness
  - Kitchen and bathroom facilities, including refrigeration
  - Availability and type of soap for handwashing
  - Presence of pets, especially cats, rodents, or reptiles

---

them and obtain a return demonstration. Teach patients and families to notify the health care provider immediately if fever or other signs of infection appear. General recommendations for Infection Precautions for patients at risk for sepsis are listed in Chart 22-4 in Chapter 22.

◆ Evaluation: Outcomes

Evaluate the care of the patient with sepsis or septic shock. The expected outcome is that the patient will maintain normal aerobic cellular metabolism. Specific indicators for these outcomes are listed for the priority patient problem under the *Planning and Implementation* section (see earlier).

⚲ CLINICAL JUDGMENT CHALLENGE

Patient-Centered Care; Evidence-Based Practice; Safety QSEN

The patient is a 70-year-old man undergoing chemotherapy for lymphoma who was brought to the hospital by his wife because he was confused. His vital signs are: T = 95.7° F (35.4°C); P = 112; R = 28; BP = 96/50; SpO$_2$ = 84%. His health history includes type 2 diabetes, a myocardial infarction 10 years ago (he now has an "on-demand" pacemaker), and hypertension. In addition to chemotherapy, his current oral medications include metformin (Glucophage) 850 mg twice daily, losartan (Cozaar) 50 mg daily, and aspirin 81 mg daily. When you ask whether there have been any changes lately, the wife tells you that he had a "touch" of fungal pneumonia 6 weeks ago and still has a cough with sputum. He has been very uncomfortable for the past week with a "boil" near his rectum. When you assess his perianal region, you find a large raised red bump with an open area draining purulent fluid.

1. What risk factors does this man have for sepsis? Explain why each factor increases his risk.
2. What stage of the sepsis spectrum is he at this time and why?
3. Should you apply oxygen to him before he is seen by the health care provider? Why or why not?

The health care provider evaluates the patient and orders: IV with dextrose 5% in normal saline; IV amikacin (Amikin); cultures of the urine, blood, sputum, his central line, and any open skin areas; complete blood count with differential; and blood values for glucose and lactic acid.

4. Which intervention do you perform first and why?
5. What do you do next and why?

NURSING CONCEPTS AND CLINICAL JUDGMENT REVIEW

What might you NOTICE if the patient is experiencing inadequate oxygenation and tissue PERFUSION as a result of hypovolemic shock?

- Pulse rapid and thready
- Pulse pressure narrowed
- Respirations rapid and shallow
- Oxygen saturation by pulse oximetry decreased
- Skin cyanosis or pallor (for lighter-skinned patients)
- Skin cool and clammy
- Cyanosis or pallor of the lips and oral mucous membranes (for patients of any skin color)
- Patient is restless or anxious
- Patient has a urine output that is less than expected compared with fluid intake
- Patient states he or she is thirsty

What should you INTERPRET and how should you RESPOND to a patient experiencing inadequate oxygenation and tissue PERFUSION as a result of hypovolemic shock?

Perform and interpret physical assessment, including:
- Taking vital signs
- Auscultating all lung fields
- Monitoring oxygen saturation by pulse oximetry
- Assessing cognition
- Checking incisions, body orifices, and under the patient for signs of active bleeding
- Assessing the skin for bruises and petechiae

- Examining all body areas for swelling or discoloration that could indicate internal bleeding

Interpret laboratory values:
- Arterial blood gas values: pH lower than 7.35
- Elevated serum lactate levels
- Hemorrhage
  Decreased hematocrit and hemoglobin
  Decreased total red blood cells and platelets
- Dehydration
  Elevated red blood cell count, hematocrit, and hemoglobin
  Elevated white blood cell count

Respond by:
- Applying oxygen
- Assisting the patient to shock position (head and chest flat or elevated to no more than 30 degrees; legs elevated)
- Notifying the Rapid Response Team
- Ensuring placement of venous access
- Increasing IV fluid infusion rate

On what should you REFLECT?
- Observe patient for evidence of improved circulation and oxygenation (see Chapter 33).
- Think about what may have caused the hypovolemia.
- Think about how you may have identified the problem sooner.

GET READY FOR THE NCLEX® EXAMINATION!

KEY POINTS

Review these Key Points for each NCLEX Examination Client Needs Category.

Safe and Effective Care Environment
- Ensure vital sign measurements are accurate, and monitor them for changes indicating the presence of shock. **Safety QSEN**
- Identify patients at high risk for infection due to age, disease, or the environment. **Safety QSEN**
- Use the recommended criteria to assess for the presence of sepsis (see Table 37-3). **Evidence-Based Practice QSEN**
- Use strict aseptic techniques when performing invasive procedures, administering IV medications, changing dressings, and handling nonintact skin. **Safety QSEN**
- Use good handwashing techniques before providing any care to a patient who is either immunocompromised or immune deficient. **Safety QSEN**
- Assign a registered nurse rather than a licensed practical nurse/licensed vocational nurse (LPN/LVN) or unlicensed assistive personnel (UAP) to assess the vital signs of a patient who is at risk for or suspected of having hypovolemic shock. **Safety QSEN**
- Use only normal saline for infusion with blood or blood products.

Health Promotion and Maintenance
- Teach all people how to avoid dehydration. **Patient-Centered Care QSEN**
- Teach all people to use safety devices to avoid trauma. **Patient-Centered Care QSEN**
- Instruct all patients going home after surgery or invasive procedures to seek immediate attention for persistent manifestations of early shock. **Patient-Centered Care QSEN**
- Teach all patients who have a local infection to seek medical attention when manifestations of systemic infection appear. **Patient-Centered Care QSEN**

Psychosocial Integrity
- Assess all patients at risk for shock for a change in affect, reduced cognition, altered level of consciousness, and increased anxiety. **Patient-Centered Care QSEN**
- Stay with the patient in shock. **Patient-Centered Care QSEN**
- Reassure patients who are in shock that the appropriate interventions are being instituted. **Patient-Centered Care QSEN**

Physiological Integrity
- Be aware of the role of the systemic inflammatory response syndrome (SIRS) in the manifestations and progression of sepsis and septic shock. **Safety QSEN**

- Assess the immunocompromised patient every shift for infection. **Safety** **QSEN**
- Assess the skin integrity of the patient with reduced immune function at least every shift. **Patient-Centered Care** **QSEN**
- Immediately assess vital signs of patients who have a change in level of consciousness, increased thirst, or anxiety. **Evidence-Based Practice** **QSEN**
- Assess for changes in pulse rate and quality or a decrease in urine output rather than blood pressure as an indicator of shock. **Evidence-Based Practice** **QSEN**

- Give oxygen to any patient in shock. **Evidence-Based Practice** **QSEN**
- Assess hourly urine output to evaluate the adequacy of treatment for hypovolemic shock. **Evidence-Based Practice** **QSEN**
- Before administering prescribed antibiotics, obtain blood cultures and cultures of urine, wound drainage, and sputum for any patient suspected to have sepsis. **Evidence-Based Practice** **QSEN**
- Administer prescribed antibiotics within 1 hour of a diagnosis of sepsis. **Evidence-Based Practice** **QSEN**

CHAPTER 38

Care of Patients with Acute Coronary Syndromes

Laura M. Dechant

http://evolve.elsevier.com/Iggy/

PRIORITY CONCEPTS

- PERFUSION
- PAIN

LEARNING OUTCOMES

Safe and Effective Care Environment
1. Explain the role of the interdisciplinary team in cardiac rehabilitation.

Health Promotion and Maintenance
2. Differentiate between modifiable and nonmodifiable risk factors for coronary artery disease (CAD).

Psychosocial Integrity
3. Assess patient and family responses to acute coronary events, especially myocardial infarction (MI).

Physiological Integrity
4. Compare and contrast the clinical manifestations of stable angina, unstable angina, and MI.

5. Interpret physical and diagnostic assessment findings in patients who have CAD.
6. Prioritize nursing care for patients who have chest PAIN.
7. Teach patients and families about drug therapy for CAD.
8. Explain the nursing care for patients who have thrombolysis for an MI.
9. Develop a plan of care for the patient who has a percutaneous coronary intervention (PCI) to promote PERFUSION.
10. Plan postoperative care for the patient who has coronary artery bypass graft (CABG) surgery based on patient preferences, clinical expertise, and current evidence.
11. Identify the postoperative needs of adults having CABG surgery.

Coronary artery disease (CAD), also called *coronary heart disease (CHD)* or simply *heart disease,* is the single largest killer of American men and women in all ethnic groups. When the arteries that supply the myocardium (heart muscle) are diseased, the heart cannot pump blood effectively to adequately perfuse vital organs and peripheral tissues. The organs and tissues need oxygen in arterial blood for survival. When PERFUSION is impaired, the patient can have life-threatening clinical manifestations and possibly death.

The incidence of CAD has declined over the past decade (Go et al., 2013). This decline is due to many factors, including increasingly effective treatment and an increased awareness and emphasis on reducing major cardiovascular risk factors (e.g., hypertension, smoking, high cholesterol). Some coronary events occur in patients without common risk factors.

❖ PATHOPHYSIOLOGY

Coronary artery disease (CAD) is a broad term that includes chronic stable angina and acute coronary syndromes. It affects the arteries that provide blood, oxygen, and nutrients to the myocardium. When blood flow through the coronary arteries is partially or completely blocked, ischemia and infarction of the myocardium may result. Ischemia occurs when *insufficient oxygen* is supplied to meet the requirements of the myocardium. Infarction (necrosis, or cell death) occurs when severe ischemia is prolonged and decreased PERFUSION causes irreversible damage to tissue.

Chronic Stable Angina Pectoris

Angina pectoris is chest PAIN caused by a temporary imbalance between the coronary arteries' ability to supply oxygen and the cardiac muscle's demand for *oxygen*. Ischemia (lack of oxygen) that occurs with angina is limited in duration and does not cause permanent damage of myocardial tissue.

Angina may be of two main types: stable angina and unstable angina. Chronic stable angina (CSA) is chest discomfort that occurs with moderate to prolonged exertion in a pattern that is familiar to the patient. The frequency, duration, and intensity of symptoms remain the same over several months. CSA results in only slight limitation of activity and is usually associated with a *fixed* atherosclerotic plaque. It is usually relieved by nitroglycerin or rest and often is managed with drug therapy. Rarely does

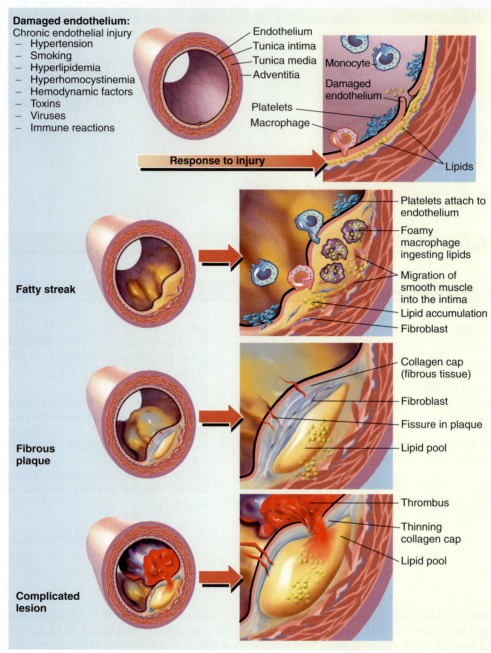

Damaged endothelium:
Chronic endothelial injury
– Hypertension
– Smoking
– Hyperlipidemia
– Hyperhomocystinemia
– Hemodynamic factors
– Toxins
– Viruses
– Immune reactions

Endothelium
Tunica intima
Tunica media
Adventitia

Monocyte

Damaged
endothelium

Platelets
Macrophage

Response to injury

Lipids

Platelets attach to
endothelium

Foamy
macrophage
ingesting lipids

Migration of
smooth muscle
into the intima

Lipid accumulation

Fibroblast

Fatty streak

Collagen cap
(fibrous tissue)

Fibroblast

Fissure in plaque

Lipid pool

**Fibrous
plaque**

Thrombus

Thinning
collagen cap

Lipid pool

**Complicated
lesion**

FIG. 38-1 A cross section of an atherosclerotic coronary artery.

CSA require aggressive treatment. *Unstable* angina is discussed in the following Acute Coronary Syndrome section.

Acute Coronary Syndrome

The term **acute coronary syndrome (ACS)** is used to describe patients who have either *unstable* angina or an acute myocardial infarction. In ACS, it is believed that the atherosclerotic plaque in the coronary artery *ruptures,* resulting in platelet aggregation ("clumping"), thrombus (clot) formation, and vasoconstriction (Fig. 38-1). The amount of disruption of the atherosclerotic plaque determines the degree of coronary artery obstruction (blockage) and the specific disease process. The artery has to have at least 40% plaque accumulation before it starts to block blood flow (McCance et al., 2014).

Historically, an acute myocardial infarction (MI) was diagnosed by the presence of ST-segment elevation on the 12-lead electrocardiogram (ECG) (see discussion of the normal ECG in Chapter 34). However, all patients do not present with this finding. Instead, they are classified into one of three categories according to the presence or absence of ST-segment elevation on the ECG and positive serum troponin markers:

- ST-elevation MI (STEMI) (traditional manifestation)
- Non–ST-elevation MI (NSTEMI) (common in women)
- Unstable angina pectoris

Unstable Angina Pectoris. Unstable angina (the most commonly used term) is chest pain or discomfort that occurs at rest or with exertion and causes severe activity limitation. An increase in the number of attacks and in the intensity of the pressure indicates unstable angina. The pressure may last longer than 15 minutes or may be poorly relieved by rest or nitroglycerin. Unstable angina describes a variety of disorders, including *new-onset angina, variant (Prinzmetal's) angina,* and *pre-infarction angina. Patients with unstable angina present with ST changes on a 12-lead ECG but do not have changes in troponin or creatine kinase (CK) levels.*

New-onset angina describes the patient who has his or her first angina symptoms, usually after exertion or other increased demands on the heart. **Variant (Prinzmetal's) angina** is chest pain or discomfort resulting from coronary artery spasm and typically occurs after rest. **Pre-infarction angina** refers to chest pain that occurs in the days or weeks before an MI.

Myocardial Infarction. The most serious acute coronary syndrome is myocardial infarction (MI), often referred to as *acute MI* or *AMI.* Undiagnosed or untreated angina can lead to this very serious health problem. **Myocardial infarction (MI)** occurs when myocardial tissue is abruptly and severely deprived of oxygen. When blood flow is quickly reduced by 80% to 90%, ischemia develops. Ischemia can lead to injury and necrosis of myocardial tissue if blood flow is not restored. Patients presenting with **non–ST-segment elevation myocardial infarction (NSTEMI)** typically have ST and T-wave changes on a 12-lead ECG. This indicates myocardial necrosis, or cell death. Cardiac enzymes may be initially normal but elevate over the next 3 to 12 hours. Causes of NSTEMI include coronary vasospasm, spontaneous dissection, and sluggish blood flow due to narrowing of the coronary artery.

Patients presenting with **ST-elevation myocardial infarction (STEMI)** typically have ST elevation in two contiguous leads on a 12-lead ECG. This indicates myocardial infarction/ necrosis. STEMI is attributable to rupture of the fibrous atherosclerotic plaque leading to platelet aggregation and thrombus formation at the site of rupture (McCance et al., 2014). *The thrombus causes an abrupt 100% occlusion to the coronary artery, is a medical emergency, and requires immediate revascularization of the blocked coronary artery.*

Often MIs begin with infarction of the subendocardial layer of cardiac muscle. This layer has the longest myofibrils in the heart, the *greatest* oxygen *demand,* and the *poorest* oxygen *supply.* Around the initial area of infarction (zone of necrosis) in the subendocardium are two other zones: (1) the zone of injury—tissue that is injured but not necrotic; and (2) the zone of ischemia—tissue that is oxygen deprived. This pattern is illustrated in Fig. 38-2.

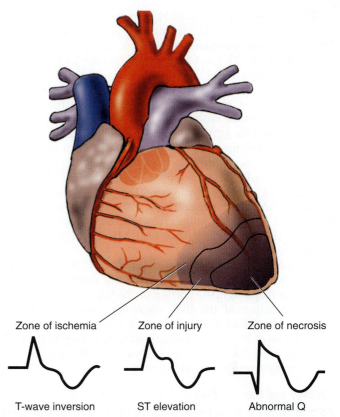

FIG. 38-2 Electrocardiographic changes and patterns associated with myocardial infarction.

Infarction is a dynamic process that does not occur instantly. Rather, it evolves over a period of several hours. Hypoxemia from ischemia may lead to local vasodilation of blood vessels and acidosis. Potassium, calcium, and magnesium imbalances, as well as acidosis at the cellular level, may cause changes in normal conduction and contractile functions. Catecholamines (epinephrine and norepinephrine) released in response to hypoxia and pain may increase the heart's rate, contractility, and afterload. These factors increase *oxygen* requirements in tissue that is already oxygen deprived. This may lead to life-threatening ventricular dysrhythmias. The area of infarction may extend into the zones of injury and ischemia. The actual extent of the zone of infarction depends on three factors: collateral circulation, anaerobic metabolism, and workload demands on the myocardium.

Obvious physical changes do not occur in the heart until 6 hours after the infarction, when the infarcted region appears blue and swollen. *These changes explain the need for intervention within the first 4 to 6 hours of symptom onset!* After 48 hours, the infarcted area turns gray with yellow streaks as neutrophils invade the tissue and begin to remove the necrotic cells. By 8 to 10 days after infarction, granulation tissue forms at the edges of the necrotic tissue. Over a 2- to 3-month period, the necrotic area eventually develops into a shrunken, thin, firm scar. Scar tissue permanently changes the size and shape of the entire left ventricle, called **ventricular remodeling.** Remodeling may decrease left ventricular function, cause heart failure, and increase morbidity and mortality. The scarred tissue does not contract, nor does it conduct electrically. Thus this area is often the cause of chronic ventricular dysrhythmias surrounding the infarcted zone (McCance et al., 2014).

GENDER HEALTH CONSIDERATIONS

Patient-Centered Care QSEN

Many women with symptomatic ischemic heart disease or abnormal stress testing do not have normal coronary angiography. Studies implicate microvascular disease or endothelial dysfunction or both as the causes for risk for CAD in women. Endothelial dysfunction is the inability of the arteries and arterioles to dilate due to lack of nitric oxide production by the endothelium. Nitric oxide is a relaxant of vascular smooth muscle.

Women typically have smaller coronary arteries and frequently have plaque that breaks off and travels into the small vessels to form an embolus (clot). Positive remodeling, or outward remodeling (lesions that protrude outward), is more common in women (McCance et al., 2014). This outpouching may be missed on coronary angiography.

The patient's response to an MI also depends on which coronary artery or arteries were obstructed and which part of the left ventricle wall was damaged: anterior, septal, lateral, inferior, or posterior. Fig. 33-3 in Chapter 33 shows the location of the major coronary arteries.

Obstruction of the left anterior descending (LAD) artery causes *anterior* or *septal* MIs because it perfuses the anterior wall and most of the septum of the left ventricle. Patients with anterior wall MIs (AWMIs) have the highest mortality rate because they are most likely to have left ventricular failure and dysrhythmias from damage to the left ventricle.

The circumflex artery supplies the lateral wall of the left ventricle and possibly portions of the posterior wall or the sinoatrial (SA) and atrioventricular (AV) nodes. Patients with obstruction of the circumflex artery may experience a *posterior* wall MI (PWMI) or a *lateral* wall MI (LWMI) and sinus dysrhythmias.

In most people, the right coronary artery (RCA) supplies most of the SA and AV nodes, as well as the right ventricle and inferior or diaphragmatic portion of the left ventricle. Patients with obstruction of the RCA often have **inferior wall MIs (IWMI)**. About half of all inferior wall MIs are associated with an occlusion of the RCA, causing significant damage to the right ventricle. *Thus it is important to obtain a "right-sided" ECG to assess for right ventricular involvement.*

Etiology and Genetic Risk

Atherosclerosis is the primary factor in the development of CAD. Numerous risk factors, both nonmodifiable and modifiable, contribute to atherosclerosis and subsequently to CAD (see Chapter 36).

Nonmodifiable risk factors are personal characteristics that cannot be altered or controlled. These risk factors, which interact with each other, include age, gender, family history, and ethnic background. People with a family history of CAD are at high risk for developing the disease.

🌐 CULTURAL CONSIDERATIONS

Patient-Centered Care   QSEN

Several groups have a higher genetic risk for CAD than others. For example, African-American and Hispanic women have higher CAD risk factors than white women of the same socioeconomic status. Of American Indians and Alaskan Natives 18 years of age and older, about 46.7% have one or more CAD risk factors (hypertension [HTN], smoking, high cholesterol, excess weight, or diabetes mellitus). The leading cause of death for both men and women in the Euro-American population is cardiovascular disease, even though they may not have genetic predispositions to developing cardiovascular risk factors (Go et al., 2013).

GENDER HEALTH CONSIDERATIONS

Patient-Centered Care   QSEN

Age is the most important risk factor for developing CAD in women. The older a woman is, the more likely she will have the disease. When compared with men, women are usually 10 years older when they have CAD. In addition, women who have MIs have a greater risk for dying during hospitalization. When they are older than 40 years, women are more likely than men to die within 1 year after their MI. If women do survive, they are less likely to participate in cardiac rehabilitation programs (Go et al., 2013).

Modifiable risk factors are lifestyle choices that can be controlled by the patient (with possible medical intervention), such as:

- Elevated serum lipid levels
- Smoking/tobacco use
- Limited physical activity
- Hypertension
- Diabetes mellitus
- Obesity
- Excessive alcohol
- Excessive stress/decreased coping skills

These risk factors are described in more detail in Chapters 33 and 36.

Incidence and Prevalence

The average age of a person having a first MI is 64.7 years for men and 72.2 years for women (Go et al., 2013). Every 34 seconds, a person in the United States has a major coronary event, and every minute, an American will die from CAD (Go et al., 2013). Many people die from coronary heart disease without being hospitalized. Most of these are sudden deaths caused by cardiac arrest.

GENDER HEALTH CONSIDERATIONS

Patient-Centered Care   QSEN

Premenopausal women have a lower incidence of MI than men. However, for postmenopausal women in their 70s or older, the incidence of MI equals that of men. Family history is also a risk factor for women; those whose parents had CAD are more susceptible to the disease. Women with abdominal obesity (android shape) and metabolic syndrome (described on p. 760) are also at increased risk for CAD. Because lesbian and bisexual women have a higher incidence of overweight and obesity than women who are not lesbian or bisexual, they should be considered an especially high-risk group for CAD. The reasons for these trends are not known (Pettinato, 2012).

Many patients who survive MIs are not able to return to work. CAD is the leading cause of premature, permanent disability in the United States and the world.

Health Promotion and Maintenance

Ninety-five percent of sudden cardiac arrest victims die before reaching the hospital, largely because of ventricular fibrillation ("v fib"). To help combat this problem, automatic external defibrillators (AEDs) are found in many public places, such as in shopping centers and on airplanes. Employees are taught how to use these devices if a sudden cardiac arrest occurs. Some patients with diagnosed CAD have AEDs in their homes or at work. The procedure for using this device is described on p. 671 in Chapter 34.

Health promotion efforts are directed toward controlling or altering modifiable risk factors for CAD. For patients at risk for coronary artery disease (CAD), especially MI, assess specific risk factors and implement an individualized health teaching plan. Teach people who have one or more of these risk factors the importance of modifying or eliminating them to decrease their chances of CAD (Chart 38-1). Chapter 36 describes health teaching and evidence-based interventions for preventing and

CHART 38-1 Patient and Family Education: Preparing for Self-Management

Prevention of Coronary Artery Disease

Smoking/Tobacco Use
- If you smoke or use tobacco, quit.
- If you don't smoke or use tobacco, don't start.

Diet
- Consume sufficient calories for your body to include:
  - 5% to 6% from saturated fats
  - Avoiding *trans* fatty acids
- Limit your cholesterol intake to less than 200 mg/day.
- Limit your sodium intake as specified by your health care provider, or under 1500 mg/day, if possible.

Cholesterol
- Have your lipid levels checked regularly.
- If your cholesterol and LDL-C levels are elevated, follow your health care provider's advice, including taking statin medications as indicated.

Physical Activity
- If you are middle-aged or older or have a history of medical problems, check with your health care provider before starting an exercise program.
- Exercise periods should be at least 40 minutes long with 10-minute warm-up and 5-minute cool-down periods.
- If you cannot exercise moderately 3 to 4 times each week, walk daily for 30 minutes at a comfortable pace.
- If you cannot walk 30 minutes daily, walk any distance you can (e.g., park farther away from a site than necessary; use the stairs, not the elevator, to go one floor up or two floors down).

Diabetes Mellitus
- Manage your diabetes with your health care provider.

Hypertension
- Have your blood pressure checked regularly.
- If your blood pressure is elevated, follow your health care provider's advice.
- Continue to monitor your blood pressure at regular intervals.

Obesity
- Avoid severely restrictive or fad diets.
- Restrict intake of saturated fats, sweets, sweetened beverages, and cholesterol-rich foods.
- Increase your physical activity.

LDL-C, Low-density lipoprotein–cholesterol.

TABLE 38-1 Indicators of Risk Factors for Metabolic Syndrome

RISK FACTOR	INDICATOR
Hypertension	**Either** blood pressure of 130/85 mm Hg or higher **or** taking antihypertensive drug(s)
Decreased HDL-C (usually with high LDL-C) level	**Either** HDL-C <45 mg/dL for men or <55 mg/dL for women **or** taking an anticholesterol drug
Increased level of triglycerides	**Either** 160 mg/dL or higher for men or 135 mg/dL or higher for women **or** taking an anticholesterol drug
Increased fasting blood glucose (due to diabetes, glucose intolerance, or insulin resistance)	**Either** 100 mg/dL or higher **or** taking antidiabetic drug(s)
Large waist size (excessive abdominal fat causing central obesity)	40 inches (102 cm) or greater for men or 35 inches (89 cm) or greater for women

HDL-C, High-density lipoprotein–cholesterol; *LDL-C,* low-density lipoprotein–cholesterol.

managing atherosclerosis and hypertension. Smoking cessation is discussed in Chapter 27.

Using Complementary and Alternative Therapies

Teach patients that adding omega-3 fatty acids from fish and plant sources has been effective for some patients in reducing lipid levels, stabilizing atherosclerotic plaques, and reducing sudden death from an MI. The preferred source of omega-3 acids is from fish 3 times a week or a daily fish oil nutritional supplement (1-2 g/day) containing eicosapentaenoic acid (EPA) and docosahexaenoic acid (DHA) (American Heart Association [AHA], 2013). Plant sources (flaxseed, flaxseed oil, walnuts, and canola oil) contain α-linolenic acid, and the conversion of α-linolenic acid to EPA and DHA is not as efficient in patients who consume a typical Western diet. Lovaza (omega-3 fatty

acids) is a medication used to reduce very high triglycerides (>500 mg/dL) levels. However, it has not been proven to prevent MIs or stroke.

Garlic supplements may also have a small effect on reducing lipid levels, but they have not been shown to prevent MI. Patients often take a number of other supplements, such as vitamin E, coenzyme Q10, Pantesin, and vitamin B complex to decrease the risk for heart disease. However, studies do not show that these substances are helpful in reducing coronary artery disease.

Managing Metabolic Syndrome

Metabolic syndrome, also called *syndrome X*, has been recognized as a risk factor for cardiovascular (CV) disease and is being aggressively researched. Patients who have three of the factors in Table 38-1 are diagnosed with metabolic syndrome. This health problem increases the risk for developing diabetes and CAD. About a third of adults older than 20 years in the United States have metabolic syndrome (Go et al., 2013). This increase is likely due to physical inactivity and the current obesity epidemic. Management is aimed at reducing risks, managing hypertension, and preventing complications.

❓ NCLEX EXAMINATION CHALLENGE
Health Promotion and Maintenance

An older client has a history of coronary artery disease. Which modifiable risk factors will the nurse assess to guide the client's teaching plan? **Select all that apply.**
A. Older age
B. Tobacco use
C. Female
D. High-fat diet
E. Family history
F. Obesity

❖ *PATIENT-CENTERED COLLABORATIVE CARE*

◆ *Assessment*

History. If symptoms of CAD are present at the time of the interview, delay collecting data until interventions for symptom relief, vital sign instability, and dysrhythmias are started and discomfort resolves. If the patient had PAIN, ask about how he or she has managed the discomfort and other symptoms and which drugs he or she may be taking. When the patient is pain-free, obtain information about family history and modifiable risk factors, including eating habits, lifestyle, and physical activity levels. Ask about a history of smoking and how much alcohol is consumed each day. Collaborate with the dietitian to assess current body mass index (BMI) and weight as needed.

Physical Assessment/Clinical Manifestations. *Rapid assessment of the patient with chest pain or other presenting symptoms is crucial.* It is important to differentiate among the types of chest PAIN and to identify the source. Question the patient to determine the characteristics of the discomfort. Patients may deny pain, however, and report that they feel "pressure." Appropriate questions to ask concerning the discomfort include onset, location, radiation, intensity, duration, and precipitating and relieving factors.

🌐 CULTURAL CONSIDERATIONS
Patient-Centered Care `QSEN`

African Americans and women tend to delay seeking treatment for MI and therefore have higher mortality rates than Euro-Americans. One contributing factor to this delay is a greater incidence of dyspnea as an acute symptom among these groups rather than the classic PAIN more typical of other groups (Go et al., 2013).

If PAIN is present, ask the patient if the pain is in the chest, epigastric area, jaw, back, shoulder, or arm. Ask him or her to rate the pain on a scale of 0 to 10, with 10 being the highest level of discomfort. Some patients describe the discomfort as tightness, a burning sensation, pressure, or indigestion. A complete pain assessment is described in Chapter 3.

GENDER HEALTH CONSIDERATIONS
Patient-Centered Care `QSEN`

Many women of any age experience atypical angina. **Atypical angina** manifests as indigestion, pain between the shoulders, an aching jaw, or a choking sensation that occurs with exertion. These symptoms typically manifest during stressful circumstances or during activities of daily living. Women may curtail activity as a result of angina, and health care providers need to ask about changes in routine. Symptoms in women typically include fatigue, sleep disturbance, and dyspnea (Go et al., 2013).

Chart 38-2 compares and contrasts angina and infarction PAIN. Because angina pain is ischemic pain, it usually improves when the imbalance between oxygen supply and demand is resolved. For example, rest reduces tissue demands and nitroglycerin improves oxygen supply. Discomfort from a

---

CHART 38-2	**Key Features**

Angina and Myocardial Infarction

ANGINA	MYOCARDIAL INFARCTION

• Substernal chest discomfort:
  ▪ Radiating to the left arm
  ▪ Precipitated by exertion or stress (or rest in variant angina)
  ▪ Relieved by nitroglycerin or rest
  ▪ Lasting less than 15 min
• Few, if any, associated symptoms
	• Pain or discomfort:
	  ▪ Substernal chest pain/pressure radiating to the left arm
	  ▪ Pain or discomfort in jaw, back, shoulder, or abdomen
	  ▪ Occurring without cause, usually in the morning
	  ▪ Relieved only by opioids
	  ▪ Lasting 30 min or more
	• Frequent associated symptoms:
	  ▪ Nausea/vomiting
	  ▪ Diaphoresis
	  ▪ Dyspnea
	  ▪ Feelings of fear and anxiety
	  ▪ Dysrhythmias
	  ▪ Fatigue
	  ▪ Palpitations
	  ▪ Epigastric distress
	  ▪ Anxiety
	  ▪ Dizziness
	  ▪ Disorientation/acute confusion
	  ▪ Feeling "short of breath"

CONSIDERATIONS FOR OLDER ADULTS
Patient-Centered Care `QSEN`

The presence of associated symptoms without chest discomfort is significant. In up to 40% of all patients with MI, primarily older women and patients with diabetes, chest pain or discomfort may be mild or absent. Instead, they have associated symptoms. Some older patients may think they are having indigestion and therefore not recognize that they are having an MI. Others report shortness of breath as the only symptom. The major manifestation of MI in people older than 80 years may be disorientation or acute confusion because of poor cardiac output and due to inadequate coronary perfusion.

In some older adults with MI, absence of chest pain may be due to cognitive impairment or inability to verbalize pain sensation. However, in most cases it is probably the result of increased collateral circulation. Silent myocardial ischemia increases the incidence of new coronary events and should be treated aggressively.

myocardial infarction (MI) does not usually resolve with these measures. Ask about any associated symptoms, including *nausea, vomiting, diaphoresis, dizziness, weakness, palpitations, and shortness of breath.*

Assess *blood pressure* and *heart rate.* Interpret the patient's cardiac rhythm and presence of *dysrhythmias.* Sinus tachycardia with premature ventricular contractions (PVCs) frequently occurs in the first few hours after an MI.

Next assess *distal peripheral pulses* and *skin temperature.* The skin should be warm with all pulses palpable. In the patient with unstable angina or MI, poor cardiac output may be manifested by cool, diaphoretic ("sweaty") skin and diminished or absent pulses. *Auscultate for an S₃ gallop, which often indicates heart failure—a serious and common complication of MI.* In adults, the S₃ heart sound is heard with the bell of the stethoscope over the apex of the heart (Jarvis, 2016).

Assess the *respiratory rate* and breath sounds for signs of heart failure. An increased respiratory rate is common because of anxiety and pain, but *crackles or wheezes* may indicate *left-sided* heart failure. Assess for the presence of jugular venous distention and peripheral edema.

The patient with MI may experience a *temperature elevation* for several days after infarction. Temperatures as high as 102° F (38.9° C) may occur in response to myocardial necrosis, indicating the inflammatory response.

Psychosocial Assessment. *Denial* is a common early reaction to chest discomfort associated with angina or MI. On average, the patient with an acute MI waits more than 2 hours before seeking medical attention. Often he or she rationalizes that symptoms are due to indigestion or overexertion. In some situations, denial is a normal part of adapting to a stressful event. However, denial that interferes with identifying a symptom such as chest discomfort can be harmful. Explain the importance of reporting any discomfort to the health care provider.

Fear, depression, anxiety, and anger are other common reactions of many patients and their families. Assist in identifying these feelings. Encourage them to explain their understanding of the event, and clarify any misconceptions.

Laboratory Assessment. Although there is no single ideal test to diagnose MI, the most common laboratory tests include troponins T and I and creatine kinase-MB (CK-MB). These cardiac markers are specific for MI and cardiac necrosis. Troponins T and I rise quickly. CK-MB is the most specific marker for MI but does not peak until about 24 hours after the onset of pain. These tests are described in more detail in Chapter 33. If serial enzymes are negative, the patient has a nuclear medicine test such as those described in the next section.

Imaging Assessment. Unless there is associated cardiac dysfunction (e.g., valve disease) or heart failure, a chest x-ray is not diagnostic for angina or MI. A chest x-ray may be performed to assist with ruling out aortic dissection, which may mimic a MI. If the x-ray demonstrates a widened mediastinum, further testing for aortic dissection with either transesophageal echography (TEE) or computed tomography (CT) scan is needed.

Thallium scans use radioisotope imaging to assess for ischemia or necrotic muscle tissue related to angina or myocardial infarction (MI). Areas of decreased or absent perfusion, referred to as *cold spots,* identify ischemia or infarction. Thallium may be used with the exercise tolerance test. Dipyridamole (Persantine) thallium scanning (DTS) may also be used.

Contrast-enhanced cardiovascular magnetic resonance (CMR) imaging may also be done as a noninvasive approach to detect CAD. *Echocardiography* may be used to visualize the structures of the heart.

Use of the 64-slice **computed tomography coronary angiography (CTCA)** has been found to be helpful in diagnosing coronary artery disease in symptomatic patients identified as having a "low- or intermediate-pretest probability" risk for CAD. This new generation of high-speed computed tomography (CT) scanners is becoming a highly reliable, noninvasive way to evaluate CAD (Weustink et al., 2010).

Other Diagnostic Assessment. *Twelve-lead electrocardiograms (ECGs)* allow the health care provider to examine the heart from varying perspectives. By identifying the lead(s) in which ECG changes are occurring, the health care provider can identify both the occurrence and the location of ischemia (angina) or necrosis (infarction). In addition to the traditional 12-lead ECG, the health care provider may request a "right-sided" or 18-lead ECG to determine whether ischemia or infarction has occurred in the right ventricle. *The ECG should be obtained within 10 minutes of patient presentation with chest discomfort!*

An ischemic myocardium does not repolarize normally. Thus 12-lead ECGs obtained during an angina episode reveal ST depression, T-wave inversion, or both. **Variant angina,** caused by coronary vasospasm (vessel spasm), usually causes elevation of the ST segment during angina attacks. These ST and T-wave changes usually subside when the ischemia is resolved and pain is relieved. However, the T wave may remain flat or inverted for a period of time. If the patient is not experiencing angina at the moment of the test, the ECG is usually normal unless he or she has evidence of an old MI.

When infarction occurs, one of two ECG changes is usually observed: ST-elevation MI (STEMI), or non–ST-elevation MI (NSTEMI). An abnormal Q wave (wider than 0.04 seconds or more than one-third the height of the QRS complex) may develop, depending on the amount of myocardium that has necrosed. Women having an MI often present with an NSTEMI.

The Q wave may develop because necrotic cells do not conduct electrical stimuli. Hours to days after the MI, the ST-segment and T-wave changes return to normal. However, when the Q wave exists, it may become permanent. The Q waves may disappear after a number of years, but their absence does not necessarily mean that the patient has not had an MI.

After the acute stages of an unstable angina episode, the health care provider often requests an *exercise tolerance test (stress test)* on a treadmill to assess for ECG changes consistent with ischemia, evaluate medical therapy, and identify those who might benefit from invasive therapy. Pharmacologic stress-testing agents such as dobutamine (Dobutrex) may be used instead of the treadmill. Treadmill exercise testing is only moderately accurate for women when compared with men. The results are also not as reliable in tall, obese men when compared with short, thinner men. In women with suspected CAD, stress echocardiography or single photon emission computed tomography (SPECT) should be performed.

Cardiac catheterization may be performed to determine the extent and exact location of coronary artery obstructions. It allows the cardiologist and cardiac surgeon to identify patients who might benefit from percutaneous coronary intervention (PCI) or from coronary artery bypass grafting (CABG). Each of these diagnostic tests is described in detail in Chapter 33.

◆ *Analysis*

The patient with coronary artery disease (CAD) may have either stable angina or acute coronary syndrome (ACS). If ACS is suspected or cannot be completely ruled out, the patient is admitted to a telemetry unit for continuous monitoring or to a critical care unit if hemodynamically unstable.

The priority NANDA-I nursing diagnoses and collaborative problems for most patients with CAD include:

1. Acute Pain related to imbalance between myocardial oxygen supply and demand (NANDA-I)
2. Inadequate tissue perfusion (cardiopulmonary) related to interruption of arterial blood flow
3. Activity Intolerance related to fatigue caused by imbalance between oxygen supply and demand (NANDA-I)
4. Ineffective Coping related to effects of acute illness and major changes in lifestyle (NANDA-I)
5. Potential for dysrhythmias

6. Potential for heart failure
7. Potential for recurrent symptoms and extension of injury

◆ Planning and Implementation

Astute assessment skills, timely analysis of troponin, and analysis of the 12-lead ECG (or 18-lead ECG for a suspected right ventricular infarction) are essential to ensure appropriate patient care management. This is particularly important since the average time a patient waits before seeking treatment is over 2 hours. This delay lessens the 4- to 6-hour window of opportunity for the most advantageous treatment with percutaneous intervention.

Managing Acute Pain. Patients with *diabetes mellitus* and coronary artery disease (CAD) may not experience chest PAIN or pressure because of diabetic neuropathy. In this patient population, the onset of ACS may be signaled by new onset of atrial fibrillation. With new-onset atrial fibrillation, a cardiac workup should be done to rule out ACS.

Planning: Expected Outcomes. The expected outcome is that the patient will verbalize a report of decreased PAIN and discomfort as a result of prompt collaborative interventions.

Interventions. The purpose of patient-centered collaborative care is to eliminate discomfort by providing PAIN relief measures, decreasing myocardial oxygen demand, and increasing myocardial oxygen supply.

Emergency Care: Myocardial Infarction. Evaluate any report of pain, obtain vital signs, ensure an IV access, and notify the health care provider of the patient's condition. Chart 38-3 summarizes the emergency interventions for the patient with symptoms of CAD.

Pain relief helps increase the oxygen supply and decrease myocardial oxygen demand. The American Heart Association (AHA) recommends several pain management strategies, including morphine sulfate and oxygen. *Give morphine as the priority in managing pain in patients having an ACS!*

Drug Therapy. At home or in the hospital, the patient may take nitroglycerin to relieve episodic anginal pain. Aspirin 325 mg,

an antiplatelet drug, may also be taken daily to prevent clots that further block coronary arteries.

Nitroglycerin (NTG), a nitrate often referred to as "nitro," increases collateral blood flow, redistributes blood flow toward the subendocardium, and dilates the coronary arteries. In addition, it decreases myocardial oxygen demand by peripheral vasodilation, which decreases both preload and afterload.

! NURSING SAFETY PRIORITY (QSEN)
Drug Alert

Before administering NTG, ensure that the patient has not taken any phosphodiesterase inhibitors for erectile dysfunction such as sildenafil (Viagra, Revatio) or tadalafil (Cialis) within the past 24 to 48 hours. Concomitant use of NTG with these inhibitors can cause profound hypotension. Remind patients not to take these medications within 24 to 48 hours of one another.

Teach the patient to hold the NTG tablet under the tongue and drink 5 mL (1 teaspoon) of water, if necessary, to allow the tablet to dissolve. NTG spray is also available and is more quickly absorbed. Pain relief should begin within 1 to 2 minutes and should be clearly evident in 3 to 5 minutes. After 5 minutes, recheck the patient's pain intensity and vital signs. If the blood pressure (BP) is less than 100 mm Hg systolic or 25 mm Hg lower than the previous reading, lower the head of the bed and notify the health care provider.

If the patient is experiencing some but not complete relief and vital signs remain stable, another NTG tablet or spray may be used. In 5-minute increments, a total of three doses may be administered in an attempt to relieve angina PAIN. If the patient uses NTG spray instead of the tablet, teach him or her to sit upright and spray the dose under the tongue. NTG topical patches should be placed below the nipple line to decrease discomfort.

Angina usually responds to NTG. The patient typically states that the PAIN is relieved or markedly diminished. When simple measures, such as taking three sublingual nitroglycerin tablets one after the other, do not relieve chest discomfort, the patient may be experiencing an MI.

! NURSING SAFETY PRIORITY (QSEN)
Critical Rescue

If the patient is experiencing an MI, prepare him or her for transfer to a specialized unit where close monitoring and appropriate management can be provided. If the patient is at home or in the community, call 911 for transfer to the closest emergency department.

In a specialized unit, the health care provider may prescribe IV NTG for management of the chest PAIN. Begin the drug infusion slowly, checking the BP and pain level every 3 to 5 minutes. The nitroglycerin dose is increased until the pain is relieved, the BP falls excessively, or the maximum prescribed dose is reached (Chart 38-4).

When PAIN or other symptoms have subsided and the patient is stabilized, the health care provider may change the drug to an oral or topical nitrate. During administration of long-term

---

CHART 38-3 Best Practice for Patient Safety & Quality Care (QSEN)

Emergency Care of the Patient with Chest Discomfort

- Assess airway, breathing, and circulation (ABCs). Defibrillate as needed.
- **Provide continuous ECG monitoring.**
- Obtain the patient's description of pain or discomfort.
- Obtain the patient's vital signs (blood pressure, pulse, respiration).
- Assess/provide vascular access.
- Consult chest pain protocol or notify the physician or Rapid Response Team for specific intervention.
- Obtain a 12-lead ECG within 10 minutes of report of chest pain.
- Provide pain-relief medication and aspirin (non–enteric coated) as prescribed.
- Administer oxygen therapy to maintain oxygen saturation ≥95%.
- Remain calm. Stay with the patient if possible.
- Assess the patient's vital signs and intensity of pain 5 minutes after administration of medication.
- Remedicate with prescribed drugs (if vital signs remain stable), and check the patient every 5 minutes.
- Notify the physician if vital signs deteriorate.

ECG, Electrocardiogram.

CHART 38-4 Common Examples of Drug Therapy

Coronary Artery Disease (Nitrates, Beta Blockers, and Antiplatelet Agents)

DRUG	USUAL DOSAGE	NURSING INTERVENTIONS	RATIONALES
Nitrates			
Nitroglycerin (Nitrostat, NitroQuick)	0.3-0.4 mg sublingually every 5 min; up to 3 tablets over 15 min	Instruct patients to lie down with the head of the bed at a level of comfort when taking the sublingual form.	Hypotension can be dramatic, immediate, and intensified by the upright position.
Nitrolingual translingual spray	0.4 mg/metered spray	Monitor BP. Pay attention to orthostatic changes.	A decrease in BP occurs with vasodilation.
		Instruct patients to allow the sublingual tablet to dissolve and to avoid swallowing the tablet.	The sublingual dose is absorbed through the sublingual mucous membranes.
		Check the expiration date on sublingual tablets and sprays. Tablets should be replaced every 3-5 mo.	The efficacy of the tablets decreases with time.
		Determine whether pain is relieved.	Additional medication may be required to relieve pain.
		Monitor for headache.	Vasodilation is generalized.
		Do not administer to patients taking drugs used to treat sexual dysfunction (e.g., sildenafil, tadalafil, vardenafil).	Very serious (possibly fatal) interactions may occur.
Isosorbide dinitrate (Isordil, Iso-Bid)	2.5 mg sublingually every 4-6 hr; 5-40 mg orally four times daily 40-80 mg sustained-release tablet every 8-12 hr	Instruct patients taking sublingual forms to lie down before administration. Monitor BP, and assess for dizziness.	The hypotensive effect can be dramatic and immediate with sublingual administration. A decrease in BP occurs with vasodilation.
Isosorbide mononitrate (Imdur)	60-mg extended-release tablet daily	Schedule sustained-release form with an 8- to 12-hr dose-free interval.	Tolerance may develop.
Nitroglycerin patch (Minitran, Nitro-Dur, Nitrek)	Transdermally started at 5 mg/24 hr (10-cm^2 system)	Remove the patch from the patient before defibrillation.	The patient may develop a burn.
		Rotate application sites.	Rotation prevents skin irritation.
		Apply the patch to a clean, dry, hairless area.	The drug is better absorbed when the skin is clean, dry, and hairless.
		Remove patch after 12-14 hr each day.	Removal prevents drug tolerance.
Beta Blockers			
Carvedilol (Coreg, Coreg CR)	12.5-25 mg orally twice daily for Coreg; 40-80 mg orally once daily for Coreg CR	Assess heart rate before administration.	Beta-blocking effects cause a decrease in heart rate.
		Monitor BP.	The hypotensive effect is due to a decrease in cardiac output, suppressed renin activity, and beta-blocking effects.
		Observe for signs of heart failure.	Heart failure may occur as a result of a decrease in cardiac output.
		Assess for shortness of breath and wheezing.	Beta$_2$-blocking effects in the lungs can cause bronchoconstriction.
Metoprolol (Lopressor, Toprol XL, Betaloc ✿), a cardioselective beta-adrenergic blocker	*Angina:* 25-100 mg orally daily *MI:* 100 mg orally twice daily; 5 mg IV over 2 min may be repeated twice for a total of 15 mg	Assess heart rate before administration; do not administer if heart rate <50-60 beats/min.	Beta blockers may cause further decreases in heart rate.
		Monitor BP, and hold for systolic <90-100 mm Hg.	Decreased BP pressure is an anticipated effect.
		Assess patients for cough, shortness of breath, edema, and weight gain.	These are indications of heart failure.
Antiplatelet Agents			
Aspirin (Empirin, Apo-ASA ✿, Ecotrin)	81-325 mg orally daily	Suggest that patients take the daily dose with food.	Gastric irritation may occur.
		Question patients about ringing in the ears.	Tinnitus may occur with aspirin toxicity.
		Emphasize to patients that aspirin is an important cardiac medication and should be continued unless they are told to stop.	Studies document significantly better survival rates for patients with coronary artery disease receiving aspirin.

Continued

CHART 38-4 Common Examples of Drug Therapy—cont'd

Coronary Artery Disease (Nitrates, Beta Blockers, and Antiplatelet Agents)

DRUG	USUAL DOSAGE	NURSING INTERVENTIONS	RATIONALES
P2Y12 Platelet Inhibitors			
Clopidogrel (Plavix) **Do not confuse Plavix with Paxil**	*Acute coronary syndrome or after stent implantation:* 300-600 mg orally loading dose, then 75-150 mg daily	Teach patients to take drug with food. Inform patients to report any unusual bleeding or bruising.	Drug can cause diarrhea and other GI disturbances. Drug prevents platelet aggregation, thus slowing down clot formation.
Prasugrel (Effient)	*Acute coronary syndrome or after stent implantation:* 60 mg orally loading dose, then 10 mg daily	Inform patients to report any unusual bleeding or bruising.	Contraindicated in patients with history of prior stroke or >75 yrs of age, due to increased risk for bleeding. If patient weighs <60 kg, consider lowering dose to 5 mg daily.
Ticagrelor (Brilinta)	*Acute coronary syndrome or after stent implantation:* 180 mg load with 325 mg aspirin, then 90 mg daily with 81 mg of aspirin	Inform patients to report any unusual bleeding or bruising. Teach patients to avoid over-the-counter pain relievers that contain aspirin. Teach patients to take no more than 100 mg of aspirin in a 24 hour period.	May cause dyspnea or bradycardia that is self-limiting. May not work as effectively with high-dose aspirin; use 81 mg of aspirin.

BP, Blood pressure; *MI,* myocardial infarction.

oral and topical nitrates, an 8- to 12-hour nitrate-free period should be maintained to prevent tolerance. The patient may initially report a headache. Give acetaminophen (Tylenol, Exdol ♦) before the nitrate to ease some of this discomfort.

The health care provider usually prescribes *morphine sulfate (MS)* to relieve discomfort that is unresponsive to nitroglycerin. Morphine relieves MI PAIN, decreases myocardial oxygen demand, relaxes smooth muscle, and reduces circulating catecholamines. It is usually administered in 2- to 10-mg doses IV every 5 to 15 minutes until the maximum prescribed dose is reached or the patient experiences relief or signs of toxicity. Monitor for adverse effects of morphine, which include respiratory depression, hypotension, bradycardia, and severe vomiting. Treatment for morphine toxicity is naloxone (Narcan) 0.2 to 0.8 mg IV, vasopressor drugs, IV fluids, and oxygen therapy. Monitor the patient's vital signs and cardiac rhythm every few minutes.

These strategies are often enough to relieve the PAIN. If they are not adequate, additional interventions identified in the Improving Cardiopulmonary Tissue Perfusion section below may be attempted.

Other Interventions. Several other interventions may be used with drug therapy to relieve chest PAIN. Supplemental oxygen increases the amount of oxygen available to myocardial tissue. Therefore oxygen is usually prescribed and administered at a flow of 2 to 4 L/min by nasal cannula titrated to maintain an arterial oxygen saturation (Sao_2) of 95% or higher. If the BP is stable, assist the patient in assuming any position of comfort. Placing the patient in semi-Fowler's position often enhances comfort and tissue oxygenation. A quiet, calm environment and explanations of interventions often reduce anxiety and help relieve chest pain. If needed, remind the patient to take several deep breaths to increase oxygenation.

Improving Cardiopulmonary Tissue Perfusion

Planning: Expected Outcomes. The primary outcome is that the patient will have increased myocardial PERFUSION as evidenced by an adequate cardiac output, normal sinus rhythm, and vital signs within normal limits.

💡 CLINICAL JUDGMENT CHALLENGE

Patient-Centered Care; Evidence-Based Practice; Informatics **QSEN**

An 82-year-old man living alone at home had a sudden onset of chest pain. He called 911 and was taken to the emergency department (ED).
1. As his ED nurse, what is your first action in response to his report of chest pain? What evidence supports this decision?
2. The physician prescribes IV nitroglycerin for pain. What assessment will you perform prior to administering this drug and why? For what adverse effects will you monitor during and after morphine administration?
3. What other drugs might the physician prescribe at this time and why?
4. The physician prescribed oxygen at 3 L/min via nasal cannula. What is the purpose of this intervention for managing chest pain?
5. What will you document in the electronic health record about this patient's care?

Interventions. Because myocardial infarction (MI) is a dynamic process, restoring PERFUSION to the injured area (usually within 4 to 6 hours for NSTEMI and 60 to 90 minutes for STEMI) often limits the amount of extension and improves left ventricular function. Complete, sustained reperfusion of coronary arteries after an ACS has decreased mortality rates.

Drug Therapy. *Aspirin (ASA)* therapy is recommended by the American College of Cardiology (ACC) and the American Heart Association (AHA) (Cayla et al., 2012). It inhibits both platelet aggregation and vasoconstriction, thereby decreasing the likelihood of thrombosis. *If the patient has new-onset angina at home, teach him or her to chew aspirin 325 mg (4 "baby aspirins" that are 81 mg each) immediately and call 911!* The antiplatelet effect of ASA begins within 1 hour of use and continues for several days. In the hospital setting, The Joint Commission

Acute Myocardial Infarction Core Measure Set requires that aspirin be given upon arrival to the emergency department or when an MI occurs in the hospital. Administer 162 to 325 mg non–enteric-coated aspirin every day to all patients with suspected CAD unless absolutely contraindicated. Instruct the patient to chew and swallow the drug and continue taking the drug as prescribed unless adverse effects occur.

> **! NURSING SAFETY PRIORITY** (QSEN)
> **Drug Alert**
>
> For patients taking aspirin every day, observe for bleeding tendencies, such as nosebleeds or blood in the stool. Aspirin should be discontinued if bleeding occurs.

Glycoprotein (GP) IIb/IIIa inhibitors target the platelet component of the thrombus. Abciximab (ReoPro), eptifibatide (Integrilin), or tirofiban (Aggrastat) may be administered IV to prevent fibrinogen from attaching to activated platelets at the site of a thrombus. These medications are used in unstable angina and NSTEMI. They are also given before and during percutaneous coronary intervention (PCI) to maintain patency of an artery with a large clot and are given with fibrinolytic agents after STEMI. If the GP IIb/IIIa inhibitors are used with a fibrinolytic agent, the dose of the thrombolytic is reduced by 25% to 50% to decrease the risk for bleeding.

> **! NURSING SAFETY PRIORITY** (QSEN)
> **Drug Alert**
>
> When giving GP IIb/IIIa inhibitors, assess the patient closely for bleeding or hypersensitivity reactions. If either occurs, notify the health care provider or Rapid Response Team immediately. Monitor the platelet level 4 hours after starting the drug and daily after that. Notify the cardiologist if the patient experiences a significant decrease in platelet count per agency protocol.

Once-a-day *beta-adrenergic blocking agents* (e.g., metoprolol XL [Toprol XL], carvedilol CR [Coreg CR]), sometimes just called *beta blockers (BBs)*, decrease the size of the infarct, the occurrence of ventricular dysrhythmias, and mortality rates in patients with MI. The physician usually prescribes a cardioselective beta-blocking agent within the first 1 to 2 hours after an MI if the patient is hemodynamically stable. Beta blockers slow the heart rate and decrease the force of cardiac contraction (see Chart 38-4). Thus these agents prolong the period of diastole and increase myocardial PERFUSION while reducing the force of myocardial contraction. With beta blockade, the heart can perform more work without ischemia. During beta-blocking therapy, monitor for:

- Bradycardia
- Hypotension
- Decreased level of consciousness (LOC)
- Chest discomfort

Assess the lungs for crackles (indicative of heart failure) and wheezes (indicative of bronchospasm). Hypoglycemia, depression, nightmares, and forgetfulness are also problems with beta blockade, especially in older patients. Many of these side effects

decrease with time. Unless contraindicated, all patients experiencing NSTEMI and STEMI should be discharged on beta blocker therapy.

> **! NURSING SAFETY PRIORITY** (QSEN)
> **Drug Alert**
>
> Do not give beta blockers if the pulse is below 55 or the systolic BP is below 100 without first checking with the health care provider.

Health care providers frequently prescribe *angiotensin-converting enzyme inhibitors (ACEIs)* or *angiotensin receptor blockers (ARBs)* within 48 hours of ACS if ejection fraction is equal to or less than 40% to prevent ventricular remodeling and the development of heart failure. Both ACEIs and ARBs increase survival after an MI. Monitor the patient for decreased urine output, hypotension, and cough. Check for changes in serum potassium, creatinine, and blood urea nitrogen. (Chapter 36 provides a more detailed discussion of ACEIs and ARBs.)

For patients with angina, the health care provider may prescribe calcium channel blockers (CCBs) to promote vasodilation and myocardial PERFUSION. These drugs are indicated for patients with variant angina or for those who are hypertensive and continue to have angina despite therapy with beta blockers (unstable angina). They are *not* indicated after AMI. Monitor the patient for hypotension and peripheral edema, and review the frequency of angina episodes.

Calcium channel blockers are also used for chronic stable angina (CSA). When they are not successful in managing CSA, *ranolazine (Ranexa)* may be added to the drug regimen. This drug has anti-angina and anti-ischemic properties and is often effective in relieving the pain associated with CSA.

Reperfusion Therapy. As time passes, myocardial tissue can become increasingly ischemic and necrotic. Therefore, based on the location and skill set within the health care institution, one of two reperfusion strategies are employed to open a blocked artery in a patient experiencing AMI: thrombolytic therapy or percutaneous coronary intervention (PCI).

Thrombolytic Therapy. Thrombolytic therapy using **fibrinolytics** dissolves thrombi in the coronary arteries and restores myocardial blood flow. Examples of these agents, which target the fibrin component of the coronary thrombosis, include:

- Tissue plasminogen activator (t-PA, alteplase [Activase]) (IV or intracoronary)
- Reteplase (Retavase) (IV or intracoronary)
- Tenecteplase (TNK) (IV push [IVP])

Intracoronary fibrinolytics may be delivered during cardiac catheterization. Thrombolytic agents are most effective when administered within the first 6 hours of a coronary event. They are used in men and women, young and old.

Thrombolytic therapy is given in a unit where the patient can be continuously monitored. It is indicated for chest pain of longer than 30 minutes' duration that is unrelieved by nitroglycerin, with *indications of STEMI by the ECG*. It is *not* indicated for the NSTEMI patient population. The goal is to start the infusion of fibrinolytics within 30 minutes of ED admission. Contraindications include recent abdominal surgery or stroke, because bleeding may occur when fresh clots are lysed (broken down or dissolved). Table 38-2 lists the current contraindications to thrombolytic therapy.

TABLE 38-2 Contraindications to Thrombolytic Therapy

Absolute
- Any prior intracranial hemorrhage
- Known structural cerebral vascular lesion (e.g., arteriovenous malformations)
- Known malignant intracranial neoplasm (primary or metastatic)
- Ischemic stroke within 3 months EXCEPT acute ischemic stroke within 3 hours
- Suspected aortic dissection
- Active bleeding or bleeding diathesis (excluding menses)
- Significant closed-head or facial trauma within 3 months

Relative
- History of chronic, severe, poorly controlled hypertension
- Severe uncontrolled hypertension on presentation (SBP >180 mm Hg or DBP >110 mm Hg)*
- History of prior ischemic stroke within 3 months, dementia, or known intracranial pathology not covered in contraindications
- Traumatic or prolonged (≥10 minutes) CPR or major surgery (within 3 weeks)
- Recent (within 2-4 weeks) internal bleeding
- Noncompressible vascular punctures
- For streptokinase/anistreplase: prior exposure (>5 days ago) or prior allergic reaction to these agents
- Pregnancy
- Active peptic ulcer
- Current use of anticoagulants; the higher the INR, the higher risk for bleeding

CPR, Cardiopulmonary resuscitation; *DBP*, diastolic blood pressure; *INR*, international normalized ratio; *MI*, myocardial infarction; *SBP*, systolic blood pressure.
*Could be an absolute contraindication in low-risk patients with MI.

! NURSING SAFETY PRIORITY (QSEN)
Drug Alert

During and after thrombolytic administration, immediately report any indications of bleeding to the health care provider or Rapid Response Team. Observe for signs of bleeding by:
- Documenting the patient's neurologic status (in case of intracranial bleeding)
- Observing all IV sites for bleeding and patency
- Monitoring clotting studies
- Observing for signs of internal bleeding (Monitor hemoglobin, hematocrit, and blood pressure.)
- Testing stools, urine, and emesis for occult blood

Patients who weigh less than 143 pounds (65 kg) may need to have their dose of thrombolytic adjusted to lessen the likelihood of bleeding.

Percutaneous Coronary Intervention. For some patients having an ACS, primary percutaneous coronary intervention (PCI) may be used to reopen the clotted coronary artery and restore PERFUSION. Percutaneous intervention has been associated with excellent return of blood flow through the coronary artery when it can be performed by an interventional cardiologist within 2 to 3 hours of the onset of symptoms. Many community hospitals can now perform emergent PCI. When primary PCI is not available, patients should receive immediate thrombolytic agents if they are appropriate candidates and then be transferred to a facility that can perform PCI. This procedure is described in detail on p. 772 of this chapter. After PCI with stent

placement, the patient requires dual antiplatelet therapy, explained later in the chapter.

Patients who receive fibrinolytics require PCI for more definitive treatment such as stent placement. Therefore, if criteria for PCI are met, it is more advantageous to go directly to the catheterization laboratory where definitive treatment, not just clot resolution, can be performed.

Monitor the patient for indications that the clot has been lysed (dissolved) and the artery reperfused. These indications include:
- Abrupt cessation of pain or discomfort
- Sudden onset of ventricular dysrhythmias
- Resolution of ST-segment depression/elevation or T-wave inversion
- A peak at 12 hours of markers of myocardial damage

After clot lysis with thrombolytics, large amounts of thrombin are released into the system, increasing the risk for vessel reocclusion. To maintain the patency of the coronary artery after thrombolytic therapy, the health care provider usually prescribes aspirin and IV heparin, a *high-alert drug*. Maintain the heparin infusion via pump for 3 to 5 days as prescribed, and monitor the activated partial thromboplastin time (aPTT). The target aPTT range is usually $1\frac{1}{2}$ to $2\frac{1}{2}$ times the control sample. The heparin antifactor Xa assay (heparin assay) test may be used instead of the aPTT in some clinical facilities. Low–molecular-weight heparin (LMWH) (enoxaparin [Lovenox]) may be substituted for IV heparin. Therapeutic dosing of LMWH in this patient population should be based on weight (1 mg/kg). Chapter 36 describes care of the patient receiving heparin or LMWH in detail.

? NCLEX EXAMINATION CHALLENGE
Physiological Integrity

A client weighing 174 pounds had thrombolytic therapy followed by a one-time dose of IV Lovenox 30 mg. The physician prescribes Lovenox 1 mg/kg subcutaneously after the IV administration. The nurse will give ____ mg of Lovenox to the client.

Increasing Activity Tolerance

Planning: Expected Outcomes. The patient is expected to increase activity without chest PAIN and the need for supplemental oxygen as a result of a collaborative cardiac rehabilitation program.

Interventions. Activity intolerance is reduced by a planned program of cardiac rehabilitation implemented primarily by the nurse and physical therapist and continued after discharge.

Cardiac rehabilitation is the process of actively assisting the patient with cardiac disease in achieving and maintaining a vital and productive life while remaining within the limits of the heart's ability to respond to increases in activity and stress. It can be divided into three phases. *Phase 1* begins with the acute illness and ends with discharge from the hospital. *Phase 2* begins after discharge and continues through convalescence at home. *Phase 3* refers to long-term conditioning.

In the acute phase (phase 1), promote rest and ensure limited mobility. Assistance may be needed for some ADLs, such as ambulation to the bathroom. Patients progress at their own rate to increasing levels of activity depending on their clinical status, age, and physical capabilities.

The next step in phase 1 is independent ambulation of the patient in the room and to the bathroom. Encourage progressive ambulation in the hallway, usually 50, 100, and then 200 feet 3 times a day. In addition, the patient may begin showering for 5 or 10 minutes with warm water. A chair should be available to facilitate rest and maintain balance.

! NURSING SAFETY PRIORITY (QSEN)
Action Alert

During cardiac rehabilitation, assess the patient's heart rate, blood pressure (BP), respiratory rate, and level of fatigue with each higher level of activity. Decreases greater than 20 mm Hg in the systolic BP, changes of 20 beats per minute in the pulse rate, and/or reports of dyspnea or chest pain indicate intolerance of activity. If these manifestations develop, notify the health care provider and do not advance the patient to the next level. Older adults with CAD often have needs and concerns different from those of younger adults, as described in Chart 38-5.

All patients with ACS should be referred to a phase 2 cardiac rehabilitation program upon discharge from the hospital. Collaborate with the case manager to plan for the patient's continuing care.

Promoting Effective Coping
Planning: Expected Outcomes. The patient is expected to learn to cope with the cardiac event and identify effective coping strategies with the help of support systems.

Interventions. Assess the patient's level of anxiety while allowing expressions of any apprehension, and attempt to define its origin. Simple, repeated explanations of therapies, expectations, and surroundings, as well as patient progress, may help relieve anxiety.

Identify the patient's current *coping* mechanisms. The most common are denial, anger, and depression. Denial allows

---

CHART 38-5 Nursing Focus on the Older Adult
Coronary Artery Disease

- Recognize that chest pain may not be evident in the older patient. Examples of associated symptoms are unexplained dyspnea, confusion, or GI symptoms.
- Although older adults have a greater reduction in mortality rate from myocardial infarction (MI) with the use of thrombolytics, they also have the most severe side effects. Monitor older patients receiving thrombolytics extremely carefully.
- Dysrhythmia may be a normal age-related change rather than a complication of MI. Determine whether the dysrhythmia is causing significant symptoms. Then notify the physician.
- If beta blockers are used, assess the patient carefully for the development of side effects. Exacerbation of the depression some older adults have is a significant problem with beta blockade.
- Plan slow, steady increases in activity. Older adults with minimal previous exercise show particular benefit from a gradual increase in activity.
- Older adults should plan longer warm-up and cool-down periods when participating in an exercise program. Their pulse rates may not return to baseline until 30 minutes or longer after exercise.

---

the patient to decrease a threat and use problem-focused coping mechanisms. The patient may avoid discussing what has happened and yet comply with treatment regimens. This type of denial decreases anxiety and should not be discouraged. *However, denial that results in a patient who refuses to follow treatment regimens can be harmful.* Because this behavior is usually due to extreme anxiety or fear, threats only worsen the behavior. Remain calm, and avoid confronting the patient. Clearly indicate when a behavior is not acceptable and is potentially harmful as a result of noncompliance.

Anger may represent an attempt to regain control of life. Encourage the patient to verbalize the source of frustration, and provide opportunities for decision making and control. Collaborate with the certified spiritual chaplain or social worker in the hospital to help the patient cope with the situation based on his or her preferences, values, and beliefs. Help the patient identify support systems, such as family, friends, church, or social group.

Depression may be a response to grief and loss of function. Listen as the patient verbalizes feelings of loss, being careful not to offer false or general reassurances. Acknowledge depression, but encourage the patient to perform ADLs and other activities within restrictions.

Identifying and Managing Dysrhythmias
Planning: Expected Outcomes. The most desired outcome for the patient is that he or she will be free of dysrhythmias. If dysrhythmias occur, they will be identified and managed early to prevent complications or death.

Interventions. *Dysrhythmias are the leading cause of prehospital death in most patients with ACS.* Even in the early period of hospitalization, most patients with ACS experience some abnormal cardiac rhythm. When a dysrhythmia develops:
- Identify the dysrhythmia.
- Assess hemodynamic status.
- Evaluate for discomfort.

Dysrhythmias are treated when they cause hemodynamic compromise, increase myocardial oxygen requirements, or predispose the patient to lethal ventricular dysrhythmias.

Typical dysrhythmias for the patient with an *inferior* ACS are bradycardias and second-degree AV blocks resulting from ischemia of the AV node. These rhythms tend to be intermittent. Monitor the cardiac rhythm and rate and the hemodynamic status. If the patient becomes hemodynamically unstable, a temporary pacemaker may be necessary.

The patient with an *anterior* ACS is likely to exhibit premature ventricular contractions (PVCs) caused by ventricular irritability. Third-degree or bundle branch block is a serious complication in this patient because it indicates that a large portion of the left ventricle is involved. The health care provider may insert a pacemaker. Observe the patient closely to detect the development of heart failure. Appropriate interventions for dysrhythmias are described in Chapter 34.

Monitoring for and Managing Heart Failure
Planning: Expected Outcomes. The most desired outcome for the patient is that he or she will be free of heart failure. However, if it occurs, the outcome is that the heart failure will be identified and treated early to prevent further complications.

Interventions. Decreased cardiac output related to heart failure is a relatively common complication after an MI resulting from left ventricular dysfunction, rupture of the intraventricular septum, papillary muscle rupture with valvular dysfunction, or right ventricular infarction. The most severe form of acute heart failure, *cardiogenic shock,* discussed later in this chapter, causes most in-hospital deaths after an ACS. The type of management used to increase cardiac output depends on the location of the ACS and the type of heart failure that resulted from the infarction.

Managing Left Ventricular Failure. When a patient with ACS experiences damage to the left ventricle, rupture of the intraventricular septum, or tear of a papillary muscle, the amount of blood that the heart can eject is reduced. When volume and pressure are markedly increased in the pulmonary vasculature, pulmonary complications can develop.

Assess for manifestations of left ventricular failure and pulmonary edema by listening for crackles and identifying their location in the lung fields. Wheezing, tachypnea, and frothy sputum may also occur with pulmonary edema. Auscultate the heart, paying particular attention to the presence of an S_3 heart sound.

! NURSING SAFETY PRIORITY (QSEN)

Critical Rescue

Monitor for, report, and document these signs of inadequate organ PERFUSION that may result from decreased cardiac output:
- A change in orientation or mental status
- Urine output less than 0.5-1 mL/kg/hr
- Cool, clammy extremities with decreased or absent pulses
- Unusual fatigue
- Recurrent chest pain

In specialized units, hemodynamic monitoring requiring the insertion of a pulmonary artery catheter may be started to assess the patient's preload, afterload, and cardiac output.

Hemodynamic Monitoring. Hemodynamic monitoring is an invasive system used in critical care areas to provide quantitative information about vascular capacity, blood volume, pump effectiveness, and tissue PERFUSION. It directly measures pressures in the heart and great vessels. These procedures are usually performed for more seriously ill patients and can provide more accurate measurements of blood pressure, heart function, and volume status. Although medical-surgical nurses do not manage these systems on general hospital units, they should be familiar with the interpretation of some of the major hemodynamic pressures as they relate to patient assessment.

Hemodynamic monitoring does involve significant risks, although complications are uncommon. Therefore informed consent is required. After obtaining consent, the critical care nurse prepares a pressure-monitoring system. The components of this system are a catheter with an infusion system, a transducer, and a monitor. The catheter receives the pressure waves (mechanical energy) from the heart or the great vessels. The transducer converts the mechanical energy into electrical energy, which is displayed as waveforms or numbers on the monitor. Patency of the catheter is maintained with a slow continuous flush of normal saline, usually infused at 3 to 4 mL/hr under pressure to prevent the backup of blood and occlusion of the catheter.

To prepare the transducer, balance and calibrate it according to hospital policy and the manufacturer's specifications. Finally, identify the phlebostatic axis (Chart 38-6) and level the

---

CHART 38-6 Best Practice for Patient Safety & Quality Care (QSEN)

Identification of the Phlebostatic Axis

1. Position the patient supine.
2. Palpate the fourth intercostal space at the sternum.
3. Follow the fourth intercostal space to the side of the patient's chest.
4. Determine the midway point between anterior and posterior.
5. Find the intersection between the midway point and the line from the fourth intercostal space, and mark it with an X in indelible ink. This is the phlebostatic axis.

---

transducer to it. The physician inserts a balloon-tipped catheter percutaneously through a large vein, usually the internal jugular or subclavian, and directs it to the right atrium (RA). When the catheter tip reaches the RA, the physician inflates the balloon. The catheter advances with the flow of blood through the tricuspid valve, into the right ventricle, past the pulmonic valve, and into a branch of the pulmonary artery. The balloon is deflated after the catheter tip reaches the pulmonary artery. Waveforms are viewed on the monitor as the pulmonary artery catheter is advanced (Fig. 38-3). A chest x-ray is used to check the location of the catheter.

A pulmonary artery catheter is a multi-lumen catheter with the capacity to measure right atrial and indirect left atrial pressures or pulmonary artery wedge pressure (PAWP), also known as the **pulmonary artery occlusive pressure (PAOP)**. A cardiac output measurement may also be obtained, as well as cardiac index and systemic and pulmonary vascular resistance.

Right atrial pressure is measured by a pressure sensor on the catheter inside the RA. Normal RA pressure ranges from 1 to 8 mm Hg. *Increased RA pressures may occur with right ventricular failure, whereas low RA pressures usually indicate hypovolemia.*

Normal pulmonary artery pressure (PAP) ranges from 15 to 26 mm Hg systolic/5 to 15 mm Hg diastolic (mean, 15) and is constantly visible on the monitor. When the balloon at the catheter tip is inflated, the catheter advances and wedges in a branch of the pulmonary artery. The tip of the catheter can sense pressures transmitted from the left atrium, which reflect left ventricular end-diastolic pressure (LVEDP). The pressure measured during balloon inflation is called the **pulmonary artery wedge pressure (PAWP)**. PAWP closely reflects left atrial pressure and LVEDP in patients with normal left ventricular function, normal heart rates, and no mitral valve disease. The PAWP is a mean pressure and normally ranges between 4 and 12 mm Hg.

Elevated PAWP measurements may indicate left ventricular failure, hypervolemia, mitral regurgitation, or intracardiac shunt. A decreased PAWP is seen with hypovolemia or afterload reduction. Individual values may be less important than the trend in values.

The critical care nurse obtains and records RA pressure, PAP, and PAWP at appropriate intervals (usually every 1 to 4 hours). Single values of these measurements are less significant than the trend of values combined with the patient's clinical manifestations. They help health care providers identify heart failure and guide the administration of fluids and vasoactive drugs. During pressure recording, it is important that the transducer be at the level of the phlebostatic axis. The patient is usually supine with

Catheter placement for pulmonary artery pressure

Pulmonic valve

Right ventricle

Tricuspid valve

Catheter placement for pulmonary artery wedge pressure

Typical pulmonary artery pressure tracing

Typical pulmonary artery wedge pressure tracing

FIG. 38-3 Cardiac pressure waveforms can be seen on the monitor.

the head elevated up to 45 degrees during hemodynamic readings, although the position may not affect results. If the balloon remains in the wedge position after PAWP measurement, try to change the catheter's position by asking the patient to cough or by changing his or her position. *If these methods are not successful, notify the physician immediately.*

Change the occlusive sterile dressing over the catheter according to hospital policy. Inspect the insertion site for redness, induration, swelling, drainage, and intactness of the sutures. Detailed discussion of the management and care of patients with pulmonary artery catheters can be found in textbooks on critical care nursing.

Be sure to assess for a number of complications associated with pulmonary artery catheters. For example, pulmonary infarction or pulmonary rupture may occur if the catheter remains in the wedge position. Air embolism is possible if the balloon has ruptured and repeated attempts are made to inflate it. Ventricular dysrhythmias may occur during insertion or if the catheter tip slips back into the right ventricle and irritates the myocardium. Thrombus and embolus formation may occur at the catheter site. Infection may result, and bleeding may be pronounced if the infusion system becomes disconnected.

Direct measurement of *arterial BP* is done by invasive arterial catheter in critically ill patients. The physician or specially trained health care professional inserts an intra-arterial catheter into the radial or femoral artery. After the catheter is inserted, it is attached to pressure tubing. A normal saline flush solution is infused constantly under pressure to maintain the integrity of the system. A transducer attached to the tubing allows continuous direct monitoring of the arterial BP. Direct measurements of BP are usually 10 to 15 mm Hg greater than indirect (cuff) measurements. The arterial catheter may also be used to obtain blood samples for arterial blood gas values and other blood tests.

Because the arterial vasculature is a high-pressure system, frequent assessment of the arterial site and infusion system is

TABLE 38-3	**Killip Classification of Heart Failure**
CLASS	**DESCRIPTION**
I	Absent crackles and S$_3$
II	Crackles in the lower half of the lung fields and possible S$_3$
III	Crackles more than halfway up the lung fields and frequent pulmonary edema
IV	Cardiogenic shock

essential. *Note any bleeding around the intra-arterial catheter or any loose connections, and correct the situation immediately.* Collateral circulation must be assessed by Doppler before and while the arterial catheter is in place. Carefully monitor color, pulse, and temperature distal to the insertion site for any early signs of circulatory compromise. Complications of systemic intra-arterial monitoring include pain, infection, arteriospasm, or obstruction at the site with the potential for distal infarction, air embolism, and hemorrhage.

Classification of Post–Myocardial Infarction Heart Failure. Several classification systems may be used to categorize heart failure after an MI. For example, the classic Killip system identifies four classes based on prognosis (Table 38-3). This system complements the ACC/AHA heart failure classification of function assessment discussed in Chapter 35.

Patients with *class I* heart failure often respond well to reduction in preload with IV nitrates and diuretics. Monitor the urine output hourly, check vital signs hourly, continue to assess for signs of heart failure, and review the serum potassium level.

Patients with *class II* and *class III* heart failure may require diuresis and more aggressive medical intervention, such as afterload reduction and/or enhancement of contractility. IV nitroprusside or nitroglycerin may be used to decrease both preload and afterload. These drugs are given as continuous infusions in specialized units where the PAWP and BP can be closely monitored. The BP can drop in response to excessive vasodilation.

Patients in *classes II* and *III* are usually started on once-a-day beta blockers (usually Toprol XR or Coreg CR). Dosing is titrated depending on goal achievement and drug tolerance. Other drugs, including ACE inhibitors and ARBs, are commonly prescribed to promote ventricular remodeling. These drugs are described in Chart 38-4 and in Chapter 36.

Positive inotropes, such as dobutamine (Dobutrex) and milrinone (Primacor), increase the force of cardiac contraction. They are administered by continuous IV infusion. The effects of these drugs on the blood vessels and heart rate vary and may be dose dependent. The infusions are titrated to promote cardiac output.

> ### ! NURSING SAFETY PRIORITY (QSEN)
> #### *Drug Alert*
>
> Use caution when giving positive inotropes because of the potential risk for increasing myocardial oxygen consumption and further decreasing cardiac output. Monitor the patient frequently, paying particular attention to the development of chest pain.

Class IV heart failure is cardiogenic shock. In **cardiogenic shock,** necrosis of more than 40% of the left ventricle occurs. Most patients have a stuttering pattern of chest pain, resulting in piecemeal extension of the ACS.

> ### ! NURSING SAFETY PRIORITY (QSEN)
> #### *Critical Rescue*
>
> Monitor for, report, and document manifestations of cardiogenic shock immediately. These signs and symptoms include:
> * Tachycardia
> * Hypotension
> * Systolic BP less than 90 mm Hg or 30 mm Hg less than the patient's baseline
> * Urine output less than 0.5-1 mL/kg/hr
> * Cold, clammy skin with poor peripheral pulses
> * Agitation, restlessness, or confusion
> * Pulmonary congestion
> * Tachypnea
> * Continuing chest discomfort
> *Early detection is essential because undiagnosed cardiogenic shock has a high mortality rate!*

Drug Therapy. Medical interventions aim to relieve pain and decrease myocardial oxygen requirements through preload and afterload reduction (see Chart 38-4 and Chart 38-7). The health care provider prescribes IV morphine, which is used to decrease pulmonary congestion and relieve pain. Oxygen is administered. Intubation and mechanical ventilation may be necessary.

Use the information gained from hemodynamic monitoring to titrate drug therapy. Preload reduction may be cautiously attempted with diuretics or nitroglycerin, as described for patients with Killip class III heart failure. (See Chapter 35 for a complete discussion of preload and afterload.) Monitor systolic pressure continuously because vasodilation may result in a further decline in BP. Vasopressors and positive inotropes may be used to maintain organ perfusion, but these drugs increase myocardial oxygen consumption and can worsen ischemia. Use extreme caution in giving drug therapy.

Other Interventions for Left-Sided Heart Failure. When patients do not respond to drug therapy with improved tissue perfusion, decreased workload of the heart, and increased cardiac contractility, an **intra-aortic balloon pump (IABP)** may be inserted. The IABP is an invasive intervention that is used to improve myocardial perfusion during an acute MI, reduce preload and afterload, and facilitate left ventricular ejection.

The health care provider can insert the device percutaneously or through a surgical cutdown. Inflation of the IABP during diastole augments the diastolic pressure and improves coronary perfusion by increasing blood flow to the arteries. Deflation of the balloon just before systole reduces afterload at the time of systolic contraction. This action facilitates emptying of the left ventricle and improves cardiac output. The balloon catheter is attached to a pump console, which is triggered by an ECG tracing and arterial waveform.

In patients undergoing high-risk percutaneous coronary intervention (PCI) or those at risk for cardiogenic shock, a *percutaneous ventricular assist device* may be used. These devices are temporary to decrease the myocardial workload and oxygen consumption of the heart and increase cardiac output and peripheral perfusion.

Immediate reperfusion is an invasive intervention that shows some promise for managing cardiogenic shock. The patient is taken to the cardiac catheterization laboratory, and an emergency left-sided heart catheterization is performed. If he or she has a treatable occlusion or occlusions, the interventional cardiologist performs a percutaneous coronary intervention in the catheterization laboratory or the patient is transferred to the operating suite for a coronary artery bypass graft (CABG).

Managing Right Ventricular Failure. Conditions other than left ventricular failure may result in decreased cardiac output after an ACS. In about a third of patients with inferior MIs, right ventricular infarction and failure develop. In this instance, the right ventricle fails independently of the left. Decreased cardiac output with a paradoxical pulse, clear lungs, and jugular venous distention occurs when the patient is in semi-Fowler's position.

A right ventricular MI may be documented by echocardiography and by an ECG using right-sided precordial leads. The desired outcome of management is to improve right ventricular stroke volume by increasing right ventricular fiber stretch or preload. To enhance right ventricular preload, give sufficient fluids (as much as 200 mL/hr) to increase right atrial pressure to 20 mm Hg. In the critical care unit, *monitor the pulmonary artery wedge pressure (PAWP)—attempting to maintain it below 15 to 20 mm Hg—and auscultate the lungs to assess for left-sided heart failure. If symptoms of this complication occur, notify the health care provider immediately.*

Monitoring for and Managing Recurrent Symptoms and Extension of Injury

Planning: Expected Outcomes. The most desired outcome is that the patient will not have recurrent symptoms or an

CHART 38-7 Common Examples of Drug Therapy

Commonly Used Intravenous Vasodilators and Inotropes

DRUG	USUAL DOSAGE	NURSING INTERVENTIONS	RATIONALES
Nitrates			
Nitroprusside sodium (Nipride, Nitropress)	IV only by infusion device Begin with 0.4-0.5 mcg/kg/min May increase gradually to 10 mcg/kg/min	Monitor BP every 2-5 min when initiating therapy. If BP drops excessively, elevate the legs, decrease the dose, and increase fluids per unit policy. Monitor PAWP, SVR, BP, heart rate, urine output frequently. Titrate medication to obtain the desired effect. Protect from light. Maintain dose at less than 3 mcg/kg/min if possible. In patients requiring doses higher than 3 mcg/kg/min for longer than 24-36 hr, monitor for metabolic acidosis, confusion, or hyperreflexia. Examine blood thiocyanate level.	This agent is a potent, rapidly reversible vasodilator acting on both peripheral venous and arterial musculature. BP may drop in 2 min. This agent is light sensitive. Doses higher than 3 mcg/kg/min are associated with thiocyanate or cyanide toxicity. These are indications of the toxic effects of cyanide.
Nitroglycerin (Tridil)	IV only by infusion device Begin with 5 mcg/kg/min and gradually increase in increments of 5 every 3-5 min If no response after 20 mcg/kg/min, increase by 10-20 mcg until desired response	Monitor BP every 1-3 min when initiating therapy. If BP drops excessively, elevate the legs and decrease the dose according to unit policies. Monitor RAP, PAWP, SVR, BP, heart rate, and urine output frequently. Titrate medication to obtain the desired effect. Intermittent administration of IV nitroglycerin should be considered. Monitor patients for headache.	This agent dilates coronary arteries. It is a more potent systemic vasodilator than an arterial vasodilator. BP may drop in 1 min. Tolerance may develop rapidly to nitroglycerin administered by continuous IV. Headache is a frequent side effect of initial nitroglycerin therapy.
Milrinone (Primacor)	IV bolus 50 mcg/kg given over 10 min; start infusion of 0.375-0.75 mcg/kg/min; reduce dose in renal impairment	Assess BP and pulse every 5 min. If systolic BP drops 30 mm Hg, stop infusion and call health care provider. Monitor I&O and weight.	Hypotension is a common adverse effect. The drug causes diuresis.
Fenoldopam (Corlopam)	0.01-1.6 mcg/kg/min IV	Assess BP and pulse every 5 min, then every 1 hr × 2, then every 4 hr, or according to agency policy. Monitor I&O, and assess for signs of dehydration. Observe IV site for extravasation.	Same as for milrinone.
Sympathomimetics			
Dopamine (Intropin)	IV only by infusion device Starting dose 2-5 mcg/kg/min Titrate up to 50 mcg/kg/min	Determine the reason for use and the expected result. Observe the patient's heart rate, ECG, BP, PAWP, SVR, cardiac output, and urine output every 5 min to every 1 hr. Titrate the dose carefully to maintain the dose range and obtain the desired effect. Infuse through a central catheter. Monitor patients for ectopy and angina.	This agent is a dose-dependent activator of alpha, beta, and dopaminergic receptors. 2-5 mcg/kg/min stimulates dopaminergic receptors, which promotes renal and mesenteric blood flow. 5 mcg/kg/min stimulates beta receptors. This increases heart rate and contractility more than 10-15 mcg/kg/min; alpha effects predominate. This causes peripheral constriction. Extravasation can cause tissue necrosis and sloughing. These are adverse effects.
Dobutamine (Dobutrex)	IV only by infusion device, 2-10 mcg/kg/min. May increase to 40 mcg/kg/min.	Observe patients continuously during administration. Titrate the drug on the basis of adequate tissue perfusion: mentation, skin temperature, peripheral pulses, PAWP, cardiac output, SVR, and urine output. Monitor for atrial and ventricular ectopy.	This agent is a very strong beta$_1$-receptor activator and a moderately strong beta$_2$-receptor activator. Dysrhythmias are an adverse effect.

BP, Blood pressure; ECG, electrocardiogram; I&O, input and output; PAWP, pulmonary artery wedge pressure; RAP, right atrial pressure; SVR, systemic vascular resistance.

1. The balloon-tipped catheter is positioned in the artery.

2. The uninflated balloon is centered in the obstruction.

3. The balloon is inflated, which flattens plaque against the artery wall.

4. The balloon is removed, and the artery is left unoccluded.

FIG. 38-4 Percutaneous coronary intervention.

extension of myocardial injury. If these problems occur, they will be identified and treated early to prevent further complications or death.

Interventions. *Recurrent discomfort despite medical therapy is one of the major indications for surgical management of CAD.* Patients who continue to have chest discomfort despite medical therapy or who have ischemia during a stress test may require invasive correction by PCI or CABG to resolve angina or prevent MI. Before invasive treatment, a left-sided cardiac catheterization with coronary angiogram is performed to document that the lesions are correctable and that left ventricular pump function is adequate.

Percutaneous Coronary Intervention. **Percutaneous coronary intervention (PCI)** is an invasive but nonsurgical technique that is performed within 90 minutes of an acute MI (AMI) diagnosis. Hospitals are required to report how many patients with AMI receive a PCI within that time frame per the AMI Core Measure Set. It is performed to reduce the frequency and severity of discomfort for patients with angina and to bridge patients to coronary artery bypass graft (CABG) surgery. It combines clot retrieval, coronary angioplasty, and stent placement. Under fluoroscopic guidance, the cardiologist performs initial coronary angiography. In the STEMI patient, if a clot is seen, a clot retrieval device is inserted over the guidewire and the clot is removed. Once the clot is removed in the STEMI patient or area of narrowing is identified in the NSTEMI patient, a balloon-tipped catheter is introduced through a guidewire to the coronary artery occlusion. The physician activates a compressor that inflates the balloon (angioplasty) to force the plaque against the vessel wall, thus dilating the wall, and reduces or eliminates the occluding clot. Balloon inflation may be repeated until angiography indicates a decrease in the stenosis (narrowing) to less than 50% of the vessel's diameter (Fig. 38-4). The balloon catheter is then withdrawn, and a balloon catheter with stent is introduced. Once the stent and balloon are in position, the stent is deployed by the balloon inflation. The balloon is deflated and the stent stays in place acting as scaffolding to hold the diseased artery open. **Stents** are expandable metal mesh devices that are used to maintain the patent lumen created by angioplasty or atherectomy. Bare metal or drug-eluting stents (DES) (drug-coated) may be used. By

FIG. 38-5 A coronary stent open after balloon inflation.

providing a supportive scaffold, these devices prevent closure of the vessel from arterial dissection or vasospasm. Fig. 38-5 shows a stent positioned in a coronary artery.

Patients who are most likely to benefit from PCI have single- or double-vessel disease with discrete, proximal, noncalcified lesions or clots. This procedure often does not work for complex clots. When identifying which lesions are treatable with PCI, the cardiologist considers the clot's complexity and location, as well as the amount of myocardium at risk. Although treating lesions located in the left main artery places a large amount of myocardial tissue at risk if the vessel closes quickly, these lesions are now being treated more with PCI. In the past, coronary artery bypass grafting (CABG) was the intervention used for these patients. PCI may also be used for the patient with an evolving acute MI, either alone or with thrombolytic therapy or glycoprotein (GP) IIb/IIIa inhibitor, to reperfuse the damaged myocardium.

Without stent placement, the artery often reoccludes due to the artery's normal elasticity and memory. Patients who undergo PCI are required to take dual antiplatelet therapy (DAT) consisting of aspirin and a P2Y12 inhibitor (see Chart 38-4). Before the procedure, the patient receives an initial dose of a P2Y12 platelet inhibitor (clopidogrel [Plavix]) or ticagrelor [Brilinta]) and aspirin. If prasugrel (Effient) is the preferred P2Y12 platelet inhibitor, it is given immediately after PCI. If there are any concerns that the patient may require CABG, the P2Y12 inhibitor may be held until after the procedure. The inhibition of the platelets is permanent and increases the risk for postoperative bleeding. Patients should wait 5 (clopidogrel and ticagrelor) to 7 (prasugrel) days before undergoing CABG. If the patient has received thrombolytic therapy, clopidogrel (Plavix) is the preferred drug.

During the procedure, the patient may receive boluses of IV heparin or a continuous infusion of bivalirudin (Angiomax). Heparin is used to maintain an elevated activated clotting time and prevent clotting on wires and catheters during the procedure. Heparin is discontinued before removal of the catheters. Bivalirudin (Angiomax) is a direct thrombin inhibitor and is frequently used as an alternative to IIb/IIIa inhibitors and heparin. Bivalirudin has a short half-life (25 minutes) and is less dependent on renal function. IV or intracoronary nitroglycerin or diltiazem (Cardizem) is given to prevent coronary vasospasm. PCI initially reopens the vessel in most appropriately selected patients. Within the first 24 hours, however, a small percentage of patients have re-stenosis. At 6 months, a larger number have one or more blockages.

> ## ! NURSING SAFETY PRIORITY (QSEN)
> ### *Critical Rescue*
>
> After PCI, monitor for potential problems including acute closure of the vessel (causes chest pain), bleeding from the insertion site, and reaction to the contrast medium used in angiography. Also monitor for and document hypotension, hypokalemia, and dysrhythmias. Document and report any of these findings to the physician or Rapid Response Team immediately!

The health care provider also prescribes a long-term nitrate and beta blocker, and an ACE inhibitor or ARB is added for patients who have had primary angioplasty after an MI. Some patients may experience hypokalemia after the procedure and require careful monitoring and potassium supplements. The nursing interventions for patients receiving these drugs are described in Chart 38-4. Provide careful explanations of drug therapy and any recommended lifestyle changes.

Other Procedures. Other techniques being used to ensure continued patency of the vessel are laser angioplasty (the laser breaks up the clot) and atherectomy. Atherectomy devices can either excise and retrieve plaque or emulsify it. One of the advantages of this procedure is that it creates a less bulky vessel with better elastic recoil. Another procedure that may be performed is rheolytic thrombectomy (e.g., AngioJet, Vortex), which uses low-pressure, high-speed saline jets to break up the clot. The EndiCOR X-SIZER lances and aspirates a clot simultaneously.

Injecting vascular endothelial growth factor (VEGF) during angioplasty has increased PERFUSION to the wall of the heart. Also, VEGF helps initiate new blood vessel growth and development, which results in increased blood supply to cardiac muscle.

Traditional Coronary Artery Bypass Graft Surgery. Over 500,000 traditional open coronary artery bypass graft (CABG) surgeries are performed in the United States each year (Go et al., 2013). It is the most common type of cardiac surgery and the most common procedure for older adults. Almost half of all CABGs are done for patients older than 65 years. The occluded coronary arteries are bypassed with the patient's own venous or arterial blood vessels or synthetic grafts. The internal mammary artery (IMA) is the current graft of choice because it has an excellent patency rate many years after the procedure.

CABG is indicated when patients do not respond to medical management of CAD or when disease progression is evident.

Because of the development of drug-eluting stents (DESs), patients who previously had no option other than CABG have been able to have their vessels revascularized without surgery. The decision for surgery is based on the patient's symptoms and the results of cardiac catheterization. Candidates for surgery are patients who have:

- Angina with greater than 50% occlusion of the left main coronary artery that cannot be stented
- Unstable angina with severe two-vessel disease, moderate three-vessel disease, or small-vessel disease in which stents could not be introduced
- Ischemia with heart failure
- Acute MI with cardiogenic shock
- Signs of ischemia or impending MI after angiography or percutaneous transluminal coronary angioplasty (PTCA)
- Valvular disease
- Coronary vessels unsuitable for PCI

The vessels to be bypassed should have proximal clots blocking more than 70% of the vessel's diameter but with good distal runoff. Bypass of less occluded vessels may result in poor perfusion through the graft and early obstruction. CABG is most effective when adequate ventricular function remains and the ejection fraction is close to or greater than 50%. Patients with lower ejection fractions are subject to develop more complications.

For most patients, the risk is low and the benefits of bypass surgery are clear. Surgical treatment of CAD does not appear to affect the life span. Left ventricular function is the most important long-term indicator of survival. CABG improves the quality of life for most patients. Most are pain-free at 1 year after surgery and remain so at 5 years after the procedure. The percentage of patients experiencing some PAIN increases sharply after 5 years.

Preoperative Care. CABG surgery may be planned as an elective procedure or performed as an emergency. It may be done as a *traditional* operative technique or performed as a *minimally invasive surgical (MIS)* technique, discussed later on p. 777. Patients undergoing elective surgery are admitted on the morning of surgery. Preoperative preparations and teaching are completed during prehospitalization interviews. Teach patients that their drugs will be changed after surgery. Ensure that the necessary drugs have been administered before surgery.

Familiarize the patient and family with the cardiac surgical–critical care unit (sometimes referred to as the "open heart" unit), and prepare them for postoperative care. If the procedure is elective, demonstrate and have the patient return a demonstration of how to splint the chest incision, cough, deep breathe, and perform arm and leg exercises. Stress that:

- The patient should report any PAIN to the nursing staff.
- Most of the pain will be in the site where the vessel was harvested. (With the use of endovascular vessel harvesting [EVH] and one or two small incisions, the pain and edema are less than for previously performed procedures.)
- Analgesics will be given for pain.
- Coughing and deep breathing are essential to prevent pulmonary complications.
- Early ambulation is important to decrease the risk for venous thrombosis and possible embolism.

For the traditional surgical procedure, explain that the patient will have a sternal incision; possibly a large leg incision; one, two, or three chest tubes; an indwelling urinary catheter; pacemaker wires; and hemodynamic monitoring. An endotracheal tube will be connected to a ventilator for several hours postoperatively. Tell the patient and family that the patient will not be able to talk while the endotracheal tube is in place. When describing the postoperative course, emphasize that close monitoring and the use of sophisticated equipment are standard treatment.

Preoperative anxiety is common. An appropriate nursing assessment should identify the level of anxiety and the coping methods patients have used successfully in the past. Some patients may find it helpful to define their fears. Common sources of fear include fear of the unknown, fear of bodily harm, and fear of death.

In elective procedures, patients may benefit from detailed information about the surgery, depending on individual preferences and cultural practices. Others may feel overwhelmed by so much material. Some patients need to discuss their feelings in detail or describe the experiences of people they know who have undergone CABG. Assess patients' anxiety level and help them cope.

Operative Procedures. Coronary artery bypass surgery is performed with the patient under general anesthesia for both cardiopulmonary bypass and off-pump surgery. For the *traditional operative procedure,* the cardiac surgical team begins the procedure with a median sternotomy incision and visualization of the heart and great vessels. Another surgical team may begin harvesting the vein if it is to be used for the graft. Synthetic grafts may be used instead.

Cardiopulmonary bypass (CPB) is used to provide oxygenation, circulation, and hypothermia during induced cardiac arrest. Blood is diverted from the heart to the bypass machine, where it is heparinized, oxygenated, and returned to the circulation through a cannula placed in the ascending aortic arch or femoral artery (Fig. 38-6). During bypass, the patient's core temperature remains between 95° F (35° C) (cold cardioplegia) and normal temperature (warm cardioplegia). Although cooling decreases the rate of metabolism and demand for oxygen, keeping the heart "warm" decreases postoperative complications that were more common when cold cardioplegia was used. The heart is perfused with a potassium solution, which decreases myocardial oxygen consumption and causes the heart to stop during diastole. This process ensures a motionless operative field and prevents myocardial ischemia.

Once the heart is arrested, the grafting procedure can begin. The surgeon uses the internal mammary artery (IMA), a saphenous vein, and/or a radial artery to bypass blockages in the coronary arteries (Fig. 38-7). The distal end of the vessel graft is dissected and attached below the clot in the coronary artery. If the surgeon uses a venous graft or the radial artery, it is anastomosed (sutured) proximally to the aorta and distally to the coronary artery just beyond the occlusion, thus improving myocardial perfusion. After flow rates through the grafts are measured, the heart is rewarmed slowly. The cardioplegic solution is flushed from the heart. The heart regains its rate and rhythm, or it may be defibrillated to return it to a normal rhythm. When the procedure is completed, the patient may be rewarmed (if cold cardioplegia was used) and weaned from the bypass machine while the grafts are observed for patency and leakage. The surgeon may place atrial and ventricular pacemaker wires and mediastinal and pleural chest tubes. Finally, the surgeon closes the sternum with wire sutures.

Postoperative Care. After traditional surgery, the patient is transported to a post–open heart surgery unit and undergoes mechanical ventilation for 3 to 6 hours. He or she requires highly skilled nursing care from a nurse qualified to provide post–cardiac surgery care, including routine postoperative care described in Chapter 16. *Be sure to use sterile technique when changing sternal or donor-site dressings.*

Connect the mediastinal tubes to water seal drainage systems, and ground the epicardial pacer wires by connecting them to the pacemaker generator. Monitor pulmonary artery and arterial pressures, as well as the heart rate and rhythm, which are displayed on a monitor.

FIG. 38-6 Heart-lung bypass circuitry used during cardiopulmonary bypass.

FIG. 38-7 Two methods of coronary artery bypass grafting. The procedure used depends on the nature of the coronary artery disease, the condition of the vessels available for grafting, and the patient's health status.

Closely assess the patient for dysrhythmias, such as brady-dysrhythmias, atrial fibrillation, or heart block. Manage symptomatic dysrhythmias according to unit protocol or the health care provider's prescription. Hypoxemia and hypokalemia are frequent causes of ventricular dysrhythmias. If the patient has symptomatic bradydysrhythmias or heart block, turn on the pacemaker and adjust the pacemaker settings as prescribed. Monitor for, report, and document other complications of CABG, including:

- Fluid and electrolyte imbalance
- Hypotension
- Hypothermia
- Hypertension
- Bleeding
- Cardiac tamponade
- Decreased level of consciousness
- Anginal pain

Managing Fluid and Electrolyte Imbalance. Assessing fluid and electrolyte balance is a high priority in the early postoperative period. Edema is common. However, decisions concerning fluid administration are made on the basis of BP, pulmonary artery wedge pressure (PAWP), right atrial pressure, cardiac output, cardiac index, systemic vascular resistance, blood loss, and urine output. An experienced specialized nurse interprets the assessment findings and adjusts fluid administration on the basis of standing unit policies or specific prescription from the physician.

Serum electrolytes (especially calcium, magnesium, and potassium) may be decreased postoperatively and are monitored carefully. Because the serum potassium level can fluctuate dramatically, electrolyte levels are checked frequently, since imbalances can cause dysrhythmias. Potassium and magnesium depletions are common and may result from hemodilution or diuretic therapy. Calcium replacement is based on the *ionized* serum calcium. The desired potassium level is 4.0 mEq/L, and the magnesium level should be 2.2 mEq/L.

If the serum potassium level is decreased, the health care provider may prescribe IV potassium replacement. The dose of potassium given exceeds the usual recommended level of no more than 20 mEq of potassium per hour. For potassium replacement, as much as 40 to 80 mEq may be mixed in 100 mL of IV solution and given at a rate up to 40 mEq per hour. The drug must be given through a central catheter and controlled by an infusion pump. The patient is placed on a cardiac monitor for intense, focused nursing observation.

Managing Other Complications. Hypotension (systolic BP <90 mm Hg) is a major problem because it may result in the collapse of the coronary graft. Decreased preload (decreased PAWP) can result from hypovolemia or vasodilation. If the patient is hypovolemic, it might be appropriate to increase fluid administration or administer blood. The health care provider may manage the patient with volume replacement followed by vasopressor therapy to increase the BP. However, if hypotension is the result of left ventricular failure (increased PAWP), IV inotropes might be needed.

Hypothermia is a common problem after surgery. Although warm cardioplegia is now the usual operative procedure used, it is not uncommon for the body temperature to drift downward after the patient leaves the surgical suite. Monitor the body temperature, and institute rewarming procedures if the temperature drops below 96.8° F (36° C). Rewarming may be accomplished with warm blankets, lights, or thermal blankets. The danger of rewarming patients too quickly is that they may begin shivering, resulting in metabolic acidosis, increased myocardial oxygen consumption, and hypoxia. To prevent shivering, rewarming should proceed at a rate no faster than 1.8° F (1° C) per hour. Discontinue the procedure when the body temperature approaches 98.6° F (37° C) and the patient's extremities feel warm.

Hypothermia is a significant risk for the patient after CABG surgery because it promotes vasoconstriction and *hypertension.* Other factors contributing to hypertension in the CABG patient include CPB, drug therapy, and increased sympathetic nervous system activity.

After surgery, many patients experience *hypertension* (hypertension is defined as a systolic BP greater than 140 to

150 mm Hg). Hypertension is dangerous because increased pressure promotes leakage from suture lines and may cause bleeding. Drugs such as nitroprusside (Nipride) or fenoldopam (Corlopam) may be given to decrease afterload, ease the workload of the heart, and prevent heart failure.

⚠ NURSING SAFETY PRIORITY (QSEN)

Action Alert

Bleeding after CABG surgery occurs to a limited extent in all patients. Measure mediastinal and pleural chest tube drainage at least hourly. Report drainage amounts over 150 mL per hour to the surgeon. Patients with internal mammary artery (IMA) grafts may have more chest drainage than those with saphenous vein grafts (from the leg).

To access the IMA, the pleural space has to be entered and requires a pleural chest tube with the mediastinal tubes, making pulmonary assessment crucial. An autotransfusion of chest drainage to assist with volume management when 500 mL has accumulated or 4 hours has elapsed may be done, depending on the clinical pathway or the health care provider's protocol. Maintain the patency of the mediastinal and pleural chest tubes. One effective way of promoting chest tube drainage is to prevent a dependent loop from forming in the tubing.

If the patient is bleeding and the mediastinal tubes are not kept patent, fluid (blood) may accumulate around the heart. The myocardium is then compressed, and cardiac tamponade results. The fluid compresses the atria and ventricles, preventing them from filling adequately and thus reducing cardiac output.

⚠ NURSING SAFETY PRIORITY (QSEN)

Critical Rescue

Assess for, document, and report manifestations of cardiac tamponade immediately, including:

- Sudden cessation of previously heavy mediastinal drainage
- Jugular venous distention but clear lung sounds
- Pulsus paradoxus (BP more than 10 mm Hg higher on expiration than on inspiration)
- An equalizing of PAWP and right atrial pressure
- Cardiovascular collapse

Prepare the patient for echocardiogram or chest x-ray to confirm the diagnosis. Pericardiocentesis (withdrawal of fluid from the pericardium via a large needle) may not be appropriate for tamponade after coronary artery bypass graft (CABG) because the blood in the pericardium may have clotted. Volume expansion and emergency sternotomy with drainage are the treatments of choice.

The patient may also demonstrate *changes in level of consciousness*, which may be permanent or transient (temporary, short-term). Transient changes related to anesthesia, cardiopulmonary bypass (CPB), air emboli, or hypothermia occur in many patients. Assess for neurologic deficits, which may include slowness to arouse, memory loss, and new-onset confusion.

Patients with transient neurologic deficits usually return to baseline neurologic status within 4 to 8 hours. *Permanent*

deficits associated with an intraoperative stroke may be manifested by:

- Abnormal pupillary response
- Failure to awaken from anesthesia
- Seizures
- Absence of sensory or motor function

⚠ NURSING SAFETY PRIORITY (QSEN)

Action Alert

After a CABG, check the patient's neurologic status every 30 to 60 minutes until he or she has awakened from anesthesia. Then check every 2 to 4 hours or per agency policy.

❓ NCLEX EXAMINATION CHALLENGE

Physiological Integrity

The nurse assesses a client who had a coronary artery bypass graft yesterday. Which assessment finding will the nurse report to the surgeon immediately?

A. Incisional pain
B. Blood pressure of 136/76
C. Decreased level of consciousness
D. Apical pulse of 88

Managing Pain. Differentiate between *sternotomy pain*, which is expected after CABG, and *anginal pain*, which might indicate graft failure. Typical sternotomy PAIN is localized, does not radiate, and often becomes worse when the patient coughs or breathes deeply. He or she may describe the pain as sharp, aching, or burning. Pain may stimulate the sympathetic nervous system, which increases the heart rate and vascular resistance while decreasing cardiac output. Administer enough of the prescribed analgesic in adequate doses to control pain. During the process of weaning the patient from mechanical ventilation, however, it may be necessary to use short-acting analgesics and to limit pain medication because of the respiratory depressant effects of analgesia.

Transfer from the Special Care Unit. Mechanical ventilation is usually provided for 3 to 6 hours after surgery until the patient is breathing adequately and is hemodynamically stable. During the first day, the patient usually has pacemaker wires, hemodynamic monitoring lines, and mediastinal tubes removed. He or she is then transferred to an intermediate care unit. *All CABG patients, especially those with IMA grafts, are at high risk for atelectasis, the number-one complication.* Encourage them to splint, cough, turn, and deep breathe to expectorate secretions. Early ambulation after surgery is essential. Two hours after extubation (removal of the endotracheal tube), patients should be dangled as tolerated and turned side to side. Within 4 to 8 hours after extubation, help patients out of bed into a chair. By the first day after surgery, they should be out of bed in a chair and ambulating 25 to 100 feet 3 times a day as tolerated. Continue to monitor for decreased cardiac output, pain, dysrhythmias, decreased oxygen saturation, and infection during these activities.

Many patients have supraventricular dysrhythmias (especially atrial fibrillation) during the postoperative period, usually on the second or third postoperative day. Examine the monitor

! NURSING SAFETY PRIORITY (QSEN)

Action Alert

Monitor the neurovascular status of the donor arm of patients whose radial artery was used as a graft in CABG. Assess the hand color, temperature, pulse (both ulnar and radial), and capillary refill every hour initially. In addition, check the fingertips, hand, and arm for sensation and mobility at least every 4 hours. IV nitroglycerin is often given for the first 24 hours postoperatively to promote vasodilation in the donor arm and therefore maintain circulation.

pattern for atrial fibrillation. When auscultating the heart, listen for an irregular rhythm.

Sternal wound infections develop between 5 days and several weeks after surgery in a small number of patients and are responsible for increased costs and longer hospital stays. Be alert for **mediastinitis** (infection of the mediastinum) by observing for:

- Fever continuing beyond the first 4 days after CABG
- Instability (bogginess) of the sternum
- Redness, induration, swelling, or drainage from suture sites
- An increased white blood cell count

The health care provider may perform a needle biopsy to confirm a sternal infection. Surgical débridement, antibiotic wound irrigation, and IV antibiotics are usually indicated. If sternal osteomyelitis has developed, 4 to 6 weeks of IV antibiotics are required. Prophylactic use of mupirocin (Bactroban) intranasally may be prescribed to decrease the incidence of sternal wound infection.

Postpericardiotomy syndrome is a source of chest discomfort for some post–cardiac surgery patients. The syndrome is characterized by pericardial and pleural pain, pericarditis, a friction rub, an elevated temperature and white blood cell count, and dysrhythmias. Postpericardiotomy syndrome may occur days to weeks after surgery and seems to be associated with blood remaining in the pericardial sac. Observe for the development of pericardial or pleural pain. For most patients, the syndrome is mild and self-limiting. However, they may require treatment similar to that for pericarditis. Be prepared to detect acute cardiac (pericardial) tamponade.

Minimally Invasive Direct Coronary Artery Bypass. The **minimally invasive direct coronary artery bypass (MIDCAB)** (also known as *"keyhole" surgery*) may be indicated for patients with a lesion of the left anterior descending (LAD) artery. In one of the most common MIDCAB procedures, a 2-inch left thoracotomy incision is made and the fourth rib is removed. Then the left internal mammary artery (IMA) is dissected and attached to the still-beating heart below the level of the lesion. Cardiopulmonary bypass (CPB) is not required.

After surgery, assess for chest pain and ECG changes (Q waves and ST-segment and T-wave changes in leads V_2 to V_6) because occlusion of the IMA graft occurs acutely in only a small percentage of patients. *If there is any question of acute graft closure, immediately notify the health care provider.* Patients tend to have more incisional PAIN after MIDCAB than after traditional CABG surgery, but it can usually be managed with oxycodone or codeine. Because they have a thoracotomy incision and a chest tube or smaller-lumen vacuum chest device, patients are encouraged to cough, deep breathe, and use an incentive spirometer for a week postoperatively. Most patients spend

less than 6 hours in a critical care unit and are discharged in 2 or 3 days.

Endovascular (Endoscopic) Vessel Harvesting. Regardless of whether the traditional CABG or the MIDCAB is performed, the donor vessel may be obtained using an endoscope rather than a large surgical incision. The radial artery or a vein in the leg may be taken using this method. Instead of a large, painful incision, the patient has one or two very small incisions in the leg or arm. This procedure has decreased hospital length of stay, postoperative complications, and pain.

Transmyocardial Laser Revascularization. **Transmyocardial laser revascularization** is a procedure for patients with unstable angina and inoperable CAD with areas of reversible myocardial ischemia. After a single-lung intubation, a left anterior thoracotomy is performed and the heart is visualized. A laser is used to create 20 to 24 long, narrow channels through the left ventricular muscle to the left ventricle. These channels will eventually allow oxygenated blood to flow during diastole from the left ventricle to nourish the muscle. After surgery, the patient is transported to a critical care unit, where hemodynamic monitoring is used to assess for anginal episodes and bleeding disturbances.

Off-Pump Coronary Artery Bypass. Off-pump coronary artery bypass (OPCAB) is a procedure in which open heart surgery is performed without the use of a heart-lung bypass machine. Advantages include shorter hospital stays and decreased mortality rate, risk for infection, and cost. The disadvantage of OPCAB is that it requires cardiac surgeons to have increased skill to master the technique.

Robotic Heart Surgery. Robotic heart surgery is a new step toward less invasive open heart surgery. Surgeons operate endoscopically through very small incisions in the chest wall. Use of robotics provides surgeons with capabilities that simplify the surgical process, eliminate tremors that can exist with human hands, increase the ability to reach otherwise inaccessible sites, and improve depth perception and visual acuity.

Other advantages of robotic procedures include shorter hospital stays (average stay is 2 to 3 days), less PAIN because of smaller incisions, no need for heart-lung bypass machine, less anxiety for the patient, and greater patient acceptance. The use of robotics also allows surgeons to perform telesurgery, performing heart procedures over long distances.

Disadvantages include computer failure, limited numbers of surgeons skilled in these techniques, and the length of surgery time (the time is about 50 minutes longer than the conventional surgery).

Community-Based Care

Home Care Management. Case management is most appropriate for patients who meet high-cost, high-volume, and high-risk criteria. Patients with coronary artery disease (CAD) clearly meet all these criteria. Clinical pathways and case management programs for those with CAD are used in most U.S. hospitals. By focusing on cardiovascular risk reduction and improving the continuity of care, health care professionals have reduced the length and cost of hospital stays. Posthospital case management should reduce hospital readmission rates and improve patient health.

Patients who have experienced a myocardial infarction (MI), angina, or coronary artery bypass graft (CABG) surgery are usually discharged to home or to a transitional care setting with drug therapy and specific activity prescriptions. Depending on the procedure, hospital stays may be 3 to 5 days for patients with MI or those undergoing CABG and only 1 to 3 days for those undergoing percutaneous coronary intervention (PCI) or newer surgeries. Therefore patients are still recovering when they are discharged from the hospital and need continuing care.

Patients should not be discharged to home alone. Assess whether the patient has family or friends to provide assistance. In some cases, a home care nurse may be needed (Chart 38-8). Older adults are often living alone when coronary events occur and may have a greater need for home assistance after CABG surgery (Chart 38-9). A patient who was a resident in a

long-term care facility may be returned there after hospitalization for unstable angina, MI, or CABG surgery.

Cardiac rehabilitation is available in most communities for patients after an MI or CABG surgery, but only a small percentage participate in structured rehabilitation programs. Dolansky et al. (2010) found that although post–acute care (PAC) is available for older adults, only 50% of patients who had a myocardial infarction (MI) received PAC. Only 44% of patients who had cardiac surgery participated in post–acute care. Cossette et al. (2012) found that a stepwise nursing intervention postdischarge significantly increased enrollment in cardiac rehabilitation programs over standard of care (see the Evidence-Based Practice box).

CHART 38-8 Home Care Assessment

The Patient Who Has Had a Myocardial Infarction

Assess cardiovascular function, including:
- Current vital signs (compare with previous to identify changes)
- Recurrence of discomfort (characteristics, frequency, onset)
- Indications of heart failure (weight gain, crackles, cough, dyspnea)
- Adequacy of tissue perfusion (mentation, skin temperature, peripheral pulses, urine output)
- Indications of serious dysrhythmia (very irregular pulse, palpitations with fainting or near fainting)

Assess coping skills, including:
- Is patient displaying denial, anger, or fear?
- Is caregiver providing adequate support?
- Are patient and caregiver disagreeing about treatment?

Assess functional ability, including:
- Activity tolerance (examine the patient's activity diary: review distance, duration, frequency, and symptoms occurring during exercise)
- Activities of daily living (is any assistance needed?)
- Household chores (who performs them?)
- Does patient plan to return to work? When?

Assess nutritional status, including:
- Food intake (review patient's intake of fats and cholesterol)

Assess patient's understanding of illness and treatment, including:
- How to treat chest discomfort
- Signs and symptoms to report to health care provider
- Dosage, effects, and side effects of medications
- How to advance and when to limit activity
- Modification of risk factors for coronary artery disease

CHART 38-9 Nursing Focus on the Older Adult

Coronary Artery Bypass Graft Surgery

- Be aware that perioperative mortality rates are higher for the older patient than for the patient younger than 60 years.
- Monitor neurologic and mental status carefully because older adults are more likely to have transient neurologic deficits after coronary artery bypass graft (CABG) surgery than younger adults are.
- Observe for side effects of cardiac drugs because older patients are more likely to develop toxic effects from positive inotropes (dobutamine) and potent antihypertensives (nitroglycerin or nitroprusside).
- Monitor the patient closely for dysrhythmias because older adults are more likely to have dysrhythmias such as atrial fibrillation or supraventricular tachycardia after CABG surgery.
- Be aware that recuperation after CABG surgery is slower for older patients and that their average hospital stay is longer.
- Teach the patient and family that during the first 2 to 5 weeks after discharge, fatigue, chest discomfort, and lack of appetite may be particularly bothersome for older adults.
- Teach the patient to let someone know where he or she is walking outside.

EVIDENCE-BASED PRACTICE QSEN

Can Nursing Interventions Tailored to the Acute MI Population Increase Enrollment in Cardiac Rehabilitation?

Cossette, S., Frasure-Smith, N., Dupuis, J., Juneau, M., & Guertin, M. (2012). Randomized controlled trial of tailored nursing interventions to improve cardiac rehabilitation enrollment. *Nursing Research, 61*(2), 111-120.

Cardiac rehabilitation, which is widely available, can reduce recurrence of coronary events by 25%. Due to the decreased length of stay, the nurse has limited time to provide important post-discharge education. In a randomized control trial, adults who experienced acute myocardial infarction (AMI) were contacted at three separate encounters: face to face prior to discharge, telephone call at 3 days post-discharge, and telephone call or face to face meeting at 10 days. The first call focused on the current condition of the patient, symptomology, activity, and patient's concerns. At the second call, the patient's current condition was reviewed and education and discussion about risk factor modification occurred. In addition to cardiac rehabilitation review, risk factor and lifestyle modification were the focus of the third call. The control group received the standard of care that included standard discharge instructions with encouragement to follow up with health care provider.

All participants completed baseline questionnaires: Revised Illness Perception Questionnaire, Family Care Climate Questionnaire—Patient Version, and State-Trait Anxiety Inventory. In addition, all participants received follow-up phone calls from a research assistant at 6 weeks post-discharge. A total of 242 participants were enrolled, and results revealed 45% of patients in the intervention group versus 24% of the control group enrolled in cardiac rehabilitation program (defined as attendance at one session prior to end of 6 weeks post-discharge). The time to mean first visit (day 20 post-discharge) did not differ between the groups. The intervention did not impact modification of risk factors. Limitations included lack of data on continued attendance, cost-effectiveness of the intervention, and long-term outcomes.

Level of Evidence: 1
The study was a large randomized controlled trial.

Commentary: Implications for Practice and Research
In view of the low percentages of older adults who attend cardiac rehabilitation, nurses can provide the necessary intervention to encourage attendance. Collaborate with the case manager or discharge planner to ensure that follow-up on lifestyle modification occurs after discharge because the patient is focused on immediate discharge needs at the time of discharge. More studies need to be completed to determine the nursing interventions that may be valuable post-discharge in the AMI patient population that not only improve outcomes but also are cost-effective.

MI, Myocardial infarction.

The most frequently cited reasons for nonparticipation are lack of insurance coverage, a physician's decision that it is unnecessary, and the patient's decision that it is not necessary. Those who participate in these programs report greater improvement in exercise tolerance and improved ability to control stress. However, no difference in their return to work has been seen.

Self-Management Education. The need for health teaching depends in part on the treatment plan or type of procedure that the patient received. Because hospital stays are short and patients are quite ill during hospitalization, most in-hospital education programs concentrate on the skills essential for self-care after discharge.

As part of home visits or a cardiac rehabilitation program, identify the additional educational needs of the patient and family and their readiness to learn. Develop a teaching plan, which usually includes education about the normal anatomy and physiology of the heart, the pathophysiology of angina and MI, risk factor modification, activity and exercise protocols, cardiac drugs, and when to seek medical assistance. Teach patients that myocardial healing after an MI begins early and is usually complete in 6 to 8 weeks. Remind those who have undergone traditional CABG that the sternotomy should heal in about 6 to 8 weeks, but upper body exercise needs to be limited for several months.

Patients who have undergone CABG require instruction on incision care for the sternum and the graft site. Teach them to inspect the incisions daily for any redness, swelling, or drainage. The leg of a saphenous vein donor site is often edematous. Instruct patients to avoid crossing legs, to wear elastic stockings until the edema subsides, and to elevate the surgical limb when sitting in a chair. Teach patients who have had a radial artery graft to open and close the hand vigorously 10 times every 2 hours.

Risk Factor Modification. Modification of risk factors is a necessary part of a patient's management and involves changing his or her health maintenance patterns. Such modifications may include tobacco cessation, altered dietary patterns, regular exercise, BP control, and blood glucose control.

For patients who use tobacco, explain its negative effects, especially cigarette smoking. Many patients choose to quit smoking soon after an MI. Chapter 30 also provides information on this lifestyle change.

The mainstays of cholesterol control are nutritional therapy and anti-hyperlipidemic agents, as described in Chapter 36. Teach patients to avoid adding salt when beginning a meal. A reduction of 80 mg/day of sodium can reduce the systolic blood pressure (SBP) by 5 mm Hg and 3 mm Hg for the diastolic blood pressure (DBP). Maintain adequate dietary potassium, calcium, and magnesium intake. Increasing potassium may reduce the SBP by 8 mm Hg. Booklets and cookbooks that can assist the patient in learning to cook with reduced fats, oils, and salt are available from the American Heart Association (AHA).

Collaborate with the physical therapist to establish an activity and exercise schedule as part of rehabilitation, depending on the cardiac procedure that was performed. Instruct the patient to remain near home during the first week after discharge and to continue a walking program. Patients may engage in light housework or any activity done while sitting and that does not precipitate angina. During the second week, they are encouraged to increase social activities and possibly to return to work part-time. By the third week, they may begin to lift objects as heavy as 15 pounds (e.g., 2 gallons of milk) but should avoid

---

> ### CHART 38-10 Patient and Family Education: Preparing for Self-Management
>
> #### Activity for the Patient with Coronary Artery Disease
>
> - Begin by walking the same distance at home as in the hospital (usually 400 feet) 3 times each day.
> - Carry nitroglycerin with you.
> - Check your pulse before, during, and after the exercise.
> - Stop the activity for a pulse increase of more than 20 beats/min, shortness of breath, angina, or dizziness.
> - Exercise outdoors when the weather is good.
> - Gradually increase the walking until the distance is $\frac{1}{4}$ mile twice daily (usually the end of the second week).
> - After an exercise tolerance test and with your physician's approval, walk at least 3 times each week, increasing the distance by $\frac{1}{2}$ mile every other week, until the total distance is 2 miles.
> - Avoid straining (lifting, push-ups, pull-ups, and straining at bowel movements).

lifting or pulling heavier objects for the first 6 to 8 weeks. Chart 38-10 lists suggested instructions for activity level.

Patients may begin a simple walking program by walking 400 feet twice a day at the rate of 1 mile/hr the first week after discharge and increasing the distance and rate as tolerated, usually weekly, until they can walk 2 miles at 3 to 4 miles/hr. Teach them to take their pulse reading before, halfway through, and after exercise. Teach the patient to stop exercising if the target pulse rate is exceeded or if dyspnea or angina develops.

After a limited exercise tolerance test, the physical therapist or nurse encourages the patient to join a formal exercise program, ideally one that assists him or her in monitoring cardiovascular progress. The program should include 5- to 7-minute warm-up and cool-down periods, as well as 30 minutes of aerobic exercise. The patient should engage in aerobic exercise a minimum of 3 (and preferably 5) times a week.

Complementary and Alternative Therapies. Additional therapies can aid in reducing the patient's anxiety about progressive activity both in the immediate postoperative period and during the rehabilitation phase. Many patients who have had cardiac surgery or other invasive procedures use complementary and alternative therapies. However, they often do not share with their health care providers that they use these therapies. Techniques such as progressive muscle relaxation, guided imagery, music therapy, pet therapy, and therapeutic touch may decrease anxiety, reduce depression, and increase compliance with activity and exercise regimens after heart surgery.

Sexual Activity. Sexual activity is often a subject of great concern to patients and their partners. Inform the patient and his or her partner that engaging in their usual sexual activity is unlikely to damage the heart. Patients can resume sexual intercourse on the advice of the health care provider, usually after an exercise tolerance assessment. In general, those who can walk one block or climb two flights of stairs without symptoms can usually safely resume sexual activity.

Suggest that initially these patients have intercourse after a period of rest. They might try having intercourse in the morning when they are well rested or wait $1\frac{1}{2}$ hours after exercise or a heavy meal. The position selected should be comfortable for both the patient and his or her partner so that no undue stress is placed on the heart or suture line.

Drug Therapy. Assess patients with diabetes mellitus for their ability to control hyperglycemia. Review the prescribed dosage of insulin or oral antidiabetic drugs with the patient and family. The patient and/or family should demonstrate accurate testing of blood for glucose levels and the technique for insulin administration, if used.

Teach the patient about the type of prescribed cardiac drugs, the benefit of each drug, potential side effects, and the correct dosage and time of day to take each drug. Drug regimens vary considerably. Many patients with angina are discharged while taking aspirin, a beta blocker, a calcium channel blocker, an anti-hyperlipidemic agent, and a nitrate. Those who have experienced an MI may require aspirin, a beta blocker, an anti-hyperlipidemic agent (statin drug), and an ACEI and/or an ARB. The Joint Commission Acute MI Core Measure Set requires hospitals to report whether patients with an MI are discharged on these drugs. Determine whether the patient can comply with the instructions.

⚠ NURSING SAFETY PRIORITY (QSEN)

Drug Alert

Use of sublingual or spray nitroglycerin (NTG) deserves special attention. *Teach the patient to carry NTG at all times.* Keep the tablets in a glass, light-resistant container. The drug should be replaced every 3 to 5 months before it loses its potency or stops producing a tingling sensation when placed under the tongue. Chart 38-11 gives instructions for management of chest discomfort at home.

Seeking Medical Assistance. Teach patients to notify their health care provider if they have:

- Heart rate remaining less than 50 after arising
- Wheezing or difficulty breathing
- Weight gain of 3 pounds in 1 week or 1 to 2 pounds overnight
- Persistent increase in NTG use
- Dizziness, faintness, or shortness of breath with activity

Remind them to always call 911 for transportation to the hospital if they have:

- Chest discomfort that does not improve after 5 minutes or 1 sublingual NTG tablet or spray

---

CHART 38-11 Patient and Family Education: Preparing for Self-Management

Management of Chest Pain at Home

- Keep fresh nitroglycerin available for immediate use.
- At the first indication of chest discomfort, cease activity and sit or lie down.
- Place one nitroglycerin tablet or spray under your tongue, allowing the tablet to dissolve.
- Wait 5 minutes for relief.
- If no relief results, call 911 for transportation to a health care facility.
- While waiting for emergency medical services (EMS), repeat the nitroglycerin and wait 5 more minutes.
- If there is no relief, repeat and wait 5 more minutes.
- Carry a medical identification card or wear a bracelet or necklace that identifies a history of heart problems.

- Extremely severe chest or epigastric discomfort with weakness, nausea, or fainting
- Other associated symptoms that are particular to them, such as fatigue and nausea

Health Care Resources. The American Heart Association (AHA) is an excellent source for booklets, films, CDs, DVDs, cookbooks, and professional service referrals for the patient with coronary artery disease (CAD). Many local chapters have their own cardiac rehabilitation programs.

Within the community, cardiac rehabilitation programs may be affiliated with local hospitals, community centers, or other facilities, such as clinics. Many shopping malls open before shopping hours to allow a measured walking program indoors. This opportunity is particularly popular with older patients because it provides a good support group and allows for an appropriate place to exercise in inclement weather.

Mended Hearts is a nationwide program with local chapters that provides education and support to coronary artery bypass graft (CABG) patients and their families. Smoking-cessation programs and clinics and weight-reduction programs are located within the community. Many hospitals also sponsor health fairs, BP screening, and risk factor modification programs.

❓ CLINICAL JUDGMENT CHALLENGE

Teamwork and Collaboration; Safety (QSEN)

A 55-year-old woman had a MIDCAB surgical procedure and is scheduled to begin cardiac rehabilitation on an ambulatory care basis. Her daughter plans to take her to the physical therapist for this program 3 days a week. The patient wants to return to her job as a nursing educator in a local community college as soon as possible.

1. What are the expected outcomes for this patient as a result of cardiac rehabilitation?
2. What is the role of the physical therapist in cardiac rehabilitation?
3. With what other members of the health care team will the nurse collaborate to ensure the patient's continuity of care?
4. What community resources might this patient use after the completion of her cardiac rehabilitation program?
5. For what surgical complications is she still at risk?

◆ Evaluation: Outcomes

Evaluate the care of the patient with CAD based on the identified priority patient problems. The expected outcomes are that the patient will:

- State that discomfort or other symptoms are alleviated
- Have adequate blood flow through the coronary vasculature to ensure heart function
- Walk 200 feet 4 times a day without discomfort, shortness of breath, or other symptoms of CAD
- Identify support systems and other sources to assist in effective coping with the cardiac event
- Be free of complications, such as dysrhythmias and heart failure

NURSING CONCEPTS AND CLINICAL JUDGMENT REVIEW

What might you NOTICE if the patient is experiencing inadequate GAS EXCHANGE and tissue PERFUSION as a result of coronary artery disease?

- Report of pain (chest, shoulder, arm, jaw, back, or abdomen)
- Report of persistent indigestion
- Dyspnea
- Diaphoresis
- Report of nausea
- Vomiting
- Anxious behavior
- Report of palpitations
- Report of fatigue
- Disorientation or acute confusion (especially in older adults)

What should you INTERPRET and how should you RESPOND to a patient experiencing inadequate GAS EXCHANGE and tissue PERFUSION as a result of coronary artery disease?

Perform and interpret physical assessment, including:
- Taking vital signs
- Monitoring oxygen saturation by pulse oximetry
- Taking 12-lead ECG
- Assessing level of consciousness and cognition
- Conducting complete pain assessment
- Drawing blood for laboratory assessment (e.g., troponins)

- Auscultating breath sounds for crackles or wheezes (left-sided heart failure)
- Auscultating heart for abnormal heart sounds
- Assessing for peripheral edema (right-sided heart failure)

Respond by:
- Calling 911 if patient is not in hospital setting OR notifying physician or Rapid Response Team in hospital setting
- Ensuring that patient rests
- Giving oxygen
- Giving nitroglycerin tablet
- Maintaining or starting IV line
- Administering morphine sulfate if MI suspected or diagnosed

On what should you REFLECT?
- Observe patient for decreased report of pain and associated symptoms.
- Continue to monitor oxygen.
- Continue to monitor for dysrhythmias and vital signs.
- Think about what could have precipitated this coronary event.
- Think about how you responded.
- Develop teaching plan for the patient to help prevent further episodes.

GET READY FOR THE NCLEX® EXAMINATION!

KEY POINTS

Review these Key Points for each NCLEX Examination Client Needs Category.

Safe and Effective Care Environment
- Collaborate with members of the interdisciplinary health care team members (e.g., physical therapist, case manager, home care providers) when caring for patients preparing for or participating in cardiac rehabilitation. **Teamwork and Collaboration** **QSEN**

Health Promotion and Maintenance
- Assess the patient for risk factors for coronary artery disease (CAD). Examples of modifiable risk factors that can be managed or controlled include obesity, smoking, high serum lipids, and hypertension; examples of nonmodifiable risk factors that cannot be altered include older age, being African American, and having a family history of CAD.
- Teach patients about the importance of decreasing their risk for CAD (see Chart 38-1). **Safety** **QSEN**

Psychosocial Integrity
- Allow patients to verbalize and express feelings of fear, anxiety, anger, denial, and grief regarding their CAD.

- Address the needs of the family and significant others, and provide teaching and information regarding the disease process. Clarify any misconceptions.

Physiological Integrity
- Teach patients that angina is the PAIN associated with decreased blood flow to the heart muscle. An MI indicates necrosis of heart muscle tissue (see Chart 38-2).
- Identify and interpret diagnostic values for cardiac markers, such as troponins and myoglobin, and other indicators of CAD.
- Monitor patients receiving thrombolytics and anticoagulants, such as heparin, for bleeding and bruising. **Safety** **QSEN**
- For patients undergoing invasive cardiac procedures, assess for signs and symptoms of active bleeding.
- Interpret and assess the patient with CAD for dysrhythmias.
- Evaluate the patient for PAIN characteristics (e.g., type, location, duration, cause, intensity, and measures taken to relieve symptoms).
- Teach patients and their families about drug therapy, including how to use nitroglycerin if they have chest or other cardiac-related PAIN (see Chart 38-4).
- After percutaneous cardiac intervention, monitor the patient for potential complications such as chest PAIN, bleeding from the insertion site, hypotension, hypokalemia, and

dysrhythmias. Document and report any of these findings immediately. **Safety** QSEN
- Identify and assess for complications for post–cardiac surgery patients, especially fluid and electrolyte imbalance, bleeding, hypothermia, hypertension, and angina PAIN.
- Provide emergency care for the patient with chest PAIN as described in Chart 38-3.

- For patients having coronary artery bypass graft (CABG) surgery, be sure to manage PAIN adequately, assess fluid and electrolyte balance, and monitor for potential complications. Examples of complications include fluid and electrolyte imbalances (especially hypokalemia), hypothermia, hypertension, bleeding, and neurologic deficits. **Evidence-Based Practice** QSEN

NCLEX® EXAMINATION CHALLENGES—ANSWER KEY

Chapter 2
p. 12   C
p. 15   C
p. 21   D

Chapter 3
p. 33   A, B, E
p. 34   B
p. 37   C
p. 41   0.4 mL
p. 44   B

Chapter 4
p. 62   D

Chapter 6
p. 79   D
p. 88   A

Chapter 7
p. 97   A, B, D, E
p. 99   A, B, C, E

Chapter 8
p. 112   A
p. 118   C

Chapter 9
p. 122   B
p. 132   A, B, C, D, E
p. 135   C

Chapter 10
p. 141   D
p. 144   A, B, E

Chapter 11
p. 158   D
p. 163   D
p. 165   B
p. 170   D

Chapter 12
p. 183   C

Chapter 13
p. 190   D, A, C, B
p. 193   100

Chapter 14
p. 216   C
p. 222   A
p. 225   C

Chapter 15
p. 244   D
p. 248   C

Chapter 16
p. 261   C
p. 263   D
p. 271   A

Chapter 17
p. 281   B

Chapter 18
p. 294   B, C, E
p. 300   B, D, E
p. 302   A
p. 308   B, C, E, F
p. 317   A, B, C, E
p. 320   C

Chapter 19
p. 332   B
p. 332   C
p. 340   D
p. 342   A

Chapter 20
p. 354   B
p. 355   D

Chapter 21
p. 365   C
p. 369   D

Chapter 22
p. 377   A
p. 383   C
p. 387   B
p. 394   C

Chapter 23
p. 405   C
p. 406   B, E

Chapter 24
p. 424   C
p. 430   B

Chapter 25
p. 453   B
p. 458   D
p. 461   C

Chapter 26
p. 475   D
p. 479   B
p. 485   A

Chapter 27
p. 500   C
p. 503   A
p. 506   C

Chapter 28
p. 516   D
p. 522   C
p. 527   A

Chapter 29
p. 533   C
p. 537   C
p. 539   D

Chapter 30
p. 557   B
p. 564   D
p. 569   D
p. 579   C

Chapter 31
p. 587   B
p. 593   A
p. 598   A, B, D

Chapter 32
p. 608   A, E
p. 616   A
p. 619   D

Chapter 33
p. 634   D
p. 645   C

Chapter 34
p. 663   C
p. 668   A, D
p. 669   C
p. 673   D

Chapter 35
p. 683   B, C, E
p. 686   D
p. 687   B
p. 697   B

Chapter 36
p. 709   A
p. 717   C
p. 722   B
p. 733   D
p. 735   A

Chapter 37
p. 746   C
p. 749   B
p. 753   D

Chapter 38
p. 761   B, D, F
p. 768   79
p. 778   C

Chapter 39
p. 792   B
p. 795   C

Chapter 40
p. 801   D
p. 806   A
p. 809   B
p. 814   C
p. 826   B

Chapter 41
p. 839   B
p. 848   A

Chapter 42
p. 857   C
p. 862   A, B, D
p. 876   C
p. 879   D

Chapter 43
p. 891   D
p. 897   A

Chapter 44
p. 916   A, C, D
p. 928   C

Chapter 45
p. 933   A, B, E
p. 938   B, A, D, C
p. 942   D
p. 953   D
p. 961   C

Chapter 46
p. 971   C

Chapter 47
p. 985   D
p. 989   C
p. 989   A
p. 994   C

Chapter 48
p. 1002   D
p. 1008   A
p. 1009   A

Chapter 49
p. 1023   B, E
p. 1027   D

Chapter 50
p. 1034   B
p. 1039   C

Chapter 51
p. 1061   A, C, D
p. 1066   A
p. 1073   C
p. 1075   A, B, E

Chapter 52
p. 1091   C
p. 1093   A, D, E

Chapter 53
p. 1102   A
p. 1105   C
p. 1107   A, E, F

Chapter 54
p. 1114   A
p. 1118   A, B, C, E

Chapter 55
p. 1130   C, B, A, D
p. 1131   A, C, E
p. 1141   D

Chapter 56
p. 1148   A
p. 1155   B, C, D
p. 1163   C

Chapter 57
p. 1172   C
p. 1176   A
p. 1179   D
p. 1188   C

Chapter 58
p. 1196   A, D, E
p. 1200   D
p. 1203   A

Chapter 59
p. 1218   B
p. 1220   C
p. 1226   C, E
p. 1230   A, C, D, E

Chapter 60
p. 1236   45.9
p. 1241   C, D, E, F

Chapter 61
p. 1259   D
p. 1264   C

Chapter 62
p. 1268   C
p. 1273   B
p. 1280   A

Chapter 63
p. 1288   A, D, E, F, G
p. 1291   C
p. 1298   D

Chapter 64
p. 1302   D
p. 1306   C
p. 1317   A
p. 1328   B

Chapter 65
p. 1354   B
p. 1359   D
p. 1363   C

Chapter 66
p. 1372   D
p. 1383   C
p. 1388   C
p. 1389   A

Chapter 67
p. 1397   B
p. 1399   A
p. 1406   C

Chapter 68
p. 1416   A
p. 1418   C
p. 1423   B

Chapter 69
p. 1456   B
p. 1459   A

Chapter 70
p. 1467   D
p. 1474   C

Chapter 71
p. 1485   C, D, E
p. 1490   B

Chapter 72
p. 1505   725
p. 1506   B
p. 1513   D
p. 1515   B

Chapter 73
p. 1524   C
p. 1527   C, D, E

Chapter 74
p. 1535   C
p. 1544   B

Chapter 1

1-1, From Potter, P., Perry, A., Stocker, P., & Hall, A. (2011). *Basic nursing* (7th ed.). St. Louis: Mosby; **1-2,** from Sorrentino, S. (2011). *Mosby's textbook for long-term care nursing assistants* (6th ed.). St. Louis: Mosby.

Chapter 2

2-3, From the Aging Clinical Research Center (ACRC), a joint project of Stanford University and the VA Palo Alto Health Care System, Palo Alto, CA, funded by the National Institute of Aging and the Department of Veterans Affairs.

Chapter 3

3-1, Modified from Pasero, C., & McCaffery, M. (2011). *Pain assessment and pharmacologic management.* St. Louis: Mosby; **3-2,** from Melzack, R. (1975). The McGill Pain Questionnaire: Major properties and scoring methods. *Pain, 1,* 272-281; **3-3,** Copyright 1983 Wong-Baker FACES Foundation.

Chapter 4

4-2, Modified from Nussbaum, R., McInnes, R., & Willard, H. (2007). *Thompson & Thompson: Genetics in medicine* (7th ed.). Philadelphia: Saunders; **4-5,** modified from Jorde, L., Carey, J., Bamshad, M., & White, R. (2000). *Medical genetics* (2nd ed.). St. Louis: Mosby; **4-8,** modified from Jorde, L., Carey, J., & Bamshad, M. (2010). *Medical genetics* (4th ed.). St. Louis: Mosby.

Chapter 5

5-1, © 2010. Rona F. Levin & Jeffrey M. Keefer; **5-2,** © 2010. R.E. Burke & R.F. Levin; **5-3,** © 2007. Visiting Nurse Service of New York and Rona F. Levin.

Chapter 6

6-1, From Scott, K., Webb, M., & Sorrentino, S. (2011). *Long-term caring* (2nd ed.). Sydney: Mosby Australia; **6-5,** from Potter, P., Perry, A., Stockert, P., & Hall, A. (2013). *Fundamentals of nursing* (8th ed.). St. Louis: Mosby.

Chapter 7

7-1, © 2005. National Hospice and Palliative Care Organization, 2007 Revised. All rights reserved. Reproduction and distribution by an organization or organized group without the written permission of the National Hospice and Palliative Care Organization is expressly forbidden. Visit caringinfo.org for more information.

Chapter 9

9-1, From Auerbach, P. S. (2012). *Wilderness medicine* (6th ed.). Philadelphia: Mosby; courtesy Michael Cardwell & Carl Barden Venom Laboratory; **9-2,** from Auerbach, P. S. (2012). *Wilderness medicine* (6th ed.).

Philadelphia: Mosby; courtesy Sherman Minton, MD; **9-3,** from Auerbach, P. S. (2012). *Wilderness medicine* (6th ed.). Philadelphia: Mosby; courtesy Michael Cardwell & Jude McNally; **9-4,** from Auerbach, P. S. (2012). *Wilderness medicine* (6th ed.). Philadelphia: Mosby; courtesy Indiana University Medical Center; **9-5,** from Auerbach, P. S. (2012). *Wilderness medicine* (6th ed.). Philadelphia: Mosby; courtesy Paul S. Auerbach, MD; **9-6,** from Auerbach, P. S. (2012). *Wilderness medicine* (6th ed.) Philadelphia: Mosby; **9-7,** from Auerbach, P. S. (2008). *Wilderness medicine* (5th ed.). Philadelphia: Mosby; courtesy Cameron Bangs, MD.

Chapter 10

10-2, Courtesy Meg Blair, PhD, RN; **10-3,** courtesy Jeanne McConnell, MSN, RN.

Chapter 11

11-2, 11-7, 11-9, ©1992 by M. Linda Workman. All rights reserved.

Chapter 12

12-3, 12-12, ©1992 by M. Linda Workman. All rights reserved.

Chapter 13

13-1, From Perry, A., Potter, P., & Ostendorf, W. (2014). *Clinical nursing skills & techniques* (8th ed.). St. Louis: Mosby; **13-2, 13-16,** courtesy and © Becton, Dickinson and Company; **13-3,** courtesy AccuVein, LLC; **13-7,** courtesy Edwards Lifesciences, Irvine, CA; **13-11,** courtesy NowMedical, Chadds Ford, PA; **13-12,** from Lilley, L., Collins, S., & Snyder, J. (2014). *Pharmacology and the nursing process* (7th ed.). St. Louis: Mosby; **13-14,** courtesy Kimberly-Clark Corporation; **13-15,** courtesy Venetec International, San Diego, CA; **13-17,** courtesy I.V. House, Hazelwood, MO; **13-18,** from Lopez, J. H., & Reyes-Ortiz, A. (2010). Subcutaneous hydration by hypodermoclysis. *Reviews in Clinical Gerontology, 20,* 105-113.

Chapter 14

14-1, From World Health Organization: Surgical safety checklist, ed 1. Available at www.who.int/patientsafety/safesurgery/en/. © World Health Organization, 2009. **14-2,** courtesy Christiana Care Health Services, Newark, DE; **14-4,** from Perry, A. G., & Potter, P. A. (2010). *Clinical nursing skills and techniques* (7th ed.). St. Louis: Mosby; **14-5,** from Angelo, R., Ryu, R., & Esch, J. (2010). *AANA advanced arthroscopy: the shoulder.* Philadelphia: Saunders.

Chapter 15

15-1, Courtesy Christiana Care Health Services, Newark, DE; **15-3, A,** from Patell, A., Whang, P., & Vaccaro, A. (2008). Overview of computer-assisted image-guided surgery of the spine.

Seminars in Spine Surgery, 20(3), 186-194; **15-3, B,** from Miller, R., & Pardo, M. (2011). *Basics of anesthesia* (6th ed.). Philadelphia: Saunders; **15-5,** redrawn with permission by Intuitive Surgical, Inc., 2007.

Chapter 16

16-1, Courtesy Forrest General Hospital, Hattiesburg, MS; **16-2, 16-4,** from Harkreader, H., Hogan, M. A., & Thobaben, M. (2007). *Fundamentals of nursing: Caring and clinical judgment* (3rd ed.). Philadelphia: Saunders; **16-3, A,** from Sirois, M. (2011). *Principles and practice of veterinary technology* (3rd ed.). St. Louis: Mosby; **16-3, B,** courtesy 2014 C. R. Bard, Inc. Covington, GA. Used with permission; **16-3 C, D,** courtesy C.R. Bard, Inc., Covington, GA.

Chapter 17

17-3, Modified from Goldman, L., & Schafer, A. (Eds.). (2012). *Goldman's Cecil medicine* (24th ed.). Philadelphia: Saunders.

Chapter 18

18-2, From Sainani, G. S. (2010). *Manual of clinical and practical medicine.* New Delhi: Elsevier India; **18-3, A,** from Jebson, L.R., & Coons, D.D. (1998). Total hip arthroplasty. *Surgical Technologist, 30*(10), 12-21; **B,** from Mercier, L.R. (2000). *Practical orthopaedics* (5th ed.). St. Louis: Mosby; **18-6,** from Damjanov, I. (2006). *Pathophysiology for the health professions* (3rd ed.). Philadelphia: Saunders; **18-9,** from Goldman L., & Ausiello, D. (2007). *Cecil medicine* (23rd ed.). Philadelphia: Saunders; **18-10,** from Currie, G., & Douglas, G. (2011). *Flesh and bones of medicine.* Edinburgh: Mosby Ltd.

Chapter 19

19-1, From Kumar, V., Abbas, A., & Fausto, N. (2010). *Robbins & Cotran pathologic basis of disease* (8th ed.). Philadelphia: Saunders; **19-3,** from McCance, K.L., & Huether, S.E. (2002). *Pathophysiology: The biologic basis for disease in adults and children* (4th ed.). St. Louis: Mosby; **19-4A,** adapted from New York State Department of Health AIDS Institute. Clinical Guidelines Development Program. (2013). Recommendations for non-occupational post-exposure prophylaxis for HIV infection. New York: Author. www.hivguidelines.org.; **19-4B,** adapted from New York State Department of Health AIDS Institute. Clinical Guidelines Development Program. (2012). Recommendations for occupational post-exposure prophylaxis for HIV infection. New York: Author. www.hivguidelines.org.; **19-5,** from Marks, J., & Miller, J. (2006). *Lookingbill & Marks' principles of dermatology* (4th ed.). Philadelphia: Saunders; **19-6,** from Leonard, P. C. (2012). *Building a medical vocabulary* (8th ed.). St. Louis: Saunders.

Chapter 20

20-2, Courtesy Dey, Napa, CA; **20-3,** from Auerbach, P. (2008). *Wilderness medicine* (5th ed.). Philadelphia: Mosby; courtesy Sheryl Olson.

Chapter 22

22-2, From Weinzweig, J., & Weinzweig, N. (2005). *The mutilated hand,* St. Louis: Mosby; **22-3,** from Workman, M.L., & LaCharity, L. (2011). *Understanding pharmacology: Essentials for medication safety.* St. Louis: Saunders; **22-4,** from Kee, J., Hayes, E., & McCuistion, L. (2012). *Pharmacology: A nursing process approach,* St. Louis: Saunders; **22-6,** from Forbes, C.D., & Jackson, W.F. (2003). *Colour atlas and text of clinical medicine* (3rd ed.). London: Mosby.

Chapter 23

23-1, A, From deWit, S.C. (2014). *Fundamental concepts and skills for nursing* (4th ed.). Philadelphia: Saunders; **B,** from Currance, P. (2006). *Medical response to weapons of mass destruction.* Philadelphia: Mosby/JEMS.

Chapter 24

24-10, Modified from Marks, J., & Miller, J. (2013). *Lookingbill and Marks' principles of dermatology* (5th ed.). Philadelphia: Saunders.

Chapter 25

25-3, Modified from Swaim, S.F. (1980). *Surgery of traumatized skin.* Philadelphia: Saunders; **25-5,** from Barbara Braden & Nancy Bergstrom. © 1988. Reprinted with permission; **25-6,** illustrations from the National Pressure Ulcer Advisory Panel and European Pressure Ulcer Advisory Panel. (2009). *Pressure ulcer prevention and treatment: Clinical practice guideline.* Washington, DC: NPUAP. Used with permission; **25-9,** from The Centers for Disease Control and Prevention, Atlanta, GA (www.bt.cdc.gov/agent/anthrax/anthrax-images/); **25-15,** courtesy Stevens Johnson Syndrome Foundation, Littleton, CO.

Chapter 26

26-15, from Herndon, D. N. (2012). *Total burn care* (4th ed.). Philadelphia: Saunders.

Chapter 27

27-12, From Young, A.P., & Proctor, D. (2008). *Kinn's the medical assistant: An applied learning approach* (10th ed.). St. Louis: Saunders; **27-13,** from Harkreader, H., Hogan, M.A., & Thobaben, M. (2007). *Fundamentals of nursing: Caring and clinical judgment* (3rd ed.). Philadelphia: Saunders.

Chapter 28

28-3, 28-9, 28-10, From Perry, A. G., Potter, P. A., & Ostendorf, W. R. (2014). *Clinical nursing skills and techniques* (8th ed.). St. Louis: Mosby; **28-11,** courtesy Chad Therapeutics, Chatsworth, CA; **28-13,** courtesy Mallinckrodt, Inc., Shiley Tracheostomy Products, St. Louis, MO; **28-14,** courtesy J.T. Posey Company, Arcadia, CA; **28-15,** courtesy Dale Medical Products, Inc., Plainville, MA.

Chapter 29

29-1, From Tardy, M.E. (1997). *Rhinoplasty: The art and science.* Philadelphia: Saunders. Used with permission; **29-2, A,** courtesy Invotec International, Jacksonville, FL.

Chapter 30

30-3, From Jarvis, C. (2012). *Physical examination and health assessment* (6th ed.). Philadelphia: Saunders; **30-4,** from Aehlert, B. (2011). *Paramedic practice today: Above and beyond.* St. Louis: Mosby; **30-9,** modified from Gift, A. (1989). A dyspnea assessment guide. *Critical Care Nurse, 9*(8), 79. Used with permission; **30-10,** from Swartz, M.H. (2009). *Textbook of physical diagnosis: History and examination* (6th ed.). Philadelphia: Saunders; **30-11,** courtesy Axcan Pharma, Mont-Saint-Hilaire, Quebec, Canada; **30-12,** modified © 2015 Hill-Rom Services, Inc. Reprinted With Permission—All Rights Reserved; **30-16,** courtesy Atrium Medical Corporation, Hudson, NH.

Chapter 31

31-1, Courtesy Covidien, AG, Switzerland; **31-2,** illustration from Workman, M.L., & LaCharity, L. (2011). *Understanding pharmacology.* St. Louis: Saunders; photo from Kumar, V., Abbas, A., Fausto, N., & Aster, J. (2009). *Robbins and Cotran pathologic basis for disease* (8th ed.). Philadelphia: Saunders; **31-3,** from Zitelli, B.J., McIntire, S. C., & Nowalk, A. J. (2012). *Zitelli and Davis' atlas of pediatric physical diagnosis* (6th ed.). Philadelphia: Saunders; courtesy Kenneth Schuitt, MD.

Chapter 32

32-2, A, courtesy Sims Porter, Inc.; **32-3,** © Dräger Medical AG & Co. KG, Lübeck, Germany. All rights reserved. No portion hereof may be reproduced, saved or stored in a data processing system, electronically or mechanically copied or otherwise recorded by any other means without express prior written permission; **32-4,** from McCance, K.L. Huether S.E., Brashers, V.L., & Rote, N.S. (2010). *Pathophysiology: The biologic basis for disease in adults and children* (6th ed.). St. Louis: Mosby.

Chapter 33

33-5, From Sahrmann, S. (2011). *Movement system impairment syndromes of the extremities, cervical and thoracic spines.* St. Louis: Mosby; **33-9,** From Baker, T., Nikolic, G., & O'Connor, S. (2008). *Practical cardiology,* ed 2, Sydney: Churchill Livingstone Australia.

Chapter 34

34-10, Reproduced with permission of Medtronic, Inc., Minneapolis, MN; **34-15,** courtesy Philips Medical Systems, Andover, MA.

Chapter 35

35-1, From McCance, K.L., & Huether, S.E. (2002). *Pathophysiology: The biologic basis for disease in adults and children* (4th ed.). St. Louis: Mosby; **35-2,** courtesy Abiomed, Inc., Danvers, MA; **35-4, A, B,** courtesy Medtronic, Inc., Minneapolis, MN; **C** courtesy Baxter Healthcare Corporation, Edwards CVS Division, Santa Ana, CA.

Chapter 36

36-4, From Brooks, M., & Jenkins, M.P. (2008). Acute and chronic ischaemia of the limb. *Surgery 26*(1), 17-20; **36-8,** from Forbes, C.D., & Jackson, W.F. (2003). *Colour atlas and text of clinical medicine* (3rd ed.). London: Mosby.

Chapter 38

38-1, From Huether S.E., McCance, K.L., Brashers, V.L., & Rote, N.S. (2012). *Understanding pathophysiology* (5th ed.). St. Louis: Mosby.

Chapter 40

40-3, From Feldman, M., Friedman, L., & Brandt, L. (2010). *Sleisenger and Fordtran's gastrointestinal and liver disease* (9th ed.). Philadelphia: Saunders; **40-4,** from Leonard, P.C. (2012). *Building a medical vocabulary: With Spanish translations* (8th ed.). St. Louis: Saunders; **40-7,** from deWit, S.C., & O'Neill, P. (2014). *Fundamental concepts and skills for nursing* (4th ed.). St. Louis: Saunders.

Chapter 41

41-3, Modified from Thibodeau, G.A., & Patton, K.T. (2007). *Anatomy and physiology* (6th ed.). St. Louis: Mosby.

Chapter 42

42-1, From Salvo, S.G. (2014). *Mosby's pathology for massage therapists* (3rd ed.). St. Louis: Mosby; **42-2, A,** from Mini-Mental State Examination © 1975, 1998, 2001 by MiniMental, LLC. All rights reserved. Published 2001 by Psychological Assessment Resources, Inc. May not be reproduced in whole or in part in any form or by any means without written permission of Psychological Assessment Resources, Inc., 16204 N. Florida Ave., Lutz, FL 33549; (800) 331-8378, www4.parinc.com/. **B,** from Seidel, H.M., Ball, J.W., Dains, J.E., Benedict, G.W. (2003). *Mosby's guide to physical examination* (5th ed.). St. Louis: Mosby.

Chapter 43

43-1, From Patton, K.T., & Thibodeau, G.A. (2014). *The human body in health & disease* (6th ed.). St. Louis: Mosby; **43-5,** from Harkreader, H. (2007). *Fundamentals of nursing: Caring and clinical judgment* (3rd ed.). Philadelphia: Saunders.

Chapter 45

45-3, From Seidel, H.M., Ball, J.W., Dains, J.E., Flynn, J.A., Solomon, B.S., & Stewart, R.W. (2011). *Mosby's guide to physical examination* (7th ed.). St. Louis: Mosby; **B,** modified from Stein, H.A., Slatt, B.J., & Stein, R.M. (1994). *The ophthalmic assistant* (6th ed.). St. Louis: Mosby. **45-10,** from Flint, P.W., Haughey, B.H., Lund, V.J., Niparko, J.K., Richardson, M.A.,

Robbins, K.T., et al. (2010). *Cummings otolaryngology: Head & neck surgery* (5th ed.). Philadelphia: Mosby; courtesy Elekta, Inc.

Chapter 46

46-11, Courtesy Medtronic Ophthalmics, Minneapolis, MN.

Chapter 47

47-5, from Patton, K.T., & Thibodeau, G.A. (2010). *Anatomy and physiology* (7th ed.). St. Louis: Mosby; **47-8,** from Workman, M.L., LaCharity, L., & Kruchko, S.C. (2011). *Understanding pharmacology*. St. Louis: Saunders.

Chapter 50

50-3, From Johal, S., Sawalha, S., & Pasapula, C. (2010). Post-traumatic acute hallux valgus: A case report. *The Foot, 29*(2), 87-89; **50-4,** from Hochberg, M., Silman, A., Smolen, J., Weinblatt, M., & Weisman, M. (2011). *Rheumatology* (5th ed). Philadelphia: Mosby.

Chapter 51

51-3, 51-5, 51-10, Courtesy Smith & Nephew, Inc., Orthopaedics Divisions, Memphis, TN; **51-4,** from Perry, A.G., Potter, P.A., & Elkin, M.K. (2012). *Nursing interventions & clinical skills* (5th ed.). St. Louis: Mosby; **51-6,** from McCance, K.L., Huether, S.E., Brashers, V.L., & Rote, N.S. (2010). *Pathophysiology: The biologic basis for disease in adults and children* (6th ed.). St. Louis: Mosby; **51-8,** from Douglas, G., Robertson, C., & Nicol, F. (2011). *Macleod exploración clínica* (12th ed.). Barcelona: Elsevier; **51-14,** courtesy Zimmer, Inc., Warsaw, IN; **51-15,** from Darby, M., & Walsh, M. (2010). *Dental hygiene: theory and practice* (3rd ed.). St. Louis: Saunders.

Chapter 53

53-1, From Friedman-Kien, A.E., & Cockerell, C.J. (1996). *Color atlas of AIDS* (2nd ed.). Philadelphia: Saunders.

Chapter 56

56-6, From Evans, S. (2009). *Surgical pitfalls*. Philadelphia: Saunders.

Chapter 57

57-3, B, From Perry, A.G., & Potter, P.A. (2006). *Clinical nursing skills & techniques* (6th ed.). St. Louis: Mosby; courtesy ConvaTec, Princeton, NJ; **57-5,** courtesy ConvaTec, a Bristol-Myers Squibb Company, Princeton, NJ.

Chapter 58

58-1, From Leonard, P. (2011). *Quick & easy medical terminology* (6th ed.). St. Louis: Saunders; **58-2,** from Talley, N., & O'Connor, S. (2010). *Clinical examination: a systematic guide to physical diagnosis* (6th ed.). Sydney: Churchill Livingstone Australia.

Chapter 60

60-1, From U.S. Department of Agriculture, 2011, www.ChooseMyPlate.gov; **60-2,** ® Société des Produits Nestlé S.A., Vevey, Switzerland, Trademark Owners; **60-3, A,** from Lilley, L., Rainforth Collins, S., Harrington, S., & Snyder, J. (2011). *Pharmacology and the nursing process* (6th ed.). St. Louis: Mosby; **B,** from Harkreader, H. (2007). *Fundamentals of nursing* (3rd ed.). St. Louis: Saunders; courtesy C.R. Bard, Inc., Billerica, MA; **C,** from Harkreader, H. (2007). *Fundamentals of nursing* (3rd ed.). St. Louis: Saunders; courtesy Ballard Medical Products, Draper, UT.

Chapter 61

61-4, From Guyton, A., & Hall, J. (2006). *Textbook of medical physiology* (11th ed.). Philadelphia: Saunders.

Chapter 62

62-1, Courtesy of the Group for Research in Pathology Educations (GRIPE), Oklahoma City, OK; **62-2,** from Wilson J.D., Foster, D., Kronenberg, H., & Larsen, P.R. (1998). *Williams textbook of endocrinology* (9th ed.). Philadelphia: Saunders; courtesy Dr. H. Patrick Higgins; **62-3,** from Wenig B.M., Heffess, C.S., & Adair, C.F. (1997). *Atlas of endocrine pathology*. Philadelphia: Saunders.

Chapter 64

64-4, Courtesy Medtronic Diabetes, Northridge, CA; **64-5,** courtesy Becton, Dickinson and Company, Franklin Lakes, NJ; **64-6,** from Frykberg, R.G., Zgonis, T., Armstrong, D.G., Driver, V.R., Giurini, J.M., Kravitz, S.R., et al. (2006). Diabetic foot disorders: A clinical practice guideline—2006 revision. *The Journal of Foot and Ankle Surgery, 45*(5), S1-S66.

Chapter 65

65-3, From Patton, K.T., & Thibodeau, G.A. (2014). *The human body in health & disease* (6th ed.). St. Louis: Mosby; **65-8,** modified from Patton, K.T., & Thibodeau, G.A. (2013). *Anatomy & physiology* (8th ed.). St. Louis: Mosby; **65-10,** Courtesy Verathon Corporation, Bothell, WA.

Chapter 66

66-1, A, Courtesy ConvaTec, A Bristol-Meyers Squibb Company, a Division of E.R. Squibb & Sons, Inc., Princeton, NJ; **66-2,** from Pollack, H.M. (2000). *Clinical urography* (2nd ed.). Philadelphia: Saunders; **66-3,** modified from Singal, R.K., & Denstedt, J.D. (1997). Contemporary management of ureteral stones. *The Urologic Clinics of North America, 24*(1), 59-70.

Chapter 67

67-2, From Kumar, V., Abbas, A., Fausto, N., & Aster, J. (2010). *Robbins and Cotran pathologic basis of disease* (8th ed.). Philadelphia: Saunders.

Chapter 68

68-1, Courtesy Kendall Company, Bothell, WA; **68-3, 68-4,** from Feehally, J., Floege, J., & Johnson, R. (2007). *Comprehensive clinical nephrology* (3rd ed.). Philadelphia: Mosby; **68-5,** courtesy Gambro Lundia AB, Lund, Sweden; **68-8, A,** from Geary, D.F., & Schaefer, F. (2008). *Comprehensive pediatric nephrology*. Philadelphia: Mosby; **68-12,** courtesy Baxter International, Inc., Deerfield, IL.

Chapter 70

70-1, From Swartz, M.H. (2009). *Textbook of physical diagnosis: History and examination* (6th ed.). Philadelphia: Saunders; **70-2,** from Mansel, R., & Bundred, N. (1995). *Color atlas of breast disease*. St. Louis: Mosby; **70-3,** from Gallager, H.S., Leis, H.P. Jr., Snyderman, R.K., & Urban, J.A. (1978). *The breast*. St. Louis: Mosby; **70-4, 70-5,** © 2010 Terese Winslow. U.S. Govt. has certain rights.

Chapter 72

72-2, Adapted from the American Urological Association Practice Guidelines Committee. (2003). Guideline on the management of benign prostatic hyperplasia (BPH). *Journal of Urology, 170*(2 Pt 1), 530-547.

Chapter 74

74-1, 74-2, From Morse, S., Ballard, R., Holmes, K., & Moreland, A. (2003). *Atlas of sexually transmitted diseases and AIDS* (3rd ed.). Edinburgh: Mosby.

Page numbers followed by "f" indicate figures, "t" indicate tables, and "b" indicate boxes.

I-1